# ORTHODONTICS
## Principles and Practice

# ORTHODONTICS
## Principles and Practice

### SECOND EDITION

**Basavaraj Subhashchandra Phulari** BDS MDS (Ortho) FRSH FAGE
*Formerly,* Faculty of Department of Orthodontics and Dentofacial Orthopedics
Mauras College of Dentistry, Hospital and Oral Research Institute
Republic of Mauritius

JAYPEE The Health Sciences Publisher

Philadelphia | New Delhi | London | Panama

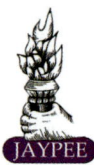

## Jaypee Brothers Medical Publishers (P) Ltd

**Headquarters**

Jaypee Brothers Medical Publishers (P) Ltd.
4838/24, Ansari Road, Daryaganj
New Delhi 110 002, India
Phone: +91-11-43574357
Fax: +91-11-43574314
E-mail: jaypee@jaypeebrothers.com

**Overseas Offices**

J.P. Medical Ltd.
83, Victoria Street, London
SW1H 0HW (UK)
Phone: +44-20 3170 8910
Fax: +44(0)20 3008 6180
E-mail: info@jpmedpub.com

Jaypee-Highlights Medical Publishers Inc.
City of Knowledge, Bld. 235, 2nd Floor, Clayton
Panama City, Panama
Phone: +1 507-301-0496
Fax: +1 507-301-0499
E-mail: cservice@jphmedical.com

Jaypee Medical Inc.
325 Chestnut Street
Suite 412, Philadelphia, PA 19106, USA
Phone: +1 267-519-9789
E-mail: support@jpmedus.com

Jaypee Brothers Medical Publishers (P) Ltd.
Bhotahity, Kathmandu, Nepal
Phone: +977-9741283608
E-mail: kathmandu@jaypeebrothers.com

Jaypee Brothers Medical Publishers (P) Ltd.
17/1-B, Babar Road, Block-B, Shaymali
Mohammadpur, Dhaka-1207
Bangladesh
Mobile: +08801912003485
E-mail: jaypeedhaka@gmail.com

Website: www.jaypeebrothers.com
Website: www.jaypeedigital.com

© 2017, Jaypee Brothers Medical Publishers

The views and opinions expressed in this book are solely those of the original contributor(s)/author(s) and do not necessarily represent those of editor(s) of the book.

All rights reserved. No part of this publication and may be reproduced, stored or transmitted in any form or by any means, electronic, mechanical, photocopying, recording or otherwise, without the prior permission in writing of the publishers.

All brand names and product names used in this book are trade names, service marks, trademarks or registered trademarks of their respective owners. The publisher is not associated with any product or vendor mentioned in this book.

Medical knowledge and practice change constantly. This book is designed to provide accurate, authoritative information about the subject matter in question. However, readers are advised to check the most current information available on procedures included and check information from the manufacturer of each product to be administered, to verify the recommended dose, formula, method and duration of administration, adverse effects and contraindications. It is the responsibility of the practitioner to take all appropriate safety precautions. Neither the publisher nor the author(s)/editor(s) assume any liability for any injury and/or damage to persons or property arising from or related to use of material in this book.

This book is sold on the understanding that the publisher is not engaged in providing professional medical services. If such advice or services are required, the services of a competent medical professional should be sought.

Every effort has been made where necessary to contact holders of copyright to obtain permission to reproduce copyright material. If any have been inadvertently overlooked, the publisher will be pleased to make the necessary arrangements at the first opportunity.

**Inquiries for bulk sales may be solicited at:** jaypee@jaypeebrothers.com

### *Orthodontics: Principles and Practices*

*First Edition:* 2011
*Second Edition:* **2017**

ISBN: 978-93-85999-89-5

*Printed at:* Sanat Printers

**Dedicated to**

My dear parents (Subhashchandra and Shivalingamma Phulari),
brothers (Sangamesh, Jagadeesh and Manjunath),
My beloved wife Dr Rashmi GS Phulari, MDS (Oral Pathology & Microbiology) and
My dearest sons (Yashas and Vrishank) for their love, support and encouragement

And to
Dear (Late) Chandu who is always in our hearts and thoughts...

# Contributors

**Aakash Shah** BDS MDS (Ortho)
Professor
Department of Orthodontics and Dentofacial Orthopedics
Faculty of Dental Sciences
Dharmsinh Desai University
Nadiad, Gujarat, India

**Aneshwar Rohanlal Bhagwandass** BDS (Manipal), DMD (USA)
Private Practioner
United States of America

**Anil Shah** BDS Master of ESOLA Academy Vienna University, Austria
President, SOLA India
Innovate Dental Center
Surat, Gujarat, India

**Basavaraj Subhashchandra Phulari**
BDS, MDS(Ortho), FRSH, FAGE
*Formerly,* Faculty
Department of Orthodontics and Dentofacial Orthopedics
Mauras College of Dentistry,
Hospital and Oral Research Institute
Republic of Mauritius

**Basti Risi Kino** DMD, MDSc, PGDip (PSM)
Director of Public Dental Services
Ministry of Health and Quality of Life
Republic of Mauritius

**Desi Moodley**
BDS, PDD-Aesthetic Dent (Stell), MSc Dent Sc (Stell), PhD (UWC)
Researcher
Oral and Dental Research Institute
University of the Western Cape
Cape Town, South Africa

**Frank Tsahannerr** Dr Med Dent (Munich University)
Implantologist
Perchastr.5
82335 Berg am starnberger see, Germany

**Mark Donald Vernon** BChD MFDSRCS (England)
Clinical Lecturer
The Barts and The London Dental Institute
United Kingdom

**Mohan Vakade** MDS (Oral and Maxillofacial Surgery)
Master of ESOLA Laser Academy, Vienna University
Professor and HOD
Department of Oral and Maxillofacial Surgery
Vaidik Dental College
Daman, Gujarat, India

**Naresh Thukral**
BDS Master of ESOLA Academy Vienna University, Austria
Founder President, SOLA India
Head, Laser Academy and a Faculty
Executive Member of Board
SOLA-International

**Ohana Gabriel**
Dentiste
7 Ar Gombetta
92400, Courbevoie
France

**Poorya Naik** BDS MDS (Ortho)
Reader
Department of Orthodontics and
Dentofacial Orthopedics
College of Dental Sciences
Davangare, Karnataka, India

**Rashmi GS** BDS MDS (Oral Pathology and Microbiology)
Professor
Department of Oral Pathology and Microbiology
Manubhai Patel Dental College and Hospital
Vadodara, Gujarat, India

**Syed Zakaullah** BDS MDS (Oral and Maxillofacial Surgery)
Professor and Vice Principal
Department of Oral and Maxillofacial Surgery
Al-Badar Dental College and Hospital
Gulbarga, Karnataka, India

**Valentina Tsipova** BDS MDS (Ortho)
University of Tartu
Estonia

**Richard Poavin and Brulet Alain**
Graphic Designer
Rich.C.lte'e
Route co^tiere-Trou- Aux-Biches
i^le Maurice
Rue Aristide Briand
78700 conflans Ste, Honorine
France

# Preface to Second Edition

Since the first edition of this book was published in 2011, I have received an overwhelming feedback in the form of numerous email messaged and letters. I am extremely grateful for the positive response the book has received from the faculty in the field of Orthodontics and students alike.

The basic format of the book comprising of 49 chapters grouped under 15 sections is retained in the second edition as well. The book continues to give simple and logical narration of difficult orthodontic concepts in a fluid easy-to-understand language.

Numerous high-quality clinical photographs and skilfully made graphic illustrations throughout the book make it easier for the students to grasp the subject. Few pictures that lacked good resolution have been replaced in the new edition.

Innovative self-explanatory flowcharts and tables along with good pictures have come to be the hallmark of this title. In addition, summary charts given at the end of each chapter as *Chapter Overview* come handy during revision of the subject in preparation to exams.

Sample questions in both long question and short note formats are given for each chapter to prepare the students for theory examination. Chapter-wise *Multiple Choice Questions (MCQs)* are also given to aid students in preparation for viva-voce.

All the efforts have been made to present the subject in concise yet all comprehensive manner. It is hoped that the new edition will continue to be appreciated by students and staff alike.

**Basavaraj Subhashchandra Phulari**
*basavarajsp@gmail.com*

# Preface to First Edition

The fascinating field of Orthodontics has come a long way since the era of finger pressure and crude wires to the more sophisticated, state-of-art techniques and appliances of today. The oldest specialty of dentistry has witnessed immense progress in the last few decades, both in terms of technology as well as patient management. Braces are no more only for children and adolescents. More and more adult patients are seeking orthodontic treatment in the recent years. Thanks to technical advances in the appliance design, there has been increased understanding of cellular responses to orthodontic force and awareness among general public.

The ever-growing field of Orthodontics and Dentofacial Orthopedics as it is called today is fascinating and at the same time complex. Teaching orthodontics to undergraduates had never been more challenging, especially, in the view of vast literature and comparatively minimal exposure to clinical orthodontics, the undergraduate students generally have during their course. This book is a humble step towards meeting this enormous challenge of providing an all comprehensive, yet simple-to-understand text for the students of dentistry. The objective is to narrate the essentials of orthodontics in a simple and logical way, at the same time arouse interest in the minds of undergraduate dental students about this wonderful field. Furthermore, it is also hoped that the book will be of value to postgraduate students as well.

The 49 chapters, encompassing 15 sections have been compiled by an impressive bunch of academicians around the world. The chapter, *History of Orthodontics* gives a quick glance at the turning events in the evolution of the first speacialty of dentistry. Often asked and considerably difficult concepts such as *Cephalometrics* and *Model Analysis* are explained systematically with provision for quick review. Management of different types of malocclusion is narrated in simple manner with complete case records to support the text.

A separate chapter on *Preclinical Orthodontics* has been included for the first time which deals with rationale, armamentarium and step-by-step wire bending procedures, much required for undergraduate students. A working classification of basic orthodontic instruments is given with their modes of usage in chapter 27—*Orthodontic Instruments*. There is another section that covers the *Recent Advances in Orthodontics* including implants, invisalign and application of lasers in orthodontics.

Over 2,000 high quality clinical photographs and professionally done graphic illustrations with informative legends in the book make the text easy to grasp. Incorporation of tables, flow charts and boxes throughout the textbook wherever necessary will give the reader a convenient summary of key features and also make reviewing easier.

An accompanying booklet *MCQs in Orthodontics* features over 2,300 multiple choice questions given chapter-wise with answer keys. Furthermore, in each chapter, the questions follow the same order of points given in that particular chapter, thus can act as a very good means of revision of that topic/chapter and at the same time prepares the student for viva voce as well as PG entrance test and other competitive tests.

I regret any deficiencies and shortcomings that might have crept in despite our best efforts. I would also welcome comments and suggestions from both students and teachers for further improvement of the book.

**Basavaraj Subhashchandra Phulari**

# Acknowledgments

There are several people who have contributed to this project without whose cheerful cooperation the task would have been arduous if not impossible.

With profound sense of gratitude and respect, I express my heartfelt thanks to Dr Rajendrasinh Rathod MDS, Chairman of Manubhai Patel Dental College and Hospital, Vadodara, Gujarat, India; Chairman and Dean of Mauras College of Dentistry, Hospital and Oral Research Institute, Republic of Mauritius, for his timely suggestions, critical observations and above all for his inspirational support not only in this endeavor but throughout my academic career. He has been a constant source of encouragement and guidance throughout this project while providing me with all the facilities required for completion of this work. My special thanks to Dr YK Desai, Professor, Prosthodontics for support and comments he provided to this work. I would also like to thank Dr Yashraj Rathod, Trustee, Manubhai Patel Dental College and Hospital, Vadodara, Gujarat, India for his unstinting support and encouragement during this endeavor.

I have much pleasure in acknowledging the help I have received from my students of Mauras College of Dentistry, Hospital and Oral Research Institute, Republic of Mauritius in grueling sessions of spell check, and for familiarizing me with 'student's point of view'.

I am indebted to Dr Anil Shah and Dr Aakash Shah for all the help and encouragement I have received from them during the formative stages of this project. I am proud to have them as contributors.

I extend my special thanks to Mr Chitranjan Luchoo for his expert comments and suggestions regarding photography, and Mr Prakash Gopoul for providing crisp, neat line drawings for the book. I will be failing in my duty if I do not mention the affection and support I have received from Dr Goyal and family, Jayantee Raghunandan and family, Ramesh Purgus and family and Gopoul family who have always provided that moral boost much needed during compilation of the book.

I take this opportunity to thank my beloved parents Mr Subhashchandra Phulari and Mrs Shivalingamma Phulari, and brothers Sangamesh, Jagadish, and Manjunath Phulari for their constant support and cooperation during the entire course of this publication. I thank my beloved wife Dr Rashmi GS Phulari MDS (Oral Pathology and Microbiology) for being a constant source of inspiration and support throughout this project, helping me at every step right from checking the flow of text, arrangement of photographs to final proofs. I fondly acknowledge my dearest sons Yashas and Vrishank for their patience and love.

I profusely thank Shri Jitendar P Vij (Group Chairman), Mr Ankit Vij (Group President) and production team of M/s Jaypee Brothers Medical Publishers (P) Ltd, New Delhi, India for their enthusiasm, excellent cooperation and constant support in publishing the book.

Most of all, I thank God for all the kindness and mercy showered upon me.

# Contents

## SECTION 1: Introduction and History

1. Introduction.................................................................................................................1
   *Basavaraj S Phulari*

2. History.......................................................................................................................7
   *Basavaraj S Phulari*

## SECTION 2: Growth and Development

3. General Principles of Growth and Development................................................... 18
   *Rashmi GS, Valentina Tsipova*

4. Prenatal Growth and Development........................................................................ 35
   *Rashmi GS*

5. Postnatal Growth and Development ..................................................................... 44
   *Basavaraj S Phulari, Poorya Naik*

6. Development of Dentition and Occlusion ............................................................. 51
   *Basavaraj S Phulari, Rashmi GS*

## SECTION 3: Classification and Etiology

7. Occlusion—Basic Concepts .................................................................................. 63
   *Basavaraj S Phulari*

8. Classification of Malocclusions ............................................................................ 71
   *Basavaraj S Phulari, Poorya Naik*

9. General Etiological Factors of Malocclusion ....................................................... 89
   *Valentina Tsipova, Rashmi GS*

10. Local Etiological Factors ...................................................................................... 96
    *Rashmi GS*

11. Genetics in Orthodontics .................................................................................... 105
    *Rashmi GS, Basavaraj S Phulari*

12. Epidemiology of Malocclusion ........................................................................... 115
    *Basti Risi Kino, Basavaraj S Phulari*

## SECTION 4: Diagnosis and Diagnostic Aids

13. Orthodontic Diagnosis ........................................................................................ 120
    *Aakash Shah, Basavaraj S Phulari*

14. **Model Analysis** .......... 135
   *Basavaraj S Phulari*

15. **Cephalometrics** .......... 142
   *Basavaraj S Phulari*

16. **Maturity Indicators** .......... 163
   *Basavaraj S Phulari*

## SECTION 5: Biomechanics

17. **Biology of Tooth Movement** .......... 172
   *Aakash Shah, Basavaraj S Phulari*

18. **Mechanics of Tooth Movement** .......... 179
   *Aakash Shah, Basavaraj S Phulari*

## SECTION 6: Preventive and Interceptive Orthodontics

19. **Preventive Orthodontics** .......... 186
   *Basavaraj S Phulari, Ohana Gabriel*

20. **Interceptive Orthodontics** .......... 195
   *Basavaraj S Phulari, Aneshwar Roshanlal Bhagwandass*

21. **Oral Habits and Their Management** .......... 206
   *Basavaraj S Phulari*

## SECTION 7: Treatment Planning

22. **Orthodontic Treatment Planning** .......... 227
   *Basavaraj S Phulari*

23. **Anchorage in Orthodontics** .......... 231
   *Aakash Shah, Basavaraj S Phulari*

24. **Methods of Gaining Space** .......... 239
   *Basavaraj S Phulari*

25. **Arch Expansion** .......... 245
   *Valentina Tsipova, Basavaraj S Phulari*

26. **Extraction in Orthodontics** .......... 255
   *Basavaraj S Phulari, Frank Tsahannerr*

## SECTION 8: Orthodontic Instruments

27. **Orthodontic Instruments** .......... 266
   *Basavaraj S Phulari*

## SECTION 9: Pre-clinical Orthodontics

28. **Pre-clinical Orthodontics** .......... 277
   *Basavaraj S Phulari*

## SECTION 10: Orthodontic Appliances

29. **General Principles of Orthodontic Appliances** ........................................................................ 293
    *Poorya Naik, Basavaraj S Phulari*

30. **Removable Appliances** ............................................................................................................ 297
    *Basavaraj S Phulari*

31. **Fixed Orthodontic Appliances and Techniques** ...................................................................... 319
    *Poorya Naik*

32. **Functional Appliances** ............................................................................................................. 346
    *Aakash Shah, Basavaraj S Phulari*

33. **Orthopedic Appliances** ........................................................................................................... 362
    *Basavaraj S Phulari*

## SECTION 11: Corrective Orthodontics

34. **Management of Class I Malocclusion** ..................................................................................... 374
    *Basavaraj S Phulari, Aakash Shah*

35. **Management of Class II Malocclusion** .................................................................................... 390
    *Basavaraj S Phulari*

36. **Management of Class III Malocclusion** ................................................................................... 400
    *Basavaraj S Phulari*

37. **Management of Midline Diastema** ......................................................................................... 406
    *Desi Modley, Basavaraj S Phulari*

38. **Management of Open Bite** ...................................................................................................... 413
    *Basavaraj S Phulari*

39. **Management of Deep Bite** ...................................................................................................... 420
    *Poorya Naik*

40. **Management of Crossbite** ....................................................................................................... 428
    *Basavaraj S Phulari, Poorya Naik*

41. **Management of Cleft Lip and Palate** ...................................................................................... 437
    *Poorya Naik, Basavaraj S Phulari*

## SECTION 12: Surgical Orthodontics

42. **Surgical Orthodontics** .............................................................................................................. 446
    *Frank Tsahannerr, Syed Zakaullah, Basavaraj S Phulari*

## SECTION 13: Retention and Relapse

43. **Retention and Relapse** ............................................................................................................ 459
    *Basavaraj S Phulari*

## SECTION 14: Laboratory Procedures in Orthodontics

44. **Orthodontic Study Model** .................................................................................................................. 468
    *Basavaraj S Phulari, Valentina Tsipova*

45. **Welding and Soldering** ....................................................................................................................... 473
    *Basavaraj S Phulari*

## SECTION 15: Recent Advances in Orthodontics

46. **Adult Orthodontics** .............................................................................................................................. 478
    *Basavaraj S Phulari*

47. **Implants in Orthodontics** ................................................................................................................... 487
    *Mark Donald Vernon*

48. **Invisalign Techniques** .......................................................................................................................... 492
    *Basavaraj S Phulari*

49. **Laser in Orthodontics** ......................................................................................................................... 495
    *Anil Shah, Naresh Thukral, Mohan Vakade*

50. **MCQs in Orthodontics** ........................................................................................................................ 507
    *Basavaraj S Phulari*

    **Index** ..................................................................................................................................................... 623

# CHAPTER 1: Introduction

*Phulari BS*

## INTRODUCTION

Humans have attempted to straighten the teeth for thousands of years before orthodontics became a dental specialty in the late nineteenth century. Proper alignment of the teeth has long been recognized to be an essential factor for esthetics, function and overall preservation of dental health. Malposed/poorly aligned teeth may predispose to a number of unfavorable sequelae such as poor oral hygiene predisposing to periodontal diseases and dental caries, poor esthetics giving rise to psychosocial problems, increased risk of trauma, abnormalities of function and temporomandibular joint (TMJ) problems **(Box 1.1)**.

**Box 1.1:** Unfavorable sequelae of malocclusion

- Poor facial appearance
- Poor oral hygiene maintenance
- Risk of dental caries
- Risk of periodontal diseases
- Abnormalities of functions
- Psychosocial problems
- Risk of trauma to the teeth
- TMJ problems.

Orthodontics is the branch of dentistry concerned with the growth of the face, development of occlusion and the prevention and correction of occlusal anomalies/abnormalities. The term "orthodontics" comes from Greek: "orthos" meaning right or correct and "odontos" meaning tooth **(Flowchart 1.1)**. The term 'orthodontics' was first coined by Le Felon in 1839.

## DEFINITION

Knowing the definition is often an important initial step in understanding any subject. A number of definitions have been put forward over the years to explain what orthodontics is. Some of the widely followed definitions are given below:

In **1911, Noyes** gave the first definition of orthodontics as "The study of the relation of the teeth to the development of the face and the correction of arrested and perverted development."

In **1922, The British Society of Orthodontists** proposed that "Orthodontics includes the study of growth and development of jaws and face particularly and the body generally, as influencing the position of the teeth; the study of action and reaction of internal and external influences on the development, and the prevention and correction of arrested and perverted development."

Later, **the American Board of Orthodontics (ABO) and the American Association of Orthodontists (AAO)** stated that, "Orthodontics is that specific area of dental practice that has, as its responsibility, the study and supervision of the growth and development of the dentition and its related anatomical structures from birth to dental maturity, including all the preventive and corrective procedures of dental irregularities, requiring the repositioning of teeth by functional or mechanical means to establish normal occlusion and pleasing facial contours."

## WHAT IS MALOCCLUSION?

The term 'malocclusion' was first coined by Guilford and it refers to any irregularities in occlusion beyond the accepted range of normal category. Malocclusions are caused by hereditary or environmental factors or more commonly, by both the factors acting together. One of the most common causes of malocclusion is the disproportion in size between the jaw and the teeth or between the maxillary and the mandibular jaws. A child who inherits mother's small jaw and father's large teeth, may have teeth that are too big for the jaw, causing crowding in the arch. Abnormal oral habits, such as thumb/digit sucking, lip biting and mouth breathing may also cause malocclusion by adversely affecting the normal occlusal development.

Malocclusion can be presented in a number of ways. Some of the common characteristics of malocclusion include:
- Overcrowded teeth
- Spacing between the teeth
- Improper "bite" between maxillary and mandibular teeth
- Disproportion in the size and the alignment between the maxillary and the mandibular jaws.

It must be appreciated that not all malocclusions need treatment. Treatment of malocclusions that are mildly unesthetic and not detrimental to the health of the teeth and their supporting structures may not be needed and is not justified.

## AIMS OF ORTHODONTIC TREATMENT

Although orthodontic treatment improves facial appearance and is occasionally performed for cosmetic reasons, it should be aimed at restoration of overall dental health.

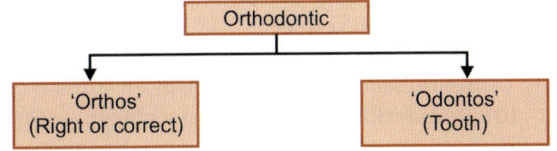

**Flowchart 1.1:** Derivation of the term orthodontics

**Jackson** has summarized the aims of orthodontic treatment that are popularly known as Jackson's Triad (**Fig. 1.1**). They are:
  i. Functional efficiency
  ii. Structural balance
  iii. Esthetic harmony.

### Functional Efficiency

The teeth along with their surrounding structures, are required to perform certain significant functions such as mastication and phonation. Orthodontic treatment should increase the efficiency of the functions performed.

### Structural Balance

Orthodontic treatment not only affects teeth but also the soft tissue envelop and the associated skeletal structures. The treatment should maintain a balance between these structures and the correction of one should not affect the health of the other.

### Esthetic Harmony

The orthodontic treatment should enhance the overall esthetic appeal of the individual. This might just require the alignment of certain teeth or movement of the complete dental arch, including its basal bone. The aim is to get results which go well with the patient's personality and make him or her look more esthetically appealing.

## BRANCHES OF ORTHODONTICS

The general field of orthodontics can be divided into the following three categories based on the nature and time of intervention:
- Preventive orthodontics
- Interceptive orthodontics
- Corrective orthodontics.

### Preventive Orthodontics

Preventive orthodontics is defined as "Action taken to preserve the integrity of what appears to be the normal occlusion at a specific time." As the name implies, preventive orthodontics includes actions undertaken prior to the onset of a malocclusion, so as to prevent the anticipated development of a malocclusion.

Preventive orthodontics encompasses all those procedures that attempt to ward off untoward environmental attacks or anything that would change the normal course of events. They include the care of deciduous dentition with restoration of carious lesions that might change the arch length; monitoring of eruption and shedding timetable of teeth; early recognition and elimination of oral habits that might interfere with the normal development of the teeth and jaws; removal of retained deciduous teeth and supernumeraries, which may impede eruption of permanent teeth and maintenance of space following premature loss of deciduous teeth to allow proper eruption of their successors.

### Interceptive Orthodontics

Interceptive orthodontics implies that an abnormal situation (malocclusion) already exists when the action is taken. Certain interceptive procedures are undertaken during the early manifestation of malocclusion to lessen the severity of malocclusion and, sometimes, to eliminate the cause.

Interceptive orthodontics is defined by the American Association of Orthodontists as "That phase of the science and art of orthodontics employed to recognize and eliminate potential irregularities and malpositions in the developing dentofacial complex."

Interceptive procedures include serial extraction, correction of developing anterior crossbite, control of abnormal oral habits, removal of supernumeraries and ankylosed teeth and elimination of bony or tissue barriers to erupting teeth.

Certain procedures undertaken may be common to both preventive and interceptive orthodontics. However, the timing of the services rendered is different. Preventive orthodontic procedures are carried out before the manifestation of a malocclusion, while the goal of interceptive orthodontics is to intercept a malocclusion that has already been developed or is developing, so as to restore a normal occlusion.

### Corrective Orthodontics

Corrective orthodontics, like interceptive orthodontics, is also undertaken after the manifestation of a malocclusion. It employs certain technical procedures to reduce or correct the malocclusion and to eliminate the possible sequelae of malocclusion.

Corrective surgical procedures may require removable or fixed mechanotherapy, functional or orthopedic appliances, or in some cases, an orthognathic/surgical approach.

## ORTHODONTIC APPLIANCES

Today orthodontists have a wide array of appliances in their armamentarium to treat malocclusions. Success of orthodontic treatment depends on the appropriate

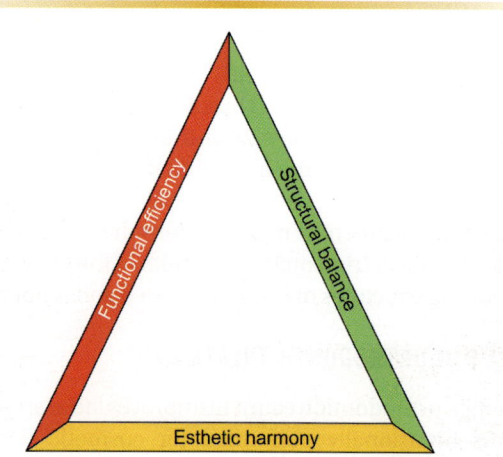

**Fig. 1.1:** Aims of orthodontic treatment (Jackson's triad)

selection of the appliances, the timing of the treatment, the type of tooth movement and/or skeletal changes desired, age of the patient and other factors. There are basically four types of orthodontic appliances, which can either be used individually or in combination to treat malocclusions.
i. Removable orthodontic appliances
ii. Fixed orthodontic appliances
iii. Functional appliances
iv. Orthopedic appliances/Extra-oral force appliances

### Removable Orthodontic Appliances

Removable orthodontic appliances are so called because they can be removed and fitted back into the mouth by the patient **(Fig. 1.2)**.

Use of removable appliances requires careful case selection for the success of the treatment. They are ideally used when simple tipping movement of teeth is sufficient to correct a certain type of malocclusion. The range of malocclusions that can be treated with removable appliances alone is limited. They can also be used as passive appliances to maintain the teeth in their corrected positions after active phase of orthodontic therapy, e.g. retainers. Removable orthodontic appliances can be used in conjunction with fixed mechanotherapy.

### Fixed Orthodontic Appliances

Fixed orthodontic appliances are so called because they are fixed to the teeth and cannot be removed by the patient. Fixed orthodontic therapy involves fixation of attachments (brackets) to the teeth and application of forces by arch wires or auxiliaries via these attachments **(Fig. 1.3)**.

Fixed appliances are indicated when multiple tooth movements are required for correction of malocclusion, such as rotations and bodily movement of the teeth. Fixed mechanotherapy allows fine finishing and settling of occlusion. There are a number of fixed orthodontic techniques such as: Begg's, Edgewise, pre-adjusted Edgewise, straight wire and lingual techniques.

### Functional Appliances

Functional appliances/myofunctional appliances are those appliances that utilize the forces of the circumoral musculature for their action to effect the desired changes **(Fig. 1.4)**. They act principally by holding the mandible away from the normal resting position to effect growth modification of the mandible.

### Orthopedic Appliances/Extraoral Force Appliances

Orthopedic appliances use extraoral forces of high magnitude (>400 g/side) to bring about skeletal changes. Intermittent application of such high forces in the growth period aids in correction of skeletal malocclusions by growth modification. Orthopedic appliances like functional appliances require good patient compliance for their success, e.g. headgears and chin cup **(Fig. 1.5)**.

## TIMING OF ORTHODONTIC INTERVENTION

Appropriate timing of orthodontic treatment is essential to accomplish the desired treatment outcome and its long-term stability. Timing of orthodontic intervention is related to the stage of dentition.

### Deciduous Dentition

Orthodontic treatment during this stage mainly includes the following:
- Parental education
- Care of deciduous dentition
- Space maintenance
- Elimination of abnormal oral habits.

### Early Mixed Dentition

Orthodontic treatment during this stage includes the monitoring of shedding timetable, serial extraction, space maintenance and control of abnormal oral habit. Although most corrective orthodontic procedures are performed in older children and adolescents, it may be advantageous in some cases to begin the treatment early before all the permanent teeth have erupted and facial growth is complete.

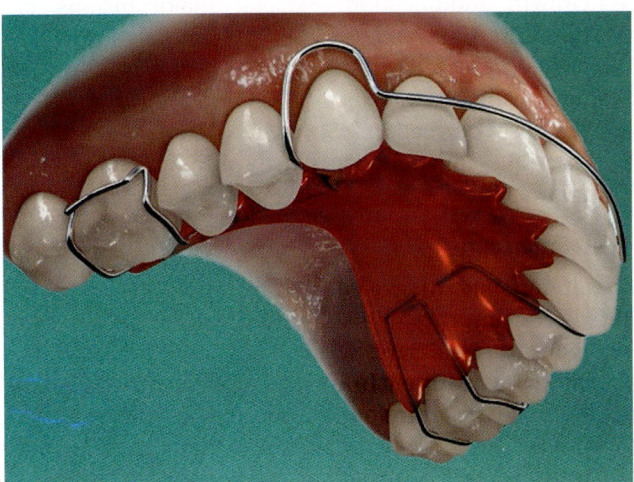

**Fig. 1.2:** Removable orthodontic appliance

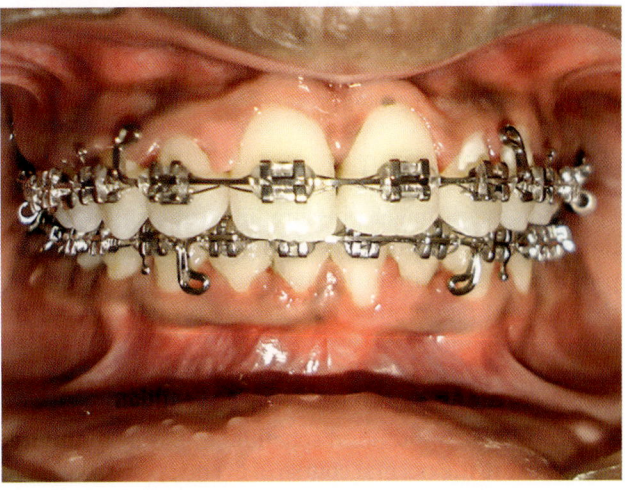

**Fig. 1.3:** Fixed orthodontic appliance

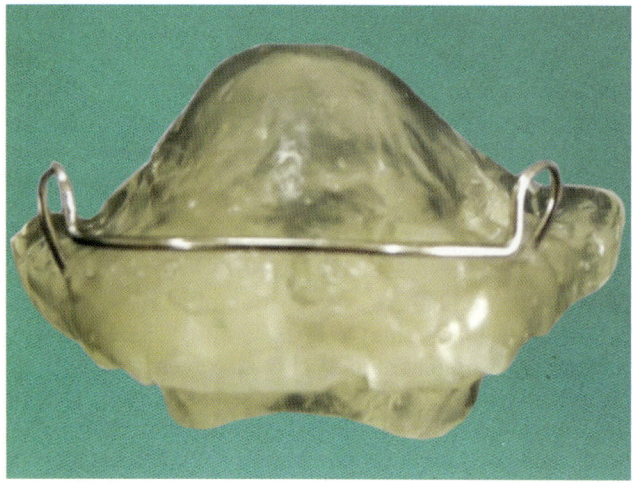

**Fig. 1.4:** Activator, a myofunctional orthodontic appliance

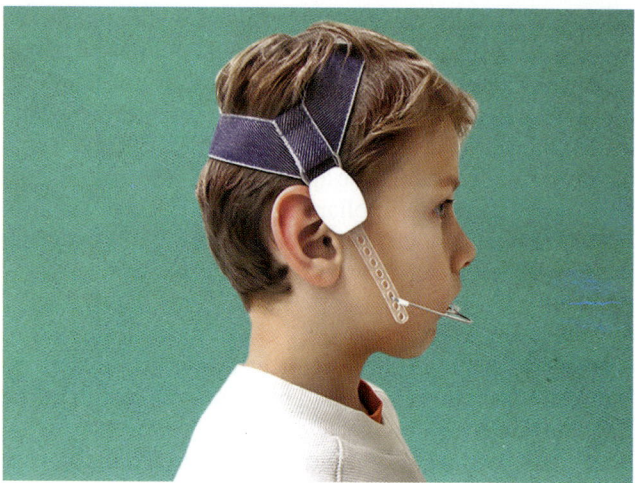

**Fig. 1.5:** Orthopedic appliance

Advantages of early orthodontic treatment include:
- Correction of bite problems by guiding jaw growth and controlling the width of the upper and lower dental arches.
- Reduction or elimination of abnormal swallowing or speech problems.
- Growth modification using functional and orthopedic appliances is best done in this period where significant growth is taking place.
- Shortening and simplification of later orthodontic treatment.
- Prevention of later tooth extractions.
- Improvements in appearance and self-esteem.
- Parental education.

### Late Mixed Dentition/Early Permanent Dentition

Most corrective orthodontic treatments are carried out in late mixed dentition or early permanent dentition stage.

### Late Treatment
- Many types of orthodontic treatments are feasible after adolescence. However, growth modification procedures to correct skeletal malocclusion may not be feasible due to cessation of growth.
- Surgical treatment involving orthognathic surgeries are best carried out in late teens/early adulthood after the cessation of growth.

## SCOPE OF ORTHODONTICS

From the era of finger pressure application to invisalign treatment, the field of orthodontics has witnessed profound development in the form of newer appliance designs and techniques, which have only increased the scope of orthodontics.

### Monitoring and Assessment of Developing Dentition
- Shedding and eruption schedule is closely monitored to ensure the normal course of events.
- Space maintainers are given in case of premature loss of primary teeth to facilitate the eruption of successor teeth.
- Habit breaking appliances are given to eliminate deleterious oral habits, such as thumb/digit-sucking and lip-biting, which can adversely affect the development of dentofacial structures.
- Planned extraction of certain deciduous and/or permanent teeth (serial extraction) done in selected cases can prevent future development of crowding by providing adequate space for the remaining teeth to erupt.

### Correcting Malocclusions of Dental Origin

Malocclusions of dental origin include abnormalities of intra-arch alignment and inter-arch relationship of teeth. They can be managed by removable or fixed orthodontic appliances.

### Correcting Malocclusions of Skeletal Origin

Skeletal malocclusions include conditions where the upper and lower jaws are abnormally related to each other.
- Growth modification: Skeletal malocclusions can be treated successfully by modifying the growth of jaws during active growth period using functional or orthopedic appliances.
- Surgical correction: Severe skeletal malocclusion in adults can be corrected by orthognathic/surgical approach.

### Adult Orthodontics

Better understanding of bone cell reactions to orthodontic forces and improvements in appliance design has made orthodontic treatment feasible in adult age as well. Orthodontic treatment in adults may involve the following:
- Adjunctive orthodontic procedures: They refer to limited orthodontic treatment carried out to facilitate other dental procedures. Adjunctive orthodontic

procedures include uprighting of tilted abutment teeth prior to bridge work, space gaining for placement of implants, etc.
- Comprehensive orthodontic treatment: It is usually carried out in young adults and involves full-fledged orthodontic treatment with or without extraction of teeth.

### Guards
- Mouthguard/Sportsguard: Mouthguards are often used during contact sports, such as boxing to prevent trauma to the teeth.
- Night guards: Night guards can be given in bruxism to prevent further loss of tooth structures by clenching of teeth.

### Management of Dentofacial Anomalies
Dentofacial anomalies such as cleft lip and cleft palate are usually associated with impaired facial appearance, speech, hearing, mastication, deglutition, and dental occlusion. Thus, management of such patients often requires a multidisciplinary approach with a long-term treatment plan and individualized rehabilitation program designed to address the treatment needs. Malocclusion is usually present and orthodontic therapy with or without corrective jaw surgery is frequently indicated.

## BENEFITS OF ORTHODONTIC TREATMENT
- Improved confidence
- Well-aligned teeth that are easier to keep clean and healthy.
- Ideally positioned teeth, which lessen the chance of gingivitis and advanced gum disease.
- Closed spaces to avoid the need for a bridge or denture.
- Better chewing and food digestion.

## BIBLIOGRAPHY
1. Ackerman JL, Profitt WR. The characteristics of malocclusion: A modern approach to classification and diagnosis. Am J Orthod 1969;56:443-54.
2. Eveleth PB, Tanner JM. World-wide variation in human growth (2nd edn), Cambridge, Mass. Cambridge University Press, 1990.
3. Foster TD. A Textbook of Orthodontics, St Louis, Blackwell Scientific Publications, 1982.
4. Graber TM, Neumann B. Removable Orthodontic Appliances. Philadelphia. WB Saunders, 1984.
5. Graber TM, Vanarsdall RL, et al. Orthodontics, Current Principles and Techniques. Diagnosis and Treatment Planning in Orthodontics. Mosby, 2000.
6. Graber TM. Orthodontics: Principles and Practice. WB Saunders, 1998.
7. Krogman WM. Child Growth Ann Arbor, Mich. The University of Michigan Press, 1972.
8. Moorrees CFA. The dentition of the growing child, Cambridge, Harvard University Press, 1959.
9. Proffit WR. Concepts of growth and development. In: Contemporary Orthodontics, 2nd edn. St Louis: Mosby Yearbook, 1999;24-62.
10. Proffit WR, Ackerman JL. Rating the characteristics of malocclusion: A systematic approach for planning treatment, Am J Orthod 1973;64(3):258-69.
11. Tanner JM, Whitehouse RH, Takaishi M. Standards from birth to maturity for height, weight, height velocity and weight velocity in British children. Arch Dis Child. 1966;41:454-71.

---

### EXAM-ORIENTED QUESTIONS

*Long Essays or Long Questions*
1. Define orthodontics. Describe aims and scope of orthodontics.
2. Describe briefly the aims, objectives, scope and limitations of orthodontic treatment.
3. What is orthodontia? Describe various sequelae of malocclusion of teeth.

*Long Note or Short Essay*
1. Aims of orthodontics and scope of orthodontics

*Short Notes*
1. Jackson's traid or aims of orthodontics
2. Branches of orthodontics
3. Benefits of orthodontic treatment
4. Unfavourable sequelae of malocclusion.

# CHAPTER OVERVIEW

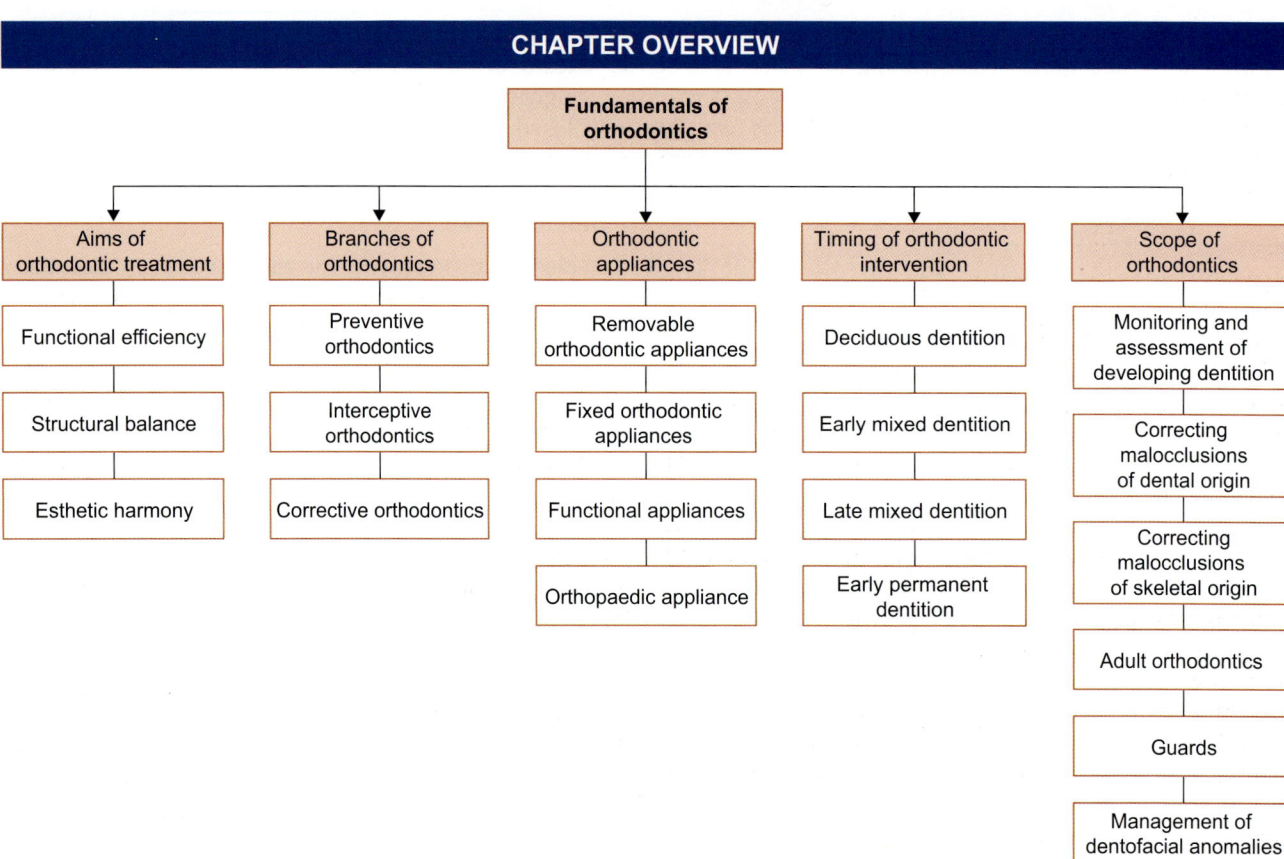

# CHAPTER 2

# History

*Phulari BS*

Since the beginning of human history, human beings have understood at a very basic level that without a proper bite, survival is very difficult. If you cannot chew well, you cannot eat well. The remains of the ancient Egyptians, Romanians and the Etruscans show that these societies used various kinds of metal and wires to straighten or adjust the teeth.

Many advances in dentistry and some pioneering efforts in teeth straightening began in the eighteenth century, but it was really in the nineteenth century that orthodontics became a science of its own.

Many inventors have significantly contributed to the fascinating science of orthodontics. The person given the most credit for pioneering modern orthodontics is **Dr Edward H Angle,** who is rightly honored as the "Father of Modern Orthodontics." Publication of Angle's classification system of malocclusion in 1899 marked a turning point in the history of orthodontics, paving way to establishment of the oldest specialty of dentistry.

The history of orthodontics is interesting and at the same time complex. It is the oldest specialty of dentistry. It would be wise to follow the development of this exciting field of science right from the era of ancient civilization to the current times. Prior to 1900s, the specialty of orthodontics was referred as "Regulation of Teeth" and as "Orthodontia" up to 1930s. The term "Orthodontics" has been used up to 1970s and currently the speciality is addressed as "Orthodontics and Dentofacial Orthopedics" **(Table 2.1).**

## ANCIENT CIVILIZATION

The history of orthodontics has been intimately interwoven with the history of dentistry for more than 2,000 years. Dentistry in turn, has its origins as a part of medicine **(Table 2.2).**

The Greek physician, **Hippocrates (460–377 BC),** was the first to separate medicine from fancy or religion. He established a medical tradition based on facts and the collected information was gathered into a text known as the "Corpus Hippocraticum." This text of the pre-Christian era contains many references to the teeth and to the tissues of the jaws as part of the medical text, which includes descriptions of irregularity and crowding of teeth.

**Aristotle (384–322 BC),** the Greek philosopher, was the first writer who studied the teeth in a broad manner. In his work entitled, "De Partibus Animalium" (On the Parts of Animals), he compared various dentitions of the known species of animals of that time.

**Aulus Cornelius Celsus (25 BC–50 AD),** the prominent Roman author of the first century, described finger pressure to move teeth in his work "De Re Medicina" (On Medicine).

"When in a child a permanent tooth appears before the fall of the milk tooth, it is necessary to dissect the gum all around the latter and extract it. The other tooth must then be pushed with the finger, day by day, towards the place that was occupied by the one extracted and this is to be continued until it reaches its proper position."

## MIDDLE AGES THROUGH SEVENTEENTH CENTURY

There is little reference to dentition during this period. An Arabic physician, **Paul of Aegina (Paulus Aeginata, 625–690)** wrote about irregularities in the dental arches caused by supernumerary teeth. He advised extraction of such teeth.

**Ambrose Paré (1517–1590),** a French surgeon, paid specific attention to the cleft palate. He was the first surgeon to devise an obturator for the treatment of cleft palate.

## EIGHTEENTH CENTURY

Eighteenth century witnessed major events in the development of **dental science dentistry.** France was the leader in dentistry throughout the world in this century. This was mainly due to one person named **Pierre Fauchard.** No one person exerted a stronger influence on the development of the profession than he did. In fact, he is referred to as the "Founder of Modern Dentistry." He created order out of chaos, developed a profession

**Table 2.1:** Evolution of term orthodontics
- Orthodontics
- Regulation prior to 1900s
- Orthodontia up to 1930s ("ia" referred to a medial condition)
- Orthodontics up to 1970s
- Currently orthodontics and dentofacial orthopedics

**Table 2.2:** Ancient civilization

| Years | Authors | Contributions to orthodontics |
|---|---|---|
| 460–377 BC | Hippocrates | Description of irregularity of teeth in "Corpus Hippocraticum". |
| 384–322 BC | Aristotle | Comparison of various Dentitions of different species of animals in his work "De Partibus Animalium". |
| 25 BC–50 AD | Aulius Cornelius Celsus | Described finger pressure to move teeth in his work "De Re Medicina." |

out of a craft and gave to this new branch of medicine a scientific and sound basis for the future. He published his two-volume book entitled "The surgeon dentist, a treatize on the teeth", which had an entire chapter on ways to straighten teeth. With reference to orthodontics, as early as 1723, he developed what is probably the first orthodontic appliance. It was called **Bandelette (Fig. 2.1)**. It was designed to expand the arch, particularly the anterior teeth and was the forerunner of the expansion arch of modern times **(Table 2.3)**.

**John Hunter (1728–1793)**, an English surgeon and a great teacher of anatomy, published his book "The Natural History of the Human Teeth" in 1771. He demonstrated the growth, development and articulation of the maxilla and the mandible and outlined the internal structure of the teeth and bone and their separate functions. He gave the basic nomenclature of dentistry incisors, bicuspids and molars.

The art of modern dentistry based on scientific foundation was first developed in Europe. It then came to the United States through the European-trained "Operators for the teeth" who came to America seeking fresh opportunities. Many native practitioners of America then began to "regulate" teeth. Malocclusion was called "irregularities" and their correction "regulation" during this period.

## NINETEENTH CENTURY

Foundations were laid in the nineteenth century to the oldest specialty of dentistry—Orthodontics. It was in the latter part of the nineteenth (1880s) century that the specialty began to emerge **(Table 2.4)**.

By the mid-nineteenth century, basic concepts of diagnosis and treatment had begun. It was a time when each practitioner attempted treatment by devising their own method based on purely mechanical principles. At that time, orthodontics was part of prosthetic dentistry and the literature on the subject described orthodontics in the area of partial or total replacement of missing teeth.

**Table 2.3:** Contribution to orthodontics in 18th century

| Year | Authors | Contributions to orthodontics |
|---|---|---|
| 1723 | Pierre Fauchard | - Father of modern dentistry<br>- He published his two-volume book entitled "The Surgeon Dentist, A Treatise on the Teeth"<br>- Developed first expansion appliance called "Bandelette" |
| 1728–1793 | John Hunter | - Natural history of teeth<br>- Growth and development of jaws<br>- Internal structure of teeth<br>- Functions of teeth |

**Table 2.4:** Contribution to orthodontics in 19th century

| Year | Authors | Contributions to orthodontics |
|---|---|---|
| 1841 | William Lintott | Introduced the use of screws |
| 1840 | JS Gunnell | Introduced chin strap |
| 1860 | Emerson C Angel | - First to introduce Arch Expansion by opening midpalatal suture<br>- Father of expansion appliances |
| 1871 | William and Magill | Developed molar bands |
| 1888 and 1889 | John Nutting Farrar | - "Father of American orthodontics"<br>- Wrote "Irregularities of the Teeth and Their Correction"<br>- Textbook was the first great work devoted exclusively to orthodontics<br>- Laid the foundation for "Scientific orthodontics" (intermittent forces, limits to amount of tooth movements) |
| 1829–1913 | Norman N Kingsley | - Treatise on oral deformities "worked on correction of cleft palate"<br>- Extraoral traction. |
| 1893 | Henry A Baker | Baker's anchorage Intermaxillary elastics) |

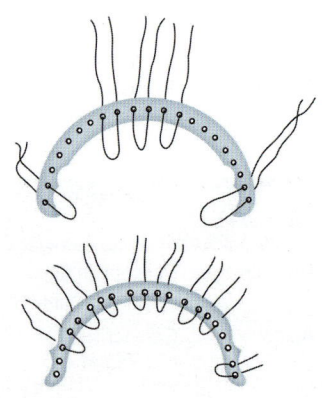

**Fig. 2.1:** Bandelette designed by Pierre Fauchard to expand dental arches

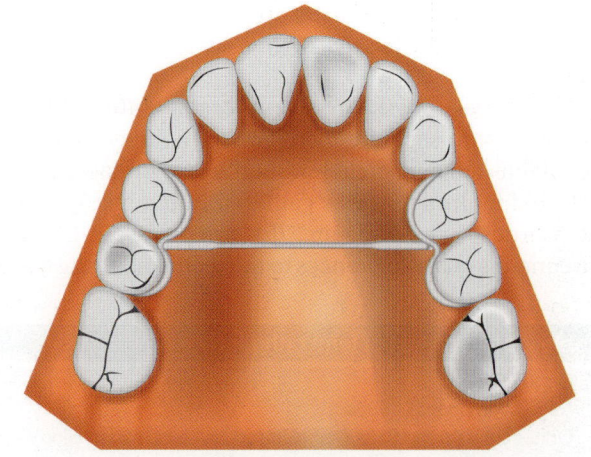

**Fig. 2.2:** Expansion appliance developed by Emerson C Angel

As early as in 1841, **William Lintott** introduced the use of screws in his work "On the teeth." He described premature loss of deciduous teeth as a cause of malocclusion, recommended that treatment be begun between the age of 14 and 25 years and also described a bite opening appliance.

**JS Gunnell, in 1840**, introduced the chin strap as occipital anchorage for the treatment of mandibular protrusion, the principle of which is used even today.

**Emerson C Angel (1823–1903)**, in 1860, was the first to advocate the opening of the median suture to provide space in the maxillary arch, since he strongly opposed extraction **(Fig. 2.2)**. This began the use of arch expansion in orthodontics.

**William and Magill** developed molar bands on the teeth as early as in 1871.

It was not until the latter part of the nineteenth century, when a few dedicated dentists gave special attention and importance to this phase of dentistry, that orthodontics began to emerge as a specialty science. It was known at that time as 'Orthodontia', the suffix 'ia' referred to a medical condition. In the last three decades of nineteenth century, some great contributors were made to the specialty by the following dentists.

**John Nutting Farrar (1839–1913)** is often referred as the "Father of American Orthodontics". It was he who gave impetus to the scientific investigations that permitted the understanding of the theory and practice of orthodontics. During his studies, he investigated the physiologic and pathologic changes occurring in animals as the result of orthodontically induced tooth movement.

He published two volumes entitled "Irregularities of the Teeth and Their Correction" in 1888 and 1889. The textbook was the first great work devoted exclusively to orthodontics. Farrar was good at designing brace appliances and was the first to suggest the use of mild force at timed intervals to move teeth "in regulating the teeth, the traction must be intermittent and must not exceed certain fixed limits." He was also the first to recommend root or bodily movement of the teeth.

Another man who also deserves much credit during this period of time is **Norman N Kingsley (1829–1913)**, a prominent dentist, artist/sculptor and orthodontist **(Fig. 2.3)**. He is known for his works on "Correction of cleft palate". As early as in 1866, he devised a technique called "Jumping the bite" with the use of a bite plane. He used vulcanite on conjunction with ligatures, elastic bands made of rubber, jackscrews and the chin cap.

**Henry A Baker** is remembered for the introduction of the so called Baker's anchorage or the use of the intermaxillary elastics with rubber bands in 1893 **(Fig. 2.4)**.

# TWENTIETH CENTURY

## Angle's Contribution to Orthodontics

One of the most dominant, dynamic and influential figures in the specialty of Orthodontics was **Edward Hartley Angle (1855–1930) (Fig. 2.5)**. He is rightly regarded as the "Father of Modern Orthodontics." **(Table 2.5)**

Edward H Angle was born on June 1, 1855, in Herrick, Pennsylvania. He completed DDS degree from Pennsylvania College of Dental Surgery in 1878. He joined the faculty of the Dental Department of the University of Minnesota in 1886. In the year 1892, He resigned from the University of Minnesota and moved to Chicago and then he became the first professor of Orthodontics at Northwestern University School of Dentistry. In 1895, Angle completed his MD degree from Marion Sims College. He moved to St. Louis, assuming the professor post first at Marion Sims College of Medicine and shortly afterwards at Washington University Dental School. It was then that he started his first orthodontic case, on his preceptor's son. Experiences in various schools led him to the conviction that orthodontia could not be properly

| Table 2.5: Angle's contribution to orthodontics | |
|---|---|
| Text book "Irregularities of the Teeth" | 1887 (1st edition) |
| Classification of malocclusion | 1899 |
| E-Arch appliance | 1900 |
| Pin and tube appliance | 1901 |
| Ribbon arch appliance | 1910 |
| Edgewise appliance | 1925 |

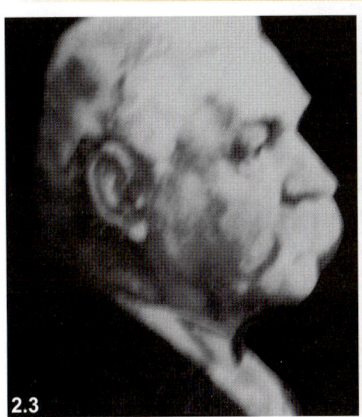
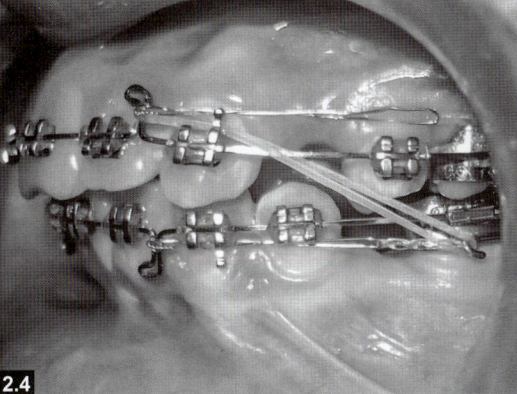
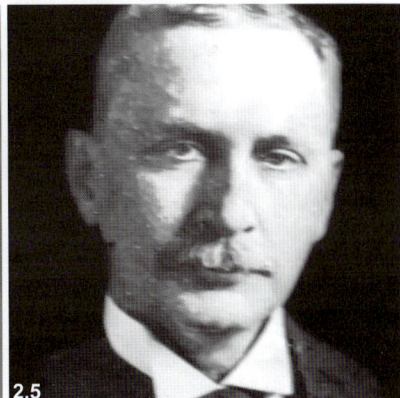

**Fig. 2.3:** Norman N Kingsley (1829–1913); **Fig. 2.4:** Intermaxillary elastics: **Fig. 2.5:** Edward Hartley Angle (1855–1930)

taught in a dental college. He started the first school of orthodontia in 1900, named as "**The Angle School of Orthodontia**" at St. Louis.

Edward H Angle organized the first orthodontic society and called it as "**The Society of Orthodontists.**" In 1935, the Society adopted the name it bears today: **The American Association of Orthodontists (AAO).** They also established the magazine, a quarterly titled **The American Orthodontist,** which we read today as the **American Journal of Orthodontics.**

**1903** — Dr. Anna Hopkins was elected the Society's first Secretary. She completed one of the early Angle courses, but was never to practice orthodontia. In 1906 she became Mrs Edward Hartley Angle.

### Appliances Contributed by Angle

- In 1900, Edward H Angle developed his first orthodontic appliance, the "E" (expansion)-arch appliance. It is also referred to as Edward Angle's E-arch. E-arch appliance consists of bands which are placed on molar teeth on either side of the arch of a heavy labial arch wire extended around the arch. The ends of labial extended arch wire threaded to the buccal aspect of the molar bands allowed the arch wire to be advanced so that the arch perimeter is increased. Individual teeth were ligated with the heavy labial extended arch wire with ligature wire of 0.010".
- Pin and tube appliance was developed in 1901. In this pin and tube appliance, all teeth are banded. Vertical tubes were welded to the bands on the labial surface in the center of the crown for all teeth in the arch. Arch wires were secured with soldered pins that inserted into the vertical tubes. Tooth movement was achieved by altering the placement of these pins.
- Angle developed Ribbon arch appliance in 1910. It is a modification of pin and tube appliance. Ribbon arch was the first appliance to use a true bracket. The bracket has a vertical slot facing occlusally. The brackets were attached to the bands at the center of labial surface of teeth.

- Edgewise appliance was developed and introduced to orthodontics by Edward H Angle in the year 1925 which formed the basis of all fixed orthodontic techniques in use today. In order to overcome the deficiencies encountered with his previous techniques Angle developed the edgewise bracket that could give a better control over individual tooth movement **(Fig. 2.6)**.

The unique feature of rectangular arch wire in a rectangular slot of the edgewise bracket enabled control of tooth movement in all three planes of space. Subsequent development of various fixed orthodontic appliances such as Straight wire appliance, pre adjusted edgewise appliance are actually modifications of the standard edgewise appliance of Angle.

### Edward H Angle's Publications and Presentations

- Angle presented his first scientific paper at the Ninth International Medical Congress in 1887.
- Published the first edition of his textbook 1887 which would go through seven editions under the following titles:
1. *Irregularities of the Teeth*, 1887.
2. *A System of Appliances for Correcting Irregularities of the Teeth*, 1890.
3. *The Angle System of Regulating and Retention of the Teeth*, 1892.
4. *The Angle System of Regulation and Retention of the Teeth—with an Addition of Treatment of Fractures of the Maxillae*, 1895.
5. *Angle System of Regulation and Retention of the Teeth and Treatment of Fractures of the Maxillae*, 1899.
6. *Malocclusion of the Teeth and Fractures of the Maxillae*, 1900.
7. *Treatment of Malocclusion of the Teeth*, 1907.
- Angle published his famous article "The Classification of Malocclusion" in the Dental Cosmos, 1899. His classification provided an intelligent and easily understood means of communication among members of the dental profession. Angle believed that the maxillary first molars were the key to occlusion and his system of classification divides malocclusions in anteroposterior/sagittal plane only. Despite this drawback, Angle's classification system has stood the test of time and is still the most commonly used method of classifying malocclusions, more than 100 years since he first proposed it.

Though Angle died in 1930 (August 11th), his influence is still felt strongly in orthodontics. His concept of normal occlusion and establishment orthodontia as a specialty science will remain Angle's greatest monument. Characteristic of the man was a remark made shortly before he died: "I have finished my work. It is as perfect as I can make it."

Another distinguished orthodontist was **Calvin S Case (1847-1923) (Fig. 2.7)**. He developed a classification of malocclusion that included 26 divisions. Case published his major work "A practical treatise on the techniques and

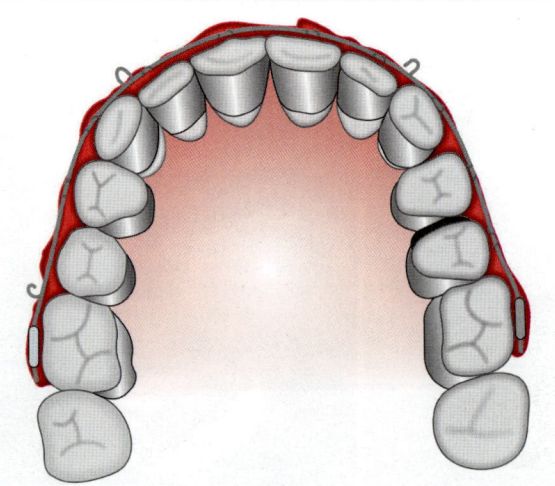

**Fig. 2.6:** Edgewise appliance

principle of dental orthopedic and prosthetic correction of the cleft palate." Case was a strong advocate of the relationship of malocclusion to facial improvement. Facial improvement was a guide to treatment. He was also a strong proponent of extraction theory in orthodontics.

**Charles A Hawley (1861–1929)** used a celluloid sheet containing a geometric figure that when adapted to a model determined the extent of proposed tooth movement (1905) and introduced the retainer appliance that bears his name (1908) **(Fig. 2.8).**

**HD Kesling (1945)** introduced his philosophy of tooth movement by using a rubber tooth positioning device in which the teeth were moved into a more ideal cuspal relationship after major correction has been accomplished.

## History of Cephalometrics

Ever since God created man in His image, man has been trying to change man into his image. Attempts to change facial appearance are recounted throughout recorded history. The question of what is a normal face, as that of what constitutes beauty, will probably never be answered in a free society. **(Table 2.6)**

Orthodontists, in their attempts to change facio-orodental deviations from accepted norms, have adopted cephalometric measurement, a method long employed in physical anthropology. With the introduction of roentgenography, it was inevitable that this procedure should be employed as a medium for the purpose of roentgenographic cephalometrics.

Cephalometric radiography was introduced to orthodontics during the 1930s.

Cephalometry had its beginnings in craniometry. **Craniometry** is defined in the Edinburgh encyclopedia of 1813 as "the art of measuring skulls of animals so as to discover their specific differences". For many years anatomists and anthropologists were confined to measuring craniofacial dimensions using the skull of dead individuals. Although precise measurements were possible craniometry has the disadvantage for growth studies.

**Cephalometry** is concerned with measuring the head inclusive of soft tissues, be it living or dead. However, this procedure had its limitations owing to the inaccuracies that resulted from having to measure skulls through varying thickness of soft tissues.

With the discovery of X-rays by Roentgen in 1895, **radiographic cephalometry** came in to being. It was defined as the measurement of head from bony and soft tissue land marks on the radiographic image (Krogman and Sassouni 1957). This approach combines the advantages of craniometry and anthropometry. The disadvantage is that it produces two-dimensional image of a three-dimensional structure.

In **1895, Professor Wilhelm Conrad Roentgen** made a remarkable contribution to the field of science with the discovery of X-rays. On December 28, 1895, he submitted a paper **"On A New Kind of Rays, A Preliminary Communication"** to the Wurzburg Physical Medical Society for publication in its journal.

**Professor Wilhem Koening and Dr Otto Walkhoff** simultaneously made the first dental radiograph in **1896**. It was clear that the use of X-rays provided the means of obtaining a different perspective on the arrangement

| Year | Authors | Contributions to orthodontics |
|---|---|---|
| 1899–1996 | William B Downs | • Cephalometric appraisal of orthodontic results<br>• Down's analysis |
| 1900–1984 | Herbert I Margolis | Tweeds triangle |
| 1913–1966 | Wendell L Wylie | Analysis based on dividing dimensions along the Frankfort plane into contributing linear components |
| 1922–1994 | Richard A Riedel | ANB angle |
| 1967 | Alexander Jacobson | The Wit's analysis |

**Table 2.6:** Cephalometry

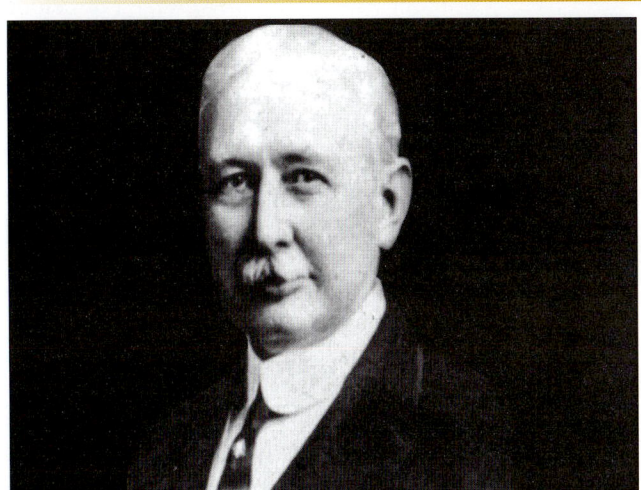

**Fig. 2.7:** Calvin S Case (1847–1923)

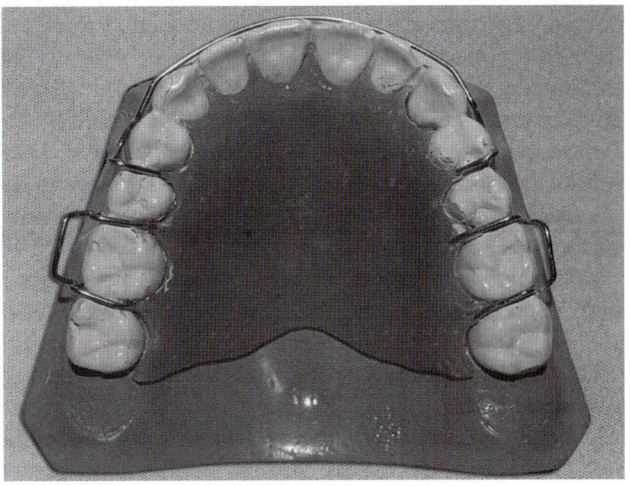

**Fig. 2.8:** Hawley's retainer introduced by Charles A Hawley

and relation of bones thus expanding the horizons of craniometry and cephalometry.

The first X-ray pictures of skull in the standard lateral view were taken by **AJ Pacini** and **Carrera in 1922**. Pacini received a research award from the American Roentgen Ray Society for a thesis entitled **"Roentgen Ray Anthropometry of the Skull"**. Pacini introduced a teleroentgenographic technique for standardized lateral head radiography and thereby opened, what proved to become a tremendous advance in cephalometry, as well as in measuring the growth and development of face. His method, which was rather primitive, involved a large fixed distance from the X-ray source to the cassette. The head of the subject, placed adjacent to a standard holding the cassette, was immobilized with a gauze bandage wrapped around both the face and the cassette after the patient's midsagittal plane was carefully oriented parallel to the cassette.

He identified the following anthropometric landmarks on the roentgenogram: gonion, pogonion, nasion, and anterior nasal spine. He also located the center of the sella turcica and the external auditory meatus. He measured the gonion angle and the degree of maxillary protrusion.

In **1931** the methodology of cephalometric radiography came to full function when **B Holly Broadbent in USA and H Hofrath in Germany** simultaneously published methods to obtain standardized head radiographs in the Angle Orthodontist (**A new X-ray technique and its application to orthodontia**) and in Fortschritte der Orthodontie, respectively.

This development enabled orthodontists to capture the field of cephalometry from the anatomists and anthropologists who had monopolized craniometric studies, particularly in nineteenth century.

## B Holly Broadbent's Contribution

**B Holly Broadbent (1931)** published an article in the first issue of the new Angle Orthodontist titled "A New X-ray technique and its application to orthodontia." It was the introduction to the specialty and to dentistry of cephalometric roentgenography **(Fig. 2.9)** and of course, cephalometric tracing and evaluation. Broadbent devised the roentgenographic cephalometer, which is the instrument that accurately positions the head relative to the film and the X-ray source. His study, supported by the Bolton family, consisted of a longitudinal study of 3,500 school children from birth to adulthood. In honor of his sponsor, Broadbent established a new point of reference on the skull, known as the Bolton point.

Broadbent's interest in craniofacial growth began with his orthodontic education under EH Angle in 1920. He continued to pursue that interest along with his orthodontic practice, working with a leading anatomist **J Wingate Todd.**

The uncertainty of locating landmarks in the skull of the living child by approaching through skin and soft tissues led him to search for a means of recording craniometric landmarks on the living child as accurately as done with a craniostat in measuring the dead skull.

During 1920s, Broadbent refined the craniostat into craniometer by the addition of metric scales. That proved to be the first step in the evolution of craniostat into a radiographic cephalostat. It did not take him much longer to convert the direct measuring instrument into a radiographic craniometer.

Meanwhile the course of Broadbent's orthodontic practice he corrected the malocclusion of **Charles Bingham Bolton,** son of **Chester** and **Francis P Bolton.** His discussions of facial growth with Congress woman Bolton led to the addition of Bolton study of facial growth to the long list of Bolton philanthropies. As Charles grew to adulthood this study became a major personal as well as financial commitment.

Cephalometrics was neither developed as a technique looking for an application nor was it developed as a diagnostic tool. Broadbent's single goal was the study of craniofacial growth. The Broadbent technique for cephalometric radiography was one of the tools that he developed for the implementation of that study.

The technique and apparatus perfected for the **Bolton Fund study of the normal developmental growth of the face**, eliminated practically all of the technical difficulties encountered in previous methods of recording dentofacial changes, and proved to be a convenient as well as scientific method of measuring orthodontic procedures.

According to Broadbent the patient's head was centered in the cephalostat with the superior borders of the external auditory meatus resting on the upper parts the two ear rods. The lowest point on the inferior bony border of the left orbit, indicated by the orbital marker, was at the level of the upper parts of the ear rods. The nose clamp was fixed at the root of the nose to support the upper part of the face. The focus film distance was set at 5 feet (152.4 cm) and the subject film distance could be measured to calculate image magnification. With the two X-ray tubes at right angles to each other in the same horizontal

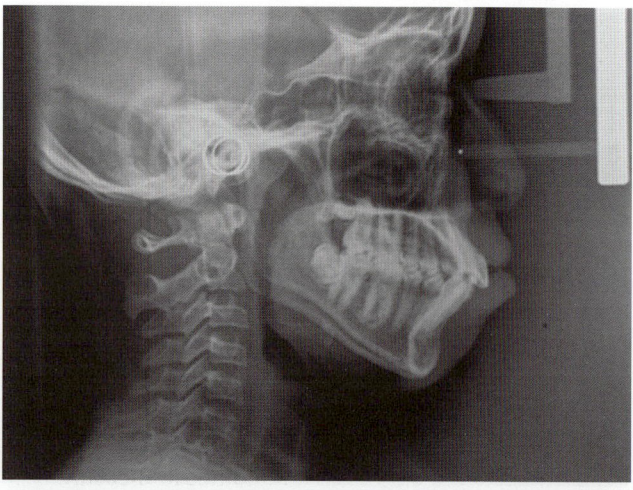

**Fig. 2.9:** Cephalometric roentgenography (Lateral cephalogram)

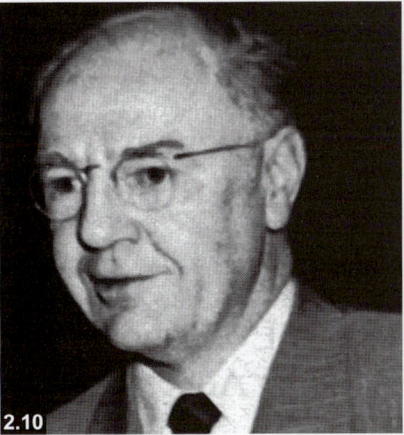 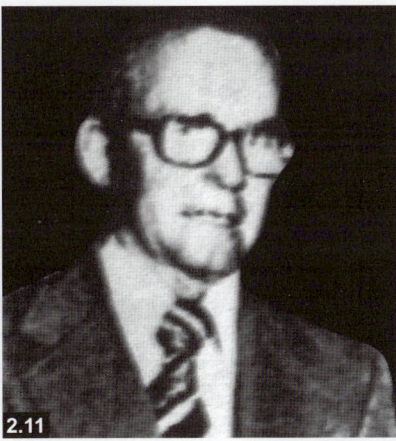 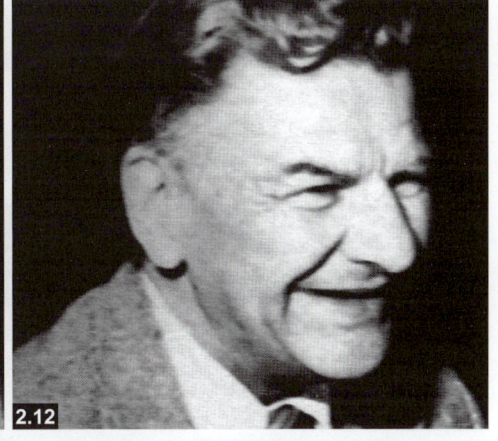

**Fig. 2.10:** William B Downs (1899–1996); **Fig. 2.11:** Herbert I Margolis (1900–1984); **Fig. 2.12:** Richard A Riedel (1922–1994)

plane, two images (lateral and posteroanterior) could be simultaneously produced.

While Germany's Hofrath's technique differed from Broadbent's in that the path of the central ray was not fixed in relation to the head and no plan was suggested for superpositioning subsequent X-rays.

**William B Downs (1899–1996) (Fig. 2.10)** was a mainstay of the teaching staff at Illinois's. With Brodie, Goldstein, and Myer, he coauthored "Cephalometric appraisal of orthodontic results" (1938).

**Margolis (1900–1984) (Fig 2.11)** wrote on the relationship between the inclination of the lower incisor and the incisor-mandibular plane angle and was the first to corroborate Tweed's clinical observation that, in normal occlusions, the lower incisors are 90° to the mandibular basal bone.

In **1947, Wylie** produced a method of assessing anteroposterior dysplasias, and, that same year, Margolis contributed his maxillofacial triangle.

## Cephalometric Analysis

The major use of radiographic cephalometry is in characterizing the patient's dental and skeletal relationships. This led to the development of a number of cephalometric analyses to compare a patient to his or her peers, using population standards. **William B Downs in 1948** developed the first cephalometric analysis. Its significance was that it presented an objective method of portraying many factors underlying malocclusion and there could be a variety of causes of malocclusion exclusive to teeth. This was followed by other analyses by Cecil C Steiner (1953), C H Tweed (1953), RM Ricketts (1958), V. Sassouni (1969), HD Enlow (1969), JR Jaraback (1970), and Alex Jacobson (1975), etc.

**Richard A Riedel (1922–1994):** Even before completing his master's requirements at Northwestern University, Richard A Riedel **(Fig. 2.12)**, introduced one of the most widely accepted diagnostic cephalometric measurement in use, that is, ANB angle.

## REMOVABLE ORTHODONTIC APPLIANCE

Removable orthodontic appliances are so called because they are designed to be fitted and removed by the patient. Removable orthodontic appliances are limited to tipping and simple rotator movements of teeth, which are sufficient for many orthodontic treatments. They depend on co-operation and a certain degree of skill on the part of the patient. Removable orthodontic appliances may be active or passive.

The use of removable orthodontic appliances was always more popular in Europe than the United States, but even there the use of fixed appliances (using bands and brackets) has largely become the primary method of treatment. Nevertheless, removable appliances are often an effective means of addressing many patients' needs and in some cases have considerable advantages over fixed appliances.

Removable orthodontic appliance consists of following three components:
1. Retentive components
2. Active components
3. Base plate.

### Retentive Components

The success of a removable orthodontic appliance mainly depends upon good retention of the appliance. Adequate retention of a removable orthodontic appliance is achieved by incorporating certain wire components, which get engaged into the undercuts on the teeth. These wires components that help in retention of a removable appliance are called clasps.

### Clasps

Clasps are the retentive components of removable orthodontic appliances. Following are the researchers, involved in the design of various types of clasps **(Table 2.7).**

### Bows

Bows are one of the active components of removable orthodontic appliance. They are usually used for overjet

**Table 2.7:** Clasps

| S. no | Types of clasp | Designed by |
|---|---|---|
| 1. | Adam's clasp | CP Adams |
| 2. | Schwartz clasp | Schwartz |
| 3. | Crozat clasp | Crozat |

**Table 2.8:** Expansion orthodontic appliances

| S. no | Type of expansion appliance | Developed by |
|---|---|---|
| 1. | Derichsweiler expansion appliance | Derichsweiler |
| 2. | Issacson's expansion appliances | Issacson |
| 3. | Hass expansion appliance | Hass |
| 4. | Coffin spring | Walter Coffin |
| 5. | Jack expansion screw | Jack |

retraction of anteriors. They can also be used for space closure in the anterior segment as well as space distal to canines. The following are some of the routinely used design of labial bows:

1. Short labial bow
2. Long labial bow
3. Split labial bow
4. Modified split labial bow
5. Reverse labial bow
6. Robert's retractor
7. Mill's retractor
8. High labial bow
9. Filled labial bow

## BASE PLATE

Base plate has a greater percentage of bulk in removable orthodontic appliance than other components. The design of base plate varies with the type of removable orthodontic appliance. Self cure or autopolymerizing acrylic resins are used for the fabrication of base plate. It joins all other (active and retentive) components of removable orthodontic appliance together into a single functional unit.

## EXPANSION ORTHODONTIC APPLIANCES

Expansion orthodontic appliances are used to relieve crowding in cases of arch length–tooth material discrepancy. Following are the researchers involved in the development of various types of expansion appliances **(Table 2.8)**.

## MYOFUNCTIONAL/FUNCTIONAL ORTHODONTIC APPLIANCES

The term functional appliance means that when the appliance is fully seated in the mouth, the mandible is forced into an eccentric/noneccentric relation position. Any such mandibular posture causes the musculature to try to move the mandible toward a centric position. This results in force systems being exerted whenever the appliance is mounted on the teeth or soft tissues of the mouth.

Although functional appliances have been used throughout the century in Europe and in the last 40 years in the United States, it was not until the late 1960s that scientific data were available to evaluate the empiric rationalization for their clinical effectiveness. This early data consisted of animal experiments demonstrating histologic and radiographic evidence of increased growth of the condylar cartilage when the mandible was held in a forward position. Petrovic suggested that the unique characteristics of the condylar cartilage, including cell division of the prechondroblast (as opposed to the chondroblast in epiphyseal cartilage of the long bones or cartilage in the synchondroses of the cranial base) make this cartilage more responsive to orthopedic devices. The animal studies of the 1960s and 1970s created enormous enthusiasm in the professional community and played an important role in the rapid acceptance and use of functional appliances in the United States that has been largely ignored up till that time.

### Activator

Norman Kingsley, an early influential American orthodontist, has been credited with the development of the first appliances to position the mandible forward as early as 1879. However, most consider Pierre Robin to have developed the earliest removable functional appliance, in fiance in 1902.

Hotz devised a "Vorbissplatte" which was a modified form of Kingsley's vulcanite palatal plate. This was used to treat retrognathism associated with deep bite.

Pierre Robin devised an appliance called Monobloc made up of a single block of vulcanite. He used it to position the mandible forward in patients with glossoptosis and severe mandibular retrognathism. By positioning the mandible forward; it reduced the risk of airway obstruction.

**Viggo Andresen** in 1908 **(Fig. 2.13)** in Denmark designed a loose filling appliance which he first used on his daughter. He made a modified Hawley type of retainer on the maxillary arch to which he added a lower lingual horse-shoe-shaped flange which helped in positioning the mandible forward. He used this appliance on his daughter who was going on a three month vacation. On her return three months later, he found a marked sagittal correction and improvement of the facial profile.

Although it was developed more than 70 years ago, the Andreson appliance, which is also known as an activator or monobloc, has been successfully used by generation of orthodontists. The thousands of cases from last 25 years, the activator is generally used in Vienna for the treatment of Class II Div I malocclusion.

During the time of Viggo Andresen and Haupl the appliances were made of vulcanized rubber, but this gave way to acrylic in the 1950s. Over the year, various modifications have been made to the original design of Andresen's appliance such as:

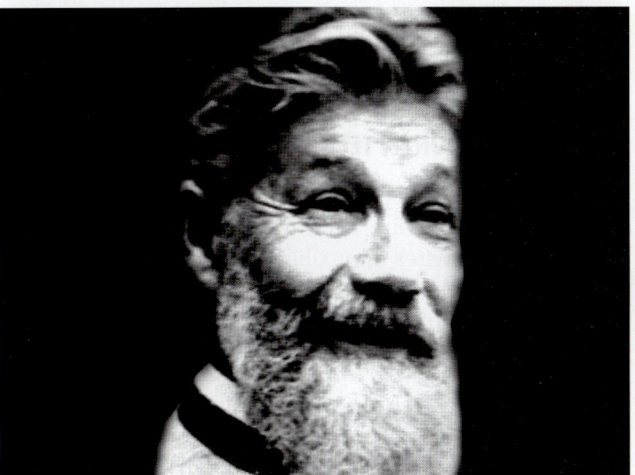

**Fig. 2.13:** Viggo Andresen

1. The bow activator of AM Schwartz
2. Wunderer's modification
3. The propulsor
4. Cutout or palate free activator
5. The reduced activator or cybernator of Schmuth
6. Kawetzky modification
7. Herren's modification of the activator.

Most of the modifications of Andresen appliance were based on Andresen's concepts. There can be advantages to using a simple design in terms of patient co-operation, case of adjustment and freedom from breakages.

*Graber observed that,*
"Numerous modifications have been made to the Andresen–Haupl monobloc and have been described in texts and periodical contributions by Petrik, Eschler, Hoffer, Grossman and others. These are surprisingly effective at times but generally a simpler design of appliance is preferred."

## Frankel Appliance

A more recent innovation in functional appliance design, the functional corrector or functional regulator or Frankel appliance was designed by Rolf Frankel in Germany and was introduced to orthodontics in 1966. This appliance was unique in that, it was principally tissue-borne, mostly supported in the vestibule rather than supported by teeth. There are five types of Frankel appliances and are used for management of Angle's class I, class II and class III malocclusions and even it is used in bimaxillary protrusion.

## Bionator

The Bionator was developed in Germany by Wilhelm Balter in the early 1950s to increase patient's comfort and facilitate daytime wear to increase the functional use of the appliance. Balter accomplished this by drastically reducing acrylic bulk of the appliance. There are three types of bionators:

1. Standard bionator.
2. Class III or reverse bionator.
3. Open bite bionator.

## Twin-block Appliance

Twin-block appliance is a functional jaw orthopedic appliance developed by Scottish orthodontist William Clark in the year 1977.

The twin-block appliance is composed of maxillary and mandibular retainers that fit tightly against the teeth, alveolus, and adjacent supporting structures. Delta clasps are used bilaterally to anchor the maxillary appliance to the first permanent molars and 0.030 inch ball clasps are placed in the interproximal areas anteriorly. The precise clasp configuration depends on the type of deciduous or permanent teeth and number of teeth present at the time of appliance construction.

Various designs are available for the lower part of the twin block appliance. The original design advocated by clark and it consists of a horse shoe of acrylic that extends anteriorly from the mesial of the first permanent molars.

The acrylic covers the lingual aspect of the premolar/deciduous molars and the canines and incisors. In this design delta clasps are used to anchor the appliance to the first premolar/first deciduous molar and ball clasp are present between the canines and lateral incisors, additional ball clasps can be placed between the incisors if appliance retention is thought to be a problem. There should not be any acrylic material touching the lower molars, this allows the lower molar to erupt vertically if the acrylic on the maxillary block is trimmed to increase the vertical dimension.

The twin block appliance has been shown to produce increase in mandibular length, incisor proclination and variations in lower anterior facial height.

The posterior bite blocks of the twin block appliance can be trimmed to facilitate the eruption of the lower posterior teeth in patient with a deep bite and an accentuated curve of Spee. The blocks also can be left untouched to prevent the eruption of the posterior teeth in patients with a tendency toward an anterior open bite.

## Herbst Appliance

The Herbst bite jumping mechanism, was developed by Emil Herbst in the early 1900s. The original banded design of this appliance was introduced at the international dental congress in Berlin (Germany) by Herbst in 1905. It was introduced by Pancherz. Pancherz used a banded Herbst design that involved the:

- Placement of bands on molar and premolar in maxilla
- Bands are connected by copper lingual wire.
- Bands on lower right first premolar and lower right first premolar
- Bands are connected by a lower lingual arch wire

The Herbst appliance is a fixed functional orthopedic appliance having passive tube and plunger system with the exact length of the tube determining the amount of

**Table 2.9:** Myofunctional/Functional orthodontic appliances

| S. no | Types of appliance | Designed by | Year |
|---|---|---|---|
| 1. | Activator | Viggo Andresen (Fig. 2.13) | 1908 |
| 2. | Frankel appliance | Rolf Frankel | 1966 |
| 3. | Bionator functional appliance | Wilhelm Balter | 1950 |
| 4. | Jasper jumper | Joseper | |
| 5. | Twin-block appliance | William Clark | 1977 |
| 6. | Herbst appliance | Emil Herbst | 1990 |
| 7. | Oral Screen | Newell | 1912 |

**Table 2.10:** Fixed orthodontic techniques

| S. no | Techniques | Formulated by |
|---|---|---|
| 1. | E–Arch | Edward H Angle |
| 2. | Pin and tube technique | Edward H Angle |
| 3. | Edge wire technique | Edward H Angle |
| 4. | Begg technique | PR Begg |
| 5. | Straight wire technique | Lawrence F Andrew |
| 6. | Lingual orthodontics | Cruz |
| 7. | Invisalign technique | Zia Chrishti |
| 8. | 3D modular orthodontics | Wilson and Wilson |

**Table 2.11:** Retainers

| S. no | Types of retainer | Designed by |
|---|---|---|
| 1. | Hawleys retainer | Hawleys |
| 2. | Begg retainer | PR Begg |
| 3. | Kesling tooth position | HD Kesling (1945) |
| 4. | Invisible retainer | Osmu |

Followings are the researchers involved in the development of various types of myofunctional appliances **(Table 2.9)**.

## FIXED ORTHODONTIC TECHNIQUES

Fixed orthodontic appliance is an orthodontic device in which attachments are fixed to the teeth and forces are applied by arch wires or auxiliaries via these attachments. Various fixed orthodontic techniques are evolved over the years and followings are the researchers involved in the formulation of fixed orthodontic techniques **(Table 2.10)**.

## RETENTION IN ORTHODONTICS

The term "retention" has been defined as "the holding of teeth in idealistic and functional positions" (Joondeph and Riedel, 1985). Followings are the researchers involved in the development of various types of retainers **(Table 2.11)**.

Changes in the areas of orthodontic practice include a resurgence of treatment of the adult patients and its concomitant expertise as the public becomes aware of personal dental health and esthetics. Included also are the invasion of areas that had not received much attention in the past, namely, orthognathic surgery and the problems associated with the temporomandibular joint. Orthodontics has achieved the status of a recognized specialty of dentistry because of a long period of craftsmanship and professional expertise.

## BIBLIOGRAPHY

1. Enlow DH, Moyers RE, Hunter WS, et al. A procedure for the analysis of intrinsic factor form and growth. Am J Orthod 1969;56:6-14.
2. Graber TM. Orthodontics: Principles and Practice. WB Saunders, 1998.
3. Profitt WR. Contemporary Orthodontics. St Louis: CV Mosby, 1986.
4. Quintero JC, et al. Craniofacial imaging in orthodontics: historical perspective, current status and future develop-ments. Angle Orthod 1999;69:491-506.

anterior mandibular development. The tube is attached to a maxillary posterior tooth, whereas the plunger is fixed anteriorly to the mandibular dentition and slides through the tube during opening and closing movements.

### EXAM-ORIENTED QUESTIONS

**Long Essay or Long Questions**

1. Define orthodontics and write in detail about history of orthodontics.
2. History of orthodontics
3. Angle's contribution to orthodontics
4. Tweed's contribution to orthodontics

**Long Note or Short Essay**

1. Orthodontics in 18th century
2. Orthodontics in 19th century
3. Orthodontics in 20th century.

# CHAPTER OVERVIEW

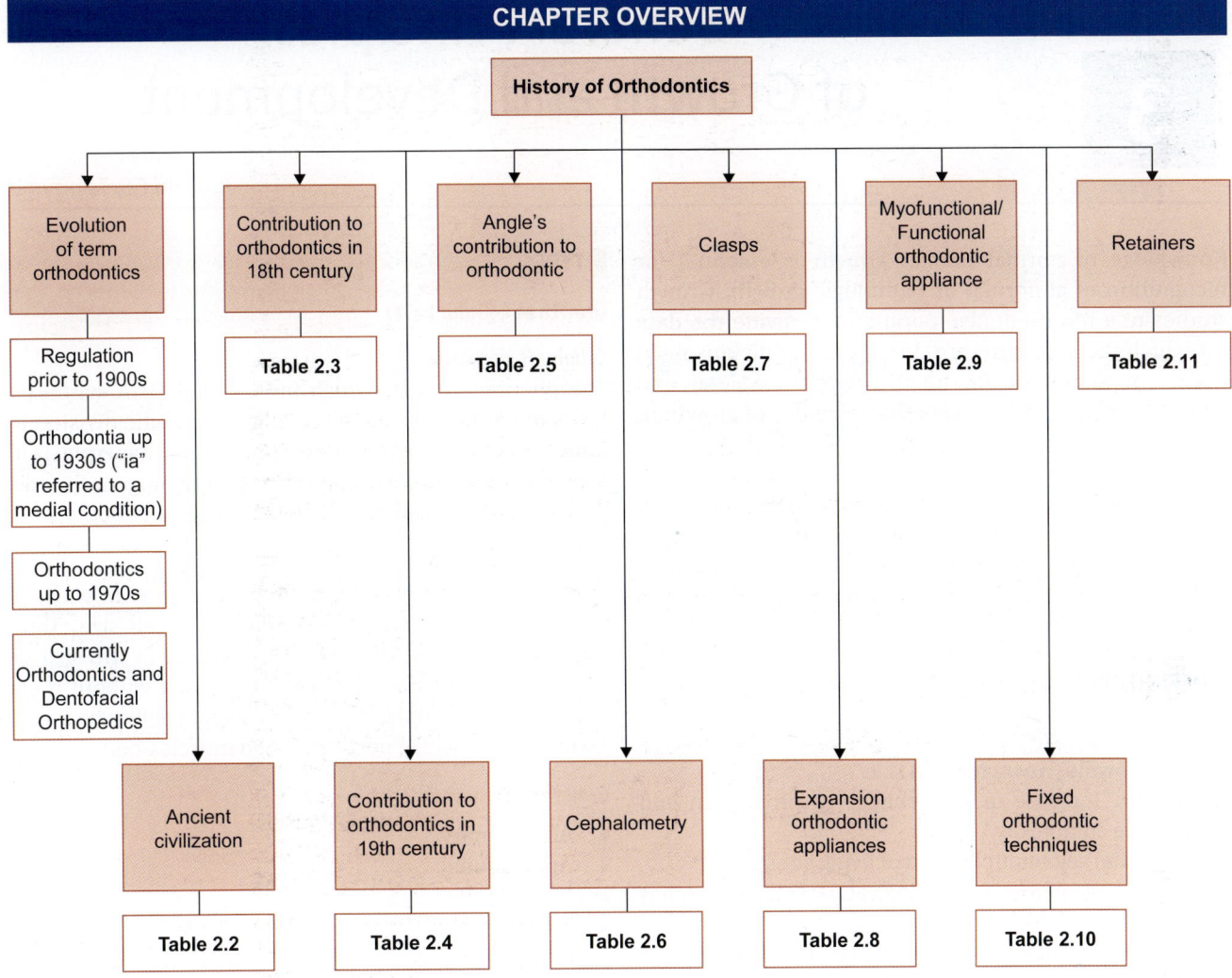

# CHAPTER 3

# General Principles of Growth and Development

*Rashmi GS, Tsipova V*

Knowledge of normal human growth is essential for recognition of abnormal or pathologic growth. Growth studies of a representative population provide the data for which the standards are developed. Clinicians need norms or standards for height, weight, skeletal and dental development to assess the normalcy of growth in patients.

Understanding the principles and complexity of craniofacial growth is of paramount importance to orthodontists, since timely recognition and intervention of an abnormal jaw growth pattern by appropriate orthodontic appliances can restore the normal occlusion and facial harmony using the active growth period.

## DEFINITION

### Growth

**Todd:** "Growth is an increase in size."
**Krogman:** "Increase in size, change in proportion and progressive complexity."
**Huxley:** "The self multiplication of living substance."
**Moss:** "Change in any morphological parameter, which is measurable."
**Moyers:** "Quantitative aspect of biologic development per unit of time."

"Entire series of sequential anatomic and physiologic changes taking place from the beginning of prenatal life to senility."

### Development

**Todd:** "Development is progress towards maturity."
**Moyers:** "All the naturally occurring unidirectional changes in the life of an individual from its existence as a single cell to its elaboration as a multifunctional unit terminating in death."

The terms "growth and development" are interrelated and some basic differences between the two can be appreciated. Growth is considered an anatomic phenomenon while development is a physiological and behavioral phenomenon. Growth is a change in size or quantity, i.e. growth is a measurable aspect of biologic life. Development on the other hand includes growth as well as differentiation.

The term "growth" simply means an increase in mass of life. However, the process of growth of cells and tissues is so complex that it is necessary to distinguish between different types of growth.

## TYPES

### Growth at Cellular Level

#### Cellular Hyperplasia

The phenomenon by which protein and DNA synthesis leads to an increase in cell number by mitotic division is known as cellular hyperplasia. For example, hyperplasia is seen during stages of embryogenesis, organogenesis, and growth in utero as well as in infancy and childhood.

#### Cellular Hypertrophy

Here, synthesis of protein and cellular material without mitotic division leads to an increase in cell size. Thus hypertrophic growth involves an increase in the size of the specific cells that characterize a tissue without their division. For example, it is usually seen in cells which can no longer divide like nerve cells and muscle fibers.

### Growth at Tissue Level

- Accretionary
- Appositional
- Interstitial
- Meristematic
- Compensatory

#### Accretionary

In this type of growth, there is an increase in the amount of extracellular matrix between tissue cells rather than an increase in either cell number or cell size.

#### Appositional

It is the specific type of growth in which new generation of cells and extracellular matrix are added to the surface of the tissue by the repeated division of cells by a cambial layer that surrounds the tissue; e.g. periosteum and perichondrium.

#### Interstitial

Interstitial growth is seen where multiplication and sometimes accretionary growth continues throughout the thickness of a tissue mass which consequently grows as a whole and expands from within.

#### Meristematic

It describes growth from a tip that contains populations of dividing cells. As division occurs, the tip moves distally leaving behind populations of cells from its earlier divisions, e.g. growth seen in limb buds in which the progress zone first produces the cells of shoulder and then is moved distally to produce cell populations of the arm and so on.

### Compensatory
A balance is maintained between loss through wear and tear and the maintenance of functional tissue integrity. For example, the regeneration of liver to gain its approximate original size after a major loss of its tissue.

## PHASES

Growth is continuous from conception to death, but it differs in rate and duration for various parts of body. Certain phases of growth can be identified as follows:
- *Prenatal growth:* It is characterized by a rapid rise in cell numbers and fast growth rates.
- *Postnatal growth:* It lasts for about the first 20 years of life and is characterized by declining growth rates and increasing the maturation of tissues.
- *Maturity:* It is a period of stability during which body achieves maximum function and growth processes are limited to the maintenance of an equilibrium state between cellular loss and gain.
- *Old age:* It is a period during which functional activity declines and growth processes slow down.

## FACTORS AFFECTING GROWTH AND MATURATION

Growths during embryonic, fetal, and postnatal periods are regulated by a variety of factors which are not completely understood. The following factors influence growth and maturation:

### Genetic Factors
The genes have the basic control of growth including rate, timing and magnitude. However, the final outcome and growth depends on the interaction between the genetic potential and environmental factors.

### Growth Hormones and Growth Factors
Probably all of the endocrine hormones have some influence on growth. In particular, postnatal growth is profoundly affected by the circulating concentration of growth hormone (somatotropin), growth hormone releasing hormone and somatostatin. All tissues respond to growth hormone and produce a proportional body growth that slows after puberty when secretion of the hormone decreases. Lack of growth hormone causes dwarfism, whereas its continued secretion produces gigantism. Abnormal secretion of growth hormone after the epiphysis plates have fused, results in acromegaly.

Other growth factors affecting growth are:
- Insulin-like growth factor - I and II (IGF-I, IGF-II)
- Platelet-derived growth factor
- Epidermal growth factor
- Vascular endothelial growth factor (VEGF)
- Transforming growth factor B (TGF -B)

The hormones of thyroid gland, thyroxine and triiodothyronine stimulate metabolism and are important in the growth of bones, teeth and the brain. The changes seen at adolescence are caused by the secretion of androgens and gonadal hormones.

### Nutrition
Poor nutrition at critical stages of life may permanently alter the normal development pattern of many organs and tissues. Proper nutrition is essential for normal postnatal growth. Apart from adequate supply of proteins, all diet should include vitamins, minerals, etc. Calcium, magnesium, phosphorous, manganese and fluorides are essential for proper bone and tooth growth. Vitamin A controls activities of both osteoclasts and osteoblasts, and its deficiency may be associated with defective bone growth. Vitamin C is necessary for proper bone and connective tissue growth. Vitamin D is also required for normal bone growth. Malnutrition results in disordered growth. However, growth process accelerates when deficient nutrient is replaced during growth period, i.e. the "catching up" growth.

### Secular Trends
There is considerable evidence that children today are growing faster than they grew in the past, for example, studies have shown that boys of 15 years of age are 5 inches taller than the same age group some decades earlier. Such secular trend may be due to decreased illness and improve health.

### Illness
Prolonged and debilitating illness can have an adverse effect on growth. However, after the period of illness, "catch up" growth normally brings the child back to the predetermined growth curve.

### Season and Circadian Rhythm
Growth in height is faster in spring than in autumn, while weight increase occurs faster in autumn than in spring. Growth also shows a circadian rhythm; growth in height and eruption of teeth appears to be greater at night than in daytime due to fluctuations in the hormone release.

### Psychological Stress
Evidence shows that psychological stress can adversely affect growth by inhibiting hormone secretion.

## METHODS OF STUDYING PHYSICAL GROWTH

The following are the two major approaches of studying physical growth. Measurement approach and experimental approach.

### Measurement Approach
This approach includes techniques that measure certain criteria on living animals/skeletal remains. These techniques are not invasive. Most growth studies on humans are conducted by measurement techniques.

Various measurement techniques can be used on living individuals or the skeletal remains including:
- Craniometry
- Anthropometry
- Cephalometric radiography

***Craniometry:*** It involves the measurement of human skulls of different age groups to appreciate the growth changes. Although it allows three-dimensional (3D) measurements, such studies can only be cross sectional.

***Anthropometry:*** It is a technique in which skeletal dimensions are measured on living individuals. Various standard landmarks established in the studies of dry skull are measured on living individuals by using soft tissue points overlying these bony landmarks. Although soft tissue thickness may vary, such techniques may be advantageous in that they allow longitudinal study of growth by repeated measurements of the same individuals over a period of life.

***Cephalometric radiography:*** This technique has contributed majorly in our study of growth and development before it became a routine practice to use the cephalogram for orthodontic diagnosis and planning. Standard cephalometric points are noted on serial radiographs of individuals and compared to analyze the growth changes occurring.

## Experimental Approach

This approach includes techniques that may be manipulative and invasive in nature and thus may harm the animal. Such studies are carried out on experimental animals. Experimental methods of study growth include the following:
- Vital staining
- Radioisotopes
- Autoradiography
- Implant radiography

### Vital Staining

Vital staining was introduced by John Hunter in the 18th century. Certain vital stains can be used to determine the sequence and amount of new bone formation as well as specific locations of bone growth by utilizing histologic sections. The method involves injecting the dyes that stain the mineralizing tissues. These stains get incorporated into the bones and teeth and thus allow the study of changes in bones and teeth. Experimental animals are then sacrificed and the mineralizing tissues are studied histologically.

By this method, detailed analysis of site, amount and rate of growth can be elicited. However, this does not allow longitudinal study. Repeated data of the same individual over time cannot be obtained. Examples of stains are Alizarin S, procion, tetracycline, trypan blue, and fluorochrome.

### Radioisotopes

Radioactive elements can be injected into tissues of experimental animals which get incorporated into the developing bone. Bone growth can be studied tracking the radioactivity emitted by those radioisotopes. For example, calcium 45, technetium 33 (Ca 45, Tc 33).

### Implant Radiography

Metallic implants are used as radiographic markers in chemical and experimental work to study bone remodelling and displacement. The technique first introduced by Bjork (1955) involves the implantation of small pieces of inert alloys into the growing bone. These implanted alloys will act as radiographic reference points. By examining the position of these implants on serial radiographs taken at regular intervals, bone growth can be monitored.

Information such as site of growth, amount of growth, rate of growth and direction of growth can be elicited accurately using implant radiography. It allows longitudinal study of growth. However, the method allows only two-dimensional (2D) study of 3D growth process. Radiation hazard is another disadvantage of this method.

### Sites of Implantation

In Mandible:
i. Symphysis in the midline below roots
ii. Right body of the mandible: One below first premolar and another below first molar
iii. Outer surface of the ramus on right side in level of occlusal plane.

In Maxilla:
i. Inferior to anterior nasal spine
ii. Bilaterally in the zygomatic process

In Hard Palate
i. Behind canines
ii. Front of first molar in the junction between alveolar process and palate.

## GROWTH DATA

### Types

The following are the different types of growth data which can be used to study growth:

***Opinion:*** It is a clever guess of an experienced person. It is not accurate and should be avoided.

***Observations:*** These are useful in studying presence or absence of certain findings such as dental caries.

***Ratings and rankings:*** They are used when it is difficult to quantify particular data. Rating uses a standard and conventionally accepted rate of classification while ranking involves arrangement of data in an orderly sequence based on the value.

***Quantitative measurements:*** The data derived from accurate quantitative measurements are the most appropriate scientifically.

Measurements can be made in the following three ways:
- Direct data is obtained from direct measurements on living individuals or skeletal remains using tapes and calipers.
- Indirect data are the measurements obtained indirectly from images/reproduction of the individual, such as photographs, radiographs or dental casts.

- Derived data are the measurements derived by comparison of two measurements, e.g. radiography and implant.

### Modes of Collection

Growth studies are of the following three types:

#### Cross-sectional Studies

A large number of individuals of different age groups are examined at one occasion to develop information on growth attained at a particular age. In a short period of time, much information can be gathered about growth at many ages. The majority of information available about growth has been obtained using cross-sectional methods. It is less time consuming and a large sample size can be included in the study due to shorter span of time.

Although mean rate of growth for a population can be estimated, variability of growth in the subjects of the sample cannot be studied.

#### Longitudinal Studies

Longitudinal studies involve repeated examination and measurements of same subjects at regular intervals over a long period during active growth. As the same subjects are followed up over long periods, the velocity pattern of development of an individual can be studied. Variability of individual growth can also be studied by this method.

Disadvantages include small sample size, difficulties in the maintenance of laboratory research, personal data storage over long periods and possible (sample decay) reduction in the sample size due to change of place and other reasons. Furthermore, inference of the study can only be obtained after analyzing the data at the end of the long study period.

#### Mixed/Semilongitudinal Studies

They are combinations of the cross-sectional and longitudinal type of studies to obtain the advantages of both methods of data collection.

Subjects at different age levels are seen longitudinally for shorter periods. For example, in a study of 6 years span, growth can be studied between birth and 6 years for 1 group, between 6 and 11 years for second group, between 10 and 16 for the third group; and between 15 and 21 years in yet another age group. In this way growth from birth to 21 years can be studied in only 6 years.

### Interpretation

Growth data is presented in the form of graph to facilitate easy understanding of the findings. The rates of growth can be indicated by increments in body length or weight which when plotted form a growth curve. There are two basic curves of growth which are described below:

#### Distance Curve/Cumulative Curve

It indicates the distance a child has traversed along the growth path. Data derived from the cross-sectional and longitudinal studies can be plotted as cumulative curve (**Fig. 3.1**).

#### Velocity/Incremental Curve

It indicates the rate of growth of the child over a period of time. The velocity curve is drawn by plotting the increments in height or weight from one age to the next. For velocity curve, data is derived from longitudinal studies. The velocity curve in **Figure 3.2** shows that the velocity of growth in height decreases from birth onwards with a marked acceleration of growth from 13–15 years — the adolescent growth spurt.

## BASIC TENETS OF GROWTH

### Pattern

Pattern of growth in human is allometric. There is a difference in the relative rates of growth between one part of the body and another. Different parts and organs of the body grow at different times and to different extents. This is termed as "differential growth."

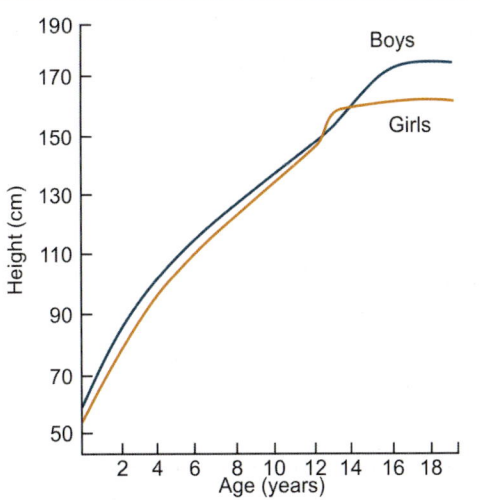

Fig. 3.1: Distance curve for height

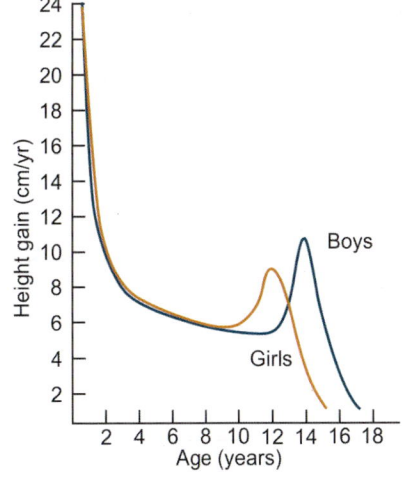

Fig. 3.2: Velocity curve for height

Differential growth in humans is reflected in:
- Cephalocaudal gradient of growth
- Scammon's curve.

### Cephalocaudal Gradient of Growth

There are differences in the relative rates of growth between one part of the body and another. Overall body proportions change as one grows from fetal life to adulthood. There is an axis of increased growth extending from the head towards the feet. The head is in advance of the trunk and the trunk in advance of the limbs regarding growth and maturity at all times. This axis of increased growth gradient extending from head towards the feet is called the cephalocaudal gradient of growth **(Fig. 3.3)**.

- In fetal life, at around 2–3 months of intrauterine life, the head is nearly one half of the total embryonic life. At this stage, limbs are rudimentary and trunk is underdeveloped.
- Subsequently, the head grows proportionally more slowly and limbs and trunk grow faster so that the proportion of entire body occupied by head is reduced to one quarter of the body length at birth.
- During childhood, this pattern of growth continues with lengthening of the torso and limbs. At adulthood, the head is reduced to one eigth of the entire body length and lower limbs occupy one half of the total length.

Cephalocaudal Growth in Face
- At birth, the face (nasomaxillary complex and mandible) is less developed with the cranium representing more than half of the total head.
- Maxilla being closer to the brain/head grows faster and its growth is completed before mandibular growth.
- Mandible being away from the brain, completes its growth later than the maxilla.

### Scammon's Growth Curve

Not all tissues of organs of the body grow at same time and to the same extent. Different body tissues show different growth rates. **Richard Scammon** described four basic growth curves **(Fig. 3.4)** of the tissues of the body: Lymphoid, neural, general, and genital. The curves span the entire postnatal period of 20 years. Normal adult size is regarded as 100% and starts from 0% at birth.

### Lymphoid Curve

- Lymphoid curve includes the thymus, pharyngeal and tonsillar adenoids, lymph nodes and intestinal lymphatic masses.
- Lymphoid tissues grow rapidly to reach 200% of adult size between 10 and 15 years of age. This is an adaptation to protect children from infections. Later their size is reduced from 200% to 100% at adult life.
- Reduction in the size is due to physiologic involution of the lymphoid tissues.

### Neural Curve

- Neural curve includes brain, spinal cord, optic apparatus related bony parts of the skull, upper face and vertebral column.
- Neural curve rises strongly during childhood with the neural tissues growing very rapidly in early years of life.
- Brain is nearly 90% its adult size by 8 years of age. Growth in size is accompanied by growth in internal structure, enabling the 8 year old child to function mentally at nearly the same level as an adult.

### General Curve

- General curve/somatic tissues include musculature, bony skeleton, respiratory and digestive organs, kidneys, liver, spleen and blood volume.
- The general tissues show an "S-shaped" growth curve.
- The curve rises steadily from birth to five years of age and then a plateau from 5 to 10 years of age followed by acceleration during puberty, and then finally, it slows down in adulthood.

### Genital Curve

- Genital curve includes the primary sex apparatus (ovary and testis) and all secondary sex characters/traits.

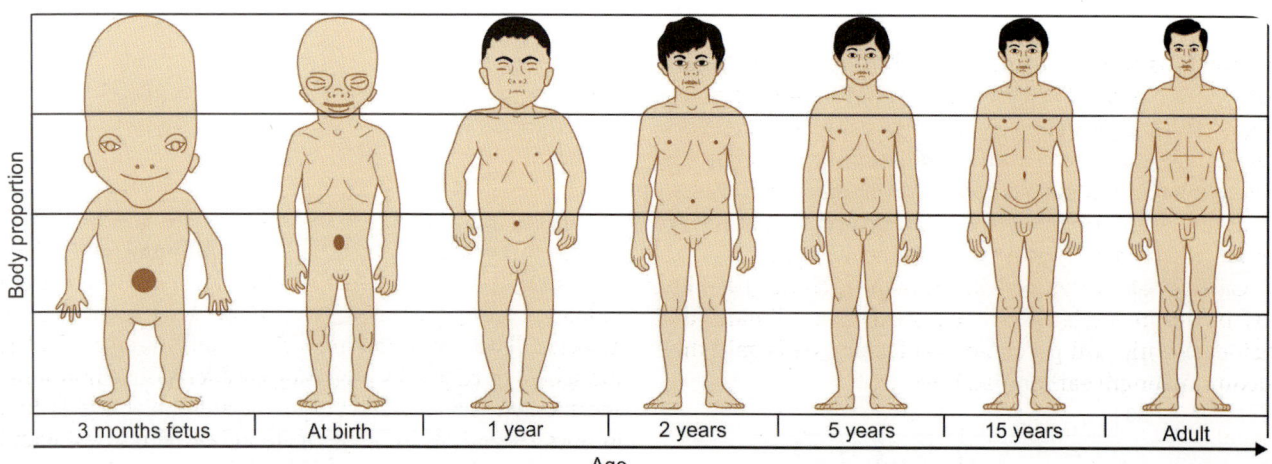

**Fig. 3.3:** Cephalocaudal gradient of growth

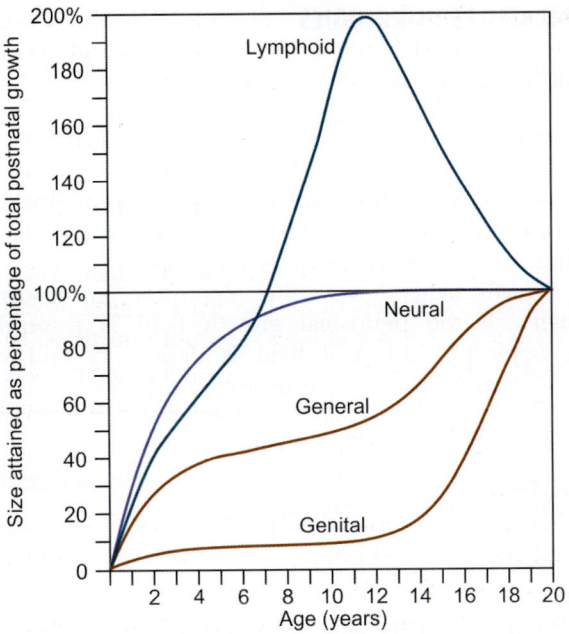

**Fig. 3.4:** Scammon's growth curve

- The genital curve has a small rise in the first year of life and then is quiescent up to around 10 years of age at which time the curve shows rapid acceleration during puberty.

### Effect of Scammon's Growth in Facial Region
- The maxilla follows neural growth pattern and its growth ceases earlier in life.
- Skeletal problems of the maxilla should be treated earlier than that of the mandible. For example, growth modification procedures (face mask) should be given earlier in life (6 years) to promote growth of maxilla.
- Mandibular growth follows general growth pattern. Its growth occurs until about 18–20 years in males. Growth modification treatment (chin cup) should be extended until cessation of mandibular growth so as to prevent relapse of class III malocclusion due to continued growth of mandible.

### Variability
Variability is the law of nature and human growth is no exception. No two individuals show the same increment of growth at a particular age. It can be appreciated in a standard growth chart that there is variability in height and weight measurements between different children.

Some children are average growers. Some are genetically tall while others are genetically short.

Causes of variability in growth include heredity, sex, nutrition, racial differences, exercise, climate, and socioeconomic and psychological factors. Girls gain their maximum length earlier than boys.

### Timing
The third and most important factor of growth in terms of clinical applications is the timing of growth. The biological clock of growth is set differently for different individuals. A particular growth event may occur at different times in different individuals.

Some children mature early. They are taller in childhood than average growers since they have matured faster than average, but they may not be particularly tall in adulthood. Late maturing children are shorter than average in childhood since they mature late. They will eventually gain normal stature at adulthood.

One important factor in timing of growth is sex of the individual. Girls attain puberty earlier than boys. Timing of menarche (attainment of sexual maturity) in girls also shows a great variation. Some girls mature faster than others. Timing of growth is an important consideration when growth modification procedures are considered in the treatment plan.

## GROWTH RHYTHM AND GROWTH SPURTS

Growth charts reveal that human growth does not proceed at a uniform rate throughout life. There appears to be a rhythm in growth process. The growth rhythm can be readily appreciated in gaining of the body height. There are periods of sudden accelerated growth interspersed with periods of relative quiescence. Such rapid increase in growth rate is termed as a "growth spurt". Three major growth spurts can be seen during postnatal development. The timing of growth spurts differ in boys and girls. Generally, girls precede boys in growth spurts by approximately two years.

1. Infantile/childhood growth spurt: Up to 3 years in both sexes
2. Mixed dentition/juvenile growth spurt: 7–9 years in females; 8–11 years in males
3. Adolescent growth spurt: 10–12 years in females; 12–14 years in males

### Infantile Growth Spurt
Body length increases from a neonatal range of 48–53 cm to about 75 cm during first year after birth and increases by 12–13 cm in second year. Thereafter, 5–6 cm is added each year.

### Childhood Growth Spurt
Growth spurt at this period is less pronounced than the other two growth spurts.

### Adolescent Growth Spurt
In longitudinal growth curves, an increase in the velocity of growth occurs between 10–12 years in girls and 12–14 years in boys. This rapid increase in growth is termed as the "adolescent growth spurt" **(Fig. 3.5)**. Accentuated growth associated with pubertal period is more dramatic and is thought to be caused by physiological alteration in hormonal secretion. Adolescent growth spurt occurs earlier in girls than in boys and it lasts for 2–2.5 years in both the sexes. Rapid raise in growth during adolescence is most obvious in the increase in height, while weight gain is more variable.

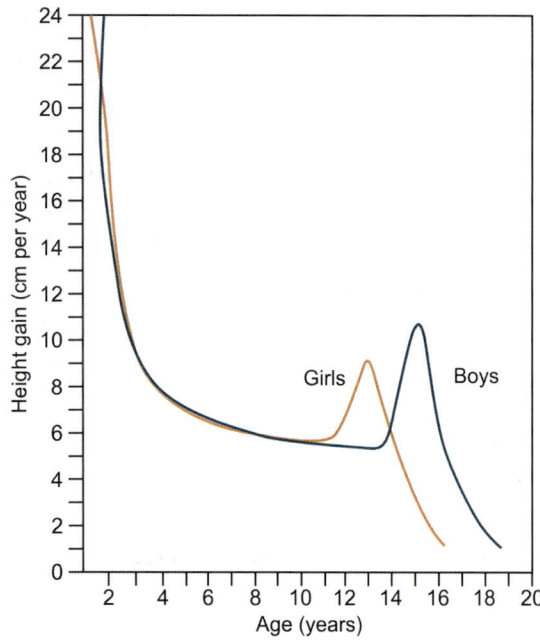

**Fig. 3.5:** Adolescent growth spurt: Accentuated growth associated with pubertal period occurs earlier in girls than in boys and it lasts for 2–2.5 years in both the sexes

Girls gain around 16 cm in height during the spurt with a peak velocity at 12 years of age. Boys gain about 20 cm in height with a peak velocity at 14 years of age. Growth rate may reach 10 cm increase in height per year. After peak height velocity (PHV) is attained, growth rate declines. Noticeable growth is believed to stop at 18 years in females and 20 years in males.

### Clinical Significance of Growth Spurts

- Adolescent growth spurt has significant clinical implications in orthodontics.
- Differences between the timing of growth spurt in males and females has to be kept in mind.
- Treatment of skeletal malocclusions by growth modification using orthopedic and functional appliances is best carried out during adolescent growth spurt, e.g. chin cup appliance to restrict mandibular advancement in treatment of class III malocclusion; Frankel functional regulator to stimulate mandibular growth in the treatment of class II malocclusion. It is advisable to continue appliance wearing until the cessation of adolescent growth spurt so as to obtain stable results.
- Expansion of dental arches (e.g. rapid maxillary expansion) responds well during adolescent growth spurt and the results are more likely to be stable.
- Certain patients with gross skeletal discrepancies may require orthognathic surgical correction and surgery is best carried out after the cessation of active growth.

## RELATED TERMINOLOGIES

### Growth Fields

Bone growth is controlled by so called "growth fields". Periosteal (outer) and endosteal (inner) surface of bones are blanketed by soft tissues and cartilage or osteogenic membrane. With this blanket of soft tissue matrix, the growth fields are disturbed in a characteristic mosaic like pattern across the surface of a given bone.

Growth fields have either depository or resorptic activity. If the periosteal growth field is resorptive, the opposing endosteal field is depository and vice versa. Depository and resorptive fields are disturbed characteristically across the entire inner and outer surfaces of the craniofacial skeleton. However, the activity of the growth field is not located in the bone itself. The genetic information resides within soft tissues.

### Growth Centers

The term "growth centers" are used to describe very active growth fields, which are significant to the growth processes/mechanisms.

*Examples*

- Cranial and facial sutures
- Synchondroses of cranial base
- Mandibular condyles
- Maxillary tuberosity
- Alveolar processes

The growth center controls the overall growth of the bone. Genetically controlled growth takes place at growth centers, i.e. they have intrinsic growth potential. Growth centers respond to functional needs; however, they show little response to external influences.

### Growth Sites

Growth sites are certain areas of a bone where significant growth of that bone takes place. Growth sites show marked response to external influences. Unlike centers, growth sites do not control the overall growth of the bone. They do not cause growth of the whole bone instead, they are simply areas of the bone where exaggerated growth takes place, e.g. mandibular condyle and maxillary tuberosity. Growth sites can occur at growth centers, but all growth sites are not growth centers.

## MODES OF BONE FORMATION

Bones develop by either of two mechanisms, namely endochondral ossification or intramembranous ossification. Bones developed from endochondral ossification are referred to as cartilaginous bones while bones formed by intramembranous ossification are called membranous bones.

### Endochondral Ossification/Indirect Ossification

In endochondral ossification, a precursor cartilage model (template) is first formed and is then replaced by bone

in an ordered sequence. Endochondral bone formation proceeds as follows:
a. The cartilage model which forms during embryogenesis (primary cartilage) acts as a miniature template for the development of cartilage bone.
b. The cartilage model becomes surrounded by a highly vascular mesenchyme: the perichondrium. The perichondrium contains osteoprogenitor cells in its deeper layer.
c. Centers of calcification appear within the cartilage primordium matrix. As calcification of cartilage matrix surrounding the cartilage cells proceeds, nutrition to the cartilage cells is cut off resulting in their death. Destruction of cartilage cells lead to formation of empty spaces within the calcifying cartilage matrix.
d. Blood vessels from surrounding perichondrium invade into the calcifying matrix, bringing undifferentiated connective tissue cells.
e. Osteoblasts get differentiated from the undifferentiated connective tissue precursor cells, and deposit (fibrous bone matrix osteoid) on the remnants of calcified cartilage matrix.
f. Osteoid tissue then gets mineralized to form bone.
g. In the craniofacial skeleton, the bones of cranial base and portions of the calvarium are derived from endochondral ossification.

### Intramembranous Ossification/Direct Ossification

Intramembranous ossification is the direct formation of bone within highly vascular sheets of membranes of condensed primitive mesenchyme. There is no precursor cartilage model here. At centers of ossification, ectomesenchymal stem cells differentiate into osteoblasts. The newly formed osteoblasts proliferate around the branches and capillary network and produce a fibrous bone matrix (osteoid). As osteoid deposition continues, osteoblast cells get encased in matrix and become osteocytes. Blood vessels are retained within the spaces and become surrounded by bone. A haversian system starts to form which nourishes the bone. Fibrous bone matrix (osteoid) eventually becomes mineralized. Entrapped blood vessels supply nutrients to osteocytes and bone tissue.

Peripheral mesenchyme condenses on the outer surface to form fibrocellular periosteum. Further bone deposition occurs from new osteoblasts differentiating from osteoprogenitor cells in the deeper layers of periostium. Membrane bones in craniofacial skeleton are cranial bones, mandible, etc. (most of the bones of craniofacial skeleton are of intramembranous origin). However, in certain membranous bones, secondary cartilages (not part of cartilaginous primordium of the embryo) develop and after initiation of intramembranous ossification contribute significantly to their growth, e.g. condylar cartilage in mandible.

### Mechanisms of Bone Growth

After osteogenesis, further growth of bone takes place by several mechanisms. Bones do not grow by simple symmetrical enlargement. Growth of craniofacial bones is complex involving differential growth mechanisms and different types of development for the individual bones. Some of the important growth mechanisms include:
- Bone remodeling
- Cortical drift
- Displacement/translation.

### Bone Remodeling

- As said earlier, bone does not grow uniformly in all directions. Selective bone resorption and deposition occurs which is called remodeling.
- Remodeling is the basic growth process providing regional changes in the shape, dimension, and proportions of the bone.
- Along with an increase in size, remodeling facilitates constant reshaping of bone while maintaining the integrity and basic shapes of the bone.
- Remodeling also provides regional adjustments in the bone needed for adapting to the changes in function.

### Cortical Drift

Cortical drift and displacement provide means of growth movement in craniofacial development.

The cortical plate can be relocated by a simultaneous apposition and resorption process occurring on the opposing periosteal and endosteal surfaces. Such a combination of simultaneous deposition and resorption resulting in a growth movement towards the depositing surface has been described as cortical drift by Enlow (1963).

The bony cortical plate drifts by depositing and resorbing the bone substance on the outer and inner surface respectively in the direction of growth.

If the resorption and deposition takes place at the same rate, the thickness of the bone remains constant with only change in location of the cortical bone. On the other hand, if bone deposition is more than resorption, thickness of the cortical bone increases along with its movement. For example, the teeth follow the drift of their alveolar bone while the jaw is growing and thus they maintain their position within the surrounding bony structures.

### Displacement/Translation

Change in the spatial position of a bone can occur by two types of displacement.
1. Primary displacement occurs where actual enlargement of the bone will change its position in space. In other words, primary displacement of the bone is brought about by its own enlargement. Primary displacement of maxilla in a forward direction occurs due to growth by maxillary tuberosity in a posterior direction **(Fig. 3.6)**. The amount of anterior displacement is equal

to the amount of posterior lengthening. Periosteal surface of the tuberosity receives continuous deposits of new bone and results in horizontal lengthening of the maxillary arch.

2. Secondary displacement, on the other hand, occurs when the growth of one bone results in a change in the spatial position of an adjacent bone. Nasomaxillary complex grows by secondary translation during primary dentition period. As the maxilla is attached to the cranial base, growth occurring at cranial base produces a passive/secondary displacement of the nasomaxillary complex in a downward and forward direction (**Fig. 3.7**).

## THEORIES OF CRANIOFACIAL DEVELOPMENT

A number of theories have evolved over the years in an attempt to understand the complex nature of craniofacial development. The major theories of growth are described below.

| | |
|---|---|
| Genetic theory | by Brodie |
| Sutural dominance theory | by Sicher |
| Cartilaginous theory | by Scott |
| Functional matrix theory | by Melvin Moss |
| Servosystem theory | by Petrovic |

Other theories related to craniofacial growth are:
  Von Limborgh's compromise theory
  Enlow's expanding 'V' principle
  Enlow's counterpart principle/growth equivalent concept
  Neurotrophism

### Genetic Theory — Brodie

This earliest theory proposed that skull growth was controlled by genetic factors and was preplanned. This theory was proposed by Brodie in 1941. According to him, genes determine the overall growth control and the persistent pattern of facial configuration is under tight genetic control.

The genetic theory was antagonized by Moss and other investigators. Primary genetic control determines only certain features and does not have complete influence on growth.

### Sutural Dominance Theory — Sicher

Sicher (1952) was the main proponent of sutural dominance theory. The sutural concept adhered to the notion that within each suture resided the genetic information that would determine the amount of growth occurring at the site of that suture.

This theory regarded suture to be a "growth center" — a center with an ability to generate tissue separating forces. The sutural theory advocated that the craniofacial suture generated tissue separating forces during growth thereby pushing apart the various bones of the craniofacial complex.

However, this theory is disproved now and the research evidence show that the sutures are adaptive. Compensatory growth mechanisms and sutures act as "growth sites" rather than as "growth centers". Thus growth in sutural area is secondary to functional needs. Thus, craniofacial sutures are now considered as important growth sites that serve to facilitate the growth of cranial vault and mid-face. Sutures respond to mild tension forces by surface deposition of bone, thereby enabling bones of the face and skull to adapt.

*Objections:* Points raised against this theory were:
- Growth does not continue after transplantation of an area of suture to another location. This shows a lack of innate growth potential of sutures.
- Suture is a tension adapted tissue and any unusual pressure on suture initiates bone resorption and not bones deposition.

### Cartilaginous Theory/Nasal Septal Theory — Scott

First proposed by James Scott, cartilaginous theory emphasizes that the intrinsic growth controlling factors are present in the cartilage and in the periosteum with sutures

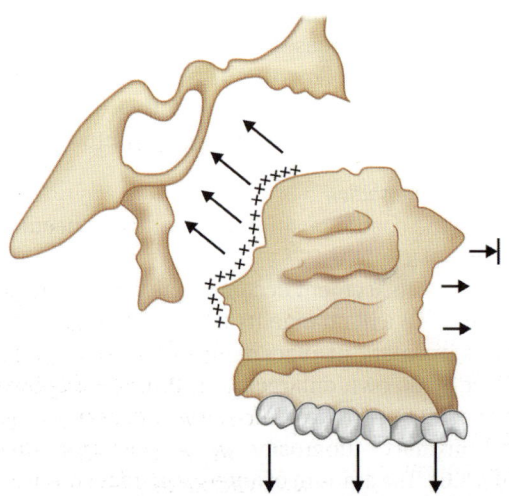

**Fig. 3.6:** Primary displacement of maxilla in a forward direction occurs due to growth by maxillary tuberosity in a posterior direction

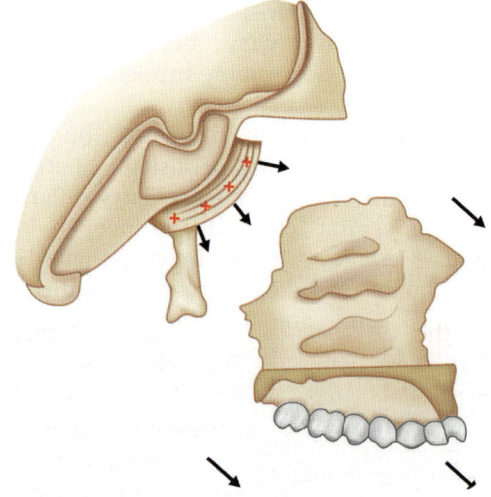

**Fig. 3.7:** Secondary displacement of bone

having only secondary adaptive role. Scott considered the cartilaginous parts of the skull as primary centers of growth. He suggested that primary cartilage present in the nasal septum is the main mechanism responsible for the growth of nasomaxillary complex. Nasal septum is considered to influence the downward and forward growth of the maxilla. In mandible, condylar cartilage is considered to be the growth center present bilaterally with the U-shaped mandible in between.

The following evidence supports the cartilaginous theory:
- Experimental studies on rats and rabbits showed retarded mid-face development when nasal septal cartilage was extirpated.
- Many bones grow by cartilaginous growth in which a precursor cartilage is replaced by bone.
- Transplantation of epiphyseal plate and synchondroses results in continued growth on transplanted area indicating intrinsic growth potential of the cartilage.

Primary cartilage found on the head and face is identical to the growth plate of long bone. It first appears in head during fifth week of gestation. By eighth week of gestation independent sites of craniofacial cartilage coalesce to form a cartilaginous mass called the chondrocranium. The chondrocranium is the precursor to the adult cranial base and nasal and otic structures. By mid-childhood, most primary cartilage is replaced by bone-endochondral bone formation. The overall influence of primary cartilage on craniofacial growth is most profound in early years of life, up to early childhood. At birth, cartilage forms a major portion of the nasal septum and cranial base. The sphenooccipital synchondrosis contributes significantly to craniofacial growth up to 6 years. After this age relative contribution of primary cartilage to craniofacial growth is small.

### Functional Matrix Theory — Melvin Moss

The functional matrix theory, as postulated by Moss (1962, 1968, and 1969), has contributed greatly to the level of understanding of growth and development. The basic principles set in the functional matrix model have provided a viable interceptive framework for many of the problems associated with the understanding of craniofacial development **(Flowchart 3.1)**.

Moss theory was influenced by the ideas of van der Klaauw (1946) who asserted that the skull was made up of units whose size, shape, and position were determined by their functions. Van der Klaauw called these units as functional cranial components.

Using the basic concept of Van der Klaauw and combining these with his research, Moss postulated his functional matrix model **(Flowchart 3.1)**. He stressed the dominance of nonosseous structures of the craniofacial complex over the bony parts. Moss regarded functional matrix as the primary requirement of growth and skeletal units as secondary responses, by stating that, "the functional matrix is primary and the origin, development and maintenance of all skeletal units is secondary, compensatory and mechanically obligatory responses to changes in shape and spatial position of its related functional matrix." According to Moss, the growth of skeletal components, whether endochondral or intramembranous in origin, is largely dependent on the growth of the functional matrices.

Moss noted that the head is a composite structure, operationally consisting of a number of vital functions such as olfaction, respiration, vision, digestion, speech, audition and neural integration. Each function is carried out by a group of soft tissues which are supported and/or protected by related skeletal elements. Taken together, the soft tissues and the skeletal elements related to a single function are termed as "functional cranial component."

A functional cranial component performing a function consists of two components:
1. *Skeletal unit:* All skeletal elements associated with a single function.
2. *Functional matrix:* All soft tissues associated with a single function.

*Skeletal unit:* The totality of all the skeletal elements associated with a single function comprises a skeletal unit. The skeletal unit may be made of bone, cartilage and tendons. The skeletal unit in turn consists of micro and macroskeletal units.

*Microskeletal unit:* The term "microskeletal unit" is used when a bone is comprised of several contiguous skeletal units. For example, maxilla and mandible are comprised of a number of microskeletal units. The mandible is made of alveolar, condylar, angular, gonial, coronoid and basal microskeletal units while the maxilla is comprised of orbital, palatal, pneumatic, alveolar and basal skeletal units.

*Macroskeletal unit:* The term "macroskeletal unit" is used when the adjoining portions of a number of neighboring bones are united to function as a single cranial component. For example, the entire cranial vault is a macroskeletal unit protecting the brain and the whole mandible is a macroskeletal unit.

*Functional matrix:* The totality of all the soft tissues associated with a single function is termed as "functional matrix".

The functional matrix has two components:
- Capsular matrix
- Periosteal matrix

*Capsular matrix:* The capsular matrices bring about spatial changes in the position of bone, i.e. translation by acting indirectly and passively on their skeletal units. These changes in the spatial position of skeletal units are brought about by the expansion of their enveloping capsules. Translative growth is not caused by apposition and resorption of bone.

Examples of capsular matrices are:
- Neurocranial capsule (skin and dura mater) which is controlled by the growing brain thrusting the bony calvarial plates outward.

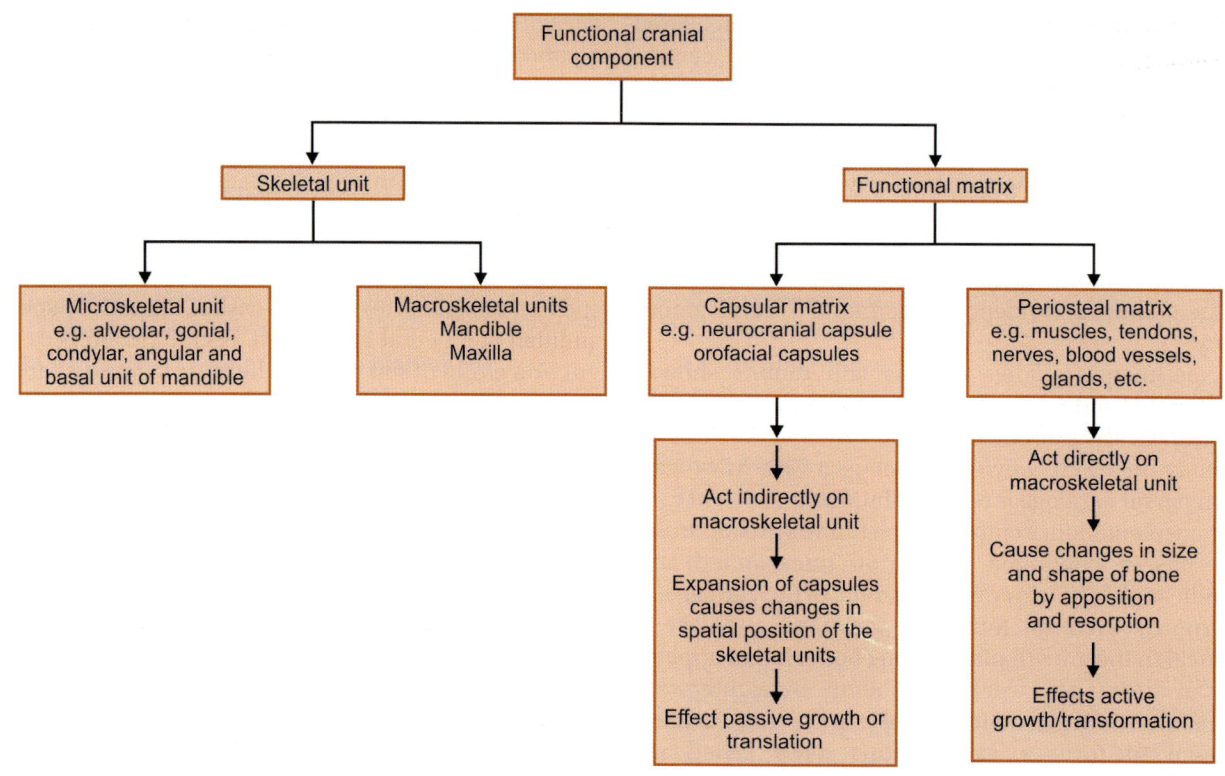

**Flowchart 3.1:** Moss's functional matrix model

- Orofacial capsules (comprising of skin and oral mucosa) within which the facial bone arise, grow and are maintained.

***Periosteal matrix:*** The periosteal matrices act directly and actively on their related skeletal units, causing more local changes in the size and shape of the skeleton, i.e. "transformation/remodeling".

The periosteal matrices bring about transformation by acting directly upon skeletal units via the periosteum and resulting in bone apposition and resorption.

Examples of the periosteal matrices include the muscles, tendon, nerves, blood vessels, glands, etc.

As stated earlier, there are a number of functions carried out by the head and all these functions require the development and maintenance of spaces. For example, neural growth and integration is an important function and space is required for the brain growth and for expansion of central and peripheral nervous system. Likewise, respiration and deglutition require development of nasal, pharyngeal and oral spaces. Repositioning of the mandible and tongue takes place to ensure patency of the nasopharyngeal spaces, i.e. patency of the airway.

Summarizing the functional matrix theory, craniofacial growth is the result of both changes in the "capsular matrices", causing spatial changes in the position of bones (translation) and by "periosteal matrices", causing more local changes in the size and shape of the bones (transformation/remodeling).

### Clinical Applications of Functional Matrix Theory

Application of force by orthodontic appliances tends to alter the functional matrix. Alteration of periosteal matrix (teeth) produces changes in microskeletal unit (alveolar bone); alteration of capsular matrix (dentofacial orthopedics) produces changes in macroskeletal unit (jaws).

- Rapid palatal expansion by widening of palatal sutures is a form of orofacial orthopedics.
- Repositioning of maxillary segments in cleft patients alter the macroskeletal unit.
- Anterior bite plane used in treatment of deep bite stimulates supraeruption of posterior teeth.
- Activator stimulates the growth of condyle.
- Frankle's functional regulator stimulates both the periosteal matrix through lip pads and buccal shields; capsular matrix by altering oropharyngeal spaces.
- Inter-arch elastics, head gears, facemask, chincup have direct effect on functional matrices by alteration of muscular behavior and spaces.

## Servosystem Theory

A new concept in understanding the process controlling postnatal craniofacial growth is the servosystem theory by Petrovic and Stutzman, 1980. Charlier and Petrovic (1967), and Stutzman and Petrovic (1970) observed some basic dissimilarities between growth of primary and secondary cartilages in their investigations. Their observations lead to the servosystem theory.

Servosystem theory is based on "cybernetic concept." Cybernetic concept states that everything affects everything and living organisms never operate in open loop mechanism. In an open loop mechanism, the input/stimulus leads to a response and there is no feedback or regulation.

Closed loop system can be expressed as follows:

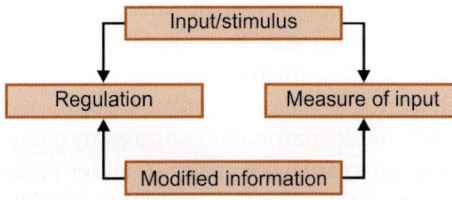

Closed loop mechanism can be of two types:
i. Regulator system in which the main input is constant
ii. Servosystem/follow-up system in which the main input varies rather than being constant.

### Components of a Servosystem

Components of a servosystem have been shown in **Figure. 3.8**.

- ***Command:*** Is a signal established independently of the feedback system under scrutiny. It affects the controlled system without being affected by the consequences of this behavior, for example, somatotropic hormone, growth hormone, testosterone and estrogen.
- ***Reference input elements:*** Establish the relationship between the command and reference input. It includes septal cartilage, septopremaxillary ligament and labionarinay muscles.
- ***Reference input:*** It is the signal established as a standard of comparison sagittal position of maxilla.
- ***Comparator:*** The configuration between the position of the upper and lower dental arch is the comparator of the servosystem.
- ***Actuating signal:*** Activity of the retrodiscal pad and lateral pterygoid constitutes the actuating signal. The elastic menisco-temporal and mensico-mandibular frenums of the condylar disc form the retrodiscal pad.
- ***Controlled system:*** It is between the actuator and controlled variable, e.g. growth of condylar cartilage through the retrodiscal pad stimulation.
- ***Controlled variable:*** It is the output signal of the servosystem. Best example is sagittal position of mandible.

### How the Servosystem Theory Explains the Growth of Jaws?

According to the Servosystem theory, the influence of somatotropic hormone on growth of primary cartilages, i.e. nasal septum, sphenooccipital synchondrosis, and other synchondroses, etc. has a cybernetic form of a "command." Growth-related hormones have a direct influence on the growth of primary cartilages. On the other hand, these hormones have both direct and indirect effects on the growth of secondary cartilages, e.g. condylar, coronoid cartilages of mandible, cartilages of midpalatal suture and some craniofacial sutures. The growth of secondary cartilages corresponds to local epigenetic and environmental factors.

In the development of jaws and face, the upper arch acts as a constantly changing reference input and the lower arch is the controlled variable. Any disturbance or confrontation between the respective positions of the upper and lower arch acts as the peripheral comparator and sends activating signals through the stimulation of retrodiscal pad and lateral pterygoid muscles.

This affects the output signal, i.e. the final sagittal position of the mandible. The inference is that, the final sagittal position of the mandible depends on the modification of condylar growth by the activity of retrodiscal pad and lateral pterygoid muscle stimulation.

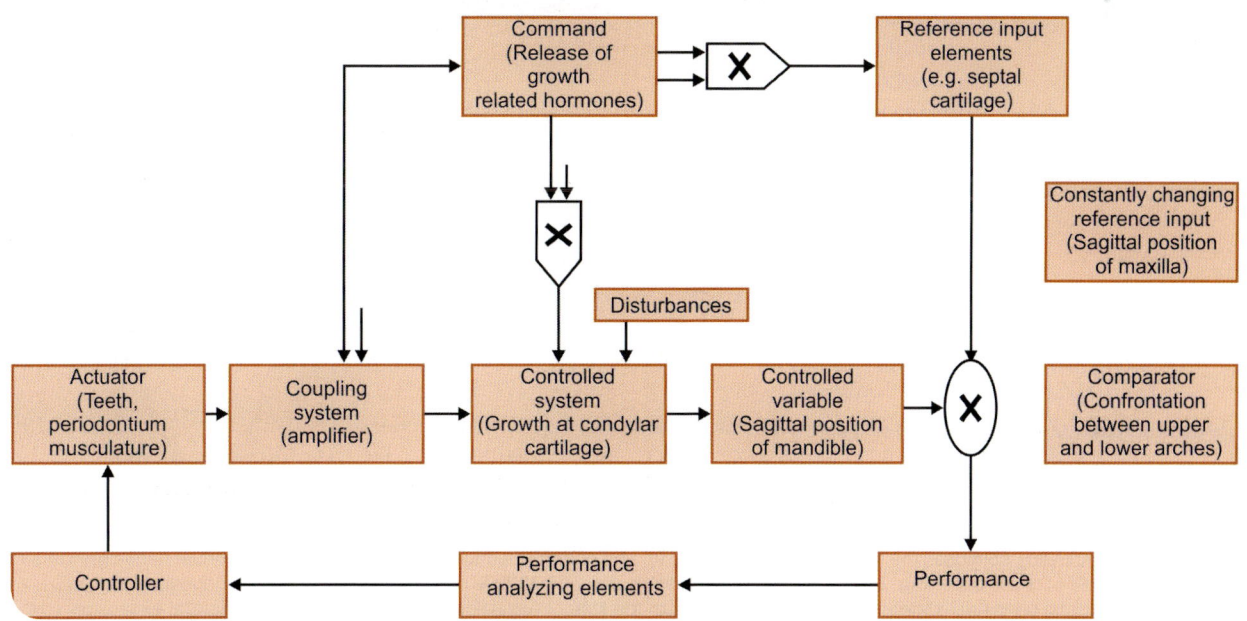

**Fig. 3.8:** Servosystem theory of growth

## OTHER THEORIES RELATED TO CRANIOFACIAL GROWTH

### Expanding 'V' Principle by Enlow

The concept of expanding 'V' principle was put forward by Enlow. The 'V' principle is an important facial skeletal growth mechanism since many facial and cranial bones have a 'V' configuration or 'V' shaped regions.

In "V" shaped bones/areas, bone resorption occurs on the outer surface of the 'V' and deposition on the inner surface. As the remodeling continues, the 'V' moves away from its tip and enlarges simultaneously. In this way growth as well as movement of the bone occurs simultaneously. Such an increase in size and the simultaneous movement of the bone in the shape of 'V' is called the expanding 'V' principle **(Fig. 3.9)**.

Such a growth process results in:
1. Enlargement in overall size of the 'V' shaped area.
2. Movement of the entire 'V' structure towards its own wider end.
3. Continuous relocation.

Most of the craniofacial bones including mandible, maxilla and palate grow on an expanding 'V'. Growth of the palate is one of the best examples of expanding 'V' principle. Deposition occurs on the palatal periosteal surface and resorption occurs on the side of nasal floor. In this way, palate expands on lateral direction and also moves downwards **(Fig. 3.10)**.

It is easier to visualize mandible as a 'V' shaped bone than maxilla because of its horse-shoe shape. Ramus of the mandible grows on an expanding 'V' and interramal width of the mandible also increases by expanding 'V' principle **(Fig. 3.11)**. The condyle remodels according to the expanding 'V' principle and the neck of the condyle gets lengthened.

### Enlow's Counterpart Principle/Growth Equivalents Concepts

According to Enlow's counterpart principle, the growth of any given craniofacial structure is related specially to certain other structural and geometric counterpart in the craniofacial complex. In other wards, growth of a given regional part can be compared with its specific counterpart, i.e. the growth equivalent.

A dimensionally balanced growth occurs when each regional part and its particular counterpart enlarge to the same extent. Imbalance can result in either protrusion or retrusion of the part of the face. Imbalance in the regional relationships can be produced by difference in:
- Amount of growth between the counterparts
- Direction of growth between the counterparts.
- Time of growth between the counterparts.

Examples of counterparts/equivalents:
- Nasomaxillary complex elongation is the counterpart for elongation of anterior cranial fossa.
- Horizontal dimension of the pharyngeal space relates to middle cranial fossa.
- Maxilla and mandibular corpus are mutual equivalents.
- Maxillary tuberosity and lingual tuberosity are mutual counterparts.

### Van Limborgh's Compromise Theory

Van Limborgh put forward a multifactorial theory in 1970 as a compromise between the existing popular three theories of growth. He accepted certain concepts of each theory which cannot be denied while negating other elements.

Van Limborgh explained the process of growth and development in a view that combines all the three theories. He accepts functional matrix theory of Moss, supports some aspects of Sutural theory of Sicher and at the same time also acknowledges genetic involvement.

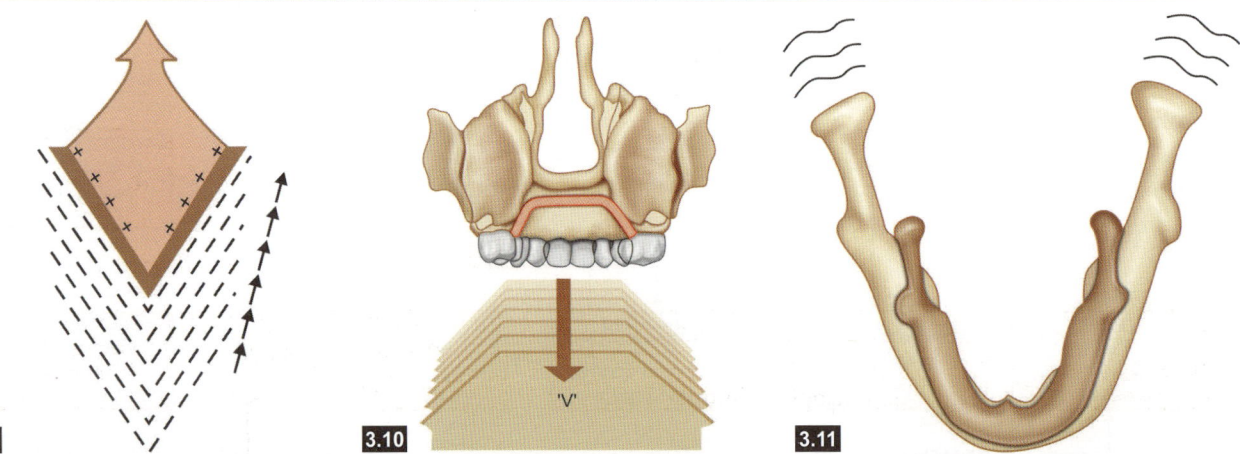

**Fig. 3.9:** Expanding 'V' principle: In "V"-shaped bones/areas, bone resorption occur on the outer surface of the 'V', and deposition on the inner surface. As the remodeling continues the 'V' moves away from its tip and enlarges simultaneously—giving rise to simultaneous growth as well as movement of the bone; **Fig. 3.10:** Growth of the palate is a good example of expanding 'V' principle. Deposition occurs on the palatal periosteal surface and resorption occurs on the side of nasal floor causing downward and lateral expansion of palate; **Fig. 3.11:** Mandibular growth follows the expanding 'V' principle

Van Limborgh proposed the following five controlling factors of growth:
1. ***Intrinsic genetic factors:*** They are the genetic factors inherent to the craniofacial skeletal tissues.
2. ***Local epigenetic factors (Capsular matrix):*** These are genetically determined influences originating from adjacent structures and spaces such as brain, eyes, etc.
3. ***General epigenetic factors:*** Genetically determined influences originating from distant structures such as sex hormones, growth hormones, etc.
4. ***Local environmental factors (periosteal matrix):*** These are local nongenetic influences from external environment, e.g. muscle force local external pressure (habit).
5. ***General environmental factors:*** General nongenetic influences from external environment, e.g. oxygen supply nutrition, etc.

### Neurotrophism in Orofacial Growth

According to functional matrix theory by Moss, the soft tissues regulate the skeletal growth through functional stimuli. The process by which the functional stimulus is transmitted to the skeletal unit interface involves neutrophism.

Neutrophism is a nonimpulse transmitive neurofunction involving axoplasmic transport providing for the long-term interactions between neurons and innervated tissues which homeostatically regulate the morphological, compositional and functional integrity of these tissues. Three types of neutrophic mechanisms are described.

#### *Neuroepithelial Trophism*

Epithelial growth regeneration is controlled by neurotrophism. The normal epithelial growth is controlled by certain neurotrophic substances by the nerve synapses. When neurotrophic process is deficient orofacial hypoplasia and malformation may occur, e.g. few patients with facial hypoplasia, cleft palate exhibit concurrent sensory deficits which clearly show neuroepithelial trophism.

#### *Neuromuscular Trophism*

According to Moss, neural innervations influence the gene expressions of the cell. The periosteal muscular functional matrices regulate the size and shape of the microskeletal units through neuromuscular trophism. It is contemplated that similar trophic influences might also exist for capsular control the position of macroskeletal unit.

#### *Neurovisceral Trophism*

Viscera such as salivary glands are regulated by neurotrophism. Salivary hyperplasia and hypertrophy is thought to be partially under neurotrophic control.

## FUNCTIONAL DEVELOPMENT

Orofacial region is associated with a variety of functions such as mastication, deglutition, respiration (ventilation) and speech. Since the functions are interrelated, normal development of orofacial region depends on normal function.

### Mastication

Mastication is the process whereby ingested food is cut or crushed into small pieces, mixed with saliva and formed into a bolus in preparation for swallowing. Mammals are heterodonts, i.e. possess teeth of different forms adapted to the communition of food. Thus the process of mastication is characteristic of mammals. In nonmammalians, teeth are mainly used for prehension of their prey before swallowing as a whole.

In humans, the process of mastication is associated with various functions, such as:
- It enables the food bolus to be easily swallowed.
- It decreases the size of food particles so that the surface area is increased for enzyme activity.
- It stimulates secretion of saliva and gastric juices by reflex action.
- It mixes food with saliva, thus initiates digestion by the activity of salivary amylase.
- It prevents irritation of gastrointestinal system by large food masses.
- It ensures healthy growth and development of the oral tissues.

Mastication occurs by the convergent movements of maxillary and mandibular teeth. During chewing cycle two processes occurs:
i. Food is first crushed by vertical movement of the mandible. The initial crushing of food does not require full occlusion of teeth.
ii. After the food is softened well by initial crushing, maxillary and mandibular teeth meet in full occlusion. The food is then sheared by lateral to medial movements of the mandible to make a bolus.

Once the cusps interdigitate the ridges on the slopes of the cusps shear the food as the mandibular teeth move across the maxillary teeth. Food is ground in the manner of mortar and pestle when the cusps move across the fossae of the opposing teeth.

#### *The Control of Mastication*

Mastication is dependent upon a complex chain of events to produce rhythmic opening and closing movements of the jaws and correlated tongue movements. Several theories are proposed to explain the origin and control of the rhythmic activity of the jaws during mastication.
i. ***Cerebral hemisphere theory:*** This theory proposed that mastication was a conscious act, a patterned set of instructions originating in the higher center of the CNS (motor cortex) and descending directly to trigeminal, facial and hypoglossal motor nervous.
ii. ***Reflex chain theory:*** Held that mastication involved a series of interacting chains of reflexes. It is negated because mastication involved prolonged bursts of

muscle activity and not the brief and abrupt behavior usually associated with reflex action of muscle.

iii. **Rhythm (pattern) generation theory:** This theory is now generally accepted. It advocates that there are central pattern generators (CGPs) within the brainstem which on being stimulated from either higher centers (motor cortex) or sensory inputs in the mouth (teeth, periodontal ligament), are driven into rhythmic activity.

### Deglutition (Swallowing)

Deglutition involves an ordered sequence of events that carry food or saliva from the mouth into the stomach. Humans swallow approximately 600 times in a day; about 150 times for swallowing foods or drinks and the rest of the times for clearing saliva from the mouth.

The swallowing pattern in infants is different from that of adults. Persistence of infantile swallow in children is a common cause of tongue thrusting habit which may lead to malocclusion.

The process of swallowing is classically divided into the following three stages for descriptive convenience:
1. **Oral stage:** Food bolus enters pharynx from mouth.
2. **Pharyngeal stage:** Bolus enters esophagus from pharynx.
3. **Esophageal stage:** Bolus enters stomach from esophagus.

*Stage 1: Oral Stage*
- It is involuntary stage
- Anterior oral seal is established by elevation of the mandible by masseter and temporalis muscles and approximation of lips by circumoral muscles.
- A longitudinal furrow is formed in the posterior dorsum of the tongue and bolus is positioned in this furrow, it is called the "preparatory position".
- The tongue is then elevated against the palate by the action of mylohyoid muscles and the groove in the tongue is progressively emptied from before backwards, moving the bolus towards the pharynx.
- Airway remains open at this stage.

*Stage 2: Pharyngeal Stage*
- It is involuntary.
- In this stage, the bolus is pushed from oropharynx into the esophagus.
- As the bolus reaches pharynx, a wave of contraction within the pharyngeal constrictor muscle arises and moves the bolus into the esophagus.
- Food entering back into the nasopharynx is prevented by elevation of the soft palate.
- Movement of bolus into larynx is prevented by approximation of vocal cords, elevation of larynx and backward movement of epiglottis to seal the laryngeal opening.
- The airway is thus closed and there is temporary arrest of breathing at this stage.

*Stage 3: Esophageal Stage*
- It is also involuntary.

- When bolus reaches the esophagus, peristaltic waves are initiated which propel the bolus into the stomach.
- The passage of bolus into the stomach requires relaxation of the lower esophageal sphincter.
- Soft palate, epiglottis and tongue return to their normal positions and the airway is re-established.

### Respiration

Respiration is an inherent reflux process that begins at birth. Breathing is evoked spontaneously at birth and is facilitated by posture of the mandible and hyoid bone. Establishment of normal nasal respiration is important for normal development of orofacial structures.

Partial or total nasal obstruction may lead to mouth breathing habit in some children. Such an alteration in breathing pattern disturbs the orofacial muscular balance because of lowered mandibular and tongue position. This may adversely affect the development of dental arches. Narrowed maxillary arch and posterior open bite are commonly observed in mouth breathers.

### Speech

Speech is probably the most complex sensorimotor developmental process in one's life. Coordinated activity of respiration, laryngeal behavior and oral structures are essential to produce effective speech.

Sounds are produced initially in the larynx by the coordinated movements of abdominal, thoracic, and laryngeal muscles. This is called as "phonation". The laryngeal note has a thin and reedy quality. The basic laryngeal sound is then modified within the resonating chambers of pharyngeal, oral and nasal cavities by the action of lips, tongue and soft palate to produce meaningful speech. This is called "articulation".

*Muscles Involved in Speech*

Although all oral structures are important, tongue has a significant role in speech. The highly complex nature of speech process is indicated by the number of muscles and nerves involved and the large areas of cerebral hemispheres of brain involved with speech.

The muscles involved in speech include:
- Muscles of chest that control breathing
- The intrinsic muscles of the larynx that are concerned with phonation
- Muscles in the pharynx and soft palate that help in resonance
- Muscles of the tongue, palate, jaws, and facial musculature that produce meaningful speech.

Although altered speech may not cause malocclusion, certain malocclusions and skeletal abnormalities (e.g. open bite, increased overjet, reverse overbite, cleft palate, etc.) may cause altered phonation of consonants and can adversely affect speech.

## TRAJECTORIAL THEORY OF BONE FORMATION

- Although bone is a hard mineralized structure, it is the most plastic connective tissue in terms of response to

functional stresses. Mature bone including jaw bones is composed of compact bone which forms the exterior and cancellous/spongy bone which forms the inner core. The cancellous bone consists of meshwork of trabecular pattern, within which, intercommunicating medullary processes are present.
- Meyer proposed the trajectorial theory of bone formation in 1867. The trajectorial theory states that the lines of orientation of the bony trabeculae correspond to the pathways of maximal pressure and tension. Bony trabeculae are thicker in the regions where the stress is greater. The lines of trabeculae (trajectories) indicate the direction of maximum stress within the bone. It is observed that most trajectories cross at a right angle which is an excellent arrangement to resist manifold stresses on the bone.
- Benninghoff did extensive study on craniofacial bones. He studied the natural lines of stress in the skull by piercing small holes into fresh skull. Later when skulls were dried, he observed that the holes assumed a linear form in the direction of the bony trabeculae. These were called the "Benninghoff lines/trajectories" which indicate the direction of the functional stresses in bone.

### Trajectories of Maxilla

Maxilla is less compact and more porous when compared to the mandible. Maxilla provides maximum strength with minimum bone material because of the trajectories. The trajectories of maxilla can be grouped into vertical and horizontal trajectories.

#### Vertical Trajectories of Maxilla
- Frontonasal buttress/pillar
- Malar-zygomatic buttress/pillar
- Pterygoid buttress/pillar

*Frontonasal buttress/pillar:* This transmits pressures from the incisors, canines and first premolars. The line originates from incisors, canine and first premolar and runs cranially along piriform aperture and crest of the nasal bones and ends in the frontal bone.

*Malar-zygomatic buttress/pillar:* Zygomatic buttress transmits stress from the posterior teeth in 3 pathways which are as follows:
- Through the zygomatic arch to the base of the skull
- Upward to the frontal bone through the lateral walls of the orbit
- Along the lower orbital margin to join the upper part of the frontonasal buttress.

*Pterygoid buttress/pillar:* This trajectory transmits stress from the second and third molars to the base of the skull.

#### Horizontal Trajectories of Maxilla
Horizontal reinforcing trajectories include:
- Hard palate
- Orbital ridges
- Zygomatic arches
- Lesser wing of sphenoid.

### Trajectories of Mandible
Mandible has major and minor trajectories to withstand the occlusal stresses.

#### Major Trajectories
Trabecular lines originate from beneath the teeth in the alveolar process and join together into a common stress pillar or trajectory system. Mandibular canal and nerve are protected by this concentration of trabeculae. The thick cortical layer of trabeculae along the lower border of the mandible offers high resistance to bending forces.

#### Minor Trajectories
These accessory trajectories are produced due to the effect of muscle attachment. They are seen at symphysis and gonial angle. One trabecular line is also seen running downwards from the coronoid process into the ramus and body of the mandible.

### Wolff's Law of Bone Transformation
In the year 1870, Julius Wolff explained the reason for the arrangement of trabecular pattern. He attributed the trabecular arrangement pattern to functional stresses. A change in the magnitude of force could produce a marked change in the internal architecture and external form of the bone. These changes are accomplished by means of selective resorption of existing bone and resorption of new bone.

These remodeling changes can take place in the compact bone under periosteum or in trabecular pattern of cancellous bone or on the walls of marrow spaces. Increase in function leads to an increase in density of bony trabeculae, while lack of function leads to a decrease in trabecular density. This is called the "Wolff's law of bone transformation".

Due to such transformation, not only the quantity of bone tissue is kept minimum that would be needed for functional requirements, but also its structure is such that it is best suited for the forces exerted on it.

## BIBLIOGRAPHY

1. Dixon AD. The development of the jaws. Dent Pract. 1953; 3:331-56.
2. Fränkel R. The functional matrix and its practical importance in orthodontics. Rep Congr Eur Orthod Soc. 1969; 207-18.
3. Graber TM. Orthodontics: Principles and Practice. WB Saunders, 1998.
4. Moss ML. The functional matrix hypothesis revisited. The role of mechanotransduction. Am J Orthod Dentofacial Orthop. 1997; 112(1):8-11.
5. Proffit WR. Contemporary Orthodontics. St Louis: CV Mosby, 1986.
6. Scott JH. Dentofacial Development and Growth, London: Pergamon Press, 1967; 65-137.

## EXAM-ORIENTED QUESTIONS

### Long Note or Short Essay

1. Growth spurts or growth spurts and two clinical importance or pubertal growth spurts
2. Methods of studying growth or what are growth studies
3. Discuss drift and displacement with example
4. Functional matrix theory
5. Neurotrophism
6. Scammon's curve
7. Safety valve mechanism
8. Endochondral and intramembranous bone formation
9. Growth site versus growth center
10. Expanding "V" Principle.

### Short Notes

1. Growth sites
2. Growth curve
3. Capsular matrix
4. Growth trends
5. Differential Growth
6. Cortical drift.

### Long Essay

1. Define growth and development. Mention various theories of growth in detail about functional matrix hypothesis.
2. Enumerate the various methods of measuring growth. Discuss the clinical importance of the knowledge of growth and development in orthodontics.
3. Define growth. Discuss briefly clinical applications of knowledge of growth and development in orthodontics.
4. Define growth and enumerate various theories of bone growth.

# CHAPTER 4
# Prenatal Growth and Development

*Rashmi GS*

Basic knowledge of embryology is essential for understanding the normal postnatal growth, as well as the development of various craniofacial abnormalities. This chapter discusses important events occurring in the prenatal development of head and neck.

## PHASES OF DEVELOPMENT

Prenatal human development is traditionally divided into the following three successive phases:
 i. Period of ovum (Fertilization to 2 weeks/14th day)
 ii. Period of embryo (3rd week to 8th week/56th day)
 iii. Period of fetus (56th day to birth).

### Period of Ovum

This period lasts for two weeks from fertilization to implantation of the ovum to the uterine wall. In this stage, rapid proliferation of cells occur with no or little differentiation.

### Period of Embryo

Cell proliferation and also differentiation occurs in this stage, which lasts from the third week to the 8th week (56th day). Organogenesis occurs in this period which is characterized by differentiation of all major organs and systems. This stage of intrauterine life is particularly vulnerable to exposure of teratogens, such as viruses and drugs. Many recognized congenital defects including cleft lip and palate develop during this period.

### Period of Fetus

From the 9th week up to birth term, the embryo is called a fetus. Further development is largely in the form of growth and maturation rather than differentiation. Overall increase in the size of the fetus occurs due to an accelerated growth. In addition to the increase in size, a change in the proportion of the structures also occurs.

## EARLY EMBRYONIC EVENTS

### Fertilization and Morula Formation

Fertilization, the process by which male and female gametes fuse, occurs in the ampullae of the uterine tube **(Fig. 4.1)**. The fertilized egg undergoes a series of rapid divisions to form a ball of cell called "morula" **(Fig. 4.2)**.

### Blastocyst Formation and its Implantation

Fluid seeps into the morula and its cells realign to form a fluid-filled hollow ball, the "blastocyst" **(Fig. 4.3)**. Two cell populations can be seen in the "blastocyst":

- "Trophoblast cells" that line the fluid-filled cavity (primitive yolk sac)
- A small cluster within the cavity, called the inner cell mass/embryoblast cells.

The inner cell mass/embryoblast cells develop into proper embryo whereas the trophoblast cells are associated with implantation of the embryo and formation of placenta. At the end of the first week, the blastocyst gets adhered to the endometrium and later gets implanted to the uterus wall.

### Bilaminar Disk

In the second week, the inner cell mass/embryoblast layer gets differentiated into a two layered disk called "bilaminar embryonic disk" **(Fig. 4.4)**. The bilaminar disk is comprised of:

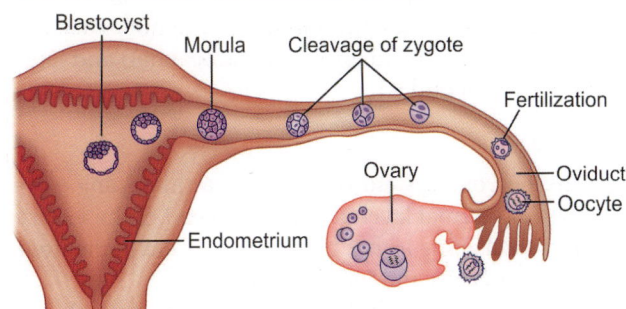

**Fig. 4.1:** Illustration depicting early developmental events occurring in the first week: Formation of zygote, morula and blastocyst

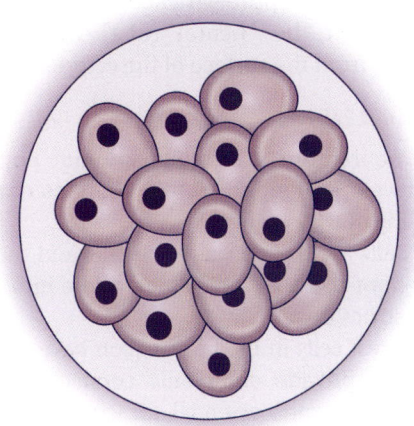

**Fig. 4.2:** Morula: The zygote undergoes a series of mitotic divisions to form a ball of cells called morula

- A dorsally situated columnar cell layer known as "the epiblast layer" and
- A cuboidal cell layer on the ventral aspect known as "the hypoblast layer."

### Trilaminar Disk

During third week, the bilaminar embryo is converted into trilaminar embryo and this process is called "gastrulation". Gastrulation begins with the formation of a structure called "primitive streak" that develops in the midline of epiblast towards the caudal end. This structure is a narrow groove with slightly bulging areas on each side and there is a small depression called "primitive node" at its cranial end **(Fig. 4.5)**.

At this stage, some cells of the epiblast migrate and invaginate into the primitive streak and primitive node. Some of these cells displace the hypoblast layer to form the "embryonic endoderm." Other cells remain between the endoderm and epiblast to form the "embryonic mesoderm." The remaining cells in the epiblast produce the "ectoderm" and thus the three germ layers are formed **(Fig. 4.6)**. In this way, all three embryonic germ layers are formed from the epiblast layer.

During the next 3–4 weeks of organogenesis period, major tissues and organs differentiate from the trilaminar embryo including the head, face, and the tissues contributing to the development of teeth.

Nervous system and neural crest tissue get differentiated from the ectoderm and the folding of the embryo occurs in two planes, along head and tail (restrocaudal) and lateral axes **(Figs 4.7A and B)**.

### Neurulation

- The nervous system develops as a thickening within the ectodermal layer at the crestal end of the embryo. This thickening is the "neural plate". Cells of the neural plate comprise the "neuroectoderm."
- The lateral edges of the neural plate become elevated to form the "neural folds." A depressed groove forms between the neural folds in the midline called "neural groove" **(Fig. 4.8)**.
- The neural folds approach each other and eventually fuse to form the "neural tube" which then gets separated from the surface of the ectoderm.

### The Neural Crest Cells

- As the neural tube is forming, a unique population of cells develops along the lateral margins of the neural plate **(Fig. 4.8)**.
- These cells are the neural crest cells and they migrate throughout the body and differentiate into numerous varied structures.
- Neural crest cells in the head region have an important role. They provide embryonic connective tissue—the "ectomesenchyme" essential for craniofacial development.
- All the tissues of the tooth and its supporting structures except enamel are derived from ectomesenchymal cells.

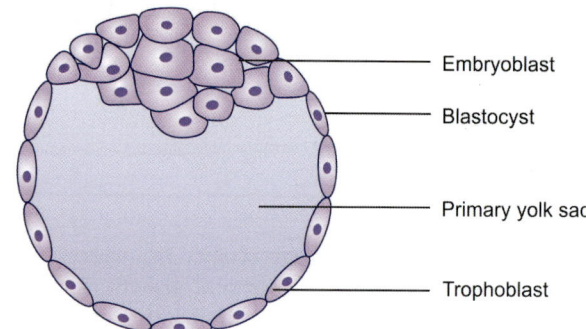

**Fig.4.3:** Blastocyst showing two distinct cell populations

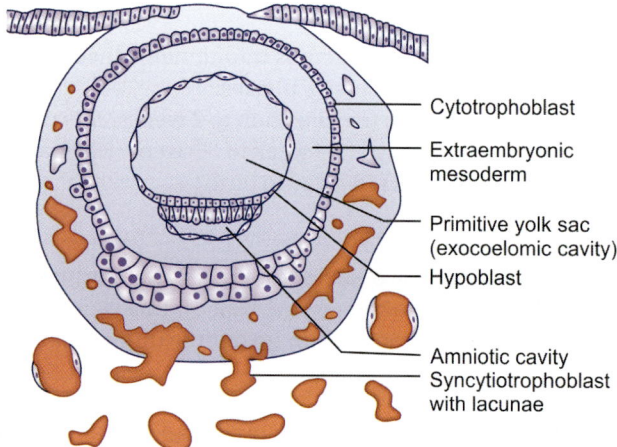

**Fig. 4.4:** Formation of bilaminar embryonic disc

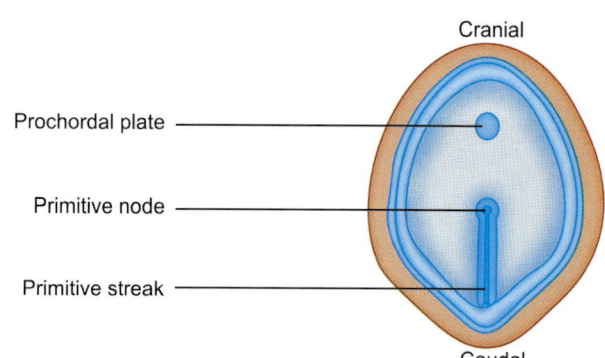

**Fig. 4.5:** Primitive streak developing in the midline of epiblast layer

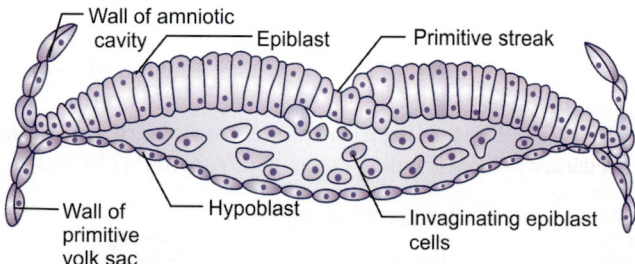

**Fig. 4.6:** Formation of bilaminar disk (Gastrulation)

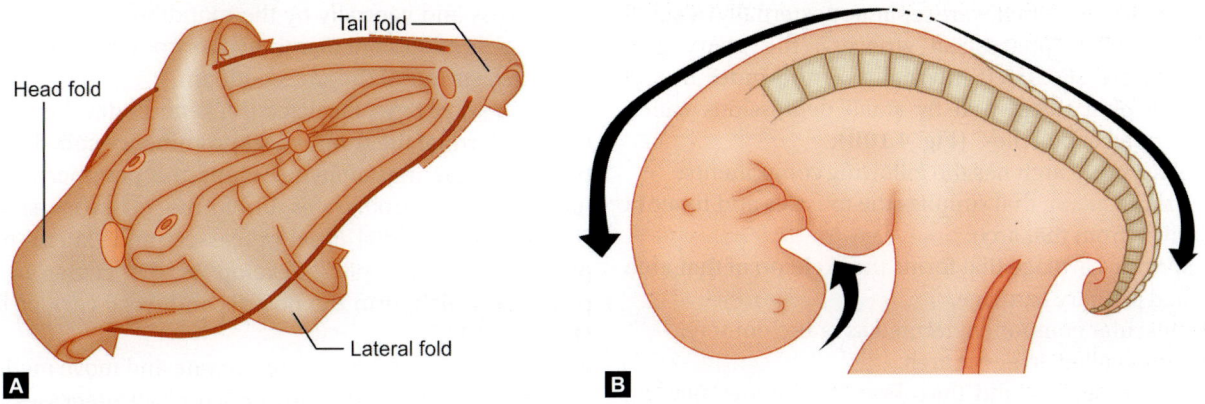

**Figs 4.7A and B:** (A) Folding of the embryo along retrocaudal and lateral axes; (B) Embryo after the completion of folding

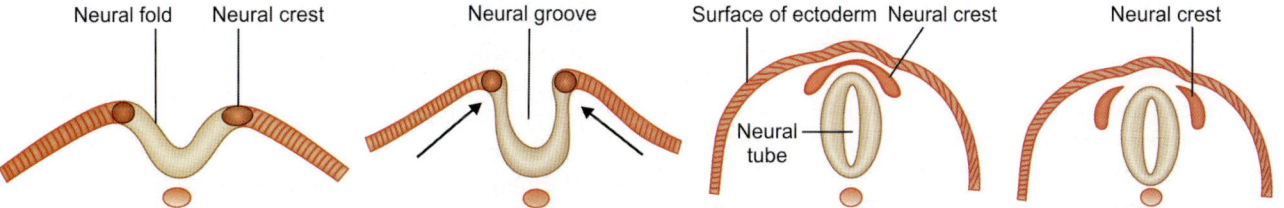

**Fig. 4.8:** Formation of neural tube and neural crest cells: Neural crest cells arise from neural folds and migrate throughout the body and differentiate into various structures. Migration of neural crest cells to head and neck region is critical for the development of teeth and jaws

- Proper migration of neural crest cells is essential for the development of face and the teeth.
- Failure of neural crest cells to properly migrate to the facial region leads to craniofacial anomalies, such as Treacher Collins syndrome.

### Pharyngeal (Branchial) Arches and Primitive Oral Cavity

- After the establishment of head fold, primitive oral cavity (stomatodeum) is formed bounded dorsally by frontal prominence and ventrally by the developing cardiac bulge. The stomatodeum is separated from the foregut by the "buccopharyngeal membrane", a bilaminar structure consisting of apposed ectoderm and endoderm **(Fig. 4.9)**. At 27th day of gestation, buccopharyngeal membrane ruptures and primitive oral cavity establishes a connection with the foregut.
- During 4th week, a series of thickenings develop in the pharyngeal wall called "pharyngeal/branchial arches." The pharyngeal apparatus gives rise to a significant number of structures of head and neck.
- The pharyngeal arches are seen as bulges on the lateral aspect of the embryo **(Fig. 4.10A)**. They are bilaterally paired and are numbered I, II, III and IV. The arches V and VI are poorly developed in humans. The fifth arch completely regresses and arch IV is the result of fusion of arches IV and VI.
- The arch I is called "mandibular arch" and arch II, the "hyoid arch." The other arches do not have any specific names.

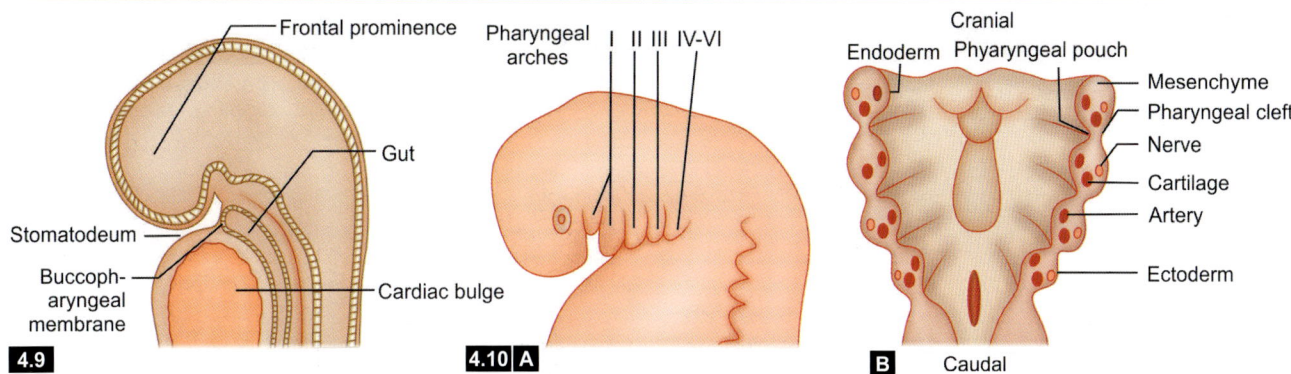

**Fig. 4.9:** Oropharyngeal development: Sagittal section through human embryo showing buccopharyngeal membrane separating the stomatodeum from foregut. Stomatodeum is bounded by frontal prominence and cardiac bulge in early stages. **Figs 4.10A and B:** (A) Development of pharyngeal arches; (B) Components of the pharyngeal arch apparatus

- The pharyngeal arches are separated externally by small clefts called "pharyngeal grooves." The pharyngeal arches are separated internally on the inner aspect of the pharyngeal wall by small depressions called "pharyngeal pouches" **(Fig. 4.10B)**.

Each pharyngeal arch has the following components:
- A specific nerve that supplies the muscles and mucosa derived from that arch.
- A specific cartilage that forms the skeleton of that arch called primary cartilage.
- A muscular component termed as branchiomere.
- Arteries called an aortic arch.

The first, second and third branchial arches play an important role in the development of face, mouth and tongue. The derivatives of pharyngeal arch system are listed in **Table 4.1**.

## Development of Face

The development of face is described in terms of the formation and fusion of several processes or prominences. Development of the face occurs primarily between 4th and 8th week of gestation. The steps in development of face are depicted in **Figs 4.11A to E**.

- At first, the stomatodeum is bounded above (cranially) by the frontonasal process, below (caudally) by the cardiac bulge and laterally by the first branchial arch. The frontonasal process develops as a downward projection of the mesoderm, covering the developing forebrain.
- Later, as the pharyngeal arches grow, the cardiac bulge is eliminated from the stomatodeum and shifts caudally. The first arch gives off a bud from its dorsal end and is called the "maxillary process." The remaining part of the mandibular arch is now called as the "mandibular process" **(Figs 4.11A and B)**. The maxillary and mandibular processes develop as a result of neural crest cells migrating and proliferating into the first pharyngeal arch.
- Thus, the stomatodeum is now bounded cranially by the frontonasal process, laterally by the maxillary process and ventrally by the mandibular process. The facial development mainly occurs from these processes which surround the stomatodeum.

At about 28 days, localized thickenings develop within the ectoderm of the frontonasal prominence called "nasal placodes." The mesenchyme, along the periphery of the nasal placodes, proliferates and forms horseshoe-shaped ridges called "medial nasal processes" and "lateral nasal processes." "Nasal pits" develop in the center of the placodes, which form the nostrils and nasal cavities later **(Fig. 4.11C)**.

- The maxillary processes proliferate and move medially approaching lateral and medial nasal processes. The medial growth of the maxillary process pushes the left and right medial nasal process toward each other which fuse in the midline **(Fig. 4.11D)**.
- In this way, the upper lip is formed from the maxillary process of each side and the medial nasal processes. The lower lip is formed by merging of the two mandibular processes **(Fig. 4.11E)**.
- The merging of medial nasal process with the frontonasal process, gives rise to the middle portion of the nose, middle portion of the upper lip, anterior portion of the maxilla carrying incisor teeth and the primary palate. Lateral nasal processes form the ala of nose.

Embryonic origin of facial structures is summarized in **Table 4.2**.

## Development of Palate

The palate develops between 6th and 9th week of gestation. The entire palate develops from the following two structures:
1. Primary palate
2. Secondary palate.

### Primary Palate

- The primary palate is the triangular-shaped part of the palate anterior to the incisive foramen. It is developed from frontonasal process. Primary palate forms the premaxilla, which carries the incisor teeth **(Fig. 4.12)**.

| Table 4.1: Derivatives of pharyngeal arches | | | |
|---|---|---|---|
| Arch | Cranial nerve | Skeletal structures: Bone, cartilage, ligaments | Muscles |
| I | Vth—Trigeminal nerve | Maxillary process: Maxilla, zygoma, zygomatic process of temporal bone | Muscles of mastication (masseter, temporalis, medial and lateral pterygoid), anterior digastric, mylohyoid, tensor veli palatine, tensor tympani |
| | | Mandibular process: Meckel's cartilage, mandible, malleus, incus, sphenomandibular ligament | |
| II | VIIth—Facial nerve | Reichert's cartilage, stapes, styloid process of temporal bone, lesser horn and superior body of hyoid bone, stylohyoid ligament | Muscles of facial expression (frontalis, orbicularis oris, orbicularis oculi, zygomaticus, buccinator, platysma), stapedius, stylohyoid, posterior belly of digastric |
| | | Greater horn and inferior body of hyoid bone | Stylopharyngeus muscle |
| III | IXth—Glossopharyngeal nerve | Laryngeal cartilages: Thyroid, cricoid and others | Cricothyroid, intrinsic muscles of larynx, constrictors of pharynx |
| IV and VI | Xth—Vagus nerve | | |

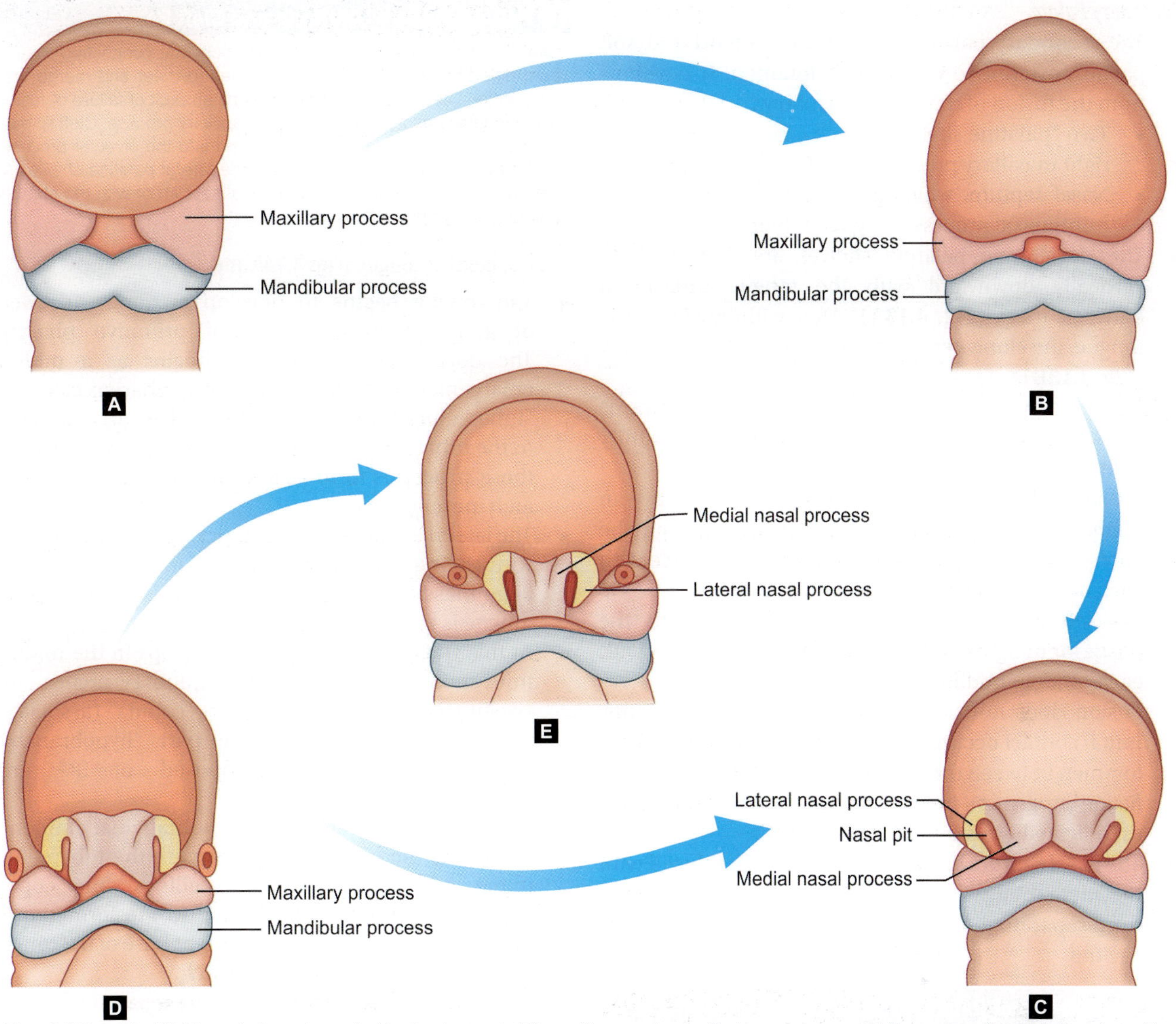

**Figs 4.11A to E:** (A) Stomatodeum bounded by frontonasal; (B) maxillary and mandibular processes; (C) Formation of nasal placodes with nasal pit surrounded by lateral and medial nasal processes; (D) Medial growth of maxillary processes, pushing the left and right medial nasal processes and leading to their fusion; (E) Fusion of various facial processes to form the face

**Table 4.2:** Derivation of facial structures

| Facial prominences | Give rise to the structure |
|---|---|
| Maxillary process | - Lateral portion of upper lip<br>- Most of maxilla including secondary palate |
| Frontonasal process | - Forehead<br>- Dorsum of bridge of the nose |
| Medial nasal process | - Midline of nose<br>- Nasal septum<br>- Philtrum of upper lip |
| Lateral nasal process | - Ala of nose |
| Mandibular process | - Entire mandible<br>- Lower lip |
| I<sup>st</sup> and 2<sup>nd</sup> branchial arches | - Muscles of mastication and facial muscles |

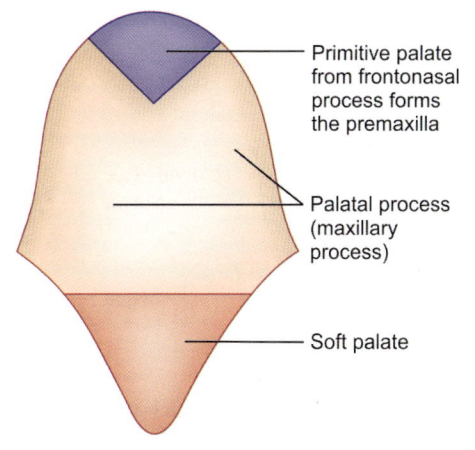

**Fig. 4.12:** Illustration showing primary and secondary palates

### Secondary Palate

- The secondary palate gives rise to the hard and soft palate posterior to the incisive foramen. It develops from the fusion of three parts as follows:
  - Two "palatine shelves" which extend from left and right maxillary process towards the midline.
  - Nasal septum, which grows downwards from the frontonasal process along the midline.
- The developing palatine shelves are first directed vertically downward with the tongue interposed between them **(Fig. 4.13A)**. After withdrawal of the tongue, the elongated shelves get oriented horizontally **(Fig. 4.13B)**.
- Horizontally oriented palatine shelves grow towards each other in the midline and are in close proximity with each other by 8 weeks of gestation.
- Initially, the palatine shelves are covered by an epithelial lining. Following epithelial degeneration, the connective tissues of palatine shelves intermingle with each other resulting in fusion.
- The left and right palatine shelves fuse with the posterior margins of the primary palate, as well as with each other in midline.
- Fusion does not occur simultaneously in all fronts. Initial contact occurs in the center posterior to incisive foramen between the palatine shelves. From this point, fusion progresses in anterior and posterior directions as indicated by arrows in **Figure 4.13C**.
- The nasal septum grows downward and gets fused with the medial edges of palatine shelves in the midline thus, separating the stomatodeum into nasal and oral cavities.

> **Ossification of Palate**
> - Later, the mesoderm of the palate undergoes intramembranous ossification to form the hard palate. Ossification of the palate begins in 8th week from a single center in the maxilla.
> - However, the most posterior portion does not get ossified and remains as soft palate.

> **Pathogenesis of Cleft Lip and Cleft Palate**
> Cleft lip and palate occur when mesenchymal connective tissues from different embryologic structures fail to meet and merge with each other. Cleft lip commonly occurs as a result of failure of fusion of the median nasal process with the maxillary process. Cleft lip may be unilateral or bilateral and may extend into the alveolar process. Cleft palate is the result of failure of the lateral palatine shelves to fuse with each other and with the nasal septum or with the primary palate (see Chapter 41).

### Development of Tongue (Figs 4.14A and B)

- The tongue begins to develop at about 4th week of gestation in the floor of primitive pharynx. The development of tongue begins as a midline enlargement in the floor of primitive pharynx called the "tuberculum impar." Two other bulges arise adjacent to the tuberculum impar called "lingual swellings." All these structures form as a result of proliferation of Ist arch mesenchyme.
- The lateral lingual swellings quickly enlarge and merge with each other and the tuberculum impar to form a large mass from which the two-thirds of the anterior tongue is formed.
- At this stage, a large swelling develops in the midline from mesenchyme of the II, III and IV arches. This swelling consists of a small part "copula" (associated with 2nd arch) and a large part "hypobranchial eminence" (primarily composed of 3rd arch mesenchyme).
- As the tongue develops, the hypobranchial eminence overgrows the copula and fuses with the tuberculum impar and lateral lingual swellings. The copula disappears without contributing to the formation of tongue. Thus, posterior one-third or base of the tongue is derived from IIIrd branchial arch.
- The body and base of the tongue are separated by a line of demarcation called "sulcus terminalis". "Foramen caecum" is found in the midline of this structure.
- The posterior part of the 4th arch gives rise to epiglottis. The muscles of the tongue have a different origin and are derived from "occipital myotomes."

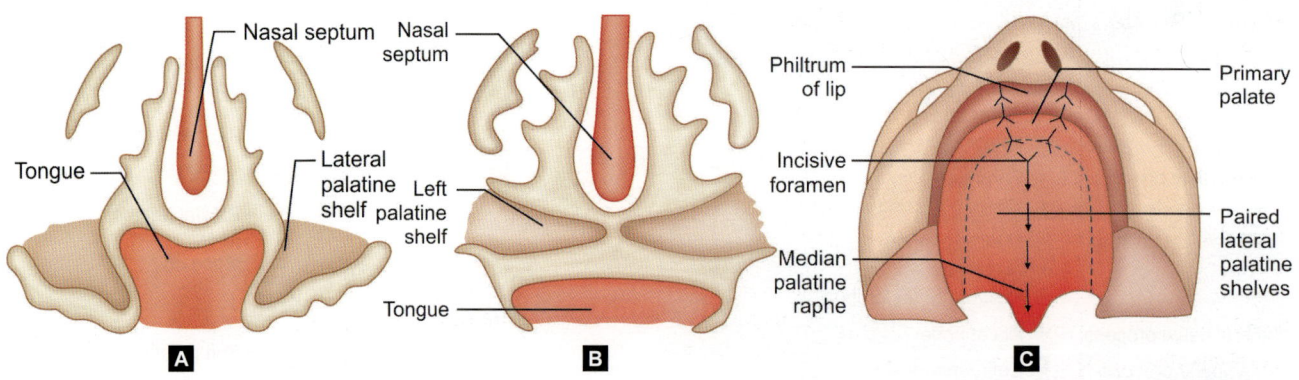

**Figs 4.13A to C:** (A) Palatine shelves are initially directed vertically downwards with tongue interposed between them; (B) After the descent of tongue, palatine shelves grow horizontally and fuse with each other in midline and with the nasal septum; (C) Fusion of primary palate and palatine processes initiate near incisive foramen and progress in anterior and posterior directions (arrows)

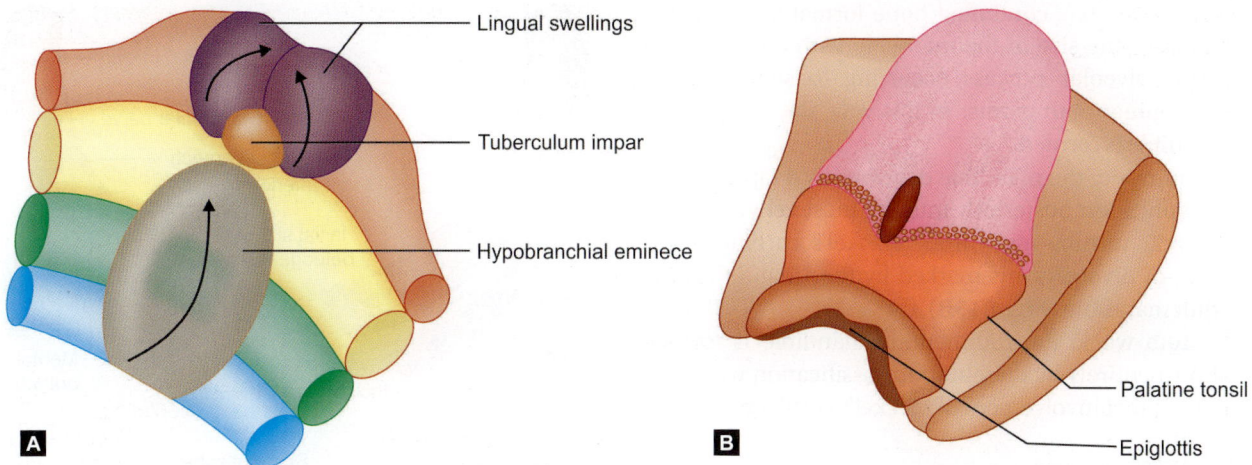

**Figs 4.14A and B:** (A) Two lingual swelling and a tuberculum impar arise from first arch to form anterior 2/3rd of tongue. Hypobranchial eminence of 3rd arch overgrows the 2nd arch and form posterior 1/3 of tongue; (B) Relative contribution of 1st, 3rd and 4th pharyngeal arches to the development of the tongue

- This unusual embryonic origin explains the innervations of tongue. Sensory innervation to the mucosa of body of the tongue is from the nerve of 1st arch, the trigeminal nerve. Sensory innervations to mucosa base of tongue are from nerve of IIIrd arch, the glossopharyngeal nerve. The motor supply to the muscles of tongue is from hypoglossal nerve, the 12th cranial nerve which is the nerve of occipital myotomes.

### Development of Skull

The skull can be divided into the following components **(Fig. 4.15)**:
  I. Neurocranium:
     - Cranial vault
     - Cranial base
  II. Viscerocranium: The facial skeleton including
     - Maxilla
     - Mandible.

The cranial vault and face develop from intramembranous ossification where bones are formed directly in mesenchyme with no cartilaginous precursors. The cranial base undergoes endochondral ossification. Some of the membranous bones may develop secondary cartilages subsequently that provide further growth.

### Development of Mandible and Maxilla

The mandible and maxilla develop from the tissues of the first branchial arch. The mandibular process gives rise to the mandible and the maxillary process forms the maxilla.

#### Mandible

The mandible initially develops intramembranously but its subsequent growth is related to the appearance of secondary cartilages. The "condylar cartilage" is the most important.

- The primary cartilage of the 1st arch, Meckel's cartilage forms the lower jaw in primitive vertebrates. However, in humans, Meckel's cartilage only has a close positional relationship to the developing mandible but makes no actual contribution to it. It merely provides a framework around which the bone of mandible forms.
- Meckel's cartilage first appears at 6th week as a solid hyaline cartilaginous rod surrounded by a fibrocellular capsule extending from the developing ear region (otic capsule) to the midsymphysis. The two cartilages of each side do not meet at midline as they are separated by a thin band of mesenchyme.
- The mandibular nerve, the nerve of 1st arch shows a close relationship to Meckel's cartilage beginning two thirds of the way along the length of the cartilage. At this point, the mandibular nerve divides into lingual and inferior alveolar branches. The inferior alveolar nerve further divides into incisive and mental nerve branches.
- A condensation of mesenchyme occurs on the lateral aspect of Meckel's cartilage in relation to the inferior alveolar nerve. At 7th week, intramembranous ossification begins in this mesenchymal condensation, at the angle formed by the division of incisive and mental nerves **(Fig. 4.15A)**.
- From this center of ossification bone formation spreads anteriorly to the midline and posteriorly towards the point where the mandibular nerve divides into lingual and inferior alveolar nerve. Bone formation spreads rapidly and surrounds the inferior alveolar nerve to form mandibular canal.
- Further spread of the developing bone in anterior and posterior directions produces a plate of bone on the lateral aspect of Meckel's cartilage, which extends toward midline where it comes into approximation with a similar bone forming on the opposite side. However, the two plates of bone remain separated by fibrous tissue mandibular symphysis until shortly after birth.

- At a later stage, continued bone formation markedly increases the size of the mandible with development of the alveolar process occurring to surround the developing tooth germs. In this way, the body of the mandible is formed.
- The ramus of the mandible develops by a rapid spread of ossification posteriorly into the mesenchyme of the 1st arch, turning away from Meckel's cartilage. This point of divergence is marked by the "lingula" in the adult mandible **(Fig. 4.15B)**.
- By 10th week, the rudimentary mandible is formed almost entirely by membranous ossification with little or no direct involvement of Meckel's cartilage.

### Fate of Meckel's cartilage

The greater part of Meckel's cartilage degenerates without contributing to the formation of mandible. It has the following fate:
- Its most posterior extremity forms the "incus" and "malleus" of the inner ear.
- Posterior portion also forms spine of sphenoid.
- Its fibrocellular capsule (perichondrium) persists as the "sphenomandibular ligament."

### Secondary Cartilages in Mandibular Development

Further growth of the mandible until birth is influenced greatly by the appearance of secondary cartilages and the development of the muscular attachments **(Fig. 4.15C)**. Between the 10th and 14th week, three secondary cartilages develop within the growing mandible. The largest and the most important of these, the condylar cartilage, which as its name suggests, appears beneath the fibrous articular layer of the future condyle. Less important transitory secondary cartilages are seen associated with the coronoid process, the coronoid cartilage and in the region of mandibular symphysis, the symphyseal cartilage. Muscular attachments also influence the growth of mandible especially in the angle of mandible and in the chin area.

The mandible develops largely from intramembranous ossification, except in the following three areas where endochondral ossification occurs aided by their respective secondary cartilages:
  I. Condylar process—condylar cartilage
  II. Coronoid process—coronoid cartilage
  III. Mental region—symphyseal cartilage

### Condylar Process

It develops from condylar cartilage, which appears as an area of mesenchymal condensation along with the developing mandible around 5th week. This area of mesenchymal condensation develops into a cone-shaped cartilage by about 10th week. The cartilage fuses with the mandibular ramus by about 4 months. As the development progresses, most of the cartilage

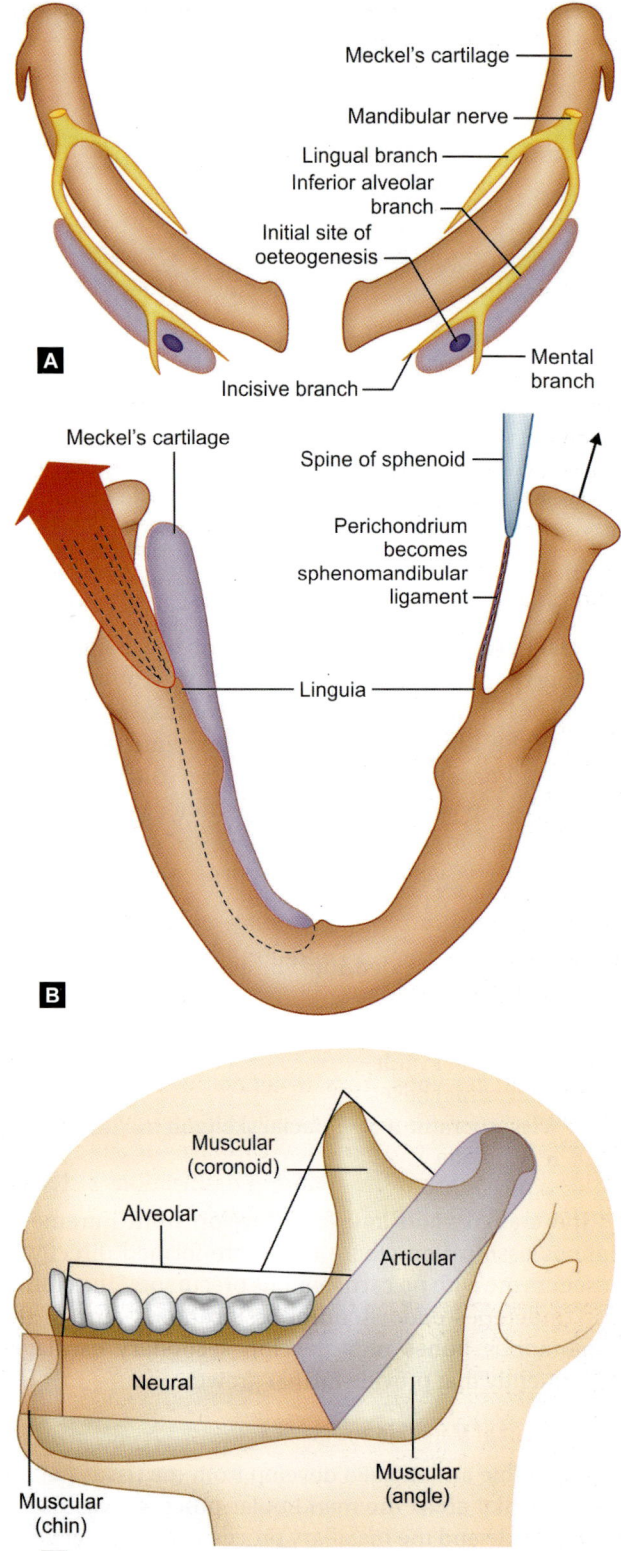

**Figs 4.15A to C:** (A) Ossification of mandible begins at the division of incisive and mental nerves and progresses posteriorly up to the point where mandibular nerve divides into lingual and inferior alveolar nerves; (B) Ossification of mandible spreads away from Meckel's cartilage at the lingual; (C) The mandibular development has neural, alveolar, articular and muscular elements. Its development is assisted by three secondary cartilages

get replaced by bone but its upper end persists into adulthood acting both as a growth cartilage and an articular cartilage.

### Coronoid Process
A secondary cartilage appears in the region of coronoid process by about 10-14th week. This cartilage of coronoid process is thought to grow as a response to the developing temporalis muscle. Coronoid cartilage becomes incorporated into the expanding intramembranous bone of the ramus and disappears before birth.

### Mental Region
Throughout the intrauterine life, left and right mandibles are separated in the midline.

Two symphyseal cartilages develop in the connective tissue between the two ends of Meckel's cartilage in the midline. In symphyseal region, small irregular bones known as "mental ossicles" develop and fuse with the mandibular body at the end of the first year after birth.

### Temporomandibular Joint
The temporomandibular joint develops from the mesenchyme lying between the developing mandibular condyle below and the temporal bone above, which develops intramembranously. During the 12th week of intrauterine life, two clefts appear in the mesenchyme producing the upper and lower joint cavities. The remaining intervening mesenchyme, surrounding the developing joint becomes the intra-articular disk. The joint capsule develops from a condensation of mesenchyme surrounding the developing joint.

### Maxilla
The maxilla develops from a center of ossification in the mesenchyme of the maxillary process of the first pharyngeal arch. No primary cartilage exists in the maxillary process but the center of ossification is closely associated with the cartilage of the "nasal capsule."

- Similar to the mandibular development, the center of ossification appears in the angle between divisions of a nerve that is between "anterosuperior alveolar" and "inferior orbital nerve." From this center, ossification spreads posteriorly towards the developing zygoma, anteriorly towards the premaxillary region and superiorly to form the frontal process of maxilla.
- Ossification also spreads into the palatine processes to form the hard palate. The medial alveolar plate develops from the junction of the palatal process and the main body of the developing maxilla.
- Median alveolar plate, together with the lateral alveolar plate forms a trough of bone around the maxillary tooth germs. The alveolar process forms containing the tooth germs in their bony crypts.
- A secondary cartilage called "zygomatic/malar cartilage" also contributes to the development of maxilla. It appears in the developing zygomatic process and adds considerably to the development of maxilla. The body of the maxilla remains relatively small at birth as the maxillary sinus is still small at birth about the size of a small pea.

### Maxillary Sinus
The maxillary sinus forms around 3rd month. It develops as an expansion of the nasal mucous membrane into the maxillary bone. Maxillary sinus is small at birth about the size of a pea. It gradually enlarges by resorption of the internal walls of maxilla to reach the adult size.

## BIBLIOGRAPHY

1. Enlow DH, Bang S. Growth and remodeling of the human maxilla. Am J Orthod 1965;51:446-64.
2. Graber TM. Orthodontics: Principles and Practice, 3rd edition. WB Saunders, 1988.
3. Moyers RE. Handbook of Orthodontics, 3rd edition. Chicago: Year Book, 1973.
4. Salzmann JA. Practice of Orthodontics. JB Lippincott Company, 1996.
5. Thompson DT. On Growth and Form. Cambridge: Cambridge University Press, 1971.

### EXAM-ORIENTED QUESTIONS

**Long Essay or Long Questionss**
1. Development of palate
2. Describe the developmental defects of maxilla
3. Postnatal growth and development of the mandible
4. Spheno-occipital synchondrosis
5. Sutural growth of maxilla
6. Development of tongue
7. Mechanism of bone growth.

**Short Notes**
1. Meckel's cartilage
2. Nasal septal cartilage
3. How does an infant and an adult mandible differ from each other?
4. Enumerate types of synchondrosis.

# CHAPTER 5

# Postnatal Growth and Development

*Phulari BS, Naik P*

Orthodontic treatment is usually carried out during growth period in adolescent age group. Patterns of growth of the jaws and development of occlusion have a strong bearing on the need for orthodontic treatment and the timing and type of the treatment prescribed.

Knowledge of growth of the skull, jaws and occlusal development is important for orthodontic treatment planning. An understanding of the growth changes is particularly important in that, the proper timing of the treatment in relation to growth may facilitate the progress of such treatment. For example, growth modification procedures using orthopedics and functional appliances must be based on sound knowledge of postnatal growth of craniofacial complex in relation to age, sex and individual variability.

Knowledge of growth changes, occurring in facial skeleton also makes treatments, such as rapid maxillary expansion possible. General aspects of postnatal growth of skull and jaws are described in this chapter.

## SKULL AND JAWS NATAL

Knowing the appearance of skull and jaws at birth is necessary to appreciate the degree and extent of their postnatal growth.

The skull at birth is far different from that of the adult skull. There are differences in shape and proportion of the face and cranium and the degree of development and fusion of the individual bones. At birth, the infant skull consists of 45 bony elements, separated by cartilage or connective tissue. This number is reduced to 22 bones in the adult life after the completion of ossification of skull. Some bones, which are single bones in adulthood, appear as separate constituent parts at birth, for example frontal, occipital and mandible bones. Other skull bones are widely separated from their neighboring bones at birth by loose connective tissues. Open spaces between the adjacent flat bones of skull are called "fontanels", which allow significant growth of brain and also provide the cranium sufficient flexibility to pass through the birth canal during parturition.

The relative sizes of face and cranium at birth and in adult life is noticeably different **(Fig. 5.1)**. The cranium grows rapidly in prenatal period, accommodating the rapidly developing brain. In contrast, the face appears small in vertical dimension when compared to that of the adult. This is because the bones, which contribute to the vertical dimension of the face (nasomaxillary complex and mandible with their alveolar bones) are relatively small at birth.

## POSTNATAL GROWTH

### Craniofacial Complex

The whole craniofacial complex skull is divided into the neurocranium and viscerocranium (face) **(Fig. 5.2)**. The growth of craniofacial complex can be studied by noting the changes occurring in the following areas:

- **Neurocranium**
  - The cranial vault
  - The cranial base
- **Viscerocranium (Face)**
  - The nasomaxillary complex
  - The mandible

Growth of the neurocranium can be divided into that of cranial vault, encasing the brain and the cranial base, which divides the craniofacial complex. The nasomaxillary complex and mandible together comprise the viscerocranium/face.

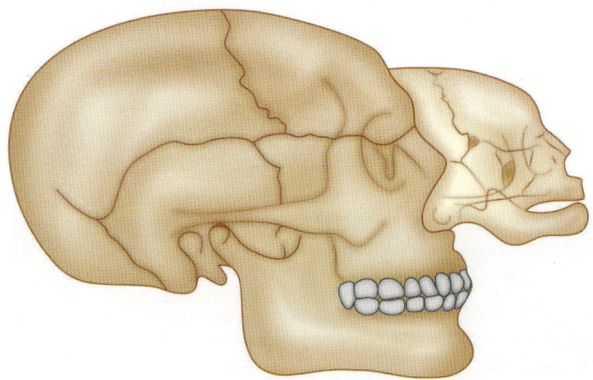

Fig. 5.1: Comparison of relative sizes of cranium and face at the birth and in adult life

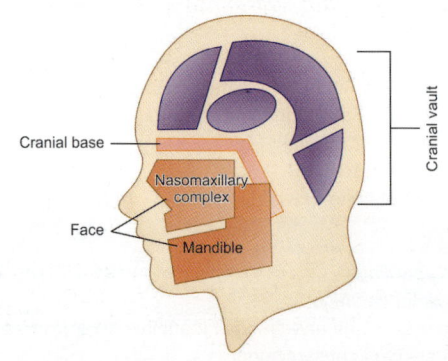

Fig. 5.2: The whole craniofacial complex/skull can be divided into neurocranium

The cranial vault and face are formed by intramembranous ossification, where bone is directly formed from undifferentiated mesenchymal tissue with no cartilaginous precursor.

On the other hand, the cranial base undergoes endochondral ossification, where a precursor/primary cartilage is converted into bone. The membranous bones may develop secondary cartilages to provide rapid growth.

Cranium and facial skeleton grow at different rates **(Table 5.1)**. Growth of the cranium being intimately associated with growth of the brain follows the neural growth curve, where most of the growth occurs in first few years of life. Growth of facial skeleton follows the general growth curve.

## Cranial Vault (Calvarium)

Cranial vault covers the upper and outer surfaces of the brain. It consists of a number of flat bones, which are formed from intramembranous ossification.

Adaptive growth occurs at the coronal, sagittal, parietal, temporal and occipital sutures to accommodate the rapidly expanding brain. As the brain expands, the separate bones of the cranial vault are displaced in outward direction. This intramembranous sutural growth replaces the fontanels that are present at birth.

Apart from growth at sutures, growth also occurs by periosteal and endosteal remodeling. Resorption at the endosteal lining and apposition at the periosteum leads to an increase in the overall thickness of the medullary space between the inner and the outer tables.

Cranial vault following the neural growth curve achieves most of its growth during first few years of life, with over 90% of growth by 5 years and 98% by 15 years of age. **Devenport (1936)** listed the percentage of growth in cranial vault in length at different ages **(Table 5.2)**.

## Cranial Base

What happens to the cranial base very much affects the structure, dimension and placement of various facial parts because the cranial base acts as a template from which the face develops.

Contrary to the cranial vault, bones of the cranial base develop from endochondral ossification. The cranial base is formed by ethmoid, sphenoid and occipital bones. The changes in the cranial base occur primarily as a result of endochondral growth through a system of synchondroses. A synchondrosis is a cartilaginous joint where the hyaline cartilage divides and subsequently is converted into bone. A series of synchondroses occurs within and between the three bones of cranial base and cartilage growth at these synchondroses leads to the growth of cranial base **(Figs 5.3 and 5.4)**.

Intraethmoidal and intrasphenoidal synchondroses—close before birth.

Intraoccipital synchondrosis—closes before 5 years of age.

Sphenoid synchondrosis—closes before 6 years of age. But the spheno-occipital synchondrosis does not ossify until 13–15 years of age. Thus, major growth occurs at spheno-occipital synchondrosis, which would increase the anteroposterior dimension of the skull base **(Fig. 5.4)** and may produce active growth up to the age of puberty.

## Nasomaxillary Complex

As stated earlier, the cranium and the facial skeleton grow at different rates. By this differential growth, the face appears to literally emerge from beneath the cranium. The upper face, under the influence of cranial base inclination, moves upward and forward, while the lower face moves downward and forward on an expanding 'V' **(Fig. 5.4)**.

As maxilla is joined to the cranial base, its growth is strongly influenced by the changes occurring at the cranial base. Thus, the position of the maxilla is dependent on the growth of the cartilaginous nasal septum, which carries the nasomaxillary complex downward and forward.

Growth of nasomaxillary complex can be attributed to the following mechanisms:

**Table 5.2:** Cranial vault at different ages (Devenport 1936)

| Stage | Growth of cranial vault (%) |
|---|---|
| At birth | 63 |
| 6 months | 76 |
| 1 year | 82 |
| 2 years | 87 |
| 3 years | 89 |
| 5 years | 91 |
| 10 years | 95 |
| 15 years | 98 |

**Table 5.1:** Craniofacial growth completed at different age (%)

| | 1–5 years | 6–10 years | 11–20 years |
|---|---|---|---|
| **Cranium** | 85% | 11% | 4% |
| **Maxilla** | 45% | 20% | 35% |
| **Mandible** | 40% | 25% | 35% |

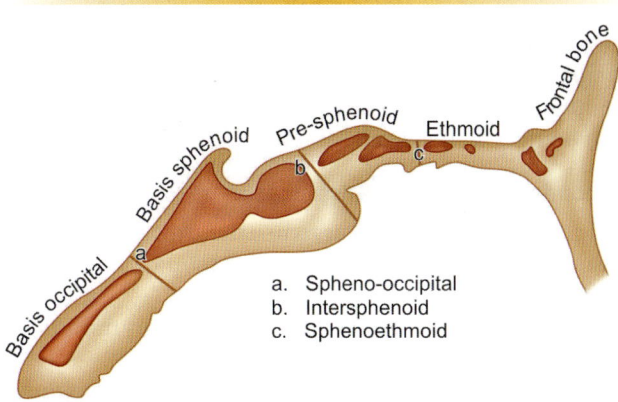

a. Spheno-occipital
b. Intersphenoid
c. Sphenoethmoid

**Fig. 5.3:** Formation of cranial base through synchondroses

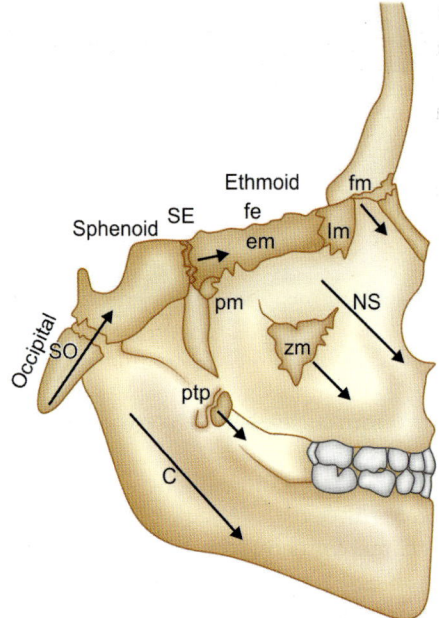

**Fig. 5.4:** During postnatal growth of face, the upper face moves in an upward and forward direction, while the lower face moves downward and forward on an expanding 'V'
SO—sphenooccipital synchondrosis; C—reflection of condylar mandibular growth; NS—nasal septum; Se—sphenoethmoid suture; ptp—pterygopalatine suture; pm—palatomaxillary suture; fe—frontoethmoidal suture; em—ethmoidal-maxillary suture; lm—lacrimal-maxillary suture; fm—frontomaxillary suture; zm—zygomaticomaxillary suture

- Translation/displacement
- Growth at sutures
- Surface remodeling.

### Translation/Displacement

Change in the spatial position of a bone can occur by two types of translation **(Figs 5.5A and B)**.

### Primary Translation/Displacement

Primary translation occurs where actual enlargement of the bone will change its position in space. In other words, primary displacement of the bone is brought about by its own enlargement.

Primary displacement of maxilla in a forward direction occurs due to the growth of maxillary tuberosity in a posterior direction **(Fig. 5.5A)**. The amount of anterior displacement is equal to the amount of posterior lengthening. Periosteal surface of the tuberosity receives continuous deposits of new bone and results in horizontal lengthening of the maxillary arch.

### Secondary Translation/Displacement

Secondary translation occurs when the growth of one bone results in a change in the spatial position of an adjacent bone.

Nasomaxillary complex grows by secondary translation during primary dentition period.

As the maxilla is attached to the cranial base, growth occurring at cranial base produces a passive/secondary displacement of the nasomaxillary complex in a downward and forward direction **(Fig. 5.5B)**.

### Growth at Sutures

The nasomaxillary complex is surrounded by a system of sutures that allows for the growth of various bones both anteroposteriorly and laterally **(Fig. 5.4)**.

These sutures include:
- Frontomaxillary suture
- Zygomaticotemporal suture
- Zygomaticomaxillary suture
- Pterygopalatine suture

According to Weinmann and Sicker, these sutures are all oblique and more or less parallel with each other. Tension produced by the downward and forward displacement of the maxillary bone stimulates the sutural bone growth at these sutures. New bone is formed on either side of the suture as a response to the tendency to displacement. Thus, as the entire maxilla is carried forward and downward by displacement, the osteogenic sutural membranes form

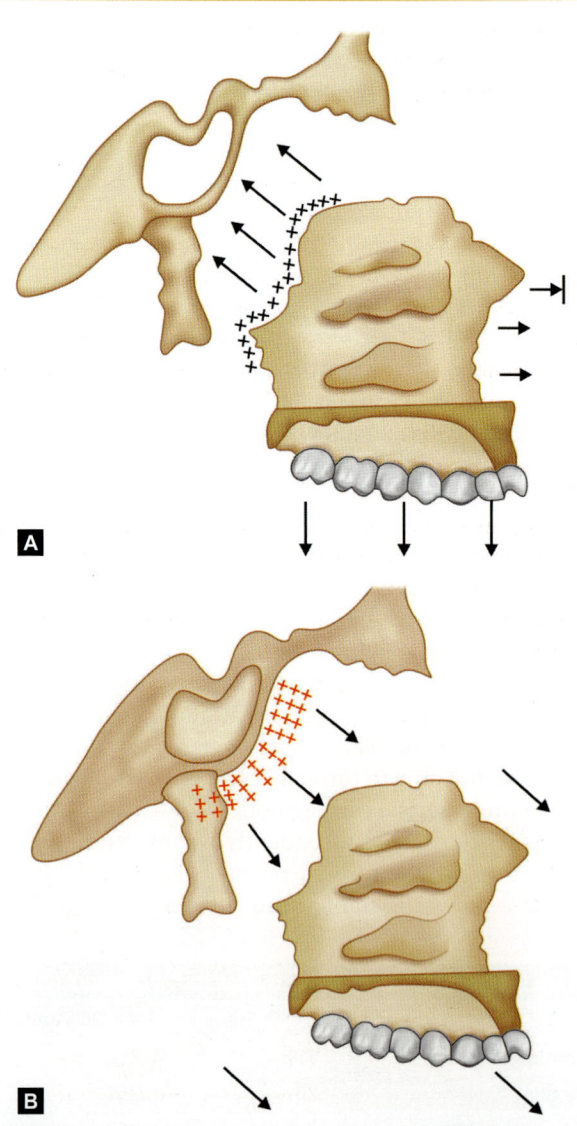

**Figs 5.5A and B:** Secondary displacement of nasomaxillary complex

new bone tissues that enlarges the overall size of the maxilla, while constantly maintaining the bone-to-bone sutural contact.

### Surface Bone Remodeling

In addition to the specific sites of bone formation, all bony surfaces undergo selective bone remodeling through deposition and resorption along with endosteal and periosteal surfaces of bone. Along with an increase in size, bone remodeling brings about changes in shape and functional relationship of the bone.

The following are some of the important remodeling changes occurring in the nasomaxillary complex (**Figs 5.6A to D**).

### Orbit

Widening of orbit occurs by resorption of inner surface of the lateral rim. Compensatory deposition occurs on the outer surface of the lateral rim and on the medial wall of the orbit (**Fig. 5.6A**).

### Nasal Cavity

To allow for the increased functional demands in the nasal cavities, resorption occurs on its lateral walls of nasal cavity. The nasal wall is lowered by resorption of floor of nasal cavity. This is accompanied by bone deposition on the oral side of palatal vault (**Fig. 5.6A**).

### Maxillary Sinus

Maxillary sinus is rudimentary at birth, about the size of a peanut. Its postnatal increase in size contributes significantly to the development of nasomaxillary complex. The lining cortical surface of maxillary sinus is all resorptive, except the medial nasal wall, which is depository, because it remodels laterally to accommodate nasal expansion (**Fig. 5.6A**).

### Maxillary Tuberosity

Deposition of periosteal bone on the posterior surface of the tuberosity increases the length of maxillary arches and provides room for erupting molars. The endosteal surface is resorptive and this contributes to maxillary sinus enlargement.

### Zygoma

The zygomatic arch moves laterally and posteriorly by deposition of bone on lateral and posterior surfaces, Compensatory resorption occurs on medial and anterior surfaces (**Fig. 5.6B**).

### Palatal Remodeling and Increase in Maxillary Height

The palatal growth follows the principle of the expanding 'V' (**Figs 5.6C and D**). Resorption occurs on the floor of the nasal cavity and deposition on the oral side of the palatal vault. This moves the palate in a downward direction. However, depth of palatal vault continues to increase with age, expanding in a 'V' shape. This is a result of growth of alveolar process that accompanies the eruption of primary and permanent teeth.

### Increase in Maxillary Height

Increase in the height of maxillary complex is mainly due to continued apposition of alveolar bone on the free borders of the alveolar process as the teeth erupt.

### Increase in Maxillary Width

Growth in width occurs during the first 5 years of life, mostly at intermaxillary and midpalatal sutures. Later, any additional increase in the width of the maxilla occurs as a result of bone deposition on the outer surface of maxilla and by the buccal eruption of permanent teeth.

## Mandible

At birth, the mandible is made of two halves, as it is not united at the midline. By the end of first year, the two halves get united to form a single mandibular bone. The rami are short and condylar development is minimal at birth.

Of the facial bones, mandible exhibits greatest amount of postnatal growth. Mandible grows in a downward and forward direction and the growth rate follows the general growth curve with significant growth spurts during puberty.

Growth of mandible largely occurs due to intramembranous ossification. However, few secondary cartilages, especially the condylar cartilage, accelerate its growth postnatally.

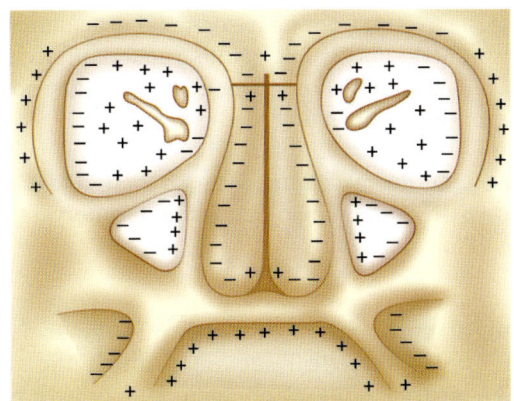

**Fig. 5.6A:** Bone remodeling changes at midface region

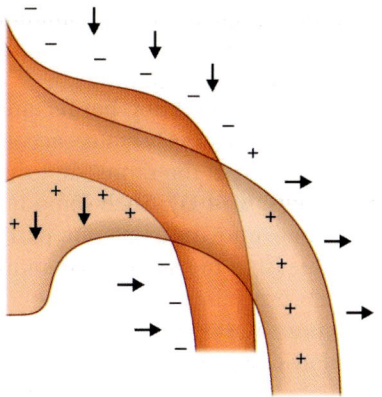

**Fig. 5.6B:** Enlargement of zygoma by bone remodeling

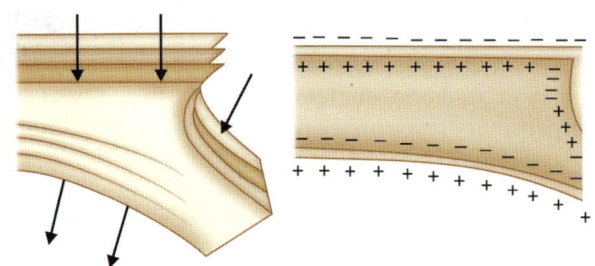

**Fig. 5.6C:** Bone remodeling of the palate resulting in its downward displacement

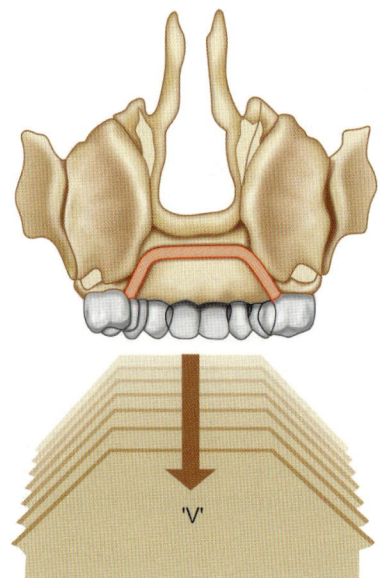

**Fig. 5.6D:** Palatal growth on an expanding 'V' occurs by resorption of nasal floor and bone deposition on oral side of palatal vault

Although a single bone, the mandible can be divided functionally and developmentally into several subunits. Postnatal development can be better understood by studying the growth of these units, which include body of mandible, alveolar process that is attached to the body, condyles, rami, lingual tuberosity with chin, and angular and coronoid processes.

Postnatal changes, occurring in the several units of mandible are described below. **Figure 5.7** depicts the overall growth, occurring at various areas of mandible. In general, the downward and forward mandibular growth follows the expanding 'V' principle (**Figs 5.7A and B**).

### Ramus

Bone resorption at the anterior border and deposition at posterior border of the ramus accounts for the anteroposterior growth of the ramus and the body of the mandible (**Figs 5.7C and D**). Such remodeling converts former ramal bone into the posterior part of the body and there by increasing the length of mandibular arch to accommodate the erupting permanent molars (**Fig. 5.7E**). 'Drift' of the ramus in a posterior direction also provides area for insertion of the increasing mass of masticatory muscles.

### Body of Mandible

Cephalometric studies indicate that the body of the mandible maintains a relatively constant angular relationship to the ramus throughout life. As the ramus 'drifts' in a posterior direction, the length of the body of mandible increases at its posterior aspect. This increase in the length of mandibular arch provides room for erupting permanent molars (**Figs 5.7C and E**).

### Angle of Mandible

Selective bone remodelling at the angle of mandible, causes flaring of the angle as age advances. On the lingual side of the angle of mandible, resorption occurs on the posteroinferior aspect, while deposition occurs on the anterosuperior aspect. On the buccal side, however, resorption occurs on the anterosuperior aspect, while deposition takes place on posterosuperior aspect, causing flaring of the angle of mandible (**Figs 5.7A and D**).

### Mandibular Condyle

The condyle shows minimum growth at birth. It is an anatomic part of special interest because it is a major site of growth of mandible, having considerable clinical significance. Growth of the condylar cartilage would increase the length and height of the mandible.

The role of condylar cartilage in mandibular growth has been a subject of controversy. There are two major schools of thought about the role of condyle:

1. Weimann and Sicker considered condyle as the major growth center of mandible with an intrinsic genetic potential. Others thought that the condylar cartilage was analogous to an epiphyseal cartilage. It was believed that condyle grows towards cranial base by deposition of bone at condylar cartilage. As the condyle pushes against the cranial base, the entire mandible gets displaced in a forward and downward direction.
2. Now, several studies have shown that the growth of the soft tissues, including muscles and connective tissues (functional matrix) carries the mandible forwards and downwards, with growth expansion of the soft tissue matrix associated with it. The condylar remodeling is not a driving force of growth, but it is rather an adaptive change secondary to the displacement of mandible by the functional matrix. Thus, as the mandible is displaced away from its basocranial articular contact, the condyle and whole ramus secondarily remodels towards the cranial base, thereby closing any potential space without an actual gap being created.

The overall mandibular length can be clinically increased or decreased to treat class II and class III individuals by physiologic or mechanic intervention, as follows (**Flowchart 5.1**):

### Coronoid Process

Growth of coronoid process follows the expanding 'V' principle. A vertical section through the ramus-coronoid process shows a characteristic growth pattern

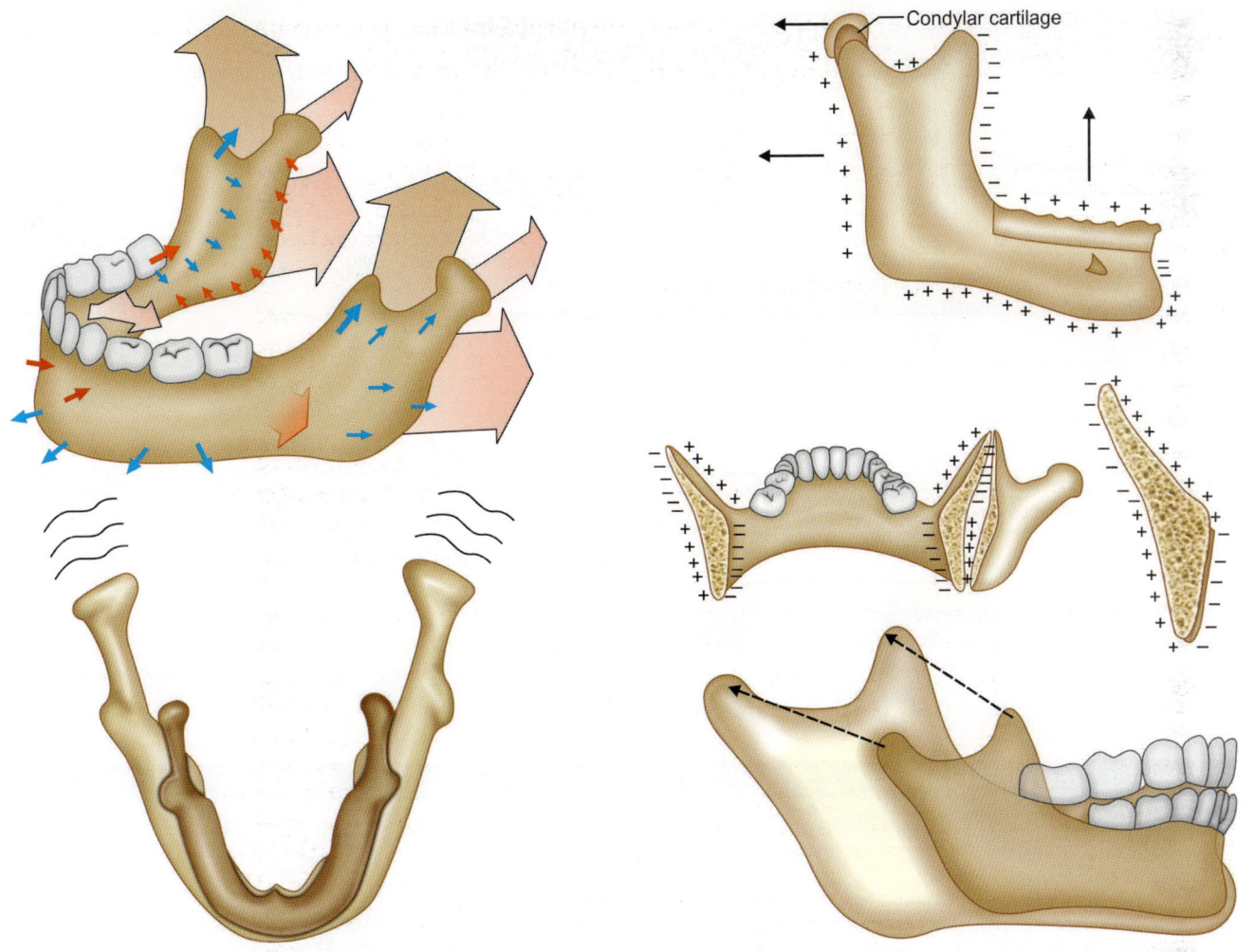

**Figs. 5.7A to E:** (A) Overall growth occurring at various areas of mandible. Red arrows bone resorption, blue arrows bone deposition; (B) Downward and forward mandibular growth follows the expanding 'V' principle; (C) Anterior-posterior growth of the ramus and the body of the mandible occurs by bone resorption at the anterior border and deposition at posterior border of the ramus; (D) Vertical section through mandibular ramus and coronoid process showing bone remodeling changes that cause expansion of the bone on a 'V' principle; (E) Increase in the length of mandibular arch, which provides room for erupting permanent molars

involving periosteal deposition on the lingual surface of coronoid processes together with resorption from buccal surface **(Fig. 5.7D)**. Basal part of ramus shows deposition on buccal side with contralateral resorption from the lingual surface. This remodeling causes an increase in height of coronoid process with their apices growing further apart.

### Alveolar Process

Alveolar growth occurs around the tooth buds. As the teeth develop and begin to erupt, alveolar process increases in size and height. This continued growth of alveolar bone with developing dentition increases the height of the mandibular body. The alveolar process grows upward and outward on an expanding arch. This permits the dental arch to accommodate the larger permanent teeth.

### Chin

The chin is not well developed at birth. Significant growth of the chin occurs at puberty as age advances, and is influenced by sexual and genetic factors. Chin becomes prominent at puberty especially in male, by selective bone remodelling. Bone resorption occurs in the alveolar region above the prominence, creating a concavity. Apposition occurs at the inferior aspect **(Fig. 5.7A)**.

In summary, the mandible literally grows as an expanding 'V'. Additive growth at the ends of this 'V' increases the distance between the terminal points. The two rami also diverge outward from below to above so that additive growth at coronoid process and condyle also increases the superior inter-ramus dimension. The condyles are not the primary sites of mandibular growth but are loci with secondary, compensatory growth potential.

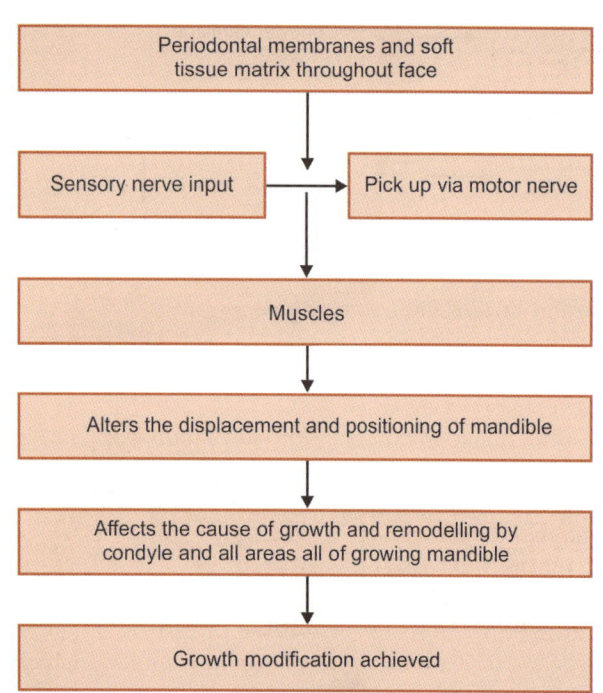

**Flowchart 5.1:** Overall mandibular length

## BIBLIOGRAPHY

1. Enlow DH, Harris DB. A study of postnatal growth of human mandible. Am J Orthod 1964; 50:25-50.
2. Graber TM. Orthodontics: Principles and Practice. WB Saunders, 1998.
3. Proffit WR. Concepts of growth and development. In: Contemporary Orthodontics, 2nd edition. St Louis: Mosby Yearbook, 1999.pp. 24-62.
4. Ten Cate AR. Oral Histology: Development, Structure & Function. St Louis: CV Mosby, 1980.

### EXAM-ORIENTED QUESTIONS

*Long Essay or Long Questions*

1. Describe in detail postnatal growth of craniofacial complex.
2. Postnatal growth of mandible

*Short Notes*

1. Growth at sutures
2. Surface remodelling.

# CHAPTER 6

# Development of Dentition and Occlusion

*Phulari BS, Rashmi GS*

Malocclusion is a reflection of disturbances that might have occurred during the normal process of occlusal development. Functional disturbances of the masticatory system may have their beginning during the development of occlusion, a period when position of the tongue, swallowing habits, chewing patterns, etc. are established. Thus, it is imperative to understand the development of dental occlusion in order to recognize and intervene in case of any abnormal development and also to treat an already existing malocclusion.

It is also important to note that certain occlusal irregularities, observed during the developing stages of occlusion are transient and thus do not require treatment. For instance, midline diastema and flaring of upper anteriors observed during ugly duckling stage at mixed entition period get self-corrected once the permanent canines erupt fully.

## DEVELOPMENT OF THE DENTITION

Humans have two sets of dentition namely, deciduous and permanent, which contain 20 and 32 teeth respectively. The formation and eruption of these teeth follow a definite pattern and fairly consistent timetable. The chronology of human dentition is given in **Tables 6.1 and 6.2**.

The primitive oral cavity or stomatodeum is lined by stratified squamous epithelium called oral ectoderm. The underlying connective tissue is called the ectomesenchyme, as these cells are formed by migration of the neural crest cells derived from ectoderm to the head region. The primitive oral cavity establishes connection with the foregut at 4th week of gestation when the buccopharyngeal membrane, which is limiting the stomatodeum, ruptures.

The first indication of tooth formation is seen at about 6th week of gestation when oral ectoderm proliferate into the underlying ectomesenchyme to form horseshoe-shaped dental lamina at the future upper and lower dental arches. The primary teeth develop directly from the dental lamina; while the permanent successor teeth develop from a lingual extension of dental lamina called successional lamina. The permanent molars, which do not have deciduous predecessors develop from a distal extension of the dental lamina.

Development of tooth occurs by a series of epithelial-mesenchymal interactions along the dental lamina. The ectoderm in certain areas of dental lamina proliferates into the underlying ectomesenchyme to form an enamel organ. Each enamel organ surrounds a local portion of ectomesenchyme called dental papilla. Condensed ectomesenchyme that limits the dental papilla and surrounds the enamel organ is called dental follicle/sac. The enamel organ forms enamel, dental papilla forms dentin and pulp and dental sac forms the supporting tissues—periodontal ligament and alveolar bone.

The enamel organ, dental papilla and dental sac together constitute a tooth bud or tooth germ. Ten such tooth germs arise in each dental arch to form the primary dentition. Tooth germs for permanent teeth arise from

| Table 6.1: Chronology of deciduous dentition | | | | | |
|---|---|---|---|---|---|
| Tooth | First evidence of calcification | Amount of enamel formed at birth | Crown completed | Eruption | Root completed |
| Primary Dentition | | | | | |
| *Maxillary* | | | | | |
| Central incisor | 4 months *in utero* | Five-sixths | 1½ months | 7½ months | 1½ years |
| Lateral incisor | 4½ months *in utero* | Two-thirds | 2½ months | 9 months | 2 years |
| Cuspid | 5 months *in utero* | One-third | 9 months | 18 months | 3¼ years |
| First molar | 5 months *in utero* | Cusps united | 6 months | 14 months | 2½ years |
| Second molar | 6 months *in utero* | Cusp tips still isolated | 11 months | 24 months | 3 years |
| *Mandibular* | | | | | |
| Central incisor | 4½ months *in utero* | Three-fifths | 2½ months | 6 months | 1½ years |
| Lateral incisor | 4½ months *in utero* | Three-fifths | 3 months | 7 months | 1½ years |
| Cuspid | 5 months *in utero* | One-third | 9 months | 16 months | 3¼ years |
| First molar | 5 months *in utero* | Cusps united | 5½ months | 12 months | 2¼ years |
| Second molar | 6 months *in utero* | Cusp tips still isolated | 10 months | 20 months | 3 years |

| Tooth | First evidence of calcification | Amount of enamel formed at birth | Crown completed | Eruption | Root completed |
|---|---|---|---|---|---|
| **Permanent Dentition** | | | | | |
| **Maxillary** | | | | | |
| Central incisor | 3–4 months | — | 4–5 years | 7–8 years | 10 years |
| Lateral incisor | 10–12 months | — | 4–5 years | 8–9 years | 11 years |
| Cuspid | 4–5 months | — | 6–7 years | 11–12 years | 13–15 years |
| First bicuspid | 1½–1¾ years | — | 5–6 years | 10–11 years | 12–13 years |
| Second bicuspid | 2–2¼ years | — | 6–7 years | 10–12 years | 12–14 years |
| First molar | At birth | Sometimes a trace | 2½–3 years | 6–7 years | 9–10 years |
| Second molar | 2½–3 years | — | 7–8 years | 12–13 years | 14–16 years |
| Third molar | 7–9 years | — | 12–16 years | 17–21 years | 18–25 years |
| **Mandibular** | | | | | |
| Central incisor | 3–4 months | — | 4–5 years | 6–7 years | 9 years |
| Lateral incisor | 3–4 months | — | 4–5 years | 7–8 years | 10 years |
| Cuspid | 4–5 months | — | 6–7 years | 9–10 years | 12–14 years |
| First bicuspid | 1¾–2 years | — | 5–6 years | 10–12 years | 12–13 years |
| Second bicuspid | 2¼–2½ years | — | 6–7 years | 11–12 years | 13–14 years |
| First molar | At birth | Sometimes a trace | 2½–3 years | 6–7 years | 9–10 years |
| Second molar | 2½–3 years | — | 7–8 years | 11–13 years | 14–15 years |
| Third molar | 8–10 years | — | 12–16 years | 17–21 years | 18–25 years |

**Table 6.2:** Chronology of permanent dentition

successional lamina and distal extension. Tooth germs undergo a series of morphological stages to eventually form respective teeth.

## Stages of Tooth Development

### Bud Stage
The enamel organ at first resembles a small bud, which is surrounded by the condensation of ectomesenchymal cells. During bud stage, the enamel organ consists of peripherally located low columnar cells and centrally located polygonal cells **(Fig. 6.1A)**.

### Cap Stage
The enamel organ then proliferates to form a cap over the dental papilla. The dental papilla and dental sac become well defined. The enamel organ differentiates to form three epithelial layers namely **(Fig. 6.1B)**.
   i. Inner dental/inner enamel epithelium
   ii. Stellate reticulum and
   iii. Outer dental/outer enamel epithelium.

### Early Bell Stage
The enamel organ acquires a bell shape due to uneven proliferation of its cells, resulting in deepening of the undersurface of the epithelial cap. Another cell layer forms between the inner dental epithelium and the stellate reticulum called stratum intermedium. Thus, the enamel organ at bell stage exhibits four different types of epithelial cells.

The inner dental epithelium differentiates into tall columnar cells called ameloblasts, which later secrete enamel. The peripheral cells of the dental papilla differentiate into odontoblasts under the organizing influence of inner dental epithelium, which later form dentin **(Fig. 6.1C)**.

### Advanced Bell Stage
First, odontoblasts form a layer of dentin and then the ameloblasts begin to secrete enamel matrix. The deposition of enamel and dentin continues until the crown formation is complete **(Fig. 6.1D)**.

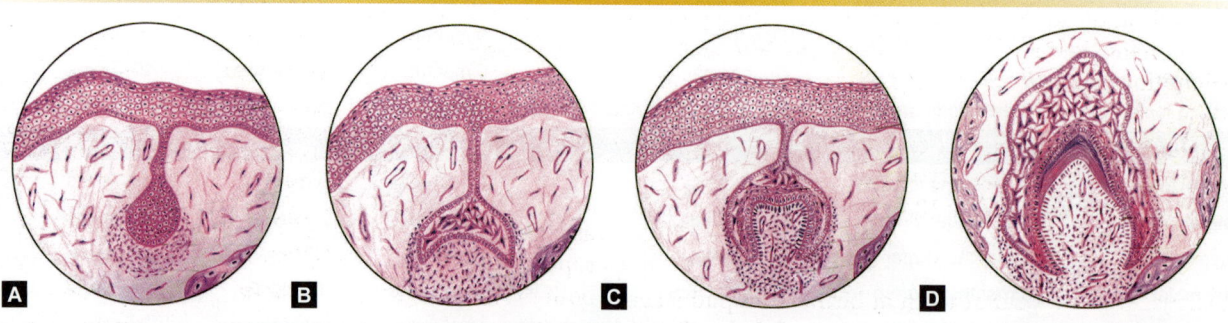

**Figs 6.1A to D:** (A) Bud stage; (B) Cap stage; (C) Early bell stage; (D) Advanced bell stage

### Root Formation

Root formation begins once the dentin and enamel reach the future cementoenamel junction. The cervical portion of the enamel organ gives rise to the Hertwig's epithelial root sheath, which molds the shape of the roots and initiates radicular dentin formation. Eruption of a tooth generally begins when two-thirds of the root is formed. Root formation is usually completed 1-3 years after the eruption of tooth.

Overlapping on these morphologic stages of tooth development are a series of physiological processes that occur in a sequential manner.

These physiological processes are:
- Initiation—dental lamina and bud stage
- Proliferation—bud and cap stage
- Histodifferentiation—early bell stage
- Morphodifferentiation—advanced bell stage
- Apposition—formation of enamel and dentin matrix.

Mineralization begins around 14th week of gestation in primary dentition and occurs first in the central incisors. The permanent tooth germs begin to form around 4th–5th month of intrauterine life and their mineralization commences at birth, beginning in the first molars.

Radiographic studies of tooth formation consider three basic stages:
I. Beginning of calcification
II. Crown completion
III. Root completion

Nolla (1960) described the tooth development in 10 stages **(Fig. 6.2)**.

### Crown

Stage 1: Absence of crypt
Stage 2: Initial calcification
Stage 3: 1/3 of crown completed
Stage 4: 2/3 of crown completed
Stage 5: Crown almost completed
Stage 6: Crown completed.

### Root

Stage 7: 1/3 of root completed
Stage 8: 2/3 of root completed
Stage 9: Root almost completed
Stage 10: Apical end of root completed.

## DEVELOPMENT OF OCCLUSION

Dental occlusion undergoes significant changes from birth until adulthood and beyond. This continuation of changes in the dental relationship during various stages of the dentition can be divided into four stages:
I. Gum pads stage: 0–6 months
II. Deciduous dentition: 6 months–6 years
III. Mixed dentition: 6–12 years
IV. Permanent dentition: 12 years and beyond.

### Gum Pad Stage (0–6 Months)

Usually jaws are devoid of teeth at birth. Gum pad stage extends from birth up to the eruption of first primary

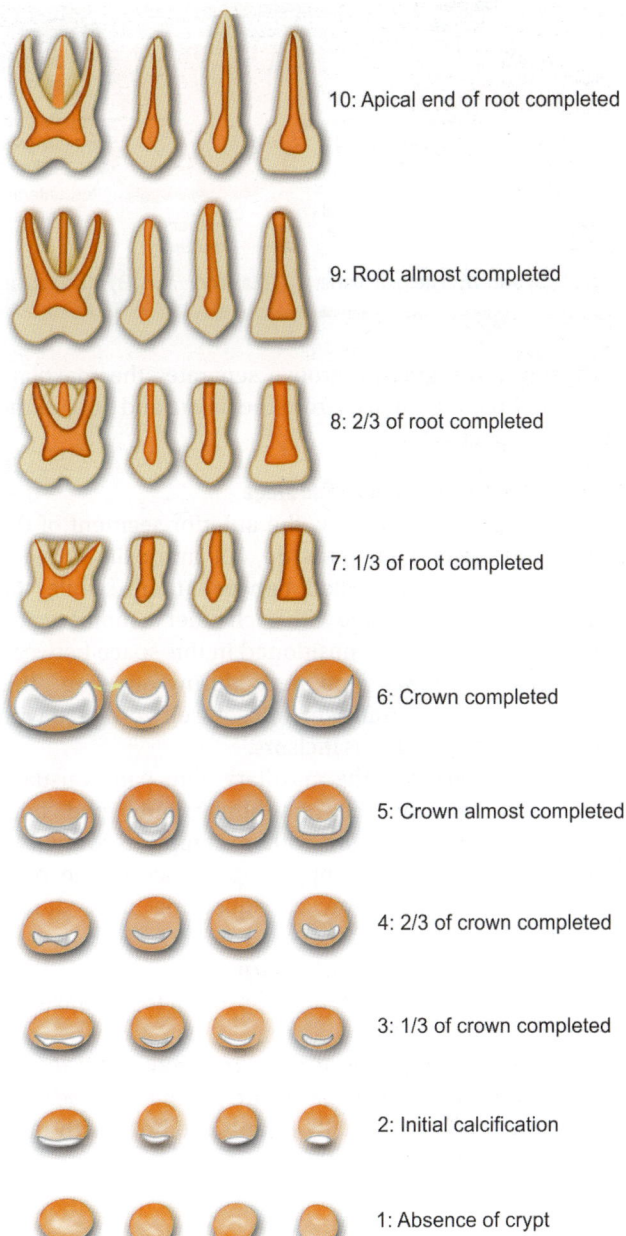

**Fig. 6.2:** Radiographic stages of tooth development by Nolla (1960)

tooth, usually the lower central incisors at around 6 months of age. The gum pads are pink in color and firm in consistency. The maxillary gum pad is horseshoe shaped and the mandibular gum pad is U/square shaped **(Figs 6.3A and B)**.

The gum pads develop in two portions, buccal and lingual, which are separated by the dental groove. The gum pads in both the arches show certain elevations and grooves that outline the portion of various primary teeth, which are still developing in the alveolar ridges. These are called as transverse grooves. The prominent transverse groove separating canine and first deciduous molar segments in both the arches is called the lateral sulcus. The lateral sulci are often used to judge the interarch relationship at a very

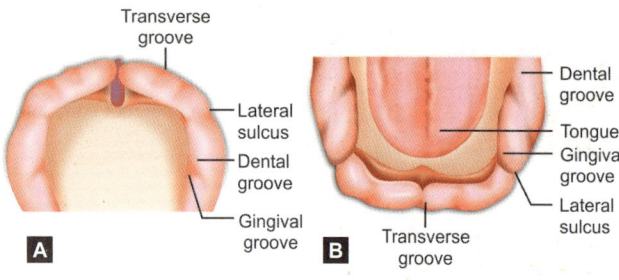

**Figs 6.3A and B:** The gum pads: (A) Maxillary; and (B) Mandibular

early stage. The gingival groove separates the maxillary and mandibular gum pads from the palate and floor of the mouth, respectively.

### Characteristic Features of Gum Pad Stage

***Infantile open bite***: Usually, the anterior segment of the upper and lower gum pads do not approximate each other with a space created between them, while the posterior segment occlude with each other at molar region **(Fig. 6.4)**. The tongue is positioned in this space between the upper and lower gum pads during suckling. This infantile open bite is transient and gets self-corrected with the eruption of deciduous incisors.

***Complete overjet***: The maxillary gum pad is usually larger and overlaps the mandibular gum pad both horizontally and vertically with a complete overjet all around. In this way, the opposing surface of the pads provides an efficient way of squeezing milk during breastfeeding.

***Anteroposterior relationship***: In general, the mandibular lateral sulci are more posterior to the maxillary lateral sulci **(Fig. 6.4)**.

***Precocious eruption of primary teeth—Natal and neonatal teeth***: Usually jaws are devoid of teeth at birth. However, occasionally infants are born with one/two erupted teeth, usually, the mandibular incisors. Such teeth present at birth are called as natal teeth **(Fig. 6.5)**. Teeth that erupt within 30 days of life are called as neonatal teeth. Familial tendency is observed in this condition and such premature eruption of teeth may cause problems during feeding. It is advised to retain them unless they are too mobile.

### Deciduous Dentition Stage (6 Months–6 Years)

The deciduous dentition stage spans from the time of eruption of primary teeth until the eruption of the first permanent tooth around 6 years of age.

### Eruption Chronology

Eruption of the primary teeth begins by 6 months of age when primary mandibular incisors erupt into oral cavity **(Fig. 6.6)**. Eruption of all the primary teeth is usually complete by two and half years by which age the deciduous dentition is in full function. Root formation of primary teeth is usually completed by three years of age.

Although considerable variation is seen in the eruption timing of deciduous teeth, there appears to be no significant gender differences. The chronology of primary teeth is presented in the **Table 6.1**.

The sequence of eruption of primary teeth may also show some variation. However, in most of the cases, the lower central incisors are the first teeth to erupt, followed by the upper central incisors. Usually, the lateral incisor, first molar and canine tend to erupt earlier in the maxilla than in the mandible.

Deciduous dentition generally shows the following order of eruption:

$$\frac{A\ B\ D\ C\ E}{A\ B\ D\ C\ E}$$

1. Central incisors
2. Lateral incisors
3. First molars
4. Canines
5. Second molars

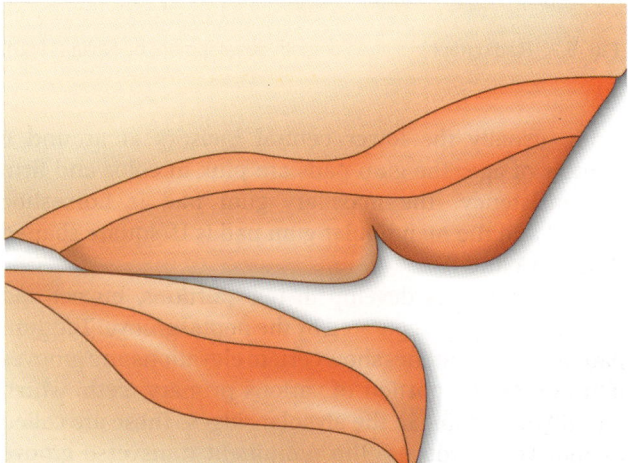

**Fig. 6.4:** Relationship between upper and lower gum pads: infantile open bite seen at birth. Also note that mandibular lateral sulcus is posterior to maxillary lateral sulcus

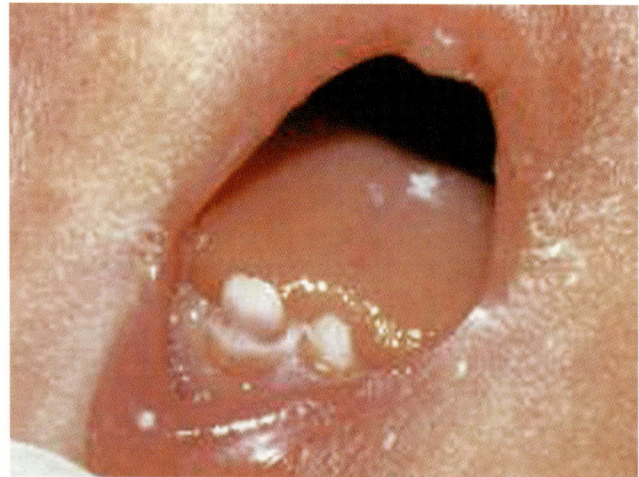

**Fig. 6.5:** Natal teeth: a child who had erupted lower central incisors at birth

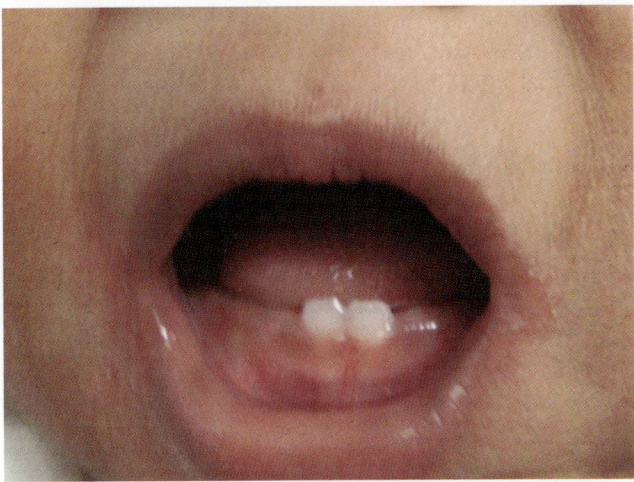

Fig. 6.6: Deciduous dentition stage is usually heralded by eruption of mandibular central incisors

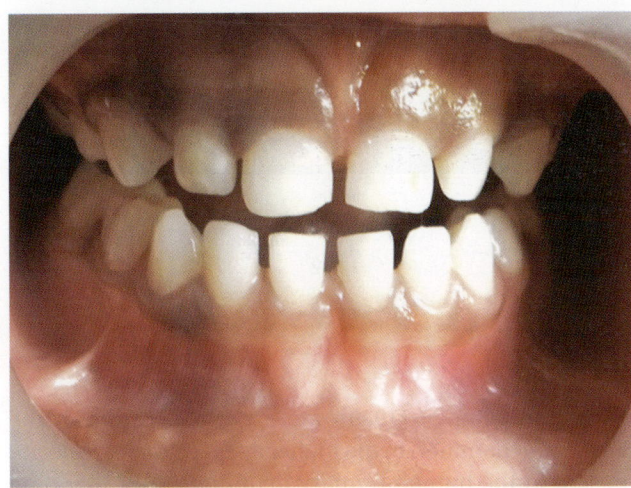

Fig. 6.7: Physiological spacing in primary dentition

By 3 years of age, the occlusion of deciduous dentition is completely established and dental arches remain relatively constant with no significant changes up to 6 years of age.

### Characteristics of Occlusion

#### Interdental Spacing

Interdental spacing, when present in permanent dentition is considered abnormal. However, presence of interdental spacing is an important and normal feature of deciduous dentition, which is required for the accommodation of larger permanent teeth at a later stage.

Spaces present between deciduous teeth are often referred to as physiologic or developmental spaces **(Fig. 6.7)**. Sufficient interdental space is needed for the permanent teeth to erupt into an uncrowded position and for the establishment of their proper alignment. Malocclusion, with crowding of teeth, can be expected in case of unspaced primary dentition **(Fig. 6.8)**. Leighton BC (1969) has given the probability of crowding of permanent dentition based, on the amount of interdental spacing available in the primary dentition **(Table 6.3)**.

Physiologic/developmental spacing in deciduous dentition includes:
- Generalized spacing between teeth
- Primate spaces.

#### Generalized Spacing

According to Foster (1982), generalized spacing occurs in almost 75% of the individuals in the primary dentition stage. Generalized spacing between the teeth are seen in both the dental arches and helps in accommodation of larger successor teeth.

#### Primate Spaces

In addition to the generalized spacing, localized spacing is often present mesial to the upper canine and distal to the lower canine. Such spaces, originally described by

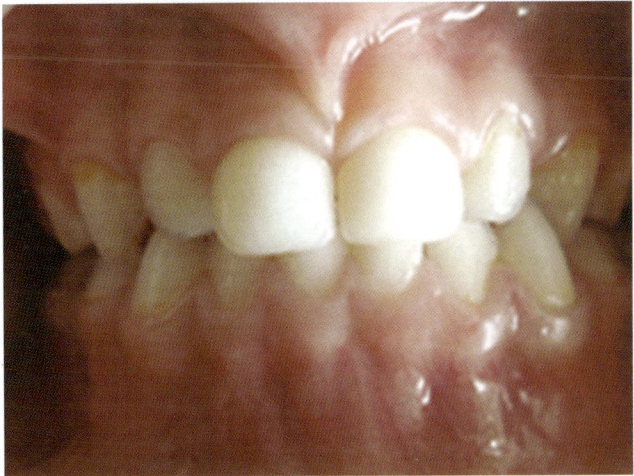

Fig. 6.8: Insufficient physiological spacing in a 5-year-old child. Inadequate interdental spacing in primary dentition often leads to crowding in permanent dentition

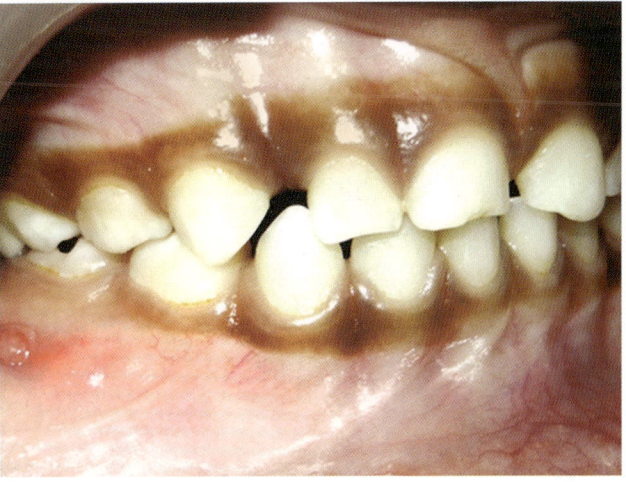

Fig. 6.9: Primate spaces

**Table 6.3:** Probability of crowding of permanent teeth based on available spaces between primary teeth—Leighton BC (1969)

| Space in Primary Teeth | Chances of Crowding of Permanent Teeth |
|---|---|
| >6 mm | None |
| 3–5 mm 1 in 5 | |
| > 3 mm | 1 in 2 |
| No spacing | 2 in 3 |
| Crowded primary teeth | 1 in 1 |

Lewis and Lehman (1929), are a normal feature of the permanent dentition in the higher apes (primates) and are present in the human primary dentition. Thus, these are usually referred to as the **anthropoid spaces**. Anthropoid spaces appear to be a more constant feature of deciduous dentition **(Fig. 6.9)**.

*Significance*: Following eruption of primary first molars, when canine teeth erupt and reach occlusion, the primate spaces facilitate proper interdigitation of the opposing canines into class I canine relationship.

### Incisor Relationship

Incisor relationship in deciduous dentition normally show:
- Increased overbite (deep bite)
- Increased overjet.

### Deep Bite

An increased overbite is usually seen in the initial stages of development with the deciduous mandibular incisors contacting the cingulum area of the deciduous maxillary incisors in centric occlusion **(Fig. 6.10)**. Deep bite may be due to the fact that the primary incisors are more vertically placed than the permanent incisors.

The ideal position of the deciduous incisors has been described as being more vertical than the permanent incisors, with a deeper incisal overbite.

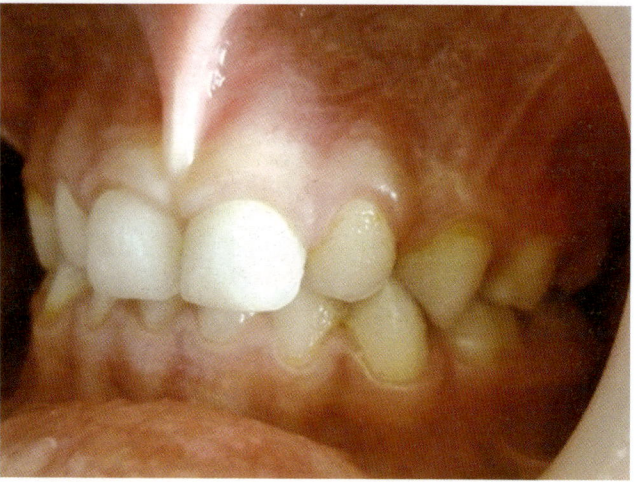

**Fig. 6.10:** Deep bite is a normal feature of deciduous dentition

This deep bite later gets self-corrected by:
- Attrition of incisors
- Eruption of deciduous molars
- Differential growth of the alveolar processes of the jaws.

### Increased Overjet

Excessive incisal overjet is often observed in deciduous dentition. 72% of children exhibited an increased overjet in a study conducted by Foster. Excessive overjet usually gets corrected later by forward growth of the mandible.

### Molar Relationship

The anteroposterior molar relationship in deciduous dentition is described in terms of the terminal planes. Terminal planes are the distal surfaces of the maxillary and mandibular second primary molars.

Moyers described three possible kinds of primary molar relationships **(Figs 6.11A to C)**:
1. Straight/Flush terminal plane
2. Mesial step
3. Distal step.

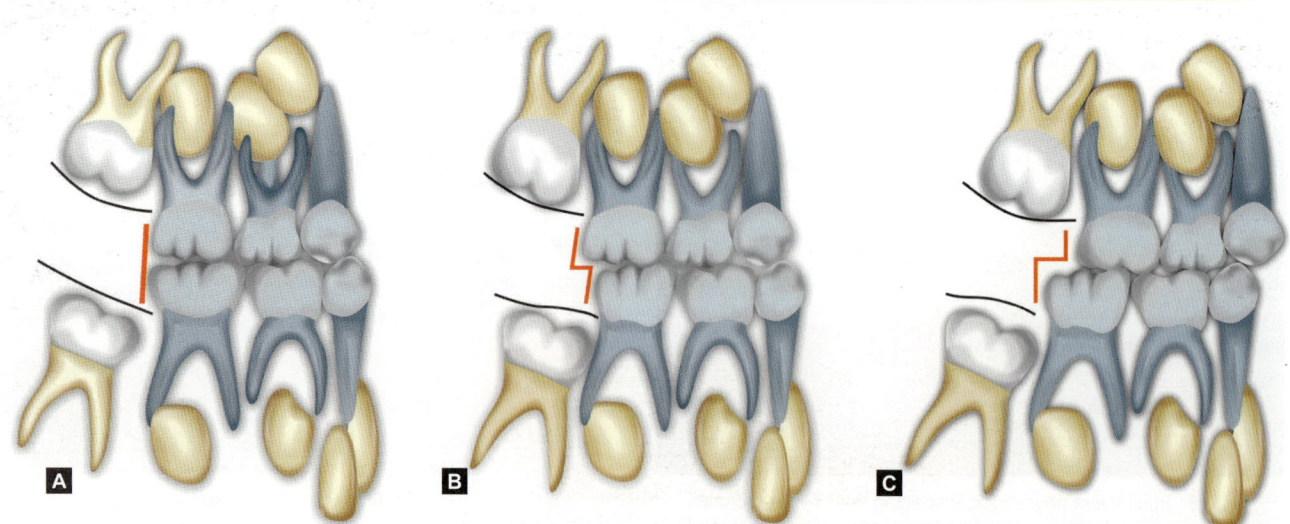

**Figs 6.11A to C:** Terminal plane relationships: (A) Flush/straight terminal plane; (B) Mesial step; (C) Distal step

### Flush Terminal Plane

In straight/flush terminal plane, the distal surfaces of the maxillary and mandibular second deciduous molars are in the same vertical plane **(Fig. 6.11A)**.

It is of significance to note that the mandibular second primary molar has a greater mesiodistal diameter than the maxillary second molar. This difference in the dimensions makes the distal surfaces of both maxillary and mandibular deciduous second molars to fall in same vertical plane in centric occlusion. Such an arrangement is called as "flush terminal plane." Flush terminal plane is considered to be the ideal kind of molar relationship in the primary dentition.

### Mesial Step

In this terminal plane relationship, the distal surface of the mandibular deciduous second molar is more mesial to the distal surface of the maxillary deciduous second molar **(Fig. 6.11B)**.

### Distal Step

Here, the distal surface of the mandibular deciduous second molar is more distal to the distal surface of the maxillary deciduous second molar. In other words, the maxillary second deciduous molar is ahead of the mandibular second deciduous molar **(Fig. 6.11C)**.

> **Significance of Terminal Plane Relationship**
>
> Determining the terminal plane relationship in the primary dentition stage is of great importance because the erupting first permanent molars are guided by the distal surfaces of the second primary molars as they erupt into occlusion. Thus, the terminal plane relationship of primary dentition largely determines the type of molar relationship in the permanent dentition to be achieved later.

### Mixed Dentition Stage (6–12 Years)

Mixed dentition stage is a transition stage when primary teeth are exfoliated in a sequential manner, followed by the eruption of their permanent successors. This stage spans from 6 years to 12 years of age, beginning with the eruption of the first permanent tooth, usually, a mandibular central incisor or a first molar. It is completed at the time, the last primary tooth is shed. Significant changes in occlusion are seen in mixed dentition period due to the loss of 20 primary teeth and eruption of their successor permanent teeth. Most malocclusions are developed at this stage.

Mixed dentition stage can be divided into the following phases:
- Early/1st transitional period
- Intertransitional period
- Late/2nd transitional period.

### Early Transitional Period (6–8 Years)

Early transitional period is concerned with the replacement of the primary incisors by their successors and the addition of four first permanent molars to the dentition. This usually occurs in the age range of 6–8 years.

### Emergence of the First Permanent Molars

The first permanent molars erupt at 6 years of age with mandibular molar preceding the maxillary molars in most cases. The first molars are considered to play an important role in the establishment of occlusion in the permanent dentition and class I molar relationship is considered as the normal anteroposterior molar relationship. The location and relationship of first permanent molars is influenced by the presence of interdental spacing and the terminal plane relationship of the primary dentition.

The erupting first permanent molars are guided by the distal surfaces of the second primary molars as they erupt into occlusion. Thus, the terminal plane relationship of primary dentition largely determines the type of molar relationship in the permanent dentition, among other factors.

The effects of terminal plane relationships are described in **Fig. 6.12**.

### Effects of Flush Terminal Plane

Flush terminal plane usually develops into class I molar relationship in the permanent dentition. Some cases of flush terminal plane may also develop into class II molar relationship if forward mandibular growth is not sufficient.

In the presence of flush terminal plane, the first permanent molars initially assume a **cusp-to-cusp or end-on molar relationship**, as they erupt distal to the second primary molars. The lower first permanent molar has to move 2–3 mm anteriorly in relation to the upper

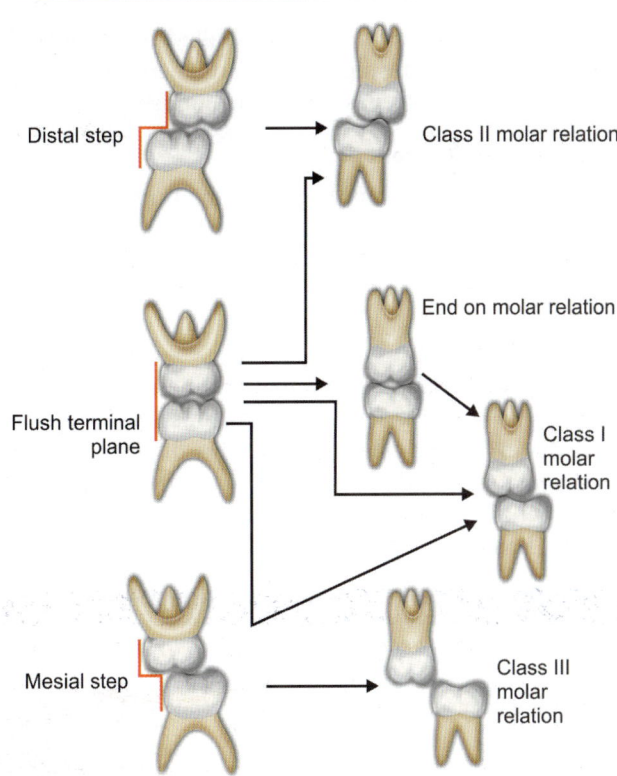

**Fig. 6.12:** The possible effects of terminal plane relationship on permanent dentition

first permanent molar in order to transform the end-on relation to class I molar relation. This transformation from end-on to class I molar relation occurs in two ways:
1. Early mesial shift
2. Late mesial shift

1. **Early mesial shift:** Early mesial shift of lower permanent first molar occurs by utilization of the physiologic spaces present between primary incisors and the primate spaces. The eruptive force of permanent molars push the deciduous molars forward into the spaces, there by establishing class I molar relationship. As this change occurs in early mixed dentition, the shift is called the "early mesial shift" **(Fig. 6.13)**.
2. **Late mesial shift:** In the absence of sufficient developmental spaces in primary dentition, the erupting permanent first molars may not be able to establish class I relationship in early mixed dentition period. In such cases, class I molar relationship can be established following the exfoliation of primary second molars; by utilizing Leeway space (Leeway space is explained later in this chapter). As this occurs in late mixed dentition, it is called as the "late mesial shift" **(Fig. 6.14)**.

### Effects of Mesial Step

When deciduous second molars are in mesial step, the first permanent molars directly erupt into class I molar relationship. Few cases may also progress to class III molar relations, if forward growth of the mandible persists.

### Effects of Distal Step

Distal step in primary dentition usually leads to Angle's class II molar relationships in the permanent dentition. A few cases may go into class I molar relationship.

### Eruption of Permanent Incisors

Permanent incisors erupt lingual to the primary incisors and mandibular central are often the first to erupt. How the larger permanent incisor teeth are accommodated is described below:

### Incisal liability

It can be readily appreciated that the mesiodistal crown dimensions of permanent incisors is considerably greater than that of the primary incisors. This difference in the mesiodistal crown dimension between the primary and permanent incisors is termed as incisal liability by Warren Mayne **(Box 6.1)**.

> **Box 6.1: Incisal liability by Warren Mayne**
> 
> ***According to the average tooth size given by Black:***
> - Incisal liability in maxillary arch is about, 7.6 mm—i.e., the maxillary permanent incisors are larger than their predecessors by 7.6 mm.
> - Incisal liability in mandibular arch is about, 6.0 mm—i.e., mandibular permanent incisors are 6.0 mm larger than their predecessors.

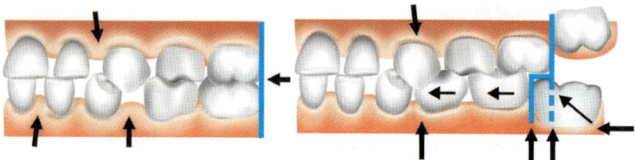

**Fig. 6.13:** Early mesial shift: Erupting lower permanent first molars shifts mesially, utilizing the primate spaces in early mixed dentition period to establish class I molar relationship

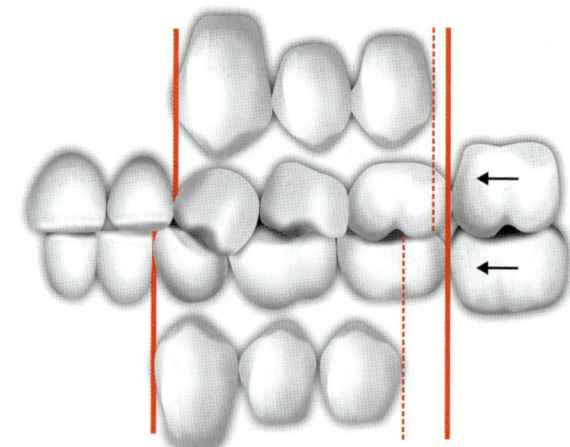

**Fig. 6.14:** Late mesial shift: In case of primate space deficiency, class I molar relationship can be achieved in late mixed dentition period following exfoliation of primary second molars, utilizing the leeway space

Thus, the amount of space available in the arch following exfoliation of the primary incisors is far less than the amount of space needed for accommodation of their permanent successors. Some degree of transient crowding may occur due to incisal liability at about 8–9 years of age and persist until the emergence of canines when the space for teeth may again become adequate.

During the course of mixed dentition period, nature makes some adjustments to achieve the fit and maintain the dynamic balance. The incisal liability is overcome by the following factors:
- *Utilization of interdental spacing between primary anteriors:* Incisal liability is partly compensated by the developmental spaces that exist in the primary dentition. Anterior crowding of permanent dentition may develop in the absence of interdental spacing.
- *Increase in the intercanine arch width:* Continuing growth of the jaws often results in an increase in the intercanine arch width during the mixed dentition period. This may significantly contribute to accommodation of the bigger permanent incisors in the arches.
- *Change in incisor inclination:* As stated previously, the deciduous incisors are more vertically positioned than the permanent incisors. Permanent incisors exhibit a more labial inclination, which tends to increase the dental arch perimeter. The change in the labiolingual

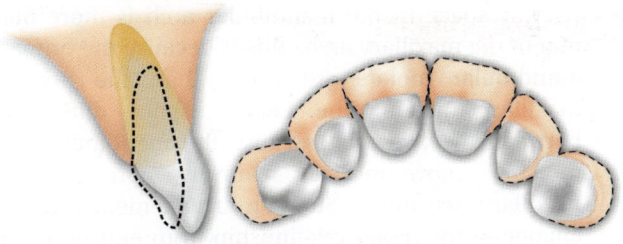

**Fig. 6.15:** Relationship of primary and permanent incisors over basal bone: Deciduous incisors are vertically placed over basal bone while permanent incisors exhibit more labial inclination that tend to increase the dental arch perimeter

inclination of incisors also contributes to overcome the incisal liability by adding 2-3 mm to the arch **(Fig. 6.15)**.

### *Intertransitional Period*

After first permanent molars and incisors establish occlusion, there is an interim period of 1-2 years before the commencement of second transitional period in which little changes in the occlusion is seen. This phase of mixed dentition stage is relatively stable with only minor changes taking place and is referred to as intertransitional period.

### *Second Transitional Period (10–13 Years)*

The second transitional period involves replacement of molars and canines by the premolars and permanent canines respectively and the emergence of second permanent molars. Exfoliation of mandibular primary canine at around 10 years of age usually makes the beginning of second transitional period.

### Eruption of Permanent Canines

Mandibular canines erupt following the eruption of the incisors at around 10 years, while the maxillary canines usually erupts after the eruption of one or both the premolars, at around 12-13 years.

### Ugly Duckling Stage

A transient malocclusion with appearance of midline diastema and flaring of upper incisors is often observed to develop in the maxillary anterior region during 8-12 years of age. This corresponds to the eruption of permanent maxillary canines. Clinicians need to recognize it as a self-correcting malocclusion and the anxious parents and children may have to be reassured. The course of events in the development of ugly duckling stage is as provided in **(Figs 6.16A and B) (Flowchart 6.1)**.

**Broadbent** described this stage of development as the ugly duckling stage as the children appear ugly with crooked teeth during this phase of development. The condition resolves by itself as the continuously erupting canines shift the pressure from roots of lateral incisors to their crowns. By the time canines are fully erupted the midline diastema is closed and laterals are realigned along the arch.

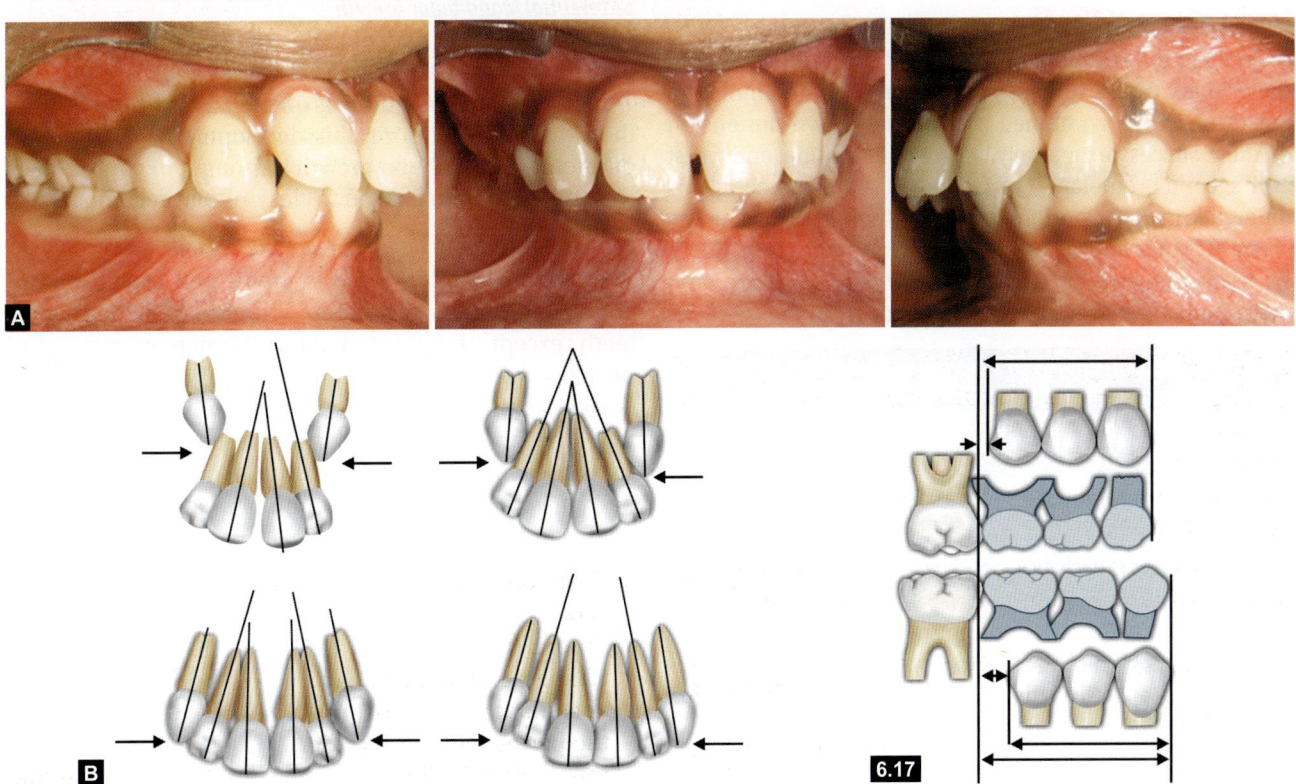

**Figs 6.16A and B:** Ugly duckling stage: clinical and schematic representation. **Fig. 6.17:** Leeway space of Nance

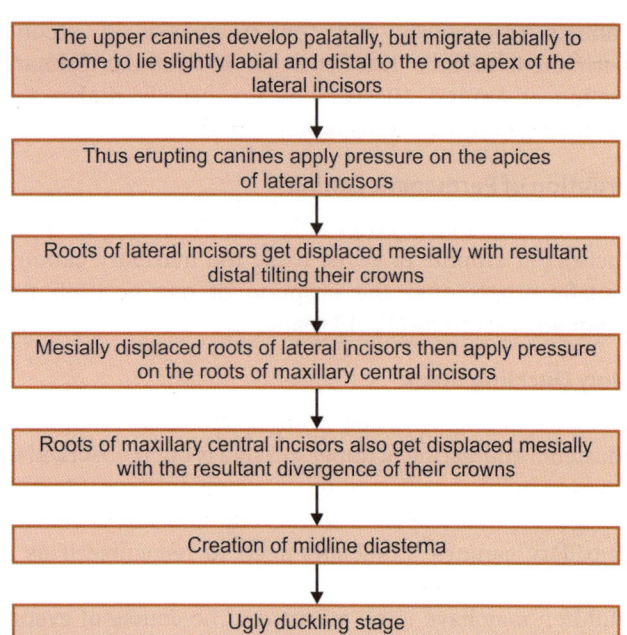

**Flowchart 6.1:** Course of events in the development of ugly duckling stage

### Eruption of the Premolars

The important portion of the dental arch in the development of occlusion is the premolar segment. This is because the erupting premolars are significantly smaller in mesiodistal dimension than the primary molars which they replace. Thus, major changes in occlusion are observed during the premolar emergence.

### Leeway Space of Nance

In general, the combined mesiodistal crown dimension of the primary canine and primary first and second molars is greater than the combined mesiodistal crown dimension of their successors namely permanent canine and first and second premolars. The amount of space gained by this difference in the posterior segments is termed as the Leeway space of Nance and is present in both the arches **(Fig. 6.17)**.

Measurement of Leeway space for maxillary and mandibular arches is given in **Box 6.2**.

**Box 6.2: Measurement of Leeway space for maxillary and mandibular arches**

*In maxilla*
- Leeway space in maxilla in each quadrant is about 0.9 mm.
- The total Leeway space in maxilla is 1.8 mm.

*In mandible*
- Leeway space in each quadrant of the mandible is about 1.7 mm.
- The total Leeway space in the mandible is 3.4 mm.

### Significance of Leeway Space of Nance
- Presence of excessive Leeway space is a favorable feature, which provides for the mesial movement of the permanent molars.
- Leeway space in the mandibular arch is more than that of the maxillary arch. This is because the primary mandibular molars are wider than the primary maxillary molars. The Leeway space differential between the two arches cause the mandibular first molar to move mesially relatively more than the maxillary first molar. Such an arrangement causes a change in the molar relationship from end-on in the early mixed dentition period to class I relation at the late mixed dentition period (late mesial shift).
- Leeway space deficiency may be seen in some individuals when size of unerupted premolars and permanent canine are larger than the space available.

### Eruption of Permanent Second Molars

Emergence of second permanent molars ideally should follow the eruption of the premolars. If the second molars erupt before the premolars erupt fully, a significant shortening of the arch perimeter occurs and malocclusion may be more likely to occur.

### Change in the Anteroposterior Molar Relationship in Mixed Dentition

To begin with, the newly erupted permanent first molars occlude in a cusp-to-cusp relation, especially when deciduous dentition exhibit flush terminal plane. Cusp-to-cusp/end-on molar relationship which is considered normal in early mixed dentition stage, changes into class I molar relationship, which is considered normal in permanent dentition stage by the following factors:
- Leeway space of Nance (Explained above in this chapter)
- Differential mandibular growth.

### Differential Mandibular Growth

During growing period, both the maxilla and the mandible grow downward and forward.

However, the mandible grows relatively more forward than the maxilla during this developmental stage. Such differential mandibular growth is thought to contribute to the transition from end-on to class I molar relationship.

### Permanent Dentition Stage (12 Years and Beyond)

Permanent dentition stage is pretty well established by about 13 years of age with the eruption of all permanent teeth except the third molars. Permanent successors develop from lingual extension of the dental lamina (successional lamina) and the permanent molar develop from the posterior extension of the dental lamina. The permanent incisors develop lingual to the primary incisors and move labially as they erupt. The premolars develop below the divergent roots of the primary molars.

Permanent dentition begins to form at birth, at which time, calcification of the first permanent molars becomes evident. Chronology of permanent dentition is depicted in **Table 6.2**.

Sequence of eruption of permanent dentition is more variable than that of the primary dentition. In addition, there are significant differences in the eruption sequences between the maxillary and the mandibular arch.

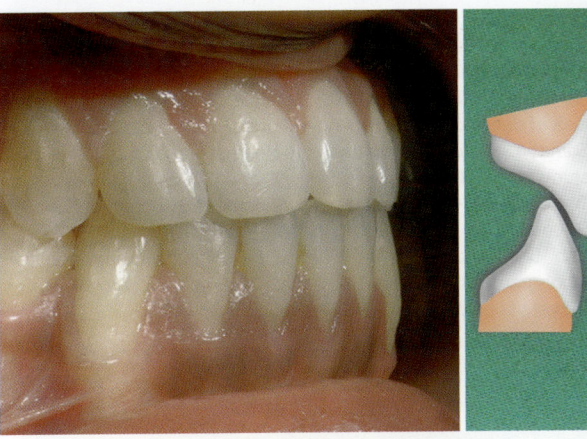

**Figs 6.18A and B:** Normal incisal relationship: (A) overbite; (B) overjet

> **Most Common Eruption Sequence in Maxilla**
> 6-1-2-4-3-5-7-8
> or
> 6-1-2-4-5-3-7-8

> **Most Common Eruption Sequence for Mandibular Arch**
> (6-1)-2-3-4-5-7-8
> or
> (6-1)-2-4-3-5-7-8

These are also the most favorable sequences for the prevention of malocclusion. It must be noted that there is a difference in eruption timing of the canines in the two arches. In the mandibular arch, the canines erupt before the premolars, whereas in the maxillary arch, the canines generally erupt after the eruption of premolars.

When second molars erupt before the premolars are fully erupted, significant shortening of the arch perimeter occurs due to mesial migration of permanent molars increasing the likelihood of malocclusion.

### Characteristics of Occlusion in Permanent Dentition

Dental occlusion is explained in detail in Chapter 7; some of the characteristics of the normal occlusion in the permanent dentition stage are listed below:

#### Overlap
The maxillary teeth overlap the mandibular teeth, both in labial and buccal segments in centric occlusion **(Fig. 6.18A and B)**.

#### Intra-arch Tooth Contacts
With the exception of the maxillary third molars and mandibular central incisors, each permanent tooth occludes with two teeth from the opposite arch. In other words, each permanent tooth has two antagonistic teeth.

#### Angulations
Permanent teeth have buccolingual and mesiodistal angulations, whereas the primary teeth are generally vertically positioned in the alveolar bone.

#### Arch Curvatures
The anteroposterior curvature exhibited by the mandibular arch is called the curve of Spee. The corresponding curve in the maxillary arch is called the compensating curve. The buccolingual curvature from one side of the arch to the others is called the curve of Monson/Curve of Wilson.

#### Incisor Relationship
The vertical overlap between maxillary and mandibular incisors is called **overbite** and is about 1–2 mm and the horizontal overlap called the **overjet** is generally between 1–3 mm **(Figs 6.18A and B)**.

#### Molar Relationship
In permanent dentition stage, the class I molar relationship is the ideal relationship. In class I molar relationship, the mesiobuccal cusp of the maxillary first molar is in the buccal groove of the mandibular first molar **(Figs 6.19A and B)**.

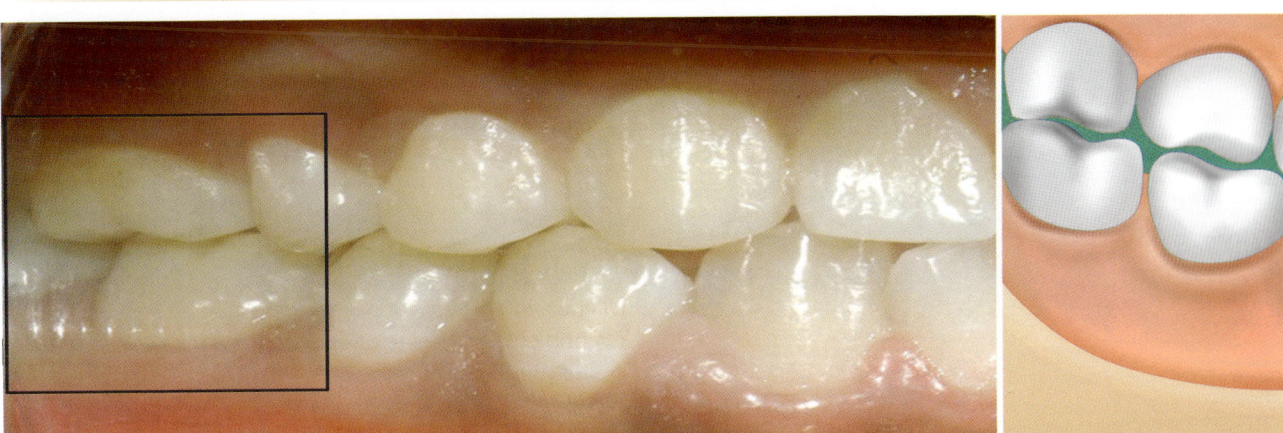

**Figs 6.19A and B:** Normal molar relationship

## BIBLIOGRAPHY

1. Angle EH. Treatment of Malocclusion of the Teeth (7th edn), Philadelphia, SS White Dental Manufacturing, 1907.
2. Bishara SE, et al. Arch width changes from 6 weeks to 45 years of age. AM J Orthod Dentofacial Orthop. 1997;111:401-9.
3. Foster TD. A Textbook of Orthodontics (2 edn), St Louis, Blackwell Scientific Publications, 1982.
4. Friel S. The development of ideal occlusion of the gum pads and teeth. Am J Orthod. 1954;40:1963.
5. Knott VB. Longitudinal study of dental arch width at four stages of dentition. Angle Orthod. 1972;42:387-94.
6. Moorrees CF, Chadha JM. Available space for the incisors during dental development. Angle Orthod. 1965;35:12-22.
7. Moorrees CF. The dentition of the growing child. A longitudinal study of dental development between 3 and 18 years of age. Cambridge, Mass: Harvard University Press, 1959.
8. Northway WM, Wainright RL, Demirjian A. Effects of premature loss of deciduous molars. Angle Orthod. 1984;54:295-329.
9. Silmann JH. Dimensional changes of the dental arches. longitudinal study from birth to 25 years. Am J Orthod. 1964;50:824-42.
10. Ten Cate AR. Oral Histology: Development Structure & Function. St Louis: CV Mosby, 1980.
11. Van Der Linden FPGM. Transition of the human dentition, Monograph no 13. Ann Arbor, Mich, Craniofacial Growth Series, University of Michigan, 1982.

## EXAM-ORIENTED QUESTIONS

### Long Essay or Long Questions

1. Discuss the development of occlusion and its significance.
2. Define normal occlusion. Describe normal occlusion in deciduous dentition and its further development till the age of 12 years.

### Short Notes

1. Gum pads
2. Flush terminal plane
3. Leeway space of nance
4. Incisors liability
5. Anthropoid space
6. Ugly duckling stage
7. Curve of spee
8. Enumerate the stages of tooth development.

# CHAPTER 7

# Occlusion—Basic Concepts

*Phulari BS*

The term occlusion has both static and dynamic aspects. Static refers to the form, alignment and articulation of teeth within and between dental arches and the relationship of teeth to their supporting structures. Dynamic refers to the function of the stomatognathic system as a whole comprising teeth, supporting structures, temporomandibular joint, and neuromuscular and nutritive systems. The term normal and malocclusion as used in orthodontics refers mainly to the static aspect or the form of the dentition.

Several concepts of an "ideal" or optimal occlusion of the natural dentition have been suggested by Angle, Schnyler, Beyron, D'Amico, Friel, Hellman, Lucia, Stallard and Stuart, and Ramfjord and Ash.

## COMMONLY USED TERMS

### Ideal Occlusion

It is a preconceived theoretical concept of occlusal structural and functional relationships that include idealized principles and characteristics that an occlusion should be. Ideal occlusion is almost never found in natural dentition. However, normal occlusion can be present.

### Normal Occlusion

Normal occlusion is a class I relationship of the maxillary and mandibular first molars in centric occlusion. Normal occlusion is an absence of large or many facets, bone loss, closed vertical dimension, bruxing habit, freedom from joint pain, and crooked and loose teeth.

### Physiological Occlusion

Physiological occlusion refers to an occlusion that deviates in one or more ways from ideal yet it is well adapted to that particular environment, is esthetic and shows no pathologic manifestations or dysfunctions.

### Functional Occlusion

Functional occlusion is defined as an arrangement of teeth, which will provide the highest efficiency during the excursive movements of the mandible, which is necessary during function.

### Balanced Occlusion

An occlusion in which balanced and equal contacts are maintained throughout the entire arch during all excursions of the mandible.

### Unilateral Balanced Occlusion

It is an occlusal relationship in which all posterior teeth on a side contact evenly as the jaw is moved towards that side.

### Bilateral Balanced Occlusion

It is an occlusal relationship in which all of the posterior teeth contact on the working side and one or more teeth contact simultaneously on the balancing side.

### Centric Occlusion

It is the maximum intercuspation or contact attained between maxillary and mandibular posterior teeth.

### Centric Relation

Centric relation is the most posterior position of the mandible relative to the maxilla at a given vertical dimension.

### Centric Relation Occlusion

Centric relation occlusion (when centric relation and centric occlusion coincide) is the simultaneous even contact between maxillary and mandibular teeth into maximum interdigitation with the mandible in centric relation (most retruded position).

### Vertical Relation of Occlusion

Vertical relation (or vertical dimension) of occlusion is the amount or separation between mandible and maxilla when teeth are in natural maximum contact (centric occlusion).

### Canine Protected Occlusion

It is an occlusal relationship in which the vertical overlap of the maxillary and mandibular canine produces a disocclusion of all the posterior teeth when the mandible moves to either side.

### Therapeutic Occlusion

It is an occlusion that has been modified by appropriate therapeutic modalities in order to change a nonphysiological occlusion to one that is at least physiologic, if not ideal.

### Traumatic Occlusion

Traumatic occlusion is an abnormal occlusal stress, which is capable of producing or has produced an injury to the periodontium.

## Trauma from Occlusion

It is defined as periodontal tissue injury caused by occlusal forces through abnormal occlusal contacts.

## Deflective Malocclusion

The mandible is deflected forward and to the left in any contact of opposing teeth, which guide or direct the mandible away from centric relation, either forward or to one side or both, as the teeth slide together into centric occlusion.

## TYPES OF CUSPS

The human dentitions present two types of cusps and are as follows:

### Centric Holding Cusp/Stamp Cusp/Supporting Cusp

The palatal cusps of the maxillary posterior teeth and the buccal cusps of the mandibular posterior teeth are referred to as supporting cusps. Supporting cusps are also called as centric holding cusps or stamp cusps and they occlude into the central fossa and marginal ridges of opposing teeth (**Fig. 7.1A and B**).

### Guiding Cusp/Shear Cusp/Non-supporting Cusp

The buccal cusps of the maxillary posterior teeth and the lingual cusps of the mandibular posterior teeth are called Non-supporting cusps. These are also called as guiding or shear cusps and they guide the mandible during lateral excursions and the shear food during mastication (**Figs 7.2A and B**).

## CENTRIC OCCLUSAL CONTACTS

One scheme of occlusal contacts, presented by Hellman included 138 points of possible occlusal contacts for 32 teeth (**Figs 7.3A and B**). Concepts of ideal occlusion are used primarily in orthodontics and even in restorative dentistry. Centric occlusal contacts are classified into anterior centric occlusal contacts and posterior centric occlusal contacts points.

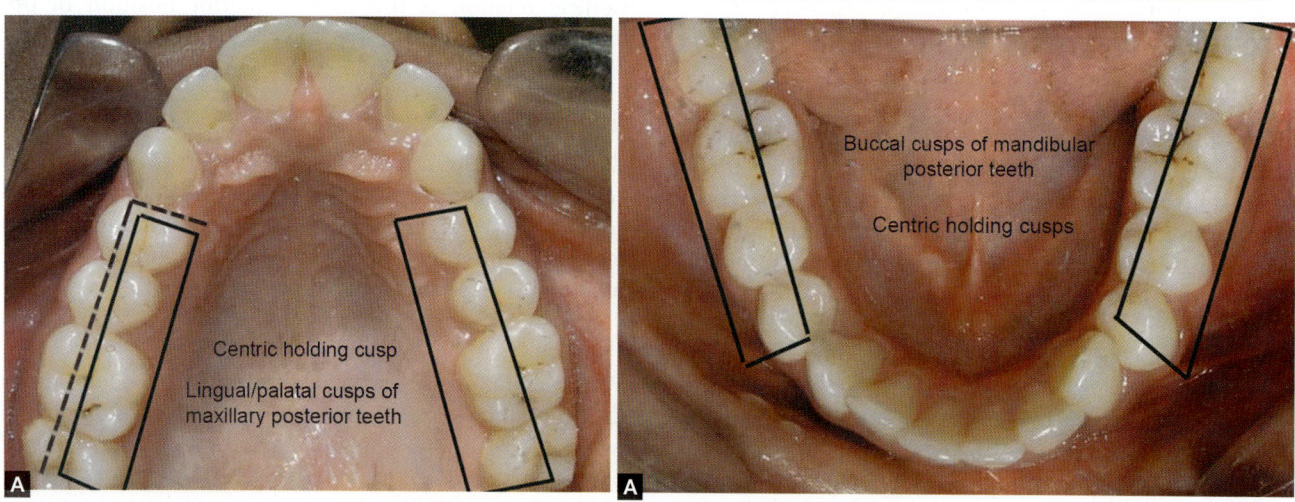

**Figs 7.1A and B:** Supporting cusp/centric holding cusp/stamp cusp

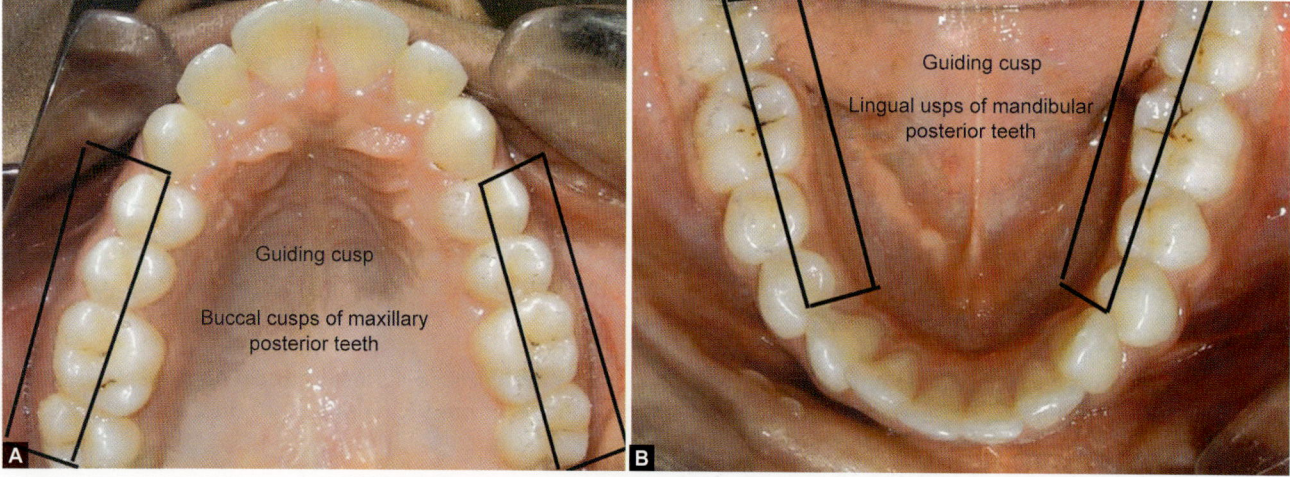

**Figs 7.2A and B:** Non-supporting cusp/guiding cusp/shear cusp

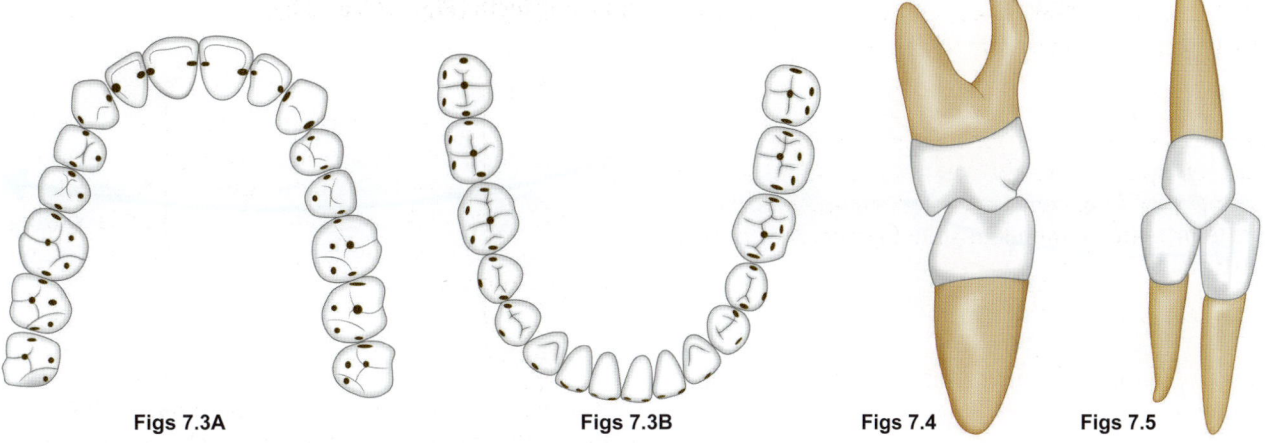

**Figs 7.3A and B:** Occlusal contacts: (A) Maxillary arch and (B) Mandibular arch; **Fig. 7.4:** Cusp-Fossa occlusion (Tooth-to-tooth); **Fig. 7.5:** Cusp-embrasure occlusion (Tooth-to-teeth)

### Anterior Centric Occlusal Contacts

Anterior centric occlusal contacts consist of the labial and lingual range of contacts of maxillary and mandibular anteriors and are in line with the buccal range of posterior centric contacts.

Anterior centric occlusal contacts are listed below:
- Palatal surfaces of maxillary incisors and canines—6
- Labial surfaces of mandibular incisors and canines—6.

### Posterior Centric Occlusal Contacts

Posterior centric occlusal contacts consist of the buccal range of contacts and the lingual range of contacts of maxillary and mandibular posteriors.

*Posterior centric occlusal contacts are listed below:*
- Triangular ridges of lingual cusps of mandibular premolars and molars—16
- Triangular ridges of buccal cusps of premolars and molars—16
- Buccal embrasure of mandibular premolar and molars—8
- Lingual embrasure of maxillary premolars and molars (including the canine and first premolar embrasure accommodating the mandibular premolar)—10
- Lingual cusp points of maxillary premolars and molars—16
- Buccal cusp points of mandibular premolars and molars—16
- Distal fossae of premolars—8
- Central fossae of the molars—12
- Mesial fossae of the mandibular molars—6
- Distal fossae of the maxillary molars—6
- Lingual grooves of the maxillary molars—6
- Buccal grooves of the mandibular molars—6.

### Cusp-Fossa Occlusion

The supporting cusp of one tooth occludes in a single fossa of a single opposing tooth are referred to as cusp-fossa occlusion or tooth-to-tooth arrangement **(Fig. 7.4)**.

### Cusp-Embrasure Occlusion

When a tooth occludes with two opposing teeth, it is called cusp-embrasure occlusion or tooth to two teeth occlusion **(Fig. 7.5)**.

## TOOTH GUIDANCE

Concepts of occlusion often describe idealized contact relations in lateral movements. However, in the natural dentition, a variety of contact relations may be found, including group function, cuspid disocclusion only or some combination of canine, premolar and molar contacts in lateral movements.

### Group Functions

Multiple contacts in lateral or eccentric mandibular movements are referred to as group functions.

### Cuspid guidance/canine guidance

When only upper and lower canine teeth are in contact during lateral mandibular movements, then it is refereed as canine guidance or cuspid guidance.

### Incisal Guidance

Incisal guidance refers to the contact of the anterior teeth during protrusive movements of the mandible.

### Condylar Guidance

Condylar guidance refers to the downward movement of both the condyles along with the slopes of the articular eminence during protrusive movements leading to separation of the posteriors.

## IMAGINARY OCCLUSAL PLANES AND CURVES

### Curve of Spee (Anteroposterior Curve/the Curve of Occlusal Plane)

When viewed from the buccal aspect, the cusp tips of posterior teeth follow a gradual curve anteroposteriorly

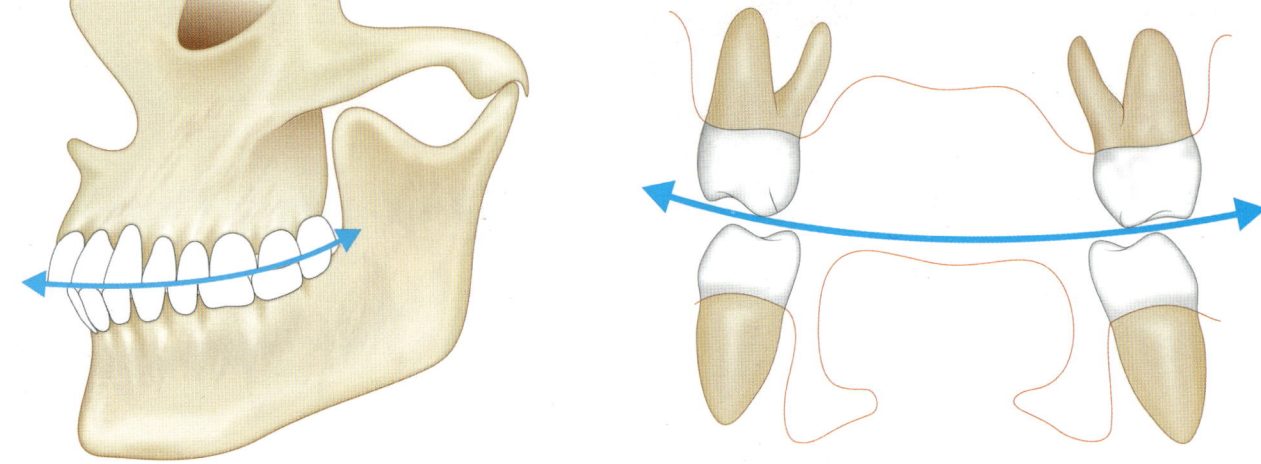

Fig. 7.6: Curve of Spee

Fig. 7.7: Curve of Wilson

(**Fig. 7.6**). The curve of the maxillary arch is convex; that of the mandibular arch.

### Curve of Wilson (Side-to-Side Curve)

When viewed from anterior aspect with the mouth slightly open, the cusp tips of the posterior teeth follow a gradual curve from the left side to the right side (**Fig. 7.7**). The curve of the maxillary arch is convex that of the mandibular arch is concave. Thus, the lingual cusps of the posterior teeth are aligned at a lower level than the buccal cusps on both sides and in both arches.

### Crest of Curvature

The crest of curvature is the highest point of a curve or greatest convexity or bulge. The crest on the facial and lingual surfaces of the crown is where this greatest bulge would be touched by a tangent line drawn parallel to the root axis (**Figs 7.8A and B**). The location of the crest of the curvature on the facial and lingual surfaces of the crowns of teeth can be seen from the mesial and distal aspects and are usually in one of the two places:

1. In the cervical third of the crown on:
   - Facial surfaces of all anterior and posterior teeth (maxillary and mandibular).
   - Lingual surfaces of all anterior teeth (maxillary and mandibular) on the cingulum.
2. In the middle-third of the crown on:
   - Lingual surface of maxillary and mandibular posterior teeth.
   - Lingual surface of all mandibular posterior teeth.

## IDEAL TOOTH RELATIONSHIPS BETWEEN ARCHES

Ideal tooth relationships were described and classified in the early 1900s by Edward H Angle. He classified ideal occlusion as class I and defined it based on the relationship between the maxillary and mandibular dental arches. When closed together, the teeth are in centric occlusion and the following relationships are seen:

### Relationship of Anterior Teeth

The maxillary anterior teeth overlap the mandibular teeth:

#### Horizontal Overlap

The incisal edges of maxillary anterior teeth are labial to the incisal edges of the mandibular teeth (**Fig. 7.9A**).

#### Vertical Overlap

The incisal edges of the maxillary anterior teeth extend below the incisal edges of the mandibular teeth (**Fig. 7.9B**).

### Relationship of Posterior Teeth

The maxillary posterior teeth are slightly buccal to the mandibular posterior teeth so that:

- The buccal cusps and buccal surfaces of the maxillary teeth are buccal to those in the mandibular arch (**Figs 7.10A to C**).

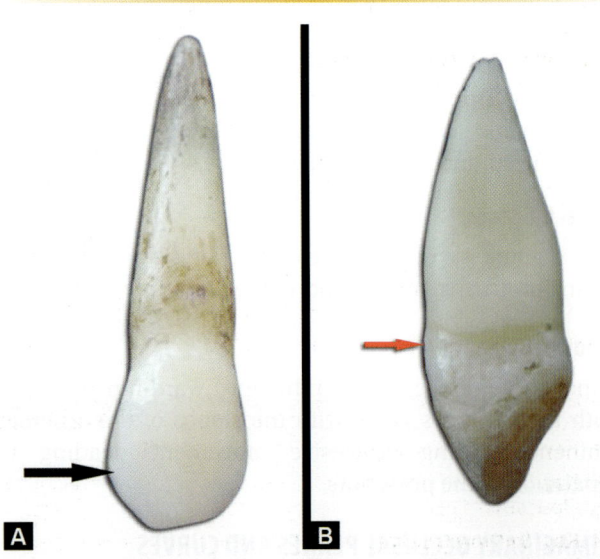

**Figs 7.8A and B:** (A) Labial surface of the maxillary right canine pictured in. The root axis is determined by bisecting the root at the cervix; (B) Mesial aspect of a right permanent maxillary canine. Crest of curvature is at cervical third on both labial and lingual surfaces of the crown of anteriors

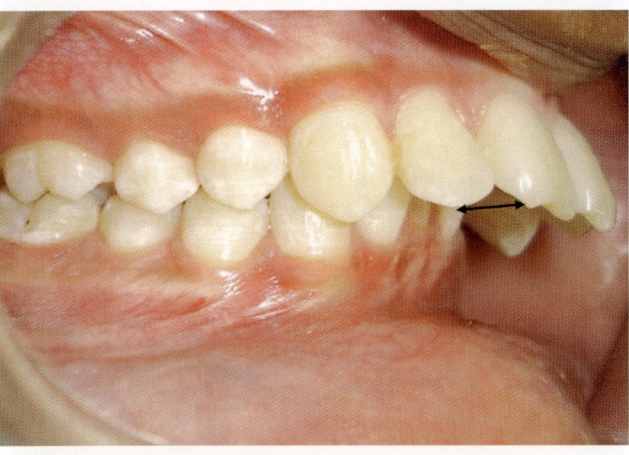

**Fig. 7.9A:** Horizontal overlap: The incisal edges of maxillary anterior teeth are labial to the incisal edges of the mandibular teeth

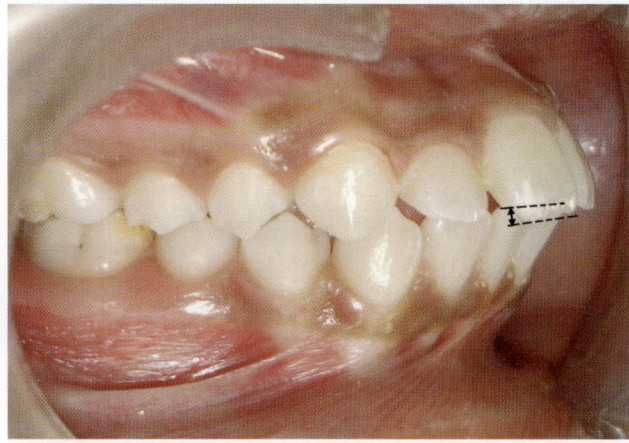

**Fig. 7.9B:** Vertical overlap: The incisal edges of the maxillary anterior teeth extend below the incisal edges of the mandibular teeth

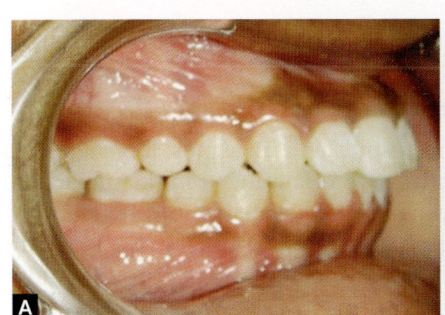
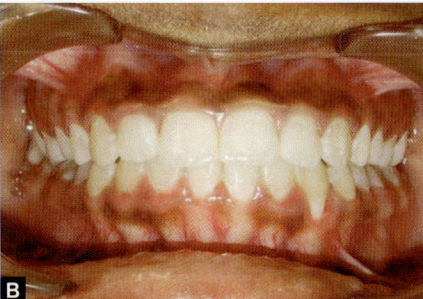
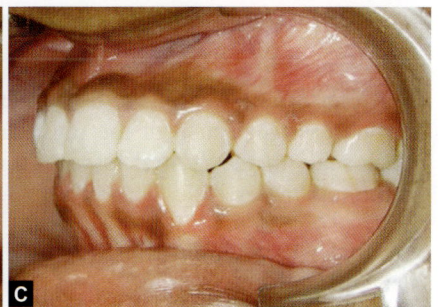

**Figs 7.10A to C:** Relationship of posterior teeth; buccal surface of buccal cusps of maxillary posterior teeth are buccal to those in the mandibular arch

- The palatal cusps of maxillary teeth rest in occlusal fossae of the mandibular teeth.
- The buccal cusps of the mandibular teeth rest in the occlusal fossae of the maxillary teeth.
- The lingual cusps and lingual surfaces of the mandibular teeth are lingual to those in the maxillary arch.

### Relative Alignment

The vertical (long) axis of each maxillary tooth is slightly distal to the vertical axis of the corresponding mandibular tooth so that:

- The tip of the mesiobuccal cusp of the maxillary first molar is aligned directly over the mesiobuccal groove on the mandibular first molar **(Figs 7.11 A and B)**. This relationship of first molar is a key factor in the definition of class I occlusion.
- The distal surface of the maxillary first molar is posterior to the distal surface of the mandibular first molar.

### Opposing Teeth

Each tooth in a dental arch occludes with two teeth in the opposing arch except the mandibular central incisors and the maxillary last molar.

### Andrew's Six Keys of Occlusion

Normal occlusion can be best defined as the contact of the upper and lower teeth in the centric relationship. But the concept of "normal occlusion" is still not clear. Different authors defined normal occlusion but no single definition could be found as yet. The concepts, which are described here are based on Lawrence F Andrew's works on 120 non-orthodontic models based upon which he gave six keys to normal occlusion and developed the "straight wire appliance."

#### Key 1—Molar Relationship (Interarch Relationship)

- The mesiobuccal cusp of the maxillary first permanent molar falls within the groove between the mesial and middle cusps of the mandibular first permanent molar **(Figs 7.12)**.
- The distal surface of the distal marginal ridge of the maxillary first permanent molar contacts and occludes with the mesial surface of the mesial marginal ridge of the mandibular second permanent molar **(Box 7.1)**.

| Box 7.1: Andrew's six keys of occlusion |
|---|
| **Key 1**: Molar Relationship (Interarch Relationship) |
| **Key 2**: Crown Angulations (Mesiodistal Crown Angula-tions/ Mesiodistal Tip) |
| **Key 3**: Crown Inclination (Labiolingual Crown Inclination, the Labiolingual or Buccolingual Torque) |
| **Key 4**: Absence of Rotations |
| **Key 5**: Presence of Tight Contacts |
| **Key 6**: Flat Occlusal Plane |

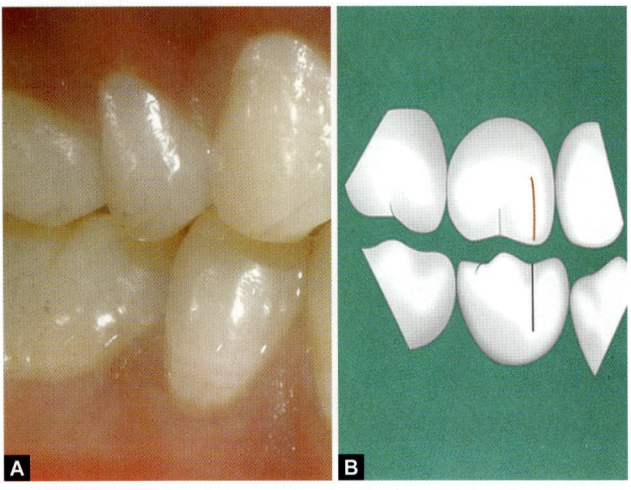

**Figs 7.11 A and B:** Class I occlusion: Mesiobuccal cusp of maxillary first permanent molar occludes in the mesiobuccal developmental groove of mandibular first permanent molar

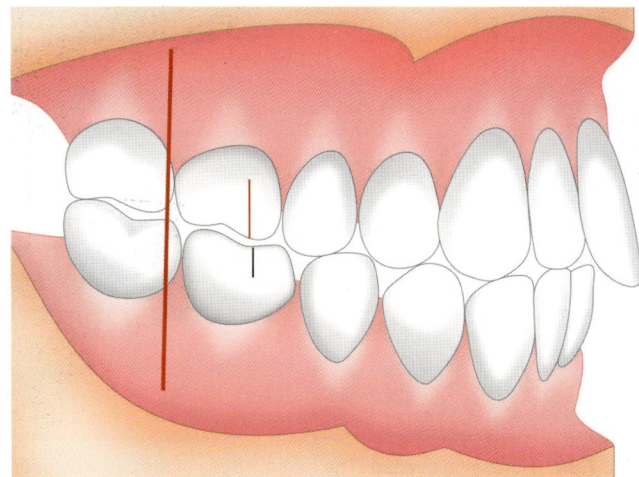

**Fig. 7.12:** Key 1—Molar relationship

### Key 1: Molar Relationship (Interarch Relationship)

The mesiolingual cusp of the maxillary first permanent molar seats in the central fossa of the mandibular first permanent molar.

### Key 2—Crown Angulations (Mesiodistal Crown Angulations/Mesiodistal Tip)

In the normal occluded teeth, the gingival portion of the long axis of each crown is distal to the occlusion portion of that axis **(Fig. 7.13)**. The degree of the angulation varies with each tooth type.

### Key 3—Crown Inclination (Labiolingual Crown Inclination, the Labiolingual or Buccolingual "Torque").

The angle between a line is 90° to the occlusal plane, as well as a line tangent to the middle of the labial or the buccal surface of clinical crown, which is referred to as crown inclination **(Fig. 7.14)**.

### Anterior Crown of Central and Lateral Incisors

In the maxillary and mandibular incisors, the incisal portion of the labial surface of the crown of the anterior teeth is labial to the gingival portion. In all the other crowns, the occlusal portion of the labial or buccal surface is lingual to the gingival portion. The average crown angle is 134° in the nonorthodontic normal models.

### Maxillary Posterior Crowns

As compared to the cuspids and bicuspids, lingual crown inclination is slightly more pronounced in the molars. In the maxillary arch, lingual/palatal inclination progressively increases from cuspids/canines to molars that is to say that the occlusal table of individual posterior teeth tilts progressively towards the palate as we move posteriorly.

### Mandibular Posterior Crowns

There is a progressive increase in the lingual inclination. In the mandibular arch, lingual inclination progressively increases from cuspids/canines to molars that is to say the occlusal table of individual posterior teeth tilts progressively towards the tongue as we move posteriorly.

### Key 4—Absence of Rotations

In order to achieve correct occlusion, none of the teeth should be rotated, rotated molars and premolars occupy more space in the dental arch than normal. Rotated incisors may occupy less space than those correctly

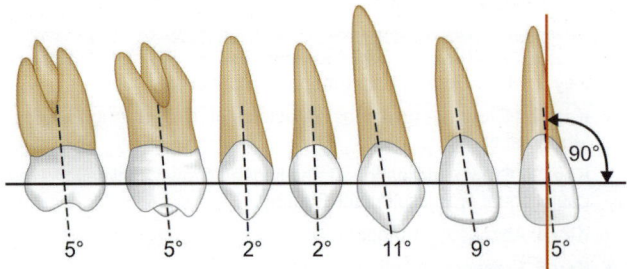

**Fig. 7.13:** Key 2—Crown angulations

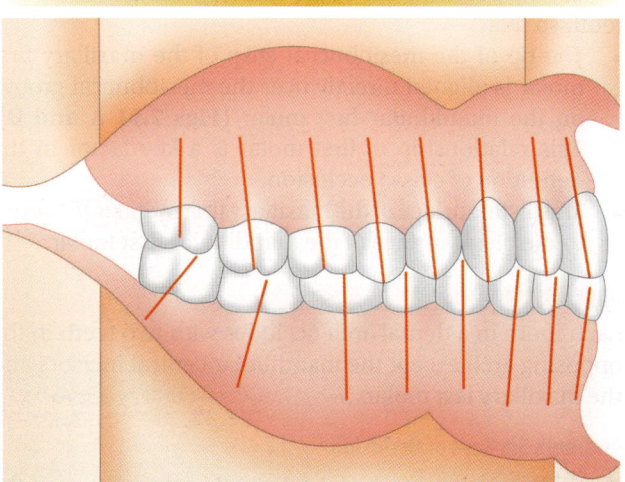

**Fig. 7.14:** Key 3—Crown inclination of teeth

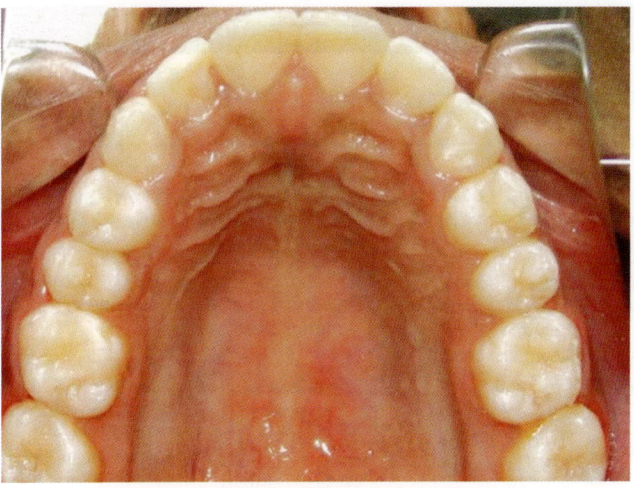
Fig. 7.15: Key 4—Absence of rotation

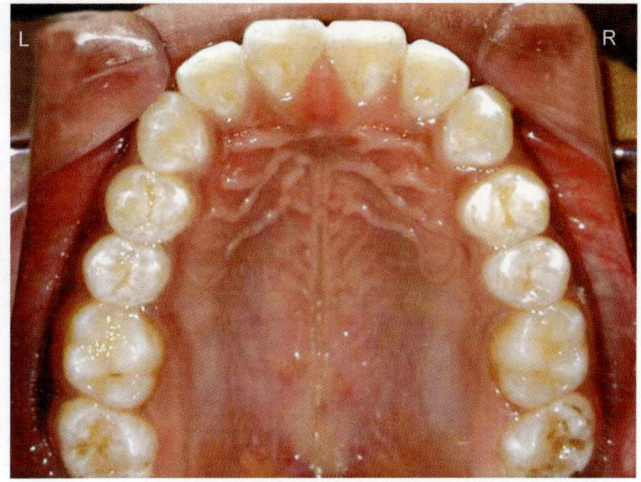
Fig. 7.16: Key 5—Presence of tight contacts

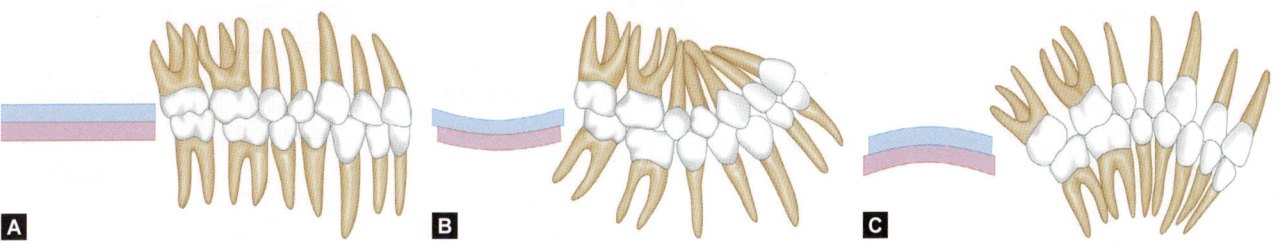
Figs 7.17A to C: **(A)** The curve of Spee, **(B)** An excessive curve of Spee **(C)** A reverse curve of Spee

aligned. Rotated canines adversely affect esthetics and may lead to occlusal interference. There should be absence of rotation in both of the dental arches to be called as normal occlusion (**Fig. 7.15**).

### Key 5—Presence of Tight Contacts
There should be tight contacts and absence of any spacing (**Fig. 7.16**). Tight contacts are an essential part to maintain the integrity of any arch form, especially the dental arches.

### Key 6—Flat Occlusal Plane
- The curve of Spee should be relatively slight or flat. The vertical distance between any tooth and a line joining the most prominent cusp tip of the mandibular molar and central incisor (curve of Spee) should not exceed 1.5 mm (**Fig. 7.17A**).
- An excessive curve of Spee restricts the amount of space available for the upper teeth, which must then move toward the mesial and distal, thus, preventing correct intercuspation (**Fig. 7.17B**).
- A reverse curve of Spee creates excessive space in the upper jaw, which prevents displacement of a normal occlusion (**Fig. 7.17C**).
- A normal occlusion has a flat occlusal plane (according to Andrew, the mandibular curve of Spee should not be deeper than 1.5 mm).

## BIBLIOGRAPHY

1. Andrews LF. The six keys to normal occlusion. Am J Orthod 1972;63:296-302.
2. Angle EH. Classification of malocclusion. Dent Cosmos 1899;41:248-64.
3. Friel S. The development of ideal occlusion of the gum pads and teeth. Am J Orthod 1954;40:1963.
4. Ramford SP, Ash MM. Occlusion. Philadelphia: WB Saunders Company. 8th Edn, 2003.

### EXAM-ORIENTED QUESTIONS

#### Short Essay or Long Notes
1. Occlusion and its basic concepts
2. What are the forces of occlusion
3. Describe six keys to normal occlusion
4. Imaginary occlusal planes and curves.

#### Short Notes
1. Curve of Spee
2. Overjet and overbite
3. Features of normal occlusion
4. Centric relation and centric occlusion.

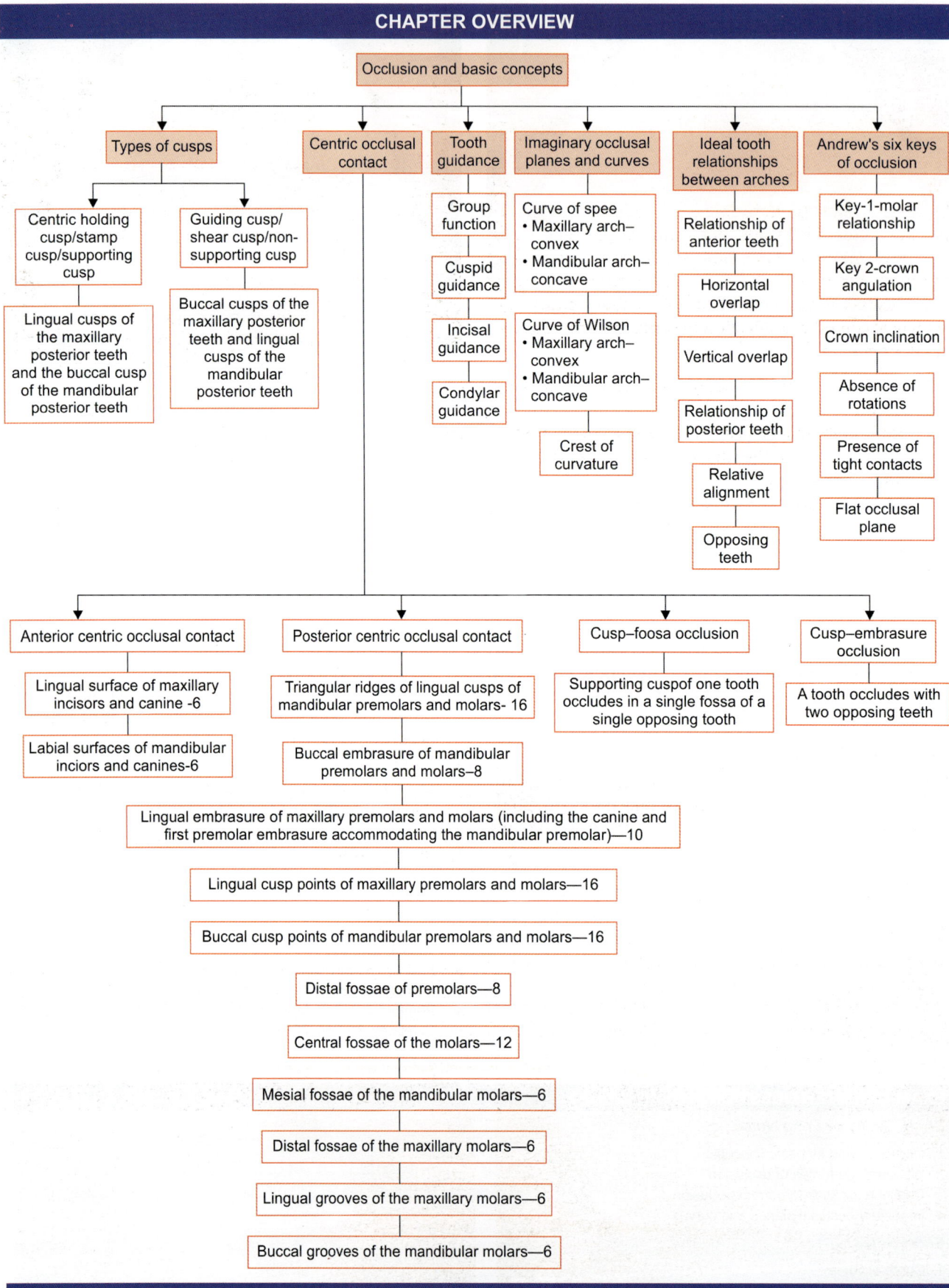

# CHAPTER 8

# Classification of Malocclusions

*Phulari BS, Naik P*

The classification or description of malocclusion is an essential prerequisite for determining prevalence or severity of malocclusion. Although numerous attempts were made throughout the nineteenth century to classify malocclusions, it was not until the end of that century that a widely accepted classification became important to the dental profession.

Malocclusions can be broadly classified into following three types:
1. Intra-arch malocclusions: Malocclusion within the same arch, i.e. either maxillary arch or mandibular arch **(Figs 8.1A and B)**.
2. Inter-arch malocclusions: Malocclusions involving both maxillary and mandibular arches **(Figs 8.2A and B)**.
3. Skeletal malocclusions: Malocclusions involving underlying skeletal structures **(Fig. 8.3)**.

## INTRA-ARCH MALOCCLUSIONS

Malalignment of individual tooth within the same dental arch are referred as intra-arch malocclusions. Intra-arch malocclusion may be in the form of abnormal inclinations, displacement, rotation, transposition or abnormal position of a tooth. Intra-arch malocclusions can be classified into following types **(Flowchart 8.1)**.

### Abnormal Inclinations

This condition involves an abnormal tilting of a crown, with the root being in normal position. A tooth may be abnormally inclined in any of the four directions.

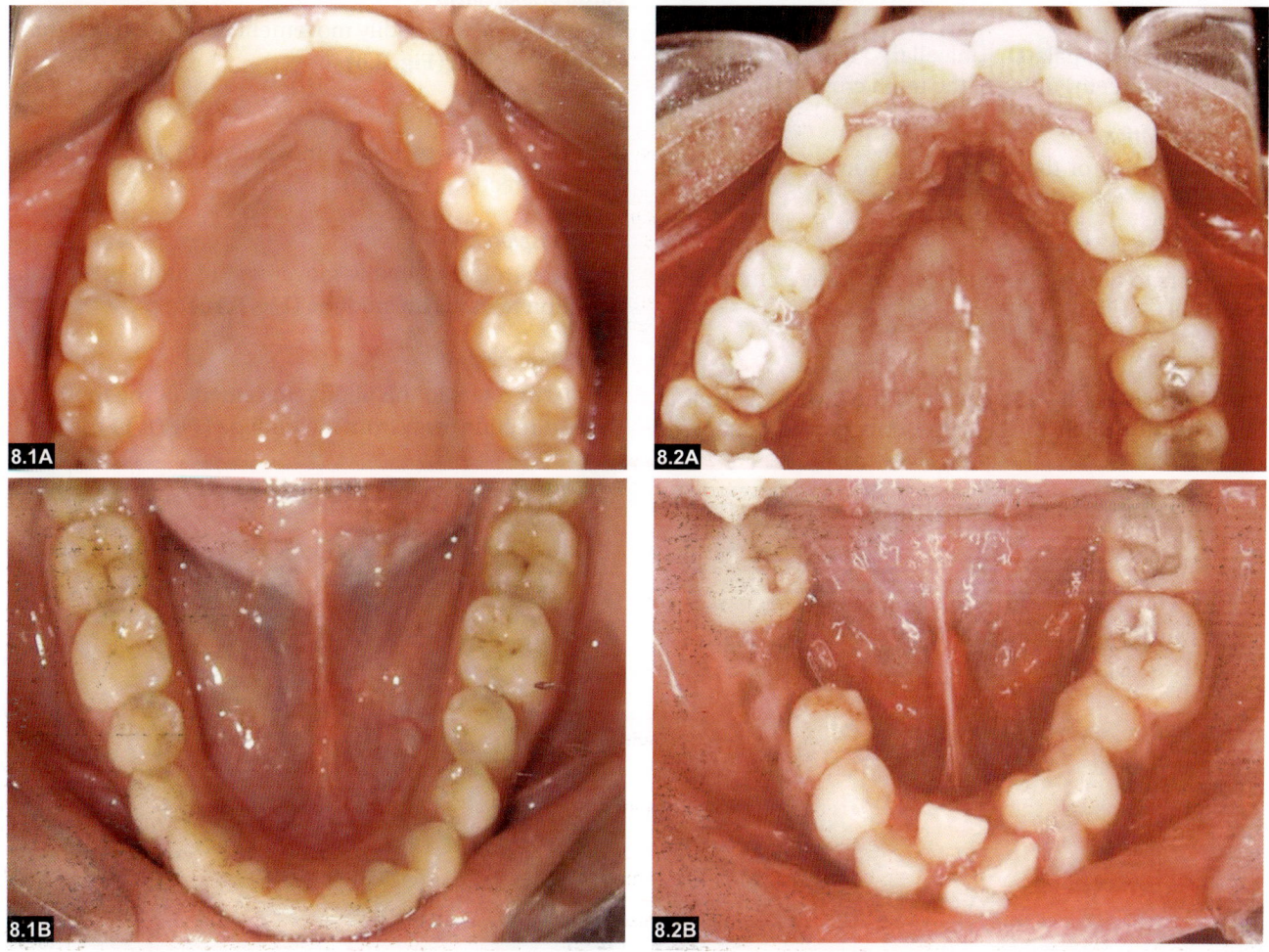

**Figs 8.1A and B:** Palatally erupting right canine due to premature loss of deciduous teeth resulting in intra-arch malocclusion
**Figs 8.2A and B:** Crowding in maxillary and mandibular arches, resulting in interarch malocclusion

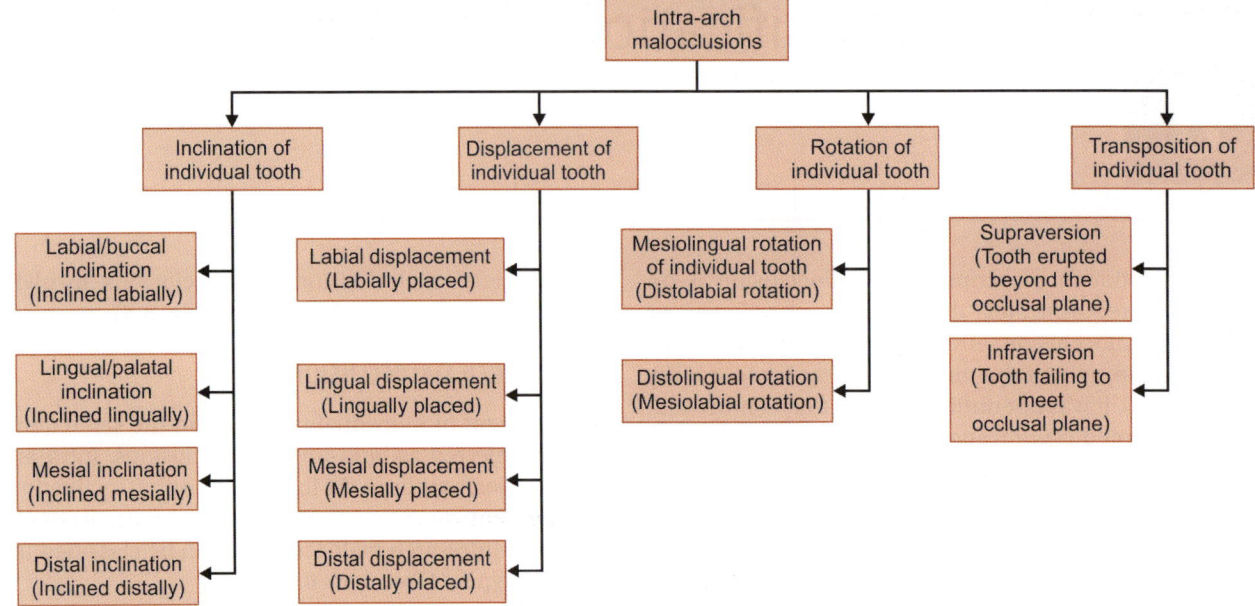

**Flowchart 8.1:** Intra-arch malocclusion

### Buccal Inclination
This refers to labial (in case of anteriors) or buccal (in case of posteriors) tilting of the tooth crown **(Fig. 8.4)**.

### Lingual Inclination
This refers to palatal (maxillary teeth) or lingual (mandibular teeth) tilting of the tooth crown **(Fig. 8.5)**.

### Mesial Inclination
Refers to tilting of the tooth crown towards the midline **(Fig. 8.6)**.

### Distal Inclination
This refers to tilting of the tooth crown away from midline **(Fig. 8.7)**.

### Displacement
This involves bodily movement of the crown, as well as the root of a tooth in the same direction to occupy an abnormal location. A tooth can be displaced in any of the four directions.

### Buccal Displacement
This term refers to bodily movement of the tooth in labial/buccal direction **(Fig. 8.8)**.

### Lingual Displacement
This term refers to bodily movement of the tooth in a lingual direction **(Fig. 8.9)**.

### Mesial Displacement
This term refers to bodily movement of tooth in a mesial direction towards the midline **(Fig. 8.10)**.

### Distal Displacement
This term refers to the bodily movement of the tooth in a distal direction away from the midline **(Fig. 8.11)**.

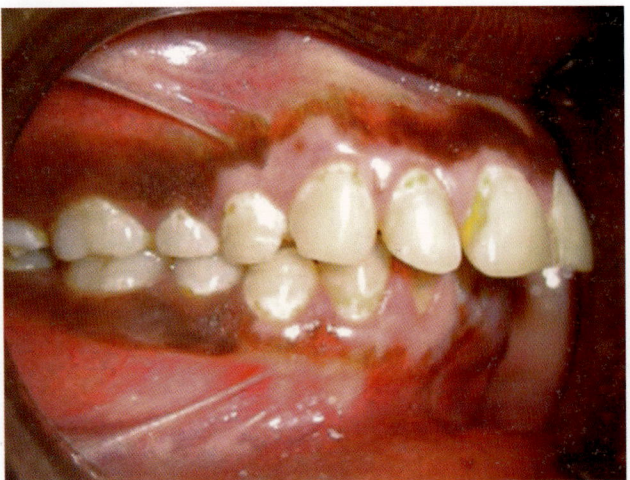

**Fig. 8.3:** Skeletal class I malocclusion

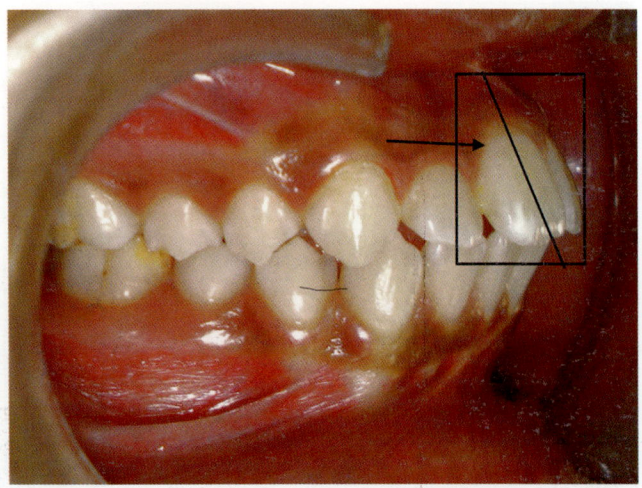

**Fig. 8.4:** Buccally inclined maxillary permanent central incisor

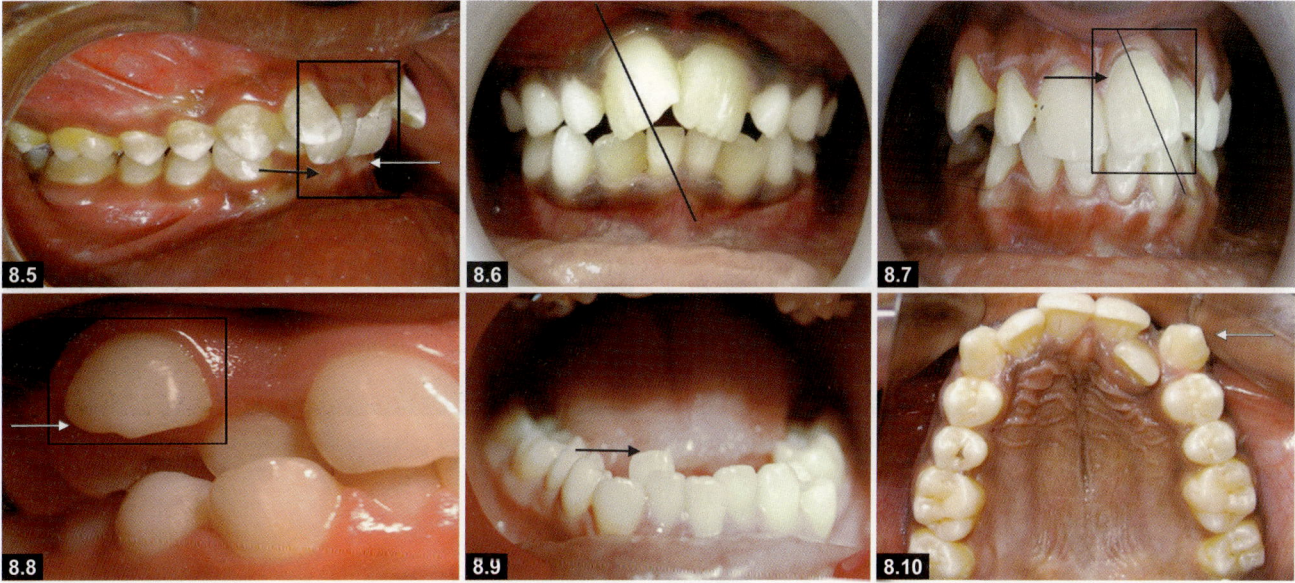

**Fig. 8.5:** Lingually inclined maxillary right and left central incisors; **Fig. 8.6:** Mesially inclined central incisor; **Fig. 8.7:** Distally inclined central incisor; **Fig. 8.8:** Buccal displacement of canine; **Fig. 8.9:** Lingual displacement of lateral incisor; **Fig. 8.10:** Mesial displacement of canine

### Rotation

This term refers to the movement of a tooth around its long axis. A tooth may be rotated in two directions:

1. Mesiolingual (distolabial) or **(Fig. 8.12A)**
2. Distolingual (mesiolabial) direction **(Fig. 8.12B)**.

### Transposition

This term refers to a condition in which two teeth have exchanged places **(Fig. 8.13)**.

### Infra/Supraversion

A tooth is said to be in infra/supraversion, when it is not at the level of occlusion as compared to other teeth in the arch depending on its rate of eruption **(Fig. 8.14)**.

## INTERARCH MALOCCLUSIONS

Such malocclusions can occur in sagittal, vertical or transverse planes of space.

### Sagittal Plane Malocclusions

This refers to conditions where the upper and lower arches are abnormally related to each other in a sagittal plane. Such malocclusions can be of two types:

1. Pre-normal occlusion: Where the lower arch is placed more anteriorly when the teeth meet in centric occlusion **(Fig. 8.15)**.
2. Post-normal occlusion: Where the lower arch is placed posteriorly when the teeth meet in centric occlusion **(Fig. 8.16)**.

### Vertical Plane Malocclusions

Vertical plane malocclusions refer to conditions where there is an abnormal vertical relationship between teeth of upper and lower dental arches. They include deep bite and open bite cases.

- Deep bite/Increased overbite: Where there is excessive vertical overlapping of upper anterior over the lower anteriors when teeth are in central occlusion **(Fig. 8.17)**.

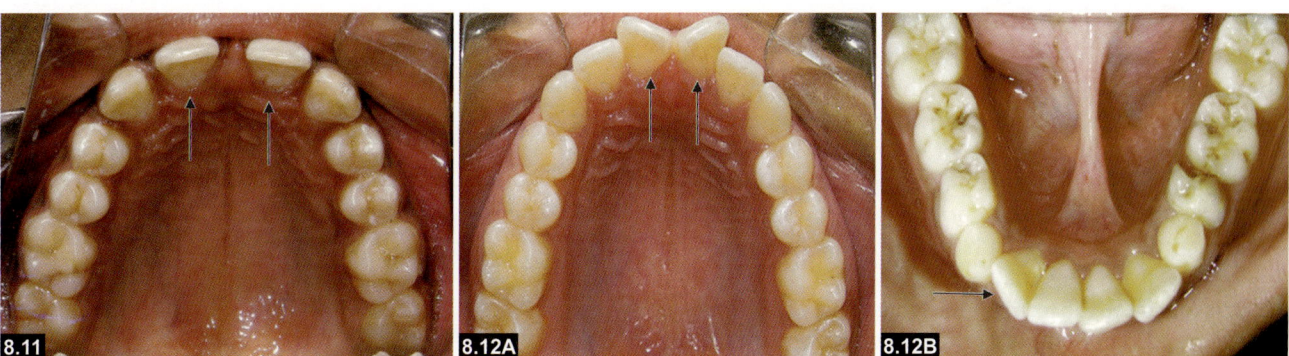

**Fig. 8.11:** Distal displacement of right and left permanent central incisors; **Figs 8.12A and B:** (A) Severe mesiopalatal rotation of right and left permanent maxillary central incisors; (B) Distolingual rotation of mandibular permanent lateral incisor

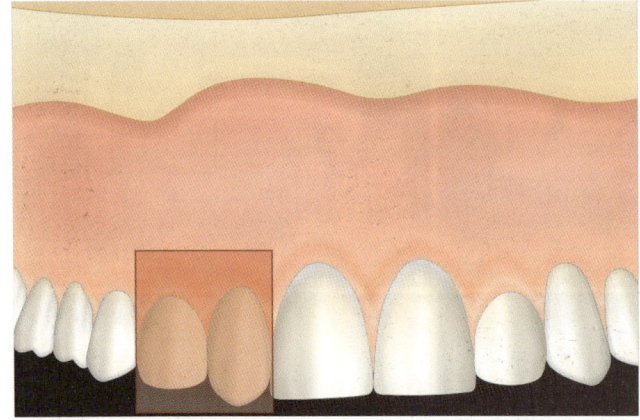

**Fig. 8.13:** Transposition in relation to canine and lateral incisor

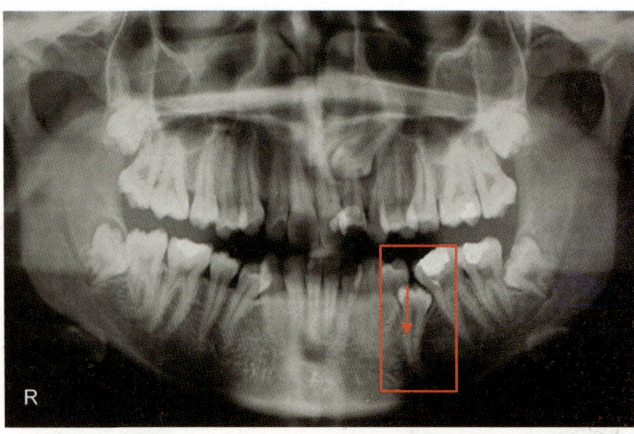

**Fig. 8.14:** Infraversion of premolar due to mesial drifting of first molar

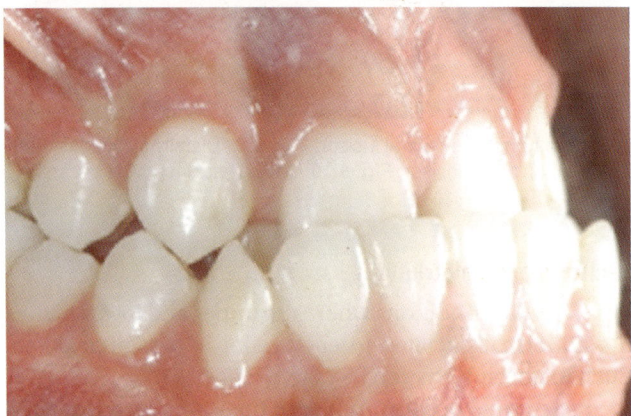

**Fig. 8.15:** Prenormal occlusion

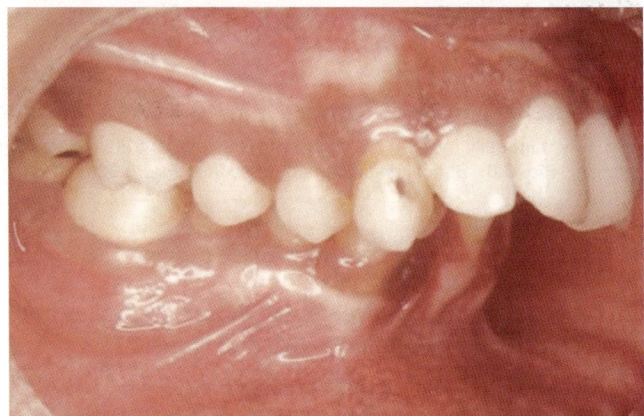

**Fig. 8.16:** Postnormal occlusion

- Open bite: Where there is lack of vertical relationship between upper and lower teeth. Open bite can be presented in the anterior or posterior regions.
  - Anterior open bite: The term refers to conditions where there is no vertical overlap of upper anterior over the lower anterior when teeth are brought to centric occlusion **(Fig. 8.18)**.
  - Posterior open bite: The term refers to a condition where there is a lack of intercuspation between upper and lower posterior teeth, when teeth are in centric occlusion. Posterior open bite can be unilateral or bilateral **(Fig. 8.19)**.

### Transverse Plane Malocclusions

Transverse plane refers to conditions where there is an abnormal transverse relationship between the upper and lower arches. These include various types of crossbites and scissor bites.

- Crossbite: The term refers to a condition where one/more teeth may be abnormally malposed buccally, lingually or labially with reference to the opposing tooth or teeth **(Fig. 8.20)**.
- Scissors bite: The term applies to total maxillary buccal (or mandibular lingual) crossbite with the mandibular dentition completely contained in habitual occlusion **(Fig. 8.21)**.

## SKELETAL MALOCCLUSION

Skeletal malocclusion can be caused by defects in size, position or relationship between the upper and lower jaws. The skeletal malocclusions can occur in sagittal, vertical and transverse planes **(Flowchart 8.2)**.

### Skeletal Malocclusions in Sagittal Planes

- These include conditions where the upper and lower jaws are abnormally related to each other in a sagittal plane.
- The term prognathism refers to forward placement of a jaw and term retrognathism is used for backward placement of a jaw.

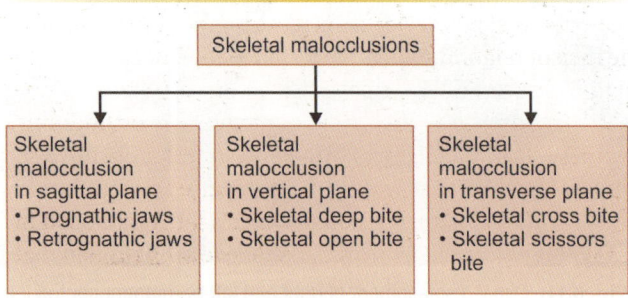

**Flowchart 8.2:** Classification of skeletal malocclusions

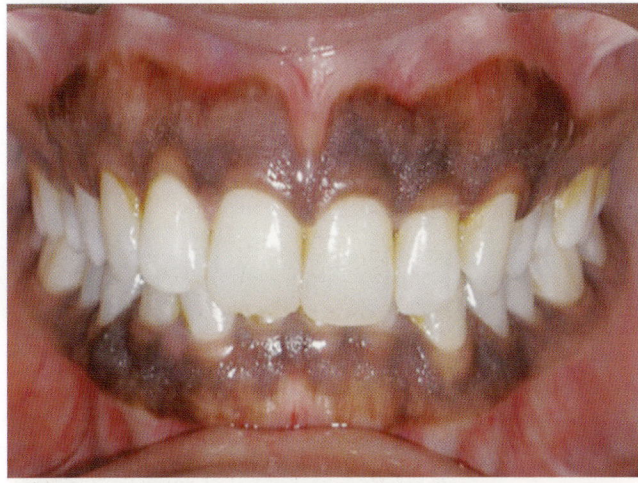

**Fig. 8.17:** Deep bite     **Fig. 8.18:** Anterior open bite

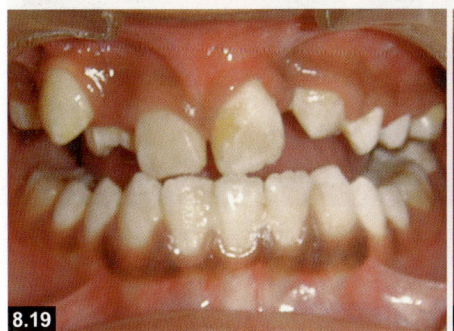 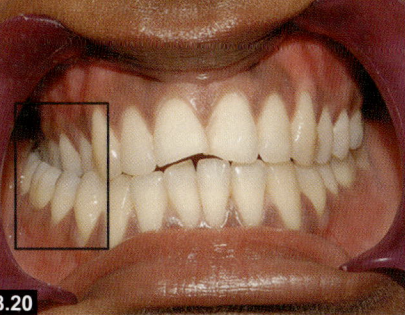 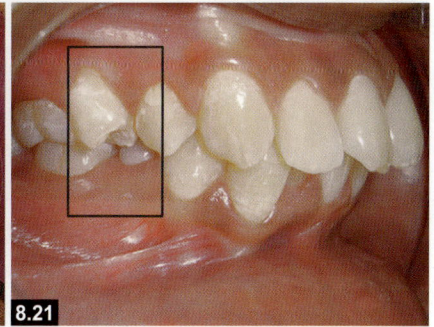

**Fig. 8.19:** Bilateral posterior open bite; **Fig. 8.20:** Unilateral posterior crossbite **Fig. 8.21:** Single tooth scissor bite

- Sagittal plane malocclusion can occur in one or both the jaws or as various combinations **(Fig. 8.22)**.

### Skeletal Malocclusions in Vertical Plane

These malocclusions include open bite and deep bite conditions **(Fig. 8.23)**.

### Skeletal Malocclusions in Transverse Plane

Narrowing or widening of the jaws may result in an abnormal relationship between upper and lower jaws in a transverse plane. These include skeletal crossbite and scissor bite conditions, which may be unilateral/bilateral **(Fig. 8.24)**.

## CLASSIFICATION OF INCISOR RELATIONSHIP

Many clinicians find it useful to classify the incisor relationship separately from buccal segment relationship. The incisor relationship may not match the buccal segment relationship and in these cases it is informative to describe both. In addition, a major objective of orthodontic treatment is to establish a normal incisor relationship and it is reasonable that a classification of malocclusion should take this into account. Although Angle's terms are used in classifying incisor relationship, it must be emphasized that this is not Angle's classification.

British standard classification of incisor relationship includes following three classes **(Flowchart 8.3)**.

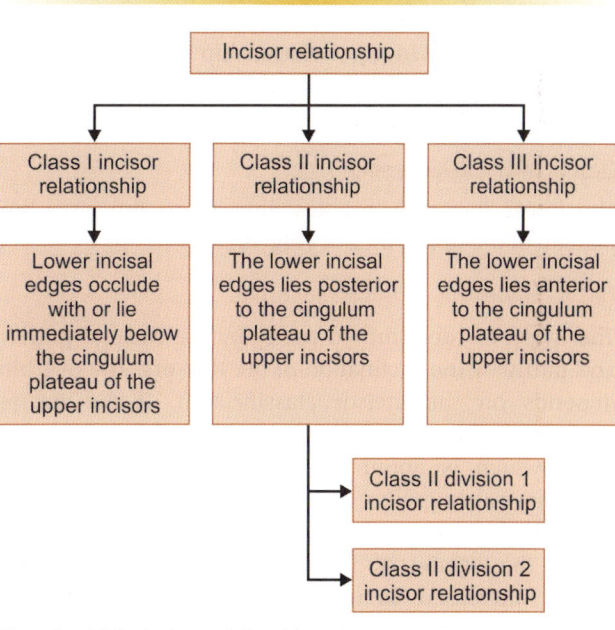

**Flowchart 8.3:** Incisor relationship

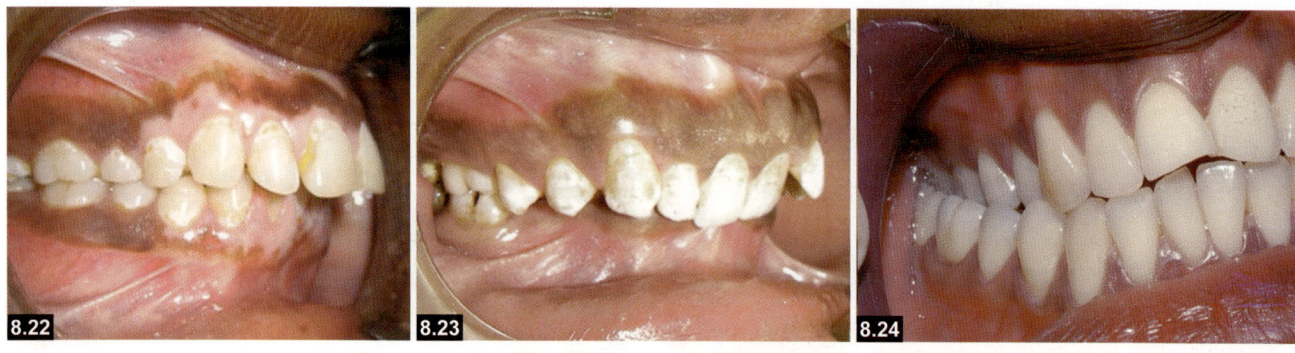

**Fig. 8.22:** Skeletal malocclusion in sagittal plane—class I. **Fig. 8.23:** Skeletal malocclusion in vertical plane
**Fig. 8.24:** Skeletal malocclusion in transverse plane—Skeletal crossbite

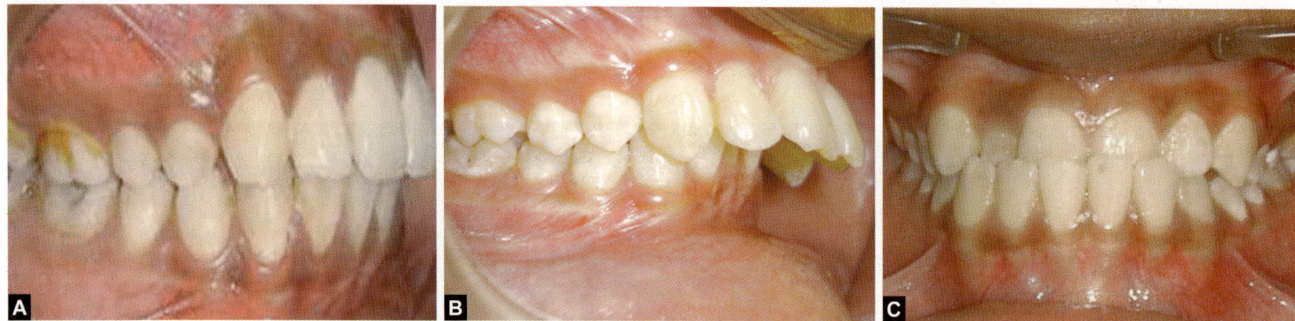

**Figs 8.25A to C:** (A) Class I incisor relationship; (B) Class II division 1 incisor relationship; (C) Class III Incisor relationship

### Class I Incisor Relationship

Lower incisal edges occlude with or lie immediately below the cingulum plateau of the upper incisors **(Fig. 8.25A)**.

### Class II Incisor Relationship

The lower incisal edge lies posterior to the cingulum plateau of the upper incisors.

Class II Division 1 Incisor Relationship: The upper central incisors are proclined or of average inclination. There is an increase in overjet **(Fig. 8.25B)**.

Class II Division 2 Incisor Relationship: The upper central incisors are retroclined. The overjet is usually minimal but may be increased.

### Class III Incisor Relationship

The lower incisal edges lies anterior to the cingulum plateau of the upper incisor **(Fig. 8.25C)**.

### Factors Influencing Incisor Relationship

The overjet is determined partly by the skeletal pattern and partly by the inclination of the incisors. The overbite depends on the incisor classification. If the overjet is normal, the depth of overbite will depend on the angle which is about 135 degree. If the interincisal angle is much greater than this, the overbite will be deep because the incisors can erupt past one another. When the overjet is increased, the overbite will be usually increased as well unless some other factors, such as a thumb sucking habit, prevents full eruption of incisors.

## CANINE RELATIONSHIP

Canine relationships are classified into following three classes **(Flowchart 8.4)**.

### Class I Canine Relationship

It means mesial inclination of the cusp of the upper canine, which overlaps the distal incline of the cusp of lower canine **(Fig. 8.26A)**.

### Class II Canine Relationship

Distal incline of the cusp of upper canine, which overlaps the mesial incline of the cusp of lower canine are termed as class II canine relationship **(Fig. 8.26B)**.

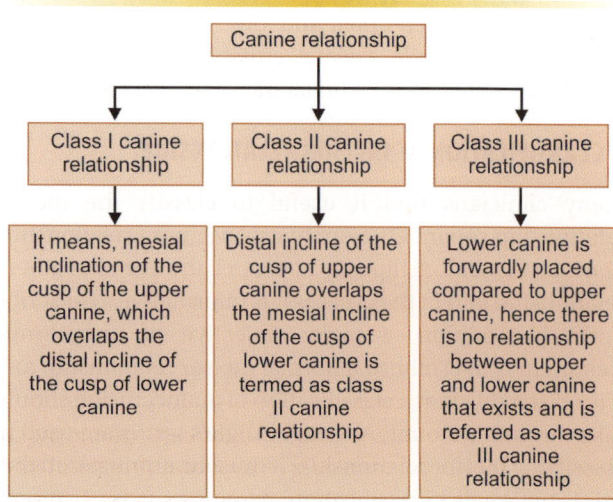

**Flowchart 8.4:** Canine relationship

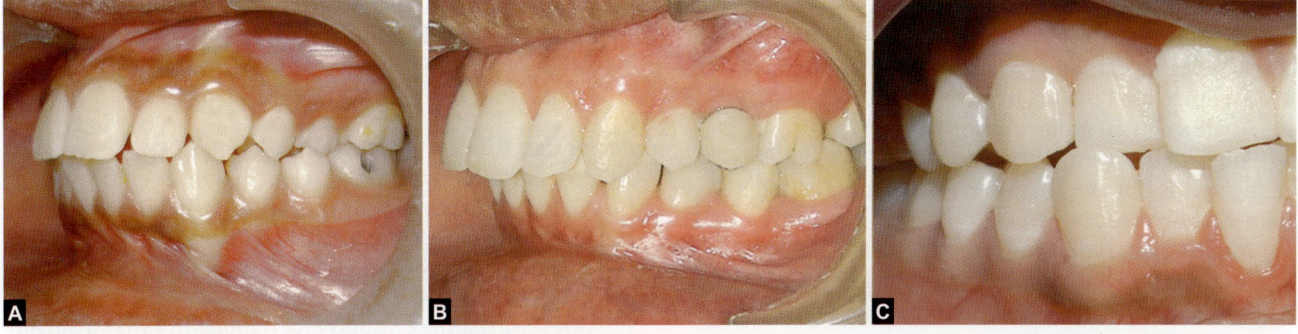

**Figs 8.26A to C:** (A) Class I canine relationship; (B) Class II canine relationship; (C) Class III canine relationship

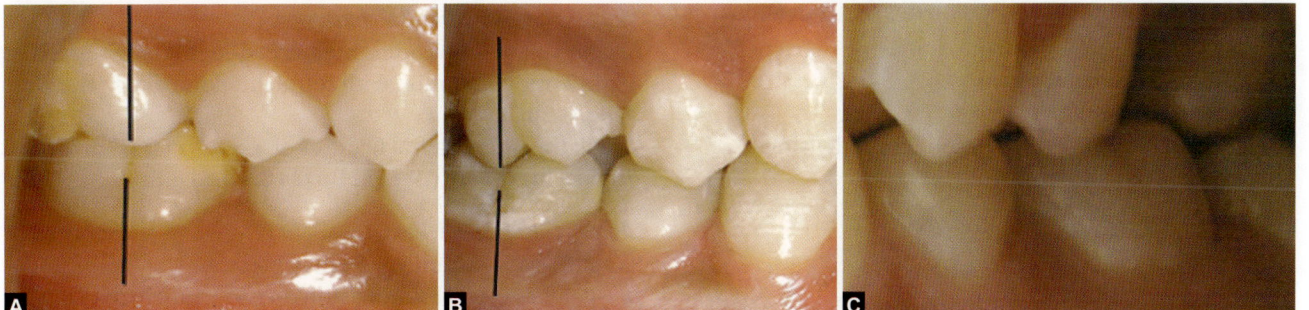

**Figs 8.27A to C:** (A) Class I molar relationship; (B) Class II molar relationship; (C) Class III molar relationship

### Class III Canine Relationship

Lower canine is forwardly placed as compared to upper canine. Hence, there is no relationship between upper and lower canine that exist and is referred as class III canine relationship **(Fig. 8.26C)**.

### MOLAR RELATIONSHIP

There are 12 permanent molars—six upper and six lower. The six permanent molar in each arch are the first, second, and third molars on either side of the arch. The permanent molars play a major role in the mastication of food (chewing and grinding to pulverize) and are the most important in maintaining the vertical dimension of the face (preventing a closing of the bite or vertical dimension, appearance). They are also important in maintaining continuity within the dental arches, thus keeping other teeth into proper alignment.

Molar relationships are classified into following three classes **(Flowchart 8.5)**.

### Class I Molar Relationship

Mesiobuccal cusp of the permanent maxillary first molar occludes in mesiobuccal developmental groove of first permanent mandibular molar, referred as Class I molar relationship **(Fig. 8.27A)**.

### Class II Molar Relationship

Distobuccal cusp of the maxillary first permanent molar occludes in the mesiobuccal development groove of first permanent mandibular molar, termed as class II molar relationship **(Fig. 8.27B)**.

### Class III Molar Relationship

Mesiobuccal cusp of maxillary first permanent molar occludes interdentally between first and second mandibular molar are said to be class III molar relationship **(Fig. 8.27C)**.

### ANGLE'S CLASSIFICATION OF MALOCCLUSION

Angle classified malocclusion based on the anteroposterior relationship of the teeth in the year 1898. He used Roman numerical I, II, III to designate the main classes, whereas Arabic numerical, 1, 2, denote the divisions of

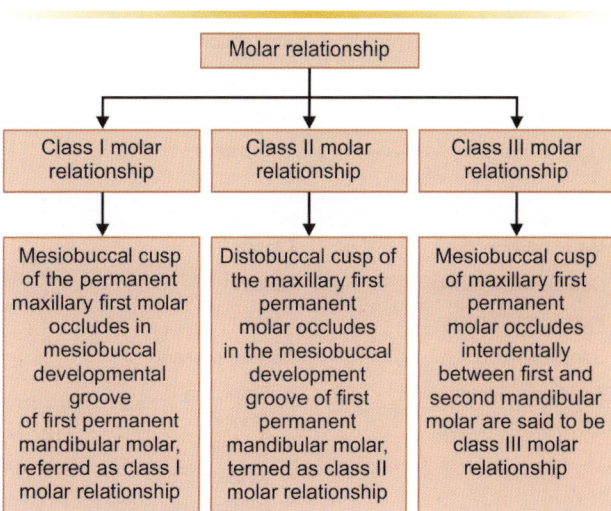

**Flowchart 8.5:** Molar relationship

the classification. Unilateral deviations were termed as subdivisions.

Angle's classes of malocclusion are given as follows:
- Angle's class I malocclusion
- Angle's class II malocclusion
- Angle's class III malocclusion

Angle's class II malocclusion is further subdivided into the following two types:
1. Angle's class II division 1 malocclusion
2. Angle's class II division 2 malocclusion

Angle's class II is classified into following types, based on subdivisions:
   a. Angle's class II subdivision division 1 malocclusion
   b. Angle's class II subdivision division 2 malocclusion

Angle's class III is classified into following two types:
1. True class III malocclusion
2. Pseudo class III malocclusion

Angle's class III is classified based on subdivisions:
Angle's class III subdivision

### Angle's Class I Malocclusion

Angle's class I malocclusion, where the mesiobuccal cusp of the maxillary permanent first molar occludes with the mesiobuccal groove of the mandibular first permanent molar **(Fig. 8.28A)**.

Extraoral features of Angle's class I malocclusion are listed in **Box 8.1**.

Intraoral features of Angle's class I malocclusion are listed in **Box 8.2**.

### Angle Class II Malocclusion

Angle class II malocclusion is characterized by class II molar relation, where the distobuccal cusp of the maxillary permanent first molar occludes with the buccal groove of the mandibular first permanent molar.

Angle's class II malocclusion has been sub-classified into the following divisions:
1. Angle class II division 1 malocclusion
2. Angle class II division 2 malocclusion

### Angle's Class II Division 1 Malocclusion

Angle's class II division 1 malocclusion is characterized by class II molar relation on either side with proclined maxillary anteriors **(Fig. 8.28B)**.

Extraoral features Angle class II division 1 malocclusion are listed in **Box 8.3**.

Intraoral features Angle class II division 1 malocclusion are listed in **Box 8.4**.

### Angle's Class II Division 2 Malocclusion

Angle's class II division 2 malocclusion is characterized by class II molar relation with retroclined maxillary anteriors **(Fig. 8.28C)**.

Extra and intraoral features of Angle's class II division 2 malocclusion are listed in **Boxes 8.5 and 8.6**.

### Angle's Class II Subdivision

Angle's class II subdivision may be:
- Angle's class II subdivision division 1 malocclusion
- Angle's class II subdivision division 2 malocclusion

### Angle's Class II Subdivision Division 1 Malocclusion

If the class II molar relation on one side of the arch and class I molar relation on the other side of the dental arch with proclined maxillary anteriors, it is termed as Angle's class II subdivision division 1 malocclusion.

### Angle's Class II Subdivision Division 2 Malocclusion

If the class II molar relation on one side of the arch and class I molar relation on the other side of the dental arch with retroclined maxillary anteriors, it is termed as Angle's class II subdivision division 2 malocclusion.

**Box 8.1:** Extraoral features of Angle's class I malocclusion

| | |
|---|---|
| Shape of the head | Mesocephalic |
| Facial form | Mesoprosopic |
| Facial profile | Straight/orthognathic |
| Facial divergence | Straight |
| Nasolabial angle | Normal |
| Lips | Competent |

**Box 8.2:** Intraoral features of Angle's class I malocclusion

| | |
|---|---|
| Molar relationship | Class I |
| Canine relationship | Class I |
| Incisor relationship | Class I |
| Spacing in arch | May be present |
| Additional features | <ul><li>Crowding</li><li>Spacing</li><li>Rotation</li><li>Missing tooth</li><li>Bimaxillary protrusion</li><li>Midline diastema</li></ul> |

**Box 8.3:** Extraoral features Angle class II division 1 malocclusion

| | |
|---|---|
| Profile | Convex |
| Nasolabial angle | Decreased |
| Lips | Incompetent |
| Mentolabial sulcus | Deep |
| Mentalis | Hyperactive |

**Box 8.4:** Intraoral features Angle class II division 1 malocclusion

| | |
|---|---|
| Molar relationship | Class II on right and left side of arch |
| Canine relationship | Class II on right and left side of arch |
| Incisor relationship | Class II division 1 incisor relationship |
| Maxillary arch | 'V' shape |
| Maxillary anteriors | Proclined |
| Overjet | Increased |
| Overbite | Increased |

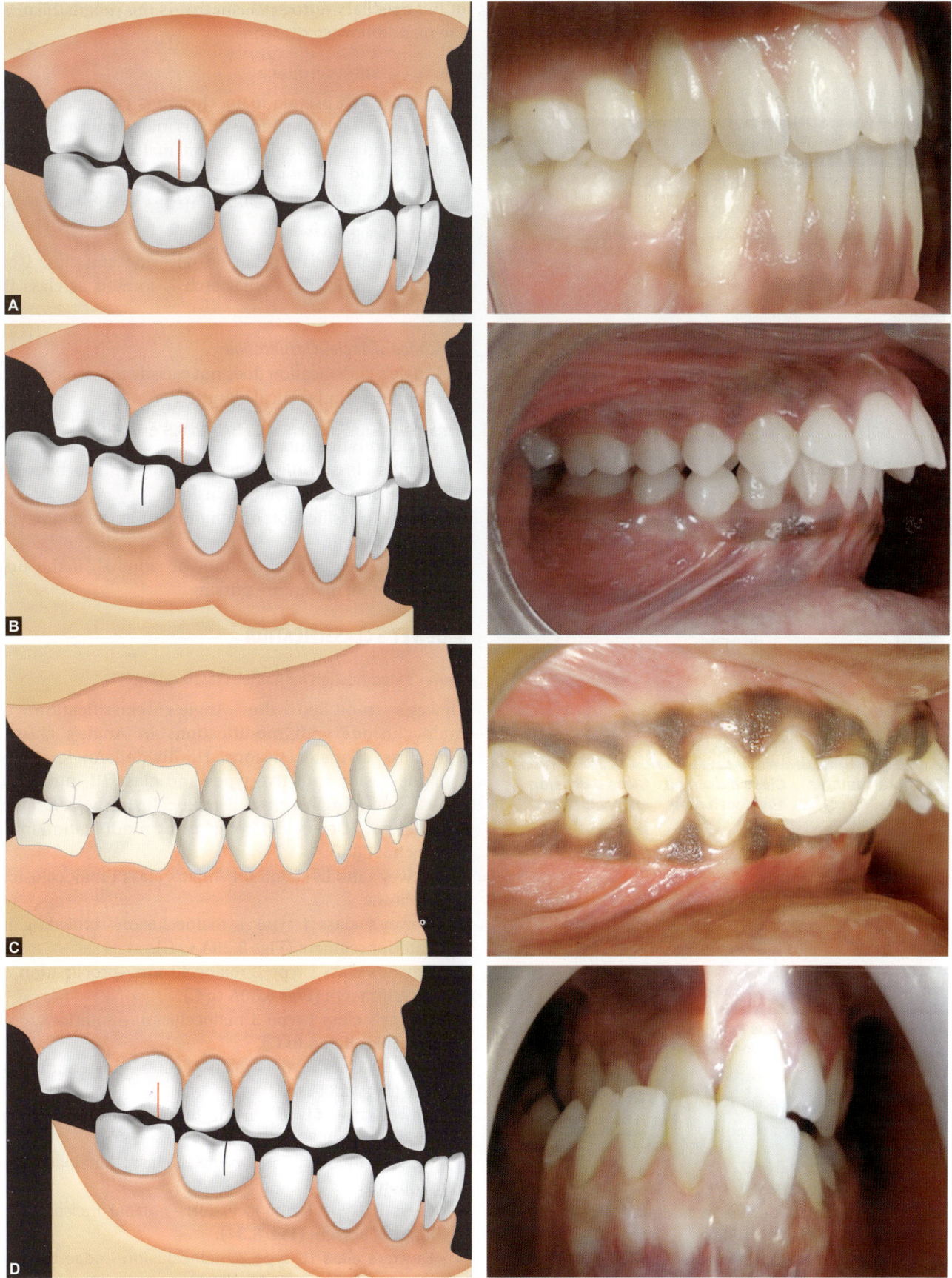

**Figs 8.28A to D:** Schematic and clinical representation of Angle's class I, class II (Division I, II ) and class III malocclusion, respectively

**Box 8.5:** Extraoral features Angle's class II division 2 malocclusion

| | |
|---|---|
| Profile | Convex |
| Nasolabial angle | Increased |

**Box 8.6:** Intraoral features Angle's class II division 2 malocclusion

| | |
|---|---|
| Molar relationship | Class II on right and left side |
| Canine relationship | Class II on right and left side |
| Incisor relationship | Class II division 2 on right and left side |
| Maxillary anterior | Crowding |
| Overjet | Decreased |
| Overbite | Increased |
| Maxillary arch | U shaped |

**Box 8.7:** Extraoral features Angle's class III malocclusion

| | |
|---|---|
| Profile | Concave |
| Lips | May be incompetent |
| Mentolabial sulcus | Shallow |
| Facial divergence | Anterior |

**Box 8.8:** Intraoral features Angle's class III malocclusion

| | |
|---|---|
| Molar relationship | Class III |
| Canine relationship | Class III |
| Incisor relationship | Class III |
| Overjet | Reversed |
| Mandibular arch | Prognathic |
| Maxillary arch | Retrognathic |

**Box 8.9:** Extraoral differences between Angle's class II division 1 and division 2 malocclusion

| Extraoral features | Class II division 1 malocclusion | Class II division 2 malocclusion |
|---|---|---|
| Profile | Convex | Straight |
| Lips | Incompetent | Incompetent |
| Nasolabial angle | Decreased | Increased |
| Mentalis | Hyperactive | Normal |
| Mentolabial sulcus | Deep | Shallow |

**Box 8.10:** Extraoral differences between Angle's class II division 1 and division 2 malocclusion

| Intraoral features | Class II division 1 malocclusion | Class II division 2 malocclusion |
|---|---|---|
| Arch | "V" shaped | "U" shaped |
| Maxillary anteriors | Proclined | Retroclined |
| Overjet | Increased | Decreased |

### Angle's Class III Malocclusion

Angle's class III malocclusion is characterized by class III molar relationship where the mesobuccal cusp of the permanent maxillary first molar occludes into the interdental space between mandibular first and second permanent molar. True class III is due to the mal relationship of either the dental arches or skeletal structure of the maxillary retrognathism that is the prognathism of the mandible.

### Pseudo Class III Malocclusion

Angle's class III pseudo malocclusion is characterized by class III molar relationship, which is mainly due to habit. It is also called as habitual or postural malocclusion.

Extra and intraoral features of Angle's class III malocclusion are listed in the **Boxes 8.7 and 8.8**.

### Class III Subdivision

Class III molar relationship on one side and class I on the other side of the dental arch is termed as class III subdivision.

### Limitation of Angle's Classification

- Angle's classification does not classify malocclusion in transverse and vertical planes.
- Angle's classification cannot be applied to the deciduous dentition.
- Angle's classification does not differentiate between dental and skeletal malocclusion.
- Angle's classification does not include the etiology of malocclusion.
- Angle's classification cannot be applied, if the first permanent molars are missing.

## DEWEY'S CLASSIFICATION

### Dewey's Modification for Angle's Classification

Dewey's modified the Angle's classification of malocclusions with modifications in Angle's class I and class III malocclusions. He divided Angle's class I malocclusion into five types and class III into three types. Since Angle's class II malocclusion was already well defined, Dewey did not give any modification for it **(Flowchart 8.6)**.

Dewey's modification for Angle's class I malocclusion is as follows:
- Dewey's class I type 1 malocclusion—crowding in anterior segment **(Figs 8.29A to C)**.
- Dewey's class I type 2 malocclusion—proclination of anterior teeth **(Figs 8.30A to C)**.
- Dewey's class I type 3 malocclusion—anterior crossbite **(Figs 8.31A to C)**.
- Dewey's class I type 4 malocclusion—posterior crossbite **(Figs 8.32A to C)**.
- Dewey's class I type 5 malocclusion—mesial drifting of molars **(Fig. 8.33)**.

Dewey's modification for Angle's class III malocclusion is as follows:
- Class III type 1 malocclusion—normal incisor overlapping present **(Fig. 8.34)**.
- Dewey's class III type 2 malocclusion—edge-to-edge incisor relationship **(Fig. 8.35)**.
- Dewey's class III type 3 malocclusion—incisors are in crossbite **(Fig. 8.36)**.

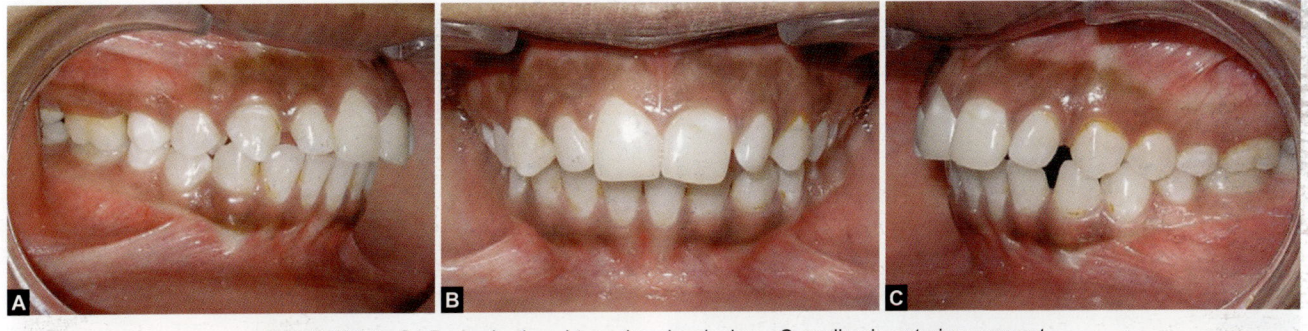

**Figs 8.29A to C:** Dewey's class I type 1 malocclusion—Crowding in anterior segment

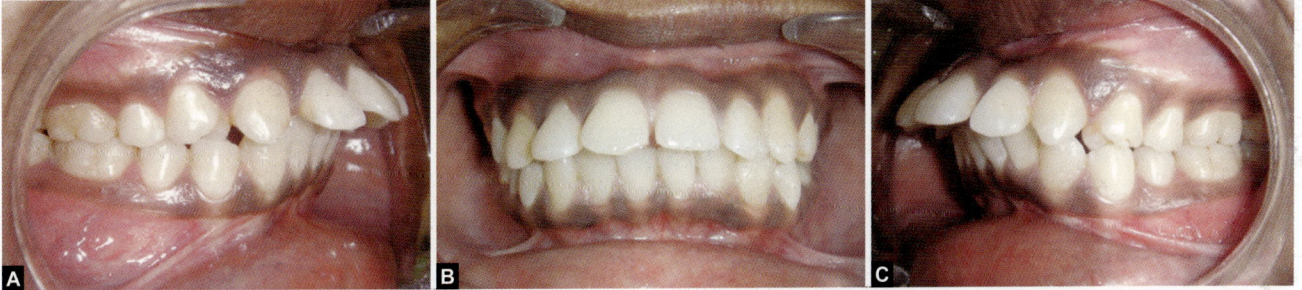

**Figs 8.30A to C:** Dewey's class I type 2 malocclusion—Proclination of anterior teeth

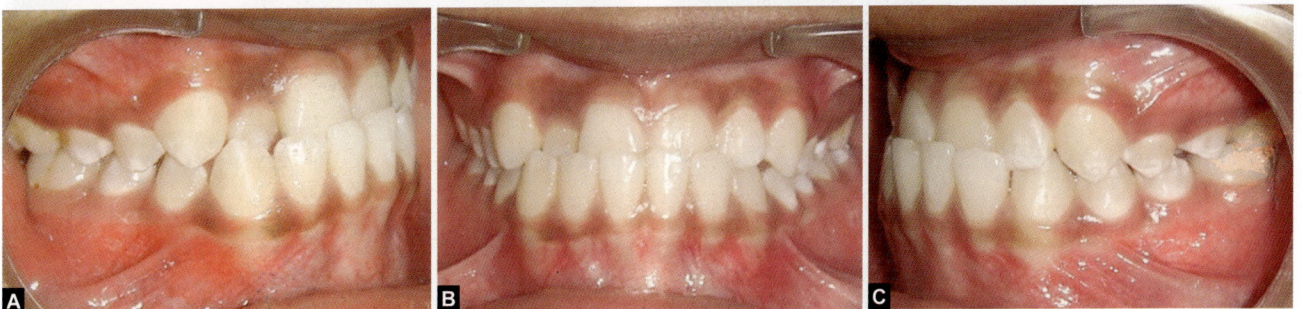

**Figs 8.31A to C:** Dewey's class I type 3 malocclusion—Anterior crossbite

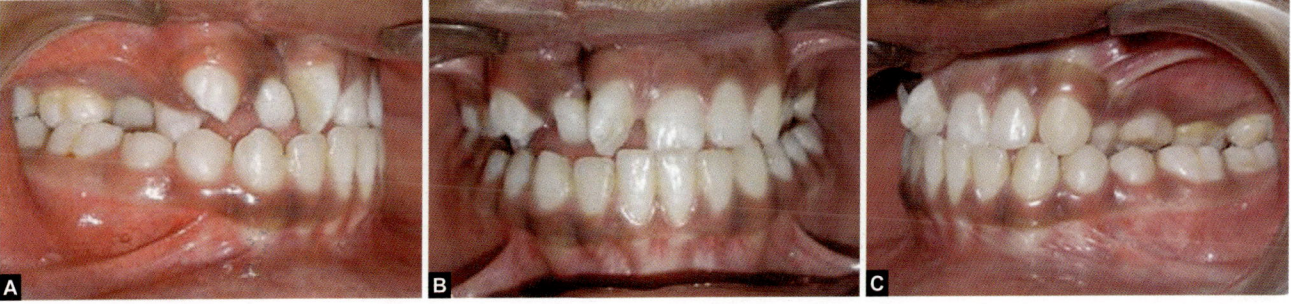

**Figs 8.32A to C:** Dewey's class I type 4 malocclusion—Posterior crossbite

## LISCHER'S CLASSIFICATION FOR MODIFICATION OF ANGLE'S CLASSIFICATION

Lischer's replaced the terms class I, II, III in Angle's classification of malocclusion, with the terms neutro-occlusion, disto-occlusion and mesio-occlusion (**Fig. 8.37**), respectively. In addition, he described other possible malpositions of a tooth or a group of teeth as listed below further.

### Neutro-Occlusion

Neutro-occlusion is the normal retention step of dental arches.

### Disto-Occlusion

Disto-occlusion is the postnormal occlusion (**Fig. 8.38**).

### Mesio-Occlusion

Mesio-occlusion is the prenormal occlusion.

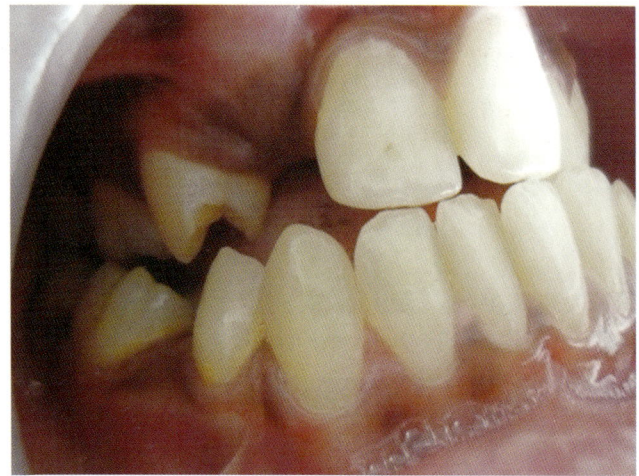

**Fig. 8.33:** Dewey's class 1 type 5 malocclusion—Mesial drifting of molars

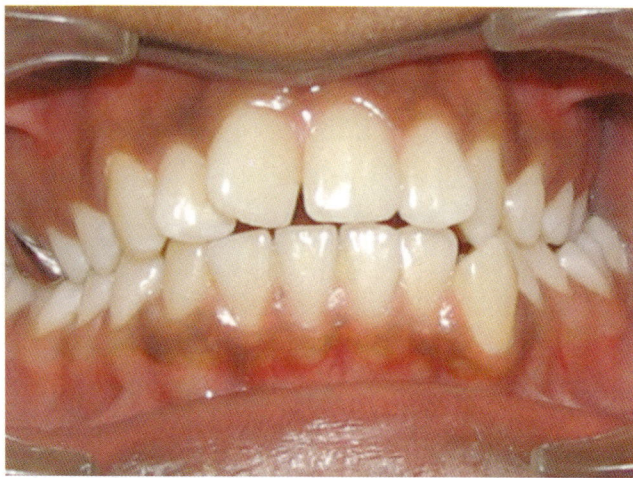

**Fig. 8.34:** Class III type 1 malocclusion—Normal incisor overlapping present

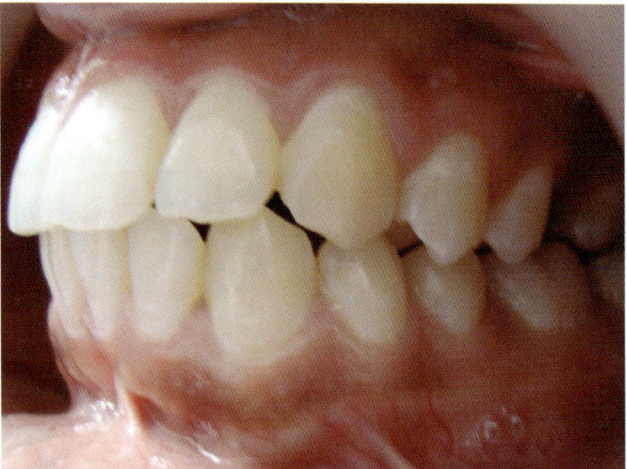

**Fig. 8.35:** Dewey's class III type 2 malocclusion—Edge-to-edge incisor relationship

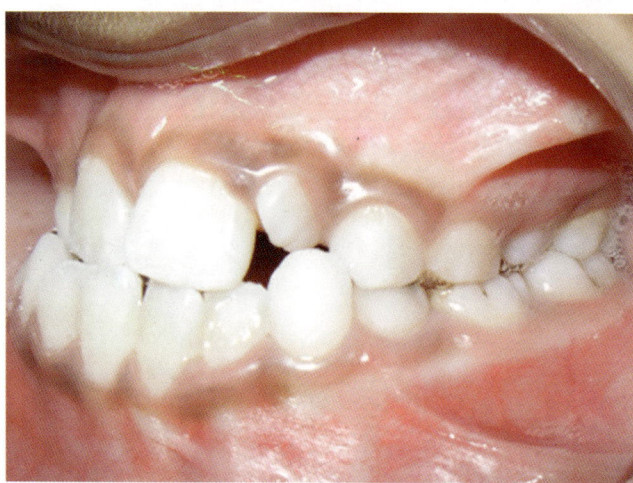

**Fig. 8.36:** Dewey's class III type 3 malocclusion—Incisors are in crossbite

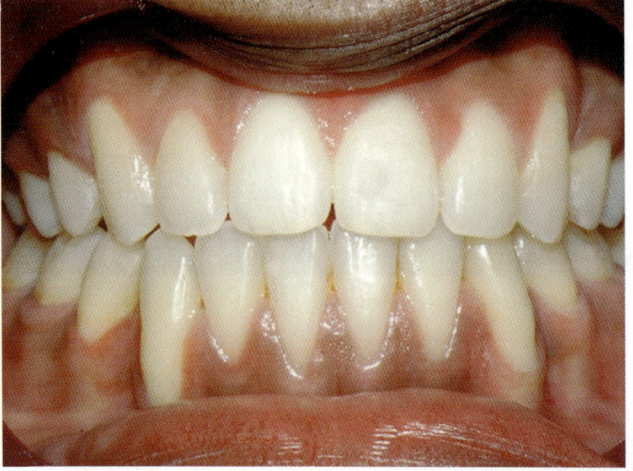

**Fig. 8.37:** Neutro-occlusion (Angle's class I malocclusion)

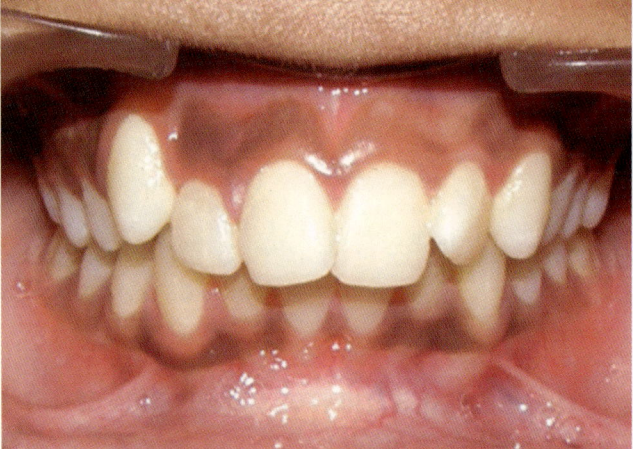

**Fig. 8.38:** Disto-occlusion (Angle's class II malocclusion)

## For Individual Teeth

- Labioverison of tooth—Movement of tooth/teeth towards the lip or cheek.
- Linguoversion of teeth—Lingual to normal position
- Mesioversion—Mesial to the normal position
- Distoversion—Distal to normal position
- Supraversion of tooth—Crossing the line of occlusion
- Infraversion of tooth—Away from the line of occlusion
- Transversion—Transposition-Wrong position in the arch
- Torsi version—Rotated on its long axis

## SIMON'S CLASSIFICATION

Simon's classification is based on anteriorposterior, transverse and vertical plane relationships of the dental arches. Simon's system of classification made use of three anthropometric, which are **(Flowchart 8.6)**:
1. Frankfort horizontal plane (FH plane)
2. Orbital plane
3. Midsagittal plane.

Simon's classification of malocclusion is based on abnormal relationship of the dental arches from their normal position in relation to anteroposterior, transverse and vertical planes.

### Frankfort Horizontal Plane (FH Plane)

This plane is from upper margin of external auditory meatus to the infraorbital margin. This plane describes the vertical relationship of the dental arches **(Fig. 8.39)**.

**Attraction:** If a dental arch or part of it is closure than normal to the Frankfort plane, then it is called as attraction.

**Abstraction:** If a dental arch or part of it is farther away from Frankfort plane, then it is called as abstraction.

### Orbital Plane

Orbital plane is perpendicular to the FH plane, dropped down from infraorbital margin of the bony orbit **(Fig. 8.40)**.

**Simon law of canine:** According to Simon, orbital plane should pass through the distal third of the maxillary canine and is called as Simon's law of cuspid.

**Protraction:** If dental arches or part of it is farther from orbital plane then it is called as protraction.

**Retraction:** If dental arches or part of it is closure to orbital plane, then it is referred as retraction.

### Midsagittal Plane

Midsagittal plane is used to describe the transverse relationship of the dental arches **(Fig. 8.41)**.

**Contraction:** If dental arch or part of it is closure to the midsagittal plane, it is referred as contraction.

**Distraction:** If dental arch or part of it is farther away from the midsagittal plane, then it is called as distraction.

## BALLARD'S CLASSIFICATION

Ballard's classification of malocclusion is based on skeletal relationship on the jaws **(Flowchart 8.7)**.

Ballard's classification includes following three classes, which are as follows.

### Skeletal Class I Malocclusion

Long axis of mandibular incisors passes through the long axis of crown of maxillary incisors **(Figs 8.42i to iii)**.

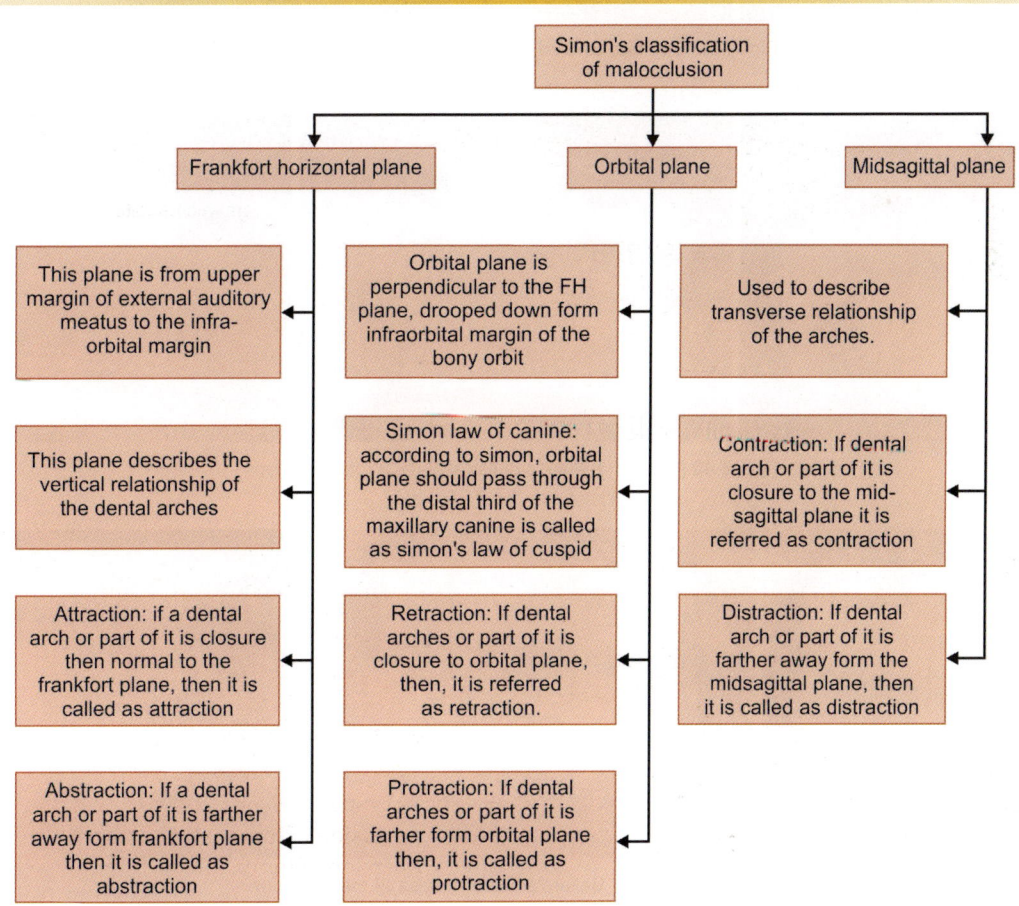

**Flowchart 8.6:** Simon's classification of malocclusion

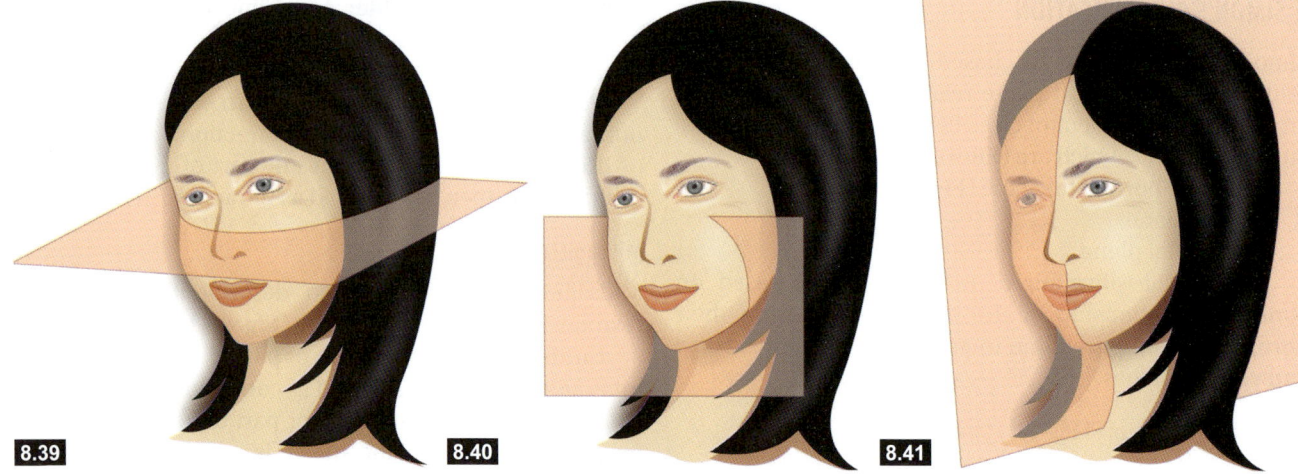

**Fig. 8.39:** Frankfort horizontal plane; **Fig. 8.40:** Orbital plane; **Fig. 8.41:** Midsagittal plane

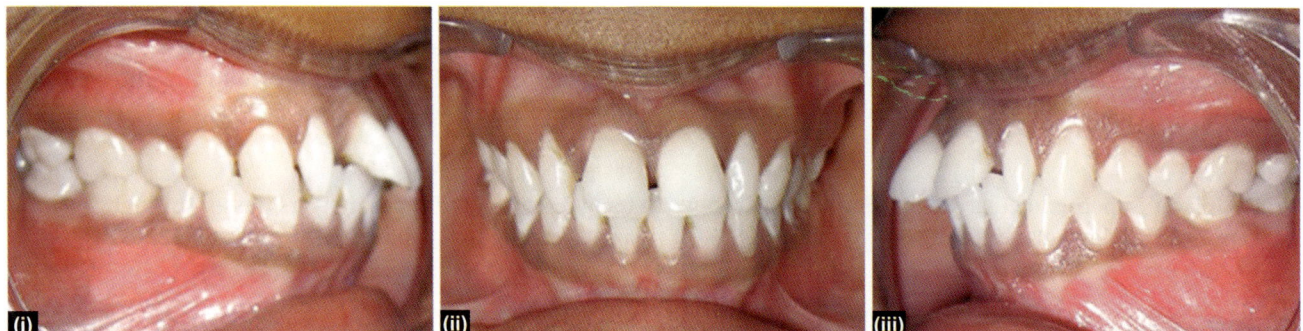

**Figs 8.42 (i to iii):** Ballard's skeletal class I malocclusion

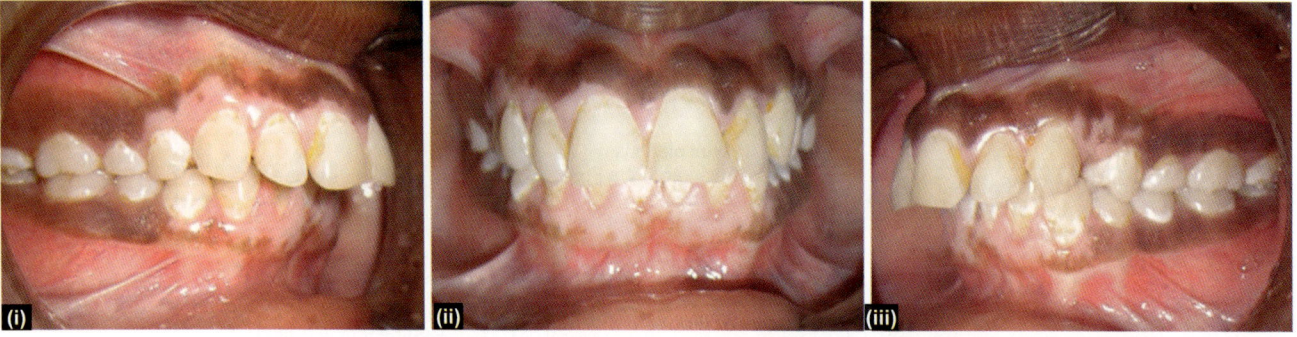

**Figs 8.43 (i to iii):** Ballard's skeletal class II malocclusion

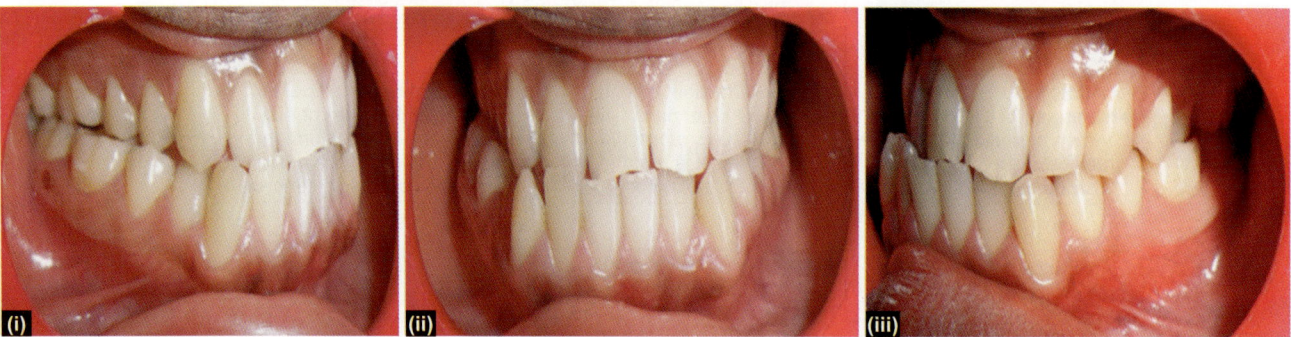

**Figs 8.44 (i to iii):** Ballard's skeletal class III malocclusion

**Flowchart 8.7:** Ballard's classification

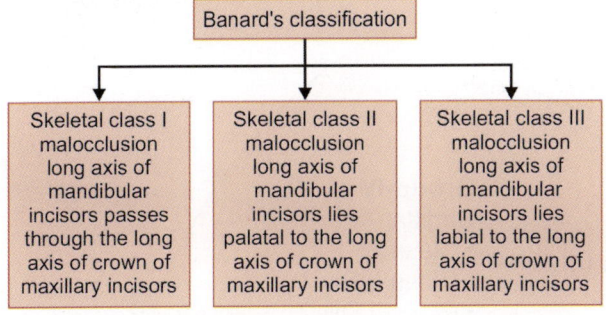

**Flowchart 8.8:** Bennett's classification

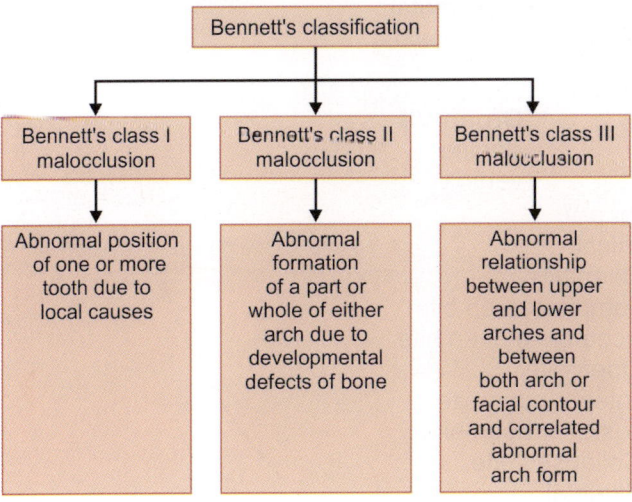

### Skeletal Class II Malocclusion

Long axis of mandibular incisors lies palatal to the long axis of crown of maxillary incisors **(Fig. 8.43i to iii)**.

### Skeletal Class III Malocclusion

Long axis of mandibular incisors lies labial to the long axis of crown of maxillary incisors **(Fig. 8.44i to iii)**.

## BENNETT'S CLASSIFICATION OF MALOCCLUSION

Sir Norman Bennett's classification of malocclusion is based on its etiology. Bennett's classification of malocclusion is as follows **(Flowchart 8.8)**:

### Bennett's Class I Malocclusion

Abnormal position of one or more tooth due to local causes.

### Bennett's Class II Malocclusion

Abnormal formation of a part or whole of either arch due to developmental defects of bone.

### Bennett's Class III Malocclusion

Abnormal relationship between upper and lower arches and between either arch or facial contour and correlated abnormal arch form.

## ACKERMAN-PROFIT SYSTEM OF CLASSIFICATION

Ackerman and Profit is the most recent of all the classifications. It is based on Venn-Diagrams. It has got 9 groups as shown in the **Figure 8.45**. Ackerman and Profit gave an all-inclusive method of diagramming and categorizing malocclusions to overcome the limitations of the Angle's classification system in which five characteristics and their interrelationships are assessed, using a modified Venn diagram.

Five characteristics assessed are:
1. Alignment
2. Profile
3. Type
4. Class
5. Bite depth.

In this classification a set theory is used where sets or groups represent malocclusions. A group contained within a larger enveloping group is a subset of the latter (enveloping group). A subset has the characteristics of its outer group also along with its own characteristics.

Since the degree of alignment and symmetry is common to all dentitions, this is presented as the outer envelope or universe (Group 1). The profile is affected by many malocclusions, so it becomes a major set within the universe (Group 2). Deviations in three planes are presented by Group 3–9 which include the overlapping or interlocking subsets.

## GROUPS AND SETS

### Group 1

Group 1 is the outer all enveloping group/universe, which represents alignment of teeth, since the degree of alignment and symmetry are common to all directions.

### Group 2

Group 2, representing the facial profile, becomes a major set within the universe (group 1), as the profile is affected by many malocclusions.

### Groups 3, 4 and 5

Groups 3, 4 and 5 represent deviations in three planes of space that is transverse (lateral), sagittal (anteroposterior) and vertical plane, respectively.

### Groups 6, 7 and 8

The overlapping groups 6, 7 and 8 at the center of the Venn diagram represent more severe problems, with characteristics from their enveloping groups.

### Group 9

The group 9 at the exact center would be the most severe, with involvement of criteria from all the groups that is alignment, profile, transverse, anteroposterior and vertical problems.

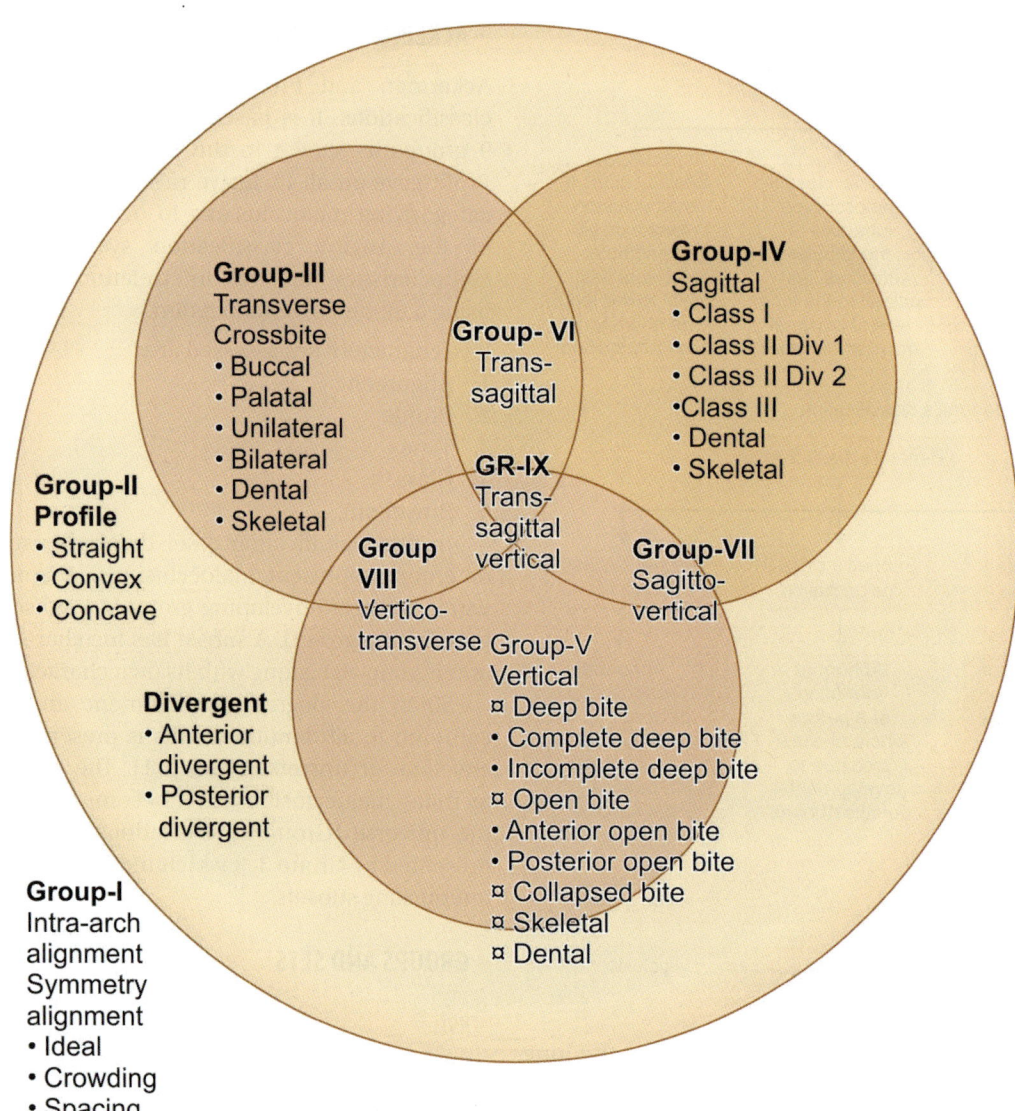

Fig. 8.45: Ackerman-Profit classifications

### Group 1/ Step 1

Group 1 involves assessment of the alignment and symmetry of the dental arch. Possibilities of alignment are:
- Ideal
- Crowding
- Spacing
- Mutilated.
Individual tooth irregularities are described.

### Group 2/Step 2

In this group, the profile is studied. The profile shows:
- Concave
- Straight
- Concave
- Anterior facial divergence
- Posterior facial divergence.

### Group 3/Step 3

Group 3 assesses lateral or transverse dental arch characteristics.

The term type is used to describe various kinds of crossbite.

### Group 4/Step 4

Step 4 involves the assessment of the sagittal relationship.

### Step 5/Bite Depth

The patient and the dentition are viewed regarding the vertical dimensions.

With bite depth used as descriptive term for vertical problems.

## Advantages of Ackerman-Profit Classification

The advantages of Ackerman-Profit classification are as follows:
1. The complexities of malocclusion are explained.
2. All three planes or dimensional problems are included.
3. Profile of the patient is given due consideration
4. This classification helps in complete diagnosis and differential treatment planning.
5. Differentiation between skeletal and dental problem is made easily with this system of classifying malocclusions.
6. Arch length problems are evaluated.
7. Ackerman: Profit introduced a new method of classification to overcome the drawbacks of traditional Angle's classification.
8. Readily adaptable to the computer processing.

## Disadvantages of Ackerman-Profit Classification

1. Etiological considerations are not included in the classification.
2. This system of classifying malocclusion is based only on static occlusion. Functional occlusion not included.

## BIBLIOGRAPHY

1. Angle EH. Classification of malocclusion. Dent Cosmos 1899;41:248-64.
2. Graber TM. Orthodontics: Principles and Practice. WB Saunders, 1998.
3. Profitt WR. Contemporary Orthodontics. St Louis: CV Mosby, 1986.
4. White TC, Gardiner JH, Leighton BC, et al. Orthodontics for Dental Students, 3rd edition. MacMillan Press Ltd, 1976. 5. White TC, Gardiner JH, Leighton BC, et al. Orthodontics for Dental Students, 4th edition. Delhi: Oxford University Press, 1998.

### EXAM-ORIENTED QUESTIONS

*Long Essay or Long Question*

1. What is classification of malocclusions and what are its advantages? Discuss different methods of classification on malocclusion.

*Short Essay or Long Notes*

1. Classify malocclusions and write in detail about any two systems (methods) classification of malocclusion in detail.
2. Define malocclusion and describe its various classification in detail.
3. Angle's classification of malocclusion
4. Dewey's classification of malocclusion
5. Lischer's classification of malocclusion
6, Simon's classification of malocclusion
7. Ackerman's-Profit system of classification of malocclusion.

*Short Notes*

1. Intra-arch malocclusion
2. Inter-arch malocclusion
3. Classification of incisor relationship
4. Canine relationship
5. Molar relationship
6. Ballard's classification of malocclusion
7. Bennett's classification of malocclusion
8. Demerit's of Angle's system of classifying malocclusion.

# CHAPTER OVERVIEW

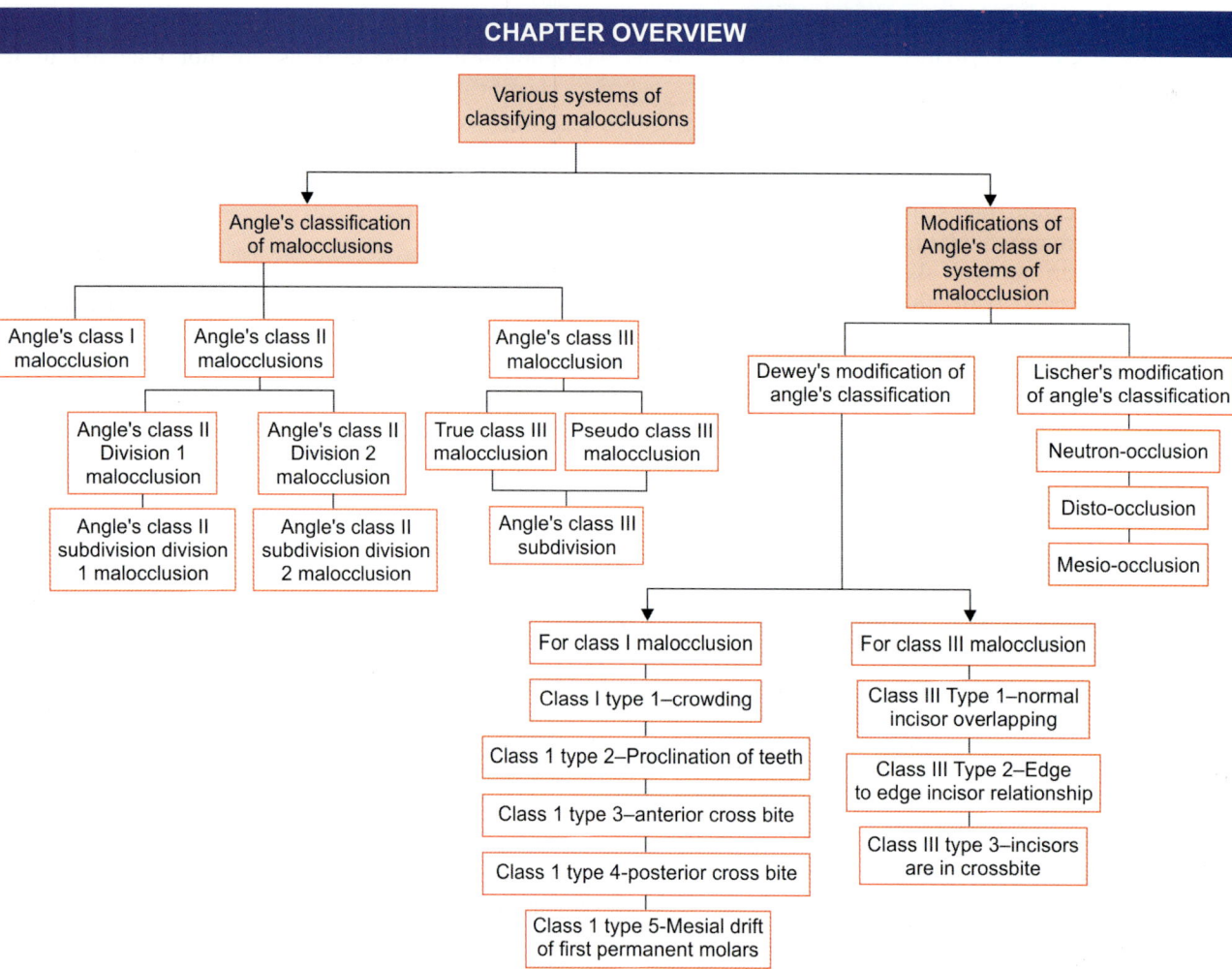

# CHAPTER 9

# General Etiological Factors of Malocclusion

*Rashmi GS, Tsipova V*

Etiology of malocclusion is the study of its causes. The factors causing malocclusion can be widely classified into two broad categories; general etiological factors and local etiological factors. A given case of malocclusion may be a result of either a single or multiple local or general factors or be caused by a combination of local and general factors. An understanding of the etiology is essential in order to prevent, intercept and correct malocclusions.

## CLASSIFICATION

Etiologic factors of malocclusion are classified in a number of ways by different authors and the most commonly referred classifications are listed in **Table 9.1**. The discussion of etiologic factors in this chapter is based on the classification given by Graber.

General aetiologic factors include the following:
- Hereditary
- Congenital
- Environmental
  - Prenatal
    - Trauma
    - Maternal diet
    - German measles
    - Maternal metabolism.
  - Postnatal
    - Birth injury
    - Cerebral palsy
    - Temporomandibular joint (TMJ) injury.
- Predisposing metabolic climate and disease
  - Endocrine imbalance
  - Metabolic disturbances
  - Infectious diseases.

**Table 9.1:** Classification

| Moyer's | Graber's |
|---|---|
| - Hereditary | - Hereditary |
|   • Neuromuscular system | - Congenital |
|   • Bone | - Environmental |
|   • Teeth |   • Prenatal (trauma, maternal diet, German measles, maternal metabolism, etc.) |
|   • Soft tissues |   • Postnatal (birth injury, cerebral palsy, TMJ injury) |
| - Developmental defects of unknown origin | - Predisposing metabolic climate and disease |
| - Trauma |   • Endocrine imbalance |
|   • Prenatal trauma and birth injuries |   • Metabolic disturbances |
|   • Postnatal trauma |   • Infectious diseases |
| - Physical agents | - Dietary problems (nutritional deficiency) |
|   • Premature extraction of primary teeth | - Abnormal pressure habits and functional aberrations |
|   • Nature of food |   • Abnormal sucking |
| - Habits |   • Thumb and finger sucking |
| - Diseases |   • Lip and nail biting |
|   • Systemic diseases |   • Abnormal swallowing habits (improper deglutition) |
|   • Endocrine disorders |   • Speech defects |
|   • Local diseases |   • Tongue thrust and tongue sucking |
|     ♦ Nasopharyngeal diseases and disturbed respiratory function |   • Respiratory abnormalities (mouth breathing, etc.) |
|     ♦ Gingival and periodontal diseases |   • Tonsils and adenoids |
|     ♦ Tumors |   • Psychogenetics and bruxism |
|     ♦ Caries | - Posture |
| - Malnutrition\**Graber's classification** | - Trauma and accidents |

*Contd...*

Contd...

| White and Gardiner's Classification | Local factors |
|---|---|
| ▪ **Dental base abnormalities** | ▪ Anomalies of number: |
| • Anteroposterior malrelationship | • Supernumerary teeth |
| • Vertical malrelationship | • Missing teeth (congenital absence or loss due to caries, accidents) |
| • Lateral malrelationship | ▪ Anomalies of tooth size |
| • Disproportion of size between teeth and basal bone | ▪ Anomalies of tooth shape |
| • Congenital abnormalities | ▪ Abnormal labial frenum: Mucosal barriers |
| ▪ **Pre-eruption abnormalities** | ▪ Premature loss of deciduous teeth |
| • Abnormalities in position of developing tooth germ | ▪ Prolonged retention of deciduous teeth |
| • Missing teeth | ▪ Delayed eruption of permanent teeth |
| • Supernumerary teeth and teeth abnormal in form | ▪ Abnormal eruptive path |
| • Prolonged retention of deciduous teeth | ▪ Ankylosis |
| • Abnormal labial frenum attachment | ▪ Dental caries |
| • Traumatic injury | ▪ Improper dental restoration |
| ▪ **Post-eruption abnormalities** | |
| • Muscular | |
| ⬥ Active muscle force | |
| ⬥ Rest position of musculature | |
| ⬥ Sucking habits | |
| ⬥ Abnormalities in path of closure | |
| • Premature loss of deciduous teeth | |
| • Extraction of permanent teeth | |

- Dietary problems (nutritional deficiency)
- Abnormal pressure habits and functional aberrations.
  - Abnormal sucking
  - Thumb and finger sucking
  - Tongue thrust and tongue sucking
  - Lip and nail biting
  - Abnormal swallowing habits (improper deglutition)
  - Speech defects
  - Respiratory abnormalities, like mouth breathing, etc.
  - Tonsils and adenoids
  - Psychogenetics and bruxism
- Posture
- Trauma and accidents.

## Hereditary Factors

Hereditary cause of malocclusion include genetic trait, inherited from the parents, which may contribute to the development of malocclusion. These genetic traits can be further influenced by prenatal or postnatal environmental factors. Since the offspring is a product of parent of dissimilar heredity, malocclusion can result, if the end product is disharmonious. Further more, studies show that the incidence of jaw size discrepancies and occlusal

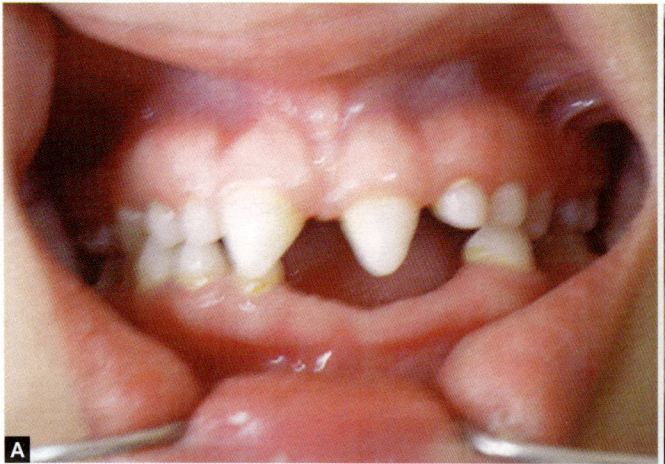
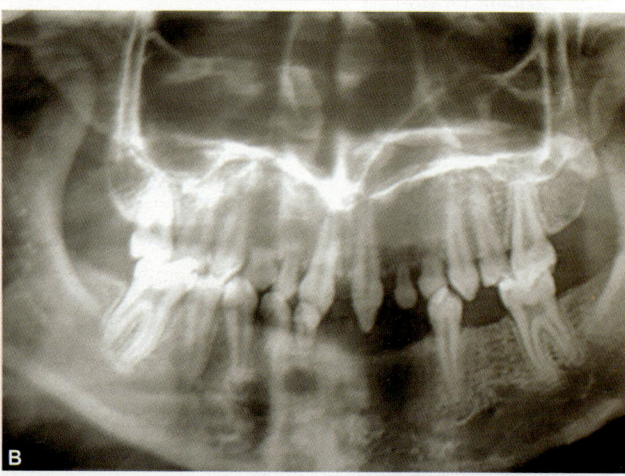

**Figs 9.1A and B:** (A) Patient with ectodermal dysplasia exhibit conical shaped incisors and several congenitally missing teeth; (B) Orthopantomogram (OPG) of the same patient

disharmonies is greater in population, where there has been a mixture of racial and ethnic strain.

The hereditary factors causing malocclusion can be those influencing the following:
- Dentition
- Skeletal structure
- Neuromuscular
- Soft tissues.

## Dentition
The following characteristics of dentition are influenced by heredity.

### Shape and Size of the Tooth
Abnormalities of the tooth size, such as macrodontia, microdontia and abnormalities of tooth shape such as peg lateral are attributed to heredity. Patients with ectodermal dysplasia exhibit conical-shaped incisors and several congenitally missing teeth **(Figs 9.1A and B)**.

### Number of Teeth
Presence of supernumerary teeth **(Figs 9.2A and B)** or congenitally missing teeth is often hereditary.

### Arch Dimension
Dental arch length and width are believed to be inherited.

### Crowding and Spacing
Arch length-tooth material discrepancy is one of the most common causes of malocclusion and is the result of the disharmonious inheritance of the tooth size from one parent and that of the jaw length from the other parent.

### Shedding Pattern of Deciduous Teeth and Sequence of Eruption of Permanent Teeth
They are to some extent under the influence of heredity.

### Inter-arch Variation
Deviation in the transverse sagittal and vertical plane relationship of upper and lower jaw can be inherited.

### Overjet
The degree of horizontal overlap of the upper anteriors over the lower anteriors called overjet and it can be inherited.

### Skeletal Structures
Skeletal malocclusion, resulting from the malposition or malformation of the jaws is often inherited. Mandibular Class III skeletal pattern with mandibular prognathism is commonly observed to show racial and familial tendencies **(Fig. 9.3)**.

### Neuromuscular System
The anomalies that have been found to possess some inherited component include deformities in size, position, tonicity, contractility and in the neuromuscular coordination pattern of facial, oral and tongue musculature.

### Soft Tissue
The following are some of the soft tissue abnormalities, which can be inherited.
- Size, shape and attachment of the labial frenum
- Ankyloglossia
- Microstomia.

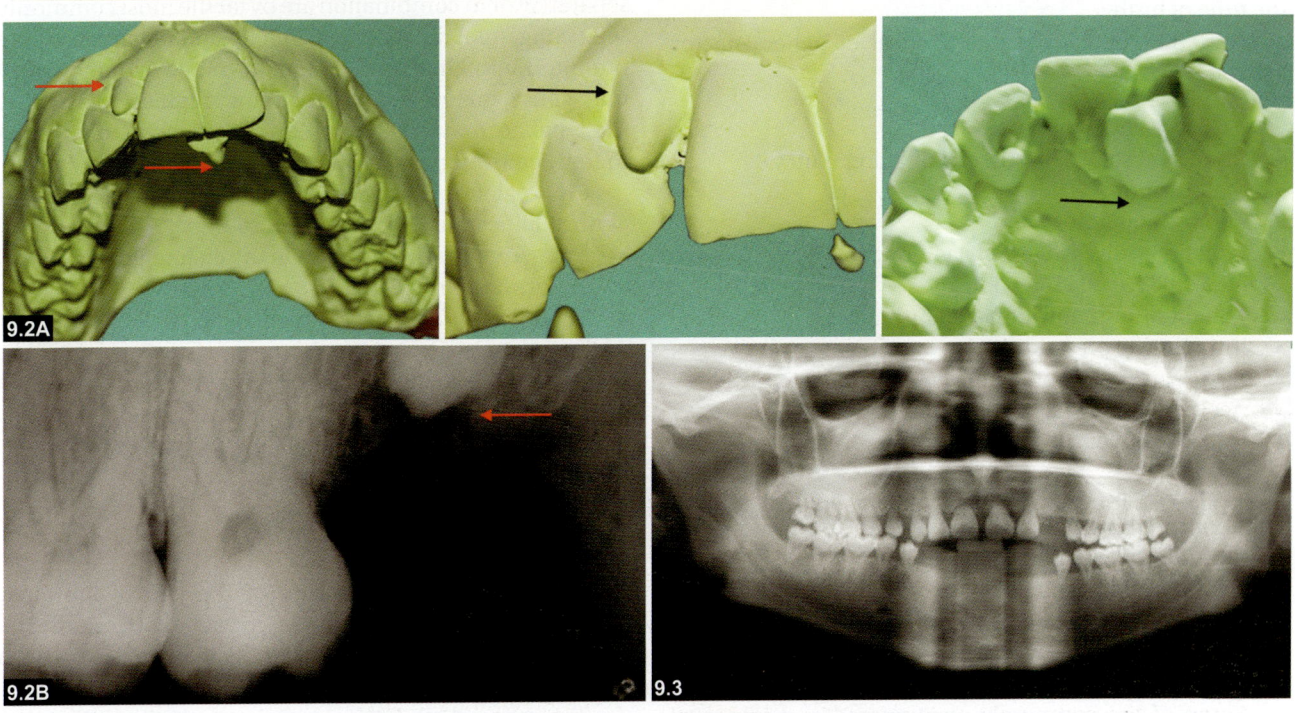

**Figs 9.2A and B:** (A) Cast showing labially erupted conical-shaped supernumerary tooth and palatally erupted mesodens with Talon cusp causing crowding in the arch; (B) Impacted distomolar; **Fig. 9.3:** Type I dentin dysplasia exhibiting extremely short conical roots with prematurely lost lower incisors

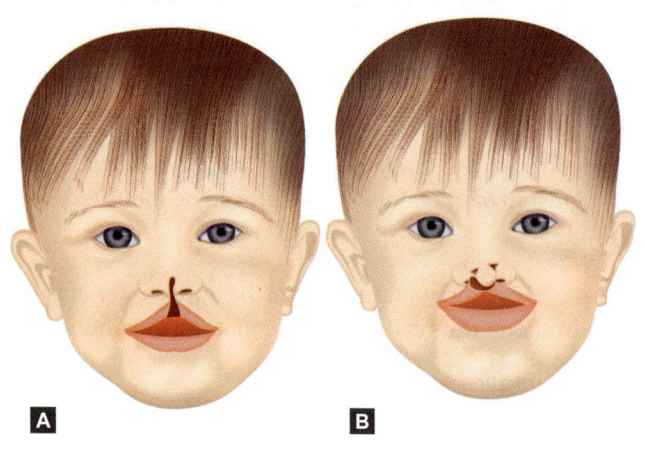

**Figs 9.4A and B:** (A) Unilateral cleft lip and (B) Bilateral cleft lip

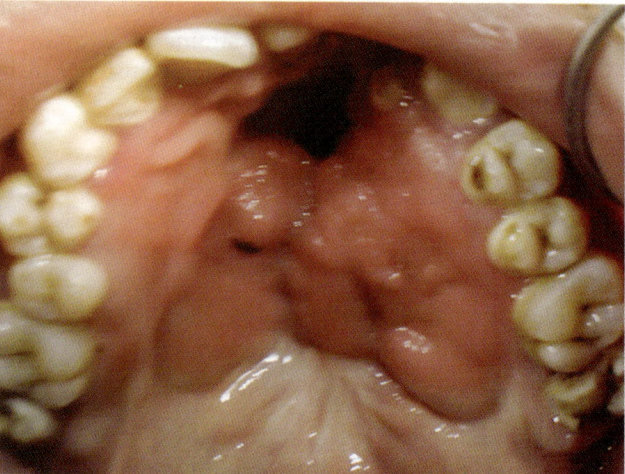

**Fig. 9.5:** Cleft palate

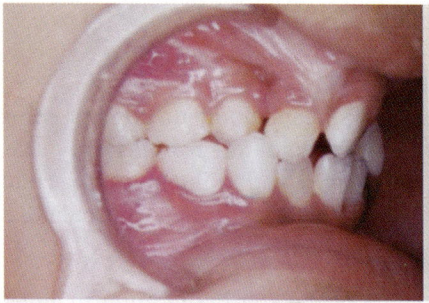 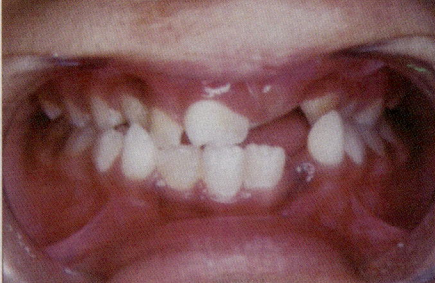 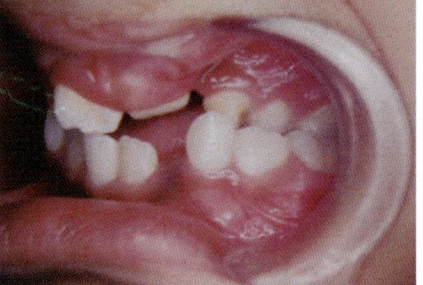

**Fig. 9.6A:** A patient with cleft palate showing a number of dental abnormalities (A) congenitally missing teeth in the cleft region

## Congenital Defects

Congenital defects are the developmental malformation at the time of birth.

They may be caused due to local or general factors listed below:

### General Congenital Factors

- Abnormal state of mother during pregnancy
- Malnutrition
- Endocrinopathies
- Infectious diseases, such as congenital syphilis and maternal rubella infection
- Metabolic and nutritional disturbances
- Intrauterine pressure
- Accidents during pregnancy and child birth
- Accidental trauma to the fetus by external forces, e.g. forceps delivery.

### Local Congenital Factors

- Abnormalities of jaw development due to abnormal intrauterine position
- Cyst of the face and palate
- Macroglossia
- Microglossia
- Cleidocranial dystosis.

Some of the commonly encountered and important congenital defects from orthodontist's point of view are discussed here:

### Cleft Lip and Palate

Cleft lip (**Figs 9.4A and B**) and palate (**Fig. 9.5**), occurring separately or in combination are by far the most commonly seen congenital deformities. Cleft lip and palate may have profound influence on the craniofacial development and may cause malocclusion of varying degrees of severity. Cleft palate may retard nomal development of maxilla thereby causing class III malocclusion.

Cleft palate may show a number of associated dental abnormalities, such as (**Figs 9.6A to E**):

- Congenitally missing teeth in the cleft region
- Supernumerary teeth
- Microdontia and peg-shaped teeth, especially upper lateral incisor
- Crowding of teeth in the area of cleft
- Insufficient development of premaxilla
- Crossbite due to narrow maxillary arch
- Rotation of teeth
- Abnormal overjet and overbites.

### Cerebral Palsy

It is characterized by paralysis or the lack of muscular coordination, attributed to an intracranial lesion. The condition is often considered to be the result of a birth injury.

The uncontrolled or aberrant activities upset the muscle balance that is necessary for establishment and maintenance of normal occlusion.

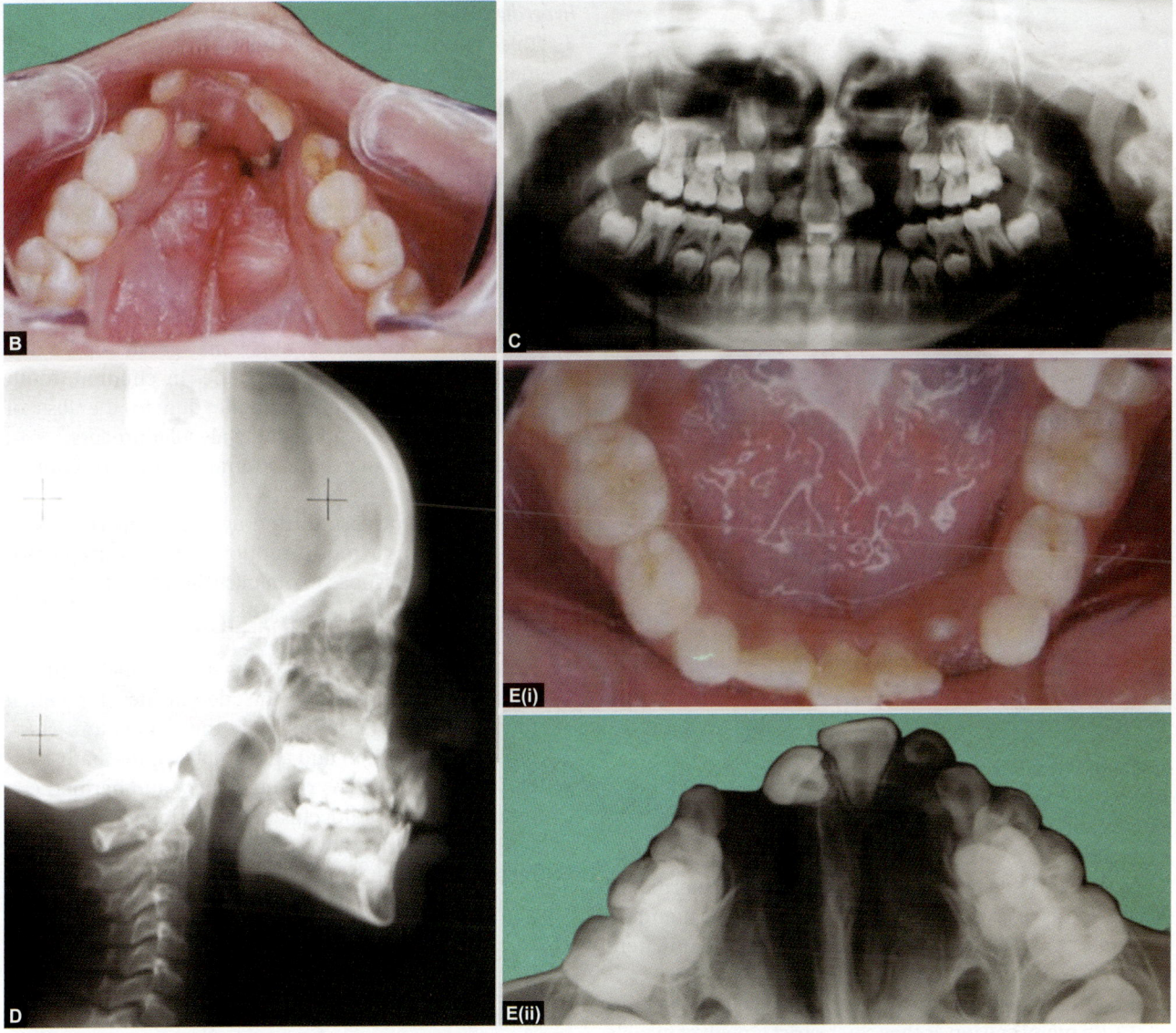

**Figs 9.6B to E:** A patient with cleft palate showing a number of dental abnormalities; (B) Supernumerary teeth; (C) Microdontia and peg shaped teeth, especially upper lateral; (D) Crowding of teeth in the area of cleft; (E) Abnormal development of premaxilla

### Cleidocranial Dysostosis

This condition is characterized by partial or complete absence of the clavicle on one or both sides. Various features that may lead to the development of malocclusion are:

- Maxillary retrusion and possible mandibular protrusion
- Retained deciduous teeth
- Retarded eruption of permanent teeth
- Numerous impacted supernumerary teeth.

### Maternal Rubella Infection during Pregnancy

Rubella infection in a pregnant mother can cause a number of dental defects in the child such as:

- Retarded eruption of teeth
- Hypoplasia of teeth **(Fig. 9.7)**
- Extensive caries.

### Congenital Syphilis

The incidence of congenital syphilis is greatly reduced in the recent years. The following features may be seen in the affected child:

- Hutchinson's incisors
- Mulberry molars
- Maxillary deficiency in relation to mandible
- Anterior crossbite
- Extensive dental caries.

## Environmental Causes

Various prenatal and postnatal environmental factors can cause malocclusion.

### Prenatal Environmental Factors

The following are some of the prenatal factors that can cause malocclusion:

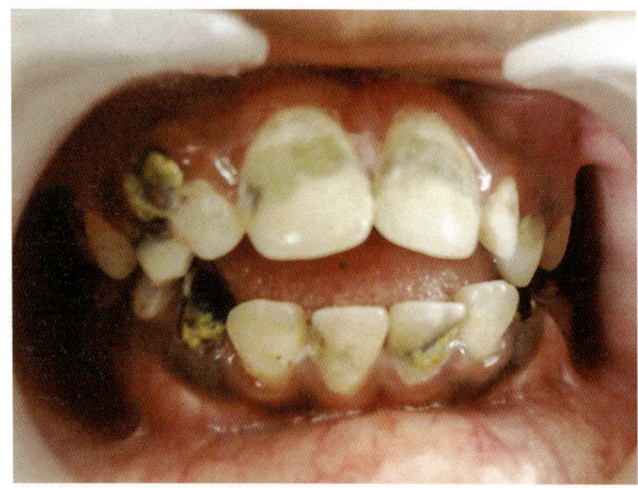

**Fig. 9.7:** Open bite with hypoplasia of teeth

- Abnormal fetal posture during gestation
- Maternal fibroids
- Amniotic lesions
- Maternal diet and metabolism
- Intake of certain drugs during pregnancy, for example thalidomide intake can cause congenital deformities, such as clefts.

### Postnatal Environmental Factors

The following are some of the postnatal factors that can cause malocclusion:

- Traumatic injuries to the condyle and the TMJ area during birth can cause mandibular growth retardation.
- Ankylosis of the TMJ may lead to hypoplastic mandible and marked facial asymmetry in case of the unilateral ankylosis.
- Presence of scar tissue, caused by cleft palate surgery may cause malocclusion as they can restrict growth of maxilla.
- Milwaukee braces used for the treatment of scoliosis derive support from the mandible, and thus can cause retardation of the mandibular growth.

### Predisposing Metabolic Climate and Diseases

Endocrinal imbalance may predispose to the development of malocclusion. Thyroid hormones play an important role in the normal development of bones and teeth. Parathormone, released from the parathyroid glands, has an active role in calcium metabolism and thus is directly involved in the development of teeth and bones.

### Hypothyroidism

It may cause the following effects:
- Retardation in the rate of calcium deposition in bone and teeth
- Delaying tooth bud formation and eruption
- Prolonged retention of primary and delayed eruption of permanent teeth
- Irregularities in tooth arrangement and crowding of teeth may occur.

### Hyperthyroidism

- This condition is associated with the increased metabolic rate and increased rate of maturation.
- Patient with hyperthyroidism may exhibit premature eruption of primary and permanent dentition.

### Hypoparathyroidism

It is often associated with delayed eruption of teeth, altered morphology and hypoplasia of teeth.

### Hyperparathyroidism

It causes an increase in blood calcium level by resorption of bone. Trabecular pattern of jaw may get disrupted due to the demineralization of the bone. In children, tooth development may become mobile due to the loss of cortical bone and resorption of the alveolar process.

Osteoporosis in such parts contraindicates orthodontic tooth movement.

Acute febrile disease during development years may cause disturbances in tooth eruption and shedding pattern and thus may predispose to malocclusion.

### Dietary Problems (Nutritional Deficiencies)

- Nutritional deficiencies may cause malocclusion primarily by upsetting the dental developmental timetable and resulting in the premature loss, prolonged retention and abnormal eruptive paths.
- Disturbances, such as rickets, scurvy and beriberi can produce severe malocclusion. Nutritional deficiencies during pregnancy have been associated with certain malformations in the child, including cretinism and cleft lip and palate.

### Abnormal Pressure Habits and Functional Aberrations

Abnormal pressure habits, such as digit sucking (**Figs 9.8A to C**), tongue thrusting, lip biting (**Fig. 9.9**) and functional aberration, such as mouth breathing may cause a variety of malocclusions. These aspects are described in detail in a separate chapter on Oral Habits (**Chapter 21**).

### Posture

Mandibular retrusion has been observed in some stoop shouldered children with head hung so that the chin rests on the chest and in some children who rest their chin on the hand to support their head. However, poor posture as a cause of malocclusion is not proved. Nevertheless, it might accentuate an existing malocclusion.

### Accident and Trauma

Traumatic injuries to the dentofacial region are quite common during early years of life when child learns to crawl, walk and even while playing. Such traumatic experiences often go unnoticed and may result in the following problems predisposing to malocclusion:
- Nonvital deciduous teeth that do not resorb.
- Deflection of permanent tooth germs.
- Abnormal eruption path of permanent successors.

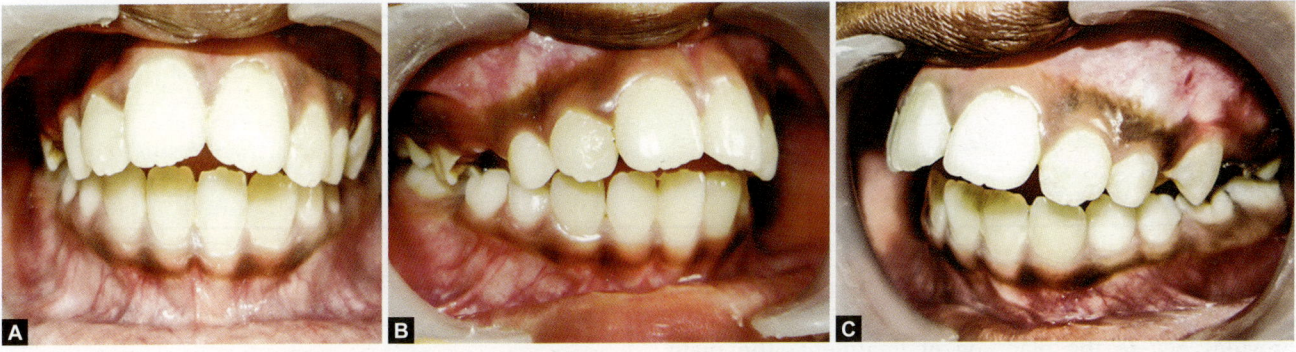

**Figs 9.8A to C:** A patient with thumb sucking habit causing skeletal class II division 1 malocclusion

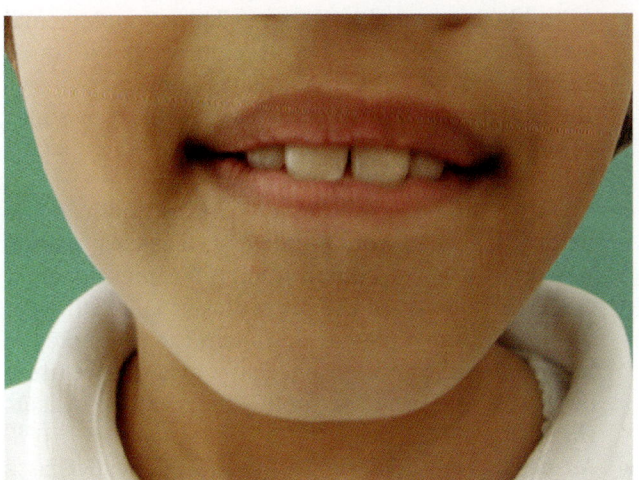

**Fig. 9.9:** A patient with lip-biting habit

## BIBLIOGRAPHY

1. Angle EH. Classification of malocclusion. Dental Cosmos 1899;41:248-64,350-7.
2. Edwards JG. A long-term prospective evaluation of the circumferencial supracrestal fiberotomy in alleviating orthodontic relapse. Am J Orthod Dentofacial Orthop. 1988;93:380-7.
3. Federation Dentaire Internationale. Commission on classification and statistics for oral conditions: a method for measuring occlusal traits. Int Dent J. 1973;23:530-7.
4. Grainger RM. Orthodontic treatment priority index. Vita Heath Stat 1967;2:1-49.
5. Harris JE, Kowalski CJ, Watnick SS. Genetic factors in the shape of the craniofacial complex. Angle Orthod. 1973;43(1):107-11.
6. Hill PA. The prevalence and severity of malocclusion and the need for orthodontic treatment in 9-,12-, and 15-year- old Glasgow school children. Br J Orthod. 1992;19:87-96.
7. Kharbanda OP, Sidhu SS. Study of the etiological factors associated with the development of malocclusion. J Clin Pediat 1994;18:80-95.
8. Larsson E, Dahlin K. The prevalence and etiology of the initial dummy- and finger-sucking habit. Am J Orthod. 1985;432-5.
9. Massler M, Frankel JM. Prevalence of malocclusion in children aged 14 to 18 years. Am J Orthod. 1951;37:751-8.
10. McNeill RW, Joondeph DR. Congenitally absent maxillary lateral incisors: treatment planning considerations. Angle Orthod. 1973; 43:24-9.
11. Punkey PJ, Sadowsky C, BeGole EA. Tooth morphology and lower incisor alignment many years after orthodontic therapy. Am J Orthod. 1984;86(4)299-305.
12. Shields TE, Little RM, Chapko MK. Stability and relapse of mandibular anterior alignment:a cephalometric appraisal of first premolar extraction cases treated by traditional edgewise orthodontics. Am J Orthod. 1985;87(1):27-38.

## EXAM-ORIENTED QUESTIONS

### Long Essay or Long Questions

1. Classify the etiology of malocclusion. Discuss general factors in detail.
2. Discuss the environmental or local causes of malocclusion.
3. Enumerate various postnatal causes of malocclusion. Elaborate endocrinal factors.

### Long Note or Short Essay

1. Moyer's classification for general etiological factors of malocclusion'.
2. Graber's classification for general etiological factors of malocclusion.

### Short Note

1. How does dental caries cause malocclusion?

# CHAPTER 10

# Local Etiological Factors

*Rashmi GS*

Etiological assessment of malocclusion is an important aspect in orthodontics as the genesis of the deformity provides key to the planning of treatment. The main etiological factors which play a part, at least to some extent in most malocclusions are—the skeletal relationship, function of oral musculature and the size of the dentition in relation to the size of the jaw bones. Less frequently, local factors may cause malocclusion, either in conjunction with or independent of other etiological factors (**Box 10.1**).

**Box 10.1:** Local factors causing malocclusion, according to Graber

- Anomalies of number
  - Supernumerary teeth
  - Missing teeth
- Anomalies of tooth size
- Anomalies of tooth shape
- Premature loss of deciduous teeth
- Prolonged retention of deciduous teeth
- Delayed eruption of permanent teeth
- Abnormal labial frenum
- Dental caries
- Improper dental restorations
- Ankylosis
- Abnormal eruptive path.

## ANOMALIES OF TOOTH NUMBER

Anomalies of tooth number include presence of extra teeth or absence of one or more teeth that can predispose to malocclusion.

### Supernumerary Teeth

- Extra teeth in relation to the normal complement of teeth are generally referred to as supernumerary teeth. These teeth usually have abnormal morphology and do not resemble normal teeth. Extra teeth, which closely resemble the normal teeth, are called as supplemental teeth, which are often observed to occur on lateral incisors (**Fig. 10.1A**) and premolar regions.
- The occurrence of supernumerary teeth may be single or multiple, unilateral or bilateral, erupted or impacted (**Fig. 10.1B**) in one or both the jaws.
- The term mesiodens is used for extra tooth in the midline between two permanent maxillary central incisors; the most common site for supernumerary teeth. Mesiodens are usually conical shaped although they can be tuberculated. Mesiodens can be erupted or impacted and when present may cause malocclusion by displacing one or both the central incisors (**Fig. 10.1C**).
- An extra tooth adjacent to the molar is called as a paramolar and when present distal to the last molar is called as distomolar. The term parapremolar is sometimes used for an extra tooth in premolar regions (**Fig. 10.1D**).
- Supernumerary teeth may cause arch length tooth material discrepancy and crowding when erupted; may delay, prevent or deviate the path of eruption of adjacent teeth.

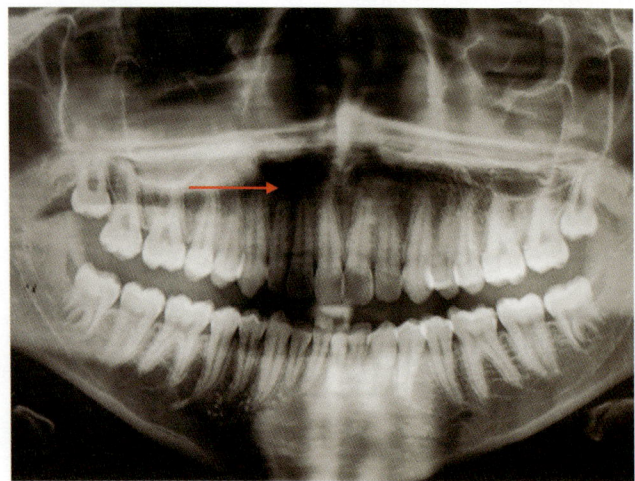

**Fig. 10.1A:** Supplemental lateral incisor causing crowding in the arch OPG of the patient

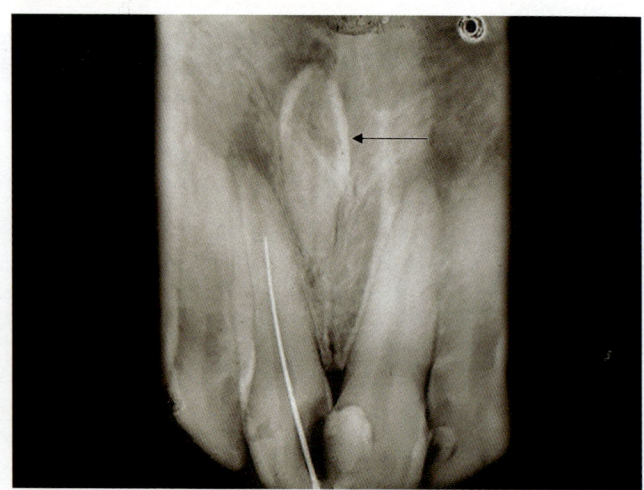

**Fig. 10.1B:** Inverted and impacted mesiodens has resulted in rotations of central incisors

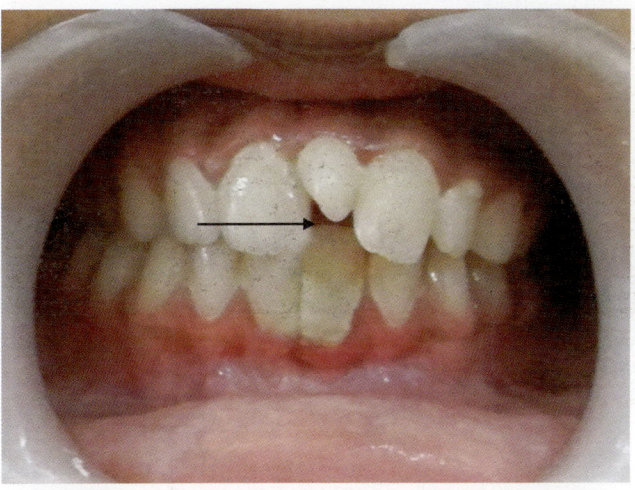

**Fig. 10.1C:** Labially erupted mesiodens causing mesiolabial or distopalatal rotation of left permanent maxillary central incisor

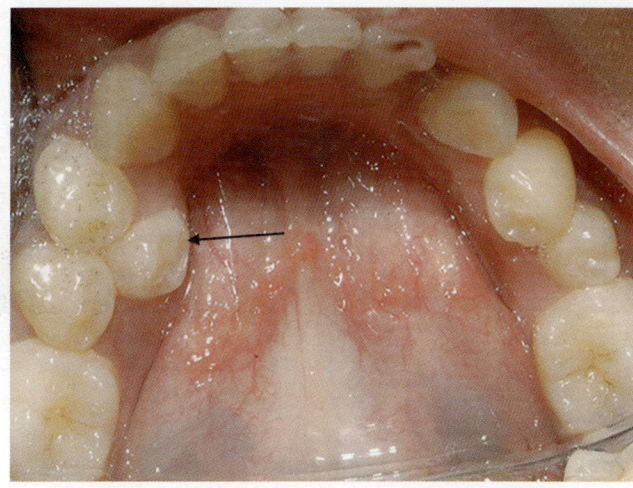

**Fig. 10.1D:** Lingually erupted parapremolar causing mild-buccal displacement of first premolar. Crowding in the posterior segment

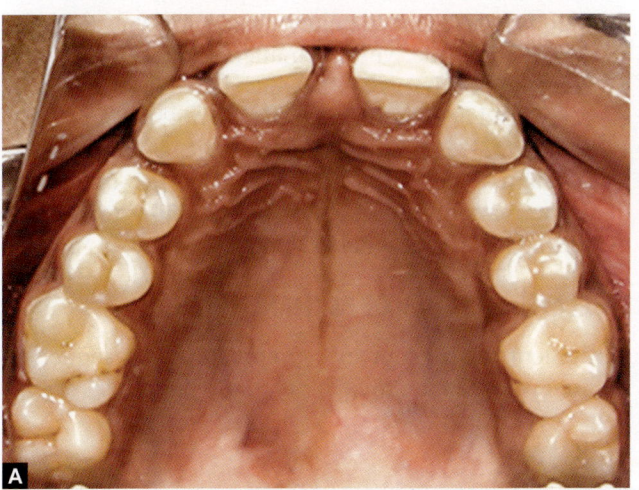
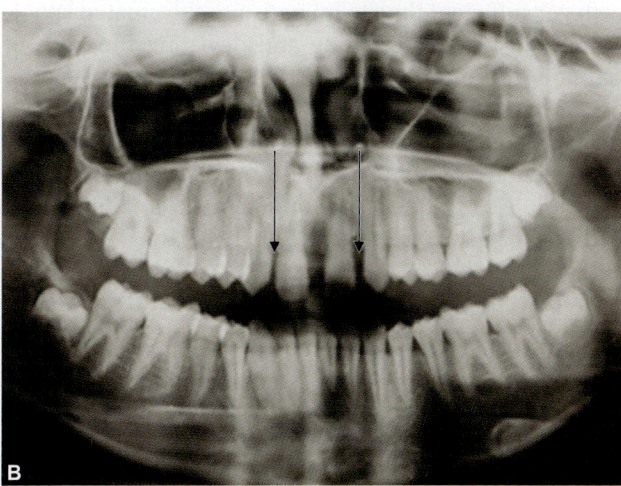

**Figs 10.2A and B:** (A) Bilateral congenitally missing permanent lateral incisors causing spacing; (B) Radiographic representation of the same

- Unerupted supernumerary teeth show a tendency for cyst formation and unerupted mesiodens can cause midline diastema.

### Congenitally Missing Teeth

- The occurrence of congenitally missing teeth may be single or multiple, unilateral or bilateral and in one or both the jaws **(Figs 10.2A and B)**.
- Anodontia or congenital absence of teeth may be of two types, total and partial. Total anodontia in which all teeth are missing may involve both deciduous and permanent teeth.
- Total anodontia is quite rare and usually occurs in association with hereditary ectodermal dysplasia whereas, partial anodontia, involving one or more teeth is rather common.
- The term hypodontia is used for absence of only few teeth; oligodontia refers to the absence of many but not all teeth.

## ANOMALIES OF TOOTH SIZE

- Anomalies of tooth size may occur as two forms: microdontia or macrodontia.
- The term microdontia is used to describe teeth, which are smaller than normal **(Fig. 10.3A)**.
- Microdontia can be generalized involving all the teeth in a dentition or localized involving a single tooth.
- Localized microdontia most commonly affects maxillary lateral incisors and third molars **(Fig. 10.3B)**.
- The term macrodontia **(Fig. 10.3C)** refers to teeth that are larger than normal. Like microdontia, macrodontia can also be generalized or localized.

## ANOMALIES OF TOOTH SHAPE

Anomalies of tooth shape often occur in association with anomalies of tooth size. Some of the anomalies of tooth shape with considerable significance in orthodontia are listed in **Table 10.1**. They may predispose to malocclusion.

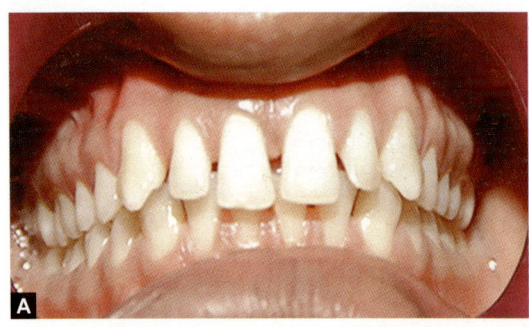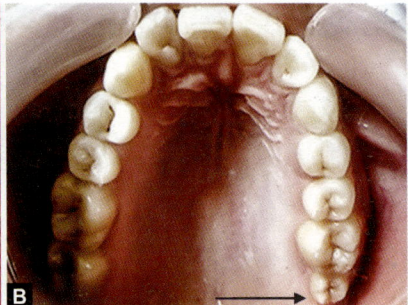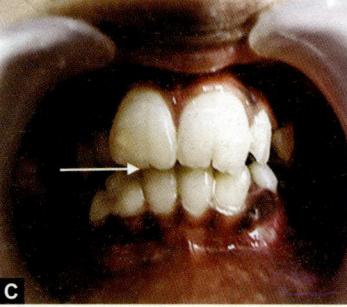

**Figs 10.3A to C:** (A) Relative microdontic causing spacing in the anterior region of the arches; (B) Microdontic right maxillary second molar; (C) Macrodontic right maxillary central incisor causing crowding in the arches—Intraoral frontal view

## PREMATURE LOSS OF DECIDUOUS TEETH

This is a condition where a primary tooth is lost before its permanent successor is ready to erupt. As the adjacent teeth get sufficient time to migrate into the created space, thereby delaying, preventing and deviating the path of eruption of the succeeding permanent tooth. Premature loss of deciduous teeth, if not intercepted often lead to malocclusion. Deciduous teeth may be lost prematurely due to dental caries, trauma and hyperthyroidism.

Possible consequences of premature loss of deciduous teeth on occlusion are listed in **Table 10.2**.

## PROLONGED RETENTION OF DECIDUOUS TEETH

This is a condition in which there is undue retention of deciduous teeth beyond the usual exception age of their permanent successor. More often than not, some parts of deciduous molar roots escape resorption as their successor.

There are number of causes for prolonged retention of deciduous teeth as listed below:
- Absence of underlying permanent tooth **(Fig. 10.9)**
- Nonvital deciduous tooth, which fail to resorb
- Ankylosed deciduous tooth that do not resorb
- Endocrinal disturbances, for example hypothyroidism.

A retained deciduous tooth may be left untouched of its permanent successor in congenitally missing as evidenced by radiographic evaluation.

## DELAYED ERUPTION OF PERMANENT TEETH

Permanent teeth erupt in a preprogrammed sequential manner throughout mixed dentition period to occupy

| Table 10.1: Anomalies of tooth shape | |
|---|---|
| **Anomalies of tooth shape** | **Effects** |
| **Talon's Cusp**<br>Anomalous structures projecting from the cingulum of maxillary permanent incisors **(Figs 10.4A and B)** | - When large, Talon's cusp may prevent establishment of normal overbite and overjet<br>- Forces from the antagonistic tooth in occlusion with Talon's cusp may cause labial tipping of the affected tooth |
| **Peg Laterals**<br>The maxillary lateral incisors with incisally converging mesial and distal surfaces to give a peg-shaped appearance **(Fig. 10.5A)** | - Spacing in the arch<br>- Migration of adjacent teeth<br>- Abnormal incisors relationship |
| **Leong Premolar**<br>An accessory cusp or a globule of an enamel on occlusal surface between buccal and lingual cusps of premolars **(Fig. 10.5B)**. | The *extra* cusp may prevent normal intercuspation with the opposing tooth |
| **Mulberry Molars/Moon's Molar**<br>In congenital syphilis, the crowns of first molars are often irregular with globules of enamel on occlusal surface rather than well-formed cusps "Screw drivers" shaped incisors with a notch by the incisal edges may also be seen in congenital syphilis | Irregular occlusal surface of molars may prevent formal intercuspation of posteriors |
| **Fusion**<br>Fusion of adjacent teeth due to union of two normally separated tooth germs | Spacing in the arch |
| **Gemination**<br>Division of a single tooth germ with resultant incomplete formations of two teeth **(Figs 10.6A and B)** | Discrepancy in arch length and tooth material that may cause crowding (if multiple teeth are affected) |
| **Dilaceration**<br>An abnormal angulation in the root of a tooth or between crown and the root **(Fig. 10.7)** | The tooth may fail to erupt up to normal level |

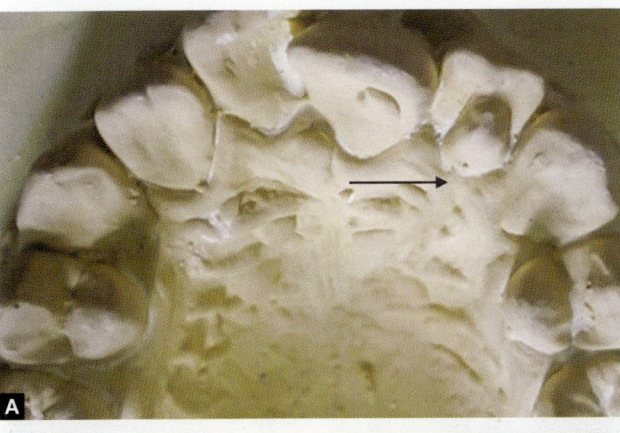 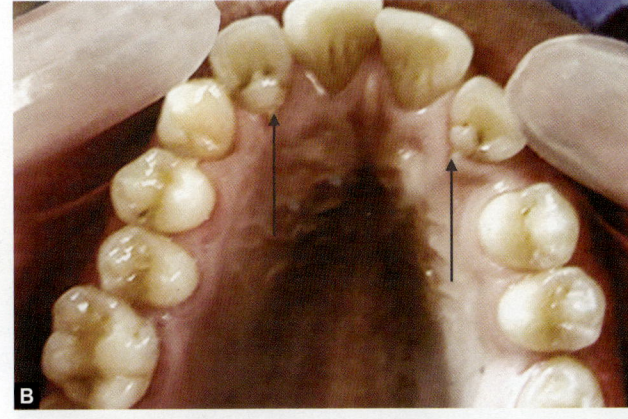

**Figs 10.4A and B:** Talon's cusp seen on the maxillary lateral incisors

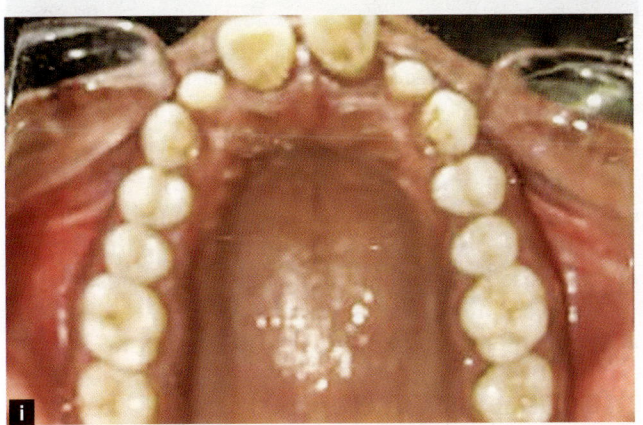 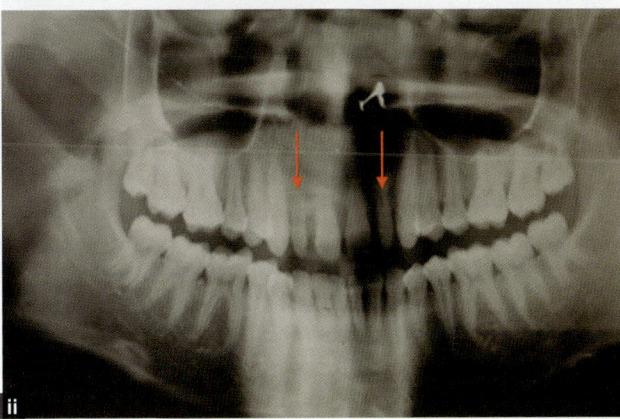

**Figs 10.5A(i and ii):** Bilateral peg-shaped lateral incisors causing spacing in the arch. (i) Intraoral photographs and (ii) OPG of the same patient

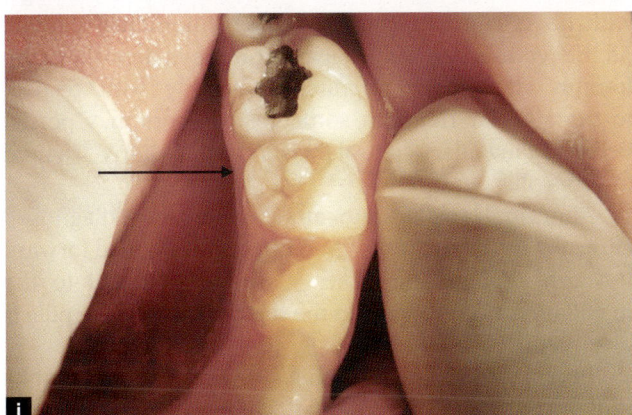 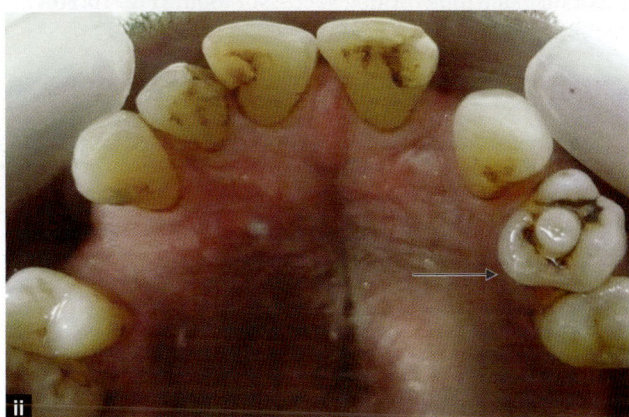

**Figs 10.5B(i and ii):** Leong's premolar/Dens evaginatus

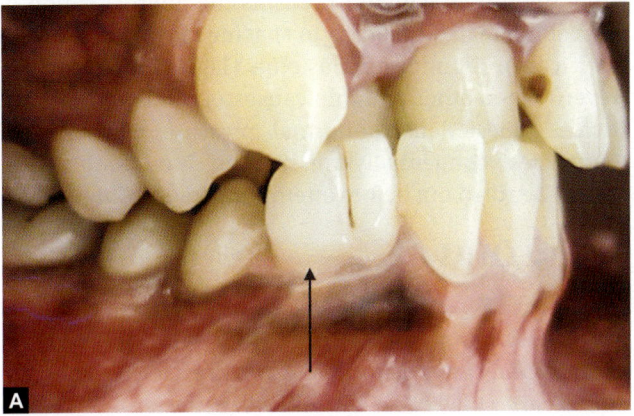 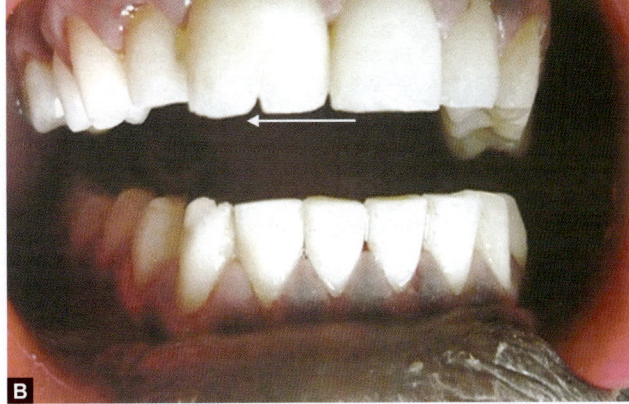

**Figs 10.6A and B:** (A) Gemination of mandibular lateral incisor causing lingual eruption of canine; (B) Gemination of right maxillary central incisor

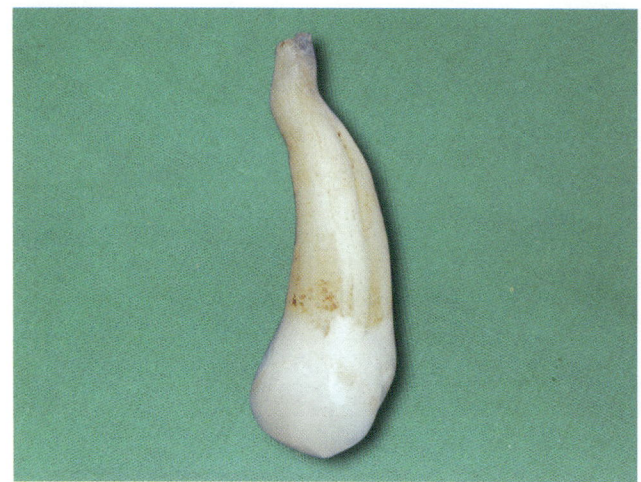

Fig. 10.7: A tooth specimen showing dilacerated root

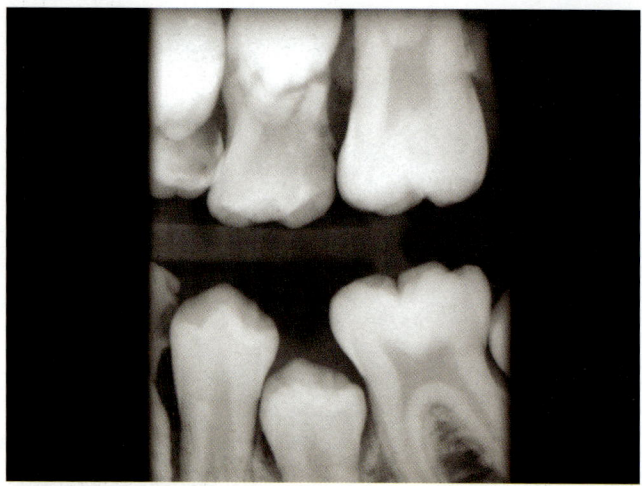

Fig. 10.8: Premature loss of mandibular deciduous second molar has resulted mesial migration of first molar

their respective places. A delay in the eruption of any of the permanent teeth, out of normal time to meet, however, can cause migration of adjacent teeth into the available space. This may result in facial/lingual eruption of the tooth involved or its complete impaction.

Some of the common causes of delayed eruption of permanent teeth are listed below:

- Presence of supernumerary teeth, for example mesiodens can delay eruption of maxillary centrals.
- Retained deciduous root fragments in the jaw may delay or displace the erupting successor tooth (**Fig. 10.10A**).
- Presence of thick mucosal barrier overlying the erupting permanent tooth (**Fig. 10.10B**).
- Premature loss of deciduous tooth can delay eruption of its successor due to formation of bony barrier.
- Ankylosed deciduous tooth that do not resorb can delay eruption of its successor.
- Endocrinal disturbances like hypothyroidism.

## ABNORMAL LABIAL FRENUM

At birth, the labial frenum is attached to the alveolar ridge, with fibers running into the lingual interdental papilla. As the teeth erupt and as alveolar bone is deposited, the frenum attachment migrates superiorly with respect to the alveolar ridge. In some cases, fibers may persist below the maxillary central incisors and in the "V" shaped intermaxillary suture.

Abnormal labial frenum attachment can be diagnosed clinically by blanch test. When upper lip is pulled forward upward, a blanching of the tissue just lingual to the maxillary central incisors in the region of incisive papilla is observed.

Radiographic examination reveals a notch like radiolucency seen interdentally between two maxillary centrals near the alveolar crest. Presence of an abnormal labial frenum attachment prevents the approximation of two central incisors leading to spacing between these two teeth called as midline diastema (**Figs 10.11A and B**). Nevertheless, other possible causes of midline diastema, such as mesiodens, abnormal pressure habits, racial tendencies, congenitally missing or microdontic teeth should be ruled out before attempting frenectomy.

## DENTAL CARIES

Dental caries is one of the most common local causes of malocclusions.

Proximal caries or complete loss of affected tooth with dental caries may cause the following effects:

**Table 10.2:** Consequences of premature loss of deciduous teeth

| Premature loss of | Possible consequences |
|---|---|
| Deciduous anterior teeth | • Spacing in the arch.<br>• A shift in the midline, if primary canine is lost from one side of the arch only |
| Deciduous molars | Premature loss of deciduous second molar<br>↓<br>Mesial migration of the permanent first molar<br>↓<br>Loss of arch length<br>↓<br>Lack of space for permanent second premolar to erupt (**Fig. 10.8**)<br>↓<br>Permanent second premolar forced to erupt lingually/buccally<br>↓<br>Crowding in the posterior segment |
| Premature loss of deciduous Maxillary second molar | Mesial migration of permanent molars<br>↓<br>Loss of arch length<br>↓<br>Maxillary canine, the last anterior tooth to erupt may cause changes its path of eruption and erupt labially<br>↓<br>Crowding in anterior segment |

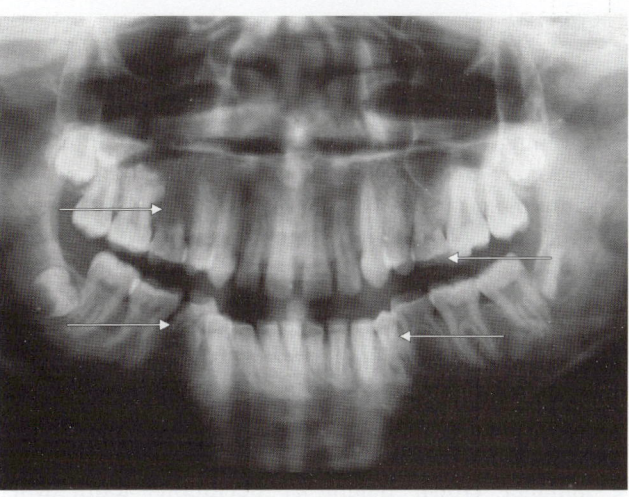

**Fig. 10.9:** Prolonged retention upper and lower second deciduous molars due to congenital missing second premolars

- Premature loss of the affected tooth or proximal caries.
- Proximal caries can cause drifting of adjacent teeth into space created with resultant loss of arch length **(Figs 10.12A and B)**.
- Premature loss of affected tooth can cause migration of adjacent teeth into the space.
- Abnormal inclination of adjacent teeth.
- Over eruption of antagonistic teeth.

## IMPROPER DENTAL RESTORATIONS

While restoring any tooth, it is important to restore the normal occlusal anatomy and proximal contours, so as to maintain normal intercuspation of the teeth and their mesiodistal dimension. Improper restoration of proximal contours may result in an increased arch length and occlusal irregularities. Possible consequences of improper dental restorations are listed in **Table 10.3**.

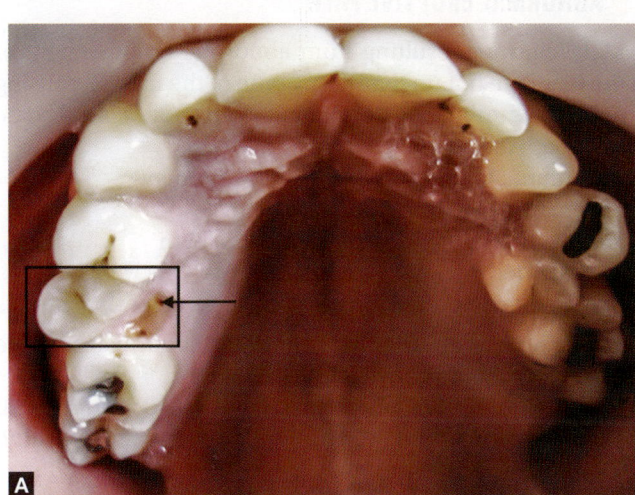
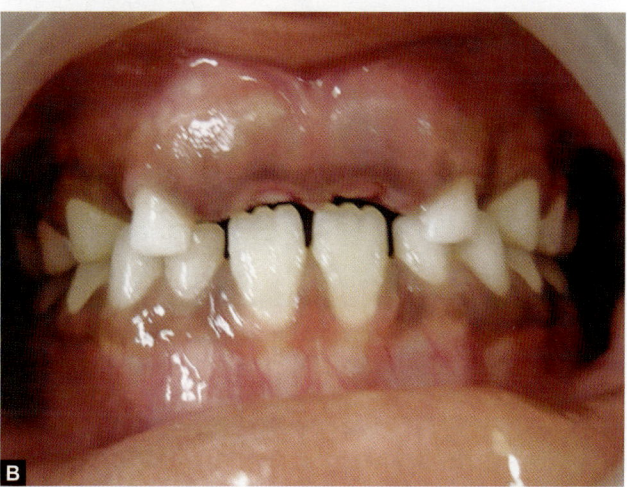

**Figs 10.10A and B:** (A) Delayed eruption of permanent teeth: Retained deciduous root fragments of second molar has resulted in disto-buccal rotation of left permanent second premolar; (B) Delayed eruption of permanent teeth: Presence of thick mucosal barrier overlying the erupting maxillary permanent central incisors

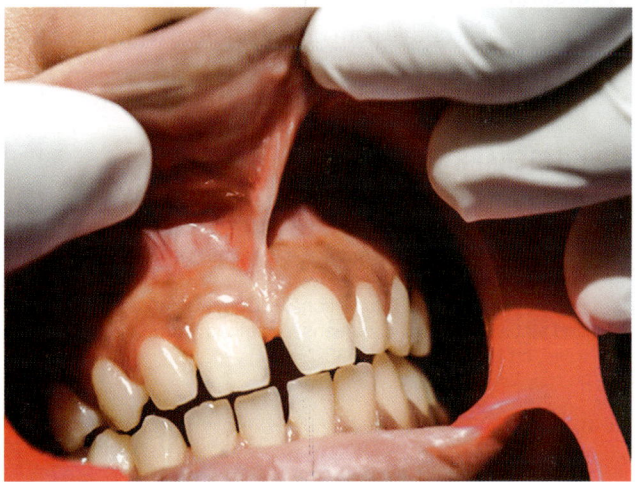

**Fig. 10.11:** Heavy fibrous labial frenum preventing approximation of both the centrals causing "Midline Diastema"

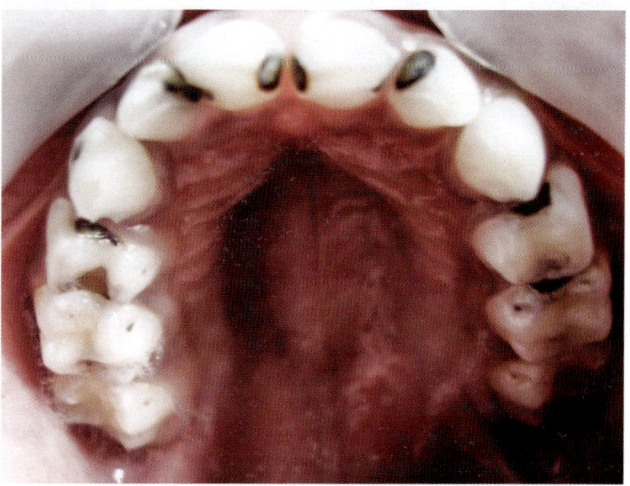

**Fig. 10.12:** Proximal caries can cause drifting of adjacent teeth into the space created with resultant loss of arch length

**Table 10.3:** Possible consequences of improper dental restoration

| | |
|---|---|
| Over contoured proximal restorations | • Too tight proximal contact leading to elongation of restored tooth or adjacent teeth<br>• Overcontoured restoration in a segment can cause increase arch length |
| Under contoured proximal restoration | Loss of arch length due to drifting adjacent teeth into the space |
| Overfilled occlusal restoration | • Functional occlusal prematurities<br>• Intrusion of antagonistic tooth—pseudo class III |
| Underfilled restoration | Supraeruption of antagonistic tooth<br>Functional occlusal disturbances |

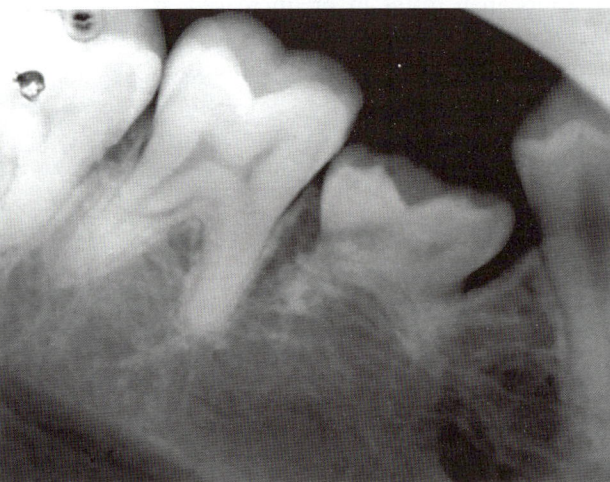

**Fig. 10.13:** Ankylosed mandibular deciduous second molar associated with, the congenitally missing predecessor tooth, the second premolar

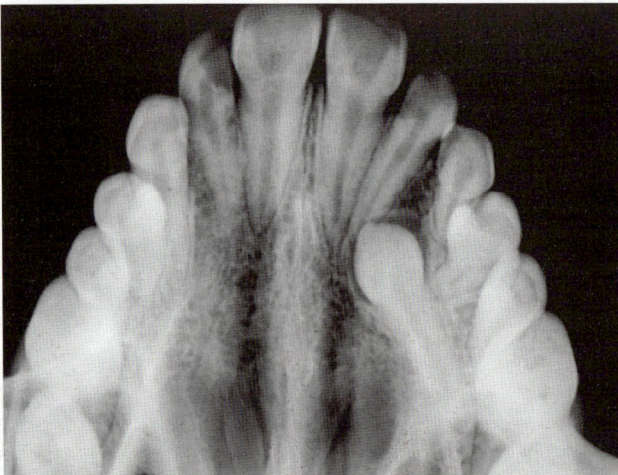

**Fig. 10.14:** Ectopically erupted maxillary left permanent canine causing crowding in the arch. Note distobuccal rotation of left second permanent premolar

# ANKYLOSIS

The tooth is said to be ankylosed when a part or whole of its root surface is directly fused to the bone without intervening periodontal ligament. The term submerged teeth often refers to the ankylosed deciduous teeth. Deciduous second molars are most commonly affected.

Ankylosis of deciduous teeth prevents their natural exfoliation and replacement by their successional permanent teeth. Once the adjacent permanent teeth erupt to their normal level, the ankylosed tooth appears to be submerged below the level of occlusion **(Fig. 10.13)**. This occlusion or submersion is created due to:
- Continued growth of alveolar process in relation to adjacent permanent teeth.
- Smaller crown height of deciduous tooth when compared to that of adjacent permanent teeth.

The antagonistic tooth may supraerupt leading to malocclusion.

# ABNORMAL ERUPTIVE PATH

Malocclusions resulting from abnormal eruptive path of the teeth are not uncommon. Some of the factors, causing delayed eruption of permanent teeth may also deviate their path of eruption, such as:
- Trauma to the tooth during development
- Presence of supernumerary teeth
- Prolonged retention of deciduous teeth
- Retained deciduous root fragments
- Deficiency of arch length and excess of tooth material.

Maxillary canine often shows an abnormal eruptive pathway possibly due to following factors:
- It has to travel a long distance from its developmental position near the floor of the orbit to its final position in the oral cavity.
- The sequence of its eruption is after the eruption of one or both of the maxillary premolars.
- After premature loss of primary canines, the premolars may migrate mesially depriving the canine of its erupting space.

Abnormal eruptive path of one or more teeth can cause:
- Crowding in the arch **(Fig. 10.14)**.
- Crossbite when more anteriors erupt palatally.

# BIBLIOGRAPHY

1. Adler-Herdecky C, Adler P. Partial anodontia as an orthodontic problem. Oset Z Stomat 1969;66:294-7.
2. Edwards JG. The diastema, the frenum, the frenectomy. Am J Orthod 1977;71:489-508.
3. Federation Dentaire Internationale. Commission on classification and statistics for oral conditions: A method for measuring occlusal traits, Int Dent J 1973;23:530-7.

4. Graber TM. The three "Ms": Muscles, Malformation & Malocclusion. Am J Orthod 1963;49:418-50.
5. Graber TM. Thumb and finger sucking. Am J Orthod 1959;45:258-64.
6. Grainger RM. Orthodontic treatment priority index. Vita Heath Stat 1967;2:1-49.
7. Hill PA. The prevalence aqnd severity of malocclusion and the need for orthodontic treatment in 9-, 12-, and 15-year-old Glasgow schoolchildren, Br J Orthod 1992;19:87-96.
8. Larsson E, Dahlin K. The prevalence and etiology of the initial dummy- and finger-sucking habit. Am J Orthod 1985;432-5.
9. Massler M, Frankel JM. Prevalence of malocclusion in children aged 14 to 18 years. Am J Orthod 1951;37:751-8.
10. McNeill RW, Joondeph DR. Congenitally absent maxillary lateral incisors: Treatment planning considerations. Angle Orthod 1973;43:24-9.
11. Proffit WR, Norton LA. Influences of tongue activity during speech and swallowing, ASHA Reports, no 5. Washington, 1970;106-15.
12. Punkey PJ, Sadowsky C, BeGole EA. Tooth morphology and lower incisor alignment many years after orthodontic therapy, Am J Orthod 1984;86(4):299-305.
13. Taylor GS. Characteristics of supernumerary teeth in primary and permanent dentition. Dent Practit 1972;22:203-8.

## EXAM-ORIENTED QUESTIONS

### Long Essay or Long Question
1. Local factors in etiology of malocclusion.

### Short Notes
1. How does ankylosis causes malocclusion?
2. How does dental caries causes malocclusion?
3. Prolonged retention of deciduous teeth.
4. How does premature loss of deciduous teeth causes malocclusion?
5. How does delayed eruption of permanent teeth causes malocclusion?

# CHAPTER OVERVIEW

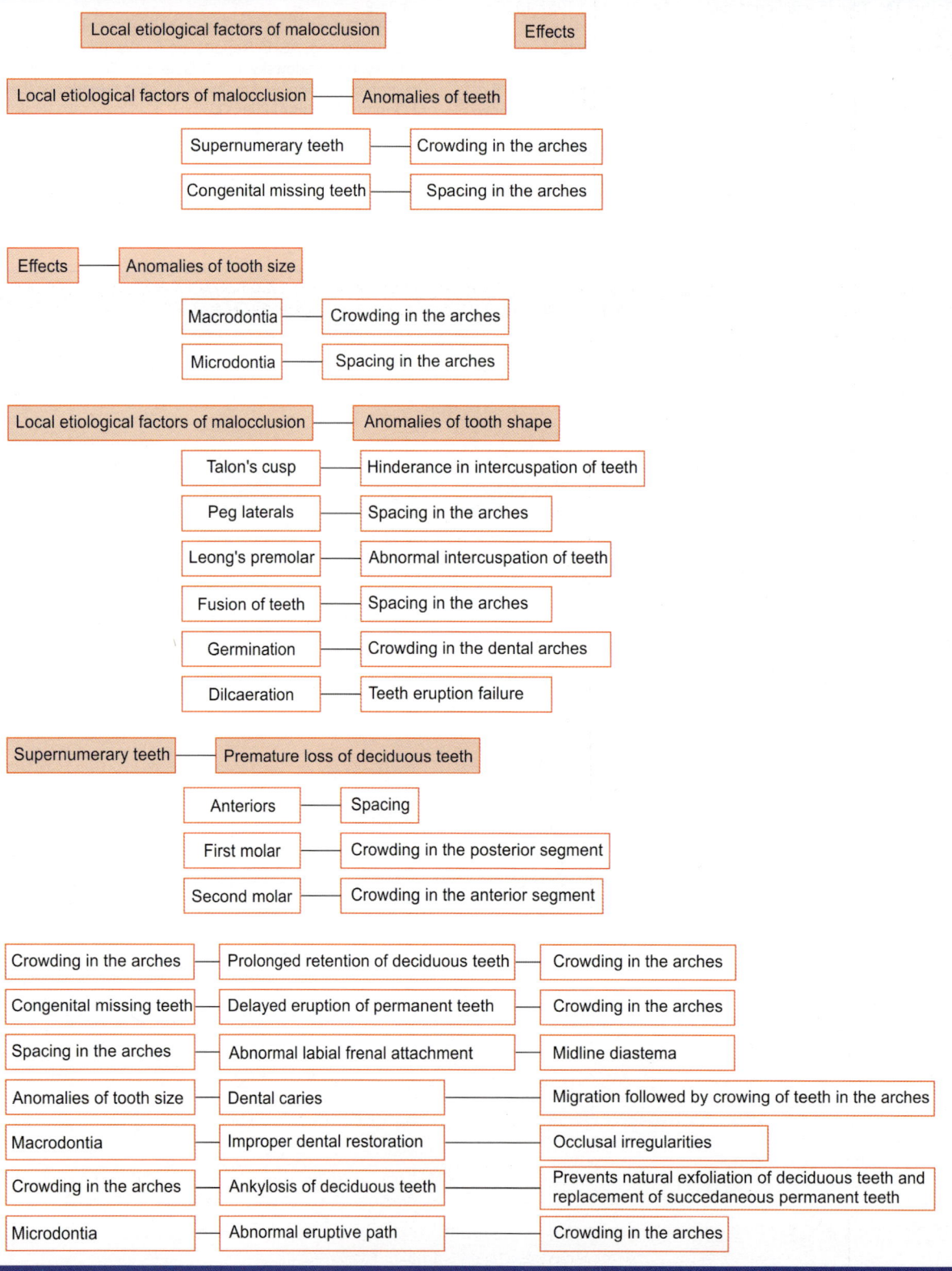

# Genetics in Orthodontics

*Rashmi GS, Phulari BS*

Growth is the combined result of interaction between several genetic and environmental factors over time and malocclusion is a manifestation of genetic and environmental interaction on the development of the orofacial region. It is important to consider genetic factors in orthodontic diagnosis, in order to understand the cause of existing problem, which may also have an influence on the final outcome of orthodontic treatment.

Generally, malocclusions with a genetic cause are thought to be less amenable to treatment than those with an environmental cause. Greater the genetic component, worse the prognosis for a successful outcome by means of orthodontics intervention. Knowing the relative influence of genetic and environmental factors would greatly enhance the clinician's ability to treat malocclusions successfully.

## BASIC TERMINOLOGIES

Before proceeding further, an understanding of the basic terminologies used in genetics is necessary.

### Chromosomes and Genes

Genes are the smallest structural functional units of inheritance. A gene is a segment of a DNA molecule that contains all the information required for synthesis of a product—a polypeptide chain or RNA molecule. Each gene has a specific position (locus) on the chromosome map. All humans normally have 22 homologous pairs of chromosomes called autosomes.

In addition, one pair of sex chromosomes is present. Females have 2 X chromosomes while males have one X and one Y chromosome. Genes at the same locus on a pair of homologous chromosomes are called as alleles. When both the members of a pair of alleles are identical, the individual is homozygous for that locus and if the two alleles at a specific locus are different, then the individual is heterozygous for that locus.

### Genome

Genome is the entire genetic content of a set of chromosomes present within a cell or an organism.

### Genotype and Phenotype

*Genotype:* Genotype is defined as the genetic constitution of an individual and may refer to specified gene locus or to all loci in general.

*Phenotype:* Phenotype on the other hand, refers to a specified character or to all the observable physical characteristics of an individual. The phenotype is determined by the individual's genotype and the environment in which the individual develops over a period of time.

## MODES OF INHERITANCE

### Trait

A trait is a particular aspect or characteristic of the phenotype, e.g. number of teeth, arch length and arch width.

Depending on the genetic influence on traits, the traits can be considered to be of three types:
   i. Monogenic
  ii. Polygenic
 iii. Multifactorial.

### Monogenic Traits

Traits that develop because of the influence of a single gene locus are monogenic. The monogenic traits can be expressed by any of the following modes of inheritance:

#### (i) Autosomal dominant type of inheritance

If having only one particular allele of the two alleles on a homologous pair of autosomes, it is sufficient to lead to the expression of the trait, the mode of inheritance of the trait is called autonomic dominant, e.g. dentinogenesis imperfecta and Marfan's syndrome.

#### (ii) Autosomal recessive type of inheritance

If expression of the trait does not occur with only one particular allele of the two alleles on autosome, and both the alleles are required for expression of the trait, then the trait is called "autosomal recessive".

#### (iii) X-linked traits

Females have two X chromosomes, while males have one X and Y chromosomes. Because of this, males have only half of the X-linked genes. Thus, when a trait present on the X chromosome is responsible for the disease, males are almost exclusively affected, although females can be occasionally affected, e.g. hemophilia is an X-linked recessive disease.

### Polygenic/Multifactorial Inheritance

Expression of some traits cannot be associated with only a single gene. In other words, traits that are resulted from complex interaction of multiple genes are called as polygenic traits.

However, as polygenic traits are also influenced by environmental factors along with multiple genetic factors, they are also referred to as multifactorial, meaning they are influenced by the interaction of multiple genes, as well as environmental factors.

### Malocclusion Traits

Depending on mode of transmission of malocclusion, three types of traits are described:

#### (i) Repetitive traits

The recurrence of a single dentofacial deviation within the immediate family and in the progenitors is referred to as repetitive trait. The same trait is repeatedly seen generation after generation.

#### (ii) Discontinuous traits

The tendency for a malocclusion trait to reappear within the family background over several generations is termed as discontinuous trait. The trait is seen in the family tree but not in all generations.

#### (iii) Variable traits

The occurrence of different but selected types of malocclusion within several generations of the same family is called variable trait. These traits are seen with a variable expression.

### Penetrance and Expressivity

Variable gene expressions are described in terms of penetrance and expressivity.

#### Penetrance

It is the proportion of individuals that show an expected phenotype. The gene is said to be having incomplete penetrance, if it is expressed only in some individuals and not in others. When a gene is completely penetrant, it is always expressed.

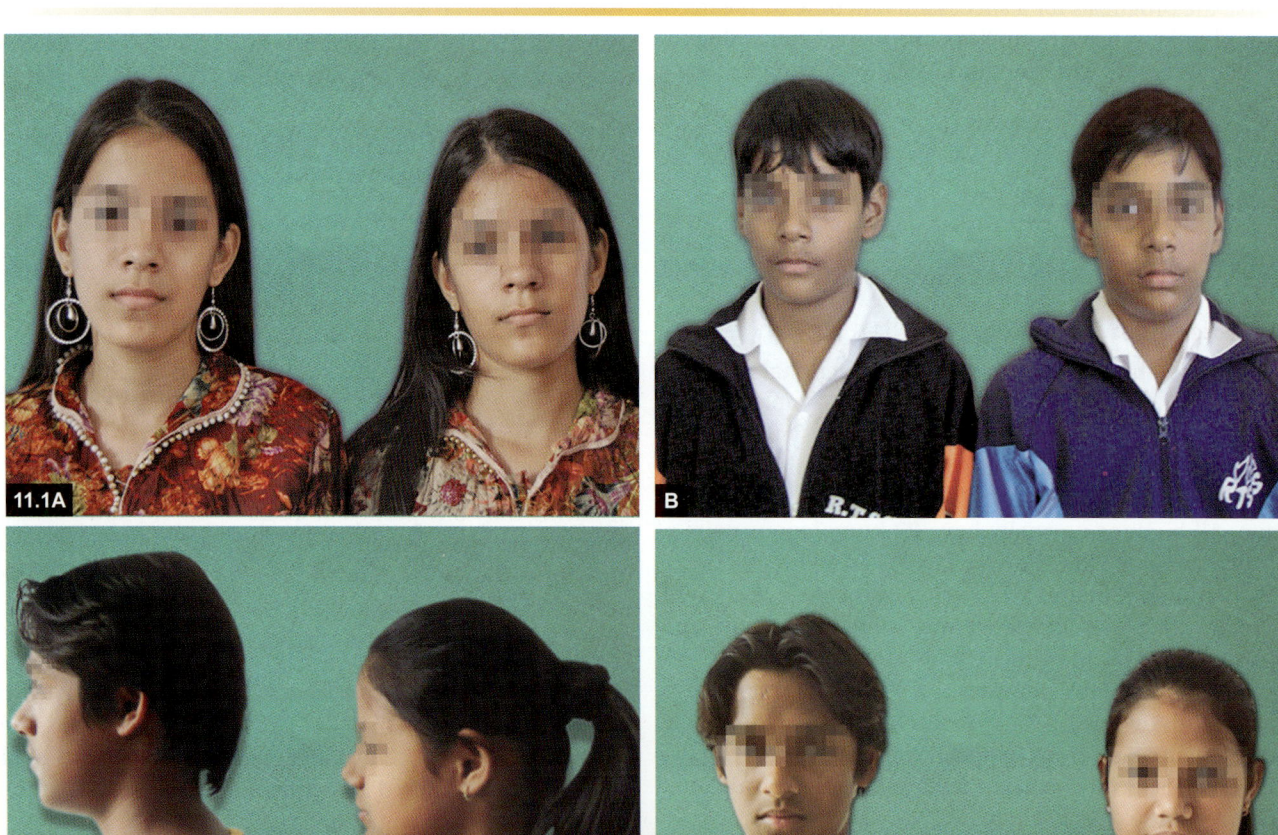

**Figs 11.1A and B:** Identical twins; **Figs 11.2A and B:** Dizygotic twins

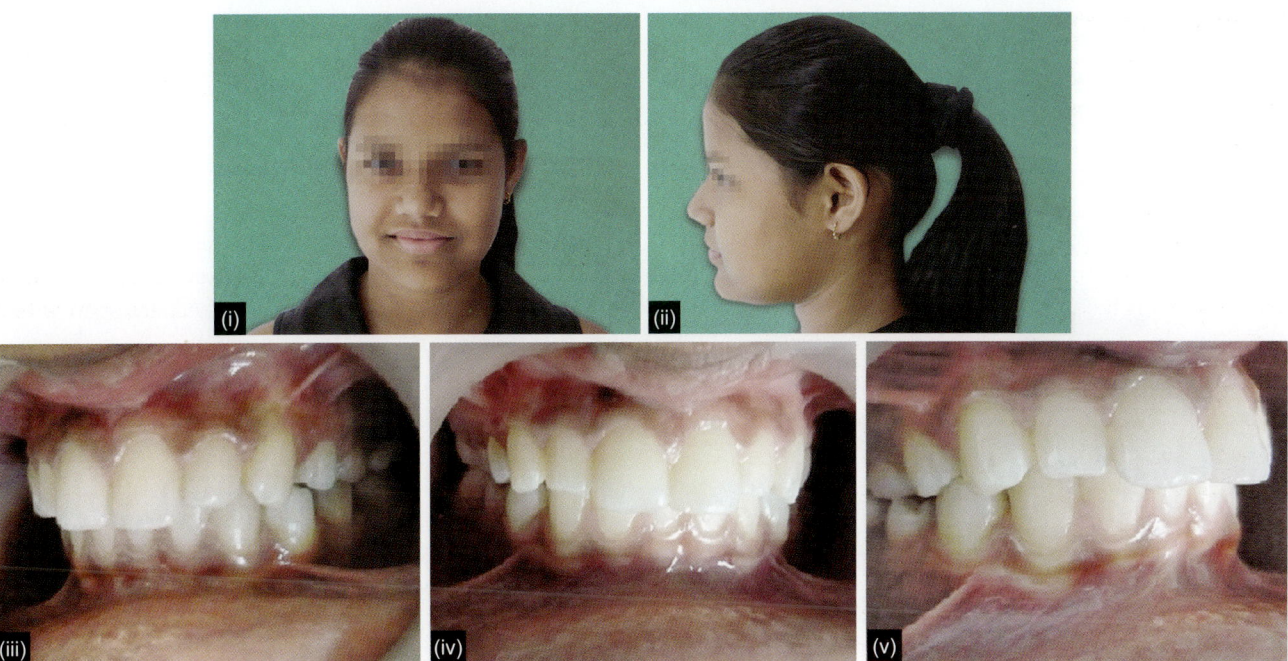

**Figs 11.2C (i to v):** Dizygotic twins

## Expressivity

It is the degree to which a gene is expressed in the same/different individuals. In other words, when a trait is present, it may vary in its severity/expression. Thus, not all individuals with the trait may have it to the same extent and may express, varying degrees of severity.

For example, osteogenesis imperfecta shows variable expression. Clinical features include multiple fractures, blue sclera, dentinogenesis imperfecta and hearing loss. Variation occurs in different clinical types of osteogenesis imperfecta and affected persons in a single family may show varying degree of disease severity. One may have only blue sclera while another may have severe form of disease with fatal bone fractures.

## Estimation of Heritability

A trait with a heritability estimate of one, theoretically, indicates that the trait is expressed without any environmental influence; whereas, a trait with a heritability of 0.5 would have half of its variability influenced by environmental factors and half by genetic factors.

## GENETIC BASIS OF MALOCCLUSION

There is dental anthropological evidence that population groups are genetically homogeneous tend to have normal occlusion. Malocclusion is almost nonexistent in pure racial stocks/ethnic groups, such as the Melanesians of the Philippine Islands. However in heterogeneous population, the incidence of malocclusion is significantly high. Although increased occurrence of malocclusion in urbanized populations has been attributed to racial interbreeding the most likely explanation may be the changed environment, such as food and airway effects.

### Methods of Studying Heritability of Malocclusion

The bulk in the evidence for the heritability of various types of malocclusion comes from familial and twin studies. The methods to estimate heritability are based on correlation and measurements of the traits between various kinds of pairs of individuals in families, including:
- Monozygotic Twins
- Dizygotic Twins
- Parent-Child
- Sib-Sib (Sibling Pairs).

### Familial Studies/Pedigree Studies

The nature of inheritability of traits can be studied by constructing family trees called pedigrees in which males are denoted by squares and females by circles and by noting who in the family has the trait and who does not. A particular trait is observed in successive generation to assess its mode of inheritance. Autosomal recessive traits are best studied in consanguineous marriages where interbreeding (marriage into a family) is permitted.

### Twin Studies

Twin studies offer the best evidence in establishing the relative contribution of genes and environment in the development of malocclusion.

Twins are of two kinds:
  i. Monozygotic twins
  ii. Dizygotic twins

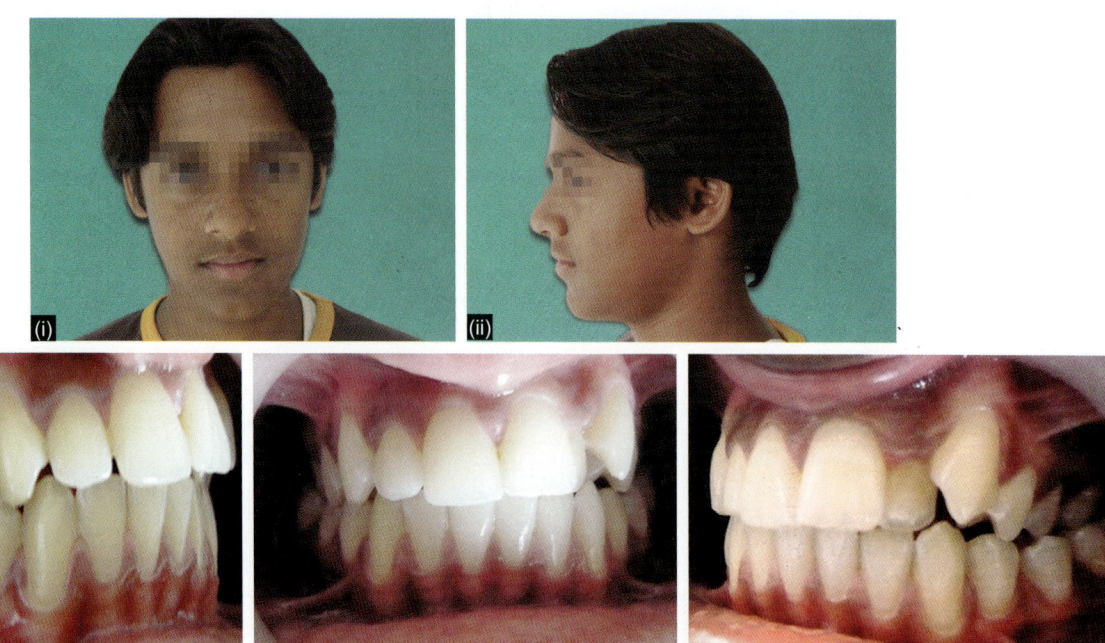

**Figs 11.2D (i to v):** Dizygotic twins

***Monozygotic twins:*** The identical twins develop from single fertilized egg that later divides into two zygotes at an early stage of development. They are identical in genetic makeup and sex, i.e. genotype is identical **(Figs 11.1A and B)**.

***Dizygotic twins:*** Dizygotic twins develop from two separately fertilized eggs at the same time. Dizygotic twins share only 50% of their total gene complement **(Figs 11.2A to D)**.

The underlying principle of twin studies is that:
- The observed difference within a pair of monozygotic twins (whose genotype is identical) is due to environmental factors.
- Differences observed within a pair of dizygotic twins, (who share 50% of their total gene complement) are due to both environment and genetic makeup.

### Craniofacial Disorders and Genetic Etiology with Malocclusion

Some of the craniofacial abnormalities, which have genetic cause and have malocclusion as one of their features are listed in **Box 11.1**.

### Genetic Influence on Skeletal and Dental Malocclusion

In general, heritability estimates of craniofacial skeletal structures are greater than those for dentoalveolar traits, such as tooth position, number and size. In other words, studies have shown that skeletal malocclusions are more influenced by genetics whereas dental malocclusions are more often due to environmental factors.

Studies of Lundstrom (1948) and Krausetal (1959) concluded that although genetic factors appear to govern the base skeletal forms and size, environmental factors in their multitudinous facets have much influence on the bony elements, and both the genetic and environmental factors combine to achieve the harmonious/disharmonious head and face.

According to Hughes and Moore (1941), mandible and maxilla are under separate genetic controls and certain positions of individual bones, such as ramus, body and symphisis of the mandible are under different genetic and environmental influences. Various familial and twin studies indicate that class II division 1 and class II division 2 malocclusions are multifactorial (interaction of both environmental factors) while class III malocclusion is heavily influenced by genetics. Class II division 2 malocclusion is often considered as a genetic trait and class III malocclusion resulting from mandibular prognathism often runs in families as an autosomal dominant trait.

### Class II Division 1 Malocclusion

Class II division I malocclusion appears to have a polygenic/multifactorial inheritance as explained below.
- Extensive cephalometric studies have showed that in class II division 1, the mandible is significantly extended than in class I patients with the body of the mandible smaller and overall mandibular length reduced.
- Higher correlation between the parts and their immediate family than in unrelated siblings is noted.

**Box 11.1:** Craniofacial disorders and genetic etiology with malocclusion

- Facial clefts, cleft lip and cleft palate
- Cleidocranial dysplasia
- Gardner's syndrome
- Down's syndrome
- Osteogenesis imperfecta.

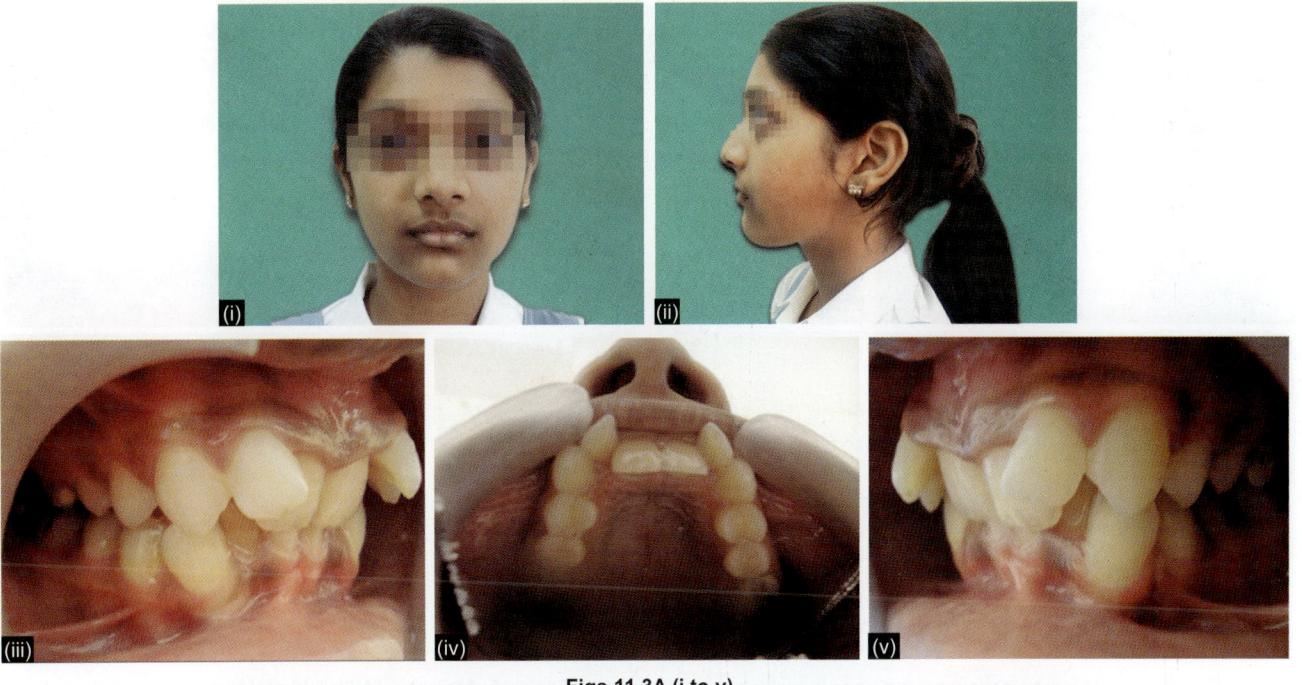

**Figs 11.3A (i to v)**

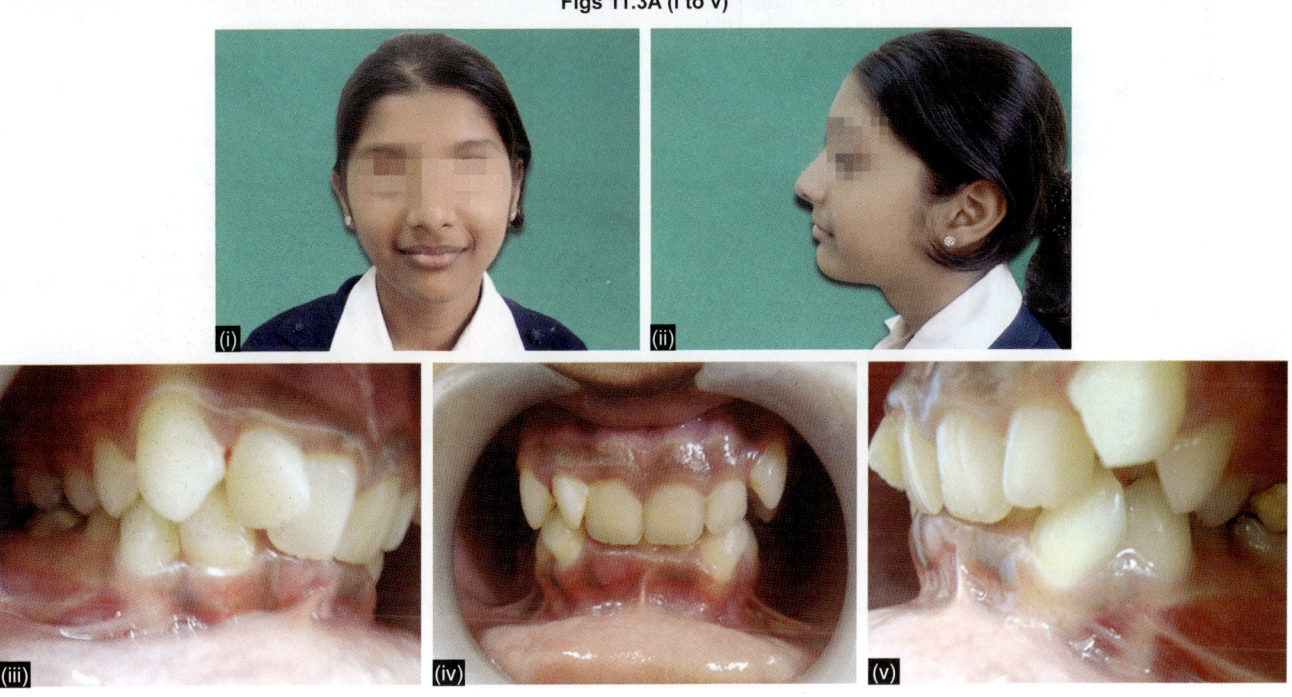

**Figs 11.3B (i to v):** Class II division 2 malocclusion in identical twins

- However, environmental factors, such as tongue pressure, digit sucking habit can also contribute to class II division 1 malocclusion.

## Class II Division 2 Malocclusion

Class II division 2 malocclusion exhibits high genetic influence and is often considered as a genetic trait (**Figs 11.3A** and **B**).

Familial occurrence of Class II division 2 malocclusion has been documented in several published reports, including twin and triplet studies and in family pedigrees [Ckloeppel (1953), Markovic (1992,) Korkhaus (1930), Peck (1998)].

Markovic (1992) carried out a clinical and cephalometric study of 114 Class II division 2 malocclusion (48 twin pairs and six sets of triplets). The results of his study showed that there was 100% concordance for class II division 2 malocclusion in monozygotic twin pairs. This gives a strong evidence for genetics as main ethological factor in development of class II division 2 malocclusion.

Results of various family pedigree studies suggest the possibility of autosomal dominant inheritance with incomplete penetrance. High lip line, lip morphology and behavior are also considered to be causing class II division 2 malocclusion.

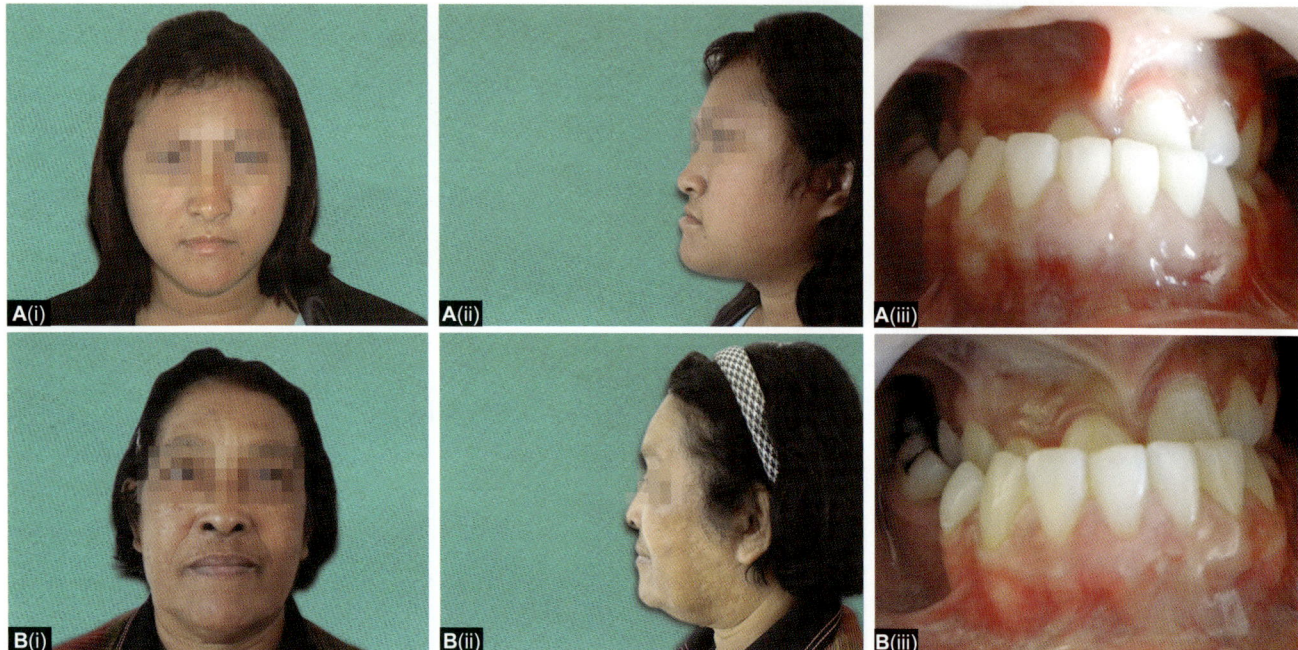

**Case 1:** A 19-year-old female patient having class III malocclusion, **(Ai and ii)**: Facial photographs, **(Aiii)**: Intraoral frontal view. Mother of the patient having class III malocclusion; **(Bi and ii)**: Facial photographs; **(Biii)**: Intraoral frontal view

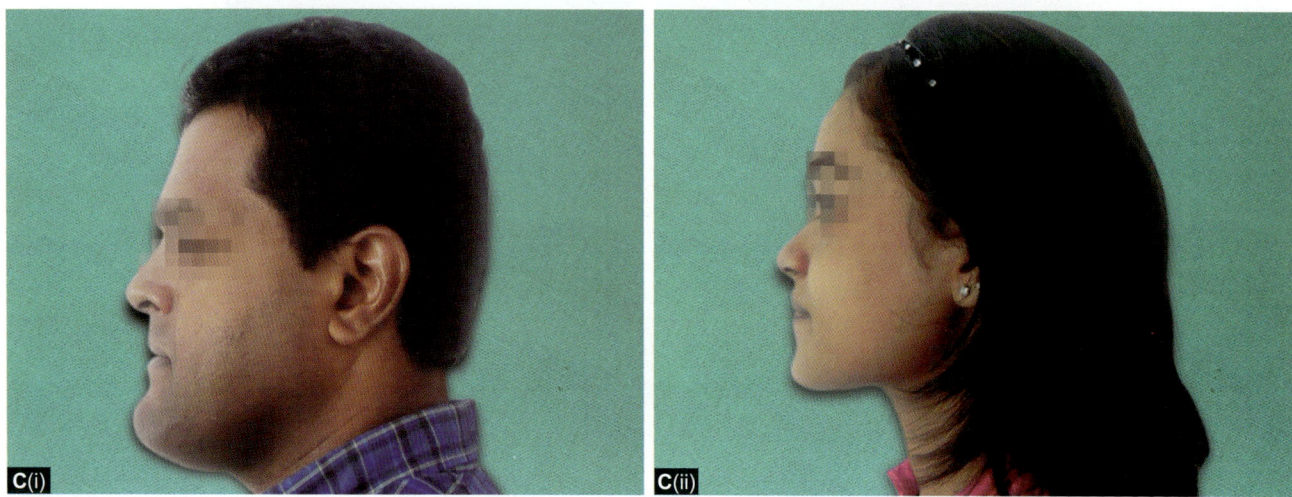

**Case 2: (Ci and Cii):** Father and daughter showing mandibular prognathism. Both have Angle's class III malocclusion

**Figs 11.4A to C:** Class III malocclusion with mandibular prognathism often runs in families

In general, simultaneous and synergistic influence of genetics and environment (multifactorial inheritance) is attributed to the development of class II division 2 malocclusion, also it has a strong genetic influence.

**Extraoral features—all features are same in both girls**

- Endomorphic physique
- Shape of the head brachycephalic
- Facial form—euryprosopic
- Facial symmetry—bilateral symmetrical
- Facial profile—convex
- Facial divergence—posterior facial divergence
- Mentolabial sulcus—deep
- Lips—competent
- Nasolabial angle—increased
- Lower facial height—decreased

**Intraoral features—all features are same in both girls**

- Class I molar relationship
- Class I canine relationship
- Class II division 2 incisor relationship
- Mandibular anterior crowding
- Maxillary anterior crowding
- von der Linden's type B
- Hypoplastic teeth in relation to 11, 21, 31, 41
- Dental caries—16, 36 and 46

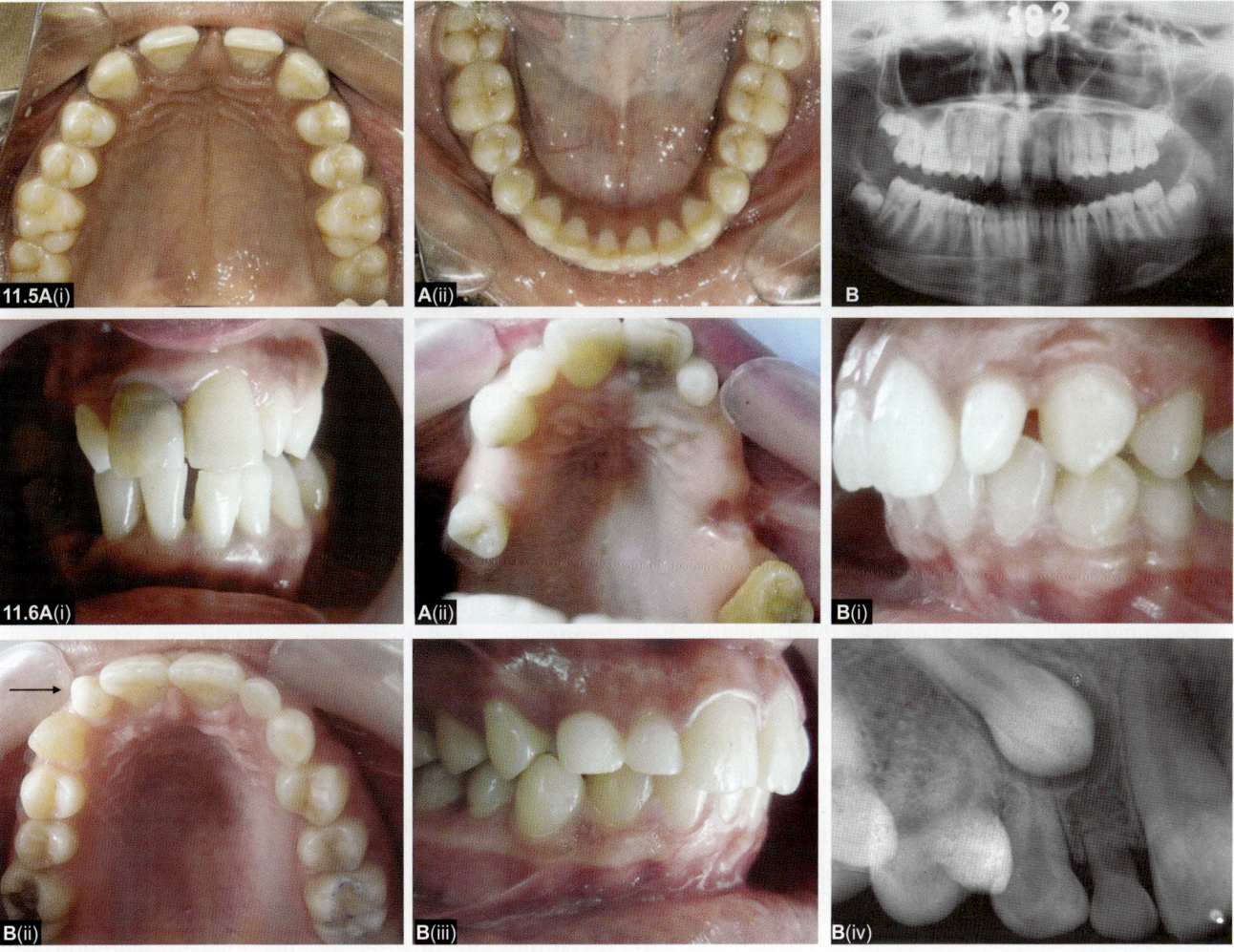

**Figs 11.5A and B:** Bilateral congenitally missing lateral incisors.; (A) Occlusal view of maxillary arch and mandibular arch; (B) OPG of the same patient; **Figs 11.6A and B:** Abnormalities in lateral incisor region varies from peg-shaped to microdont to missing teeth, all of which have familial trends, female preponderance and association with other dental anomalies, suggesting a polygenic etiology. (Ai and ii): Mother with bilateral peg-shaped lateral incisors; (Bi to iv): Daughter showing peg lateral incisor on one side and congenitally missing lateral with retained deciduous lateral incisor and canine and impacted permanent right canine

## Class III Malocclusion

Class III malocclusion with mandibular prognathism often runs in families **(Figs 11.4A to C).**

The most famous example of a genetic trait in humans passing through several generations is probably the pedigree of the so-called "Hapsburg Jaw." This was the famous mandibular prognathism demonstrated by several generations of the Hungarian/Austrian dual monarchy.

Strohmayer (1937) from his detailed pedigree analysis of Hapsburg family concluded that mandibular prognathism was an autosomal dominant trait. Other studies, such as Suzuki's (1961) study on 243 Japanese families and twin studies have also suggested strong genetic basis for mandibular prognathism. Although various environmental factors, such as enlarged tonsils, nasal blockage, posture, premature loss of permanent molars due to trauma can also cause class III malocclusion, the overall inheritance pattern best fits an autosomal dominant model.

## Genetic Influences on Tooth Size, Number, Morphology, Position and Eruption

### Tooth Size

Twin studies have shown that tooth crown dimensions are strongly determined by heredity. Butler's field theory, explained later in this chapter supports this. As dietary habits in humans adapt from a hunter/gatherer to a defined food culture, evolutionary selection pressures are tending to reduce tooth volume, which is manifested in third molar, second premolar and lateral incisor "fields." Hypodontia of the above mentioned teeth shows a familial tendency and fits polygenic models of inheritance.

### Tooth Number

Supernumerary teeth, most frequently seen on premaxillary region, also appears to be genetically determined. Mesiodens are more commonly present in parents and

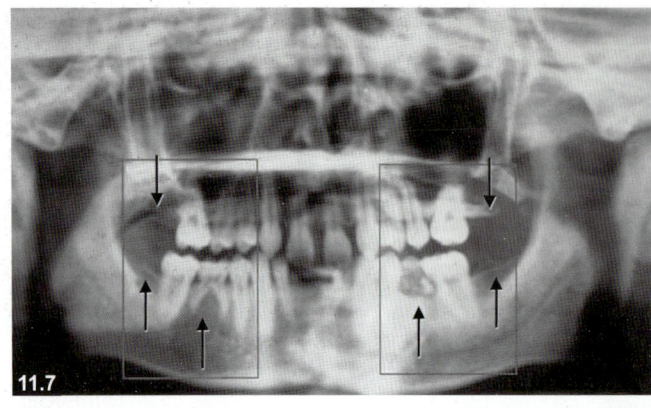
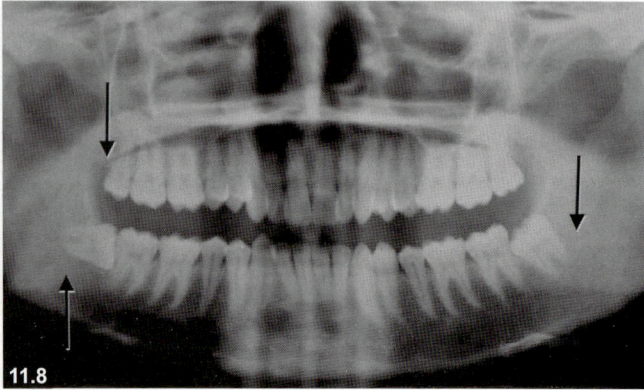

**Fig. 11.7:** Butler's field theory. Note the following features within molar/premolar field: (1) Congenitally missing permanent second and third molars in all four quadrants, (2) Congenitally missing mandibular second premolars;
**Fig. 11.8:** Microdontic third molar and impacted mandibular molars

siblings of the patients who exhibit them. Hereditary nature of hypodontia is revealed in familial and twin studies. Maxillary lateral incisor, the most common tooth to be congenitally missing next to third molars often exhibit familial occurrence **(Figs 11.5A and B)**.

### Abnormal Tooth Shape
Abnormalities in lateral incisor region varies from peg-shaped to microdont to missing teeth, all of which have familial trends, female preponderance and association with other dental anomalies (missing teeth, ectopic canines, transposition), suggesting a polygenic etiology. Carabelli trait also appears to be strongly influenced by genes.

### Ectopic Maxillary Canine
Various studies have indicated a genetic tendency for ectopic maxillary canine **(Figs 11.6A and B)**. Pecketal (1991) concluded that palatally ectopic canines have an inherited trait, being one of the anomalies in a complex and genetically related dental disturbances, often occurring in combination with missing teeth, microdontia, supernumerary teeth and other ectopically positioned teeth.

Studies (Mossy, et al in 1994 and others) have also shown an association between ectopic maxillary canines and class II malocclusion, which has a strong basis. In addition, tooth transposition most commonly affects maxillary canine/first premolar class position and shows a familial occurrence.

### Submerged Primary Molars
Primary molars, especially in mandibular arch, are the commonly submerged teeth.

## Hereditability and Functional Component of Occlusion
Balance between external and internal functional matrices is important for the establishment of normal occlusion. During diagnostic process, it is also important to consider the possible role of functional components of occlusion. Evidence from recent studies has indicated strong genetic influence on certain aspects of masticator muscle behavior.

Soft tissue morphology and behavior have a genetic component and they have a significant influence on the dentoalveolar morphology. For example, in class II division 1, a short upper lip and low lip level with flaccid lip tone will favor proclination of upper incisors. The external matrix (lip morphology and behavior, cheeks) is thought to be strongly genetically determined, while internal matrix (tongue posture and behavior) can be influenced by both genetic and environmental factors.

## Butler's Field Theory
According to this theory, mammalian dentition can be divided into several developmental fields. The developmental fields include molar/premolar field, the canine field and the incisor field. Within each developmental field, there is a key tooth, which is more stable developmentally and on either side of this key tooth, the remaining teeth within the field become progressively less stable.

***Example 1:*** Within Molar/Premolar Field: Within molar/premolar field, according to Butler's field theory, maximum variability will be seen for the third molars. Third molars are the most common teeth to be congenitally absent and to be impacted **(Fig. 11.7)**.

Variability of third molars includes:

### Variable in Size
Third molars can be small appearing as microdonts **(Fig. 11.8)**. They can have small roots and small cusps.

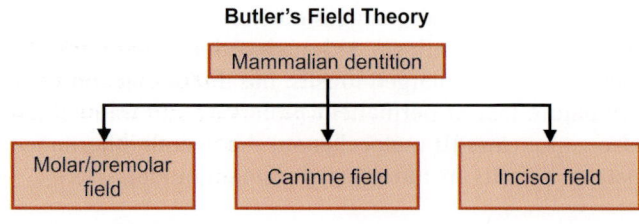

Butler's Field Theory

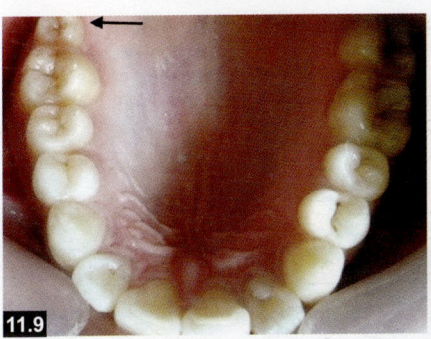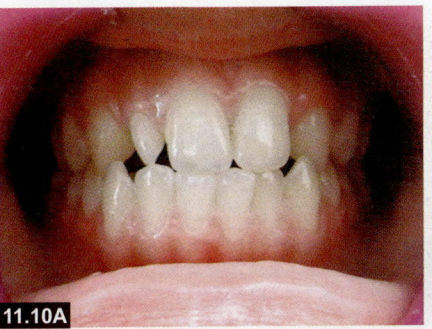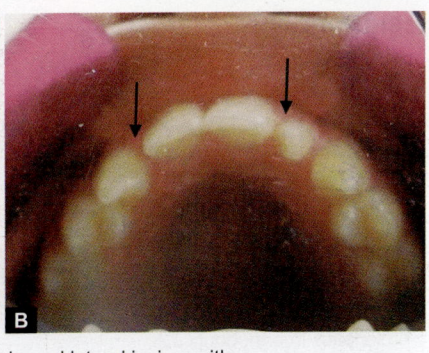

**Fig. 11.9:** Microdontic second molar; **Figs 11.10A and B:** Unilateral peg-shaped lateral incisor with congenitally missing lateral incisor on the other side

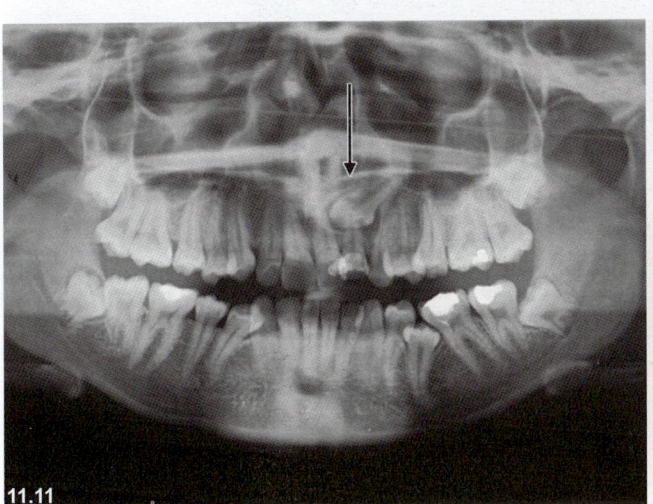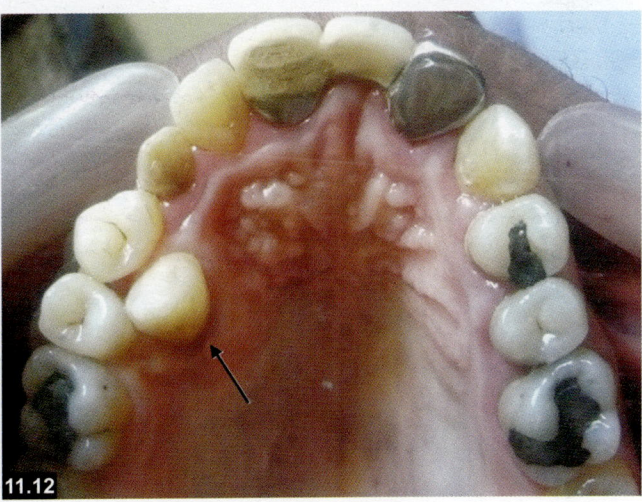

**Fig. 11.11:** A female patient having impacted left permanent canine and retained left deciduous canine; **Fig. 11.12:** Ectopically erupted canine in relation to premolars on palatal aspect with retained deciduous canine

### Variable in Form
1. They may have well-formed cusps or several small tubercles.
2. Some maxillary third molars may not resemble any of the teeth and appear like abnormalities.
3. The roots can be very short, long often fused, may be separate and sometimes an extra root can be seen.

Second molar can also show variation, such as microdontic tooth **(Fig. 11.9)**. When premolars are congenitally absent, the second premolars are more commonly affected than the first premolars **(Fig. 11.7)**.

***Example 2:*** **Within Incisor Field:** Within incisor field, according to Butler's field theory, the maximum variability will be seen for the lateral incisor.

Variability of lateral incisor includes:
a. Peg-shaped lateral incisor **(Figs 11.5 and 11.10A and B)**
b. Congenitally missing laterals **(Fig. 11.5)**.

***Example 3:*** Within Canine Field

Canines, especially in maxillary arch, can be impacted **(Fig. 11.11)** or ectopically erupted **(Fig. 11.12)**.

### Clinical Implications of Genetics in Orthodontics
- Malocclusion with a "genetic cause" is generally thought to be less amenable to treatment than those with an "environmental cause". The greater the genetic component, the worse the prognosis for a successful outcome by means of orthodontic intervention.
- However, knowing exactly the relative contribution of genetic and environmental factors is not always possible.
- In recent times, malocclusions of genetic origin (skeletal discrepancies) when detected in growing period, are being successfully treated using orthopedic and functional appliances, except in extreme cases where surgical intervention is required.
- When malocclusion is primarily of genetic origin, for example, severe mandibular prognathism then treatment will be palliative or surgical.
- Examination of parents and older siblings can give information regarding the treatment need for a child and treatment can be begun at an early age.

## BIBLIOGRAPHY

1. Horowitz SL, Osborne RH, Degeorge FV. A Cephalometric Study of Craniofacial Variation in Adult Twins. Angle Orthod. 1960;30:1-5.
2. King L, Harris EF, Tolley EA. Heritability of skeletal odental relationships. Am J Orthod. 1993;121-31.
3. Litton SF, Ackerman LV, Isaacson RJ, et al. A genetic study of class III malocclusion. Am J Orthod. 1970;58:556-77.
4. Wolff G, Weinker TF, Sander H. On the genetics of mandibular prognathism: analysis of large European noble families. J Med Genet. 1993;30:112-6.

### EXAM-ORIENTED QUESTIONS

#### Long Essay or Long Questions
1. Genetics in orthodontics
2. Importance of genetics in orthodontics
3. Role of genetics in aetiology of malocclusion.

#### Long Note
1. Methods of genetic studies.

#### Short Notes
1. Butler's field theory
2. Teratogens
3. Pedigree studies
4. Mutations
5. Dentofacial disturbances of genetic origin.

# CHAPTER 12

# Epidemiology of Malocclusion

*Kino BR, Phulari BS*

Malocclusion is a common oral disorder, which manifests itself during childhood and the correction of malocclusion (orthodontic treatment) is frequently carried out during childhood. With the growing demand for orthodontic treatment, a variety of clinician-based indices have been developed to classify various types of malocclusion and determine their orthodontic treatment need, prioritizing of treatment requirement in patients, referred for orthodontics, particularly where there are limited resources for orthodontics among public health care services and safeguarding for the patients.

The most commonly employed malocclusion indices are the Dental Aesthetic Index (DAI), Index of Orthodontic Treatment Need (IOTN), Peer Assessment Rating (PAR) and Index of Complexity, Outcome and Need (ICON).

Generally, among the commonly used indices, IOTN (AC, DHC), DAI and ICON are used to assess the orthodontic treatment needs while ICON and PAR are used to assess the treatment outcome. In some ways, the indices of IOTN, DAI and ICON are similar. All include two components—morphological and esthetic. The difference is that for the IOTN and the esthetic component is separated from the dental health component. All the three indices measure similar traits, such as overjet, reverse overjet, open bite, overbite, anteroposterior molar relationship and displacement. However, the weights of these traits are rated differently by each index. The four indices are described below.

## INDEX OF ORTHODONTIC TREATMENT NEED

Brook and Shaw, in 1989, developed a valid and reproducible index (Index of Orthodontic Treatment Need (IOTN) to determine orthodontic treatment need. This index attempts to rank malocclusion in terms of the significance of various occlusal traits for an individual's dental health and perceived aesthetic impairment. It intends to identify those individuals who would most likely benefit from orthodontic treatment. The index has two components, the Aesthetic and the dental health components, which rank malocclusion in increasing priority according to Aesthetic considerations and dental health implication.

### Aesthetic Component

Aesthetic component (AC) consists of a scale of ten color photographs, showing different levels of dental attractiveness. The dental attractiveness of prospective patients can be rated with reference to this scale. Grade 1 represents the most and grade 10, the least attractive arrangement of teeth. The score reflects the aesthetic impairment. aesthetic Component value indicates patient's Aesthetic concern and reflects sociopsychological needs.

- Grades 1, 2, 3 and 4—no or slight need for treatment.
- Grades 5, 6 and 7—moderate or borderline need for treatment.
- Grades 8, 9 and 10—need for orthodontic treatment.

### Dental Health Component

Dental Health Component (DHC) involves features that might impair the health and function of the dentition. It records the various occlusal traits of a malocclusion that would increase the morbidity of the dentition and the surrounding structures. The traits of malocclusion are: overjet, reverse overjet, overbite, open bite, crossbite, displacement of teeth, impeded eruption of teeth, buccal occlusion, hypodontia, and defects of cleft lip and palate. Functional disturbances are also recorded, which included lip competency, mandibular displacement, traumatic occlusion and masticatory or speech difficulties. Only the worst occlusal feature is recorded. The components of DHC are shown in **Table 12.1**. There are five grades:

- Grades 1 and 2—no need or slight need for treatment.
- Grade 3—moderate or borderline need for treatment.
- Grades 4 and 5—need for orthodontic treatment.

### Limitations

Aesthetic component cannot be used accurately in mixed dentition. There is a shortage of scientific information regarding the long-term effects of malocclusion. Nonetheless, the DHC of IOTN provides a structured method for assessment of malocclusion.

## PEER ASSESSMENT RATING

The peer assessment rating (PAR) index, previously referred to as the index of treatment standards, was described by S Richmond, WC Shaw, KD O'Briene, IB Buchaman, R Joes, CD Stephens and M Andrew in 1992. The PAR index is a quantitative occlusal index, measuring how much a patient deviates from normal alignment and occlusion. This index is designed to measure the efficacy or the outcome of orthodontic treatment by comparing the severity of occlusion on pretreatment and post-treatment casts. The PAR index has five components.

### Upper and Lower Anterior Segments

Scores are recorded for both upper and lower anterior segment alignment. The features recorded are crowding, spacing and impacted teeth.

**Table 12.1:** The dental health components of the index of orthodontic treatment need (IOTN) (Shaw et al, 1989)

| | **Grade 5 (Need treatment)** |
|---|---|
| 5.a | Impeded eruption of teeth (except for third molars) due to crowding, displacement, presence of supernumerary teeth, retained deciduous teeth and any pathological cause. |
| 5.b | Extensive hypodontia with restorative implications (more than 1 tooth missing in any quadrant), requiring prerestorative orthodontics. |
| 5.c | Increased overjet greater than 9 mm. |
| 5.d | Reverse overjet greater than 3.5 mm with reported masticatory or speech difficulties. |
| 5.e | Defects of cleft lip and palate and other craniofacial anomalies. |
| 5.f | Submerged deciduous teeth. |
| | **Grade 4 (Need treatment)** |
| 4.a | Less extensive hypodontia, requiring prerestorative orthodontic or orthodontic space closure to obviate the need for prosthesis. |
| 4.b | Increased overjet greater than 6 mm but less than or equal to 9 mm. |
| 4.c | Reverse overjet greater than 1 mm but less than 3.5 mm with reported masticatory or speech difficulties. |
| 4.d | Anterior or posterior crossbites with greater than 2 mm discrepancy between retruded contact position and intercuspal position. |
| 4.e | Posterior lingual crossbite with no functional occlusal contact in one or both buccal segments. |
| 4.f | Severe contact point displacements greater than 4 mm. |
| 4.g | Extreme lateral or anterior open bite greater than 4 mm. |
| 4.h | Increased and completed overbite with gingival or palatal trauma. |
| 4.i | Partially erupted teeth, tipped and impacted against adjacent teeth. |
| 4.j | Presence of supernumerary teeth. |
| | **Grade 3 (Borderline need)** |
| 3.a | Increased overjet greater than 3.5 mm but less than or equal to 6 mm with incompetent lips. |
| 3.b | Reverse overjet greater than 1 mm but less than or equal to 3.5 mm. |
| 3.c | Anterior or posterior crossbites with greater than 1 mm but less than or equal to 2 mm discrepancy between retruded contact position and intercuspal position. |
| 3.d | Contact points displacements greater than 2 mm but less than or equal to 4 mm. |
| 3.e | Lateral or anterior open bite greater than 2 mm but less than or equal to 4 mm. |
| 3.f | Deep overbite complete on gingival or palatal tissues but no trauma. |
| | **Grade 2 (Little need)** |
| 2.a | Increased overjet greater than 3.5 mm but less than or equal to 6 mm with incompetent lips. |
| 2.b | Reverse overjet greater than 0 mm but less than or equal to 1 mm. |
| 2.c | Anterior or posterior crossbites with greater than 1 mm but less than or equal to 1 mm discrepancy between retruded contact position and intercuspal position. |
| 2.d | Contact point displacements greater than 1 mm but less than or equal to 2 mm. |
| 2.e | Anterior or posterior open bite greater than 1 mm but less than or equal to 2 mm. |
| 2.f | Increased overbite greater than or equal to 3.5 mm without gingival contact. |
| 2.g | Prenormal or postnormal occlusions with no other anomalies (includes up to half a unit discrepancy). |
| | **Grade 1 (None)** |
| 1 | Extremely minor malocclusions, including contact points displacements less than 1 mm. |

## Buccal Occlusion

The buccal occlusion is recorded for both left and right sides. The recording zone is from the canine to the last molar. All discrepancies are recorded when teeth are in occlusion.

## Overjet

Positive overjet, as well as teeth in crossbite is recorded. The most prominent aspect of any one incisor is recorded. If the two lateral incisors are in crossbite while the centered incisors are with increased overjet of 4 mm, the score will be 3 for crossbite and 1 for the positive overjet, 4 in total.

## Overbite

The vertical overlap or open bite of the anterior teeth is recorded.

## Centerline Assessment

The centerline discrepancy between the upper and lower dental midline is recorded in relation to lower central incisors.

The PAR index is applied to an individual's pre- and post-treatment study casts. Scores are assigned to each component. The individual scores are calculated in each component and multiplied by a weight of each component. Scores are summed to obtain a total score that represents the degree a case deviates from normal alignment and occlusion. The degree of improvement as a result of orthodontic intervention is obtained by calculating the difference between the pre- and post-treatment PAR scores. The degree of improvement can be assessed, using two different methods:

### Nomogram
The degree of change is separated into three sections:
1. Worse or no difference
2. Improved
3. Greatly improved.

### Percentage Improvement
This method gives a more sensitive assessment than the nomogram, which only provides three broad bands of treatment change. A change of score from 40 to 10 would represent an 80% improvement as would a change from 15 to 3. However, the actual reduction in PAR scores is also relevant as in the first case, where there has been a much greater change with a 30 point reduction as opposed to the second case in which the degree of change is less with only a 12 point reduction.

## INDEX OF COMPLEXITY, OUTCOME AND NEED

The Index of Complexity, Outcome and Need (ICON) has been developed recently and claims among other things, to evaluate orthodontic treatment complexity. ICON is based on the subjective judgements of 97 orthodontists from nine countries. It is a single assessment method to quantify orthodontic treatment complexity, outcome and need. The ICON consists of following five weighted components **(Table 12.2)**.

### Aesthetic Component
The dental Aesthetic Component (AC) of the IOTN is used. Once this score is obtained, it is multiplied by the weighting of 7.

### Crossbite
Crossbite is deemed to be present, if a transverse reaction of cusp-to-cusp or worse exists in the buccal segment. This includes buccal and lingual crossbites, consisting of one or more teeth with or without mandibular displacement.

### Anterior Vertical Relationship
This trait includes both open bite (excluding development conditions) and deep bite. If both traits are present only the highest scoring raw score is counted. Scoring protocol is given in **Table 12.2**.

### Upper Arch Crowding and Spacing
The sum of the mesiodistal crown diameters is compared to the available arch circumference, mesial to the last standing tooth on either side.

### Buccal Segment Anteroposterior Relationship
The anteroposterior cuspal relationship is scored, according to the protocol given in **Table 12.2** for each side in turn. The raw scores for both sides are added together.

### Calculation of the Final Scores
Once all of the raw scores have been obtained and multiplied by their respective weights, they are added together to yield a weighted summary score for a particular cast. The summed score is interpreted as following: pretreatment scores give the treatment needs and complexity grades;

| Table 12.2: Protocol for occlusal trait scoring (Daniel and Richmond, 2000) | | | | | | | |
|---|---|---|---|---|---|---|---|
| | Score | 0 | 1 | 2 | 3 | 4 | 5 |
| Aesthetic | 1–10 as judged using IOTN AC | | | | | | |
| Upper arch crowding | Score only the highest trait either spacing or crowding | Less than 2.0 mm | 2.1–5.0 mm | 5.1–9.0 mm | 9.1–13.0 mm | 13.1–17.0 mm | >17.0 mm or impacted teeth |
| Upper spacing | Transverse | Up to 2.0 mm | 2.1–5.0 mm | 5.1–9.0 mm | >9.0 mm | | |
| Crossbite | Relationship of cusp to cusp or worse | No crossbite | Crossbite present | | | | |
| Incisor open bite | Score only the highest trait either open bite or overbite | Complete bite | Less than 1 mm | 1.1–2.0 mm | 2.1–4.0 mm | >4 mm | |
| Incisor over bite | Lower incisor coverage | Up to 1/3 tooth | 1/3–2/3 coverage | 1/3 up to full covered | Fully covered | | |
| Buccal segment anteroposterior | Left and right added together | Cusp to embrasure relationship only, class I, II or III | Any cusp relation up to but not including cusp to cusp | Cusp to cusp relationship | | | |

end of treatment scores gives the acceptability; while (pretreatment scores) – (4 × post-treatment scores) gives the degree of improvement.

### Limitations

PAR is based solely on study models and does not account for changes in facial profile, iatrogenic damage, tooth inclination, arch width or posterior spacing and is not appropriate for the assessment of mixed dentition treatment.

## DENTAL AESTHETIC INDEX

The Dental Aesthetic Index (DAI) was developed by NC Cons, J Jenny and FJ Kohaut in 1986 to assess orthodontic treatment need. It is an orthodontic index, based on socially defined aesthetic norms.

The Dental Aesthetic Index (DAI) has been adopted by the World Health Organization as a cross-cultural index. It identifies deviant occlusal traits and mathematically derives a single score. Its structure consists of 10 occlusal features of malocclusion; overjet, underjet, missing teeth, diastema, anterior openbite, anterior crowding, anterior spacing, largest anterior irregularity (mandible and maxilla) and anteroposterior molar relationship. The ten occlusal features are weighted on the basis of their relative importance according to a panel of lay judges. The codes and criteria are as follows:

### I. Missing Incisor, Canine and Premolar Teeth

The number of missing permanent incisor, canine and premolar teeth in the upper and lower arches should be counted and recorded.

### II. Crowding in the Incisal Segments

Both the upper and lower incisal segments should be examined for crowding. Crowding in the incisal segments is recorded as following:
- 0-no crowding
- 1-one segment crowded
- 2-two segments crowded.

### III. Spacing in the Incisal Segments

Both the upper and lower incisal segments should be examined for spacing. Spacing in the incisal segments is recorded as following:
- 0-no spacing
- 1-one segment spaced
- 2-two segments spaced.

### IV. Diastema

A midline diastema is defined as the space, in millimeters, between the two permanent maxillary incisors at the normal position of the contact points.

### V. Largest Anterior Maxillary Irregularity

Irregularities may be either rotation out of or displacements from normal alignment. The four incisors in the maxillary arch should be examined to locate the greatest irregularity.

### VI. Largest Anterior Mandibular Irregularity

The measurement is the same as on the upper arch except that it is made on the mandibular arch.

**Table 12.3:** Severity of malocclusion and decision of treatment need

| Severity of malocclusion | Treatment indication | DAI scores |
|---|---|---|
| No abnormality or minor malocclusion | No or slight need | < 25 |
| Definite malocclusion | Elective | 26–30 |
| Severe malocclusion | Highly desirable | 31–35 |
| Very severe or handicapping malocclusion | Mandatory | > 36 |

### VII. Anterior Maxillary Overjet

The largest maxillary overjet is recorded to the nearest whole millimeter.

### VIII. Anterior Mandibular Overjet

Mandibular overjet is recorded when any lower incisor is in crossbite.

### IX. Vertical Anterior Openbite

### X. Anteroposterior Molar Relation

The right and left sides are assessed with the teeth in occlusion and only the largest deviation from the normal molar relation is recorded.

The following codes are used:
- 0-normal
- 1-half cusp
- 2-full cusp.

### Calculation of DAI Scores

The regression equation used for calculating standard DAI scores is as follows: (missing visible teeth × 6) + (crowding) + (spacing) + (diastema × 3) + (largest anterior maxillary irregularity) + (largest anterior mandibular irregularity) + (anterior maxillary overjet × 2) + (anterior mandibular overjet × 4) + (vertical anterior openbite × 4) + (anteroposterior molar relation × 3) + 13. The severity of malocclusion is classified on the basis of the DAI scores as shown in the **Table 12.3**.

## BIBLIOGRAPHY

1. Brook PH, Shaw WC. The development of an index of orthodontic treatment priority. Eur J Orthod. 1989;11:309-20.
2. Daniels C, Richmond S. The development of the index of complexity, outcome and need (ICON). J Orthod. 2000;27:149-62.
3. Fox NA, Daniels C, Gilgrass T. A comparison of the index of complexity outcome and need (ICON) with the peer assessment rating (PAR) and the index of orthodontic treatment need (IOTN). Br Dent J. 2002;193:225-30.
4. Proffit WR, Fields HW. Contemporary Orthodontics. St. Louis: Mosby, 2000.
5. Richmond S, Shaw WC, O'Brien KD, et al. The development of the PAR Index (Peer Assessment Rating): reliability and validity. Eur J Orthod. 1992;14:125-39.
6. Richmond S, Shaw WC, Roberts CT, et al. The PAR Index (Peer Assessment Rating): methods to determine outcome of orthodontic treatment in terms of improvement and standards. Eur J Orthod. 1992;14:180-7.
7. Shaw WC, Richmond S, O'Brien KD. The use of occlusal indices: a European perspective. Am J Orthod Dentofacial Orthop. 1995;107:1-10.

## EXAM-ORIENTED QUESTIONS

*Long Question*

1. Epidemiology of malocclusion.

*Long Notes*

1. Index of Complexity, Outcome and Need
2. PAR.

*Short Note*

1. Dental aesthetic index (DAI).

# CHAPTER 13

# Orthodontic Diagnosis

*Shah A, Phulari BS*

Diagnosis is the most critical part of orthodontic treatment. In the diagnostic phase, it is important to take the following factors into consideration which can aid in planning the treatment:
- Initial malocclusion
- Growth
- Patient's primary concern (esthetics, etc.)
- Treatment limitations
- Treatment objectives.

## DIAGNOSTIC AIDS

Data required for orthodontic diagnosis are derived from routine essential diagnostic aids and also from supplemental aids when needed. Graber has categorized the diagnostic aids into essential and supplemental diagnostic aids.

### Essential

As the name suggests, these aids are indispensable for appraisal of the condition and it's etiology for treatment planning. Essential diagnostic aids include:
- Case history
- Clinical examination
- Study models
- Certain radiographs
  - Periapical radiographs
  - Bitewing radiographs
  - Orthopantomograms
- Facial photographs and intraoral photographs.

### Supplemental

Supplemental diagnostic aids may be needed in certain cases and these aids usually require specialized equipment. These include:
- Specialized radiographs
  - Occlusal views of maxilla and mandible
  - Selected lateral jaw views
  - Lateral cephalograms
- Hand-wrist radiographs and other maturity indicators.
- Electromyography to assess muscle activity
- Endocrine tests
- Estimation of basal metabolic rate
- Occlusograms.

## CASE HISTORY

A complete case history includes all the relevant information derived from the patient and the parents and is an essential prerequisite for planning and executing any orthodontic treatment.

The case history must include the following data.

### Personal Details

#### Name
- Knowing patient's name is the first important step towards understanding patient's concern and treatment needs.
- Calling the patient by his/her name not only establishes a good rapport but also imparts confidence in the patient's mind about the treatment provider.
- In case of children, it might help to know their pet names.

#### Age
- Patient's chronological age should be recorded, which will have a bearing on diagnosis, treatment planning, as well as the outcome of planned treatment.
- Certain malocclusions occurring during growth period are transient and self correcting.
- Growth modification procedures such as, functional and orthopedic orthodontic therapy can be carried out only during growth periods.
- Surgical resective procedures such as orthognathic surgeries are best carried out after cessation of growth.
- Chronological age is important for the maintaining of shedding and eruption timetables as well.

#### Sex
- Recording gender of the patient is important for treatment planning. Females are observed to precede males in growth related events such as, onset of growth spurts, eruption of teeth and onset of puberty.
- Gender may also have a bearing on patient's compliance towards certain types of orthodontic treatment.

#### Occupation and Address
- Occupation of patient and/or parent gives an idea about socioeconomic condition, which might influence the selection of orthodontic appliances for the patient.
- Address is needed for future correspondence and for maintaining the record.

### Chief Complaint
- It is the complaint for which patient seeks orthodontic care. It reflects what outcome he/she expects from the orthodontic treatment.

- Patient's primary concern must be given priority during treatment planning.

## Medical History

A thorough medical history should be taken. Conditions which might affect orthodontic treatment include the following:

### Rheumatic Fever
- Invasive procedures such as extractions, band placement and removal should be covered with the recommended antibiotic regime.
- A chlorhexidine rinse prior to the adjustment of a fixed appliance is a useful adjunct, although daily long-term use of chlorhexidine may lead to bacterial resistance.
- If the patient's oral hygiene deteriorates during the treatment, it may be advisable to discontinue appliance treatment.

### Epilepsy
Because of the risk of damage to the mouth caused by a broken appliance during an epileptic attack, it is prudent to delay treatment in this group of patients until the condition is well controlled.

### Recurrent Aphthous Ulcerations (RAU)
In patients with history of recurrent aphthous ulceration, it may be prudent to carry out a thorough investigation first, including referral for blood tests if indicated and to determine the effect of appliance before irreversible steps such as extraction is taken.

### Hay Fever
Atopic children may experience problems with a functional appliance during the summer months.

### Dental History
- Regular dental care and good oral health are essential prerequisites to orthodontic treatment.
- Patient's past dental history should include details of any previous appliance therapy.
- If permanent teeth have been extracted, the timing of these extractions and the reason for removal should be ascertained, if possible.

### Prenatal History
- Relevant information regarding the condition of the mother during pregnancy must be recorded. Infections like German measles and intake of certain drugs like thalidomide may cause congenital deformities in child.
- Type of delivery must also be noted as injury to TMJ by way of forceps delivery may adversely affect mandibular growth of patient.

### Postnatal History
Type, duration of feeding, milestones of normal development and presence of any habits such as, thumb sucking, tongue thrusting and lip biting must be recorded.

### Family History
Certain malocclusions such as Angle's class III malocclusions and conditions like cleft lip and cleft palate are often observed to be inherited. Details of other family members with similar conditions must be recorded.

## Clinical Examination

### General Examination
General examination includes general appraisal of the patient, which begins as soon as the patient enters the clinic.

#### Height and Weight
Recording of the weight and height aids in assessing the physical growth and maturation of the patient.

#### Gait
Any abnormality in gait is recorded, which may be due to an underlying neuromuscular disorder.

#### Posture
Sometime abnormal posture of patient may be accentuating the existing malocclusion.

### Extraoral Examination

#### Physique
Physique of an individual may fall into one of the three categories in either of the classifications given below **(Table 13.1)**.

#### According to General Classification
- Athletic—Average physique with normal-sized dental arches.
- Plethoric—Short physique with broad dental arches.
- Esthetic—Thin physique with narrow dental arches.

#### According to Sheldon
According to Sheldon, physique of an individual is classified into following three types:
1. Mesomorphic—Average physique.
2. Endomorphic—Short and obese physique.
3. Ectomorphic—Tall and thin physique.

#### Cephalic and Facial Examination
Shape of the head and facial form may give an idea about the dentoalveolar arch form of an individual.

| Table 13.1: General & Sheldon's classification of physique | | |
|---|---|---|
| **General** | **Sheldon's** | **Definition** |
| Athletic | Mesomorphic | Average physique |
| Plethoric | Endomorphic | Short and obese |
| Esthetic | Ectomorphic | Tall and thin |

| Table 13.2: Cephalic index value | | | |
|---|---|---|---|
| **Shape of the head** | **Meaning** | **Dental arch** | **Fig. citation** |
| Mesocephalic | Normal | Normal | Fig. 13.1A |
| Brachycephalic | Short and broad | Broad | Fig. 13.1B |
| Dolichocephalic | Long and narrow | Narrow | Fig. 13.1C |

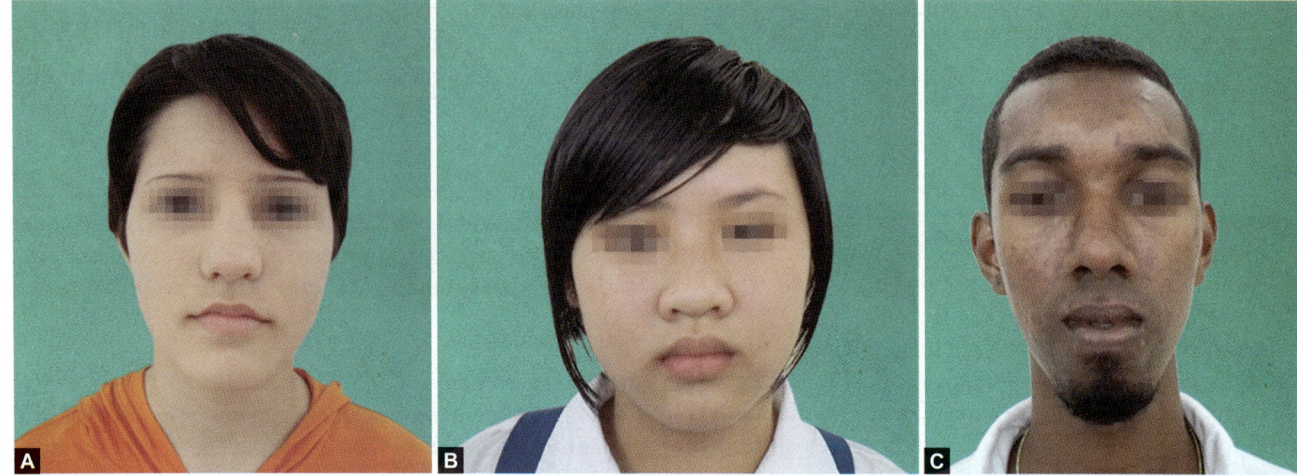

**Figs 13.1A to C:** Shape of the head: (A) Mesocephalic head and mesoprosopic face; (B) Brachycephalic head and euryprosopic face; (C) Dolichocephalic head and leptoprosopic face

Martin and Saller in 1957, formulated cephalic and facial indices to evaluate shape of the head and the facial form respectively.

### Shape of the Head (Cephalic Index)

$$\text{Cephalic index of the head (I)} = \frac{\text{Maximum skull width}}{\text{Maximum skull length}}$$

Depending on the cephalic index value, shape of the head may fall into one of the three categories **(Table 13.2)**.
i. Mesocephalic—Average shape of the head.
ii. Brachycephalic—Broad and short shape of the head.
iii. Dolichocephalic—Long and narrow shape of the head.

### *Facial Form*

Assessment of shape of face (facial form)
It is done by morphologic facial index values, which was given by Martin and Saller in the year 1957.

Facial index value = Morphologic facial height (Distance between nasion and gnathion)/Bizygomatic width (distance between the zygomatic points)

Depending on facial index values obtained, facial form of an individual may be categorized into one of the following types **(Table 13.3)**:
i. Mesoprosopic—Average facial form
ii. Euryprosopic—Short and broad facial form
iii. Leptoprosopic—Long and narrow facial form

### Assessment of Facial Asymmetry

Right and left halves of the human body, including the face are in symmetry with each other although a certain degree of asymmetry may be considered normal. Gross asymmetry of the face must be noted, which may occur in the following conditions:
- Hemi-facial hypertrophy
- Hemi-facial atrophy
- First arch syndrome
- Congenital defects, such as cleft lip and palate
- Unilateral condylar hyperplasia
- Unilateral ankylosis
- Facial palsy.

### Facial Profile

Facial profile helps in diagnosing gross deviation in the maxillomandibular relationship. For example, an individual with concave profile may exhibit Angle's class III malocclusion. Examination of facial profile is done by viewing the patient from the side.
Facial profile is assessed by joining two reference lines.
1. **First reference line:** It is the line joining the forehead to the soft tissue point A.
   *Note:* Soft tissue point A is the deepest point in the curvature of upper lip.
2. **Second reference line:** It is the line joining point A to the soft tissue pogonion
   Following are three types of facial profiles **(Table 13.4)**:
   i. Straight or orthognathic facial profile
   ii. Convex facial profile
   iii. Concave facial profile.

### Facial Divergence

Examination of facial divergence is done by viewing the patient from the side. Facial divergence is often influenced by patient's ethnicity and racial background. For instance, convex profile with an anterior facial divergence is a normal feature of negroid race groups.

Facial divergence is defined as an anterior or posterior inclination of mandible (lower face) relative to the forehead. Assessment of facial divergence is done by a line

| Table 13.3: Facial form | | |
|---|---|---|
| **Facial form** | **Definition presentation** | **Figures** |
| Mesoprosopic | Average face | Fig. 13.1A |
| Euryprosopic | Broad and short face | Fig. 13.1B |
| Leptoprosopic | Long and narrow face | Fig. 13.1C |

**Table 13.4:** Facial profile

| Facial profile | Definition: Using the two reference lines— Forehead to Point A, Point A to pogonion 1. | Figures presentation | Possible type of malocclusion |
|---|---|---|---|
| Straight/Orthognathic facial profile | Two lines form an almost straight line | Fig. 13.2A | Class I malocclusion |
| Convex facial profile | The soft tissue point A is well ahead of soft tissue point Pogonion, although the degree may vary from individual to individual. | Fig. 13.2B | Class II division I malocclusion |
| Concave facial profile | The soft tissue point A is well behind the soft tissue point Pogonion, although the degree may vary from individual to individual. | Fig. 13.2C | Class III malocclusion |

drawn from the forehead to the chin. Facial divergence of an individual may fall into any one of the following three types **(Figs 13.3A to C** and **Table 13.5)**:
1. Straight/orthognathic—A line drawn from forehead to chin is almost straight.
2. Anterior facial divergence—The line drawn from forehead to the chin is inclined anteriorly.
3. Posterior facial divergence—The line drawn from forehead to the chin is inclined posteriorly.

### Assessment of Anteroposterior Jaw Relationship

Ideally, maxillary skeletal base is 2–3 mm anterior to the mandibular skeletal base in centric occlusion. The sagittal skeletal relationship can be clinically assessed by two finger test.

### Two-finger Test

Clinical assessment of anteroposterior jaw relationship can be done by using the examiner's index and middle fingers placed approximately at point A and point B, respectively **(Fig. 13.4)**.
- Index finger—at point A
- Middle finger—at point B

*Inference of the test:* The sagittal skeletal relationship of the patient can be guessed by relative position of the two fingers.
- If the index finger is slightly ahead of middle finger—it indicates class II skeletal base pattern.
- If the middle finger is ahead of the index finger—it indicates class III skeletal base pattern.

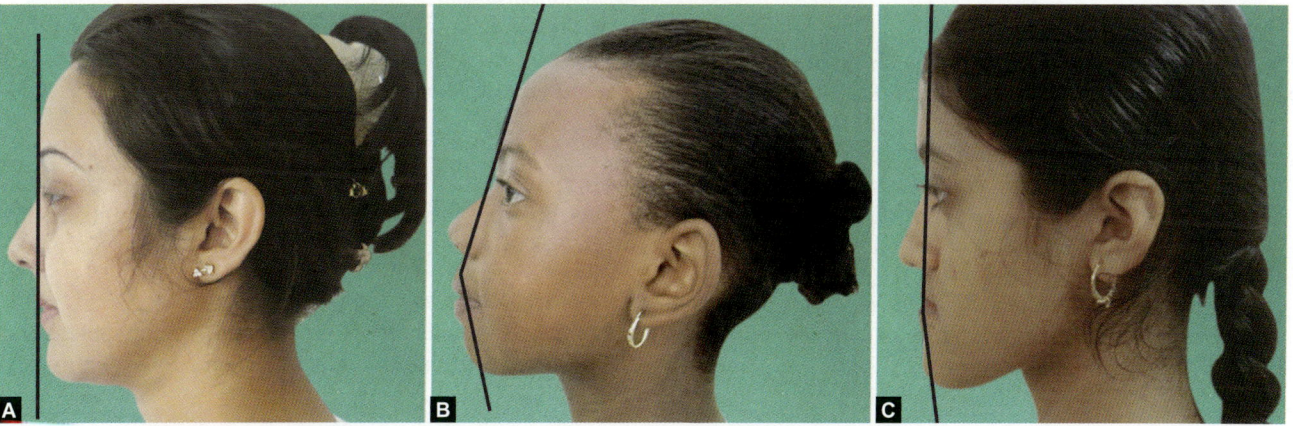

**Figs 13.2A to C:** Facial profile: (A) Straight/Orthognathic profile; (B) Convex facial profile; (C) Concave facial profile

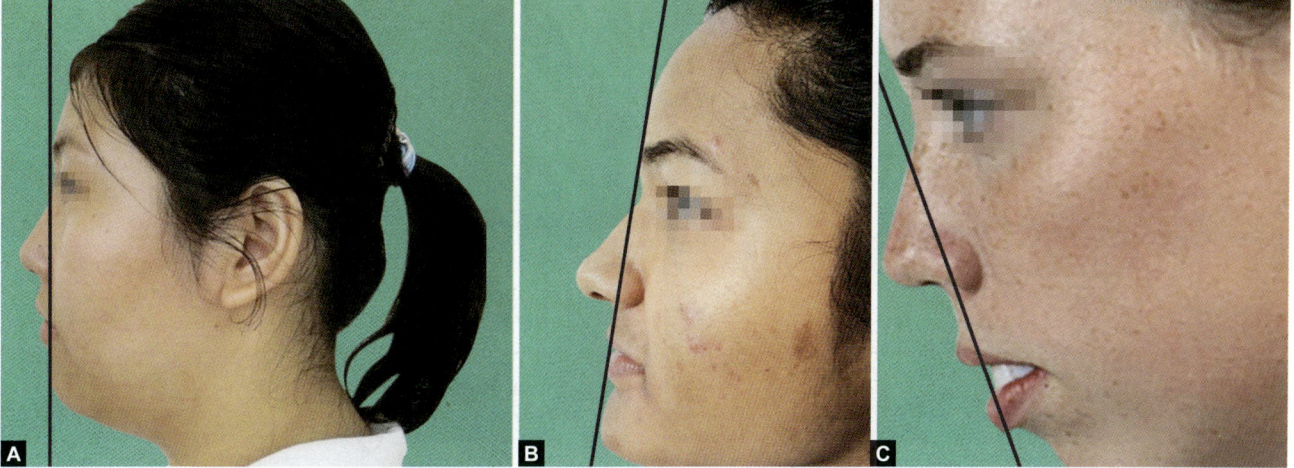

**Figs 13.3A to C:** Facial divergence: (A) Straight facial divergences; (B) Anterior facial divergences; (C) Posterior facial divergences

**Table 13.5:** Facial divergence

| Facial divergence type | Definition: Reference line | (Malocclusion) | Figures presentation |
|---|---|---|---|
| Straight/orthognathic | Straight line | Class I | Fig. 13.3A |
| Anterior divergence | Anterior inclination | Class III | Fig. 13.3B |
| Posterior divergence | Posterior inclination | Class II | Fig. 13.3C |

**Table 13.6:** Assessment of vertical skeletal relationship

| Relationship | Definition | Assessment |
|---|---|---|
| Average FMA angle | FH and mandibular planes intersect at the occipital region | Average growth |
| Low FMA angle | FH and mandibular meet far beyond the occipital region | Horizontal growth |
| High FMA angle | FH and mandibular meet anterior to the occipital region | Vertical growth |

### Assessment of Vertical Skeletal Relationship

In an ideal skeletal relationship, the distance between the glabella (a point between the eyebrow in the midline) and subnasale (base of the nose) is equal to the distance from the subnasale to the underside of the chin (**Table 13.6**).

### Assessment

Assessment of vertical skeletal relationship is done by measuring the FMA angle (**Fig. 13.5**).

*Note:* The FMA angle is defined as the angle formed by the following two reference planes:
i. FH plane (Frankfort horizontal plane—A line between the most superior point of the external auditory meatus and inferior border of the orbit).
ii. Mandibular plane (a line from menton to gonion).

### Evaluation of Facial Proportions

A well proportioned face can be divided into three vertical thirds using four horizontal planes at the level of the hairline, the supraorbital ridge, the base of nose and the inferior border of the chin. Within the lower face, the upper lip occupies a third of the distance while the chin occupies the rest of the space (**Figs 13.6A** and **B**).

### Examination of Nose

Nose has a greater significance in the esthetic appearance of a face, and its form may aid in the assessment of breathing pattern of the patient.

### Size of the Nose

Ideally, length of the nose is equal to one-third of the total facial height (**Fig. 13.7**).

### Shape of the Nose

Shape of the nose can be straight, convex or crooked (**Figs 13.8A** and **B**).

### Shape of the Width of the Nostrils

Normally nostrils should be oval and bilaterally symmetrical. The width of the nostril should be approximately 70% the length of the nose. Stenosis of the nostrils may indicate impaired nasal breathing.

### Examination of Chin

Position and prominence of the chin should be recorded. Examination of the chin should also include assessment of mentolabial sulcus.

### Mentolabial Sulcus

Mentolabial sulcus is a shallow depression seen below the lower lip. The mentolabial sulcus can be normal, shallow or deep (**Table 13.7** and **Fig. 13.11**).

### Mentalis Muscle Activity

Normally, mentalis muscle contraction is not seen at rest. Hyperactivity of the mentalis muscle may be seen in class

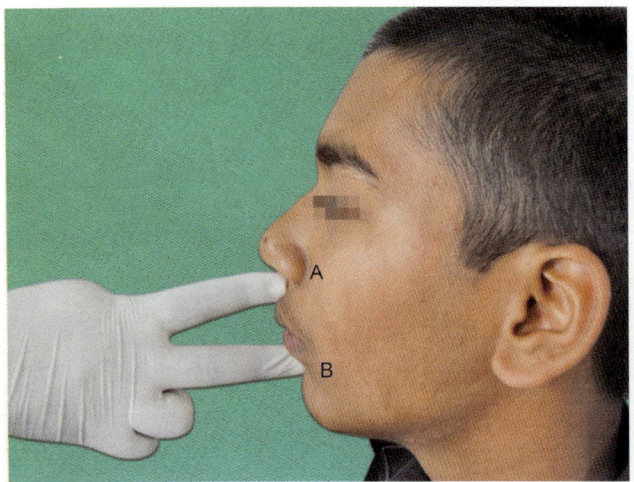

**Fig. 13.4:** Assessment of anteroposterior jaw relationship by using the index and middle fingers placed at point A and point B

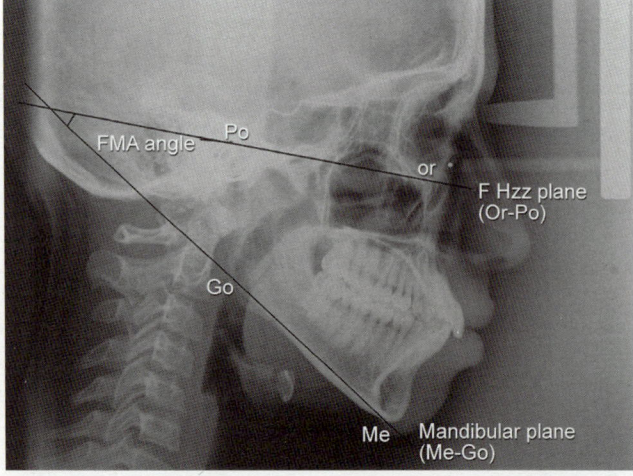

**Fig. 13.5:** Assessment of vertical skeletal relationship is done by measuring the FMA angle

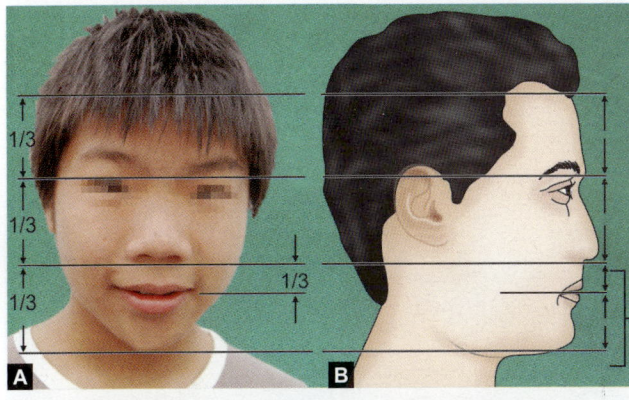

Figs 13.6A and B: Evaluation of facial proportions

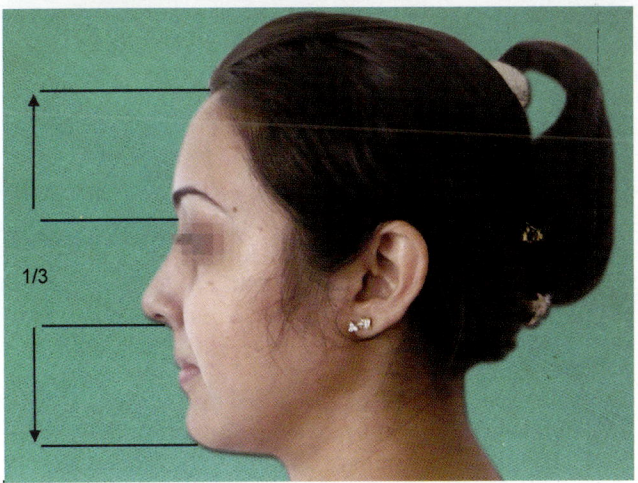

Fig. 13.7: Length of the nose is equal to one-third of the total facial height

II division 1 malocclusion and in patients with deleterious oral habits, such as thumb sucking **(Fig. 13.10)**.

### Chin Position and Prominence

Prominent chin is usually seen in class III malocclusion and recessive chin is observed in class II malocclusions **(Table 13.8** and **Fig. 13.13)**.

| Table 13.7: Mentolabial sulcus |  |  |
| --- | --- | --- |
| *Type* | *Figure* | *Condition* |
| Normal | **Fig. 13.9A** | Angle's class I malocclusion |
| Shallow | **Fig 13.9B** | Bimaxillary protrusion |
| Deep | **Fig 13.9C** | Angle's class II division 1 malocclusion |

| Table 13.8: Chin position and prominence |  |  |
| --- | --- | --- |
| *Type* | *Figure* | *Condition seen* |
| Prominent chin | **Fig. 13.11A** | Angle's class III malocclusion |
| Recessive chin | **Fig. 13.11B** | Angle's class II malocclusion |

| Table 13.9: Nasolabial angle |  |  |
| --- | --- | --- |
| *Nasolabial angle* | *Figure* | *Clinical condition* |
| Normal | **Fig. 13.12A** | Angle's class I malocclusion |
| Increased | **Fig. 13.12B** | Angle's class II division 2 malocclusion |
| Decreased | **Fig. 13.12C** | Angle's class II division 1 malocclusion |

### Nasolabial Angle

Nasolabial angle is the angle formed between the lower border of the nose and a line connecting the intersection of the nose and upper lip with the tip of the upper lip (Labiale superius) **(Table 13.9)**.

### Normal Value and Significance

Normally, the nasolabial angle ranges from 90–110 degrees **(Figs 13.12A to C)**.
i. An increased nasolabial angle (i.e. > 110 degree) may suggest maxillary anterior retroclination.
ii. A decreased nasolabial angle (i.e. < 90 degree) may indicate maxillary proclination.

### Examination of Lips

Lips may be competent, potentially competent or incompetent **(Table 13.10** and **Fig. 13.15)**.

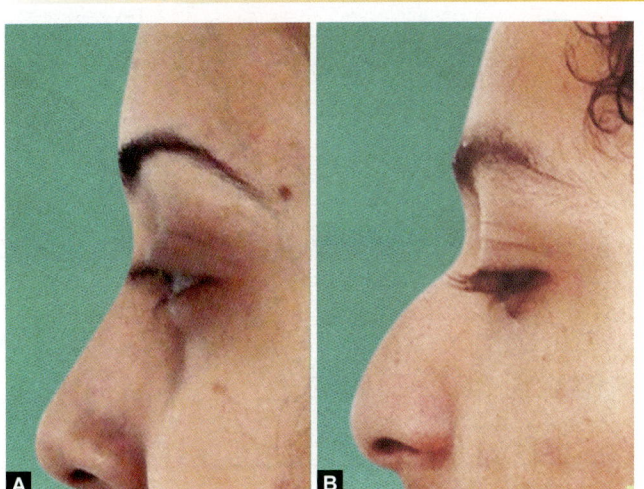
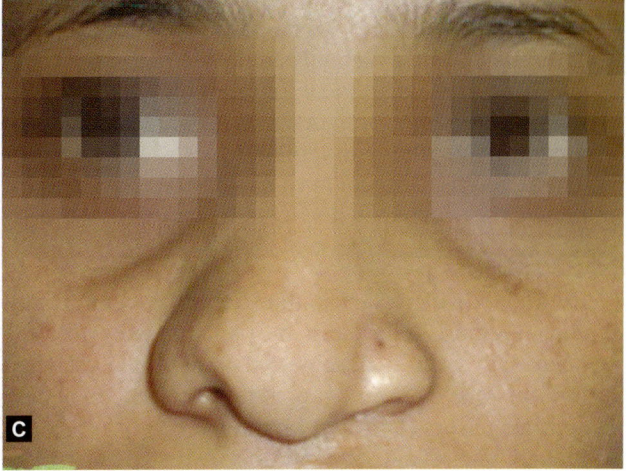

Figs 13.8A and C: Shape of the nose: (A) Straight nose; (B) Convex nose; (C) Crooked nose

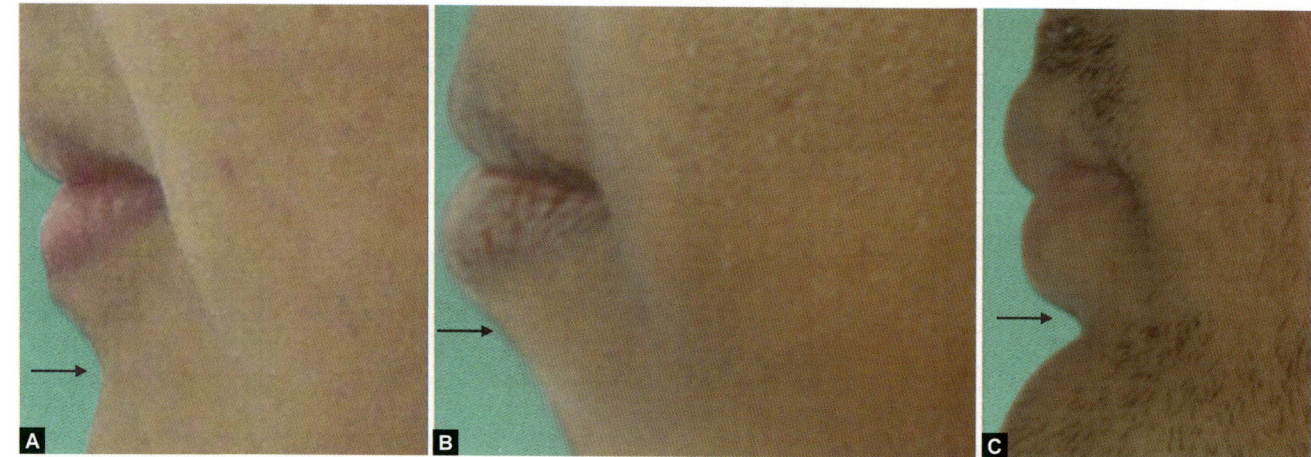

**Figs 13.9A to C:** Mentolabial sulcus. (A) Normal depth of mentolabial sulcus in a patient with Angle's class I malocclusion; (B) Shallow mentolabial sulcus in a female patient with bimaxillary protrusion; (C) Deep mentolabial sulcus in a male patient with Angle's class II division 2 malocclusion

### Competent Lips

When patient is at rest, the upper and lower lips meet each other without muscle exertion and can be seen in class I malocclusion.

### Potentially Incompetent Lips

Lip seal can be achieved with muscle exertion. It can be seen in class I malocclusion.

### Incompetent Lips

When patient at rest, upper and lower lips fail to meet each other. It can be seen in open bite cases and bimaxillary proclination.

### Intraoral Examination

#### Tongue

- A state of equilibrium between intraoral (tongue) and perioral musculatures (lips and other facial muscles) is essential for the normal development of dentofacial structures and malocclusion may result when this balance is disturbed.
- Microglossia may cause narrow and collapsed dental arches, while macroglossia may cause flaring of anteriors and spacing between the teeth.
- The tongue is examined for abnormalities in size, shape, color and configuration. An abnormally large tongue may exhibit indentations of the teeth at its lateral margin. Lingual frenum must be examined for tongue tie, which may restrict tongue movements.

#### Frenal Attachments

- Examination of maxillary labial frenum is an important consideration, especially in patients with midline diastema. A thick, fibrous and abnormally attached frenum may prevent approximation of maxillary central incisors (**Figs 13.14A and B**).
- Blanch test is a useful adjunct, which aids in the diagnosis of abnormal labial frenum attachment.
- Intraoral periapical radiograph of the area may show notch like radiolucency in the alveolar crest region between two maxillary central incisors.
- Abnormal attachment of mandibular labial frenum may cause recession of gingiva in that area.

#### Palate

The palate is examined for the following findings:
- Depth and form of the palate may be correlated with the facial form of the patient. For example, brachycephalic patients generally have broad palate (**Fig. 13.15A**) whereas, narrow palate (**Fig. 13.15B**) is usually seen in dolichocephalic patients.
- Palatal swelling may be indication of an impacted tooth, cyst or other pathologies.
- Mucosal ulceration and indentations may reveal traumatic deep bite.
- Presence of clefts in the palate causes malocclusion (**Fig. 13.15C**). Postsurgical scar tissue may restrict maxillary growth.

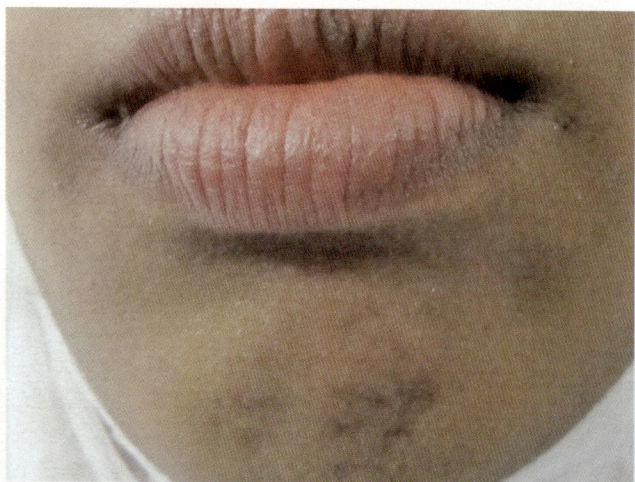

**Fig. 13.10:** Puckering of the chin indicative of hyperactive mentalis muscle activity

| Table 13.10: Different forms of lips | | | |
|---|---|---|---|
| Type | Figure showing lip | Meaning | Clinical condition |
| Competent lip | Fig. 13.13A | Lips are in contact on muscle relaxation | Angle's class I malocclusion |
| Potentially incompetent lips | Fig. 13.13B | Lips are in contact on muscle exertion | Deway's class I type 1 malocclusion |
| Incompetent lips | Fig. 13.13C | No lip contact present | Open bite cases |
| Everted lips | Fig. 13.13D | Hypertrophied lips | Angle's class II division 1 malocclusion |

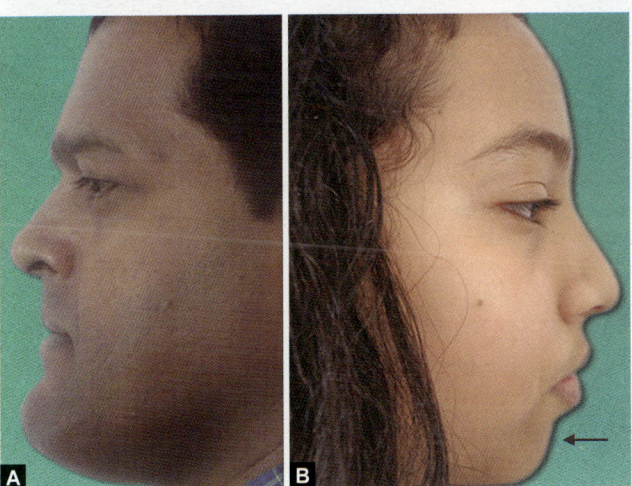

**Figs 13.11A and B:** Examination of the chin. (A) Prominent chin; (B) Recessive chin

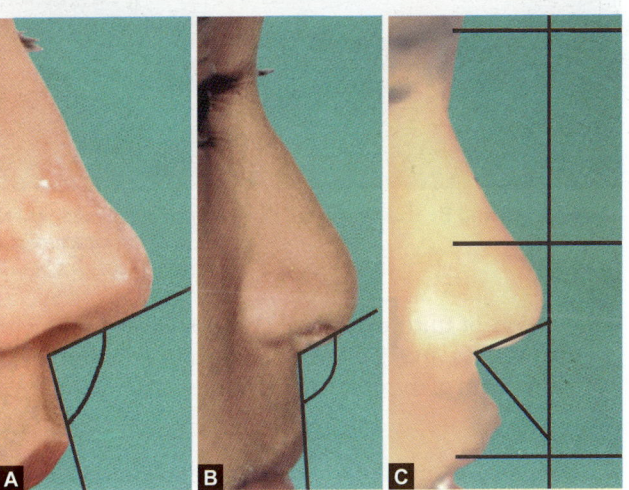

**Figs 13.12A to C:** Nasolabial angle: (A) Normal nasolabial angle; (B) Increased nasolabial angle; (C) Decreased nasolabial angle

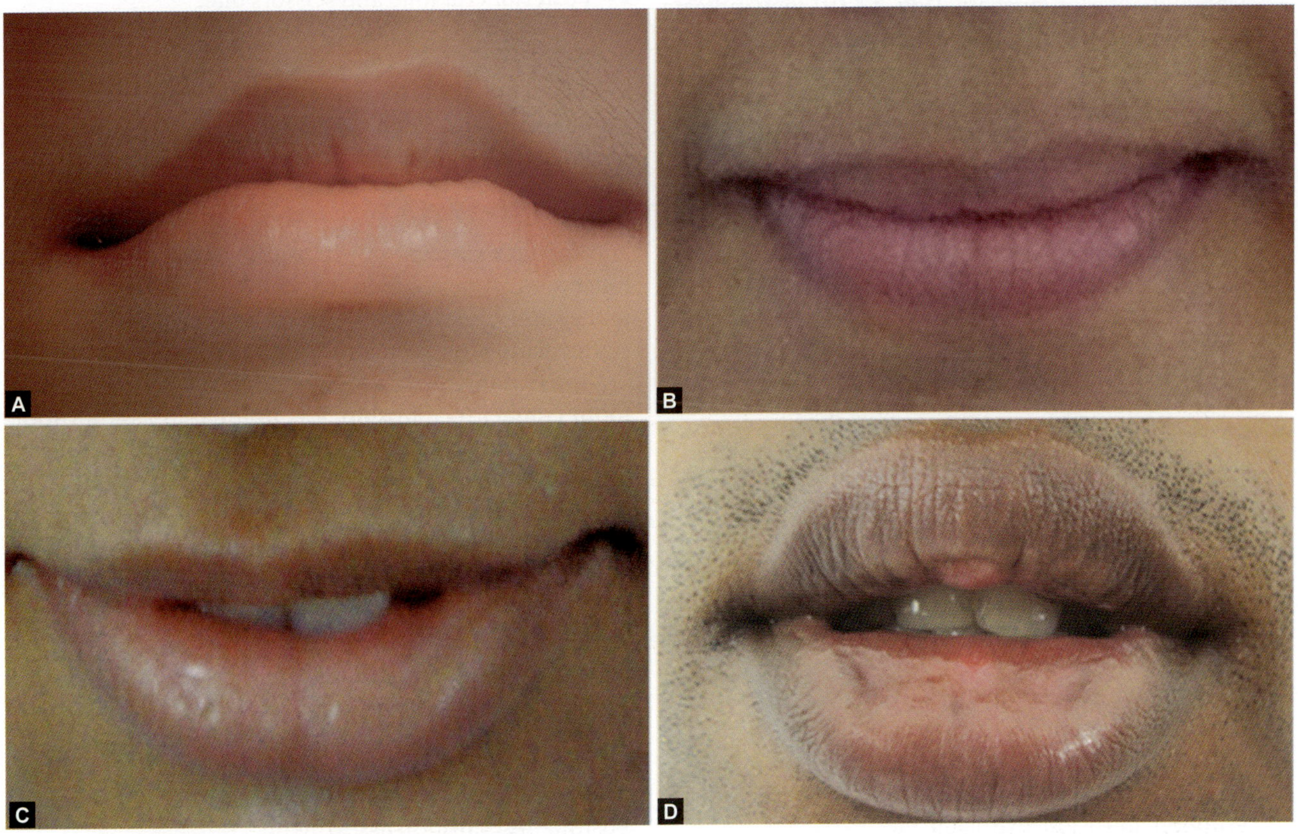

**Figs 13.13A to D:** Examination of lips: (A) Competent lips; (B) Potentially incompetent lips; (C) Incompetent lips; (D) Everted lips

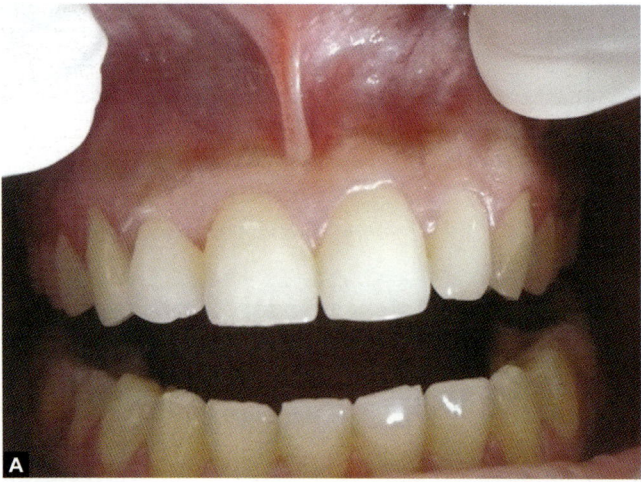 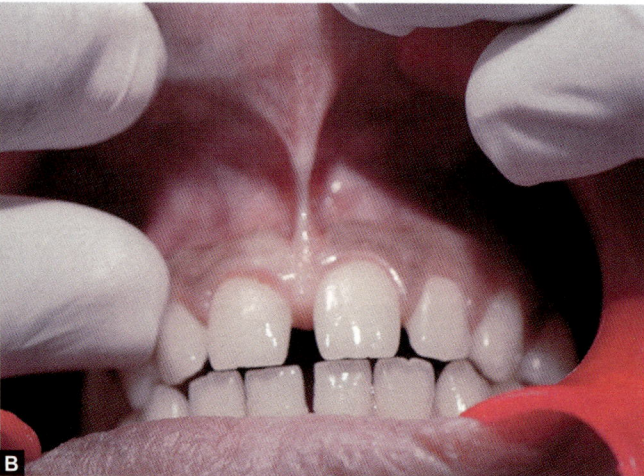

**Figs 13.14A and B:** Examination of labial frenum attachment: (A) Normal attachment of labial frenum; (B) Thick, fibrous abnormal high labial frenum attachment causing midline diastema

- Position of third rugae, which is usually in line with the canines, may be used as a useful adjunct in the assessment of maxillary anterior proclination.

### Gingiva
- Gingiva is examined for inflammation, recession and other mucogingival lesions.
- Good oral hygiene and health of gingiva is a prerequisite for successful orthodontic treatment.
- Marginal anterior gingivitis **(Fig. 13.16)** may indicate mouth breathing habit. Localized gingival recession may be the indication of traumatic occlusion and hyperplastic gingiva may suggest that the patient is under certain medications like dilatin sodium.

### Examination of Tonsils and Adenoids
Inflammation of the tonsils can cause alteration in tongue and jaw posture, thereby disturbing the orofacial balance, leading to malocclusion.

### Examination of the Dentition
Dentition is examined for the following:
- Stage of dentition.
  - Primary
  - Early mixed/late mixed
  - Permanent.
- Eruption status
  - Premature loss of any deciduous teeth
  - Number of erupted permanent teeth and whether eruption status is correlating with chronological age of the patient.
- Developmental anomalies, dental caries and restorative status of teeth.
- and symmetry of individual dental arches.
- Individual tooth malpositions such as rotation, ectopic eruption, intrusion, extrusion, etc.
- Assessment of interarch relationships in all three planes of space.

### Anteroposterior Plane
- Molar relationship whether it is class I, class II division 1, class II division 2 or class III
- Incisor overjet whether it is normal, edge-to-edge or reverse overjet (anterior crossbite).

### Transverse Plane
- Any shift of midline in anterior segment
- Posterior crossbite and scissors bite.

### Vertical Plane
- Assessment of incisors overbite—whether normal, deep bite and anterior open bite.
- Posterior open bite.

### Functional Examination
The modern concept of occlusion views occlusion as an integrated system of functional units involving teeth, joints, and muscles of the head and neck rather than a static relation between maxillary and mandibular teeth.

Thus along with evaluation of static, morphologic tooth contact relationship, it is prudent to assess various functional units of the stomatognathic system as well.

The functional examination should include the following:
- Assessment of postural rest position and interocclusal space
- Path of closure of mandible
- Examination of TMJ
- Assessment of respiration
- Swallowing pattern
- Phonation.

### Postural Rest Position and Interocclusal Space
Postural rest position assessment
- Postural rest position is the position of the mandible at which the muscles that close the jaw and those that

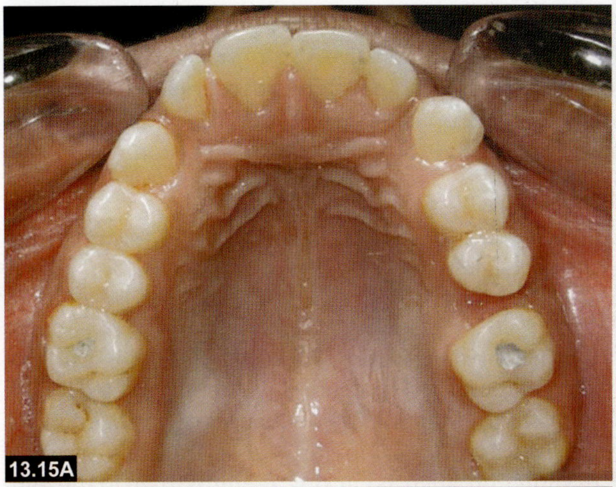

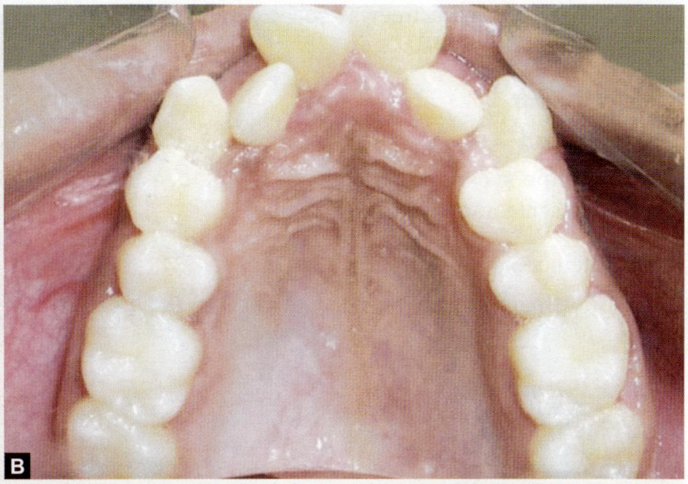

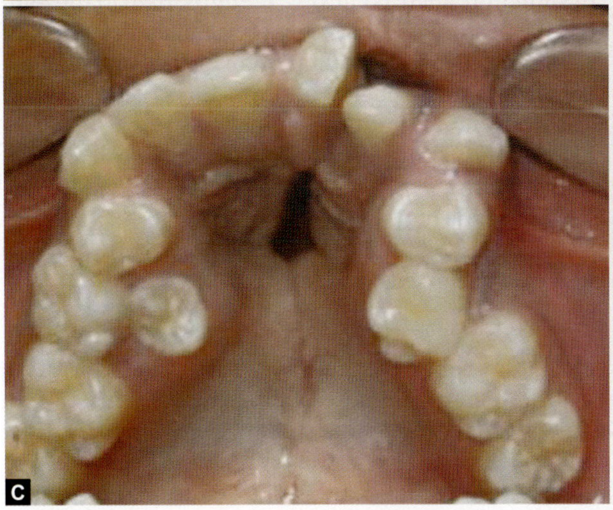

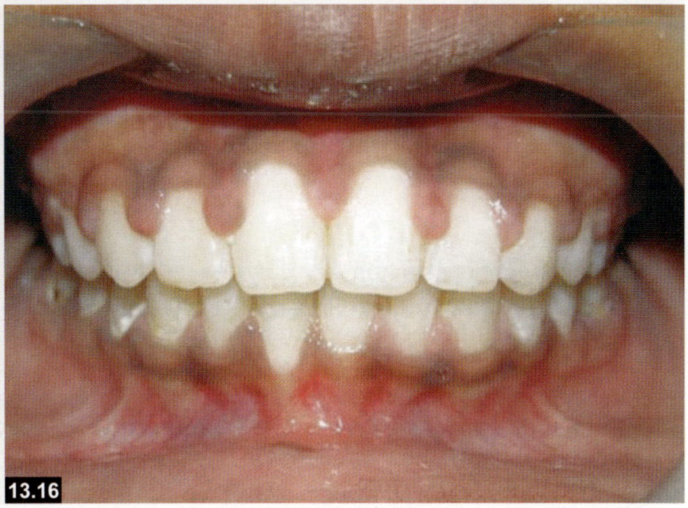

**Figs 13.15A to C:** Examination of the palate: (A) Broad palate seen in a brachycephalic patient; (B) Narrow palate in dolichocephalic patient; (C) Cleft palate causing severe malocclusion; **Fig. 13.16:** Examination of gingiva—Marginal gingivitis in a male patient with mouth-breathing habit

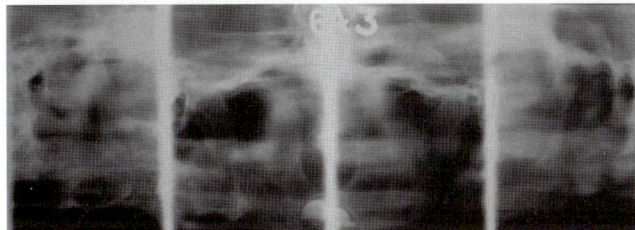

**Fig. 13.17:** TMJ projection

open them are in a state of minimal contraction just sufficient into maintain their posture of the mandible.
- Various methods can be used to assess postural rest position as described below.
- During assessment the patient must be seated upright with his/her back unsupported and looking straight ahead.

## Phonetic Method

- Phonetic method involves encouraging to the patient to pronounce certain consonants, such as "M" by asking the patient to repeat words like "swim" or "Mississippi."

- The mandible returns to its postural rest position 1-2 seconds after the exercise. The patient is asked not to change the jaw, lip or tongue posture after exercise and clinician studies the interocclusal space by parting the patient's lips.

### Command Method

Patient is asked to perform certain functions, such as swallowing at the end of which the mandible spontaneously returns to rest position.

### Noncommand Method

In this method, the clinician diverts patient's mind by engaging the patient in conversation about unrelated topics so as to relax him/her. The clinician observes the patient as he/she speaks or swallows.

### Interocclusal Clearance/Freeway Space Assessment

At postural rest position, maxillary and mandibular teeth are not in contact and the existent space between the upper and lower jaws is referred to as the interocclusal clearance or the freeway space. Normally the freeway space is in the range of 3 mm in the canine region.

Interocclusal clearance/freeway space can be assessed by following ways:

### Intraoral Methods
#### Direct Method
Vernier calipers can be directly used to measure the interocclusal clearance in canine region.

#### Indirect Method
Impression material can be used to register the freeway space.

### Extraoral Methods
#### Direct Method
- Two reference points are marked, using sticky plaster, one on nose and the other on the chin in mid-sagittal plane.
- The distance between these two reference points is measured at rest position and at centric occlusion. The difference between the two measurements is the freeway space.

#### Indirect Method
- Cephalometric registration
- Lateral cephalograms, one taken at rest position and the other at centric occlusion, are taken to determine the freeway space.
- Kinesiographic registration
- This method uses a magnet, fixed on the lower anterior, and mandibular mounts are recorded by scissors and are then processed in the kinesiograph.

### Evaluation of the Path of Closure
The path of closure is the movement of the mandible from rest position to habitual occlusion. In certain malocclusions, the path of closure of mandible may be deviated.

### Forward Path of Closure
- A forward path of closure may be seen in patients with mild skeletal prenormalcy or edge-to-edge incisor contact.
- The mandible is guided to a more forward position by such patients so as to bring the mandibular incisors labial to the upper incisors.

### Backward Path of Closure
Patients with class II division 2 malocclusion exhibit premature incisor contact due to retroclined maxillary incisors. In such patients, mandible is guided to a more backward position so as to establish occlusion.

### Lateral Path of Closure
Mandible may be deviated to left or right side during closure due to occlusal prematurities or posterior cross-bites.

### Examination of TMJ
- Clinical examination of TMJ should include auscultation and palpation of temporomandibular joint (TMJ), examination of muscles of mastication.
- The patient is examined for symptoms of TMJ dysfunction, such as clicking, crepitus, pain in the joint or masticatory muscles, hypermobility, deviation of mandible, dislocation, limitation of jaw movements and other morphological abnormalities.
- The maximum mouth opening can be determined by measuring the distance between maxillary and mandibular incisal edges with the mouth wide open. Normally, the mouth opening is about 40–45 mm.
- Specific radiographic projections of TMJ may be needed in selected cases (**Fig. 13.17**).

### Assessment of Swallowing Patterns
At birth, the tongue is relatively large and protrudes between the gum pads to establish lip seal. This kind of swallow is called as infantile swallow, which persists until the age 1–2 years. Infantile swallow is gradually replaced by mature swallow as the deciduous teeth erupt. Persistence of infantile swallow may lead to the development of tongue thrusting habit and causes malocclusion.

### Assessment of Respiration
Oral or oronasal mouth breathing habit may be a contributing factor of the existing malocclusion in the patient. Breathing pattern of the patient can be examined by the following four methods (**Fig. 13.18A to C**):

### Visual Observation
In nasal breathers the external nares may dilate during inspiration, although this is not a rule. In mouth breather,

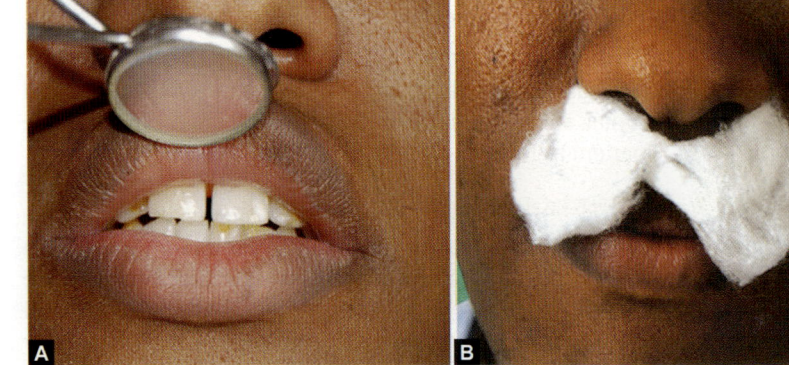
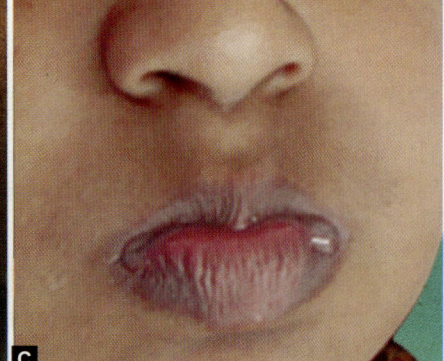

**Figs 13.18A to C:** Assessment of respiration: (A) Mirror test; (B) Cotton test; (C) Water test

there is no lip seal at rest and the external nares may constrict or unchanged during inspiration.

### Mirror Test
A double-sided mirror is held between the nose and the mouth. Presence of fogging on the mirror towards the nose indicates nasal breathing while fogging on the other side indicates mouth breathing **(Fig. 13.18A)**.

### Cotton Test
A small butterfly-shaped piece of cotton is placed above the upper lip, near the nostrils. In nasal breathers, the cotton flutters as patient respires **(Fig. 13.18B)**.

### Water Test
The patient is asked to fill and retain water in his/her mouth for a period of time.

Mouth breathers find this task difficult while nasal breathers can easily perform it **(Fig. 13.18C)**.

### Assessment of Phonation
Phonation may be affected in certain malocclusion. The patient is observed while he/she reads from book or counts numbers from 1-10. Patients with anterior open bite and tongue thrusting habit may tend to lisp while cleft palate patients may have a nasal tone.

### Facial Photographs
#### Frontal
a. ***Frontal at rest***: If lip competence is present, the lips should be in repose of the mandible in rest position **(Fig. 13.19A)**.
b. Frontal view with the teeth in maximal intercuspation, with the lips closed even if this strains the patient **(Fig. 13.19B)**.
c. ***Frontal dynamism (Smile)***: This type of frontal facial photographs help in the assessment of amount of incisors shown on smile (percentage of maxillary incisors display on smile) and any excessive gingival display **(Fig. 13.19C)**.
d. ***A close-up image of the posed smile***: A close-up image of the posed smile is used for careful analysis of the smile relationship **(Fig. 13.19D)**.

### Oblique (Three quarter, 45 degree)
In this type of facial photograph, the patient in natural head position, looking 45 degrees to the camera. Oblique facial photographs are taken in the following three

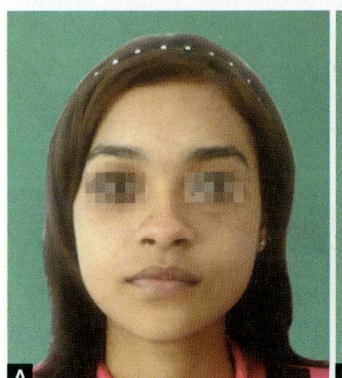 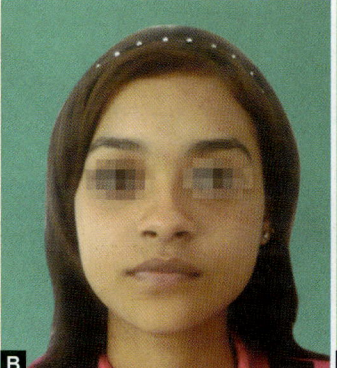 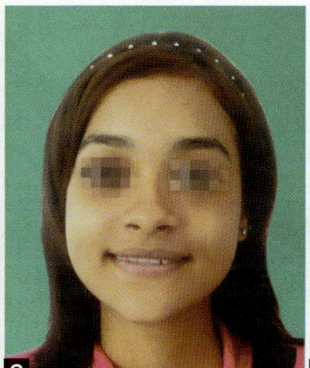 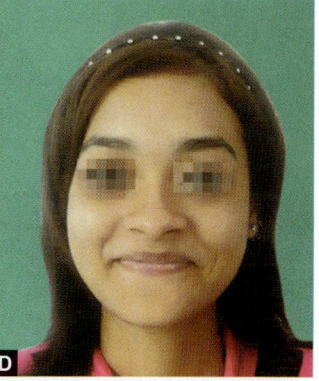

**Figs 13.19A to D:** Frontal facial photographs: (A) Frontal facial photograph at rest; (B) Frontal view with the teeth in maximal intercuspation, with the lips closed; (C) Frontal facial photograph with smile; (D) A close-up image of the posed smile

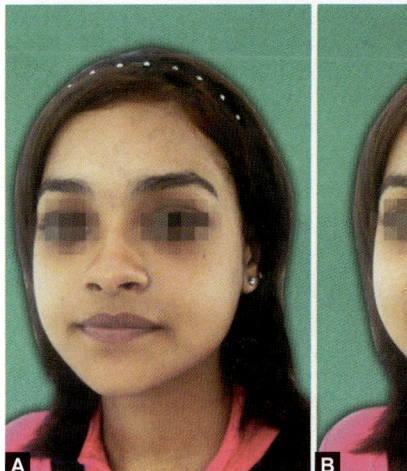 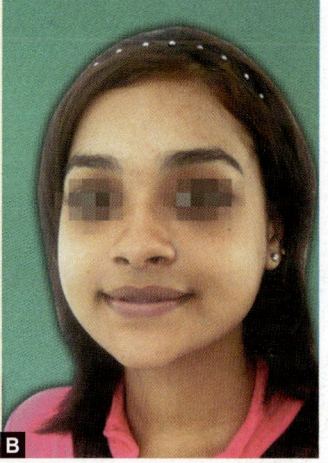 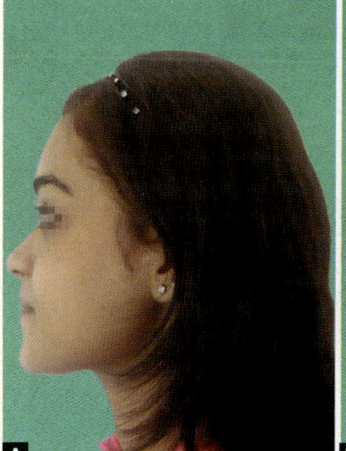 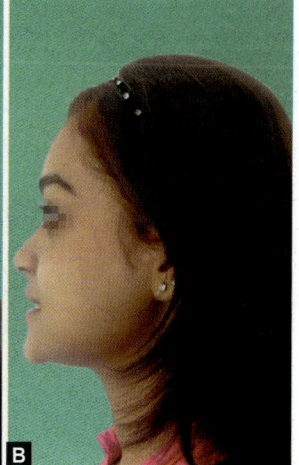

**Figs 13.20A and B:** (A) Oblique facial photograph at rest; (B) Oblique facial photograph with smile

**Figs 13.21A and B:** (A) Profile facial photograph at rest; (B) Profile facial photograph with smile

views, which are helpful in the orthodontic diagnosis **(Fig. 13.20A)**.

a. ***Oblique at rest:*** Oblique at rest photograph is useful for the examination of the midface and is particularly informative of midface deformities, including nasal deformity.
b. ***Oblique on smile:*** Oblique on smile reveals characteristics of the smile not obtainable on the frontal view and certainly not obtainable through any cephalometric analysis **(Fig. 13.20B)**.
c. ***Oblique close-up smile:*** Oblique close-up smile view helps in more precise evaluation of the lip relationship of the teeth and jaw that is possible using the full oblique view.

### Profile Facial Photograph

a. ***Profile at rest:*** In this view, the lips should be relaxed **(Fig. 13.21A)**.
b. ***Profile smile:*** This view helps in the assessment of angulations of the maxillary incisors **(Fig. 13.21B)**.

### An Optional Sub-Mental View

An optional sub-mental view helps in the assessment of mandibular asymmetry.

### Digital Photography

Digital view of computer technology currently enables the clinician to record anterior tooth, display during speech and smiling at the equivalent of 30 frames per second.

### Intraoral Photographs

The intraoral photographs include the following five views:
1. Right lateral view **(Fig. 13.22A)**
2. Left lateral view **(Fig. 13.22C)**
3. Anterior/frontal view **(Fig. 13.22B)**
4. Maxillary occlusal view **(Fig. 13.22D)**
5. Mandibular occlusal view **(Fig. 13.22E)**

The purpose of the intraoral photographs are listed below:
- To record type of malocclusion.
- To record any soft tissue abnormalities, such as gingival abscess, hypertrophy, ulcers, cysts and tumors.
- To record any hard tissue pathologies, such as caries, fracture, discoloration and odontomes.

### Panoramic and Intraoral Radiographs

The panoramic radiograph helps to assess dental age and development and bony pathologies, such as root resorption, odontomes, impactions, jaw fracture, tumors and ankylosis, etc. **(Fig. 13.23)**. The intraoral radio-graphs are necessary for adult patients with periodontal disease.

### Cephalometric Radiograph

Purpose of having cephalometric radiographs is listed below:
- They reveal details of skeletal and dental relationship that cannot be obtained in other ways.
- They allow a precise evaluation of response to treatment.

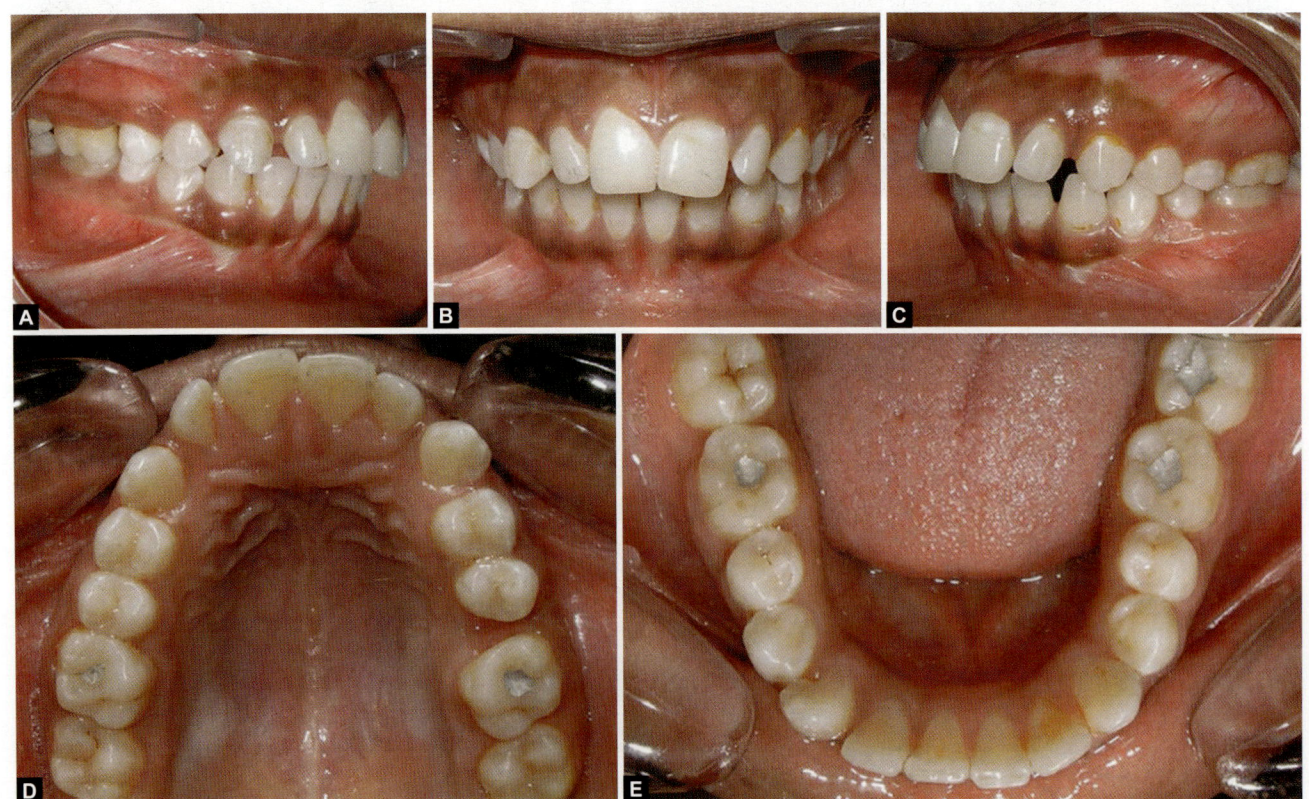

Figs 13.22A to E: Intraoral photographs

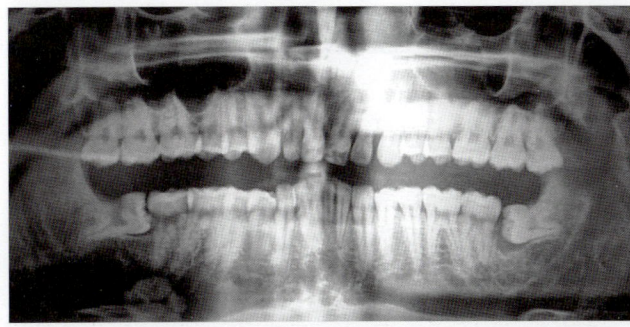

**Fig. 13.23:** OPG showing bilateral horizontally impacted mandibular third molars

## BIBLIOGRAPHY

1. Ackerman JL, Profitt WR: The characteristics of malocclusion: a modern approach to classification and diagnosis. Am J Orthod. 1969;56:443-54.
2. Andrews LF. The six keys to normal occlusion. Am J Orthod. 1972;62:296-309.
3. Begg PR. Begg orthodontic theory and technique, Philadelphia. WB Saunders, 1965.
4. Downs WB. Analysis of the dentofacial profile. Angle Orthod. 1956;26:191.
5. Graber TM, Vanarsdall RL. Orthodontics Current Principles and Techniques. Mosby Year Book Inc, 1994.
6. Graber TM. Orthodontics: Principles and Practice, 3rd edition. WB Saunders, 1988.
7. Jacobson. Introduction to Radiographic Cephalometry. Philadelphia: Lea and Febiger; 1985.
8. Koski K: The norm concept in dental orthopaedics. Angle Orthod. 1955;25:113-7.
9. Profitt WR, Ackerman JL. Rating the characteristics of malocclusion: A systematic approach for planning treatment. Am J Orthod. 1973;64(3):258-69.
10. Quintero JC, et al. Craniofacial imaging in orthodontics: Historical perspective, current status and future developments. Angle Orthod. 1999;69:491-506.
11. Tung AW, Kiyak HA. Psychological influences on the timing of orthodontic treatment. Am J Orthod Dentofacial Orthop. 1998;113:29-39.
12. Whaties E. Essentials of Dental Radiography and Radiology, 2nd edn. London: Churchill Livingstone, 1996.

## EXAM-ORIENTED QUESTIONS

### Long Essay or Long Questions
1. Discuss various diagnostic aids used in orthodontics.
2. Enumerate diagnostic aids used in orthodontics and write in detail essential diagnostic aids.

### Short Essay or Long Notes
1. Electromyography
2. Uses of radiographs in orthodontics
3. Hand wrist radiographs
4. Advanced diagnostic aids.

### Short Notes
1. Supplemental diagnostics aids
2. Facial divergence
3. Facial profile
4. Nasolabial angle
5. Mentolabial sulcus
6. Examination of TMJ
7. Examination of lips
8. Two finger test used to assess jaw relationship
9. Cephalometric index value.

# CHAPTER OVERVIEW

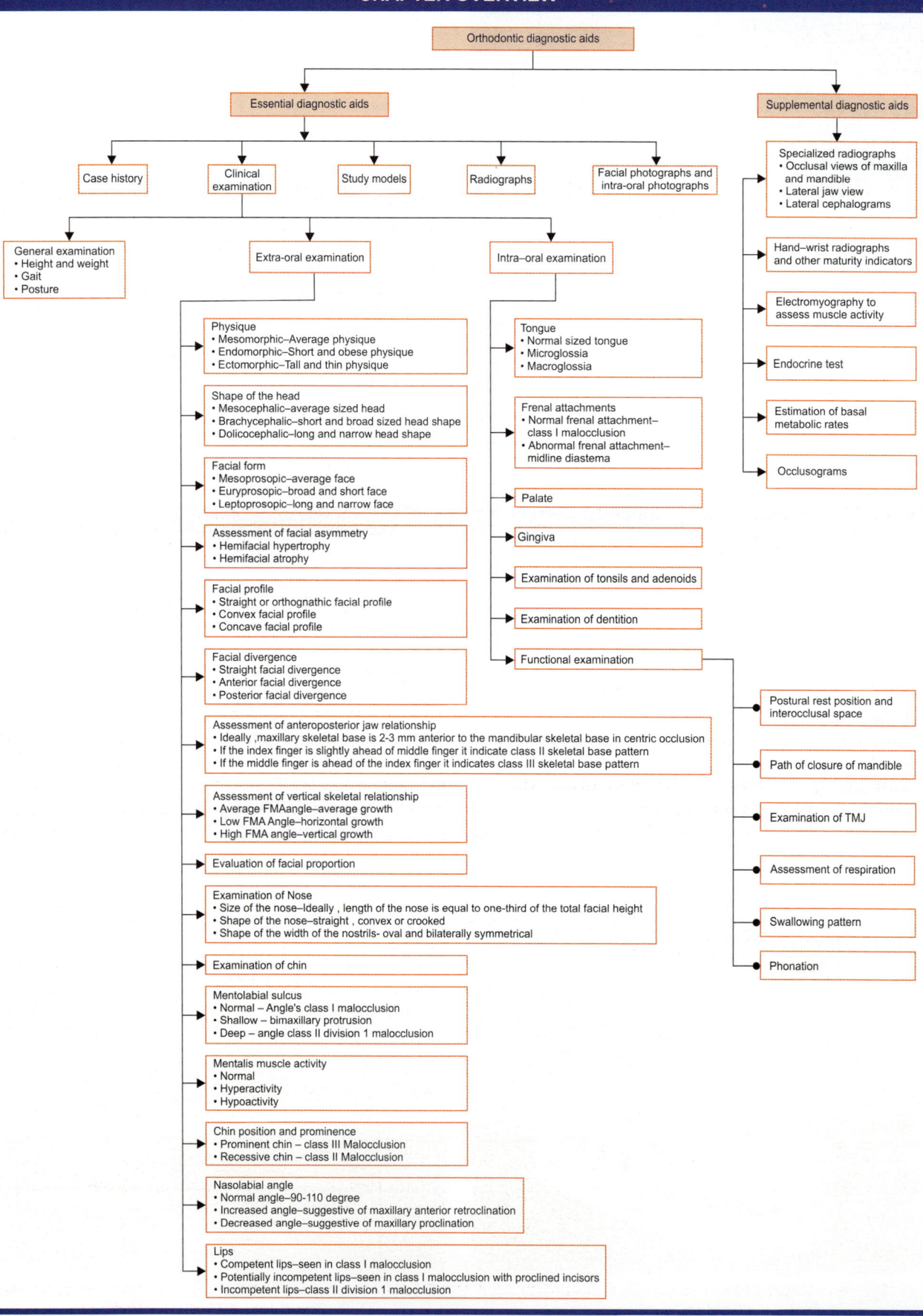

# CHAPTER 14

# Model Analysis

*Phulari BS*

Orthodontic diagnosis and treatment planning is done by taking into consideration, the tooth material, skeletal and muscle balance and the growth potential. Among the various decisions taken, an important decision is the one taken for or against the extraction of certain teeth to achieve the desired results. Model analysis is an essential diagnostic tool, which can aid in making up this important decision of opting for arch expansion or extraction in a given case.

Among other benefits, model analysis provides a means of evaluating the amount of space required for proper alignment of teeth by allowing the accurate assessment of arch length-tooth material discrepancy.

Various methods of model analysis have been described and appropriate analysis must be selected for a given case. A working classification is given in **(Table 14.1)** for the ease of understanding.

## ARMAMENTARIUM

The following things are needed to carryout model analysis:
- Maxillary and mandibular study casts of the patient **(Fig. 14.1)**.
- 0.012 inch soft round brass wire—to measure the arch length **(Fig. 14.2A)**.
- Bow divider—to measure the mesiodistal width of teeth and arch width **(Fig. 14.2B)**.
- Scale—to record the measurements, obtained by the bow divider **(Fig. 14.2C)**.

**Table 14.1:** Different types of model analysis and their use in specific conditions

**Analyses used to assess the need of extraction**
- Analysis used for maxillary arch:
  • Arch perimeter analysis
- Analysis used in mandibular arch:
  • Nance Carey's analysis
- Analyses used to assess the need of arch expansion
  • Pont's analysis
  • Linder Harth index
  • Korkhaus analysis
  • Ashley Howe analysis
- Analysis used to assess the tooth material excess
  • Bolton's analysis
- Analysis used in mixed dentition
  • Mixed dentition analysis

- Marking pencil to mark on the brass wire **(Fig. 14.2D)**.
- Measured with using bow divides is then transferred to the scale **(Fig. 14.2E)**.

## CAREY'S ANALYSIS

Arch length-tooth material discrepancy is one of the important causative factors of malocclusion. Carey's analysis is aimed at determining the extent of the discrepancy. Carey's analysis is performed on the mandibular cast. If the same analysis is carried out on the maxillary arch then it is called as *arch perimeter analysis*.

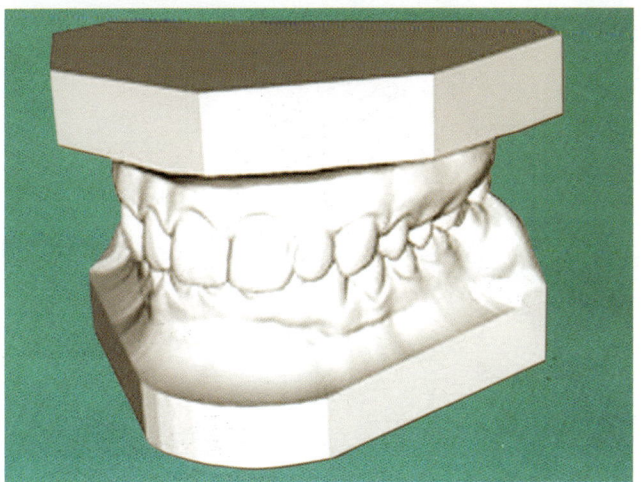

**Fig. 14.1:** Maxillary and mandibular study casts of the patient

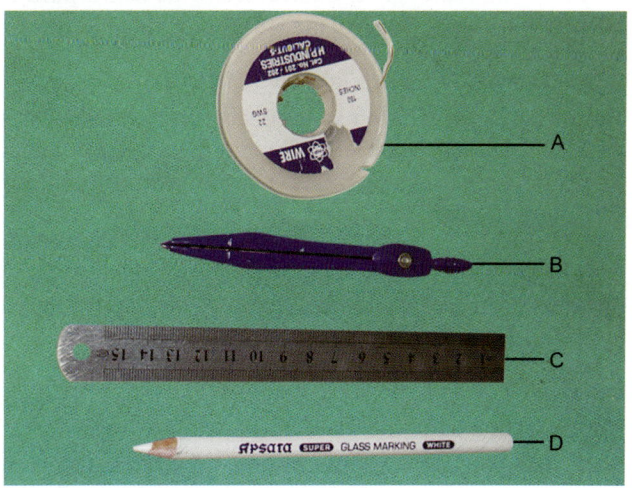

**Figs 14.2A to D:** Armamentarium. (A) 0.012 inch soft round brass wire; (B) Bow divider; (C) Scale; (D) Marking pencil

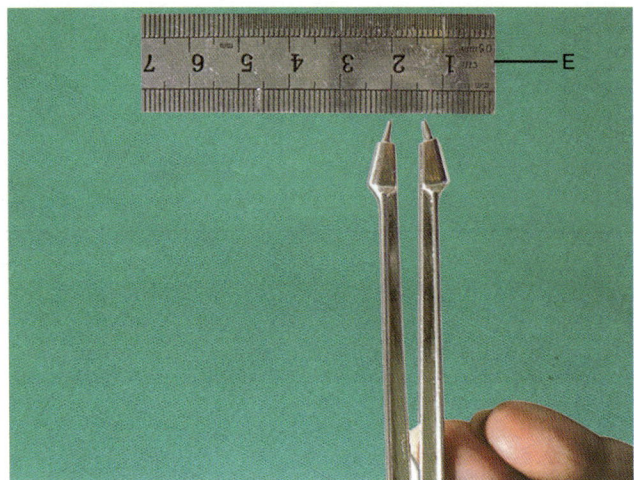

**Fig. 14.2E:** Armamentarium measured width from bow divider is transferred to scale

## Procedure

### Determination of Arch Length

The arch length, anterior to the mandibular first molars is measured using a 0.012 inch soft round brass wire. The wire is adapted to the model of the mandibular arch so that one end engages first permanent lower molar near the marginal ridge.

The wire is next passed over the buccal cusps of the premolars, then over the normal cuspal position of the cuspid, then over the anterior teeth at ridge center and finally around the same course on the opposite side, ending in the mesiobuccal line angle of the lower first permanent molar of the other side **(Fig. 14.3)**. The wire is cut at this point and straightened and the length is recorded.

- In case of proclined anteriors, the brass wire is passed along the cingulum of anterior teeth.
- In case of retroclined anteriors, the brass wire is passed labial to the anterior teeth.
- In case of well-aligned anterior teeth, the wire is passed over the incisal edges of the anterior teeth.

### Determination of Arch Width/Total Tooth Material (TTM)

Tooth material is determined by measuring the mesiodistal width of the teeth anterior to the first permanent molars (incisors, canines and premolars) at the maximum contour using bow divider.

### Determination of the Discrepancy

The discrepancy refers to the difference between the arch length and total tooth material.

### Inference

Nonextraction case

If the discrepancy is 2.5 mm or less, it indicates minimal tooth material excess, which can be managed by proximal stripping.

### Extraction of second premolar

If the discrepancy is 2.5–5 mm, second premolar may need to be extracted.

### Extraction of first premolar

If the discrepancy is more than 5 mm then extraction of first premolar is advised.

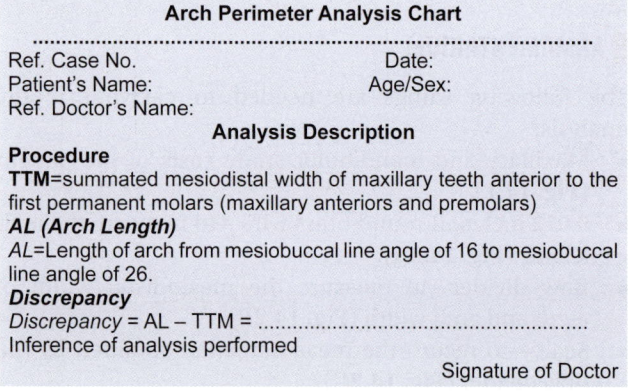

## ARCH PERIMETER ANALYSIS

Arch perimeter analysis is similar to the Carey's analysis, but it is performed on the maxillary cast.

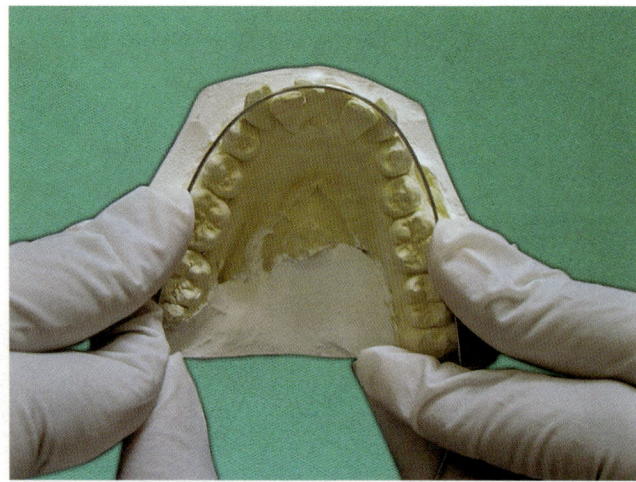

**Fig. 14.3:** Determination of arch length using 0.012 inch round soft brass wire, the lower right first permanent molar to lower left first permanent molar

## PONT'S ANALYSIS

Pont reported his analysis in the year 1909 and proposed that the measurement of four maxillary incisors will automatically establish the width of the arch in premolar and molar regions. Pont's analysis helps in the following:
- Determining whether the dental arch is narrow or wide.
- Determining the need for the lateral arch expansion.
- Determining how much expansion is possible at the premolar and molar region.

### Procedure

#### Determination of Sum of Incisors (SI)

The mesiodistal width of the four maxillary incisors is measured and values summed up. This is called the sum of incisors, i.e. mesiodistal width of following teeth:
- Right maxillary central incisor (11)
- Right maxillary lateral incisor (12)
- Left maxillary central incisor (21)
- Left maxillary lateral incisor (22)

Sum of incisors (SI) = Mesiodistal width of (teeth 11 + 12 + 21 + 22). *Note:* FDI system of tooth notation is used.

#### Determination of Measured Premolar Value (MPV)

The width of arch in the premolar region from the distal pit of one upper first premolar to the distal pit of the first premolar on the opposite side is measured. It is called as measured premolar value.

#### Determination of Measured Molar Value (MMV)

The width of the arch in the molar region from the mesial pit of one upper first molar to the mesial pit of the opposite side first molar is measured. This value is called the measured molar value.

#### Determination of Calculated Premolar Value (CPV)

Calculated premolar value or the expected arch width in the premolar region is determined by the formula,

$$CPV = \frac{SI \times 100}{80}$$

#### Determination of Calculated Molar Value (CMV)

Calculated molar value or the expected arch width in the molar region is determined by the formula,

$$CMV = \frac{SI \times 100}{64}$$

### Inference

If the measured value is less than the calculated value, then expansion is indicated.

How much expansion is needed in the premolar region is determined by the following formula:

**Amount of expansion needed in the premolar region = CPV − MPV**

How much expansion is needed in molar region is determined by,

**Amount of expansion needed in the molar region = CMV − MMV**

---

### Pont's Analysis Chart

Ref. Case No.:     Date:
Patient's Name:     Age/Sex:
Ref. Doctor's Name:

**Analysis Description**

**Procedure**

**Sum of Incisors (SI)**
SI = Mesiodistal width of Maxillary Incisors (11+12+21+22) =

**MPV (Measured Premolar Value):**
MPV = Distal pit of 14 to that of 24 =

**MMV (Measured Molar Value):**
MMV = Mesial pit of 16 to that of 26 =

**CPV (Calculated Premolar Value):**

$$CPV = \frac{SI \times 100}{80}$$

**CMV (Calculated Molar Value):**

$$CPV = \frac{SI \times 100}{64}$$

**Result of analysis performed**
*Amount of Expansion Needed*
- In premolar region:
  CPV − MPV =
- In molar region
  CMV − MMV =

Signature of Doctor

---

## LINDER HARTH INDEX

Linder Harth index is a modification of Pont's analysis where the formula for calculated premolar value is modified. However, the formula for calculated molar value is not changed.

**Formula for CPV (Calculated Premolar Value)**

$$CPV = \frac{SI \times 100}{80}$$

Formula for CMV (Calculated Molar Value)

$$CMV = \frac{SI \times 100}{64}$$

### Linder Harth's Analysis Chart

Ref. Case No.:     Date:
Patient's Name:     Age/Sex:
Ref. Doctor's Name:

**Analysis Description**

**Procedure**

**Sum of Incisors (SI)**
SI = Mesiodistal width of maxillary incisors (11+12+21+22) =

**MPV (Measured Premolar Value):**
MPV = Distal pit of 14 to that of 24 =

**MMV (Measured Molar Value):**
MMV = Mesial pit of 16 to that of 26 =

*(contd.)*

*(contd.)*

**CPV (Calculated Premolar Value):**

$$CPV = \frac{SI \times 100}{80}$$

**CMV (Calculated Molar Value):**

$$CPV = \frac{SI \times 100}{64}$$

**Inference of the analysis performed**
*Amount of Expansion Needed*
- In premolar region
  CPV – MPV
- In molar region
  CMV – MMV

Signature of Doctor

## KORKHAUS ANALYSIS

Korkhaus analysis is also similar to the Pont's analysis and uses Linder Harth's formula to determine the ideal arch width in premolar and molar regions. However, this analysis uses an additional parameter, a measurement made from the midpoint of the interpremolar line to the point between the two maxillary central incisors **(Fig. 14.4)**.

Korkhaus advocated that for a given width of upper incisors, a specific value of the distance between the midpoint of interpremolar line to the point between two maxillary incisors should exist. An increase in this measurement is seen in the case of upper anterior proclination and this value is decreased in the case of anterior retroclination.

## ASHLEY HOWE'S ANALYSIS

Ashley Howe believed that crowding results due to a deficiency in arch width rather than that of the arch length. He established a relationship between total widths of the 12 teeth anterior to the second molars to the width of the dental arch in the first premolar region.

Canine fossa is found distal to the canine eminence. Measurement of the width from canine fossa of one side to the other gives an estimate of basal arch width at the premolar region. Howe states that, in a normal case, the apical base above the first premolar in canine fossa region always has same width or a little wider than the premolar arch width and he has shown that there is safety in the assumption that this premolar arch width must be at least 43% of the maxillary tooth material. He further adds that, if this be true, we may assume that the canine fossa measurement hereafter known as canine fossa (CF), must be slightly greater or at least 44% of the maxillary tooth material, if it is to be considered normal **(Table. 14.2)**.

### Procedure

*Determination of Total Tooth Material (TTM)*
The mesiodistal width of all the teeth mesial to the second permanent molar is measured with the help of bow divider and all the values are summed up. This value is called as "total tooth material (TTM)."

*Determination of Premolar Dimension (PMD)*
Premolar dimension (PMD) is the arch width determined from the tip of buccal cusp of left first permanent premolar to the right first permanent premolar in the same arch **(Fig. 14.5)**.

*Determination of Premolar Basal Arch Width (PMBAW)*
Premolar basal arch width (PMBAW) is measured from left canine fossa to the right canine fossa **(Fig. 14.6)**.

### Exception Cases

If the canine fossa is not clearly distinguishable, the measurements are made from a point that is 8 mm apical the crest of the interdental papilla distal to the canine.

**Ashley Howe's Analysis Chart**

Ref. Case No.                           Date:
Patient's Name:                         Age/Sex:
Ref. Doctor's Name:

**Analysis Description**

**Procedure**
**TTM (Total Tooth Material) =**
**PMD (Premolar Dimension) =**
**PMBAW (Premolar Basal Arch Width) =**
Formula

$$PMBAW\ (\%) = \frac{PMBAW \times 100}{TTM}$$

**Inference of the analysis performed**

Signature of Doctor

*Formula*

$$PMBAW\ (\%) = \frac{PMBAW \times 100}{TTM}$$

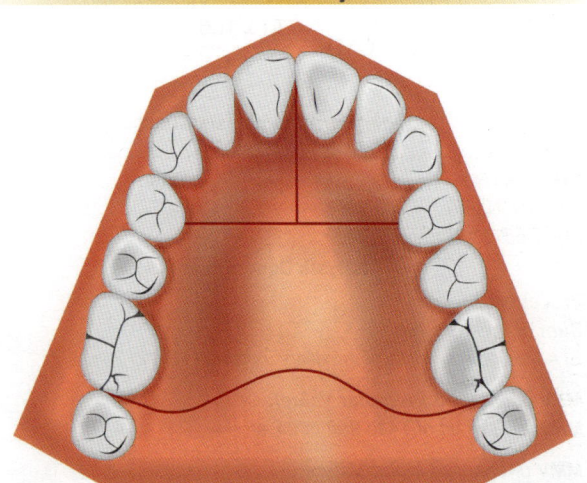

**Fig. 14.4:** Measurement made from the midpoint of the inter premolar line to the point between the two maxillary incisors

Table 14.2: Ashley Howe's analysis inference

| PMBAW (%) | Inference |
|---|---|
| 44 or more | Treatment by nonextraction |
| 37–44 | Borderline cases |
| 37 or less | Need for extraction |

### Inference
- Expansion of an arch is possible, if PMBAW is greater than PMD.
- Expansion is not possible, if PMBAW is less than PMD.

Howe divided the cases analyzed into three groups (**Table. 14.2**):
- If PMPAW (%) is 44 or more, such cases can be treated without extraction of any teeth.
- If PMPAW (%) is 37–44, they are considered as borderline cases.
- If PMPAW (%) is 37 or less, it indicates a need for extraction.

## BOLTON'S ANALYSIS

Bolton analysis gives significance to tooth size. According to Bolton, there exists a ratio between the mesiodistal width of maxillary and mandibular teeth. Malocclusion occurs when there is disparity between the mesiodistal dimensions of maxillary and mandibular teeth. Bolton's analysis helps in determining disproportion in size between maxillary and mandibular teeth.

### Procedure

#### Sum of Mandibular 12 Teeth
The mesiodistal width of all the teeth mesial to the mandibular second permanent molars is measured and summed up.

#### Sum of Maxillary 12 Teeth
The mesiodistal width of all the teeth mesial to the maxillary second permanent molars is measured and summed up.

#### Sum of Mandibular 6 Teeth (Anteriors)
The mesiodistal width of all the teeth mesial to the mandibular first permanent premolars, i.e. mandibular anteriors is measured and summed up.

#### Sum of Maxillary 6 Teeth (Anteriors)
The mesiodistal width of all the teeth mesial to the maxillary first permanent premolars, i.e. maxillary anteriors is measured and summed up.

### Determination of Overall Ratio

According to Bolton's study, the sum of mesiodistal width of the mandibular teeth anterior to second permanent molars should be 91.3% of the mesiodistal width of maxillary teeth anterior to the second permanent molar.

The overall ratio is determined by the formula,

$$\text{Overall Ratio} = \frac{\text{Sum of mandibular 12}}{\text{Sum of maxillary 12}} \times 100$$

### Inference
If the ratio is less than 91.3%, then it indicates maxillary tooth material excess.

Amount of maxillary tooth excess is determined by the formula,

$$\text{Sum of maxillary 12} = \frac{\text{Sum of mandibular 12}}{91.3} \times 100$$

If the ratio is more than 91.3%, then it indicates mandibular tooth material excess.

Amount of mandibular excess is determined by the formula,

$$\text{Sum of mandibular 12} = \frac{\text{Sum of maxillary 12}}{100} \times 91.3$$

### Determination of Anterior Ratio

According to Bolton's study, the sum of mesiodistal widths of mandibular anteriors should be 77.2% of the mesiodistal width of maxillary anteriors. The anterior ratio is obtained by the formula,

$$\text{Anterior ratio} = \frac{\text{Sum of mandibular 6}}{\text{Sum of maxillary 6}} \times 100$$

### Inference
If the ratio is less than 77.2%, then it indicates maxillary tooth material excess.

Amount of maxillary excess is determined by the formula,

$$\text{Sum of maxillary 6} = \frac{\text{Sum of mandibular 6}}{77.2} \times 100$$

If the ratio is more than 77.2%, then it indicates mandibular tooth material excess.

Amount of mandibular excess is determined by the formula,

$$\text{Sum of mandibular 6} = \frac{\text{Sum of maxillary 6}}{100} \times 77.2$$

---

**Bolton's Analysis Chart**

Ref. Case No.   Date:
Patient's Name:   Age/Sex:
Ref. Doctor's Name:

**Analysis Description**

**Procedure**
Sum of mandibular 12 teeth =
Sum of maxillary 12 teeth =
Sum of mandibular 6 teeth (anterior) =
Sum of maxillary 6 teeth (anterior) =

$$\text{Overall ratio} = \frac{\text{Sum of mandibular 12}}{\text{Sum of maxillary 12}} \times 100$$

**Determination of anterior ratio**

$$\text{Anterior ratio} = \frac{\text{Sum of mandibular 6}}{\text{Sum of maxillary 6}} \times 100$$

**Inference of analysis performed**

Signature of Doctor

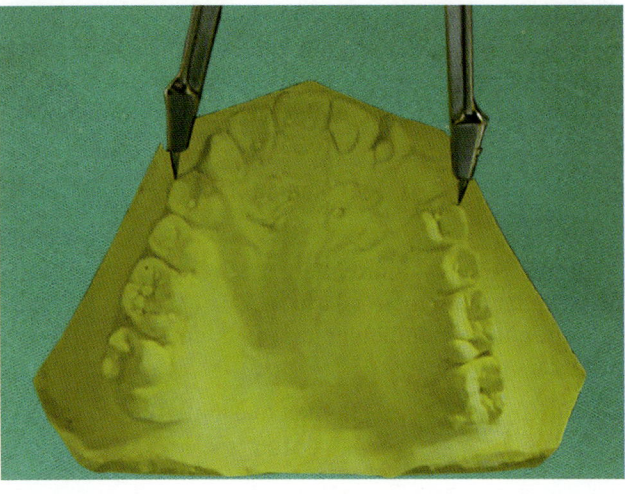

**Fig. 14.5:** Premolar dimension is determined from the tip of buccal cusp of left first permanent premolar to the right first permanent premolar in the same arch

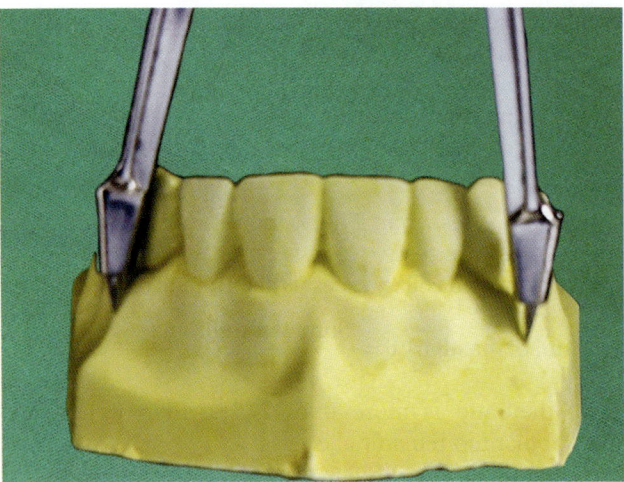

**Fig. 14.6:** Premolar basal arch width is measured by placing tip ends of the divider at around approximately 8 mm apical to the gingival margin of canines

## MIXED DENTITION ANALYSIS (RADIOGRAPHIC METHOD)

This technique makes use of radiographs, as well as study cast model to determine the width of the unerupted teeth. Radiographic measurement of an unerupted tooth may not be precise because of distortion and thus is unreliable. However, it is possible to predict the width of unerupted tooth by comparing the measurement of an already erupted permanent tooth on the cast as well as on the radiograph.

The formula is,

$$Y1 = \frac{X1 \times Y2}{X2}$$

where,

Y1 = Width of unerupted tooth whose measurement is to be determined.
Y2 = Width of unerupted tooth on the radiograph.
X1 = Width of a tooth that has erupted on the cast.
X2 = Width of a tooth that has erupted measured on the radiograph.

---

**Mixed Dentition Analysis (Radiographic Method)**

Ref. Case No.                                 Date:
Patient's Name:                                Age/Sex:
Ref. Doctor's Name:

**Analysis Description**
**Procedure**
Y1 = Width of unerupted tooth whose measurement is to be determined =
Y2 = Width of unerupted tooth on the radiograph =
X1 = Width of a tooth that has erupted on the cast =
X2 = Width of a tooth that has erupted measured on the radiograph =

$$Y1 = \frac{X1 \times Y2}{X2}$$

**Result of analysis performed**
**Inference:**

Signature of Doctor

---

## BIBLIOGRAPHY

1. Bolton WA. Dishormony in tooth size and its relation to the analysis and treatment of malocclusion. Angle Ortho 1958; 28:113-30.
2. Bolton WA. The clinical evaluation of tooth size analysis. Am J Orthod 1962; 48:504-29.
3. Carey CW. Linear arch dimension and tooth size. Am J Orthod 1949; 35:764-6.
4. Howes JH. A polygon portrayal of coronal and basal arch dimensions in the horizontal plane. Am J Orthod 1954; 40:811-31.
5. Martinek, Edward E. A comparison of various sur+veys on the adequacy of basal bone. Am J Orthod 1956; 42:244-54.
6. Pont A. Der Zahn Index in der Orthodontic. Ztschr f. Zahnarzt Orthopodic 1909; 3:306-21.
7. Suwannee. The effects of premolar-extraction: A long-term comparison of outcomes in "clear-cut" extraction and nonextraction Class II patients.
8. Tanaka MM, Johnston LE. The prediction of the size of the unerupted canines and premolars in a contemporary orthodontic Population. J Am Dent Assoc 1974; 88:798-801.

# EXAM ORIENTED QUESTIONS

## Long Essay or Long Questions
1. Describe in detail about various methods of model analysis used for orthodontic treatment planning.
2. Carey's model analysis
3. Arch-perimeter model analysis
4. Linder harth model analysis
5. Karhan's model analysis
6. Ashley Howe's model analysis
7. Bolton's model analysis
8. Mixed Dentition Analysis.

## Short Notes
1. Compare and contrast between Pont's and Linder-Harth analysis
2. Mixed Dentition Analysis.

## CHAPTER OVERVIEW

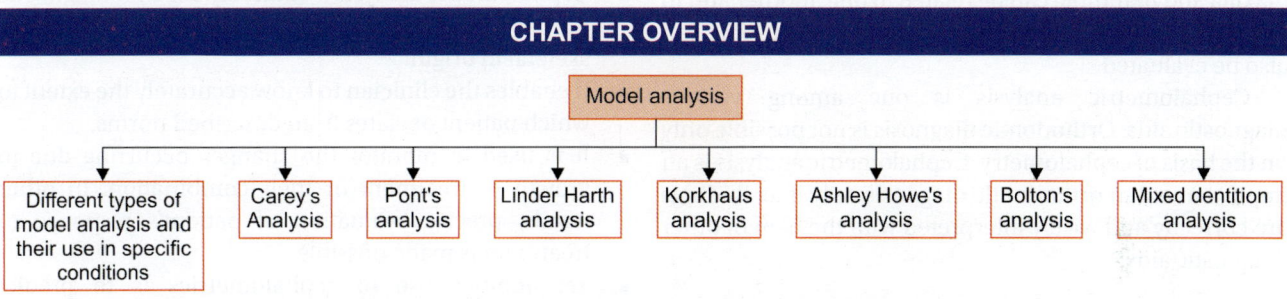

# CHAPTER 15

# Cephalometrics

*Phulari BS*

Cephalometric radiographs are used in orthodontic diagnosis to evaluate the pretreatment dental and facial relationship of the patient. They are also used to evaluate changes during treatment and to assess tooth movement and facial growth at the end of the treatment. On the cephalometric film, teeth can be related to one another, to the jaw in which they reside and to cranial structures. The maxilla and mandible can be related to one another and to other structures in the cranium. The soft tissue profile can also be evaluated.

Cephalometric analysis is one among various diagnostic aids. Orthodontic diagnosis is not possible only on the basis of cephalometry. Cephalometric analysis is an important aid in orthodontic diagnosis only if its findings are correctly and wisely interpreted with the help of other diagnostic aids.

## TYPES

There are following two types of cephalograms:

### Lateral Cephalogram

Lateral cephalogram provides a lateral view of the skull (**Fig. 15.1A**). It is taken with the head in a standardized reproducible position at a specified distance from the source of the X-ray. Lateral cephalogram is commonly used for cephalometric analysis.

### Frontal Cephalogram

This provides an anteroposterior view of the skull (**Fig. 15.1B**). It is generally used to assess symmetry of the face.

## USES

- Cephalometric analysis is routinely used for diagnostic purpose to assess whether malocclusion is dental or skeletal in origin.
- It enables the clinician to know accurately the extent to which patient deviates from described norms.
- It is used to monitor the changes occurring due to growth or treatment or their combination. In other words, precise evaluation of patient's response to treatment is made possible.
- Yet another use of cephalometrics is to predict changes that should occur in future for the patient after orthodontic treatment. An architectural plan/blueprint of orthodontic treatment can be made.

## TECHNICAL ASPECTS

The cephalometric radiographs are taken using an apparatus that consists of an X-ray source and a head-holding device called "cephalostat" (**Fig. 15.1C**). The cephalostat consists of two ear rods that prevent the

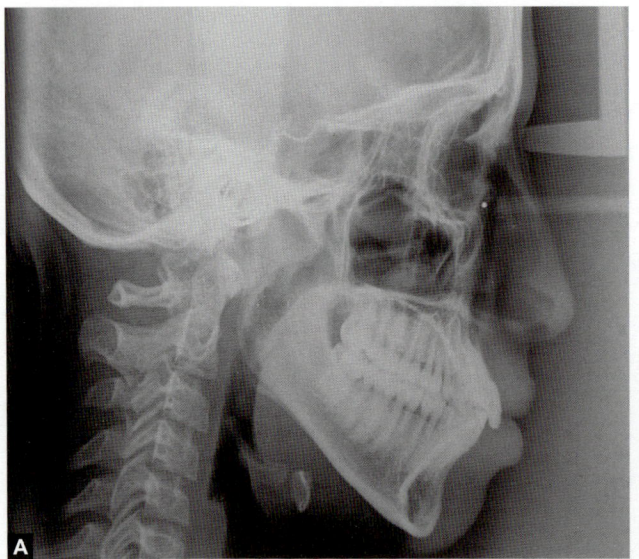
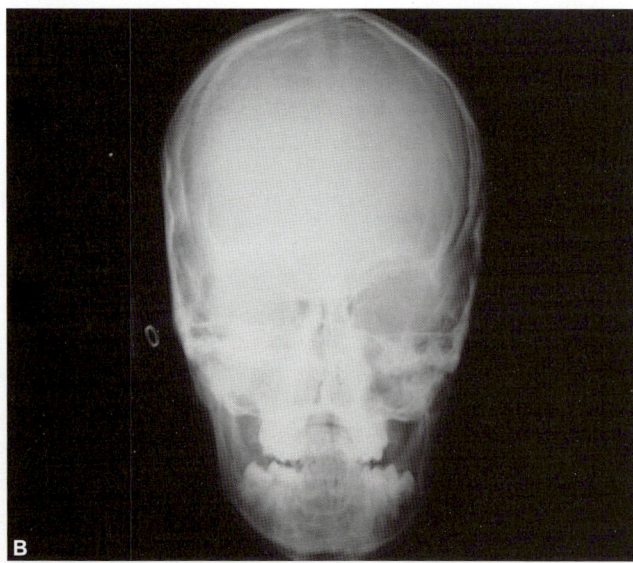

**Figs 15.1A and B:** (A) Lateral cephalogram and (B) Frontal cephalogram

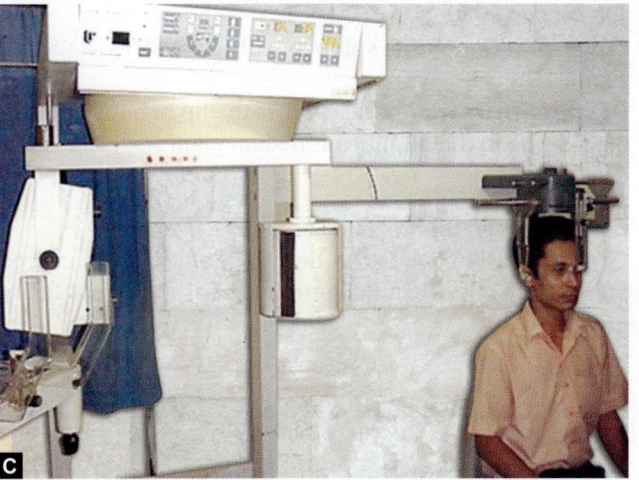

**Fig. 15.1C:** The cephalostat with the patient in position. The patient head position is constant and X-ray sources to film distance is fixed at 5 feet

movement of the head in the horizontal plane. Vertical stabilization of the head is brought about by an orbital pointer that contacts the lower border of the left orbit. The upper part of the face is supported by the forehead clamp positioned above the region of the nasal bridge. The distance between the X-ray source and the mid-sagittal plane of the patient is fixed at 5 feet (152.4 cm). Thus, the equipment helps in standardizing the radiographs by use of constant head position and source-film distance, so that serial radiographs can be compared.

There are many systems of cephalometric analysis, which utilize various points and outline on the lateral cephalogram radiograph.

## CEPHALOMETRIC X-RAY TRACING TECHNIQUES

Masking tape is used to attach the cephalometric X-ray to the acrylic acetate tracing paper sheet. Tracing is made on the frosted surface of acetate tracing sheet.

The tracing is begun by marking the hard and soft tissue points needed for the analysis on the tracing sheet. Soft tissue profile is traced and then the sella turcica going forward to the planum sphenoid ale along the floor of the anterior cranial fossa of the shadows of the greater wings of sphenoid bone are traced. The anterior surface of the frontal and nasal bones are then traced followed by tracing the outline of the maxilla and from the anterior nasal spine along the floor of the nasal cavity back to posterior nasal spine.

## CEPHALOMETRIC LANDMARKS

Cephalometry makes use of certain landmarks or points on the skull, which are used for quantitative analysis and measurements. The landmarks used in cephalometrics are of two broad categories: hard tissue landmarks and soft tissue landmarks. The hard tissue landmarks can be anatomic or derived. Some of the hard tissue landmarks are unilateral while others are bilateral. Cephalometric landmarks are classified as follows **(Flowchart 15.1 and Table 15.1)**:

- Anatomic cephalometric landmarks
- Derived cephalometric landmarks.

### Anatomic

These landmarks represent the actual anatomic structures of the skull. They may be unilateral or bilateral.

### Derived

These are landmarks that have been obtained secondarily from anatomic structures in a lateral cephalogram.

**Flowchart 15.1:** Cephalometric landmarks

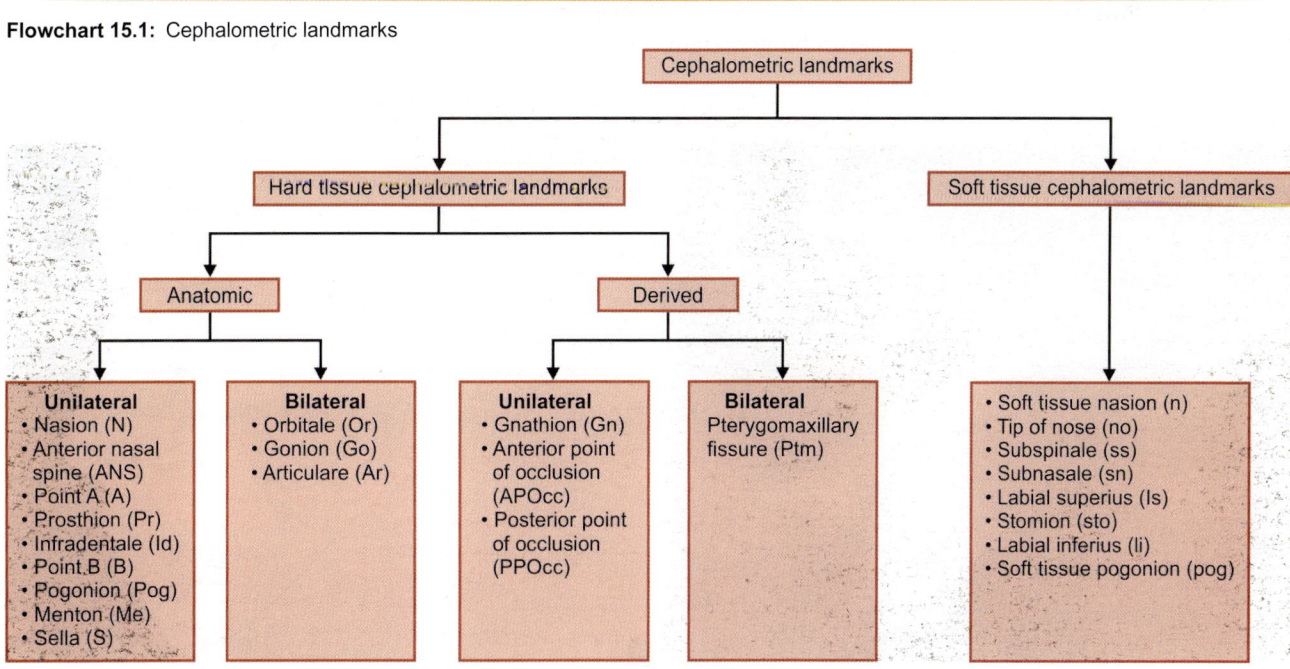

| Table 15.1: Hard tissue cephalometric landmarks | |
|---|---|
| **Anatomic** | |
| Nasion | N |
| Anterior nasal spine | ANS |
| Point A | A |
| Prosthion | Pr |
| Infradentale | Id |
| Point B | B |
| Pogonion | Pog |
| Menton | Me |
| Sella | S |
| Orbitale | Or |
| Gonion | Go |
| Articulare | Ar |
| **Derived** | |
| Gnathion | Gn |
| Anterior point of occlusion | APOcc |
| Posterior point of occlusion | PPOcc |
| Pterygomaxillary fissure | Ptm |

## Hard Tissue Landmarks

Some important hard tissue landmarks are described here (**Figs 15.2A** and **B**):

### Nasion (N)
*Code/Abbreviation:* Nasion is abbreviated as N (Capital alphabet)
*Definition:* Nasion is the most anterior point of frontonasal outline in the midline.

### Orbitale (Or)
*Code/Abbreviation:* Orbitale is abbreviated as Or (Capital alphabet O followed by small r)
*Definition:* The lowest point on the inferior bony margin of the orbit.

### Anterior Nasal Spine (ANS)
*Code:* Anterior nasal spine is abbreviated as ANS (all capital letters).
*Definition:* Anterior nasal spine is the tip of bony anterior nasal spine in the midline or median plane.

### Point A (A)
*Code:* Point A is abbreviated as point A itself.
*Definition:* Point A is the deepest point on the curved bony outline between the anterior nasal spine (ANS) and prosthion.

### Prosthion (Pr)
*Code:* Prosthion is abbreviated as Pr (Capital P followed by small r).
*Definition:* It is the lower most anterior point of alveolar process of pre-maxilla in the midline between two central incisors.

### Anterior Point of Occlusion (APOcc)
*Code:* APOcc (Capital APO followed by double small c).
*Definition:* Anterior point of occlusal plane is the midpoint in the incisors overbite in the occlusion.

### Infradentale (Id)
*Code:* Infradentale is abbreviated as Id (Capital I followed by small d).
*Definition:* Infradentale is the highest anterior point of the alveolar process of mandible between two central incisors in midline.

### Point B
*Code:* Point B is abbreviated as point B itself.
*Definition:* It is the deepest point of curvature on the contour of mandibular alveolar process in the middle between infradentale and pogonion.

### Pogonion (Pog)
*Code:* Pogonion is abbreviated as Pog (Capital P followed by small o and g).

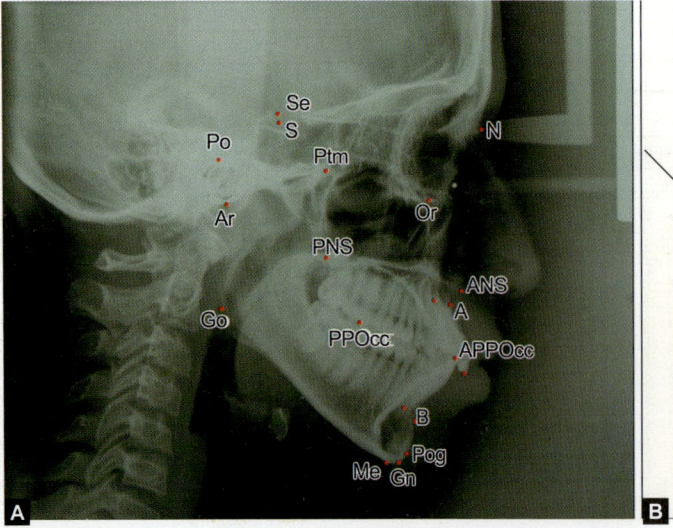
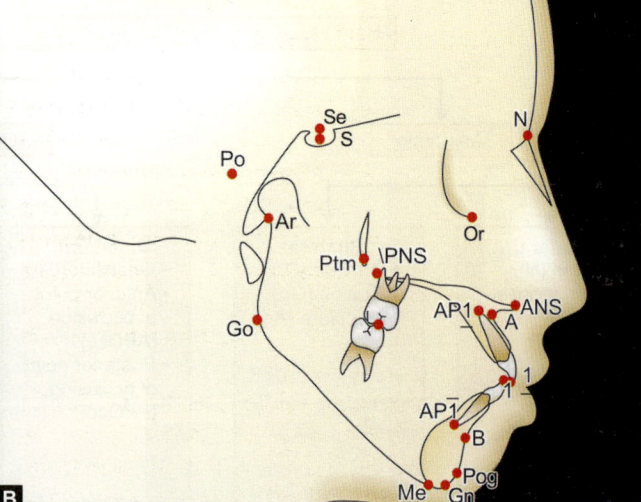

**Figs 15.2A and B:** Hard tissue cephalometric landmarks

*Definition:* Pogonion is the most anterior point of the bony chin in the midline.

### Gnathion (Gn)
*Code:* Gnathion is abbreviated as Gn (Capital G followed by small n).
*Definition:* It is the most anterior and inferior point of the bony chin. It is constructed by intersecting a line drawn perpendicularly to the line connecting menton and pogonion with bony outline.
*According to Graig:* Gnathion is the point of intersection of two planes.
*According to Muzi and May:* Gnathion is the lower point of the chin.
*According to AM Schwarz:* Gnathion is the lowest point of the chin.
*According to Martin Saller:* It is located in the midline of the mandible, where the anterior line in the outline of the chin merges with the body of the mandible.

### Menton (Me)
*Code:* Menton is abbreviated as Me (Capital M followed by small e).
*Definition:* According to Krogman and Sassouni, Menton is the most caudal point in the outline of the symphysis. It is regarded as the lowest point of the mandible.

### Sella (S)
*Code:* Sella is abbreviated as S (capital letter 'S').
*Definition:* Sella is the midpoint of sella turcica or hypophyseal fossa or pituitary fossa.

### Se
*Code:* Se is abbreviated as Se (Capital S followed by small e).
*Definition:* Se is the mid-entrance point of sella turcica or pituitary fossa.

### Pterygomaxillary Fissure (Ptm)
*Code:* Pterygomaxillary fissure is abbreviated as Ptm (Capital P followed by small t and m).
*Definition:* It is the intersection of the inferior border of the foramen rotundum with the posterior wall of the pterygomaxillary fissure.

### Posterior Nasal Spine (PNS)
*Code:* Posterior nasal spine is abbreviated as PNS (all capital letters).
*Definition:* It is the intersection of a continuation of the anterior wall of the pterygopalatine fossa and the floor of the nose.

### Posterior Point of Occlusion (PPOcc)
*Code:* Posterior point of occlusion is abbreviated as PPOcc (capital PPO followed by small double c).
*Definition:* Posterior point for the occlusal plane is the most distal point of contact between the most posterior molar in occlusion.

### Articulare (Ar)
*Code:* Articulare is abbreviated as Ar (capital A followed by small r). It was introduced by Bjorio (1947).
*Definition:* Articulare is the point of intersection of the posterior margin of the ascending ramus and the outer margin of the cranial base.

### Condylion (Cd)
*Code:* Condylion is abbreviated as Cd (Capital C followed by small d).
*Definition:* It is the superior most point of the head of the condyle of the mandible.

### Gonion (Go)
*Code:* Gonion is abbreviated as Go (Capital G followed by small o).
*Definition:* Gonion is the intersection of the lines tangent to the posterior margin of the ascending ramus and the mandibular base.

### Porion (Po)
*Code:* Porion is abbreviated as Po (Capital P and small o)
*Definition:* It is the midpoint on the upper edge of the porus acusticus externus located by means of the metal rods on the cephalometer.

### Basion (Ba)
*Code:* Basion is abbreviated as Ba (Capital B followed by small a).
*Definition:* Basion is the lowest point on the anterior margin of the foramen magnum in the midline.

### Soft Tissue Landmarks
The following are some of the important soft tissue cephalometric landmarks **(Table 15.2) (Figs 15.3A and B)**.

### Cephalometric Reference Planes
Reference planes are classified into the following two groups:
1. Horizontal cephalometric reference planes
2. Vertical cephalometric reference planes.

### Horizontal Cephalometric Planes
Horizontal cephalometric planes are listed below:
- S-N plane
- Se-N plane

| Table 15.2: Soft tissue cephalometric landmarks | |
|---|---|
| Soft tissue nasion | n |
| Tip of nose | no |
| Subspinale | ss |
| Subnasale | sn |
| Labial superius | ls |
| Stomion | sto |
| Labial inferius | li |
| Soft tissue pogonion | pog |

- F-H plane
- Occlusal plane
- Palatal plane
- Mandibular plane.

### Description of Horizontal Planes (Figs 15.4A and B)

#### S-N Plane

- It is the plane formed by the line connecting sella turcica (midpoint of hypophyseal fossa) and the nasion (anterior point of frontonasal suture).
- *Significance:* It represents the anteroposterior extent of anterior cranial base.

#### Se-N Plane

- It is the plane formed by the line connecting Se (mid-entrance point of pituitary fossa) and the nasion (anterior point of frontonasal suture).
- *Significance:* As S-N plane, it also expresses the anteroposterior extent of anterior cranial base.

#### F-H Plane

- Frankfort-Horizontal plane is the plane that connects the lowest point of the orbit (orbitale) to the superior point of the external auditory meatus (Porion).
- *Significance:* It is horizontal cephalometric reference plane used to assess horizontal growth during the analysis.

#### Occlusal Plane (APOcc–PPOcc)

- Occlusal plane is formed by a line connecting anterior point of occlusion (APOcc) to the posterior point of occlusion (PPOcc).
- *Significance:* It has significant role in the assessment of horizontal growth pattern.

#### Palatal Plane (ANS-PNS Plane)

- Palatal plane is formed by the line joining the point anterior nasal spine (ANS) to the posterior nasal spine (PNS).
- *Significance:* Growth pattern assessment.

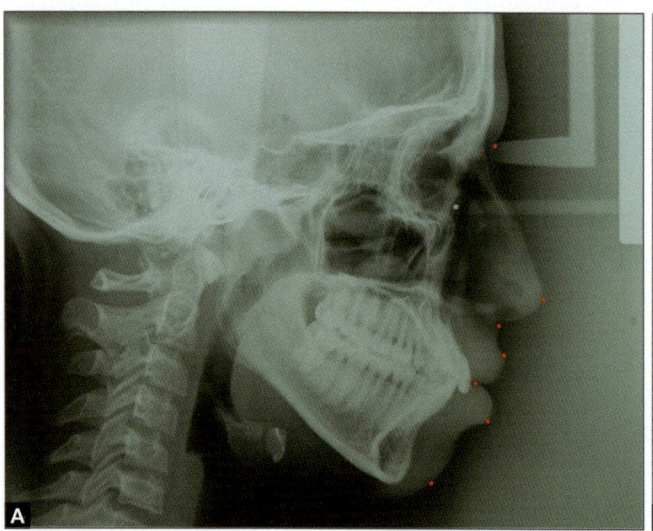
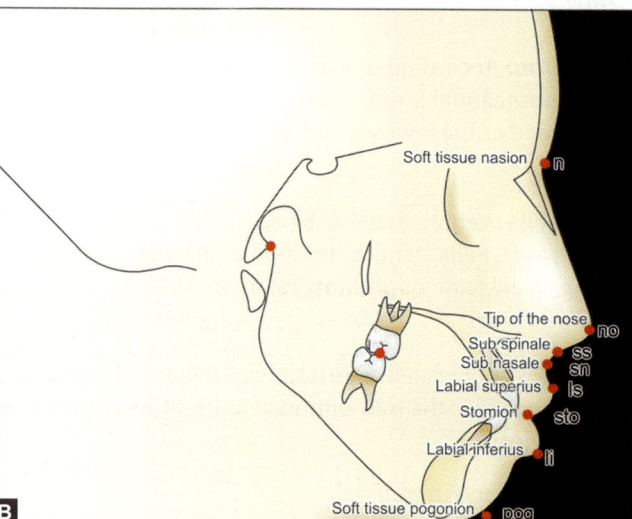

**Figs 15.3A and B:** Soft tissue cephalometric landmarks

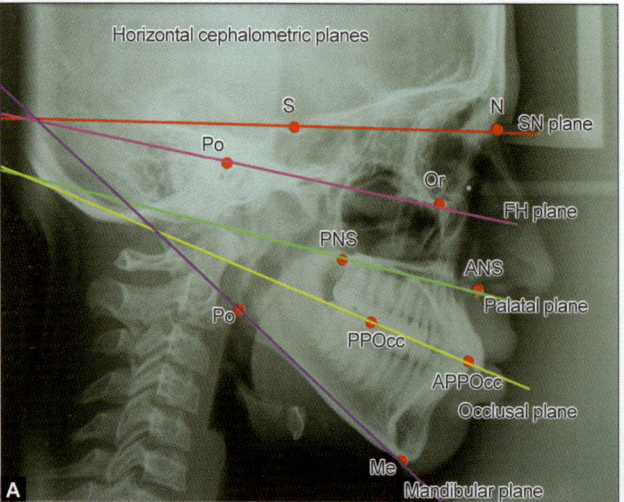
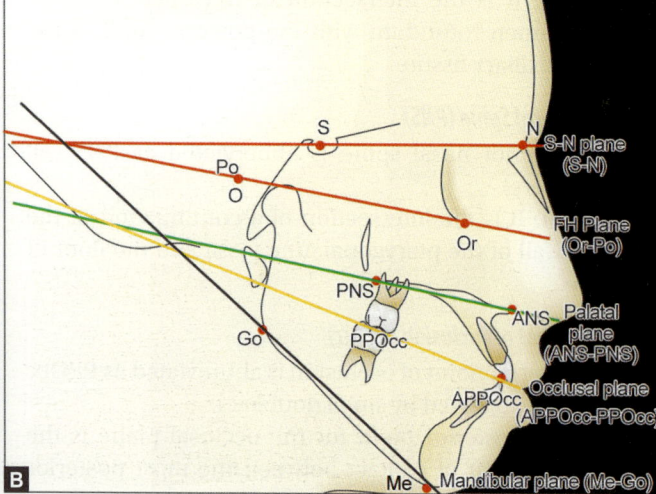

**Figs 15.4A and B:** Horizontal cephalometric planes

### Mandibular Plane/Me-Go Plane

- It is the plane that connects the point Me (Menton) to the point Go (Gonion).
- ***Significance:*** Growth pattern assessment.

### Vertical Cephalometric Reference Planes

Vertical cephalometric planes include the following **(Figs 15.5A and B)**:

- A-Pog line
- Facial plane
- Facial axis
- E-plane
- S-Ar plane
- Ar-Go plane.

### A-Pog Line

It is a line from point A on the maxilla to pogonion on the mandible.

### Facial Plane

It is a line from the anterior point of the frontonasal suture (nasion) to the most anterior point of the mandible (pogonion).

### Facial Axis

A line from Ptm point to cephalometric gnathion.

### E-Plane

E-plane is also called esthetic plane and it is a line between the most anterior point of the soft tissue nose and chin.

### S-Ar Plane

- It is the plane between the sella point (center of sella turcica) and the Ar (articulare) point.
- ***Significance:*** This plane represents the lateral extent of cranial base.

### Ar-Go Plane

- Ar-Go plane is formed by the line connecting from articulare (Ar) to the gonion (Go).
- ***Significance:*** This plane is important in the determination of length of ramus.

## CEPHALOMETRIC ANALYSES

In the cephalometric assessment, certain carefully defined points are located on the cephalometric radiograph and linear and angular measurements are made from these points. The expression of these measurements in various ways produces analysis of skeletal size and form. The Down's analysis, Steiner's analysis and Wit's appraisal are explained below:

### Down's Analysis

The Down's cephalometric analysis is one of the most frequently used analyses. It consists of the following five skeletal parameters **(Table 15.3)**:

1. Facial angle
2. Angle of convexity
3. A-B plane angle
4. Mandibular plane angle
5. Y-axis.

In addition, it consists of five dental parameters, such as:

1. Cant of occlusal plane
2. Interincisal angle
3. Incisor-occlusal plane angle
4. Incisor-mandibular plane angle
5. Upper incisor to A-pog line.

### Skeletal Parameters

#### 1. Facial Angle

Facial angle **(Fig. 15.6A)** is the angle formed by the intersection of N-pog plane and the F-H plane.

#### Planes of Facial Angle

- N-pog plane
- F-H plane.

***Significance:*** Facial value signifies the anteroposterior positioning of the mandible to the upper face.

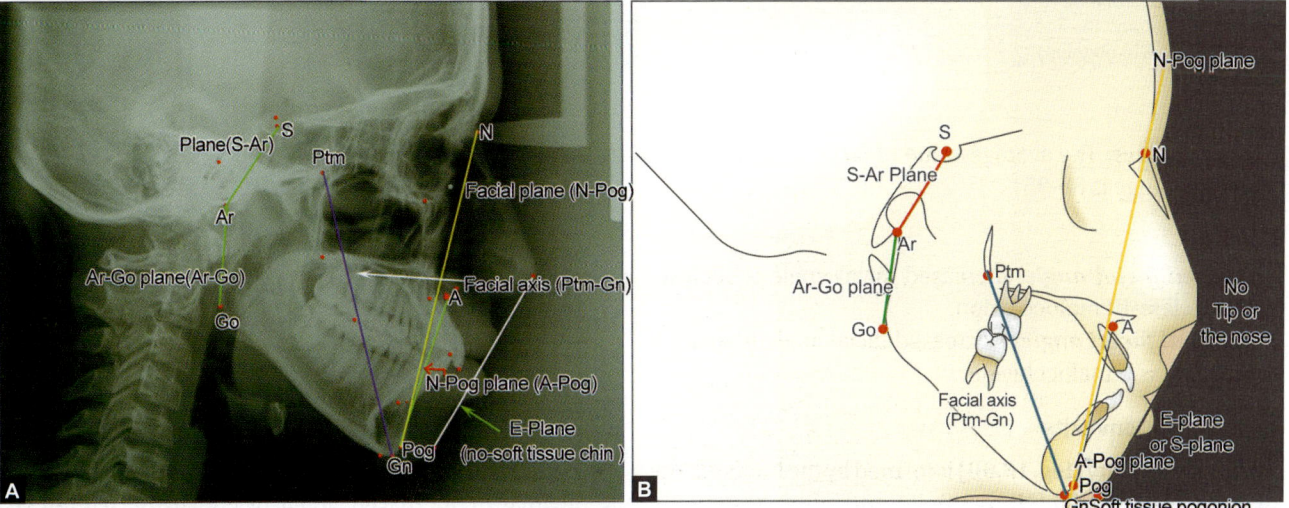

**Figs 15.5A and B:** Vertical cephalometric planes

**Table 15.3:** Down's analysis

### Skeletal Parameters

| Angle | Significance | Mean and range (Normal) | Inference | |
|---|---|---|---|---|
| | | | Increased | Decreased |
| Facial angle (intersection of F-H plane–N-Pog plane) | Anteroposterior inclination of mandible in relation to upper cranial base | 87.8° (82–95°) | Skeletal class III malocclusion | Skeletal class II malocclusion |
| Angle of convexity (intersection of NA plane–A-Pog plane) | Convexity or concavity of skeletal profile | 0° (−8.5–10°) | Prominent maxillary based relative to mandible | Prognathic profile |
| AB plane angle (intersection of AB plane – N-Pog plane) | Maxillomandibular relationship in relation to facial plane | −4.6° (−9–0°) | Class III malocclusion | Class II malocclusion |
| Mandibular plane angle (intersection of F-H plane – Go-Me plane) | Assessment of growth pattern | 21.9° (17–28°) | Vertical growth pattern (open bite) | Horizontal growth pattern (deep bite) |
| Y-axis (intersection of SGn plane – F-H plane) | Assessment of growth pattern | 59° (53–66°) | Vertical growth pattern (open bite) | Horizontal growth pattern (deep bite) |

### Dental Parameters

| Angle | Mean and Range (Normal) | Inference | |
|---|---|---|---|
| | | Increased | Decreased |
| Cant of occlusal plane (intersection of occlusal plane and F-H plane) | 9.3° (1.5–14°) | Vertical growth pattern | Horizontal growth pattern |
| Interincisal angle (intersection of upper and lower central incisors) | 135.6° (130–150.5°) | Class II division 2 malocclusion | Class II division 1 malocclusion |
| | | | Class I bimaxillary protrusion |
| Incisor occlusal plane angle (intersection of long axis of lower central incisor and occlusal plane angle) | 14.5° (3.5–20°) | Lower incisor retroclination | Lower incisor proclination |
| Incisor mandibular plane angle (intersection of long axis of lower incisor and mandibular plane) | 1.4° (−8.5–7°) | Lower incisor proclination | Lower incisor retroclination |
| Upper incisor to A-Pog line (linear measurement between the incisal edge of maxillary central incisor and the line joining point A to pognion) | 2–7 mm (−1–5 mm) | Upper incisor proclination | Upper incisor retroclination |

***Normal values:*** The average value of facial angle is 87.8°, while the range is 82–95°.

### Variation

***Increased facial angle:*** Increased facial angle is seen in skeletal class-III malocclusion.

***Decreased facial angle:*** Decreased facial angle is seen in skeletal class II malocclusion.

### 2. Angle of Convexity

Angle of convexity **(Fig. 15.6B)** is formed by the intersection of a line from nasion (N) to point A and a line from point A to pogonion.

### Planes of Angle of Convexity

- N—point A plane
- Point A—Pog plane.

***Significance:*** Angle of convexity helps in determining convexity or concavity of the skeletal profile.

***Mean value:*** The average value of angle of convexity is 0°, while the range is −8.5 to 10°.

### Variation of Angle

***Positive angle or increased angle:*** When angle of convexity is more than its normal value, then it is referred as positive or increased angle of convexity. It indicates prominent maxillary base relative to mandible.

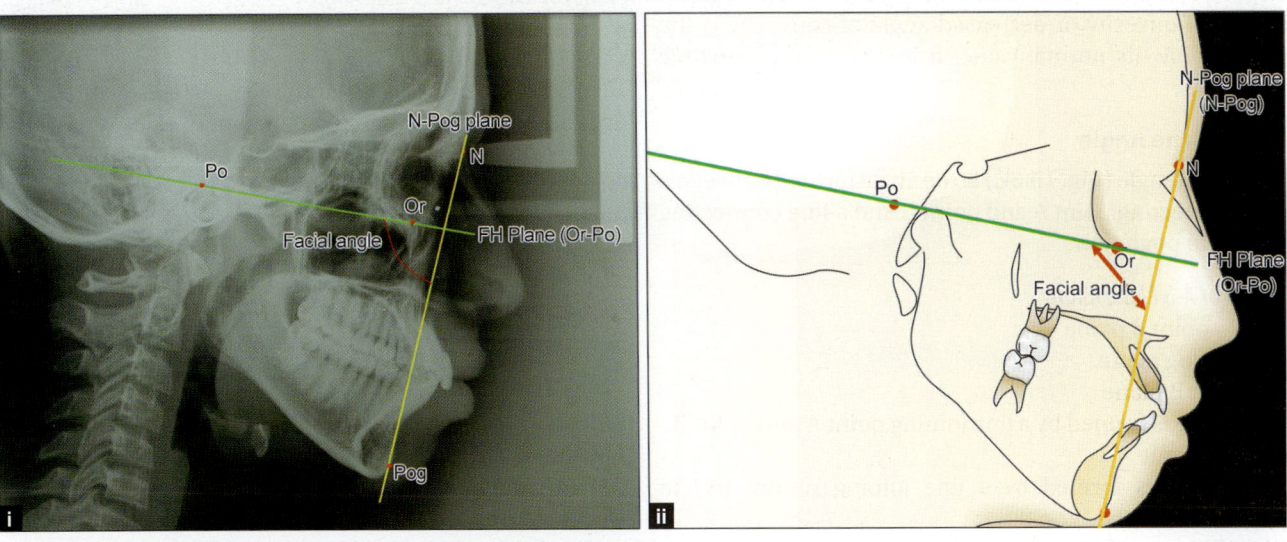

**Figs 15.6A (i and ii):** Facial angle. The average value of facial angle is 87.8°, while the range is 82 to 95°

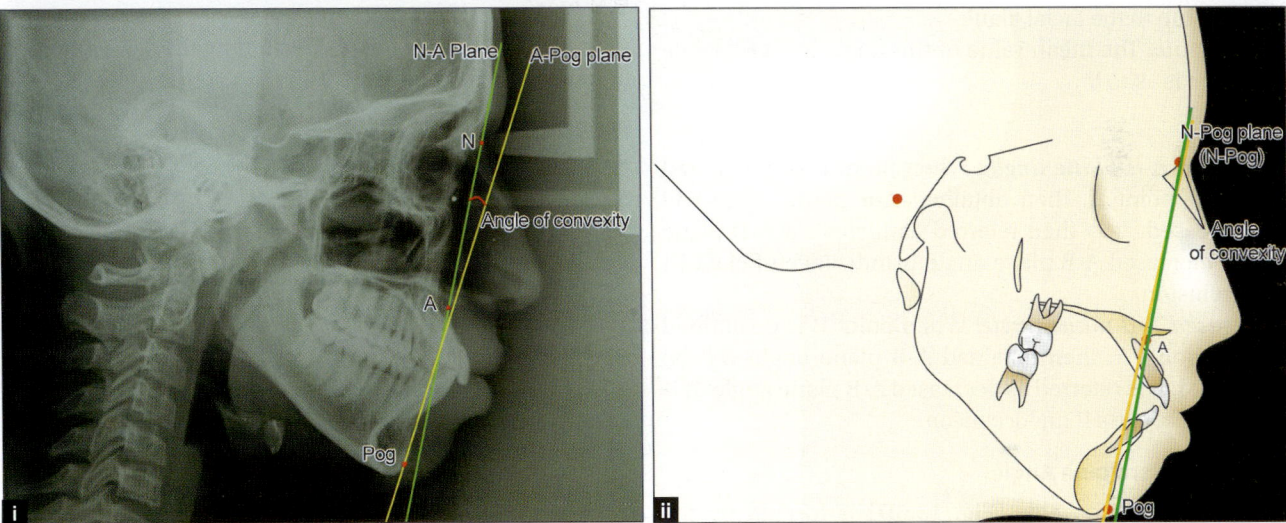

**Figs 15.6B (i and ii):** Angle of convexity. The average value of angle of convexity is 0°, while the range is –8.5 to 10°

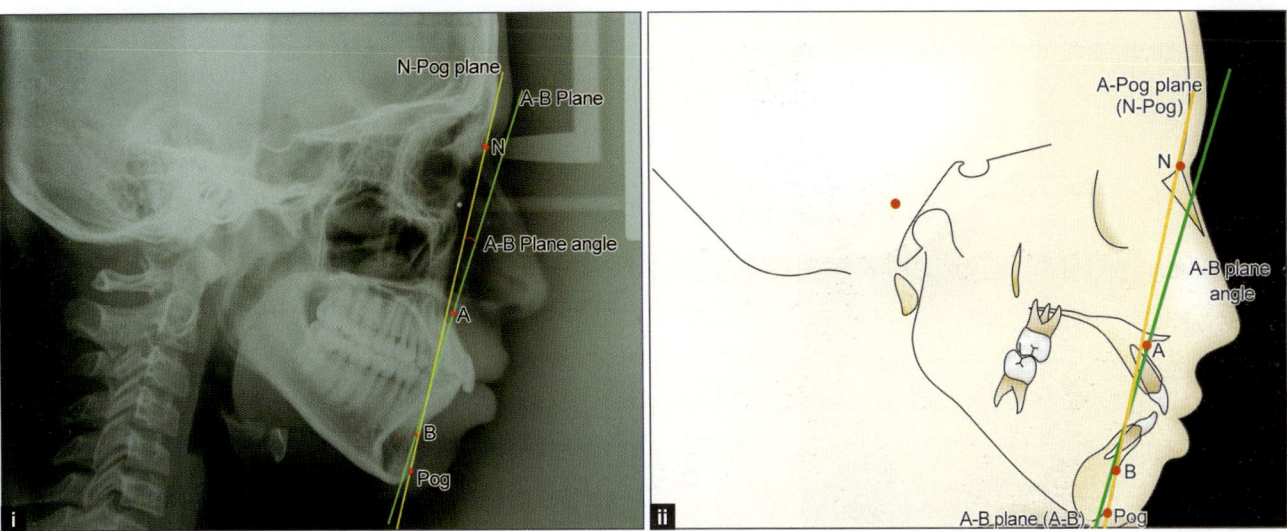

**Figs 15.6C (i and ii):** AB plane angle. The mean value of this angle is 4.6°, while the range is 9 to 0°

*Negative angle or decreased angle of convexity:* Negative angle of convexity or decreased angle of convexity is the angle below its normal value. It indicates of prognathic profile.

### 3. A-B Plane Angle

A-B plane angle **(Fig. 15.6C)** is the angle formed between a line connecting point A and point B and a line connecting nasion to pogonion.

#### Planes of A-B Plane Angle
- A—point B plane
- N—Pog plane.

A—point B plane
This plane is formed by a line joining point A and point B.
N—Pog plane
This plane is formed by a line joining nasion (N) to pogonion (Pog).
*Significance of this angle:* Significance of A–B plane angle is that it is the indication of maxillomandibular relationship to the facial plane.
*Mean value:* The mean value of this angle is—4.6°, while the range is –9 to 0°.

#### Variation
*Increased A-B plane angle:* When point B is positioned ahead to point A, then obtained A-B plane angle will be increased. It is then referred as increased A-B plane angle. Increased A-B plane angle is indicative of class III malocclusion.
*Decreased A-B plane angle:* When point B is positioned behind point A, then obtained A-B plane angle will be decreased. It is referred as decreased A-B plane angle. It is indicative of class II malocclusion.

### 4. Mandibular Plane Angle

Mandibular plane angle **(Fig. 15.6D)** is formed by the intersection of the mandibular plane with F-H plane.

#### Planes of Mandibular Plane Angle
- Mandibular plane
- F-H plane.

*Mandibular plane:* Mandibular plane is formed by a line joining point gonion (Go) to menton (Me).
*F-H plane:* F-H plane (Frankfort-horizontal plane) is formed by a line joining orbital (O) to external auditory meatus.
*Mean value:* The average value of mandibular plane angle is 21.9°, while the range is 17–28°.
*Significance of this angle:* Mandibular plane angle helps in assessing whether the growth pattern is horizontal or vertical.

#### Variation
*Increased mandibular plane angle:* It is indicative of vertical growth pattern.
*Decreased mandibular plane angle:* It is indicative of horizontal growth pattern.

### 5. Y-Axis

y-axis **(Fig. 15.6E)** is formed by joining the sella-gnathion line with the F-H plane.

#### Planes of y-Axis
- Sella-gnathion
- F-H plane

#### Sella-Gnathion Plane (S-Gn plane)
S-Gn plane (sella-gnathion plane) is formed by a line joining sella to gnathion.

#### F-H Plane
F-H plane (Frankfort-horizontal plane) is formed by a line joining orbital (Or) to external auditory meatus.
*Mean value:* The mean value of y-axis is 59° and its range is 53–66°.
*Significance of y-axis:* y-axis helps in the diagnosis of growth pattern of the individual.

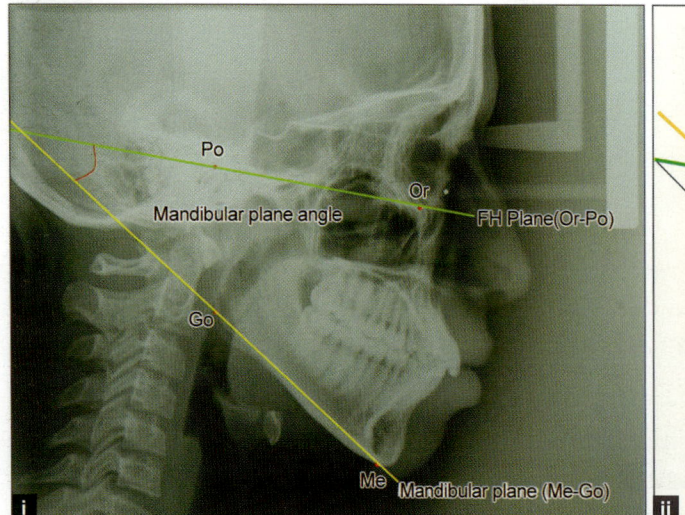 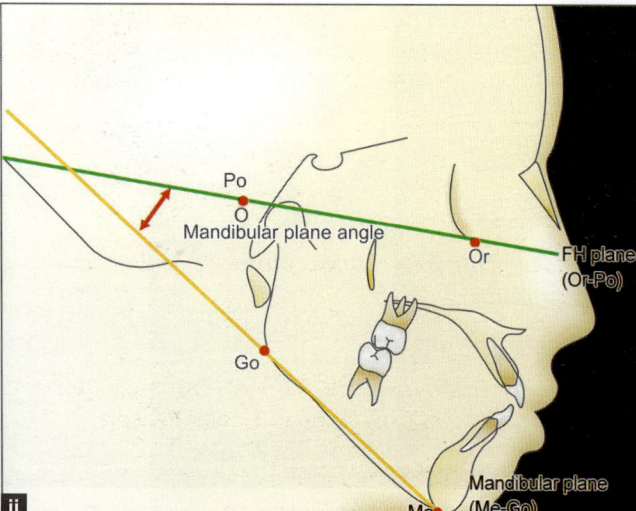

**Figs 15.6D (i and ii):** Mandibular plane angle. The average value of mandibular plane angle is 21.9°, while the range is 17 to 28°

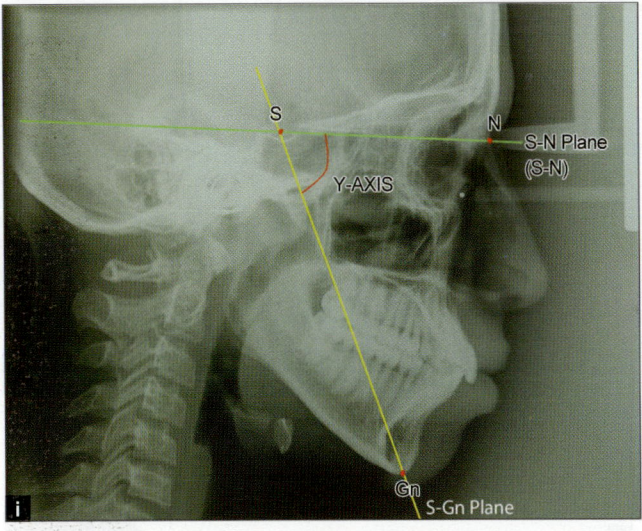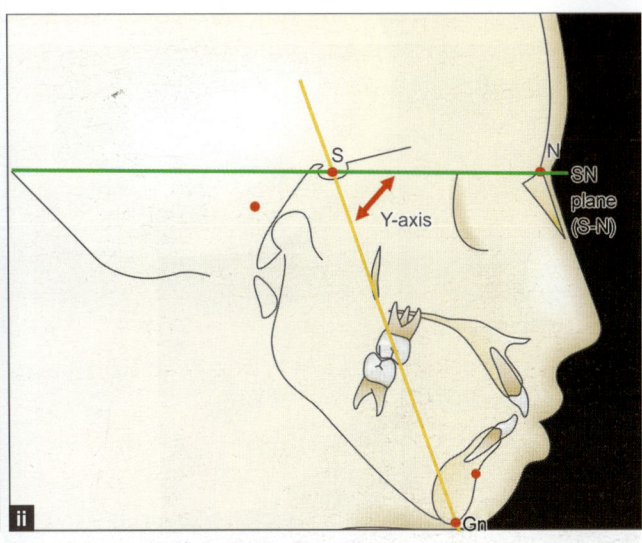

**Figs 15.6E(i and ii):** Y-axis. The mean value of y-axis is 59°, while the range is 53 to 66°

**Figs 15.6A to E:** Skeletal parameters of Down's analysis

### Variation

***Increased Y-axis:*** It is indicative of vertical growth pattern.
***Decreased Y-axis:*** It is indicative of horizontal growth pattern.

### Dental Parameters

#### 1. Cant of Occlusal Plane

Cant of occlusal plane **(Fig. 15.7A)** is formed by the intersection of occlusal plane with F-H plane.

#### Planes of Cant of Occlusal Plane
- Occlusal plane
- F-H plane.

#### Occlusal Plane
Occlusal plane is formed by a line joining APOcc to PPOcc.

#### F-H Plane
Frankfort-horizontal plane is formed by a line joining orbital (Or) to external auditory meatus.

***Significance:*** Cant of occlusal plane gives a measure of the slope of the occlusal plane relative to the F-H plane.
***Mean value:*** The mean value of cant of occlusal plane is 9.3°, while the range is 1.5–14°.

#### Variation
***Increased cant of occlusal plane:*** It is indicative of vertical growth pattern of the individual.
***Decreased cant of occlusal plane:*** It is indicative of horizontal growth pattern.

#### 2. Inter-incisal Angle

Inter-incisal angle **(Fig. 15.7B)** is the angle formed between the long axis of upper and lower incisors.

#### Planes of Inter-incisal Angle
- Long axis of upper incisor
- Long axis of lower incisor.

***Long axis of upper incisor:*** It is a line drawn from tip of the crown to the apex of the root of upper incisor.
***Long axis of lower incisor:*** Long axis of lower incisor is a line drawn from tip of incisal edge of the crown to the root apex of lower incisor.
***Significance:*** Relationship of upper incisor with lower incisor can be assessed.
***Mean value:*** The mean value of interincisal angle is 135.4°, while the range is 130–150.5°.

#### Variations
***Increased interincisal angle:*** Increased interincisal angle indicates class II division 2 malocclusion (retroclination of upper and lower incisor).
***Decreased interincisal angle:*** Decreased interincisal angle indicates bimaxillary protrusion (proclination of both upper and lower incisor).

#### 3. Incisor Occlusal Plane Angle

Incisor occlusal plane angle **(Fig. 15.7C)** is the angle formed by the intersection between the long axis of lower central incisor and the occlusal plane.

#### Planes of Incisor Occlusal Plane Angle
- Long axis of lower central incisor
- Occlusal plane.

#### Long Axis of Lower Central Incisor
Long axis of lower central incisor is from tip of incisal edge to the tip of root apex of lower central incisor.

#### Occlusal Plane
Occlusal plane is formed by a line joining anterior point of occlusion to posterior point of occlusion.
***Significance:*** Inclination of lower permanent central incisor.
***Mean value:*** The mean value of incisor occlusal plane angle is 14.5°, while the range is 3.5–20°.

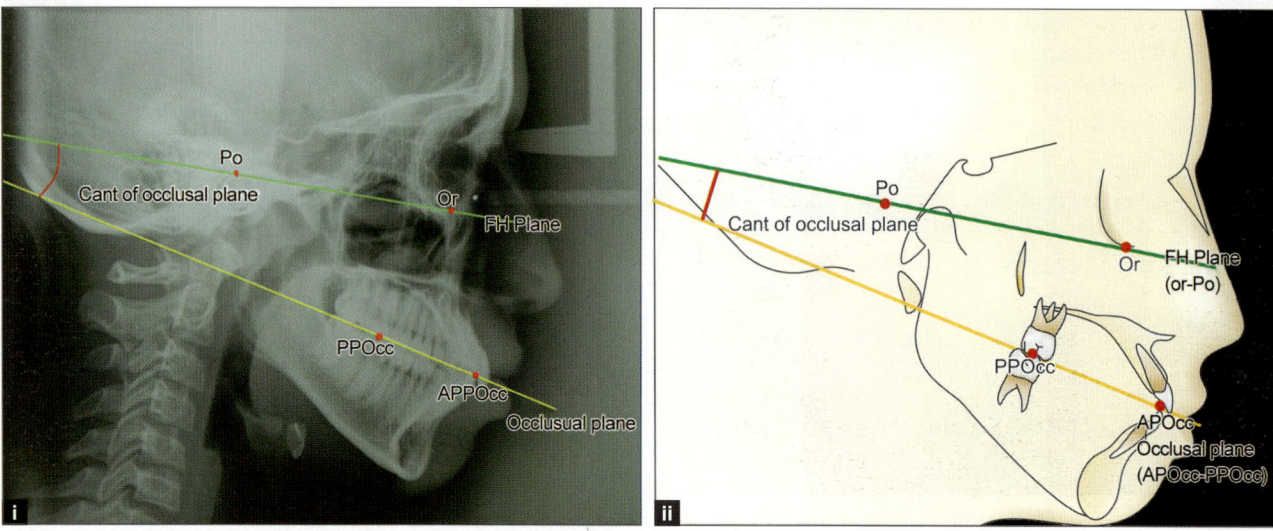

**Figs 15.7A (i and ii):** Cant of occlusal plane. The mean value of cant of occlusal plane is 9.3°, while the range is 1.5 to 14°

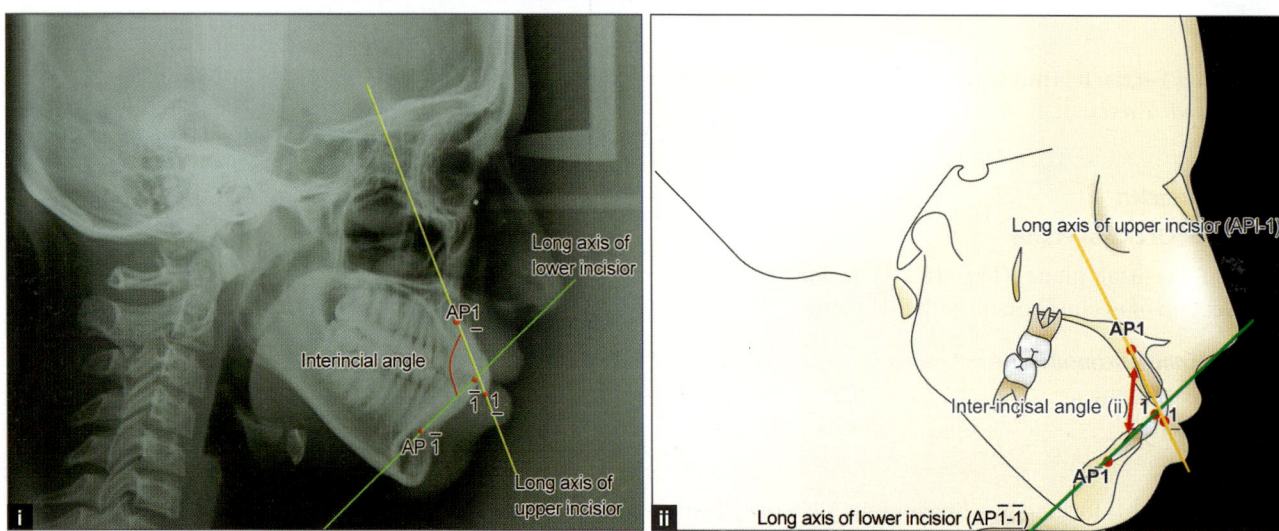

**Figs 15.7B (i and ii):** Interincisal angle. The mean value of interincisal angle is 135.4°, while the range is 130 to 150.5°

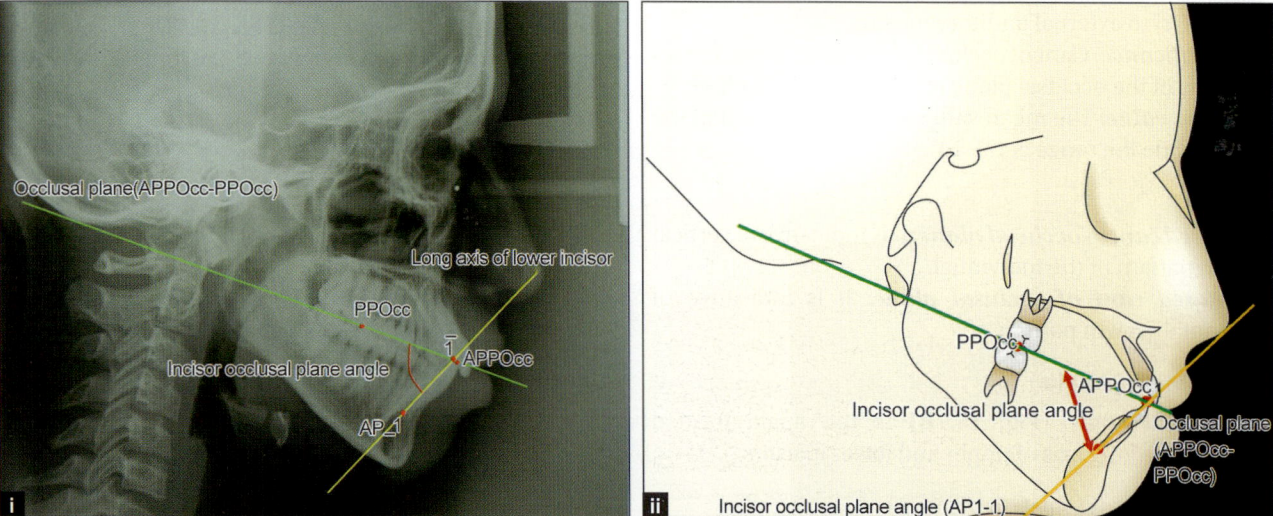

**Figs 15.7C (i and ii):** Incisor occlusal plane angle. The mean value of incisor occlusal plane angle is 14.5°, while the range is 3.5 to 20°

## Variations

***Increased incisor occlusal plane:*** It indicates incisor retroclination.

***Decreased incisor occlusal plane:*** It indicates incisor proclination.

### 4. Incisor Mandibular Plane Angle

Incisor mandibular plane angle **(Fig. 15.7D)** is the angle formed by intersection of the long axis of the lower incisor and the mandibular plane.

### Planes of Incisor Mandibular Plane Angle

- Long axis of lower incisor
- Mandibular plane.

### Long Axis of Lower Incisor

Long axis of lower incisor is line drawn from tip of incisal edge of crown of incisor to the tip of root apex of incisor.

### Mandibular Plane

It is a line joining gonion to menton.

***Significance of incisor-mandibular plane angle:*** It shows inclination of lower incisor to the mandibular plane.
***Mean value:*** Mean is 1.4°. Range is –8.5 to 7°.

### Variations

***Increased incisor-mandibular plane angle:*** It indicates lower incisor-proclination.

Decreased incisor-mandibular plane angle: It indicates lower incisor retroclination.

### 5. Upper Incisor to A-Pog Line

Upper incisor to A-Pog line **(Fig. 15.7E)** is a linear measurement between the incisal edge of the maxillary central incisor and the line joining point A to pogonion.
***Mean value:*** The mean value is 2.7 mm and the range is –1 to 5 mm.

### Variation

***Increased measurement:*** When distance is more than 2 mm, then it is suggestive of upper incisor proclination.

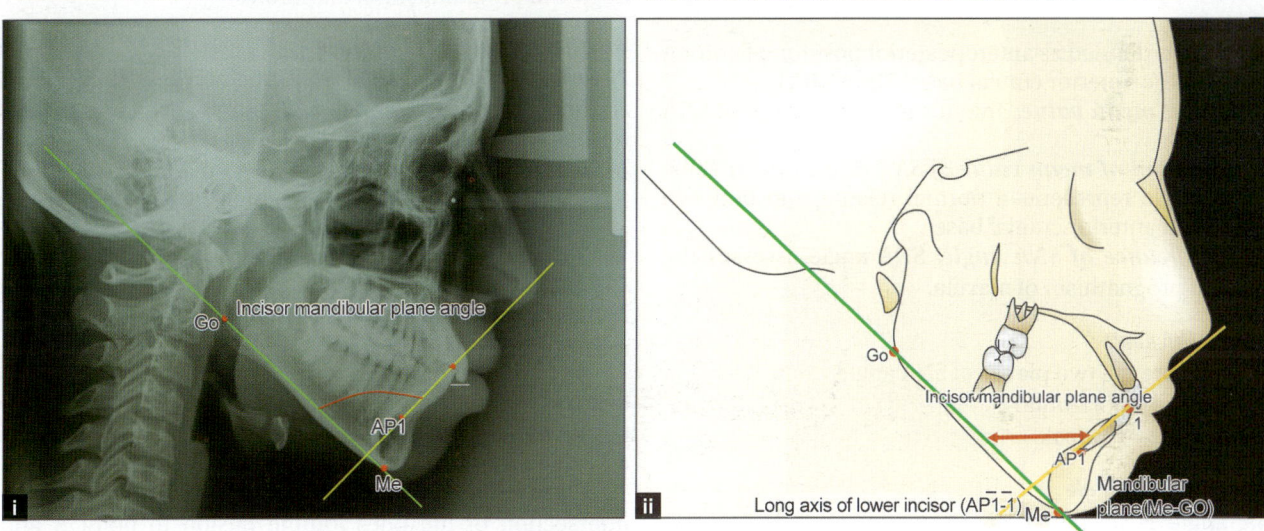

**Figs 15.7D (i and ii):** Incisor mandibular plane angle. The mean value of incisor mandibular plane angle is 1.4°, while the range is –8.5 to 7°

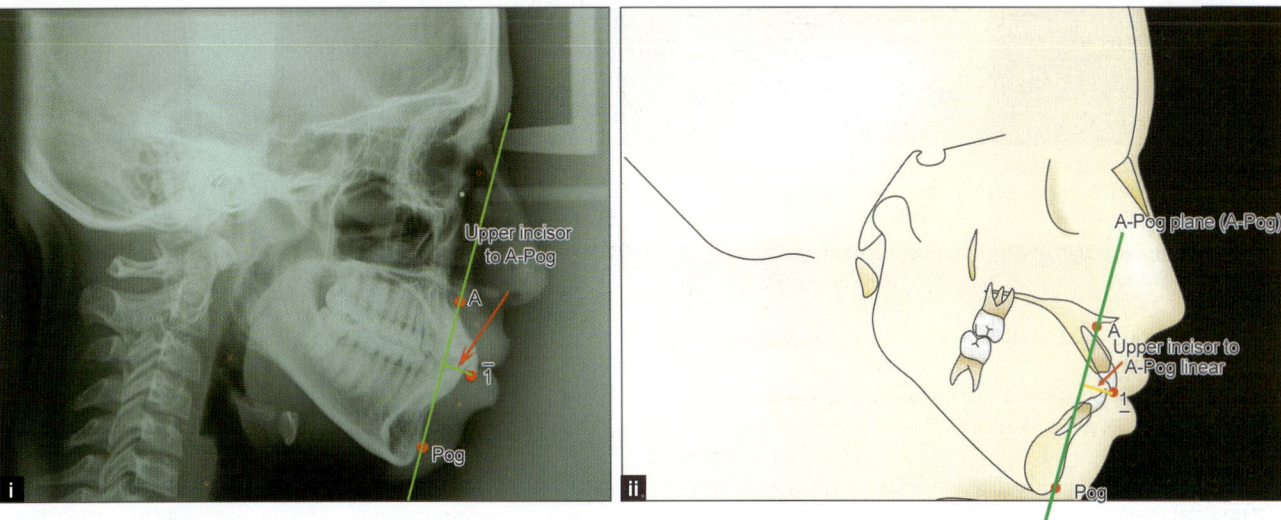

**Figs 15.7E (i and ii):** Upper incisor to A-Pog line. The mean value is 2.7 mm and the range is –1 to 5 mm

**Figs 15.7A to E:** Dental parameters of Down's analysis

***Decreased measurement:*** When distance is less than 2 mm, then it is suggestive of upper incisor retroclinaton.

## STEINER'S ANALYSIS

Cecil C Steiner in the year 1930 developed this analysis with the idea of providing maximal clinical information with the least number of measurements. This analysis has three components:
1. Skeletal analysis
2. Dental analysis
3. Soft tissue analysis

### Skeletal Analysis

Following are the parameters of skeletal analysis of Steiner's analysis **(Table 15.4)**:
- SNA angle
- SNB angle
- ANB angle
- Mandibular plane angle
- Occlusal plane angle.

### SNA Angle

SNA angle is defined as anteroposterior position of point A relative to the anterior cranial base **(Fig. 15.8A)**.

***Normal mean value:*** The normal mean value of SNA angle is 81°.

***Indication of mean value of SNA angle:*** Mean value of SNA angle represents a normal relationship between maxilla and anterior cranial base.

***Siginificance of SNA angle:*** SNA angle assesses the degree of prognathism of maxilla.

### Planes of SNA Angle

Following are the two planes of SNA angle:
1. SN plane—horizontal
2. NA plane—vertical.

### Formation of SNA Angle

SNA angle is formed by SN horizontal plane and NA vertical plane.

### Variation/Deviation of SNA Angle

***Increased SNA angle:*** If the SNA angle is more than the mean value, then it indicates that maxilla lies more anteriorly in relation to the cranial base.

***Decreased SNA angle:*** If SNA angle is less than normal, then it indicates that maxilla lies more posterior in relation to the cranial base.

### SNB Angle

SNB angle defines the anteroposterior position of the mandible in relation to the anterior cranial base **(Fig. 15.8B)**.

***Normal mean value:*** The mean value of SNB angle is 79°.

### Planes of SNB Angle
- SN plane—horizontal
- NB plane—vertical.

***Formation of SNB angle:*** SNB angle is formed by the intersection of SN plane—horizontal and NB plane—vertical.

***Significance of SNB angle:*** SNB angle assesses the degree of prognathism of mandible.

### Variation/Deviation of SNB Angle

***Decreased SNB angle:*** If SNB angle is less than 79°, it is then referred as small SNB angle, which indicates retrognathism of mandible.

***Increased SNB angle:*** If SNB angle is greater than 79°, then it is called as large SNB angle. Large SNB angle—indicates prognathism of mandible.

### ANB Angle

ANB angle is defined as the mutual relationship of the maxillary and mandibular bases in sagittal plane **(Fig. 15.8C)**.

### Planes of ANB Angle
- NA plane—vertical.
- NB plane—vertical.

***Formation of ANB angle:*** It is formed by the intersection of the lines joining nasion to point A and nasion to point B.

**Table 15.4:** Steiner's skeletal analysis

| Angle | Significance | Mean and range | Inference | |
|---|---|---|---|---|
| | | (Normal) | Increased | Decreased |
| SNA angle (intersection of SN plane—NA plane) | Anteroposterior positioning of the maxilla in relation to the cranial base | 82° | Skeletal class II malocclusion | Skeletal class III malocclusion |
| SNB angle (intersection of SN plane—NB plane) | Anteroposterior positioning of the mandible in relation to the cranial base | 80° | Skeletal class III malocclusion | Skeletal class II malocclusion |
| ANB angle (intersection of NA plane—NB plane) | Position of the maxilla to mandible | 2° | Skeletal class II malocclusion | Skeletal class III malocclusion |
| Mandibular plane angle (intersection of SN plane—Go-Gn plane) | Assessment of growth pattern | 32° | Vertical growth pattern (open bite) | Horizontal growth pattern (deep bite) |
| Occlusal plane angle (intersection of occlusal plane—SN plane) | Assessment of growth pattern | 14.5° | Vertical growth pattern (open bite) | Horizontal growth pattern (deep bite) |

***Normal mean value:*** = $\dfrac{\text{Mean value of ANB angle is 2°}}{\text{ANB = SNA-SNB angle}}$

***Significance of ANB angle:*** ANB is used to assess the sagittal relationship between the maxillary and mandibular bases.

### Variation/Deviation of ANB Angle

***Increased ANB angle:*** If ANB angle is greater than normal, it is known as large ANB angle. It indicates class II skeletal tendency.

***Decreased ANB angle:*** If ANB angle is smaller than 2°, then it is referred as small ANB angle. It indicates class III skeletal tendency.

### Mandibular Plane Angle

Mandibular plane angle gives an indication of growth pattern of an individual **(Fig. 15.8D)**.

### Planes of Mandibular Plane Angle

- SN plane (S-N)
- Mandibular plane (Gn-Go).

***Formation of mandibular plane angle:*** It is the angle formed between SN plane and the mandibular plane. The mandibular plane angle is used in this analysis, which is a line connecting gonion and gnathion.

***Normal mean value:*** The average mandibular plane angle is 32°.

***Significance:*** Assessment of growth pattern.

### Variation/Deviation of Mandibular Plane Angle

***Increased mandibular plane angle:*** Increased mandibular plane angle indicates vertical growth pattern.

***Decreased mandibular plane angle:*** Decreased mandibular plane angle indicates horizontal growth pattern.

### Occlusal Plane Angle

Occlusal plane angle indicates the relation of the occlusal plane to the cranium and face **(Fig. 15.8E)**.

### Planes of Occlusal Plane Angle

- SN plane (S-N)

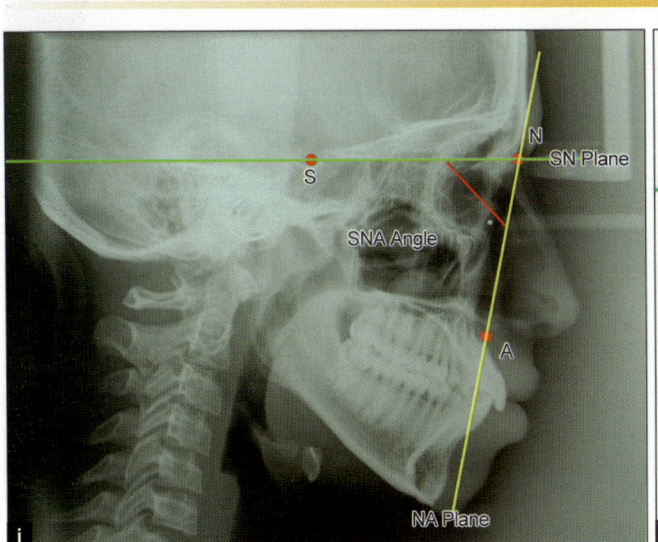
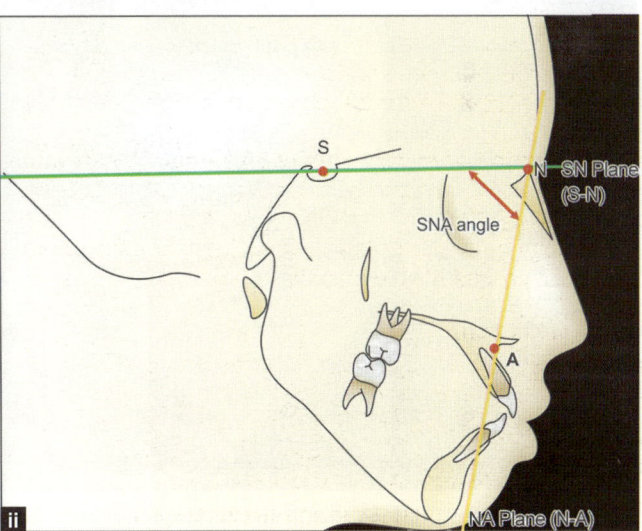

**Figs 15.8A(i and ii):** SNA angle. The normal mean value of SNA angle is 81°

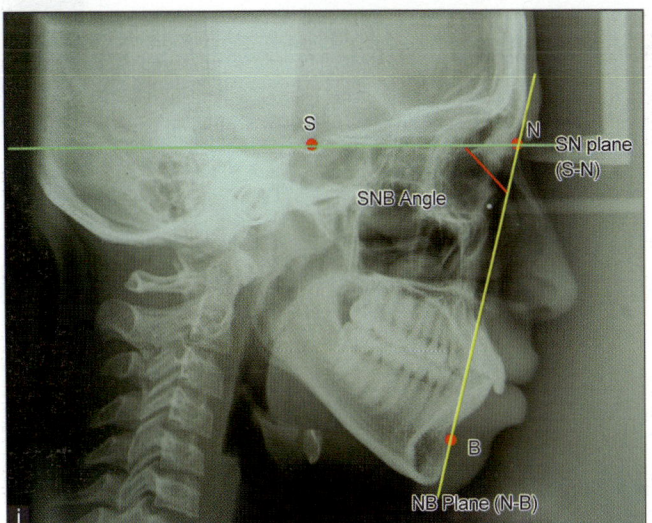
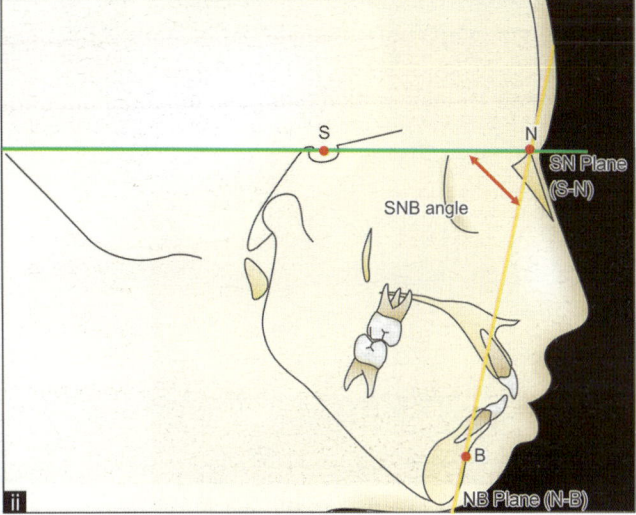

**Figs 15.8B(i and ii):** SNB angle. The mean value of SNB angle is 79°

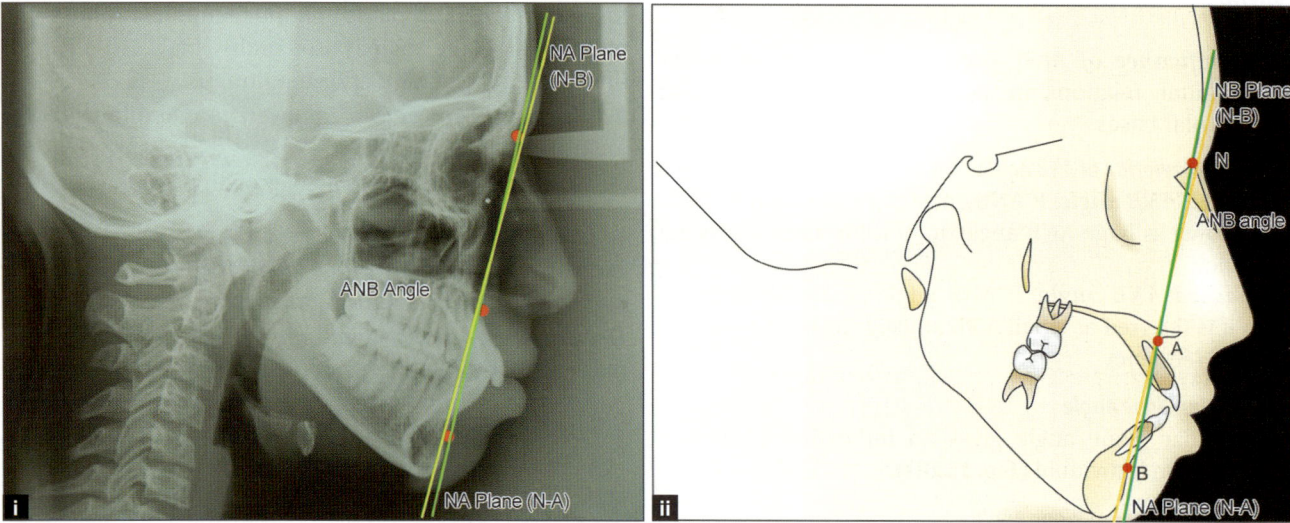

**Figs 15.8C(i and ii):** ANB angle. Mean value of ANB angle is 2°

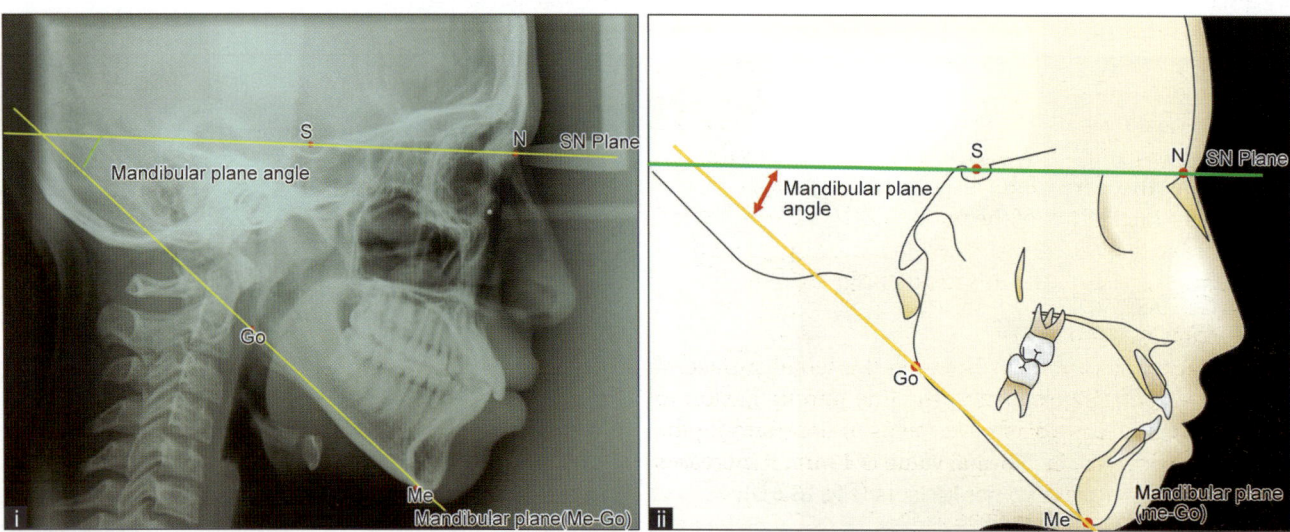

**Figs 15.8D(i and ii):** Mandibular plane angle. The average mandibular plane angle is 32°

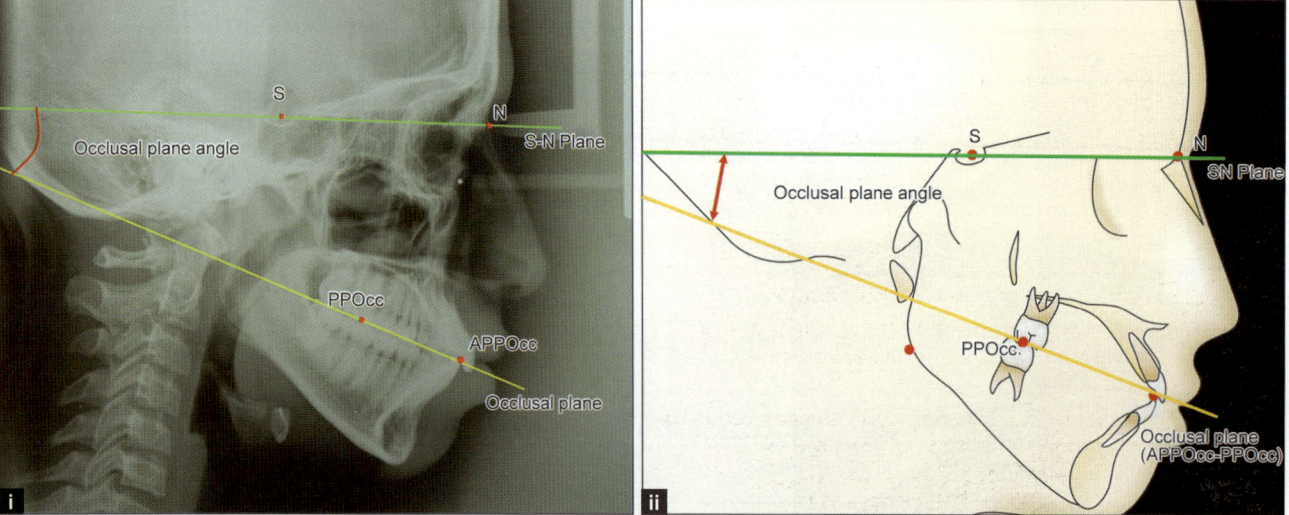

**Figs 15.8E(i and ii):** Occlusal plane angle. The average occlusal plane angle is 14.5°
**Figs 15.8A to E:** Steiner's skeletal parameters

- **Occlusal Plane:** It represents a line passing through the overlapping cusps of first premolars and first molars.

### Formation of Occlusal Plane Angle
It is the angle formed between SN plane and the occlusal plane.
***Normal mean value:*** The average occlusal plane angle is 14.5°.
***Significance:*** Assessment of growth pattern.

### Variation/Deviation of Occlusal Plane Angle
***Increased occlusal plane angle:*** Increased occlusal plane angle indicates vertical growth pattern.
***Decreased occlusal plane angle:*** Decreased occlusal plane angle indicates horizontal growth pattern.

## Dental Analysis

The parameters used in dental analysis are **(Table 15.5)**:
- Upper incisor to NA angle
- Upper incisor to NA (linear)
- Lower incisor to NB angle
- Lower incisor to NB (linear)
- Interincisor angle

### Upper Incisor to NA Angle
It is the angle formed by the intersection of the long axis of the upper central incisors and the line joining nasion to point A. The normal angle is 22°. This angle indicates the relative inclination of the upper incisors. An increased angle is seen in patients who have proclined upper incisors as in class II division 1 malocclusion **(Fig. 15.9A)**.

### Upper Incisor to NA (Linear)
It is a linear measurement between the labial surface of the upper central incisors and the line joining nasion to point A. This measurement also helps in determining the upper incisor position. Normal value is 4 mm. It increases in cases with proclined upper incisors **(Fig 15.9B)**.

### Lower Incisor to NB Angle
This angle is formed between the NB plane and the long axis of the lower incisors. This angle indicates the inclination of the lower central incisor and has a mean value of 25°. An increased value indicates proclination of lower incisors whereas a decreased value indicates upright or retroclined lower incisors **(Fig. 15.9C)**.

### Lower Incisor to NB (Linear)
It is the linear distance between the labial surface of lower central incisors and the line joining nasion to point B. This measurement also helps in assessing the lower incisor inclination. An increase in this measurement indicates proclined lower incisors. The normal value is 4 mm **(Fig. 15.9D)**.

### Inter-incisor Angle
This is an angle formed between the long axis of the upper and lower central incisors. A reduced interincisor angle is associated with a class II division 1 malocclusion or a class I bimaxillary protrusion. A larger than normal angle is seen in class II division 2 malocclusion. The mean value is 130–131° **(Fig. 15.9E)**.

## Soft Tissue Analysis

### Reference Lines of the Analysis
Reference lines of the Steiner's analysis are center point of the S-shaped curve between tip of nose and subnasale.

### Reference Line of Steiner's Lip Analysis
Reference line of Steiner's lip analysis is the line joining from center point of the S-shaped curve between the tip of nose and subnasale to the lower point (soft tissue pogonion) **(Figs 15.10A and B)**.

### Interpretation of the Analysis
***Flat lips:*** If lips lie behind the line connecting two reference points, they are too flat.
***Prominent lips:*** If lips lie anterior to the line connecting two reference points, they are too prominent.

## TWEED'S TRIANGLE

The Tweed's triangle **(Figs 15.11A and B)** makes use of three planes that form a diagnostic triangle called Tweed's triangle.

| Table 15.5: Steiner's dental analysis | | | | |
|---|---|---|---|---|
| **Angle** | **Significance** | **Mean (Normal)** | **Inference** | |
| | | | *Increased* | *Decreased* |
| Upper incisor to NA angle (intersection of long axis of upper central incisors—NA plane) | Relative inclination of the upper incisors | 22° | Proclination of upper incisors | Retroclination of upper incisors |
| Upper incisor to NA (distance between labial surface of upper incisor to NA) | Assessment of position of upper incisors | 4 mm | Proclination of upper incisors | Retroclination of upper incisors |
| Lower incisor to NB angle (intersection of NB plane— long axis of lower incisors) | Relative inclination of lower incisors | 25° | Proclination of lower incisors | Retroclination of lower incisors (upright lower incisors) |
| Lower incisor to NB (distance between labial surface of lower central incisors to NB) | Assessment of position of lower incisors | 4 mm | Proclination of lower incisors | Retroclination of lower incisors |
| Interincisor angle (intersection between long axis of upper and lower central incisors) | Relative inclination of upper incisors to lower incisors | 130–131° | Class II division 2 malocclusion | Class II division 1 malocclusion |

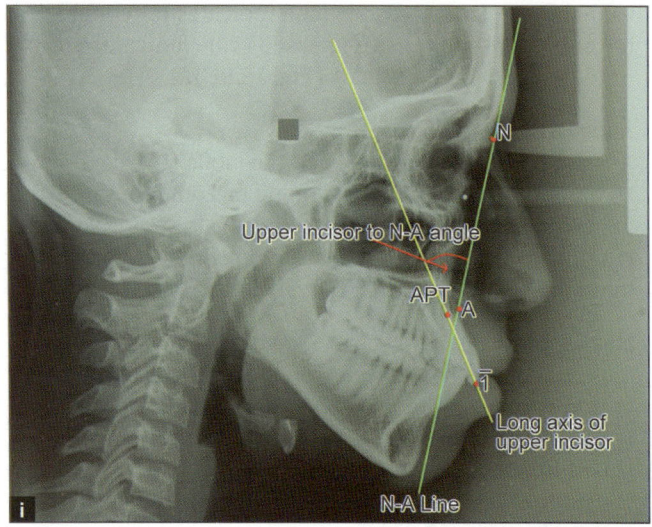 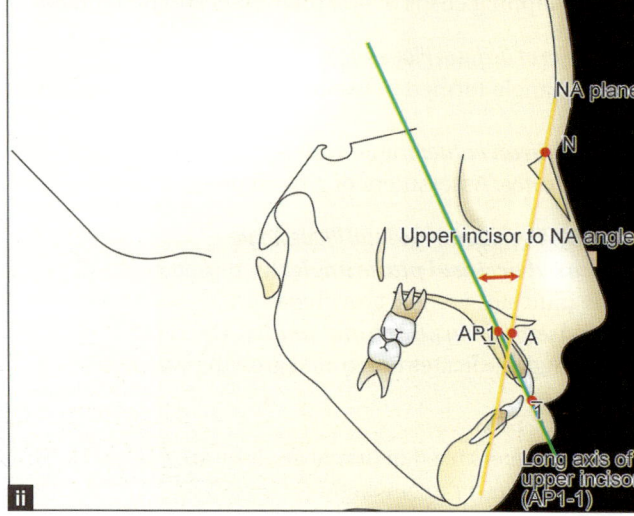

**Figs 15.9A (i and ii):** Upper incisor to NA angle. The normal angle is 22°

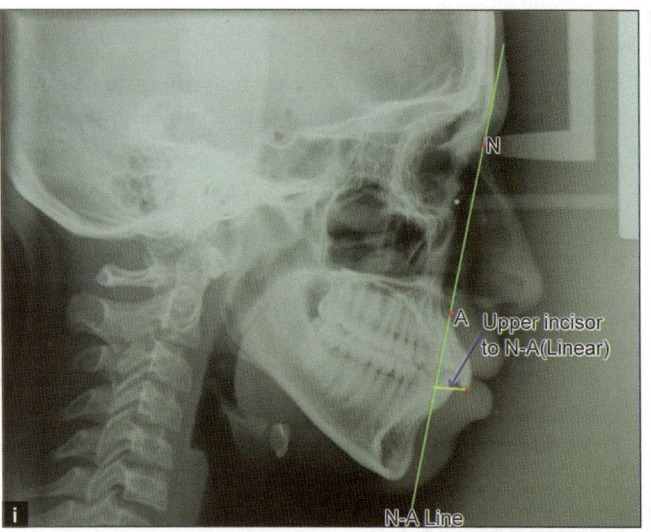 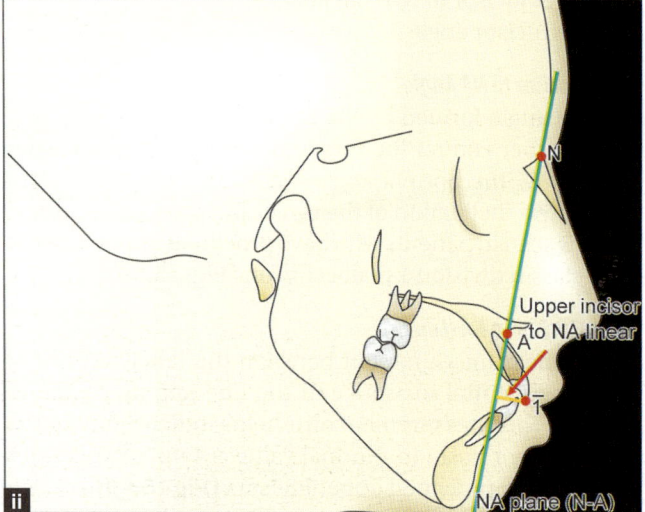

**Figs 15.9B (i and ii):** Upper incisor to NA (linear)

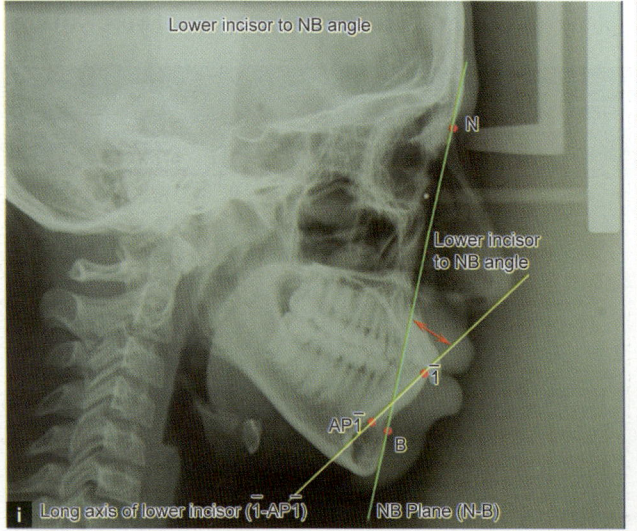 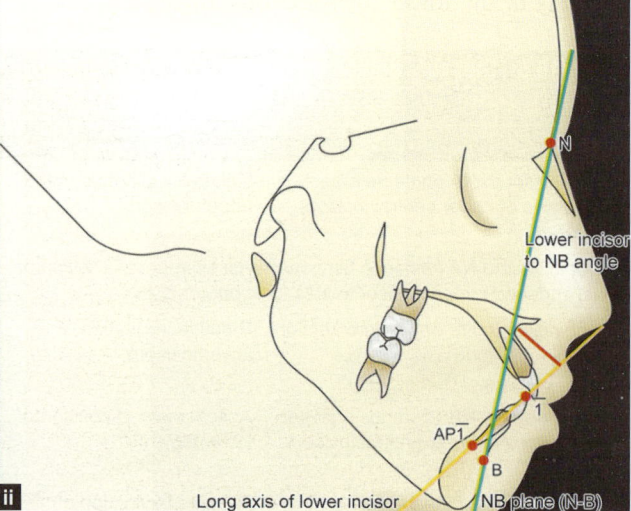

**Figs 15.9C (i and ii):** Lower incisor to NB angle. Normal value is 4 mm

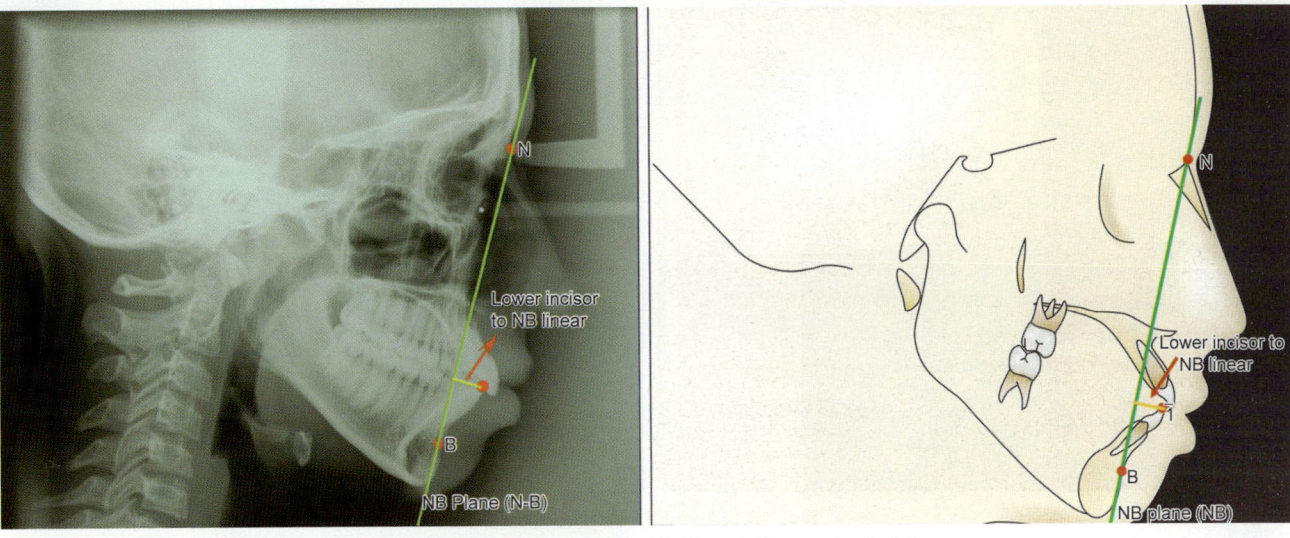

**Figs 15.9D:** Lower incisor to NB (linear). Mean value is 25°

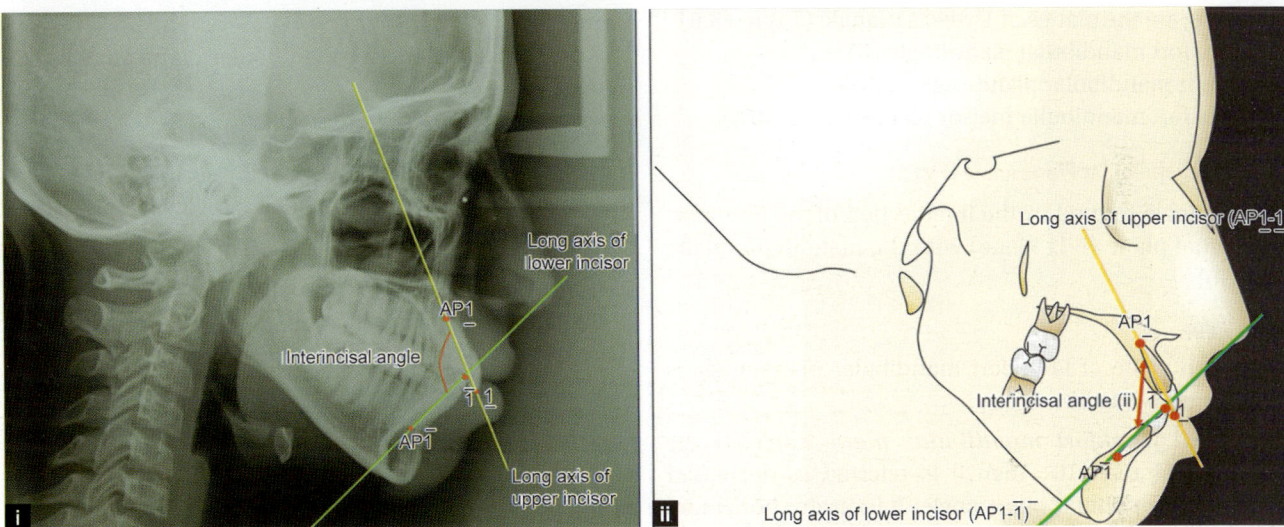

**Figs 15.9E (i and ii):** Inter-incisor angle. The mean value is 130 to 131°
**Figs 15.9A to E:** Dental parameters of Steiner's analysis

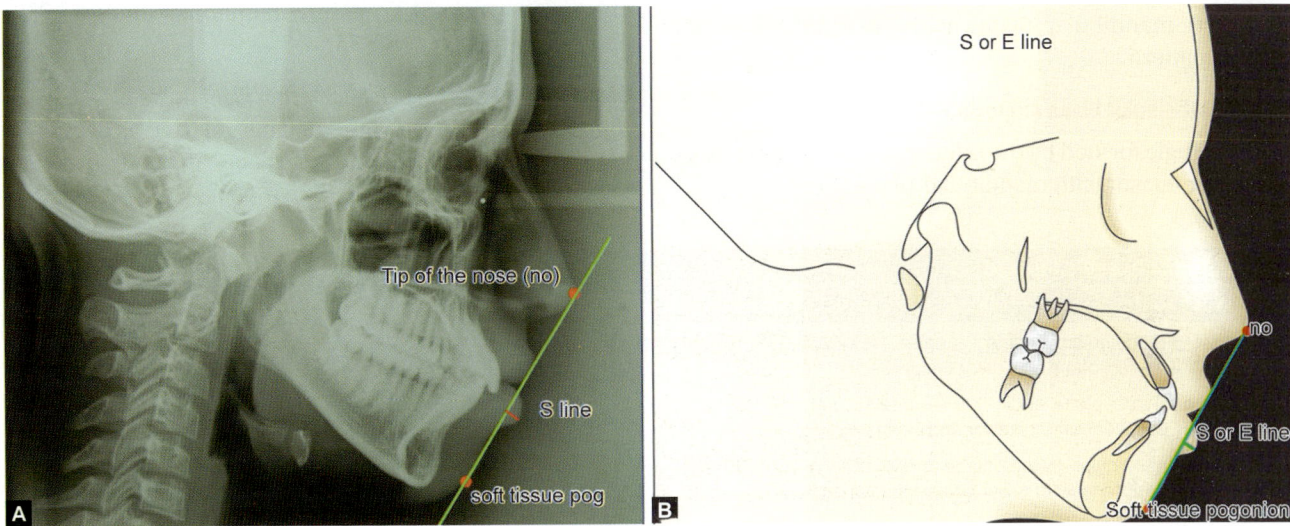

**Figs 15.10A and B:** "S" line

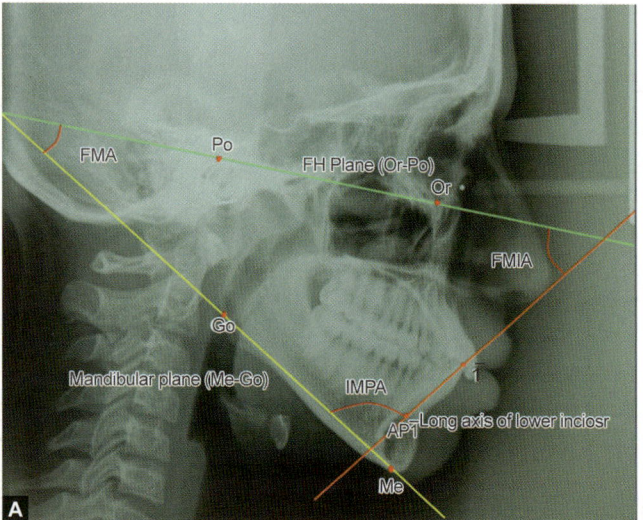 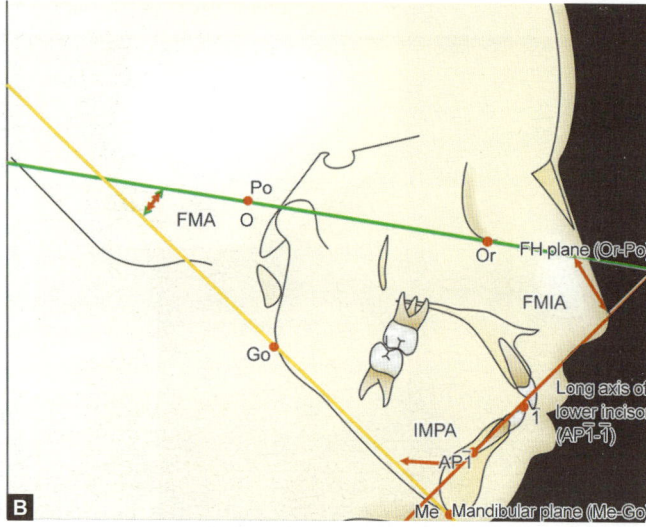

**Figs 15.11A and B:** Tweed's triangle

Following are the planes of Tweed's triangle **(Table 15.6)**:
- Frankfort mandibular plane angle (FMA)
- Incisor mandibular plane angle (IMPA)
- Frankfort mandibular incisor plane angle (FMIA).

## Frankfort Mandibular Plane Angle (FMPA)

It is the angle formed by the intersection of the Frankfort Horizontal plane (F-H Plane) with the mandibular plane (Me-Go).

### Mean Value

The mean value of Frankfort mandibular plane angle is 25º. Range is 16 to 35º.

*Decreased frankfort mandibular plane angle:* If the angle is less than 16º, then it is referred as decreased Frankfort mandibular plane angle. It indicates horizontal growth pattern.

*Increased frankfort mandibular plane angle:* If the angle is greater than 35º, then it is referred as increased Frankfort mandibular plane angle. It indicates vertical growth pattern.

## Incisor Mandibular Plane Angle (IMPA)

It is the angle formed by the intersection of the long axis of the lower incisor with mandibular plane (Me-Go).

### Mean Value

The mean value of incisor mandibular plane angle is 90º. Range is 85–95º.

### Decreased Incisor Mandibular Plane Angle

If the angle is less than 85º, then it is referred as decreased incisor mandibular plane angle. It indicates lower incisor retroclination.

### Increased Incisor Mandibular Plane Angle

If the angle is greater than 95º, then it is referred as increased incisor mandibular plane angle. It indicates lower incisor proclination.

## Frankfort Mandibular Incisor Plane Angle (FMIA)

It is the angle formed by the intersection of the long axis of the lower incisor with the Frankfort horizontal plane (F-H Plane).

### Mean Value

The mean value of Frankfort mandibular incisor plane angle is 65º. Range is 60–75 º.

### Decreased Frankfort Mandibular Incisor Plane Angle

If the angle is less than 60º, then it is referred as decreased Frankfort mandibular incisor plane angle. It indicates lower incisor proclination.

| Table 15.6: Tweed's triangle | | | |
|---|---|---|---|
| Angle | Mean and range | Decreased | Increased |
| Frankfort mandibular plane angle (FMPA) (intersection of F-H plane and mandibular plane) | 25° (16–35°) | Horizontal growth pattern | Vertical growth pattern |
| Incisor mandibular plane angle (IMPA) (intersection of long axis of lower central incisor and F-H plane) | 90° (85–95°) | Lower incisor retroclination | Lower incisor proclination |
| Frankfort mandibular incisor plane angle (FMIA) (intersection of long axis of lower central incisor and F-H plane) | 65° (60–75°) | Lower incisor proclination | Lower incisor retroclination |

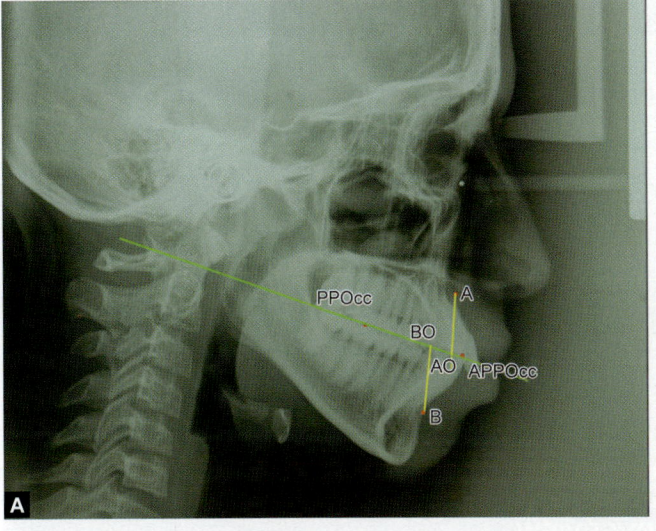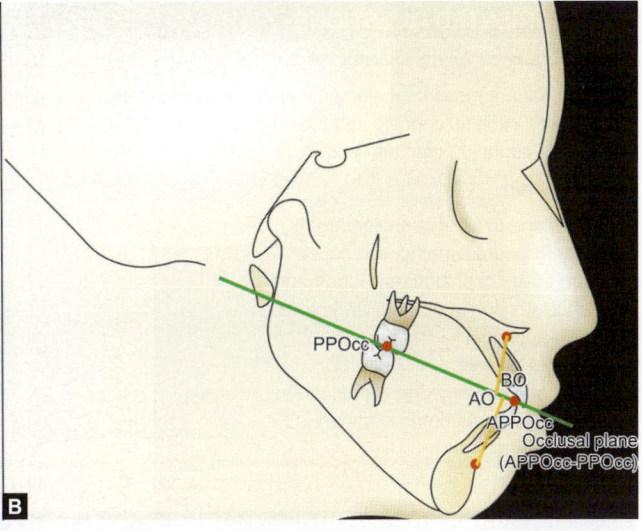

**Figs 15.12A and B:** Wit's appraisal. The point BO was approximately 1 mm anterior to point AO

### *Increased Frankfort Mandibular Incisor Plane Angle*
If the angle is greater than 75º, then it is referred as increased Frankfort mandibular incisor plane angle. It indicates lower incisor retroclination.

## WIT'S APPRAISAL

Jacobson described the Wit's (University of Witwatersrand, South Africa) appraisal.

Wit's appraisal **(Figs 15.12A and B)** measures the extent to which the jaws are related to each other anteroposteriorly.

### *Method of Assessment*
- The method of assessing the extent of jaw disharmony entails drawing perpendicular on a lateral cephalometric lead film tracing from point A and B on the maxilla and mandible, respectively into the occlusal plane, which is drawn through the region of maximum cuspal interdigitation.
- The point of contact on the occlusal plane from A and B are labeled AO and BO, respectively.

### *Normal Occlusion*
The point AO is approximately 1 mm anterior to point BO.

### *Skeletal Class II Jaw Dysplasias*
The point BO will be located well behind point AO.

### *Skeletal Class III Jaw Disharmonies*
The point BO will be ahead of point AO.

### *Deviations of Wit's Appraisal*
- 1 mm in male
- 0 mm in female.

## BIBLIOGRAPHY

1. Bennett GC, Kronman JH. A cephalometric study of mandibular development and its relationship to the mandibular and occlusal planes. Angle Orthod. 1970;40:119-28.
2. Bjork A. Prediction of mandibular growth rotation. Am J Orthod. 1969;55:585-99.
3. Broadbent BH. A new X-ray technique and its application to orthodontics. Angle Orthod.1931;1:45-66.
4. Brodie AG, Downs WB, Goldstein A, et al. Cephalometric appraisal of orthodontic results: a preliminary report. Angle Orthod1938; 8:261-5.
5. Downs WB. Analyis of the dentofacial profile. Angle Orthod. 1956; 26:191-212.
6. Downs WB. Variations in facial relationship: Their significance in treatment and prognosis. Am J Orthod. 1948;34:812-40.
7. Graber TM, Vanarsdall RL. Orthodontics, Current Principles and Techniques. Mosby Year Book, Inc, 1994.
8. Houston WJB. The analysis of error in orthodontics measurements. Am J Orthod. 1983;83:382-90.
9. Jacobson A. Radiographic Cephalometry: From Basics to Video-Imaging. Chicago: Quintessence, 1995.
10. Jacobson A. The "Wit's"appraisal of jaw disharmony. Am J Orthod. 1975;67:125-38.
11. Jacobson. Introduction to Radiographic Cephalometry. Philadelphia: Lea and Febiger, 1985.
12. Jakobsson SO. Cephalometric evaluation of treatment effect on Class II, Division 1 malocclusions. Am J Orthod. 1967;53:446-57.
13. Moorrees CFA, Lebret L. The mesh diagram and cephalometrics. Angle Orthod. 1962;32:214-31.
14. Rickets RM, Bench RW. An overview of computerized cephalometrics. Am J Orthod. 1972;61:1-28.
15. Steiner CC. The use of cephalometrics as an aid to planning and assessing orthodontic treatment. Am J Orthod. 1960;46:721-35.
16. Subtelny JD. Cephalometric diagnosis, growth, and treatment: something old something new. Am J Orthod. 1970;57:262-86.
17. Susomi R. A cephalometric evaluation of dentofacial growth in mandibular protrusion subjects. J Osaka Univ. 1969;9:25-35.
18. Tweed CH. The diagnostic facial triangle in the control of treatment objectives. Am J Orthod. 1969;55:651-7.

## EXAM-ORIENTED QUESTIONS

### Long Essay or Long Questions
1. Enumerate various cephalometric analysis used in treatment planning and write in detail any 2 cephalometric analyses.
2. Steiner's skeletal cephalometric analysis.
3. Down's cephalometric analysis.

### Short Notes
1. Types and uses of cephalogram
2. Classify cephalometric landmarks
3. Hard tissue cephalometric landmarks
4. Soft tissue cephalometric landmarks
5. Witt's appraisal
6. Tweed's triangle
7. Any 1 angle of any one cephalometric analysis
8. Derived cephalometric landmarks.

## CHAPTER OVERVIEW

```
                        Cephalometrics in orthodontics
   ┌──────────┬──────────────┬──────────┬──────────┬──────────┬──────────┐
 Types of   Cephalometric   Down's    Steiner's   Tweed's    Wits appraisal
 cephalogram  landmarks   cephalometric cephalometric cephalometric
            FLOW CHART    analysis    analysis    analysis
            NO 15.1       Table 15.3  Table 15.4  Table 15.6
                                      and table 15.5
   ┌─────┴─────┐
 Frontal    Lateral
 cephalogram cephalogram
```

- Types of cephalogram
  - Frontal cephalogram
  - Lateral cephalogram
- Cephalometric landmarks — FLOW CHART NO 15.1
- Down's cephalometric analysis — Table 15.3
- Steiner's cephalometric analysis — Table 15.4 and table 15.5
- Tweed's cephalometric analysis — Table 15.6
- Wits appraisal
  - In normal occlusion—The point AO is approximately 1mm anterior to point BO
  - Skeletal class II jaw dysplasias—The point BO will be located well behind point AO
  - Skeletal class III jaw disharmonies—The point BO will be forward of point AO
  - Deviations of Wit's appraisal
  - 1mm in male
  - 0 mm in female

# CHAPTER 16

# Maturity Indicators

*Phulari BS*

The level of maturity attained and the amount of growth potential remaining is an important consideration while treating malocclusions. The maturational status of the patient has a strong bearing on orthodontic diagnosis, treatment planning, outcome of the treatment and posttreatment stability. The prepubertal growth spurt is considered to be an advantageous period for certain types of orthodontic treatment, such as growth modification procedures using orthopedic and functional appliances; while orthognathic surgeries are best carried out after the cessation of growth.

Chronological age is an unreliable guide for the assessment of children's maturational status due to the wide individual variation observed in terms of timing, duration and velocity of growth. Children of same age may vary in their maturity status a great deal; therefore, maturity indicators have been developed using other parameters, such as height gained, secondary sex changes, dental development and skeletal ossification **(Box 16.1)**. Ideal requirements of a maturity indicator are given in **(Box 16.2)**.

Since orthodontist works primarily with teeth and bone, the skeletal age or bone age can provide reliable information while helping in accurate growth prediction. Hand-wrist radiographs have been widely used to assess skeletal maturity. However, evaluation of cervical vertebrae on lateral cephalograms is gaining popularity in the recent years.

## HAND-WRIST RADIOGRAPHS

The basis of using hand-wrist radiographs for assessing skeletal age is that the skeleton in the hand-wrist region is made of numerous small bones (27 small bones + distal ends of long bones radius and ulna); these numerous bones in the hand-wrist region are derived from a total of 51 separate growth centers **(Box 16.3)**. The development of these bones from the appearance of calcification centers to epiphyseal plate closure occurs throughout the entire postnatal growth period and therefore provides a useful means of assessing skeletal maturity.

**Correlation:** Hand-wrist radiographs have been correlated to:
- Dental development
- Peak height velocity
- Cervical vertebrae
- Cranial base outline
- Spheno–occipital synchondrosis.

### Anatomy of Hand and Wrist

Here is a brief description of the anatomy of hand-wrist, which aids in understanding the various methods. The skeleton of the hand-wrist region is made of the following four groups of bones **(Figs 16.1A and B)**:
- Distal ends of long bones of forearm (radius and ulna)
- Carpals

---

**Box 16.1:** Biologic indicators of maturity

- **Morphologic age:** It is based on height gained. Height or morphological age is useful as a maturity indicator from late infancy to early adulthood.
- **Dental age:** Dental age can be assessed by two different methods:
  - By eruption status of primary and permanent dentition
  - By radiologic assessment of calcification of crowns and development of roots of unerupted and developing teeth.
  
  Dental age maturity indicators are useful from birth to early adolescence.
- **Sexual age:** It refers to the development of secondary sex characteristics: breast development and menarche in females; penis and testes growth in males; and axillary and pubic hair development in both sexes. Sexual age as a maturity indicator is useful only for adolescent growth.
- **Skeletal age:** It is determined by accessing the development of bones in the hand and wrist or by evaluating the development of cervical vertebrae on lateral cephalograms. It provides a most useful means of assessing biologic maturity and is useful through the postnatal growth period.

---

**Box 16.2:** Ideal requirements of a maturity indicator

- It should be safe.
- It should be noninvasive.
- Radiation exposure should be minimal.
- It should be accurate.
- The stages of maturity should be well defined and easily identifiable.
- The method should be simple to perform with minimal armamentarium and personnel requirements.
- The method should be valid in both genders and in different population groups.
- It should be cost-effective.

---

**Box 16.3:** Growth centers in hand-wrist region

| | |
|---|---|
| Phalanges | 28 (14 primary and 14 secondary) |
| Metacarpals | 10 (5 primary and 5 secondary) |
| Carpals | 8 |
| Ulna | 2 |
| Radius | 2 |
| Sesamoid | 1 |
| Total | 51 separate growth centers |

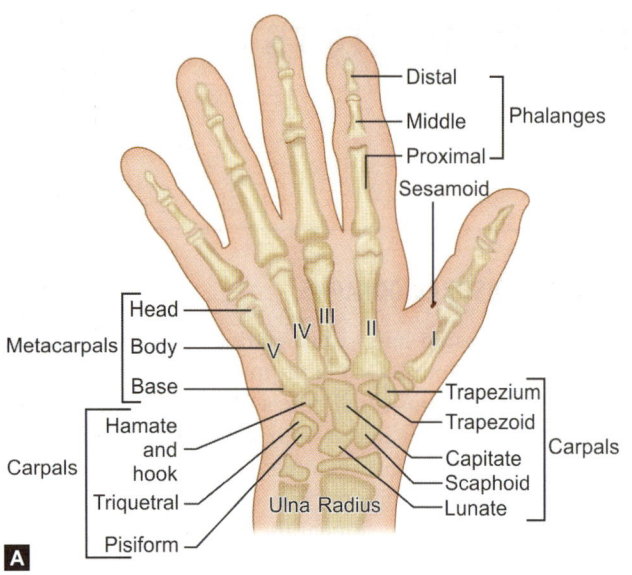
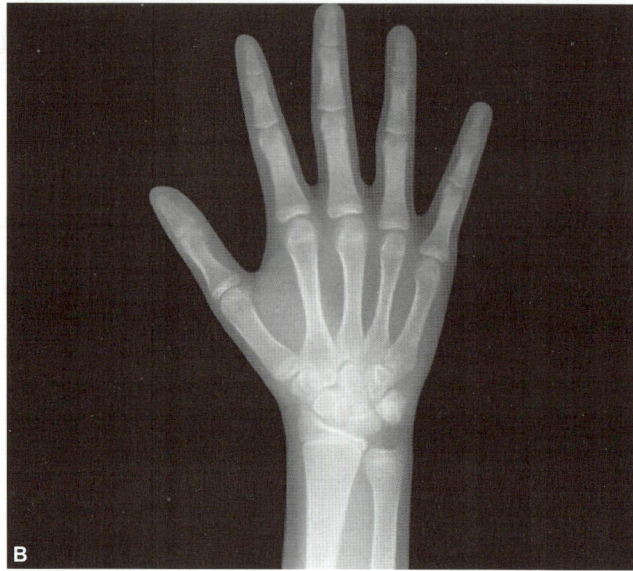

**Figs 16.1A and B:** Anatomy of hand and wrist. (A) Graphic illustration showing individual bones of hand–wrist region. (B) Hand and wrist radiograph

- Metacarpals
- Phalanges.

### Distal Ends of Bones of Forearm

The radius and ulna are the long bones of the forearm. Their distal ends with respective epiphyseal bones form the first group of bones in the hand-wrist region.

### Carpal Bones

Carpus consists of small, roughly cuboidal bones, which are arranged in two rows; proximal and distal. The carpal bones which form the proximal row in a radioulnar order (from lateral to medial order) are "scaphoid, lunate, triquetrum and pisiform." The distsal row is made up of the "trapezium, trapezoid, capitate and hamate." Hamate has a hamular process which is also called as "**hook of hamate.**" Each of these carpal bones ossifies from one primary center and their ossification follows a predictable pattern thus enabling prediction of skeletal maturation possible.

### Metacarpal Bones

- The metacarpus of hand consists of five metacarpal bones. They are conventionally numbered in radio-ulnar order (from lateral to medial side), so that the thumb has the first metacarpal bone, while the little finger has the fifth.
- The metacarpal bones are miniature long bones, with a distal head, a shaft and a base. The rounded heads articulate with the proximal phalanges, while the bases of the metacarpal bones articulate with the distal row of carpal bones.
- Each metacarpal bone ossifies from one primary center (in the shaft) and a secondary center on its distal end, except for the first metacarpal bone (thumb) where the secondary center appears at the proximal end.

### Phalanges

The phalanges are the small bones that form the skeleton of the fingers. Each digit of the hand, except the thumb, has three phalanges; proximal, middle and distal. Thus, there are a total of 14 phalanges, with 3 in each finger and 2 in the thumb. Each phalanx has a distal head, shaft and proximal base.

### Ossification of Phalanges

The phalanges are ossified from a primary center for the shaft and a proximal epiphyseal center. Ossification in the shaft (primary center) begins prenatally. The epiphyseal centers (secondary centers) appear postnatally around two to four years of age. Ossification in the epiphyses continues progressively and the fusion of the epiphyses with their respective diaphyses is completed during puberty at about 15th–16th year in females and 17th–18th year in males.

The phalanges appear to ossify in three stages **(Figs 16.2A to C)**.

- Stage 1: The epiphysis and the diaphysis are equal.
- Stage 2: The epiphysis caps the diaphysis by covering it like a cap.
- Stage 3: Fusion occurs between the epiphysis and the diaphysis.

### Ulnar Sesamoid Bone

The sesamoid is a small nodular bone, which is most often found embedded within the tendons in the region of thumb **(Figs 16.3A and B)**.

Now, it can be appreciated from the series of hand-wrist radiographs of different age groups given in **Figure 16.4** that the development of numerous small bones of the hand-wrist region (from the appearance of calcification centers to epiphyseal plate closure), occurs throughout the entire postnatal growth period and thus offers a useful means of assessing skeletal maturity.

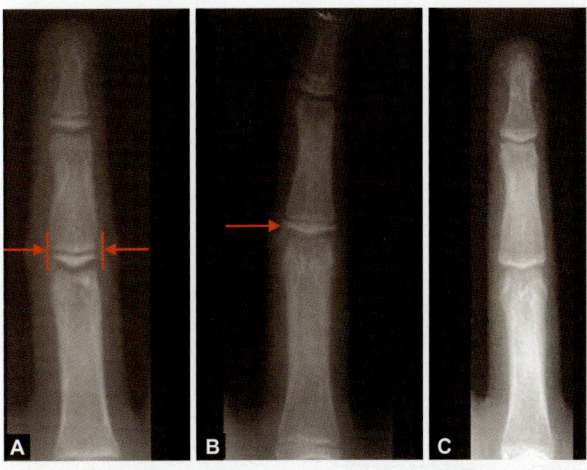

**Figs 16.2A to C:** Stages in ossification of phalanges; (A) Stage 1: The epiphysis and the diaphysis are equal; (B) Stage 2: The epiphysis caps the diaphysis by connecting it like a cap; (C) Stage 3: Fusion occurs between the epiphysis and the diaphysis

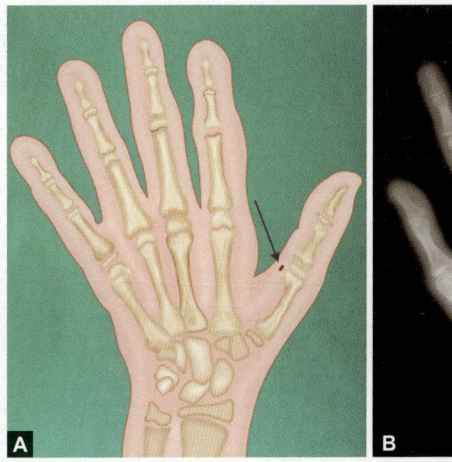

**Figs 16.3A and B:** Ossification onset of the ulnar sesamoid, a small nodular bone often found embedded in tendons in the region of thumb is a useful indication of skeletal maturity

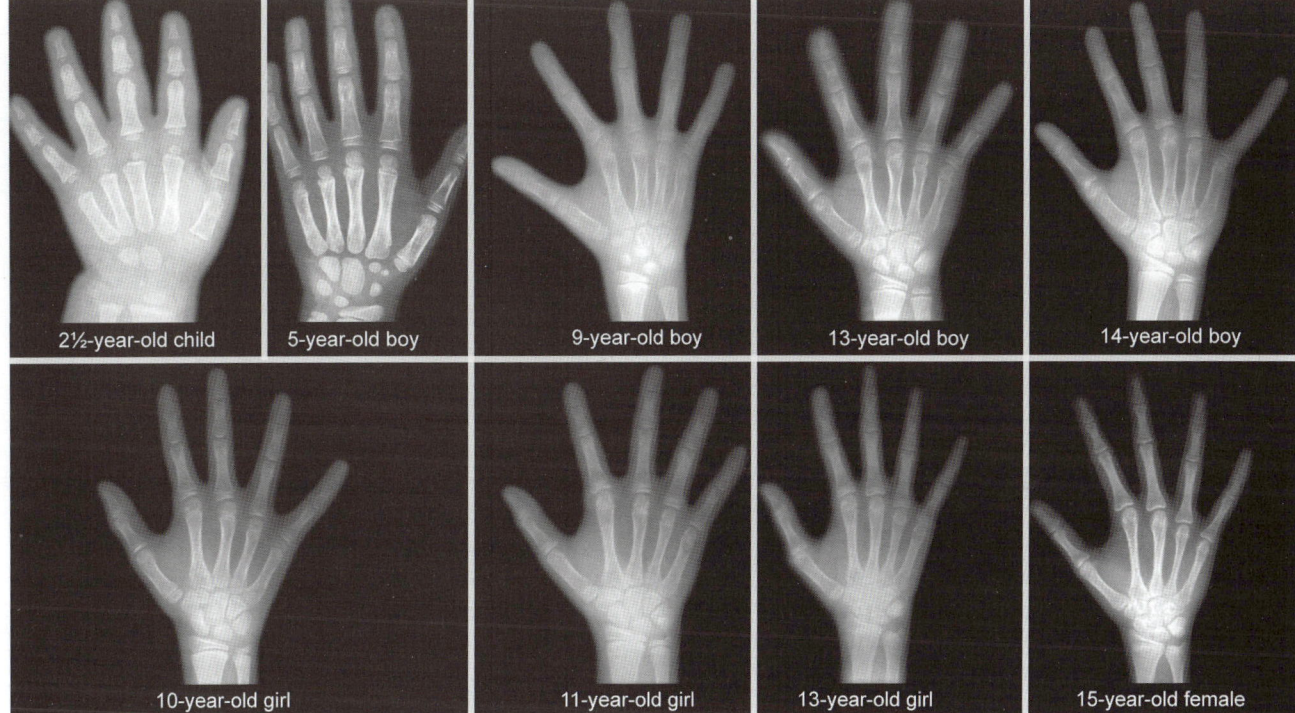

**Fig. 16.4:** Development of numerous small bones of the hand-wrist region occurs throughout the entire postnatal growth period and thus provides a useful means of assessing skeletal maturity

Different ossification centers in hand and wrist appear and mature at different times. The appearance and progression of ossification in various ossification centers follows a predictable and scheduled pattern which can be standardized. A number of methods have been developed to assess skeletal age using hand-wrist radiographs, and some of the commonly used methods are discussed here.
- Greulich and Pyle method
- Bjork, Grave and Brown method
- Fishman's skeletal maturity indicators
- Singer's method
- Hog and Taranger method.

### Greulich and Pyle Method

Greulich and Pyle published an atlas, containing ideal skeletal age pictures of the hand-wrist for different chronological ages of males and females. Each photograph in the atlas is the representative of a particular skeletal age. The skeletal age of a patient is assessed by matching the patient's radiograph on an overall basis with one of the photographs in the atlas.

### Bjork, Grave and Brown Method

Bjork, Grave and Brown divided skeletal development into nine stages **(Fig. 16.5)**. Each of these stages represents a

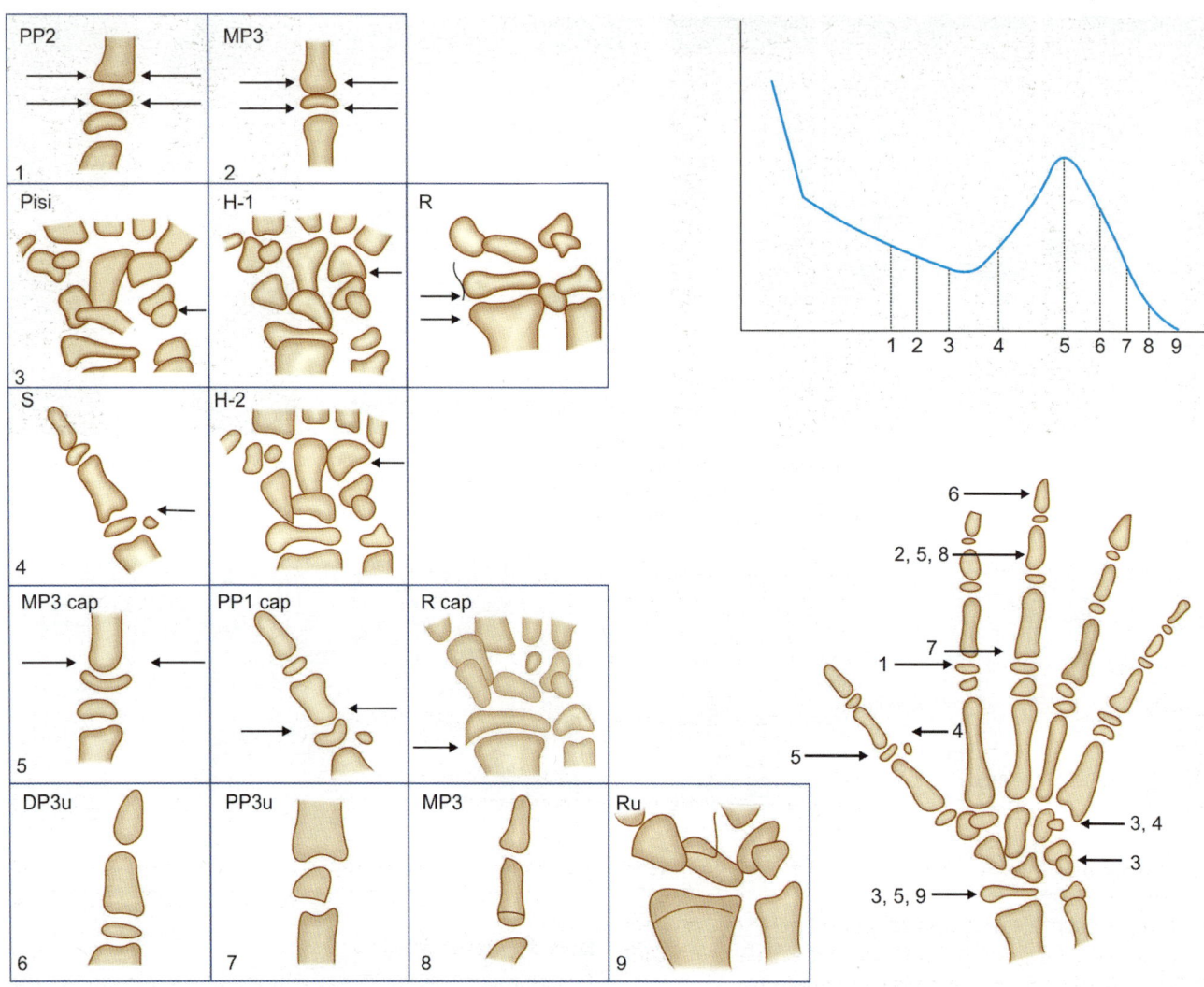

**Fig. 16.5:** Bjork, Grave and Brown method of skeletal maturity assessment using hand-wrist radiographs

level of skeletal maturity **(Table 16.1)**. Later in the year 1978, Schopf gave the appropriate chronological age for each of the stages. Skeletal age is assessed by matching the characteristics of patient's radiograph with any of these stages.

### Fishman's Skeletal Maturity Indicators

Leonard S Fishman in 1982 proposed a system of evaluation for skeletal maturation. Fishman made use of four anatomical sites, located on the thumb, third finger, fifth finger and radius **(Figs 16.6A and B)**. Eleven discrete adolescent skeletal maturity indicators (SMIs) were proposed, which covered the entire period of adolescent development **(Table 16.2)**. **Table 16.3** gives the approximate chronological age and percentage of growth that is completed corresponding to each of the eleven SMIs.

### Interpretation

The Fishman's system of interpretation uses four stages of bone maturation. They are
 i. Epiphysis is equal in width to diaphysis.
 ii. Appearance of adductor sesamoid of the thumb.
 iii. Capping of epiphysis.
 iv. Fusion of epiphysis.

### Singer's Method

A relatively rapid and easier method of skeletal maturity assessment based on hand-wrist radiographs was developed by Julian Singer in 1980. He described six progressive developmental stages of hand-wrist skeleton namely, early, prepubertal, pubertal onset, pubertal, pubertal deceleration and growth completion.

The stages are described as:

### Stage 1 (Early)

- In this stage, the pisiform and the hook of hamate are still absent and epiphysis and proximal phalanx of second finger is narrower than its diaphysis.

### Stage 2 (Prepubertal)

- This stage is characterized by initial ossification of hook of the hamate and that of pisiform. The epiphysis

**Table 16.1:** Bjork, Grave and Brown method of skeletal maturity assessment

| Stage | Male aged (years) | Female aged (years) | Characteristics | Figure |
|---|---|---|---|---|
| 1. | 10.6 | 8.1 | The epiphysis and diaphysis of the proximal phalanx of index finger are equal | Fig. 16.5 (1) PP2 |
| 2. | 12.0 | 8.1 | The epiphysis and diaphysis of the middle phalanx of the middle finger are equal | Fig. 16.5 (2) MP3 |
| 3. | 12.6 | 9.6 | Three areas of ossification:<br>• The hamular process of the hamate exhibit ossifications.<br>• Ossification of pisiform.<br>• The epiphysis and diaphysis of radius are equal. | Fig. 16.5 (3)<br>H-1<br>Pisi<br>R |
| 4. | 13.0 | 10.6 | This stage marks the beginning of the pubertal growth spurt. It is characterized by<br>• Initial mineralization of the ulnar sesamoid of the thumb.<br>• Increased ossification of the gamular process of the hamate bone. | Fig. 16.5 (4)<br>S<br>H-2 |
| 5. | 14.0 | 11.0 | In this stage heralds the peak of the pubertal growth spurt. Capping of diaphysis by the epiphysis is seen in<br>• Middle phalanx of the third finger.<br>• Proximal phalanx of the thumb.<br>• Radius. | Fig. 16.5 (5)<br>MP3 cap<br>PP1 cap<br>R cap |
| 6. | 15.0 | 13.0 | This stage signifies the end of the pubertal growth spurt. It is characterized by union between epiphysis and diaphysis of the distal phalanx of the middle finger. | Fig. 16.5 (6)<br>DP3u |
| 7. | 15.9 | 13.3 | Union of epiphysis and diaphysis of the proximal phalanx of the little finger occurs. | Fig. 16.5 (7)<br>PP3u |
| 8. | 15.9 | 13.9 | This stage shows fusion between the epiphysis and diaphysis of the middle phalanx of the middle finger. | Fig. 16.5 (8)<br>MP3 |
| 9. | 18.5 | 16.0 | This is the last stage and it signifies the end of skeletal growth. It is characterized by fusion of epiphysis and diaphysis of the radius. | Fig. 16.5 (9)<br>Ru |

and diaphysis of the proximal phalanx of second finger become equal.
- It represents the prepubertal period prior to the onset of adolescent growth spurt, during which significant amount of normal growth is still remaining.
- Growth modification procedures are best carried out during this period. For example, skeletal growth class II relationship can be corrected with considerable ease by applying maxillary orthodontic therapy in conjunction with mandibular growth modification.

### Stage 3 (Pubertal Onset)

It is characterized by the beginning of calcification of the sesamoid, increased width of the epiphysis of proximal phalanx of the second fingers and increased calcification of the hamate and pisiform.

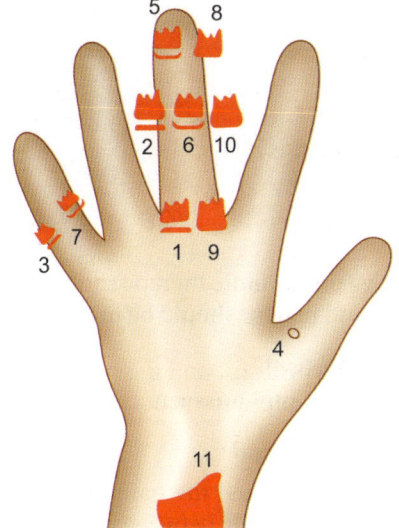
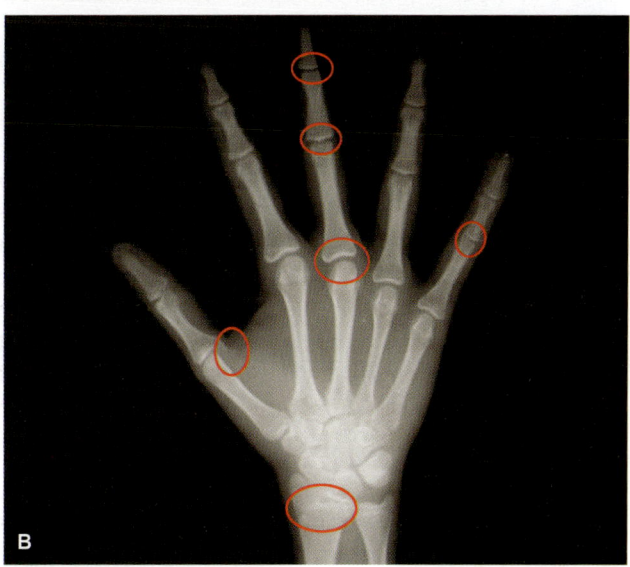

**Figs 16.6A and B:** Fishman's skeletal maturity indicators

**Table 16.2:** Fishman's skeletal maturity indicators

| | |
|---|---|
| SMI 1: | Proximal phalanx of the third finger shows equal widths of epiphysis and diaphysis. |
| SMI 2: | Width of the epiphysis is equal to that of diaphysis in the middle phalanx of the third finger. |
| SMI 3: | Width of the epiphysis is equal to that of diaphysis in the middle phalanx of the fifth finger. |
| SMI 4: | Appearance of the adductor sesamoid of the thumb. |
| SMI 5: | Capping of epiphysis seen in distal phalanx of the third finger. |
| SMI 6: | Capping of epiphysis seen in middle phalanx of the third finger. |
| SMI 7: | Capping of epiphysis in middle phalanx of the fifth finger. |
| SMI 8: | Fusion of epiphysis and diaphysis in the distal phalanx of third finger. |
| SMI 9: | Fusion of epiphysis and diaphysis in the proximal phalanx of third finger. |
| SMI 10: | Fusion of epiphysis and diaphysis in the middle phalanx of third finger. |
| SMI 11: | Fusion of epiphysis and diaphysis seen in the radius. |

**Table 16.3:** Approximate chronological age and percentage of growth completed corresponding to the skeletal maturity indicators

| SMI No. | Age in years | Percentage of adolescent growth completed | % of Max. growth completed | % of Mand. growth completed |
|---|---|---|---|---|
| **Female** | | | | |
| 1 | 9.94+/− 0.96 | | | |
| 2 | 10.58+/− 0.88 | 12.2 | 16.7 | 14.7 |
| 3 | 10.88+/− 0.99 | 22.5 | 18.5 | 25.0 |
| 4 | 11.22 +/−1.11 | 32.7 | 20.3 | 33.1 |
| 5 | 11.64 +/−0.90 | 39.8 | 28.6 | 38.3 |
| 6 | 12.06 +/−0.96 | 51.7 | 49.7 | 47.0 |
| 7 | 12.34 +/−0.90 | 73.6 | 69.0 | 58.0 |
| 8 | 13.10+/− 0.87 | 86.6 | 83.0 | 72.7 |
| 9 | 13.90 +/−0.99 | 91.9 | 89.6 | 84.0 |
| 10 | 14.77+/− 0.96 | 96.1 | 92.7 | 90.0 |
| 11 | 16.07 +/−1.25 | 100% | 100% | 100% |
| **Male** | | | | |
| 1 | 11.01+/−1.22 | | | |
| 2 | 11.68+/− 1.06 | 15 | 16.7 | 15.9 |
| 3 | 12.12+/− 1.00 | 21.6 | 18.5 | 19.5 |
| 4 | 12.33 +/−1.09 | 28.9 | 20.3 | 26.7 |
| 5 | 12.98 +/−1.12 | 34.0 | 28.6 | 30.8 |
| 6 | 13.75+/− 1.06 | 52.6 | 49.7 | 48.5 |
| 7 | 14.38+/− 1.08 | 74.3 | 69.0 | 66.7 |
| 8 | 15.11+/− 1.03 | 87.3 | 83.0 | 77.7 |
| 9 | 15.50+/− 1.07 | 92.0 | 89.6 | 84.6 |
| 10 | 16.40+/− 1.00 | 95.3 | 92.7 | 91.5 |
| 11 | 17.37+/− 1.26 | 100% | 100% | 100% |

*Stage 4 (Pubertal)*
It is characterized by calcification of the sesamoid and capping of the diaphysis of the middle phalanx of third finger by its epiphysis.

*Stage 5 (Pubertal Deceleration)*
This stage is characterized by fully calcified sesamoid, fusion of epiphysis of distal phalanx of third finger with its shaft and epiphyses of radius and ulna not fully fused with their respective shafts.

Ideally, active orthodontic therapy should be completed by this stage and patient should be in retention period.

*Stage 6 (Growth Completion)*
No remaining growth sites are seen.

### Hagg and Taranger Method

Hagg and Taranger analyzed the hand-wrist radiographs of individuals taken annually between the ages of 6 and 18 years and studied the ossification of the following bones:

- Ulnar sesamoid (S)
- Certain specified stages of 3 epiphyseal bones namely,
  - The middle and distal phalanges of the third finger (MP3 and DP3).
  - The distal epiphysis of the radius (R).

### Sesamoid (S)

Sesamoid is usually attained during the acceleration period of the pubertal growth spurt, i.e. at the onset of peak height velocity (PHV).

### Third Finger—Middle Phalanx

#### MP3—F

- The epiphysis is as wide as the metaphysis.
- This is attained before onset of peak height velocity in about 40% of the subjects and at PHV in many others.

#### MP3—FG

- The epiphysis is as wide as the metaphysis and there is distinct medial and/or lateral border of the epiphysis forming a line of demarcation at right angle to the distal border.
- This stage is attained 1 year before or at PHV.

#### MP3—G

- The sides of the epiphysis have thickened and also cap its metaphysis, forming a sharp edge distally at one or both sides.
- This stage is attained at 1 year after PHV.

#### MP3—H

- Fusion of the epiphysis and metaphysis has begun.
- This stage is attained after PHV, but before end of growth spurt by practically all boys and about 90% of the girls.

#### MP3—I

This stage is attained before or at the end of growth spurt in all subjects except in a few girls.

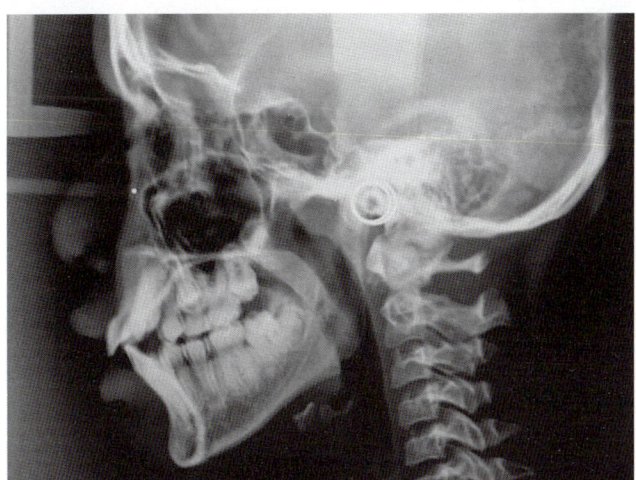

Fig. 16.7: Cervical vertebral maturation method is increasingly being used since cervical vertebrae can be examined on lateral cephalogram, which is used regularly in orthodontic diagnosis, thus precluding the need for an additional radiograph

### Third Finger—Distal Phalanx

#### DP3—I

- Fusion of the epiphysis and metaphysis is completed in distal phalanx of third finger.
- This stage is attained during the deceleration period of the pubertal growth spurt (i.e. end of PHV) by all subject.

### Radius

R—I: Fusion of the epiphysis and metaphysis has begun. This stage is attained 1 year before or at the end of growth spurt in about 80% of females and in about 90% of males.
R—IJ: Fusion is almost complete except for a small gap still remaining at one or both the margins.
R—J: This stage is characterized by the fusion of epiphysis and metaphysis.

## CERVICAL VERTEBRAE-SKELETAL MATURITY INDICATOR

Hand-wrist radiographs have been used conventionally as the standard method of evaluating skeletal maturity. Although accurate, this method necessitates additional radiation exposure to patients. Furthermore, the handwrist site is far removed from the jaw, which is the site of orthodontic correction. In recent years, evaluation of cervical vertebrae has been increasingly used to determine skeletal maturation.

A new system of skeletal maturation assessment using the cervical vertebrae was first developed by Hassel and Farman. A number of subsequent studies have shown significant correlation between developmental or maturational changes occurring in the cervical vertebrae than that of the hand-wrist region.

Cervical vertebrae maturity indicator (CMVI) method is increasingly being used in the recent years instead of the conventional hand-wrist radiograph method. One of the main reasons for the rising popularity of the method is that cervical vertebral maturation can be assessed on lateral cephalograms **(Fig. 16.7)**, which is used regularly in orthodontic diagnosis, thus, precluding the need for an additional radiograph.

In 1972, Lamparski stated that the cervical vertebrae were as statistically and clinically reliable in assessing skeletal age as the hand-wrist technique. Several authors (San-Roman et al. 2002) have reported a high correlation between cervical vertebrae maturation and skeletal maturation of the hand-wrist. It has been found that cervical vertebrae could offer an alternative method for assessing maturity without the need of hand-wrist radiographs and thus, decreasing patient's radiation exposure.

Most methods of cervical vertebral maturation are based on morphologic changes that occur in cervical vertebral bodies as growth progresses. Hassel and Farman developed a method of skeletal maturation assessment using cervical vertebrae in which there are six stages of development **(Fig. 16.8)**. They take into account the

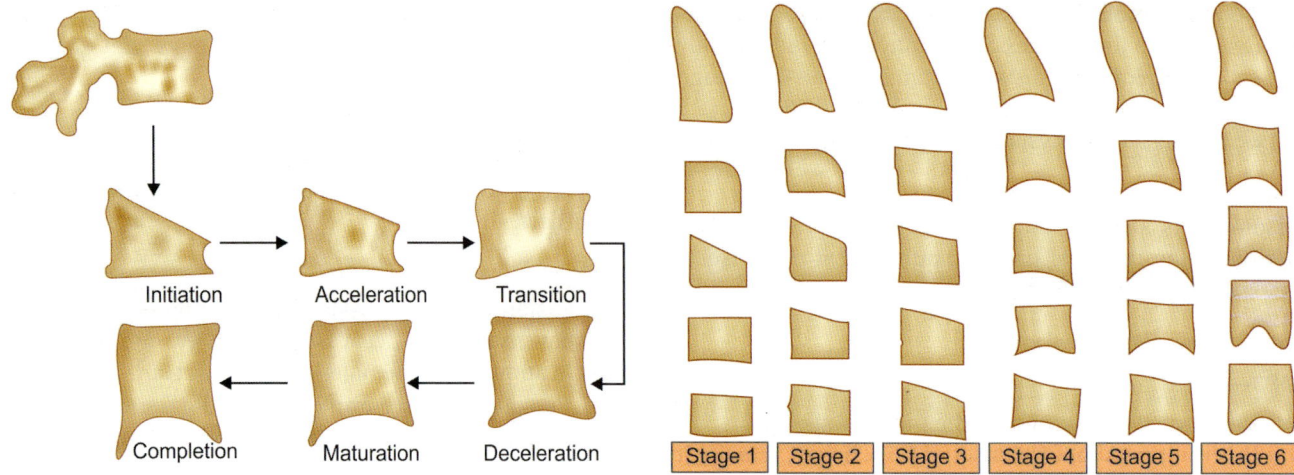

**Fig. 16.8:** Stages of development and maturation of cervical vertebrae

**Fig. 16.9:** Assessment of skeletal maturity using cervical vertebrae

morphologic characteristics of the cervical (C2, C3 and C4) vertebrae, such as:
- Shape of the vertebral bodies
- Height of the vertebral bodies
- Concavity of the lower border of the cervical bodies.

The changes in the shape of cervical vertebral bodies of C3 and C4 at each level of skeletal development are assessed **(Fig. 16.9)**.

- At first they are wedge-shaped, then changed to rectangular, next to square-shaped.
- The vertical dimensions of the cervical vertebral bodies increase with increased skeletal maturity.
- It is also observed that, the inferior borders of the cervical vertebral bodies which are flat at the beginning become concave as they mature.

**Table 16.4:** Assessment of skeletal maturity using cervical vertebrae

| Stage | Name | Changes in vertebrae |
|---|---|---|
| Stage 1 | Initiation | <ul><li>Marks the beginning of adolescent growth.</li><li>The cervical vertebral bodies and C2, C3 and C4 are wedge-shaped with their superior borders tapering posteroanteriorly.</li><li>Their inferior borders are flat.</li><li>80–95% of pubertal growth is remaining.</li></ul> |
| Stage 2 | Acceleration | <ul><li>Acceleration of growth occurs.</li><li>Concavities are developing on the lower borders of C2 and C3.</li><li>Lower border of C4 vertebral body is flat.</li><li>C3 and C4 assume rectangular shape.</li><li>65–85% of pubertal growth remains.</li></ul> |
| Stage 3 | Transition | <ul><li>Growth is accelerated to reach peak height velocity.</li><li>Distinct concavity seen in lower borders of C2 and C3.</li><li>Concavity is developing in the lower borders of C4.</li><li>C3 and C4 are more rectangular in shape.</li><li>25–65% pubertal growth is remaining.</li></ul> |
| Stage 4 | Deceleration | <ul><li>Deceleration of adolescent growth spurt begins.</li><li>Distinct concavities seen at the lower borders of all three vertebrae, that is, C2, C3 and C4.</li><li>C3 and C4 are nearly square in shape.</li><li>10–25% of pubertal growth is remaining.</li></ul> |
| Stage 5 | Maturation | <ul><li>Cervical vertebrae attain maturity.</li><li>Concavities at lower borders of C2, C3 and C4 become more accentuated.</li><li>C3 and C4 are more square in shape.</li><li>5–10% pubertal growth remaining.</li></ul> |
| Stage 6 | Completion | <ul><li>Adolescent growth is nearly complete.</li><li>More accentuated concavities are seen at lower borders of C2, C3 and C4.</li><li>Shape of C3 and C4 is square with greater vertical dimension than width.</li><li>Pubertal growth is complete with no more growth potential remaining.</li></ul> |

- The concavity of the inferior vertebral borders is seen to appear sequentially from C2 to C3 and then to C4 as the skeleton matures.

Depending on these changes observed in C2, C3 and C4 cervical vertebrae, Hassel and Farman gave 6 stages of development depicted in **Table 16.4.**

## BIBLIOGRAPHY

1. Anderson DL, Thompson GW, Popovich F. Interrelationship of dental maturity, skeletal maturity, height and weight from age 4 to 14 years. Growth. 1975;39:453-62.
2. Bowden BD. Epiphyseal changes in the hand-wrist area as an indicators of adolescent. Am J Orthod. 1976;4:87-104.
3. Demirjian, Buschang, Tanguay, a and Patters: Interrelationship among measures of somatic, skeletal, dental, and sexual maturity. Am J Orthod. 1985; vol 433-8.
4. Fishman LS. Radiographic evaluation of skeletal maturity. Angle Orthod. 1982;52:88-112.
5. Grave KC, Brown T. Skeletal ossification and adolescent growth spurt. Am J Orthod. 1976;69:611-9.
6. Hassel and Farman: Skeletal maturation evaluation. Am J Orthod. 1995;58-66.
7. Houston WJB, Miller JC, Tanner JM. Prediction of the timing of the adolescent growth spurt from ossification. Events in hand-wrist films. Brit J Orthod. 1979;6:145-52.
8. Moore, Moyer, BuBOis. Skeletal maturation and craniofacial growth. Am J Orthod. 1990;98:33-40.
9. Rassouw, Lombard, Harris. Frontal sinus and mandibular growth prediction. Am J Orthod. 1991;542-6.
10. Revelo, Fishman. Evaluation of ossification of midpalatal suture. Am J Orthod Dentofacial Orthop. 1994;105:288-92.

## EXAM-ORIENTED QUESTIONS

*Long Essay or Long Questions*

1. Enumerate various methods available to assess skeletal maturity of an individual and its implication in orthodontic diagnosis and treatment planning. Explain in detail about hand wrist radiographs.

*Short Notes*

1. Hand – wrist radiography or How hand –wrist radiographs are useful in orthodontic diagnosis and treatment planning.
2. Compare skeletal age and dental age
3. Cervical vertebrae as skeletal maturity indicators.

# CHAPTER 17
# Biology of Tooth Movement

*Phulari BS, Shah A*

Tooth movement can be induced orthodontically because of the gomphosis type of attachment of teeth where the teeth are suspended in their sockets by periodontal ligament rather than being ankylosed to the bone. By applying properly regulated forces, the teeth can be moved through the alveolar bone of jaws without causing permanent damage to either the teeth or their investing tissues. Despite a lot of research on the subject, the detailed biological mechanisms of orthodontic tooth movement are far from being completely understood.

While certain tooth movements occur naturally (physiologic tooth movement), teeth also exhibit movement in some pathologic conditions (pathologic tooth movement). In orthodontics, tooth movement is induced for therapeutic purposes. The tooth movement can be:
- Physiologic
- Pathologic
- Orthodontic.

Before proceeding further, a brief review of various physiologic tooth movements is given below which can aid in the understanding of the biologic changes that occur during orthodontic tooth movement.

## PHYSIOLOGIC TOOTH MOVEMENT

Physiologic tooth movement can be described in three phases:
1. Pre-eruptive tooth movement
2. Eruptive tooth movement
3. Posteruptive tooth movement.

### Pre-eruptive Tooth Movement

Both primary and permanent tooth germs move within the jaws after their differentiation and these movements are facilitated by the jaw growth. These movements help the teeth to occupy their preparatory positions within the jaws prior to their eruption.

### Eruptive Tooth Movement

Eruption is the movement of the teeth from their developmental position within the jaws to their functional position in occlusion. Eruptive movement generally begins when about 2/3rd portion of the root is formed and is primarily brought about by the periodontal ligament traction.

#### Mechanisms of Tooth Eruption
- Tooth eruption is the result of a number of factors, and many theories have been proposed to explain the mechanism of tooth eruption, including *bone remodeling, root formation, vascular pressure and periodontal ligament traction theories*.
- Periodontal ligament traction theory is the most accepted one and a lot of evidences suggest that the eruptive movement is brought about by the d*ental follicle—periodontal ligament complex*.
- The contractile force exerted by the periodontal ligament fibroblasts is transmitted to the properly oriented collagen fibers bundles. Summation of these contractile forces causes the tooth movement. Bone remodeling necessary for forming the eruptive pathway is facilitated by the cells of dental follicle.

### Posteruptive Tooth Movement

Even after the eruption is complete, the teeth move in order to maintain their position in occlusion until the jaw growth is completed. The teeth also exhibit movements in occlusal and mesial direction throughout a person's life to compensate for occlusal and proximal wear. Continuous deposition of cementum around the apices of the roots of teeth is believed to be sufficient to compensate for occlusal wear.

## HISTOLOGICAL CHANGES OCCURRING DURING ORTHODONTIC TOOTH MOVEMENT

A number of investigations have been carried out to know the tissue reactions to forces on the teeth. Sandstedt (1904) was probably the first to investigate the phenomenon of tooth movement by histological examination of the supporting structures. He studied the histological changes in supporting structures by using orthodontic appliances on dogs. Other investigators who have made major contributions in this area are Oppenheim (1911), Schwarz (1932), Reitan (1951), Baumrind (1960), and Buck and Church (1972) among others.

Major conclusions of these studies suggest that when a force is applied to the crown of a tooth, it is transmitted through the root of the tooth to the periodontal ligament and alveolar bone. According to the direction of the force, there will be areas of pressure and areas of tension on these supporting structures. For a tooth to move, there must be the resorption of alveolar bone in response to this stress, and at the same time, there must also be the deposition of bone in the areas of tension so as to maintain the integrity of tooth attachment. As a result of this bone remodeling, the socket of the tooth moves concomitant with movement of the tooth through the alveolar bone.

The histological changes occurring during tooth movement vary according to the magnitude and duration

**Flowchart 17.1:** Changes following application of mild force

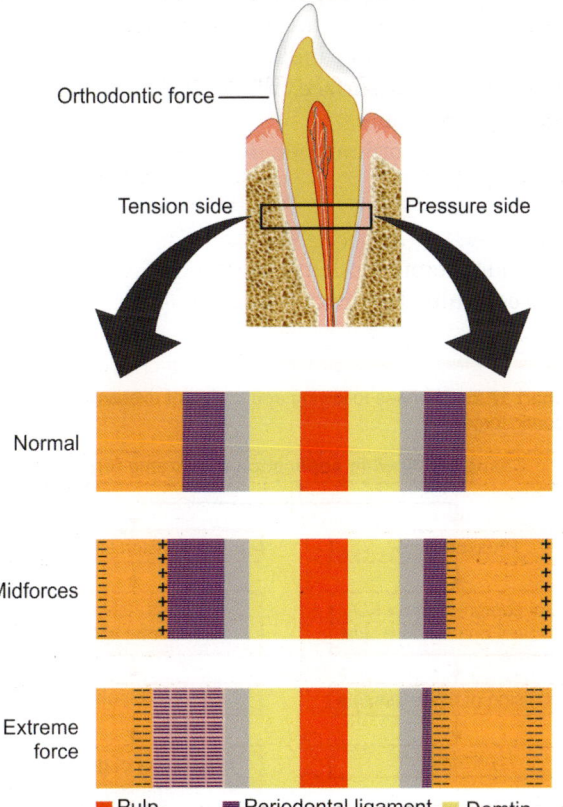

**Fig. 17.1:** The histological changes occurring during tooth movement vary according to the magnitude and duration of the force applied

of the force applied **(Fig. 17.1)**. The histological changes occurring during tooth movement can be described under the following headings:
- Changes following application of mild orthodontic forces.
- Changes following application of excessive orthodontic forces.

## Changes Following Application of Mild Orthodontic Forces

Whenever a force is applied to a tooth, areas of pressure and tension are created. The following changes occur on pressure and tension areas of the periodontal ligament **(Flowchart 17.1)**:

### Changes on Pressure Side

Periodontal ligament gets slightly compressed on the pressure side. As the mild forces are not sufficient to occlude the blood vessels of the periodontal ligament, vessels may dilate and there will be recruitment of osteoclasts to that area of periodontal ligament. The osteoclasts will cause resorption of the alveolar bone immediately adjacent to the periodontal ligament. This kind of resorption where the periosteal bone from the inner wall of the socket is resorbed is called as *frontal resorption* or *direct periosteal/ frontal resorption* **(Fig. 17.2A)**. There is no resorption of the tooth root.

### Changes on Tension Side

An area of tension is created in the supporting structure of the tooth, opposite to the direction of force. The periodontal ligament is stretched in this area and vascularity is increased. Increased vascularity leads to mobilization of osteoblasts and fibroblasts in those areas. The osteoblasts lay down a layer of osteoid bone immediately adjacent to the lamina dura, which gets matured over a period of time. In this way, the socket, as well as the tooth move due to osteoclastic and osteoblastic activity on the pressure and tension areas, respectively.

In summary, on application of mild orthodontic forces:
- Hyperemia within the periodontal ligament, dilatation of the blood vessels.
- Increased number of oteoclasts and osteoblasts.
- Lamina dura resorbed from the area next to periodontal ligament on pressure side—frontal/ Direct resorption.
- Deposition of osteoid bone on the tension side, which calcifies subsequently.
- Tooth movement occurs due to bone resorption and deposition.
- No root resorption.

## Changes Following Application of Excessive Orthodontic Forces

Although it might appear logical to think that heavier forces can bring about faster tooth movement, it is not true as explained in **Flowchart 17.2**.

### Changes on Pressure Side

On applying excessive forces, the periodontal ligament on pressure side is extremely compressed/crushed, possibly causing contact between the tooth and the alveolar bone. This leads to occlusion of blood vessels in that area. As a result, the periodontal ligament in these areas gets deprived of nutritional supply and begins to show regressive changes with cell free areas called *hyalinization*. Due to ischemia and hyalinization, there is no recruitment of osteoclasts in the pressure side. No resorption occurs on the periosteal surface of the socket, i.e., no frontal resorption and thus tooth does not move for a period of time.

After a lag period, bone resorption occurs in the adjacent marrow spaces under the hyalinized areas. Such endosteal resorption is termed as *undermining indirect* or *rearward resorption* (**Fig. 17.2B**).

If the forces are grossly excessive, resorption of the root surfaces may also occur. Nonvitality and ankylosis of the tooth are other possible consequences of extreme orthodontic forces.

### Changes on Tension Side

Periodontal ligament on the tension side gets overstretched leading to tearing of blood vessels and ischemia. When excessive force is applied, there is an increased osteoclastic activity as compared to osteoblastic activity and thus the tooth may become loosened in its socket.

Thus, if the force applied is severely excessive and prolonged, the periodontal ligament in the area of pressure will be deprived of its blood supply and there may be necrosis of the ligament, with massive underlining resorption and possibly resorption of the root surface of the tooth. Application of very heavy orthodontic forces cause pain, loosening of the tooth in its socket and healing may occur by ankylosis of the tooth to the alveolar bone.

To summarize, on applying excessive orthodontic forces:
- Compression of periodontal ligament and occlusion of blood vessels in the areas of pressure and ischemia.
- Formation of wide zones of hyalinization and extended lag period.
- No frontal resorption and no immediate tooth movement.
- Increased endosteal vascularity and endosteal resorption of the socket wall under the hyalinized area—undermining/rearward resorption.
- Eventually tooth moves as a result of this undermining resorption.
- Relatively rapid tooth movement with bone deposition in the areas of tension.
- Grossly excessive forces may cause root resorption, loosening, nonvitality and ankylosis of the tooth.

### Secondary Bone Remodeling

In addition to changes in the socket wall, bone changes also occur elsewhere. These changes are called as secondary bone remodeling. It involves the addition of bone to the endosteal surface beneath the areas of pressure and the resorption of bone from the endosteal surface beneath the areas of tension. These compensatory bone changes are necessary to maintain the thickness of the supporting alveolar process (**Figs 17.3A and B**).

### What is Optimum Orthodontic Force?

Having understood that heavy forces do not necessarily bring about faster tooth movement, it is important to know what is the optimum orthodontic force. The optimum orthodontic force is the one, which moves teeth most rapidly in the desired direction, with the least possible damage to tissues and with minimum patient discomfort.

From a series of experiments, Oppenheinm and Schwarz concluded that the optimum force for tooth movement was one that induced a pressure of around 20–26 g/cm$^2$ of root surface, which is equivalent to the capillary pulse pressure.

The optimum orthodontic force has the following characteristics:

### Clinically

- It produces rapid tooth movement.
- Causes minimal patient discomfort.

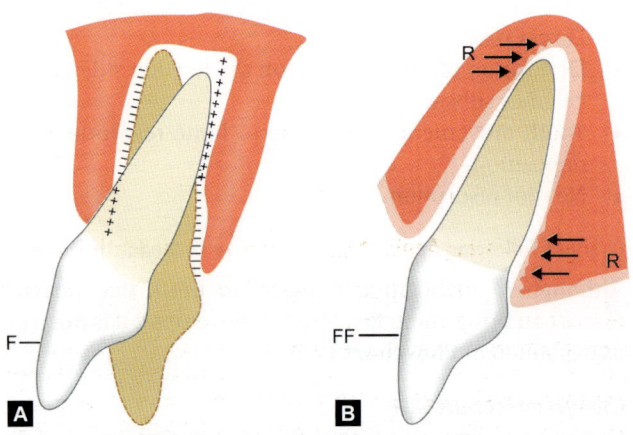

**Figs 17.2 A and B:** (A) Frontal resorption; (B) undermining/indirect resorption

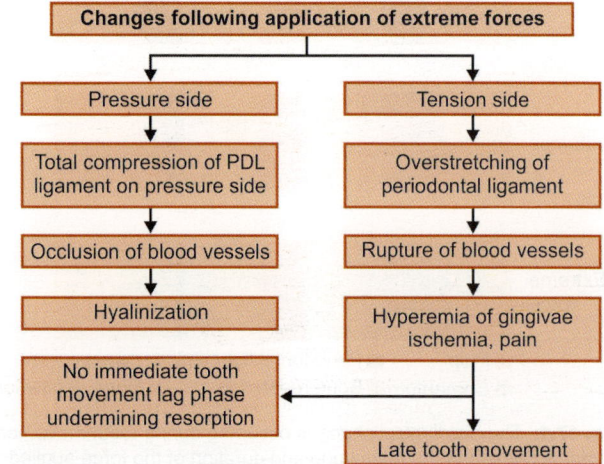

**Flowchart 17.2:** Changes following application of excessive orthodontic forces.

- Lag phase of tooth movement is shorter.
- The tooth being moved does not become loosened in its socket.

*Histologically*
- Vitality of tooth and periodontal ligament is maintained.
- Initiates maximum cellular response.
- Produces direct or frontal resorption.
- Integrity of periodontal attachment is maintained by reorganization of the fibers.

## Hyalinization

Hyalinization is a type of tissue degeneration characterized by formation of a clear, eosinophilic homogeneous substance, which is free of cellular elements. The amount and site of hyalinized zones varies in different types of tooth movement and depends on the magnitude of force applied **(Flowchart 17.3) (Figs 17.4A to C)**.

Some amount of hyalinization of periodontal ligament on the pressure side occurs inevitably in almost all forms of orthodontic tooth movement. However, area of hyalinization can be minimized by using mild continuous forces. Wider areas of hyalinization occur with extreme forces.

Hyalinized areas of periodontal ligament become nonfunctional and frontal resorption cannot occur as there are no viable cells in the area. Further tooth movement cannot occur until the local hyalinized tissue gets removed and the adjacent alveolar bone areas are resorbed.

The hyalinized tissue is eliminated by the following mechanism:
- Resorption of the alveolar bone by the osteoclasts differentiating in the peripheral intact periodontal ligament and in the adjacent marrow spaces.
- The osteoclast cells from the periphery invade the necrotic tissue. The invading cells penetrate the hyalinized tissue and eliminate unwanted fibrous tissue by enzymatic action and phagocytosis.

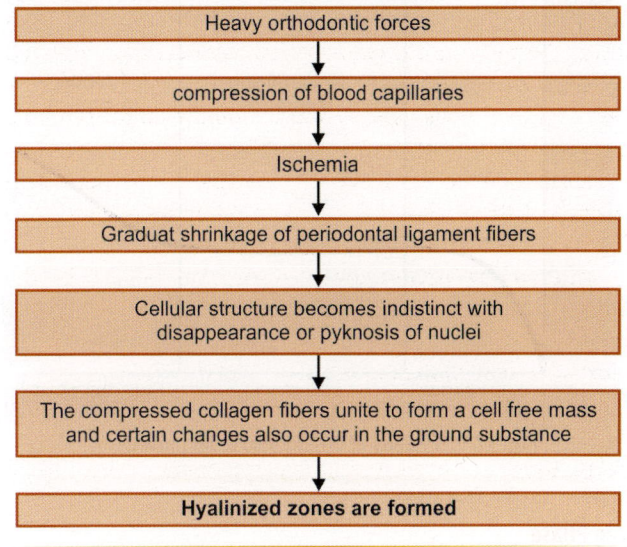

**Flowchart 17.3:** Formation of hyalinized areas

## PHASES OF TOOTH MOVEMENT

Investigations have shown that orthodontic tooth movement occurs in three stages **(Fig. 17.5)**:
1. Initial phase
2. Lag phase
3. Post lag phase.

### Initial Phase

When orthodontic therapy is begun, a rapid tooth movement occurs for a short distance, which then stops. The extent of tooth movement in this initial phase appears to be the same for both light and heavy forces. Tooth movement, occurring in initial phase, is perhaps caused by the displacement of the tooth in periodontal ligament space and also by bending of alveolar bone to some extent. Usually, an initial tooth movement of 0.4–0.9 mm occurs in a week's time.

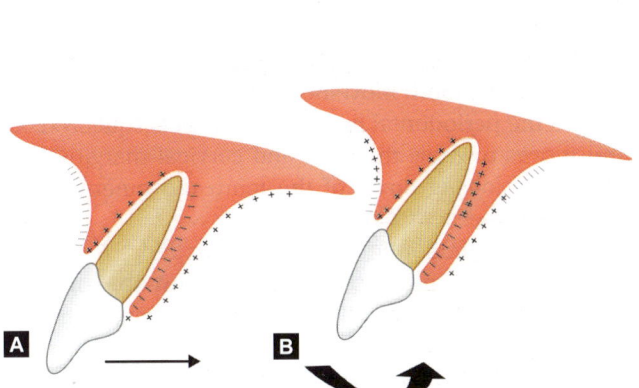

**Figs 17.3A and B:** Secondary bone remodeling changes (A) During bodily movement; (B) During tipping movement

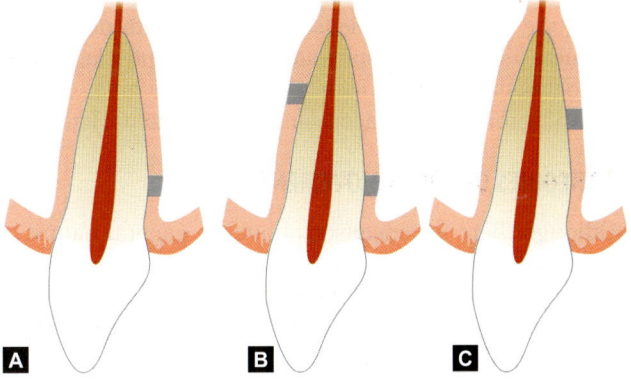

**Figs 17.4A to C:** Areas of hyalinization during tooth movement. (A) During tipping movement, hyalinization zone is close to the alveolar crest; (B) Tipping with excessive force results in two areas of hyalinization, one near the alveolar crest and the other near apical region; (C) In bodily tooth movement, hyalinization zone is near the middle third of the root

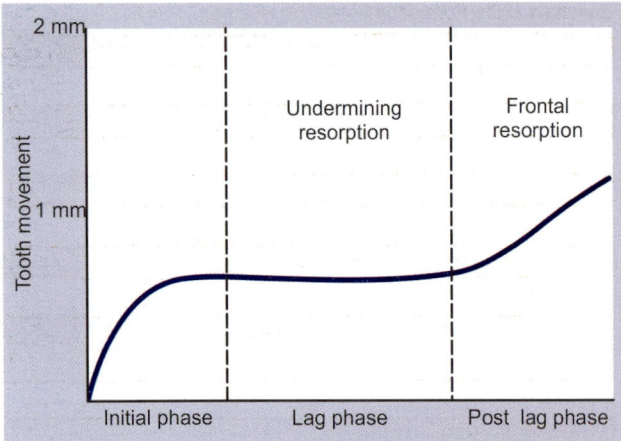

**Fig. 17.5:** Phases of orthodontic tooth movement

### Lag Phase

Following the initial phase, there is a lag period in which there is a little or no tooth movement. Lag phase occurs due to the formation of hyalinization tissue in the periodontal ligament, which has to be eliminated before tooth movement can progress further.

The duration of lag period varies in different types of tooth movement and depends on the amount of force applied. When light forces are applied, the area of hyalinization is small and frontal resorption occurs, whereas larger area of hyalinization occurs with heavy orthodontic forces. Generally, a lag period of 2–3 weeks is seen although it can extend for longer periods.

A number of factors determine the duration of lag phase including the following:
- Amount of force
- Duration of force
- Type of tooth movement and type of tooth
- Density of alveolar bone
- Age of the patient
- Extent of hyalinization.

### Post Lag Phase

Since the hyalinized tissue is eliminated, tooth movement can now progress in a rapid rate. During the post lag phase, osteoclasts are formed over a large surface area, directly resorbing the bone surface facing the periodontal ligament.

## THEORIES OF TOOTH MOVEMENT

Although there is consensus about the general nature of the cellular reactions to force on the teeth which result in bone resorption and deposition by osteoblastic and osteoclastic activities, there are different opinions about the intermediary causes of these cellular reactions. Various theories have been proposed over the years to explain the mechanism of orthodontic tooth movement among which the following are widely followed.
- Pressure/tension theory by Schwartz
- Blood flow theory by Bien
- Bone bending/Piezoelectricity by Picton, Cochran and Grimm
- Mechanochemical theory by Justus and Luft.

### Pressure/Tension Theory: Schwartz (1932)

Although Sandstedt (1904) and Oppenheim (1911) investigated the phenomenon of tooth movement by histological examination of the supporting structure, Schwartz is credited with pressure/tension theory which has been widely accepted.

According to this theory, areas of pressure and tension are created whenever a tooth is subjected to orthodontic force. The area of the periodontium in the direction of force is under pressure while the area of periodontium opposite to the direction of force is under tension. Bone resorption occurs in the areas of pressure, while new bone is deposited in areas of tension. This bone remodeling effects the movement of tooth along with its socket **(Figs 17.1 and 17.2)**.

### Blood Flow Theory/Fluid Dynamic Theory: Bien (1966)

According to this theory, tooth movement occurs as a result of alterations in fluid dynamics in the periodontal ligament space, a confined environment which is limited on either side by hard tissues that are cementum on one side and alveolar socket wall on the other. Thus, passage of fluid in and out of this confined space is limited.

It is suggested that the ligament should be considered as a continuous hydrostatic system made of:
- Blood vessels
- Interstitial fluid
- Cellular elements
- Viscous ground substance.

Because of this confined nature of the contents of periodontal ligament space, a unique hydrodynamic condition resembling a hydraulic mechanism is created.

When a force of shorter duration as in mastication is applied to the tooth, the fluid in periodontal ligament escapes through tiny vascular channels. The fluid gets replenished by diffusion from capillary walls and recirculation of the interstitial fluid as soon as the force is removed.

However, when a force of longer duration as in the case of orthodontic tooth movement is applied, the interstitial fluid in the periodontal ligament space gets squeezed out and moves towards the apex and cervical margins. This results in slowing down of the tooth movement and is called as "*squeeze film effect*" by Bien.

When orthodontic force is applied, it causes compression of periodontal ligament on the pressure side. The blood vessels of the periodontal ligament gets compressed between the principal fibers of the ligament and results in their stenosis. The blood vessels beyond the area of stenosis balloon up forming "*aneurysms.*"

The formation of aneurysms causes the blood gases to escape into the interstitial fluid, thereby creating a favorable local environment for resorption. Bien suggested

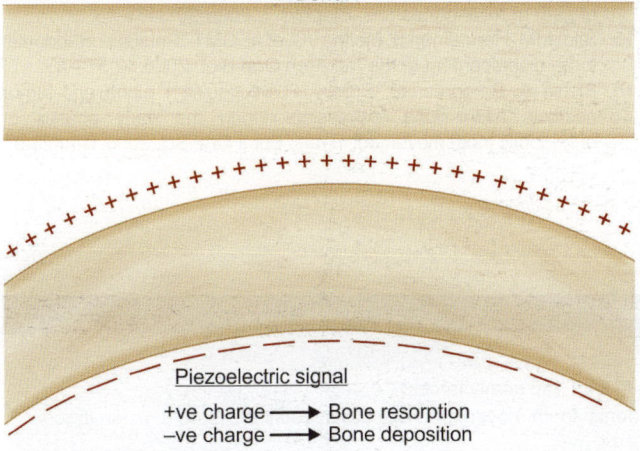

**Fig. 17.6:** Piezoelectric theory of tooth movement: When a force is applied to tooth, the distorted adjacent alveolar bone forms areas of concavity and convexity. Bone deposition occurs in the areas of concavity, which is negatively charged. Areas of convexity become positively charged and bone resorption occurs

that the chemical environment at the side of the vascular stenosis is altered due to a decreased oxygen level in the compressed areas. Such an environment with decreased level of oxygen is favorable for bone resorption.

### Bone Bending or Piezoelectric Theory

Picton (1965), Cochran (1967) and Grimm (1972) among others suggested that the effects of physical distortion of the alveolar bone by the forces from orthodontic appliance may be responsible for the cellular reactions observed during tooth movement.

When orthodontic force is applied to teeth, it causes deformation or bending of the alveolar bone. It has been shown that bone, which is deformed by stress becomes electrically charged and exhibits a phenomenon called piezoelectricity.

When a force is applied to tooth, the distorted adjacent alveolar bone forms areas of concavity and convexity. Bone deposition occurs in the areas of concavity, which is negatively charged. Areas of convexity become positively charged and bone resorpion occurs **(Fig. 17.6)**.

Many crystalline substances exhibit piezoelectricity, a phenomenon in which deformation of the crystal structure produces a flow of current as a result of displacement of electrons from one part of the crystal lattice to the other. Both hydroxyapatite and collagen fibers present in bone are crystalline materials with piezoelectricity. Furthermore, the collagen–hydroxyapatite interface and mucopolysaccharide present in the ground substance can also cause generation of electric current.

Thus, possible sources of piezoelectricity in alveolar bone are:
- Hydroxyapatite crystals
- Collagen fibers
- Collagen–hydroxyapatite interface
- Mucopolysaccharide of ground substance.

Piezoelectricity is characterized by two unique properties: Quick decay rate and reverse piezoelectricity.

### Quick Decay Rate

When forces are applied to teeth, crystalline substance of bone gets deformed and electric charges are produced as a result of migration of electrons from one location to another. As long as the force is maintained, the crystal structure is stable and no further electric effect is observed. In other words, when a force is applied piezoelectricity is generated which immediately goes to zero level, even if the force is continuously applied. This property is known as quick decay rate.

### Reverse Piezoelectricity (Production of Equivalent Current but in Opposite Direction when Force is Released)

However, when the force is released, a reverse flow of electrons occurs as the crystals return to their original shape.

### Mechanochemical Theory: Justus and Luft (1970)

Mechanochemical theory was put forward by Justus and Luft in the year 1970. According to this theory, application of physical stress to the bones changes the solubility of the hydroxyapatite crystals. Change in solubility of the hydroxyapatite results in remodeling of bone. This theory is not widely accepted.

### BIBLIOGRAPHY

1. Adachi T, Sato K, Tomita Y. Directional dependence of osteoblastic calcium response to mechanical stimuli. Biomech Model Mechanobiol. 2003;2:73-82.
2. Ajubi NE, Klein-Nulend J, Alblas MJ, et al. Signal transduction pathways involved in fluid flow-induced PGE2 production by cultured osteocytes. Am J Physiol. 1999;276:171-8.
3. Alhashimi N, Frithiof L, Brudvik P, et al. Orthodontic tooth movement and de novo synthesis of proinflammatory cytokines. Am J Orthod Dentofacial Orthop. 2001;119:307-12.
4. Anderson DM, Maraskovsky E, Billingsley WL, et al. A homologue of the TNF receptor and its ligand enhance T-cell growth and dendritic-cell function. Nature. 1997;390:175-9.
5. Apajalahti S, Sorsa T, Railavo S, et al. The in vivo levels of matrix metalloproteinase-1 and -8 in gingival crevicular fluid during initial orthodontic tooth movement. J Dent Res. 2003;82:1018-22.
6. Arai F, Miyamoto T, Ohneda O, et al. Commitment and differentiation of osteoclast precursor cells by the sequential expression of c-Fms and receptor activator of nuclear factor kappaB (RANK) receptors. J Exp Med. 1999;190:1741-54.
7. Arnoczky SP, Tian T, Lavagnino M, et al. Ex vivo static tensile loading inhibits MMP-1 expression in rat tail tendon cells through a cytoskeletally based mechanotransduction mechanism. J Orthop Res. 2004;22:328-33.
8. Bakker A, Klein-Nulend J, Burger E. Shear stress inhibits while disuse promotes osteocyte apoptosis. Biochem Biophys Res Commun. 2004;320:1163-8.
9. Bakker AD, Soejima K, Klein-Nulend J, et al. The production of nitric oxide and prostaglandin E(2) by primary bone cells is shear stress dependent. J Biomech. 2001;34:671-7.
10. Bartlett JD, Zhou Z, Skobe Z, et al. Delayed tooth eruption in membrane type-1 matrix metalloproteinase deficient mice. Connect Tissue Res. 2003;44(Suppl 1):300-4.

11. Basaran G, Ozer T, Kaya FA, et al. Interleukins 2, 6 and 8 levels in human gingival sulcus during orthodontic treatment. Am J Orthod Dentofacial Orthop. 2006;130:1-6.
12. Beertsen W, Holmbeck K, Niehof A, et al. On the role of MT1-MMP, a matrix metalloproteinase essential to collagen remodeling, in murine molar eruption and root growth. Eur J Oral Sci. 2002;110:445-51.
13. Berkovitz BK, Thomas NR. Unimpeded eruption in the root-resected lower incisor of the rat with a preliminary note on root transection. Arch Oral Biol. 1969;14:771-80.
14. Besser A, Safran SA. Force-induced adsorption and anisotropic growth of focal adhesions. Biophys J. 2006;90:3469-84.
15. Bildt MM, Henneman S, Maltha JC, et al. CMT-3 inhibits orthodontic tooth displacement in the rat. Arch Oral Biol. 2006;52:571-8.
16. Bletsa A, Berggreen E, Brudvik P. Interleukin-1 alpha and tumor necrosis factor-alpha expression during the early phases of orthodontic tooth movement in rats. Eur J Oral Sci. 2006;114:423-9.

## EXAM-ORIENTED QUESTIONS

### Long Essay or Long Questions
1. Define optimal orthodontic force. Discuss tissue changes subsequent to light and heavy forces.
2. What are the various theories that are involved in the biology of orthodontic tooth movement? Discuss in detail pressure–tension theory.
3. What are different types of tooth movement?

### Short Notes
1. Explain frontal resorption
2. Response of bone and periodontium to orthodontic force at tension zone
3. Undermining resorption
4. Enumerate various phases of tooth movements
5. Piezoelectric theory.

## CHAPTER OVERVIEW

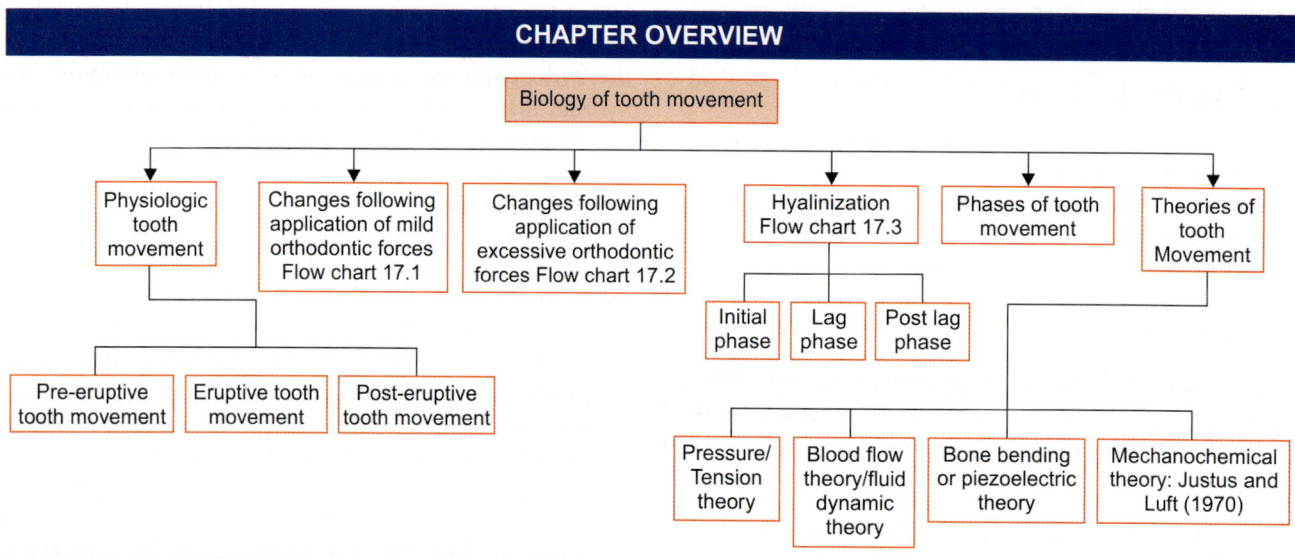

# CHAPTER 18

# Mechanics of Tooth Movement

*Shah A, Phulari BS*

Mechanics is the science that describes the effect of force on a body. In the context of orthodontics, tooth movement occurs as a response to application of a force. An understanding and proper application of the biomechanical principles enables efficient tooth movement in the shortest possible duration and with minimal tissue damage.

Sound knowledge of the fundamental principles of biomechanics is necessary:
- To understand the design of an appliance
- To know its mode of action
- To understand the response of tooth and other structures to application of force
- To select the appliance appropriate for a given case
- To use the selected appliance in an efficient manner to bring about the desired changes.

Before proceeding further, some of the terminologies used in mechanics and their implication in the field of orthodontics must be considered.

The following terms are described for the ease of explanation of the subject:
- Force
- Moment
- Couple.

## FORCE

Force can be defined as load applied to an object that will tend to move it to a different position in the space. Although force is generally expressed in unit of Newtons (N), in orthodontics, forces have been commonly expressed in grams (g).

Force is a vector having both direction and magnitude. In clinical terms, the direction may be:
- Pull (towards the source of force) or
- Push (away from the source of force).

The magnitude may be:
- Light or
- Heavy.

The point of application of force is also important for understanding tooth movements.
Theoretically, point of application of force can be at:
- Center of mass
- Center of gravity
- Center of resistance.

### Center of Mass and Gravity

A free body in space has a point in its mass, which behaves as if the whole mass is concentrated at that single point. This point is termed as center of mass in a gravity-free environment (**Fig. 18.1**).

The same is called "center of gravity" in an environment where gravity is present. Any force that is directed through this center of mass in any direction causes all points in the body to move to the same amount in the same direction as the line of force. When all points on a body (a tooth in the context of orthodontics)—move the same amount in the same direction, such a movement is called as "translation or bodily movement."

### Center of Resistance

A tooth in the oral cavity, however, is not a free body because of its supporting tissues, which would restrain its movement. Hence, tooth in the oral cavity has a point analogous to the center of mass called as "center of resistance."

The center of resistance is a point at which the resistance to tooth movement is concentrated. **Figs 18.2A to C** shows the approximate location of the center of resistance of a single tooth. Single tooth, units of teeth, complete dental arches and the jaws themselves have center(s) of resistance. The approximate location of the center of resistance for two-tooth unit is shown in **Fig. 18.3**. Studies show that the center of resistance for maxilla is about 5-10 mm inferior to the orbitale (**Fig. 18.4**).

Location of the center of resistance of a tooth depends upon several factors, such as the root length, morphology, number of roots and the level of alveolar bone support (**Figs 18.5A to C**). The center of resistance of a single-rooted tooth with normal alveolar bone level is situated at about one-fourth to one-third the distance from the CEJ to the root apex (**Fig. 18.5A**). The center of resistance shifts apically in case of alveolar bone loss (**Fig. 18.5B**), while it may shift coronally when the root is shortened due to its resorption (**Fig. 18.5C**). In case of multirooted teeth, the center of resistance is 1 to 2 mm apical to the furcation (**Fig. 18.6**).

### Forces Acting at the Center of Resistance

Any force acting through the tooth's center of resistance would bring about translation of the tooth along the line of action of the force. Such a movement when all the parts of the tooth move the same amount in the same direction is called as bodily movement (**Fig. 18.7**).

### Forces not Acting at the Center of Resistance

Bodily movement of tooth would be desirable in most cases of malocclusion. However, in orthodontics, it is seldom possible to apply a force at the tooth's center of

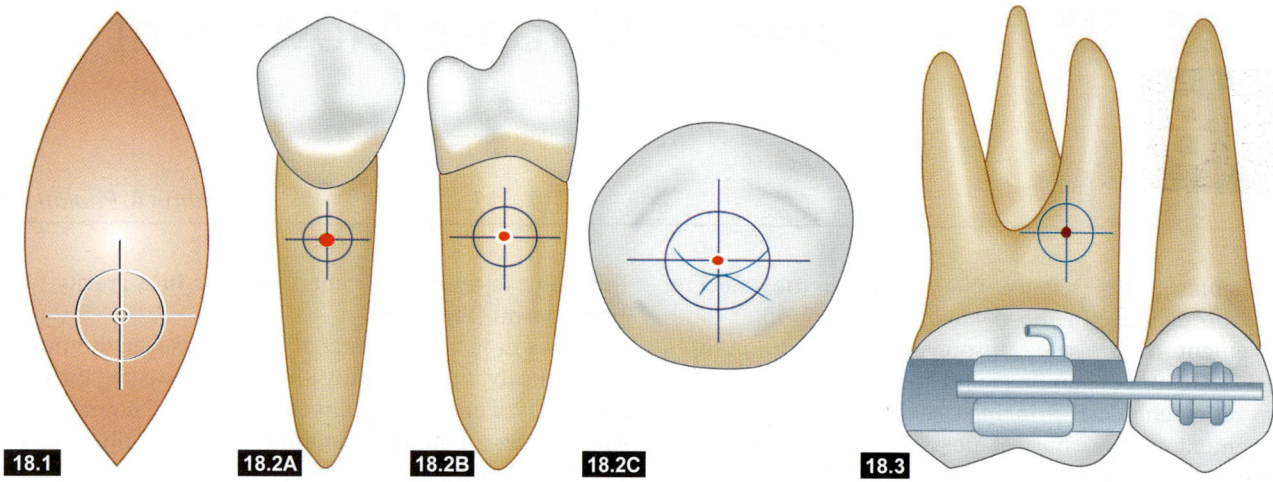

**Fig. 18.1:** Center of mass in a gravity-free body; **Figs 18.2A to C:** Center of resistance can be described in all three planes of space; **Fig. 18.3:** Center of resistance for a two cemento-enamel junction (CEJ) tooth segment

resistance, which is located on the root as the brackets can only be placed on the crown of the tooth.

If a force is applied to a body and the force does not act through the center of resistance, then the force tends to rotate the body rather than translating it. The tendency to rotate is called as "moment." Rotation can be defined as the movement of a body where no two points on the body move to the same amount in the same direction.

The total tooth movement, resulting from forces not acting through the center of resistance, is a combination of rotation and translation, occurring simultaneously. In other words, a single force applied not at the center of resistance causes the body to rotate around the center of resistance while the center of resistance simultaneously moves in the direction of the line of force **(Fig. 18.8)**.

### Center of Rotation

Should it be in heading, of application of force as well? When a body rotates, there is another point located either internal or external to the body around which, the body turns and this point is called as center of rotation. Center of rotation can be defined as an arbitrary point about which a body appears to have rotated, as determined from its initial and final position.

Location of the center of rotation varies and depends on how far the force is applied from the center of resistance **(Figs 18.9A to D)**. The center of rotation can approach but can never reach the center of resistance.

### Center of Rotation in Bodily Movement

If the force is applied at the center of resistance, the body translates and the center of rotation is at infinity.

### Center of Rotation in Uncontrolled Tipping

Here the center of rotation lies somewhere near the center of resistance of the tooth.

### Center of Rotation in Controlled Tipping

In controlled tipping, the center of rotation will be at the root apex.

### Center of Rotation in Torquing Movement

It is at incisal edge during torquing.

### Center of Rotation during Intrusion and Extrusion

It is outside the tooth during intrusion and extrusion.

## MOMENT

A moment is a measure of the tendency to rotate. From the foregoing discussion, it is understood that if a force applied to a body is not acting through its center of resistance, the force causes a tendency for the body to rotate. This tendency of a force to produce a rotation is called as the moment of the force **(Fig. 18.10)**.

The moment of the force is determined by multiplying the magnitude of the force with the perpendicular distance of the line of action of force with the center of resistance. The unit of measurement of moment is gram millimeters.

Moment of force ($M_f$) = Magnitude of force (F) × distance (d)

Thus, the clinician can achieve the desired force systems by altering these two variables, i.e. the magnitude of force and distance.

## COUPLE

A couple is a pair of concentrated forces having equal magnitude and opposite direction with parallel but noncollinear line of action. In other words, a couple is a system of two parallel forces of equal magnitude, acting in opposite directions and separated by a distance **(Fig. 18.11)**. The action of a couple is the sum of the action of two equal and opposite single force systems.

A couple brings about pure rotation of the body about the center of resistance. The control that couples provide in three planes of space is the unique feature of the original edgewise bracket and is the basic characteristic of most fixed appliances which are in use today **(Figs 18.12A and B)**.

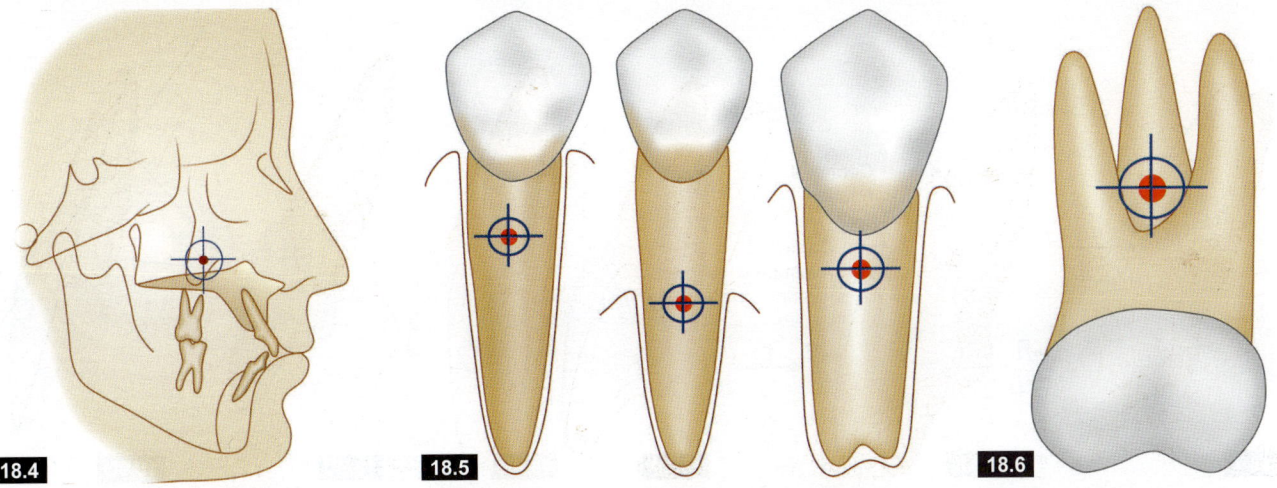

**Fig. 18.4:** Center of resistance for maxilla is about 5-10 mm inferior to the orbitale; **Figs 18.5A to C:** Location of center of resistance in a single rooted tooth, (A) with normal alveolar bone, (B) with alveolar bone loss, (C) with a shortened root; **Fig. 18.6:** Location of center of resistance in a multirooted tooth

### Moment-to-Force Ratio

The ratio of the counter balancing moment produced to the net force that is applied to the tooth will determine the type of tooth movement, which will occur. This is called the moment-to-force ratio.

## TYPES OF TOOTH MOVEMENT

Basically there are two main types of tooth movement, which can occur—translation and rotation. However, because of the nature of the attachment of teeth to alveolar bone and placement of brackets only on the crowns, all the movements in orthodontic therapy are likely to be complex. Most of the tooth movements occurring in routine clinical practice, are the combination of both translation and rotation.

### Pure Translation

A tooth is said to be translated when all points on a body move the same amount in the same direction. Such a movement can occur only when the force is acting through the center of resistance of the tooth.

Clinically, pure translation can be seen in:
- Intrusion
- Extrusion
- Bodily movement of tooth in mesiodistal or labiolingual direction.

### Pure Rotation

Forces applied at the bracket can almost never act through the center of resistance in all three planes of space. Rotation of a tooth occurs when the force is applied not through the center of resistance.

In orthodontics, the process of rotation:
- Around the long axis of the tooth is called rotation.
- Around a facio-lingual axis is called tipping.
- Around a mesiodistal axis is called torque.

### Combined Rotation and Translation

Most of the tooth movements, occurring during orthodontic treatment are neither pure rotation nor pure translation but a combination of both rotation and translation.

Clinically, the following terms are used for various types of tooth movement:
- Tipping
- Bodily movement
- Torque
- Vertical tooth movements
  - Intrusion
  - Extrusion.
- Multiple tooth movements
- Rotation.

### Tipping

Tipping is perhaps the simplest type of tooth movement and the one most readily carried out. A single force applied at one point of the crown of a tooth causes the crown to move in the direction of the force and the root in the opposite direction.

Tipping tooth movement may be of two types; uncontrolled and controlled.

#### Uncontrolled Tipping

- Uncontrolled tipping occurs when a single force is applied to the crown of the tooth and it moves about a center of rotation, which is between the center of resistance and the root apex **(Fig. 18.13)**
- In uncontrolled tipping, the crown moves in one direction, while the root moves in the opposite direction
- This is the simplest type of tooth movement to produce but is often undesirable
- Stresses in the periodontal ligament are not uniform and are concentrated near the apex and cervical area.

#### Controlled Tipping

- Controlled tipping of a tooth occurs when the center of rotation is at the root apex **(Fig. 18.14)**

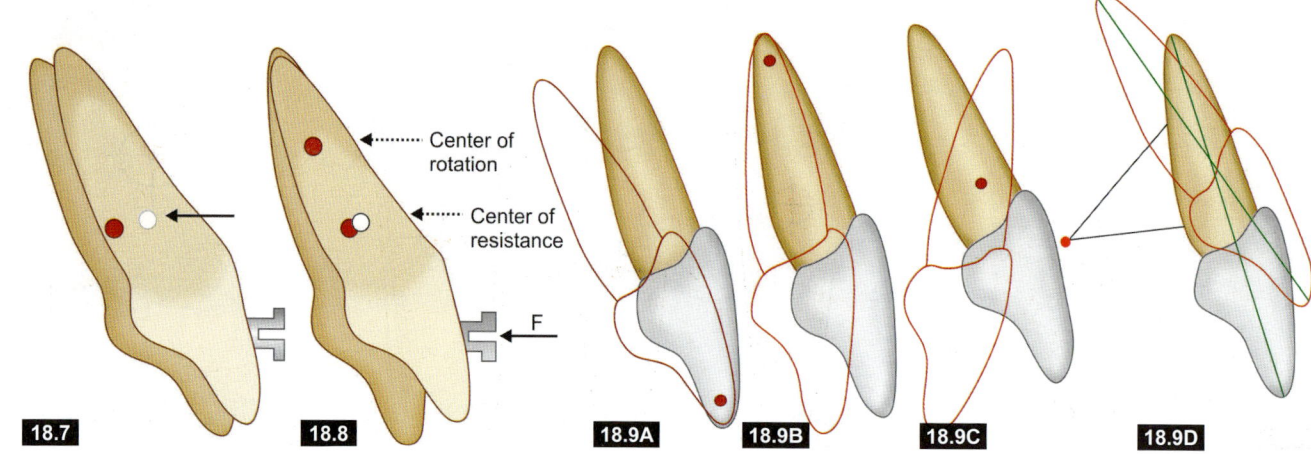

**Fig. 18.7:** Translation bodily movement of a tooth: **Fig. 18.8:** Total tooth movement caused by a force not acting through the center of resistance is a combination of rotation and translation occurring, Simultaneously; **Figs 18.9A to D:** Center of rotation: (A) At incisal edge during torquing, (B) At root apex during controlled tipping, (C) Near but not at center of resistance during uncontrolled tipping, (D) Outside the tooth during intrusion and extrusion

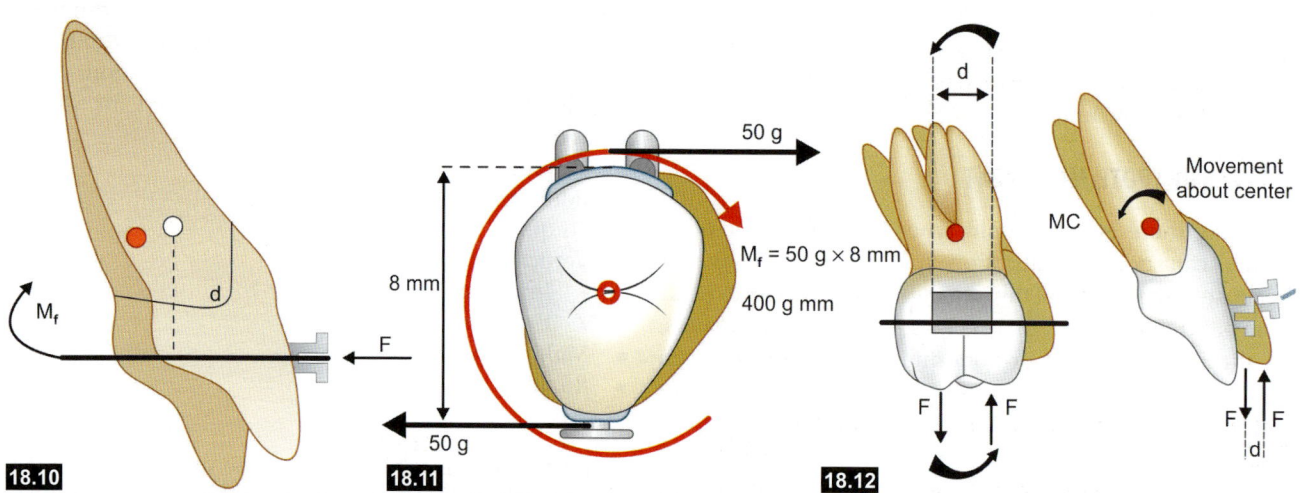

**Fig. 18.10:** Moment of force: **Fig. 18.11:** A force couple of tooth; **Figs 18.12A and B:** Clinical application of couples in fixed orthodontic appliances providing three-dimensional control during tooth movement

- Here, apart from applying force to move the crown, the movement of the root in the opposite direction of the force is controlled by application of couple at the bracket. The intention is to move the crown while maintaining the position of the root apex as it is
- Controlled tipping is a very desirable type of tooth movement
- Stress in the periodontal ligament is concentrated at the cervical area with minimal stress at the apex.

### Bodily Movement

- When a force is applied through the center of resistance of the tooth, it causes all the points on the tooth to move the same amount in the same direction as the line of force. Such type of tooth movement is called bodily movement/translation **(Fig. 18.15)**.
- The term bodily movement is used to describe the complete translation of a tooth to a new position with all parts (crown and root) of the tooth moving an equal distance
- During bodily movement, the center of rotation is at infinity
- In clinical practice, it is difficult to carry out translation as a single movement, but something close to complete bodily movement can be achieved with appropriate appliances
- Like controlled tipping, bodily movement requires simultaneous application of a force and a couple at the bracket
- The magnitude of the force applied is usually greater than the force needed for tipping movement
- The pressure is more evenly distributed over the whole length of the periodontal ligament.

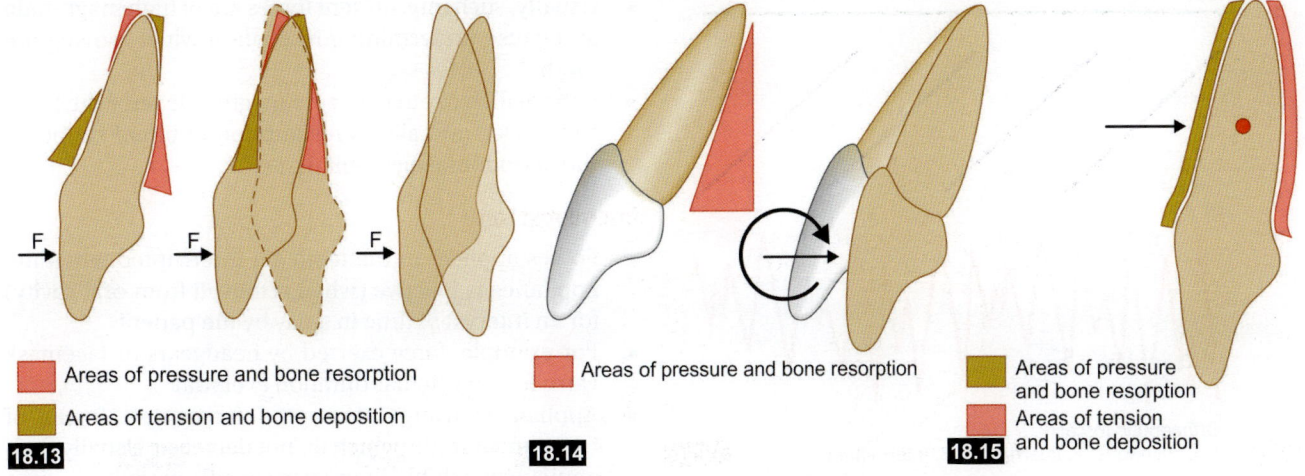

**Fig. 18.13:** Uncontrolled tipping. Stresses in the periodontal ligament are concentrated near the apex and cervical area; **Fig. 18.14:** Controlled tipping; **Fig. 18.15:** Bodily movement of the tooth

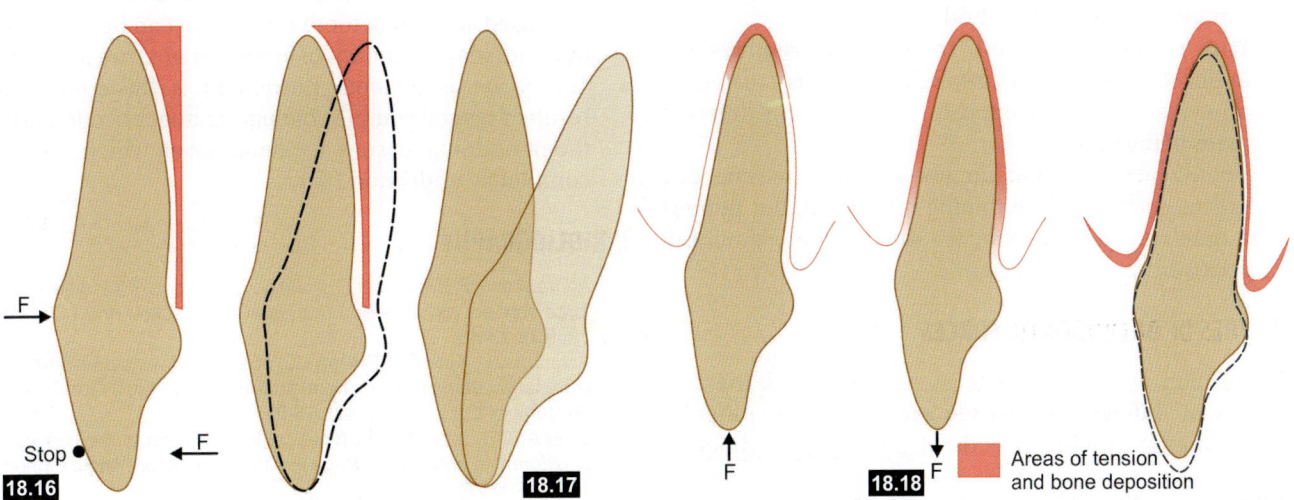

**Fig. 18.16:** Root torque; **Fig. 18.17:** Intrusive tooth movement; **Fig. 18.18:** Extrusive tooth movement

### Torque

- The term 'torque' in orthodontics refers to the differential movement of one part of a tooth, while physically restraining any movement of the other parts. **(Fig. 18.16)**
- The term is often applied to movement of root without the movement of crown
- Root torque is usually achieved by applying a force couple to the crown of the tooth, at the same time mechanically restricting crown movement in the opposite direction
- The center of rotation of the tooth is at the incisal edge or bracket
- Stresses in the periodontal ligament are more near the root apex.

### Vertical Tooth Movement

Vertical tooth movement can be in the form of intrusion or extrusion.

#### Intrusion

Intrusion of the tooth involves resorption of bone, particularly around the apex of the tooth. In this movement, the whole of supporting structures are under pressure with virtually no areas of tension **(Fig. 18.17)**.

#### Extrusion

Extrusion of the teeth from its socket can be achieved without much resorption of bone, bone deposition being required to reform the supporting mechanism of the tooth. Generally speaking, tension is induced on the whole of the supporting structure rather than pressure **(Fig. 18.18)**.

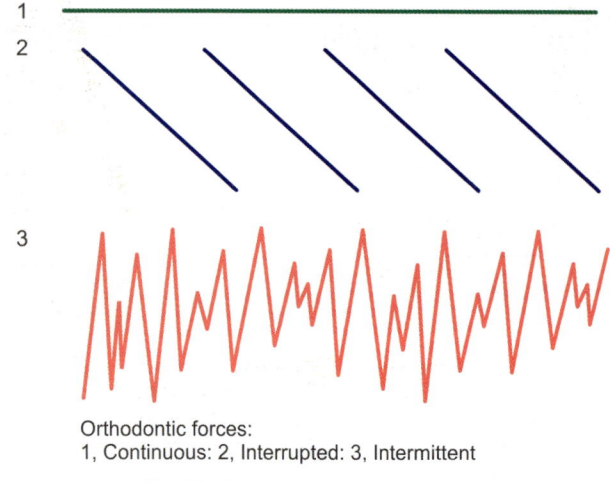

Orthodontic forces:
1, Continuous: 2, Interrupted: 3, Intermittent

**Fig. 18.19:** Types of orthodontic forces

### Rotation

- The movement of the tooth around its long axis is termed as rotation in orthodontics
- Pure rotation of a tooth in its socket requires the application of a force couple. A couple is created by applying equal and opposite forces to the different areas of the tooth
- Rotational movement do not normally require any greater force than the tipping movement, but there is a much greater tendency for rotational movement to relapse.

## TYPES OF ORTHODONTIC FORCES

Application of force is the basis of orthodontic therapy. Forces of different magnitude are applied in different directions for varying periods of time to treat different malocclusions.

Based on the duration of application, force can be divided into the following three types (**Fig. 18.19**):
1. Continuous force.
2. Intermittent force.
3. Interrupted force.

### Continuous Force

- A continuous force is the one, whose magnitude does not decrease appreciably over time. The force decay is minimal between visits to the clinician
- Ideally, light and continuous forces are most efficient as they bring about tooth movement mainly by frontal resorption
- For example, flexible wires and light elastics used in light-wire differential force technique produce continuous forces.

### Intermittent Force

- The force is said to be intermittent when it decays to zero or nearly zero magnitude prior to the next appointment.
- For example, removable appliance with an expansion screw.
- Usually, such intermittent forces are of high magnitude and cause undermining resorption while moving the tooth
- Force will decay to near zero magnitude once the tooth has moved and allows resumption of blood supply in the periodontal ligament tissue.

### Interrupted Force

- Forces applied on the teeth get interrupted when the appliance is inactive (when removed from oral cavity) for an interval of time in a day by the patient
- For example, force exerted by headgears or facemask worn for a particular duration everyday
- Appliances using interrupted forces use forces of heavy magnitude, which do not decrease. Usually such appliances exhibit, long-term specific magnitude-time pattern, for example 200-300 gm of force 14 hours a day to bring about skeletal changes
- Although it appears logical to think that, continuous forces cause continuous tooth movement and an increased amount of tooth movement can be achieved by an increased amount of force, it is not true in reality
- This is because, tooth movement is the combined result of several complex biologic changes occurring in the periodontal tissues at cellular level; which are not completely understood yet.

## BIBLIOGRAPHY

1. Andreasen GF, Zwanziger D. A clinical evaluation of the differential force concept as applied to the edgewise bracket. Am J Orthod. 1980;78:25-40.
2. Ashmore JL, Kurland BF, King GJ, et al. A 3-dimensional analysis of molar movement during headgear treatment. Am J Orthod. and Dentofacial Orthop. 2002;121:18-29.
3. Boester CH, Johnson LE. A clinical investigation of the concepts of differential and optimal force in canine retraction. Angle Orthod. 1974;44:113-9.
4. Burstone CJ. Biomechanics of the orthodontic appliance. In: Current Orthodontic Concepts and Techniques, 2nd edition. Philadelphia: WB Saunders. 1975.
5. De Lange A, Huiskes R, Kauer JMG. Measurement errors in roentgen-stereophotogrammetric joint-motion analysis. J Biomech. 1990;23:259-69.
6. DeLong R, Ko CC, Olson I, et al. Helical axis errors affect computer-generated occlusal contact. J Dent Res. 2002;81:338-43.
7. Gallo LM, Airoldi GB, Airoldi RL, et al. Description of mandibular finite helical axis pathways in asymptomatic subjects. J Dent Res. 1997;76:704-13.
8. Gallo LM, Fushima K, Palla S, et al. Mandibular helical axis pathways during mastication. J Dent Res. 2000;79:1566-72.
9. Gianelly AA, Force-induced change in the vascularity of the periodontal ligament. Am J Orthod. 1969;55:5-11.
10. Graber TM, Swain BF. Orthodontics: Current Principles and Techniques. St Louis: CV Mosby, 1985.
11. Graber TM, Vanarsdall RL. Orthodontics Current Principles and Techniques. Mosby Year Book, Inc. 1994.
12. Hayashi K, Araki Y, Uechi J, et al. A novel method for the three-dimensional analysis of orthodontic tooth movement-calculation of rotation about and translation along the finite helical axis. J Biomech. 2002;35:45-51.
13. Profitt Wr. Contemporary Orthodontics. St Louis: CV Mosby, 1986.
14. Pryputniewicz RJ, Burstone CJ. The effects of time and force magnitude on orthodontic tooth movement. J Dent Res. 1979;58:1154.

# CHAPTER 18: Mechanics of Tooth Movement

## EXAM-ORIENTED QUESTIONS

### Long Essay or Long Questions
1. Define force and add a note on point of application of force.
2. Types of tooth movement.

### Short Notes
1. Types of orthodontic forces
2. Torque
3. Moment-to-Force ratio
4. Center of resistance.

## CHAPTER OVERVIEW

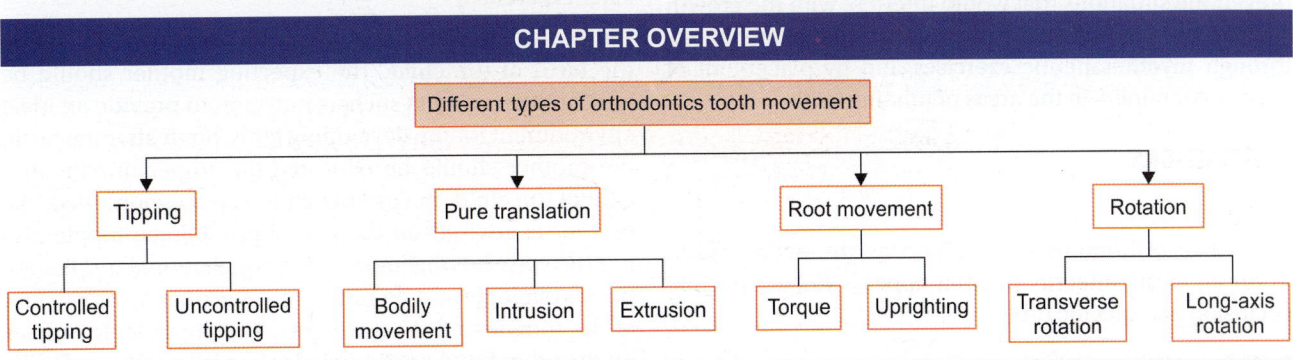

# CHAPTER 19
# Preventive Orthodontics

*Phulari BS, Gabriel O*

Preventive orthodontics includes all those procedures undertaken to preserve the integrity of normally developing occlusion by protecting current conditions or preventing situations that would interfere with the growth such as, the restoration of caries, elimination of oral habits through myotherapeutic exercises and by placement of space maintainers in the areas of missing teeth.

## DEFINITIONS

### Graber (1966)

Preventive orthodontics is defined as the action taken to preserve the integrity of what appears to be a normal occlusion at a specific time.

### Proffit and Ackerman (1980)

Preventive orthodontics is defined as the prevention of potential interference with occlusal development.

## PREVENTIVE ORTHODONTIC PROCEDURES

Following are some of the most commonly undertaken preventive orthodontic measures:
- Parent education
- Caries control
- Care of deciduous dentition
- Maintenance of shedding and eruption timetable
- Management of premature loss of deciduous teeth
- Management of ankylosis of deciduous teeth
- Management of prolonged retention of deciduous teeth
- Extraction of supernumerary teeth
- Management of oral habits
- Management of deeply locked first permanent molars
- Treatment of occlusal prematurities
- Management of abnormal frenum attachments
- Prevention of Milwaukee braces damage
- Space maintainers

### Parent Education

Preventive dentistry should ideally begin much before the birth of the child. The expecting mother should be educated on matters such as nutrition to provide an ideal environment for the developing fetus. Soon after the birth, the mother should be educated on proper nursing and care of the child. In case the child is being bottle-fed, the mother is advised on the use of physiologic nipple and not the conventional nipple. The conventional nipples are nonphysiologic and do not permit suckling by movement of the tongue and the lower jaw. The physiologic nipples on the other hand are designed to permit suckling of milk, which more or less resembles normal functional activity as in breast-feeding. The parents should also be educated on the need for maintaining good oral hygiene of the child's oral cavity.

### Caries Control

Caries involving proximal surfaces of deciduous teeth, if not treated, causes mesial migration of adjacent teeth leading to the loss of arch length **(Figs 19.1A to C)**. Later, eruption of succeeding larger permanent teeth may result in arch length-tooth material discrepancy thereby resulting in malocclusion. Therefore, early detection of such type of carious lesions plays an important role in the prevention of malocclusion.

#### Preventive Measures
- Early detection of carious lesions either by clinical or by radiographic examination should be done.
- Once the caries is detected, the affected teeth should be restored with appropriate restorative material.

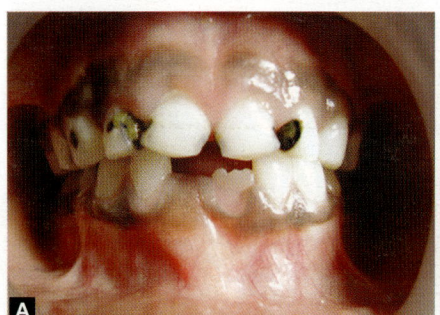
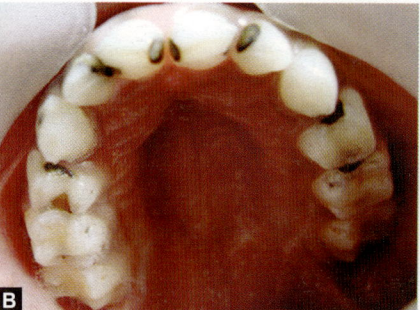
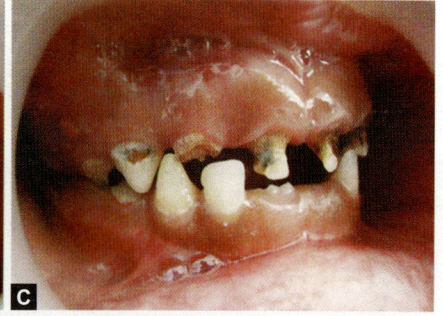

**Figs 19.1A to C:** Proximal caries of deciduous teeth, if not treated; cause mesial migration of adjacent teeth, leading to loss of arch length. On eruption of succeeding larger permanent teeth, there occurs arch length–tooth material discrepancy resulting in malocclusion

## Care of Deciduous Dentition

Deciduous teeth by themselves act as the best natural space maintainers, which not only maintain the space for their succeeding permanent teeth but also guide the latter teeth into their proper position in the dental arches **(Fig. 19.2)**.

## Maintenance of Shedding and Eruption Timetable

The pattern and schedule of primary teeth exfoliation and subsequent eruption of the permanent teeth should be closely monitored so as to intervene as and when the need arises. Generally, the deciduous teeth should exfoliate in about three months of exfoliation of their conterparts in the contralateral arch. Furthermore, the permanent succedaneous teeth should erupt within three months of exfoliation of their predecessors.

### Preventive Measures

- Regular dental checkups
- Proper oral hygiene measures.

## Premature Loss of Deciduous Teeth

Premature loss of deciduous teeth leads to the following deteriorative consequences:

- Migration of adjacent teeth into the space.
- Noneruption or altered path of eruption of the succedaneous tooth.
- Tongue thrusting may develop.
- Hampered phonation in the case of anterior tooth loss.
- Unesthetic appearance of face. Psychological effect on the child, especially in the case of anterior tooth loss **(Fig. 19.3)**.

### Preventive Measure

Space maintainers are given until the eruption of succeeding permanent teeth into the oral cavity.

## Management of Ankylosed Deciduous Teeth

Ankylosis of deciduous teeth **(Fig. 19.4)** prevents the eruption of succeeding permanent teeth.

### Preventive Measure

Surgical extraction of ankylosed deciduous teeth at an appropriate time facilitates the eruption of succeeding permanent teeth.

## Management of Prolonged Retention of Deciduous Teeth

Prolonged retention of deciduous teeth **(Figs 19.5A and B)** may be due to a number of reasons such as ankylosis, hypothyroidism, etc. Retained deciduous teeth may lead to abnormal eruptive pathway of succeeding permanent teeth.

### Preventive Measure

Extraction of retained deciduous tooth to facilitate the eruption of underlying succedaneous tooth.

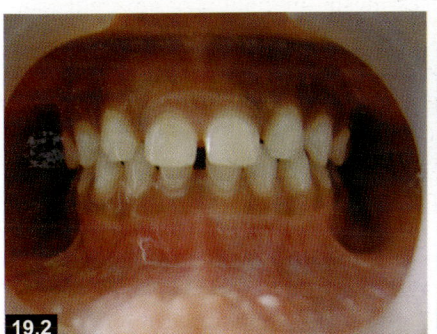
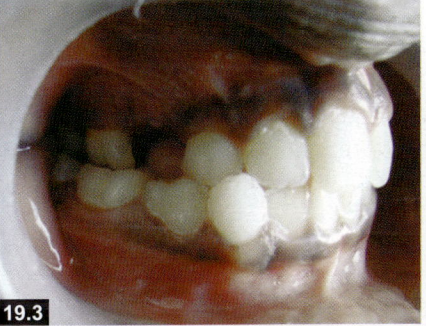
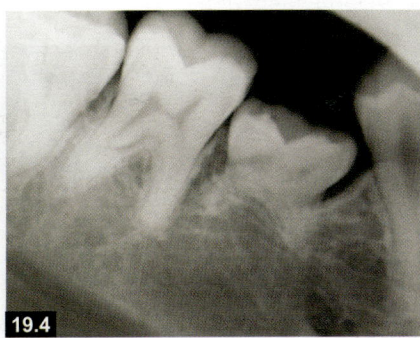

**Fig. 19.2:** Deciduous teeth acting as the best natural space maintainers;
**Fig. 19.3:** Premature loss of deciduous first molar; **Fig. 19.4:** Ankylosis of deciduous teeth

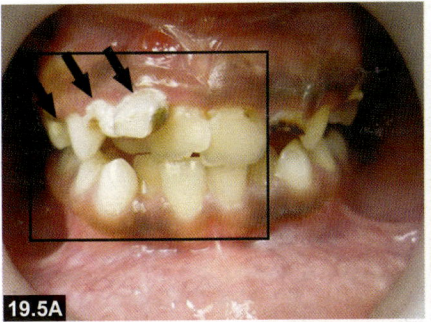
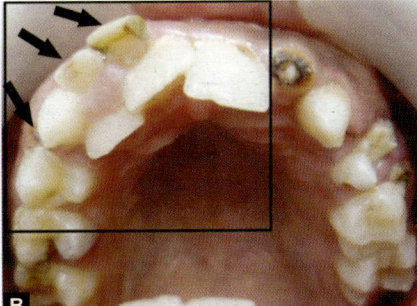
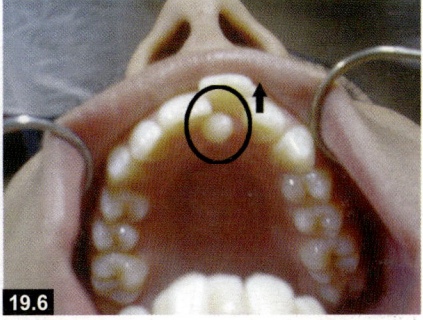

**Figs 19.5A and B:** (A) Palatally erupted maxillary permanent right incisors.
(B) Mesiolabial rotation of maxillary right permanent central incisor and retained root stumps of deciduous teeth;
**Fig. 19.6:** Palatally erupted mesiodens has resulted in the labial displacement of maxillary permanent central incisor

### Extraction of Supernumerary Teeth

Supernumerary teeth may cause the following:
a. Crowding in the arch.
b. Prevent eruption of succeeding permanent teeth.
c. If left untreated, may cause cystic formation **(Fig. 19.6)**.

*Preventive Measure*

Early diagnosis and extraction of supernumerary teeth is recommended to prevent all deleterious consequences associated with supernumerary teeth.

### Management of Oral Habits

Abnormal oral habits such as, thumb/digit-sucking **(Fig. 19.7A)**, lip-biting **(Fig. 19.7B),** tongue-thrusting and mouth-breathing habits have deleterious effects on oral health including malocclusion and gingivitis among others.

*Preventive Measures*

- Education of parents about the consequences of abnormal oral habits.
- Educating and motivating the child to stop the habit.
- Elimination of oral habits using habit-breaking appliances **(Fig. 19.8)**.

### Management of Deeply Locked First Permanent Molars

Occasionally, the first permanent molar may get deeply locked under the crest of contour of the distal surface of deciduous second molar due to distal inclination of the latter tooth.

*Preventive Measure*

Reproximation/proximal stripping to a certain extent on mesial and distal surface of second deciduous molar will guide the eruption of deeply locked first permanent molar.

### Treatment of Occlusal Prematurities

Occlusal prematurities due to over or underfilled restoration or uneven attrition of teeth causes a tendency of forward placement of mandible. This may lead to pseudo-class III malocclusion **(Figs 19.9A to C)**.

*Preventive Measures*

- Correcting the improper restoration.
- Treatment of attrition by composite restoration.

### Management of Abnormal Frenum Attachment

Abnormal frenum attachment may cause midline diastema **(Fig. 19.10A)**, which can be diagnosed clinically by Blanch test and radiographically by presence of a notch like radiolucency in the alveolar crest between permanent maxillary central incisors **(Fig. 19.10B).**

*Preventive Measure*

Surgical removal of abnormal fibrous tissue of the labial frenum is referred as Frenectomy.

### Preventing Milwaukee Brace Damage

Milwaukee brace is an orthodontic appliance used for the correction of scoliosis.

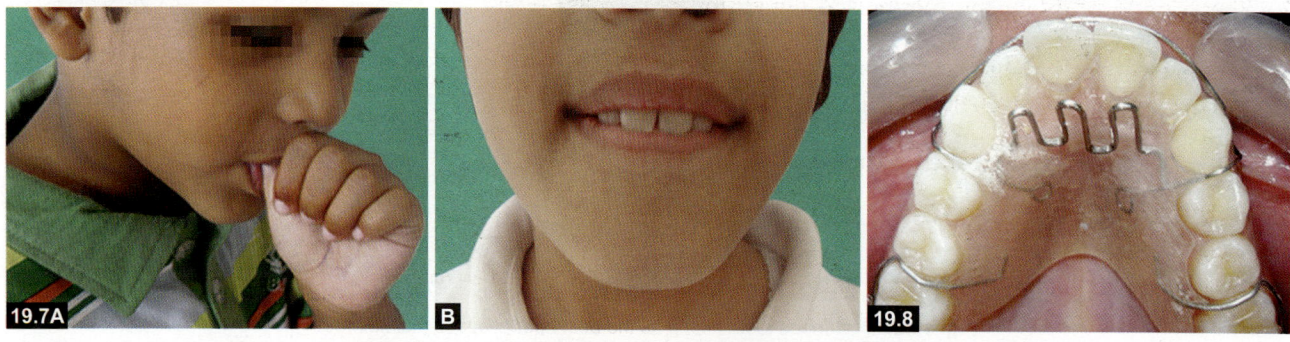

**Figs 19.7A and B:** (A) Thumb-sucking habit; (B) Lip-biting habit;
**Fig. 19.8:** Removable habit-breaking appliance with crib used to eliminate the thumb-sucking habit

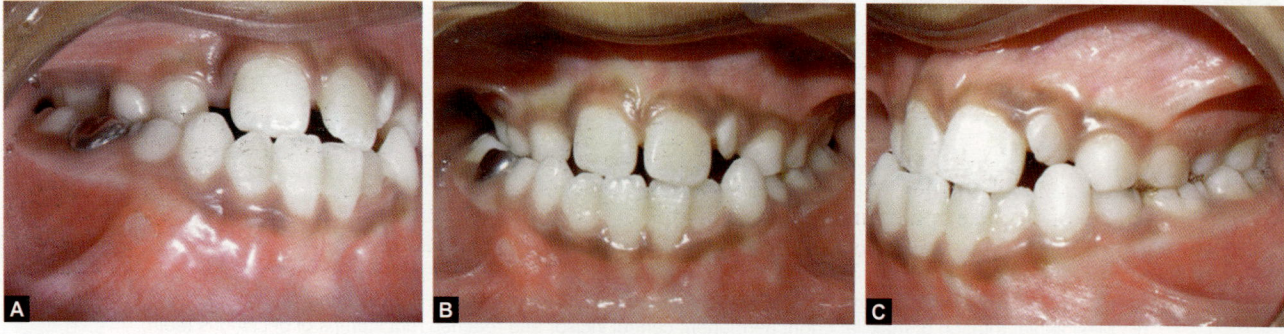

**Figs 19.9A to C:** Pseudo-class III malocclusion due to occlusal prematurities

## Effects of Milwaukee Brace

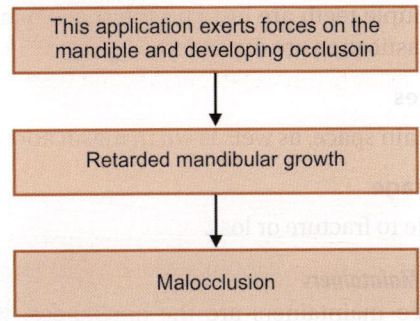

### Preventive Measures
Occlusion should be protected by using one of the following appliances:
- Functional appliances
- Tooth positioners
- Guards

### Space Maintainers
Whenever primary teeth are lost prematurely, the arch integrity is disturbed due to loss of space and decrease in arch length. Migration of adjacent primary and/or permanent teeth can occur and the available space may be reduced by an amount sufficient to cause some degree of crowding in the permanent dentition **(Table 19.1)**.

According to Boucher space maintainer is a fixed or removable appliance designed to preserve the space created by premature loss of a tooth or a group of teeth.

### Ideal Requirements for Space Maintainers
There are certain ideal requirements for all space maintainers, whether they are removable or fixed.
- They should maintain the mesiodistal dimension of the lost tooth.
- If possible, they should be functional, at least to the extent of preventing the over-eruption of the opposing tooth or teeth.
- They should be as simple and it should be as strong as possible.
- They should permit easy cleaning and maintenance of good oral hygiene.
- Their construction must be such that they do not restrict normal growth and developmental processes or interfere with such function as mastication, speech or deglutition.

### Classification of Space Maintainers
Space maintainers are generally classified into removable and fixed appliances **(Box 19.1)**. Other ways of calssifying space maintainers are given in **(Box 19.2)**.

### Indications
- The premature loss of primary molars may require the placement of a space maintainer to prevent the migration of the adjacent teeth, depending upon the teeth present and the arch length.
- When loss of a primary canine occur, the dental arch midline may be compromised and the arch length also may be reduced. The premature loss of primary canines may, therefore, require the placement of a space maintaining appliance to prevent midline deviation and/or loss of arch length, perimeter and/or circumference.
- The premature loss of primary incisors does not usually require the placement of a dental appliance for the maintenance of space because the mesial movement of the adjacent teeth is not generally expected.

**Box 19.1: Classification of space maintainers**

*Removable Appliances*
Hawley appliance/removable dentures space maintainer

*Fixed Appliances*
- Band and loop space maintainer
- Band and bar space maintainer
- Crown and loop space maintainer
- Crown and bar space maintainer
- Distal shoe space maintainer
- Lower lingual arch space maintainer
- Nance space maintainer
- Transpalatal arch

**Box 19.2: Other classification of space maintainers**

*According to Hitchcock*
- Removable or fixed or semi-fixed
- With bands or without bands
- Functional or nonfunctional
- Active or passive
- Certain combinations of the above

*According to Raymond C Thurow*
- Removable
- Complete arch
  - Lingual arch
  - Extra-oral anchorage
- Individual tooth

*According to Henrichsen*
- Fixed space maintainers

Class I
- Non-functional types
  - Bar type
  - Loop type
- Functional types
  - Pontic type
  - Lingual arch type

Class II
Cantilever type (distal shoe, band and loop)
- Removable space maintainers

Acrylic partial dentures

### Contraindications
- A space maintainer is usually not necessary, if there is sufficient amount of space present to allow for the eruption of permanent tooth/teeth.
- A space maintainer may not be recommended, if severe crowding exists, such that space maintenance is of minimal effect and subsequent orthodontic intervention is indicated.
- A space maintainer may not be necessary, if the succedaneous tooth will be erupting soon.
- When succedaneous tooth is absent.

### Pre-requisites for Space Maintainer
- Space maintainers should maintain the mesiodistal dimensions of the lost teeth.
- They must not endanger the remaining teeth by imposing excessive stresses on them.
- They must be easily cleaned and not serve as trays for debris, which might enhance dental caries and soft tissue pathologies.
- Their construction must be such that they do not restrict normal growth and development process or interfere with functions, such as mastication, speech or deglutition.

Depending on the tooth lost, the segment involved, the type of occlusion, possible speech involvements and cooperation, particular type of space maintainer may be indicated.

Removable space maintainers/Functional space maintainers/Removable acrylic space maintainers **(Fig. 19.11)**.
- Functional space maintainer is a removable type of space maintainer and is the choice of space maintainer, when there is multiple premature loss of deciduous teeth. This type of space maintainer is fabricated with acrylic material. It not only helps in esthetic but also helps in the regaining of lost masticatory functions.
- This type of space maintainer consists of acrylic plate, acrylic teeth and clasps on molars. The incisors of acrylic teeth help in regaining lost masticatory functions and esthetics. Clasps may be a simple "c" clasps on molars which aid in retention.

### Indications
When multiple teeth are lost and the space maintenance and the mastication are of concern.

### Advantages
Can maintain space, as well as aid in mastication.

### Disadvantage
Susceptible to fracture or loss.

### Fixed Space Maintainers
Fixed space maintainers are the appliances, which are fixed onto the teeth and utilize bands or crowns for their fabrication.

### Band and Loop Space Maintainer
Band and loop space maintainer is a fixed space maintainer and is one of the most commonly used space maintainers in the dental practice. It can be constructed on one side of the arch or on the both **(Figs 19.12A to C)**.

### Reverse Band and Loop Space Maintainer
This type of space maintainer is given when there is premature loss of primary second molar and the permanent molars have not erupted fully to support a band. In such cases, deciduous first molar is banded and loop is made that touches just below the marginal ridges of permanent molars.

### Mayne's Space Maintainer
Mayne's space maintainer is a type of band and loop space maintainer where the loop is halved.

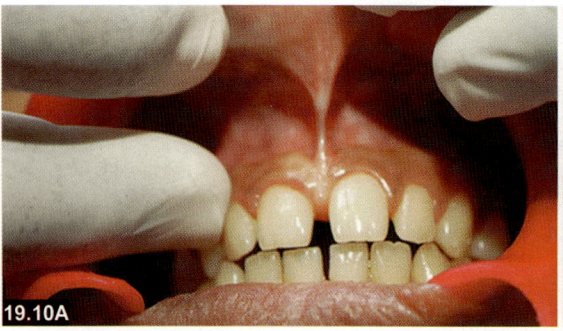
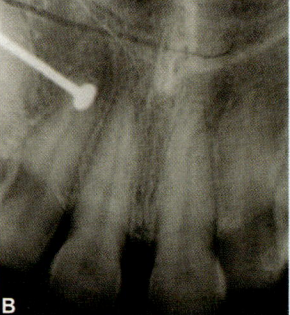
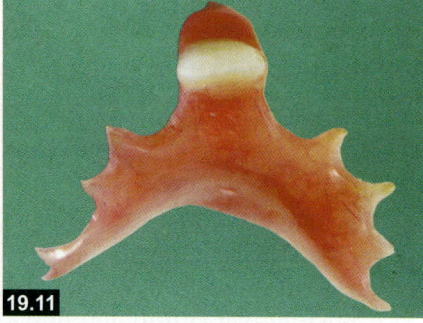

**Figs 19.10A and B:** (A) Thick, fibrous maxillary labial frenum attachment, causing midline diastema, (B) IOPA showing notch-like radiolucency in the alveolar crest between permanent maxillary centrals; **Fig. 19.11:** Removable space maintainers/functional space maintainers/removable acrylic space maintainers

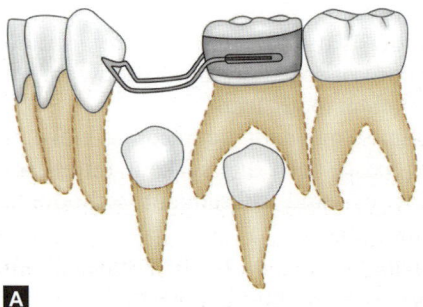
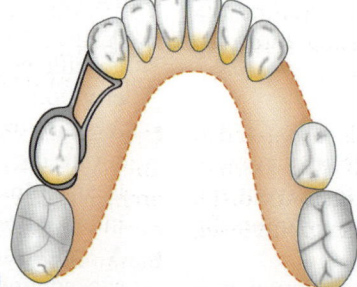
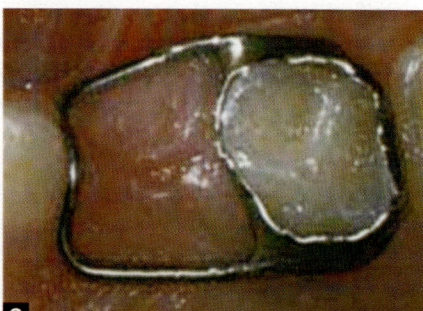

**Figs 19.12A to C:** Band and loop space maintainer

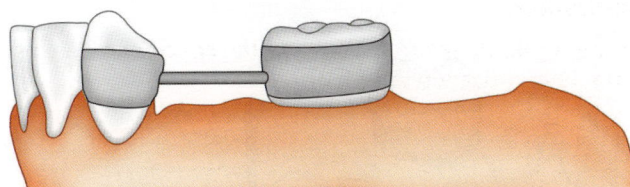

**Fig. 19.13:** Band and bar space maintainer

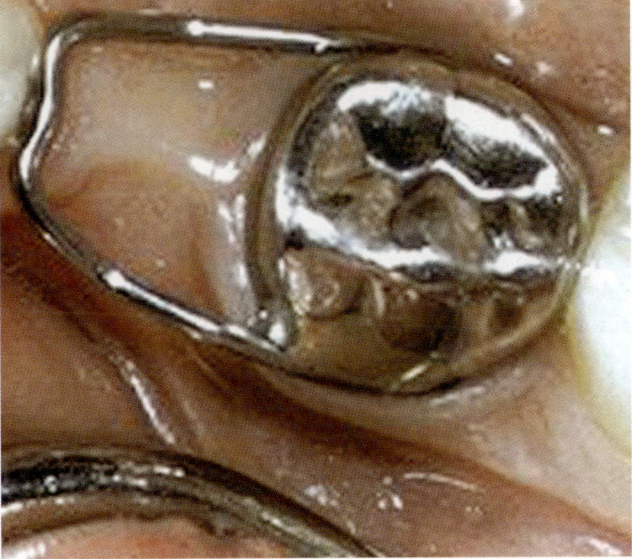

**Fig. 19.14:** Crown and loop space maintainer

## Indication

Loss of first primary molar.

## Advantage

Ease of fabrication for the clinician and ease of maintenance for the patient.

## Disadvantages

- Opposing tooth may supra-erupt.
- This type of space maintainer cannot be used for the multiple loss of deciduous teeth.

### Band and Bar Space Maintainer

- Band and bar space maintainer is a fixed type of space maintainer in which the abutment teeth on either side of the extraction space are banded and connected to each other by a bar (**Fig. 19.13**).
- Band and bar space maintainer is a fixed type of space maintainer, in which tooth mesial and distal to the extraction space are banded either using direct or indirect banding procedure and connected to each other by a bar.
- A bar is a thick stainless steel wire, its ends is soldered to the mesial surface of banded distal tooth at the contact point level and its another end is soldered to the distal surface of the banded tooth at the contact point level, which is mesial to the extraction site.
- In some cases, band and bar space maintainer may consist of only one banded tooth and a bar soldered to it.

### Crown and Loop Space Maintainer

Crown and loop space maintainer is also a fixed space maintainer. It can be constructed either unilateral or bilateral depending upon the deciduous tooth. This type of space maintainer is exactly same as band and loop type of space maintainer in all aspects except that a stainless steel crown is used instead of band on the tooth distal to the extraction space. This type of space maintainer is indicated in cases where the tooth distal to the extractions spaces (**Fig. 19.14**).

### Indication

Loss of first primary molar with significant loss of tooth substance of the abutment tooth.

### Advantage

Ease of fabrication for the clinician and ease of maintenance for the patient.

### Disadvantage

More difficult to fabricate than band and loop.

### Crown and Bar Space Maintainer

Crown and bar space maintainer is a fixed type of space maintainer in which the stainless steel crown can be used on abutment teeth (**Fig. 19.15**).

### Distal Shoe (Intra-alveolar Space Maintainer)

Distal shoe space maintainer is also known as intra-alveolar appliance. The distal surface of the second deciduous molar guides the unerupted first permanent molar when the second deciduous molar is extracted prior to the eruptions of the first permanent molar. Distal shoe space maintainer provides greater contact of the path of the eruption of the unerupted tooth and prevents undesirable migration (**Fig. 19.16**).

Distal shoe space maintainer can be removable when acrylic is used for distal extension and can be fixed when a thick stainless steel wire is soldered to the distal surface of first deciduous molar at contact point level.

### Indication

Loss of second primary molar prior to eruption of the first permanent molar.

### Advantage

Maintains the second primary molar space.

### Disadvantage

Difficult to fabricate; contraindicated in some medically compromised patients, that is, pathological heart murmur.

### Lower Lingual Holding Arch (LLHA) Space Maintainer

This type of space maintainer is used only in mandibular arch, in this type of space maintainer either first or second deciduous molar are banded using either direct or indirect banding procedure and a lingual arch is fabricated with thick stainless steel wire in such a way that it should contact the lingual surface of all mandibular incisors and

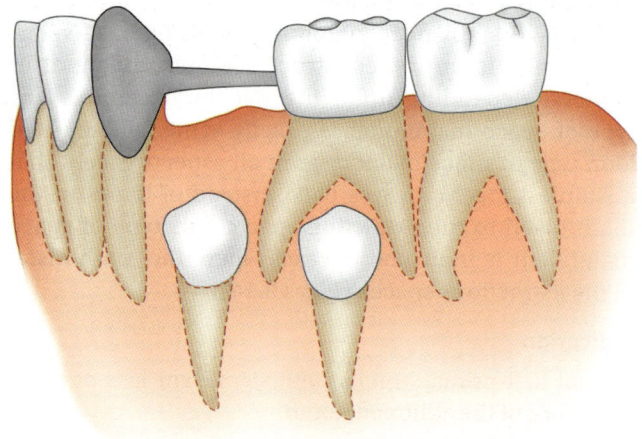

Fig. 19.15: Crown and bar space maintainer

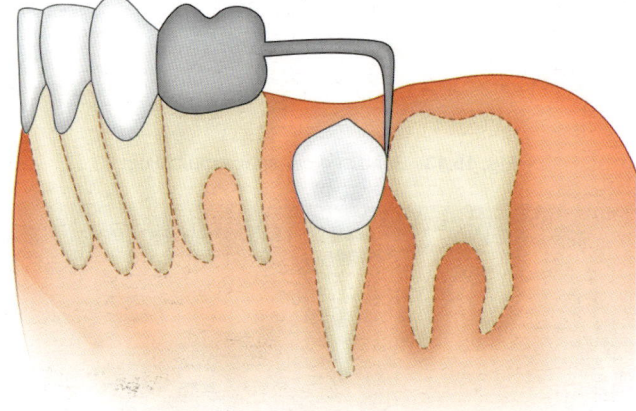

Fig. 19.16: Distal shoe (Intra-alveolar space maintainer)

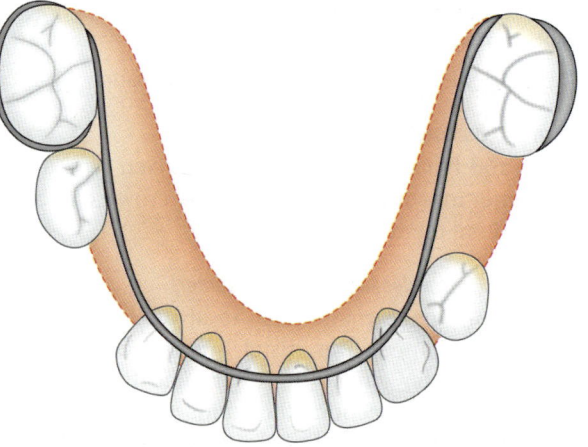

Fig. 19.17: Lower lingual holding arch (LLHA) space maintainer

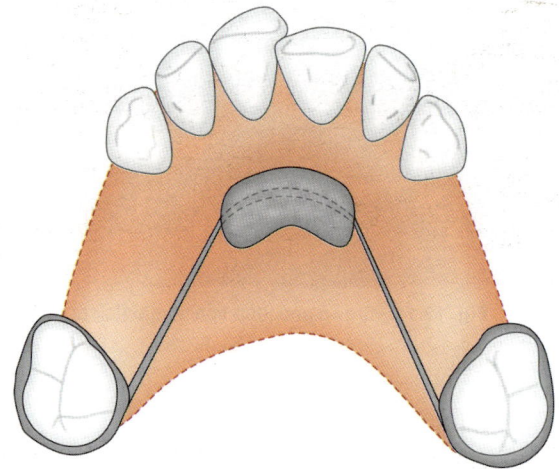

Fig. 19.18: Nance palatal arch space maintainer

is soldered to the lingual surface of band on either side of the same arch **(Fig. 19.17)**.

This type of space maintainer is used to preserve the space created by multiple loss of deciduous molars and also it helps in preventing drifting of molars, thereby help in maintaining arch perimeter.

### Indication

Loss of second primary molar in the mandible (counterpart to Nance).

### Advantages

Maintains the tooth space and the leeway space.

### Disadvantages

First permanent molars may be susceptible to decalcification; may be prone to breakage unless the patient is well-informed on maintenance.

#### Nance Palatal Arch Space Maintainer

Nance palatal arch space maintainer consists of two molar bands of a wire component (palatal arch) and acrylic or palatal button. It is used only in maxillary arch. Bands are fabricated either using direct or indirect banding procedure on maxillary molars on either side of the same arch. A wire component (palatal arch) is fabricated using 0.036-stainless steel wire like lingual arch **(Fig. 19.18)**.

Both ends of the palatal arch are soldered to the palatal surface of the band on both sides of the same arch and its anterior portion is made to get embedded in the acrylic portion or palatal button or Nance button. This type of space maintainer is used to prevent mesial migration of maxillary molars.

### Indication

Loss of second primary molar in the maxilla-counterpart to lower lingual holding arch.

### Advantage

Maintains the tooth space and the leeway space.

### Disadvantages

- Meticulous hygiene of the acrylic button is required.

| Table 19.1: Indications and uses of specific types of space maintainer | |
|---|---|
| **Indication** | **Space maintainers of choice** |
| Premature loss of deciduous incisors | <ul><li>Functional space maintainers</li><li>Removable space maintainers</li></ul> |
| **Premature loss of deciduous canines** | |
| Unilateral premature loss of deciduous canines when deciduous first molar is sound (free of caries). Unilateral premature loss of deciduous canines when deciduous first molar is decayed. Bilateral premature loss of deciduous canine in maxillary arch. Bilateral premature loss of deciduous canine in mandibular arch. | <ul><li>Band and loop space maintainers</li><li>Band and bar space maintainers</li><li>Crown and loop space maintainers</li><li>Crown and bar space maintainers</li><li>Nance palatal arch space maintainers</li><li>Lingual arch space maintainers</li></ul> |
| **Premature loss of deciduous first molar** | |
| Unilateral premature loss of deciduous first molar with sound second molar. Unilateral premature loss of deciduous first molar when second deciduous molar adjacent to missing is decayed. Bilateral premature loss of first deciduous molar in maxillary arch. Bilateral premature loss of first deciduous molar in mandibular arch. | <ul><li>Band and loop space maintainers</li><li>Band and bar space maintainers</li><li>Crown and loop space maintainers</li><li>Crown and bar space maintainers</li><li>Nance palatal arch space maintainers</li><li>Transpalatal arch</li><li>Bilaterally placed band and loop space maintainers</li><li>Lingual arch space maintainers</li><li>Bilaterally placed band and loop space maintainers</li></ul> |
| **Premature loss of deciduous second molar** | |
| Unilateral premature loss of deciduous second molar Bilateral premature loss of deciduous second molar in the maxillary arch. Bilateral premature loss of deciduous second molar in the mandibular arch. Premature loss of deciduous second molar prior to eruption of permanent first molar | <ul><li>Band and loop space maintainers</li><li>Nance palatal arch space maintainers</li><li>Transpalatal arch</li><li>Bilaterally placed band and loop space maintainers</li><li>Bilaterally placed band and bar space maintainers</li><li>Lingual arch space maintainers</li><li>Bilaterally placed band and loop space maintainers</li><li>Bilaterally placed band and bar space maintainers</li><li>Distal shoe space maintainers.</li></ul> |

- This type of space maintainer cannot be used in patients allergic to acrylic.

### Transpalatal Arch

- The transpalatal arch, as the name implies, extends from one maxillary first molar along the contour of the palate to the molar on the opposite side **(Fig. 19.19)**.

- The transpalatal arches can be either removable when they inserted into the lingual sheath welded on the lingual surface of molar band or fixed when they are soldered to the lingual surface of molar band.
- Transpalatal arches are made from 0.036-inch stainless steel wire and that is soldered to the molar bands at their mesiolingual line angles.

### Functions of Transpalatal Arch

- The major function of transpalatal arch in the mixed dentition is to prevent the mesial migration of the maxillary first molars during the transition from the second deciduous molars to the second premolars.
- The transpalatal arch can also be used for molar distalization and anchorage.
- The transpalatal arch routinely is left in place until the final comprehension phase of orthodontic therapy is completed.

### BIBLIOGRAPHY

1. Akerman JL, Proffit WR. Preventive and interceptive orthodontics: A strong theory proves weak in practice. Angle Orthod 1980;50: 75-86.
2. Foster TD. A Textbook of Orthodontics (2nd edn). St Louis, 1982, Blackwell Scientific Publication.
3. Gould JE. Space maintenance. Brit Dent J 1974;118:20-6.

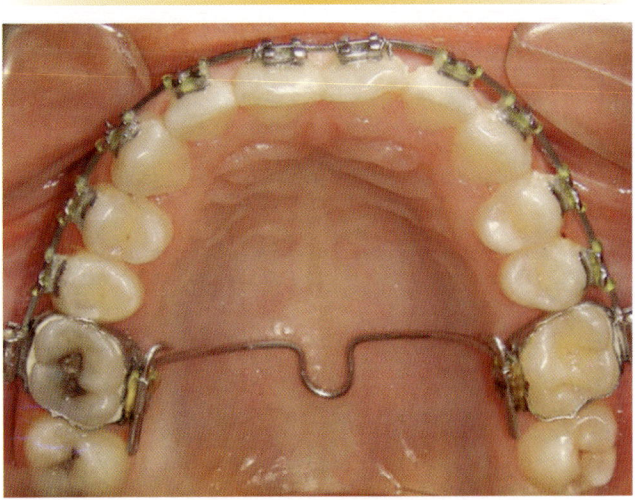

**Fig. 19.19:** Transpalatal arch

4. Northway WM, Wainright RL, Demirjian A. Effects of premature loss of deciduous molars. Angle Orthod 1984;54:295-329.
5. Norton A, Wickwire Na, Gellin ME. Space management in mixed dentition. J Dent Child 1975;42:0112-8.
6. Profitt WR. Contemporary Orthodontics, St Louis, CV Mosby, 1986.
7. Thomas M Graber, Robert L Vanarsdall. Orthodontics current principles and techniques, Mosby Year Book Inc, 1994.
8. Wright GZ, Kennedyt DB. Space control in the primary and mixed dentitions. Dent Clin North Am 1978;22:579-601.

## EXAM-ORIENTED QUESTIONS

### Long Essay or Long Questions
1. Define preventive orthodontics, enumerate preventive orthodontic measures and write in detail about any 3 measures in detail.
2. Define and classify space maintainers and write any 3 space maintainers in detail.

### Short Essay or Long Notes
1. Indications and the use of specific types of space maintainers.
2. Preventive orthodontics.

### Short Notes
1. Moyer's space maintainer
2. Transpalatal arch
3. Preventing Milwaukee brace damage
4. Lower lingual holding arch
5. Indication and contraindication of space maintainers
6. Ideal requirements of space maintainers
7. Intra-alveolar space maintainers.

## CHAPTER OVERVIEW

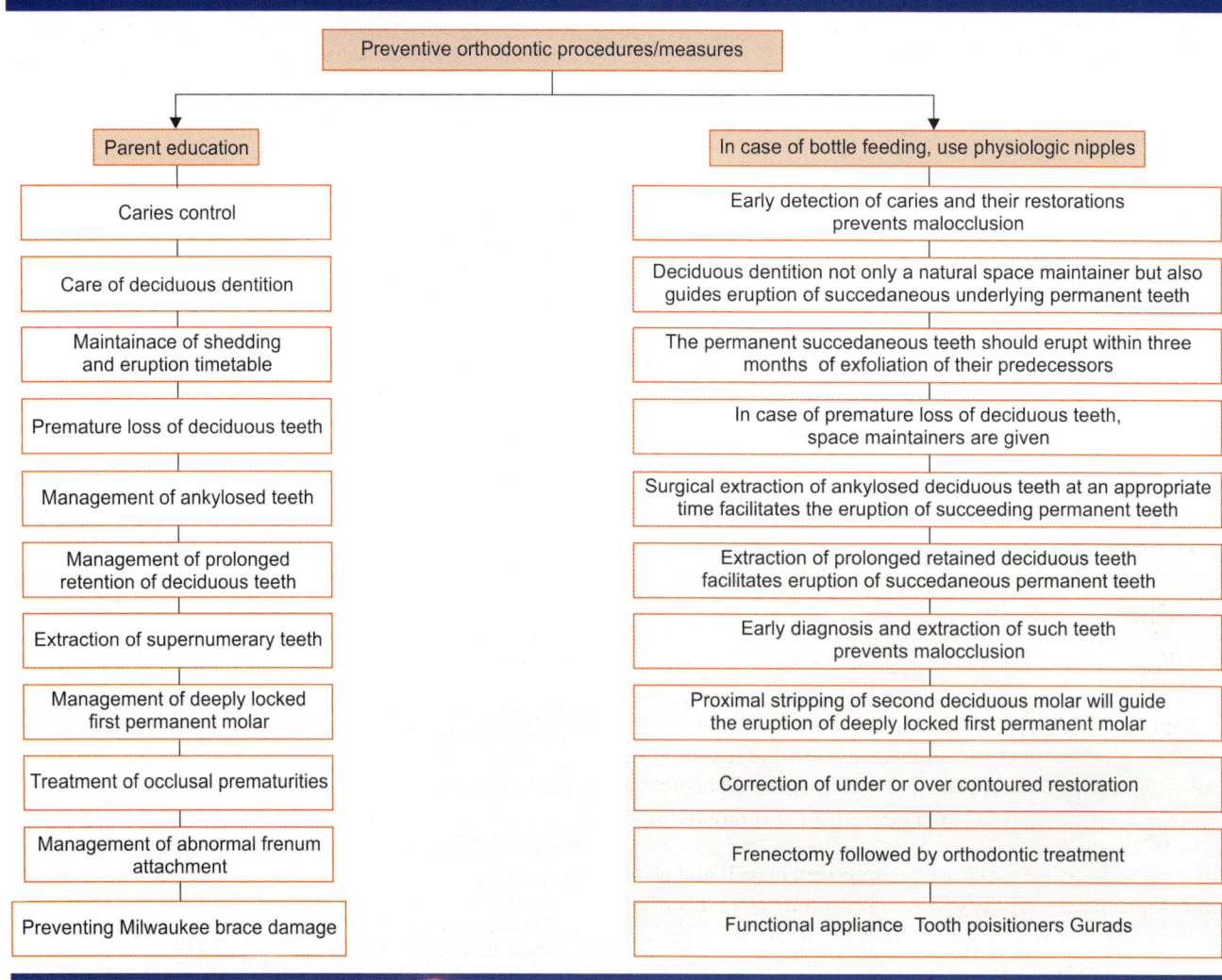

# CHAPTER 20

# Interceptive Orthodontics

*Phulari BS, Rashanal A*

Unlike preventive orthodontics which deals with the elimination of factors that may lead to malocclusion, interceptive orthodontics is undertaken at a time when malocclusion has already developed or developing. Some of the preventive measures may also be used as interceptive procedures. The difference between preventive and interceptive orthodontics lies in the timing of the services rendered. Preventive orthodontic procedures are undertaken when the dentition and occlusion are perfectly normal, while the interceptive procedures are carried out when signs and symptoms of a developing malocclusion are evident.

Various interceptive orthodontic procedures that will help in the correction or reduction of the severity of malocclusions are listed below:
- Serial extraction/guidance of occlusion
- Correction of developing crossbites
- Control of abnormal oral habits
- Proximal stripping of deciduous teeth to facilitate the eruption of adjacent permanent teeth
- Correction of occlusal interferences
- Interception of skeletal malrelations
- Space regaining
- Muscle exercises
- Removal of soft tissue and bony barriers.

## SERIAL EXTRACTION

Serial extraction is an interceptive orthodontic procedure undertaken in the (early) mixed dentition period that involves planned removal of certain primary and permanent teeth in a programmed sequence, so as to relieve crowding in the arches and to guide the remaining erupting permanent teeth into a more favorable position.

A thorough understanding of the dynamics of orofacial growth and development and that of the stomatognathic system is essential for the success of serial extraction procedures.

When executed properly in carefully selected patients with the proper assessment, skilled timing and careful monitoring, programmed serial extraction procedures can produce the best possible and the most stable results with minimal or in some cases, no further need of corrective mechanotherapy at a later stage, when all permanent teeth erupts.

Although occasionally used to intercept class II and class III malocclusions, serial extraction procedure is mainly used to intercept and/or treat class I malocclusions with crowding resulting from severe tooth size-arch length discrepancy.

### Definitions

**Tweed** defined serial extraction as the planned and sequential removal of the primary and permanent teeth to intercept and reduce dental crowding problems.

**Tondon:** The correctly timed, planned removal of certain deciduous and permanent teeth in mixed dentition cases with dentoalveolar disproportion.

### Historical Perspective (Box 20.1)

**Robert Bunon**, in the early 1743, was the first to advise the extraction of primary teeth to achieve a better alignment of permanent teeth in his work "Diseases of teeth" **(Box 20.1)**.

Later, several authors like Bourdet (1757), Hunter (1771), Robinson (1846) and Harris (1855) advocated removal of the primary canines and the premolars when permanent incisors were crowded.

The term serial extraction was first coined by **Kjellgren in 1929**. However, it was **Nance** who popularized the procedure in 1940s in England and is considered as the Father of Serial Extraction technique, practiced today.

Although popular, the term serial extraction does not stress the importance of thorough knowledge of growth and development, comprehensive analysis based on investigative records required to execute the procedure properly and thus, may be misleading.

**Hotz (1970)** recommended the term guidance of eruption. It is also sometimes referred to as guided extraction, while other authors prefer to call the procedure, guidance of occlusion.

### Indications

Serial extraction procedure is primarily indicated in developing class I malocclusions with moderate to severe arch length-tooth material discrepancy with resultant crowding of teeth. Serial extraction gives best results in patients with ideal orthognathic profile and in whom all the components of stomatognathic system (i.e. neuromuscular envelope, basal jaw bones, and teeth) are

| Box 20.1: | History of serial extraction procedures |
|---|---|
| **Robert Bunon (1743)** | First reference to the extraction of primary teeth to facilitate the alignment of permanent teeth in Diseases of Teeth |
| **Kjellgren (1929)** | First coined the term Serial Extraction |
| **Nance (1940)** | Popularised the procedure. He is called Father of Serial Extraction Technique |
| **Hotz (1970)** | Argued against the term Serial Extraction. Preferred the term Guidance of eruption. |

in balance with good facial harmony. Indications of serial extraction can be listed as the following:
1. Class I malocclusion with ideal orthognathic facial profile and good neuromuscular balance
2. Severe arch length-tooth material discrepancy of 10 mm or more in the arch.

Arch length deficiency as compared to total tooth material can be indicated by the following features:
- Absence of developmental/physiologic spacing in deciduous dentition
- Premature exfoliation of deciduous canines especially in the lower arch
- Abnormal root resorption pattern of deciduous canines–radiographic examination reveals a crescent pattern of resorption on the mesial side of the primary canine roots
- Midline shift due to displacement of lateral incisors following premature loss of unilateral deciduous canine
- Proclination of permanent upper and lower incisors, associated with crowding
- Lingual eruption of upper lateral incisors
- Extreme labial displacement of lower incisors
- Gingival recession in relation to labially placed lower incisor teeth
- Abnormal exfoliation sequence of primary teeth
- Altered eruption sequence of primary teeth
- Ankylosis of primary teeth
- Ectopic eruption of permanent teeth especially, that of upper canines. Upper canines erupt after the emergence of one or both the premolars and thus, tend to assume extreme buccal or palatal position when there is lack of space in the arch.

## Contraindications

- Class I malocclusion with minimal arch length-tooth material discrepancy which can be overcome subsequently as the jaws grow
- Class II and class III malocclusions with skeletal abnormalities and abnormal neuromuscular behavior
- Presence of midline diastema and spacing
- Congenitally missing teeth
- When there is collapsed arch
- Presence of deep bite and open bite
- In cleft lip and palate cases.

## Rationale

Serial extraction is ideally carried out in class I malocclusion, with an initial normal sagittal jaw relationship and neuromuscular balance. Here all the components of the stomatogathic system, i.e. neuromuscular envelope, basal jaw bones and teeth are in balance. But there is a malocclusion present, caused by the tooth size-arch length discrepancy. The objective of serial extraction is to correct the dental irregularities while maintaining this balance and the facial harmony.

Eruption of the permanent incisors in early mixed dentition may result in a marked crowding problem in patients with severe tooth size-arch length discrepancy of 8-10 mm or more. Arch expansion is not an ideal option here as teeth moved off their apical base into excessive neuromuscular force are unlikely to be stable in the long run. Such patients would ultimately require extraction of four premolars to provide space for proper alignment of the remaining permanent teeth.

Delaying the extraction of premolars until all permanent teeth erupt may lead to severely displaced teeth that may require prolonged corrective mechanotherapy at a later stage, often during the difficult teenage period. Rationale of serial extraction procedure is to intercept the malocclusion at early mixed dentition period by extracting certain primary and permanent teeth, and then guiding the eruption of remaining permanent teeth into the best possible occlusion by using the physiologic eruptive forces and the existing normal neuromuscular balance. By doing so, the extent and the need of corrective orthodontic treatment at a later stage can be minimized.

### Diagnosis and Planning

Extraction of any tooth is a critical step in orthodontic management. Thus the decision of resorting to serial extraction should always be based on comprehensive assessment of dental, skeletal and soft tissues. Serial extraction is not a single-decision but a multi-decisional, time-lined process where factors such as the amount of crowding, arch length requirements, whether to extract the next set of teeth or not, and when to extract are re-evaluated at each visit by the patient. Thus serial extraction is a continum of decision making process rather than a single-time diagnosis.

The following investigations are recommended after a thorough clinical examination:

#### Orthodontic Study Models

Moderate to severe arch length-tooth material discrepancy of not less than 5–7 mm should exist to undertake the serial extraction procedure.

Study models are required for:
- Assessing the morphology of teeth
- Assessing the dental arch form
- Evaluation of occlusion
- To perform model analyses—Carey's analysis in the lower arch and Arch perimeter analysis in the upper arch. Mixed dentition analysis helps in determining the space requirement for erupting posterior teeth.

#### Radiographs

Various radiographic views recommended are:
- Intraoral periapical view
- Lateral cephalogram—to analyse the skeletal relation and direction of growth using cephalometric analysis.
- Orthopantomograph (OPG)
  - To detect congenitally missing teeth and supernumerary teeth
  - To carry out radiographic mixed dentition analysis

- To assess dental age
- To assess the amount of root development and possible eruption pattern
- To detect any bony pathologies.

### Photographs

Pre, mid and post-treatment intra- and extra-oral photographs are taken. They act as permanent records of pre-treatment state, improvements during the procedure and also help in patient motivation.

### Procedure

A number of extraction sequences are in use and the choice of a particular method depends on individual case. No single extracton sequence applies to all patients. Some of the commonly used methods are described here.

- Dewel's method
- Nance method
- Tweed's method
- Grewe's method.

### Dewel's Method (1978) (Extraction of CD4)

Dewel proposed a three-step serial extraction procedure in 1978. This is the most satisfactory order in most patients even today **(Box 20.2)**.

### Step 1: Extraction of deciduous canines

In this step, the deciduous canines are extracted at around 8-9 years to create space for the alignment of the incisors **(Fig. 20.1A)**.

**Box 20.2:** Dewel's Method (Extraction of CD4)

| Steps | Tooth extracted | Purpose |
|---|---|---|
| Step 1 | Extraction of deciduous canines | To facilitate alignment of incisors |
| Step 2 | Extraction of deciduous first molars | To facilitate the eruption of first premolars before the eruption of permanent canines |
| Step 3 | Extraction of first premolars | To facilitate the eruption of permanent canines |

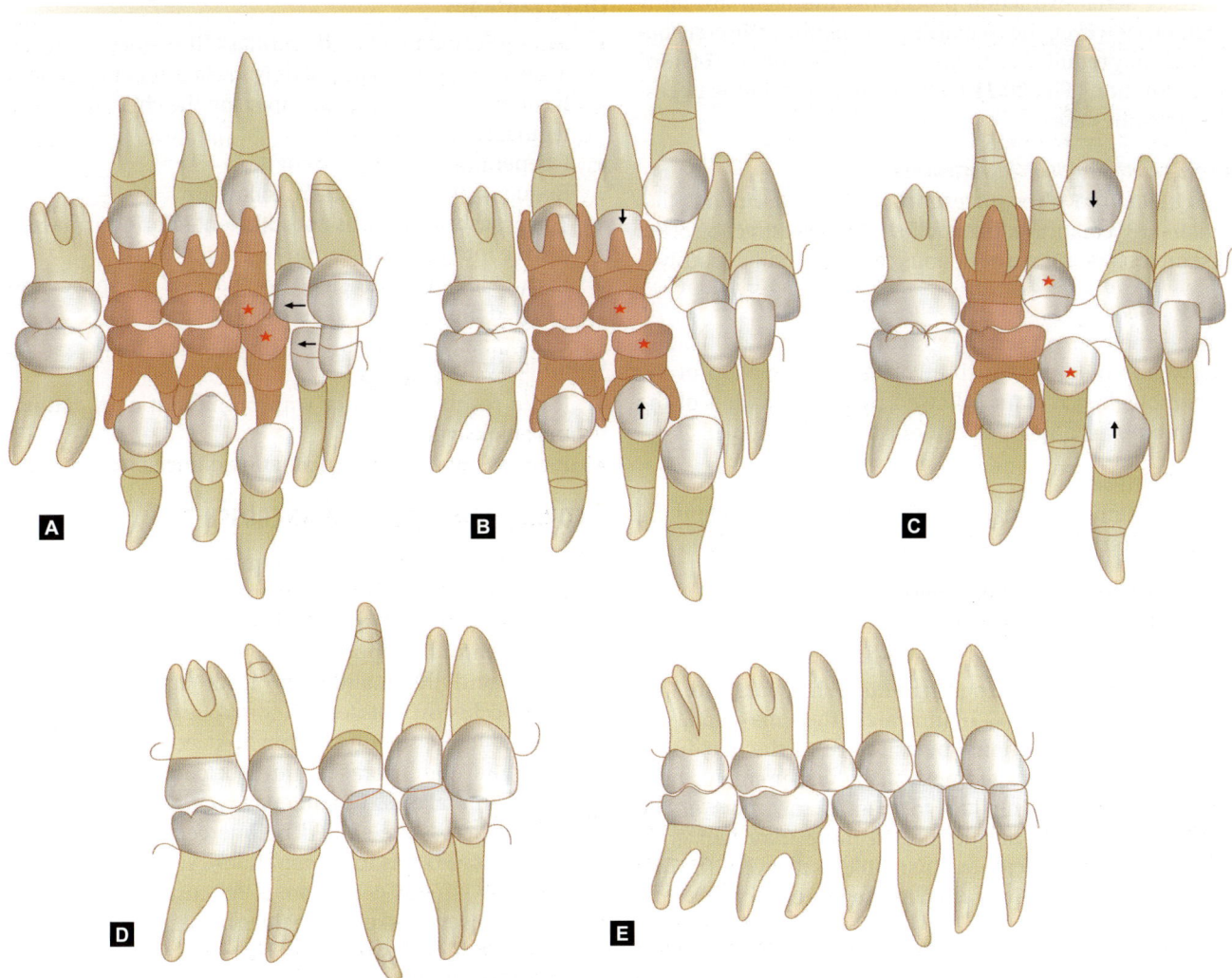

**Figs 20.1A to E:** Dewel's method of serial extraction. (A) Deciduous canines are extracted to create space for the alignment of the incisors, (B) Deciduous first molars are extracted to facilitate eruption of first premolars, (C) First premolars are extracted to facilitate the eruption of permanent canines, (D) Favorable eruption of canines after the removal of first premolars, (E) Proper occlusion after minimal period of fixed orthodontic mechanotherapy

The main objective of extracting primary canines is to establish the integrity of upper and lower incisors. This prevents the development of lingual crossbite of maxillary laterals and resultant mesial migration of maxillary canines.

### Step 2: Extraction of deciduous first molars

In this step, deciduous first molars are extracted when first premolars reach half of the root length as evidenced by radiographs. This would be some 12 months after the extraction of deciduous canines at around 9-10 years of age. The objective of deciduous first molar extraction is to accelerate the eruption of first premolars. This ensures that the first premolars emerge into oral cavity, before the eruption of permanent canines **(Fig. 20.1B)**.

### Step 3: Extraction of first premolars

In this step, first premolars are extracted as they are emerging into oral cavity and when the permanent canines have developed beyond half of the root length **(Figs 20.1C and D)**.

Extraction of first premolars facilitates proper eruption and alignment of permanent canines

After serial extraction procedure, the teeth are fairly aligned. However, the establishment of proper intercuspation usually requires orthodontic mechanotherapy of minimal duration **(Fig. 20.1E)**, although it may not be necessary in some cases.

#### Tweed's Method (1966) (Extraction of D4C)

This method involves the extraction of the deciduous first molars at 8 years of age. This is followed by the extraction of the first premolars and the deciduous canines, simultaneously.

#### Nance Method

Nance method of serial extraction is the modification of Tweed's method, which involves the extraction of the deciduous first molars, followed by the extraction of the first premolars and the deciduous canines.

#### Grewe's Method

Grewe's method of serial extraction is based on the planning of extraction sequence for different clinical conditions.

### Class I Malocclusion with Premature Loss of a Mandibular Deciduous Canine

Class I malocclusion with premature loss of a mandibular deciduous canine will result in midline shift, when the arch length discrepancy is 5-10 mm/arch, then the remaining deciduous canines should be extracted as the deciduous first molars are extracted next, if the first premolar have their roots more than half formed. If the roots of the first premolars are not developed more than half, then extractions of the deciduous first molar is delayed. The first premolars should be extracted as they emerge.

### Class I Malocclusion with Severe Mandibular Anterior Crowding

Deciduous canines are extracted, when there is arch length deficiency and more than 5 mm per quadrant. The deciduous first molars are extracted next on completion of at least half of first premolar root formation and the extraction of first premolars follow as they erupt into the oral cavity.

### Class I Malocclusion where Minimal Mandibular Anterior Crowding is 6-10 mm Arch Deficiency

In such conditions, the first premolars are extracted. The deciduous first molars are extracted when the roots of the premolars are more than half formed, as this would in turn result in premature loss or eruption of the first premolar as soon as the first premolars erupt into the oral cavity; these are extracted followed by deciduous canines. If this is bound to be the eruption of permanent canines before that of first premolar, then the deciduous canine is extracted first followed by the extraction of the deciduous first molar and enucleation of the first premolar.

#### Advantages

- It brings about early self-induced alignment of the permanent teeth
- There is improved overall oral health.

#### Disadvantages

- Not indicated for class II and class III malocclusions, if at all, extraction is carried only in class II in upper arch
- It can have psychological impact on the child, if total 12 teeth have to be extracted
- Deepening of bite can occur
- Requires prolonged patient follow-up
- The procedure alone is not sufficient to bring impacted canine into proper position
- Early extraction can lead to the loss of space and delayed the eruption of permanent teeth.

#### Complications

- It can result in flat face with prominent chin. Patient may look aged
- It can result in lingual inclination of incisors.

## CORRECTION OF DEVELOPING CROSSBITE

Occasionally, even with adequate arch-length, the maxillary lateral incisors erupt too far palatally and their crowns are forced completely to the palatal side of the crown of the opposing mandibular incisors as the maxillary and the mandibular teeth are brought into habitual occlusion. This tendency may be more commonly manifested in the so-called, straight-faced individual with less overbite than average, and is of course seen where there is a familial class III tendency.

Anterior crossbite should be intercepted and treated at an early stage so as to prevent future severe dentofacial abnormality. If the condition is left untreated, it may develop into severe skeletal malocclusion, which requires invasive orthodontic treatment. Therefore, it is desirable to intercept and treat the crossbite, as soon as it is recognized.

Anterior crossbites can be classified into following three types:
1. Dentoalveolar anterior crossbite

2. Skeletal anterior crossbite.
3. Functional anterior crossbite.

### Dentoalveolar Anterior Crossbite

Anterior crossbite is the condition in which one or more upper anterior teeth are in lingual relation to the lower anterior teeth and is referred as dentoalveolar anterior crossbite. Dentoalveolar anterior crossbite is often associated with single tooth rather than multiple teeth and usually occurs due to over retained deciduous canine teeth that deflects the erupting permanent tooth palatally. Dentoalveolar anterior crossbites are best treated using tongue blade therapy, Catlan's appliance and "Z" spring with posterior bite plane (Ref. Chapter 40).

The developing crossbite can be intercepted by use of a tongue blade. The child is instructed to place a tongue blade in such a manner that it rests on the lower incisors opposing the tooth in crossbite. With lower incisor margin as a fulcrum, the oral portion of the tongue blade is rotated upwards and forward to engage the lingual surface of the upper incisors **(Figs 20.2A to F)**. The patient is advised to bite with a constant pressure on the wood and at the same time asked to exert a slight but constant pressure with his hand on the blade, so as to prevent tongue blade displacement. The tongue blade therapy is advised for an hour or two, in a day. 10-14 days of practice is usually sufficient to deflect the lingually erupting maxillary incisors into proper relationship.

### Skeletal Anterior Crossbite

Skeletal anterior crossbite usually occurs as a result of skeletal discrepancies in the maxilla (retrognathic) or the mandible (prognathic). Skeletal anterior crossbites in growing patients can be treated by the use of either myofunctional appliances such as Frankel III appliance or orthopaedic appliances such as chin-cup appliance. On the other hand, non-growing patiens can be treated by either mandibular set back or maxillary advancement surgical procedures.

### Functional Anterior Crossbite

Functional anterior crossbites **(Figs 20.3 A to I)** is a type of pseudo class III malocclusion in which the mandible is forced in a forward position of its true centric relation. These type of crossbites are mainly due to occlusal prematurities. Functional crossbites are treated by eliminating occlusal prematurities. Interception of anterior crossbite is shown in **Table 20.1**.

### CONTROL OF ABNORMAL ORAL HABITS

Correction of deleterious oral habits, such as thumb sucking **(Figs 20.4A to C)**, tongue thrusting **(Figs 20.5A to C)**, mouth breathing, etc. should be undertaken as a part of interceptive orthodontic procedure. Not all oral habits damage the dentoalveolar structures and thus, do not require orthodontic interventions. If definite damage due to any oral habits exists, then thorough case history should be recorded.

The optimal time for appliances placement is between the age of 3½ and 4½ years. The oral habits can be intercepted by either removable orthodontic appliances, such as removable appliance with crib, oral screen or fixed orthodontic appliance, such as fixed mechanotherapy with a fixed crib.

### PROXIMAL STRIPPING OF DECIDUOUS TEETH

Proximal stripping of first or second deciduous molars often require to facilitate the eruption of adjacent succedaneous permanent teeth into normal occlusion. Proximal stripping of mesial surface of mandibular deciduous first molar can be of help in preventing mandibular anterior crowding. When there is lack of space for maxillary canine to erupt, then space can be created by disking of second deciduous molar, which leads to distal drifting of the first premolar creating space for the canine to erupt.

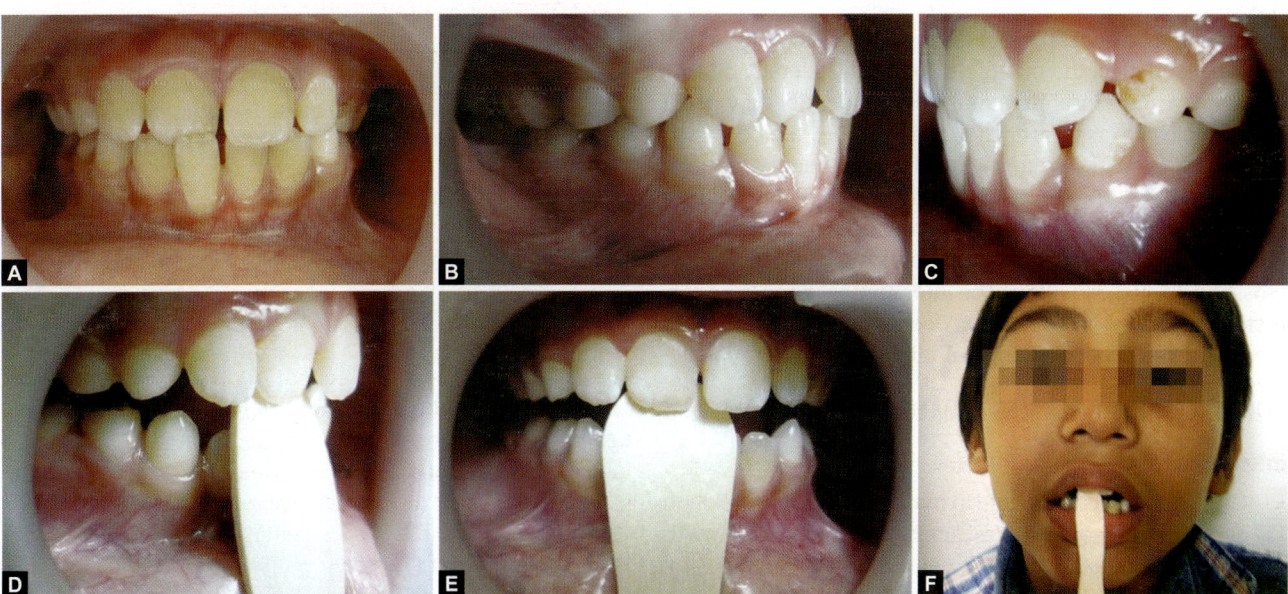

**Figs 20.2A to F:** Tongue blade therapy

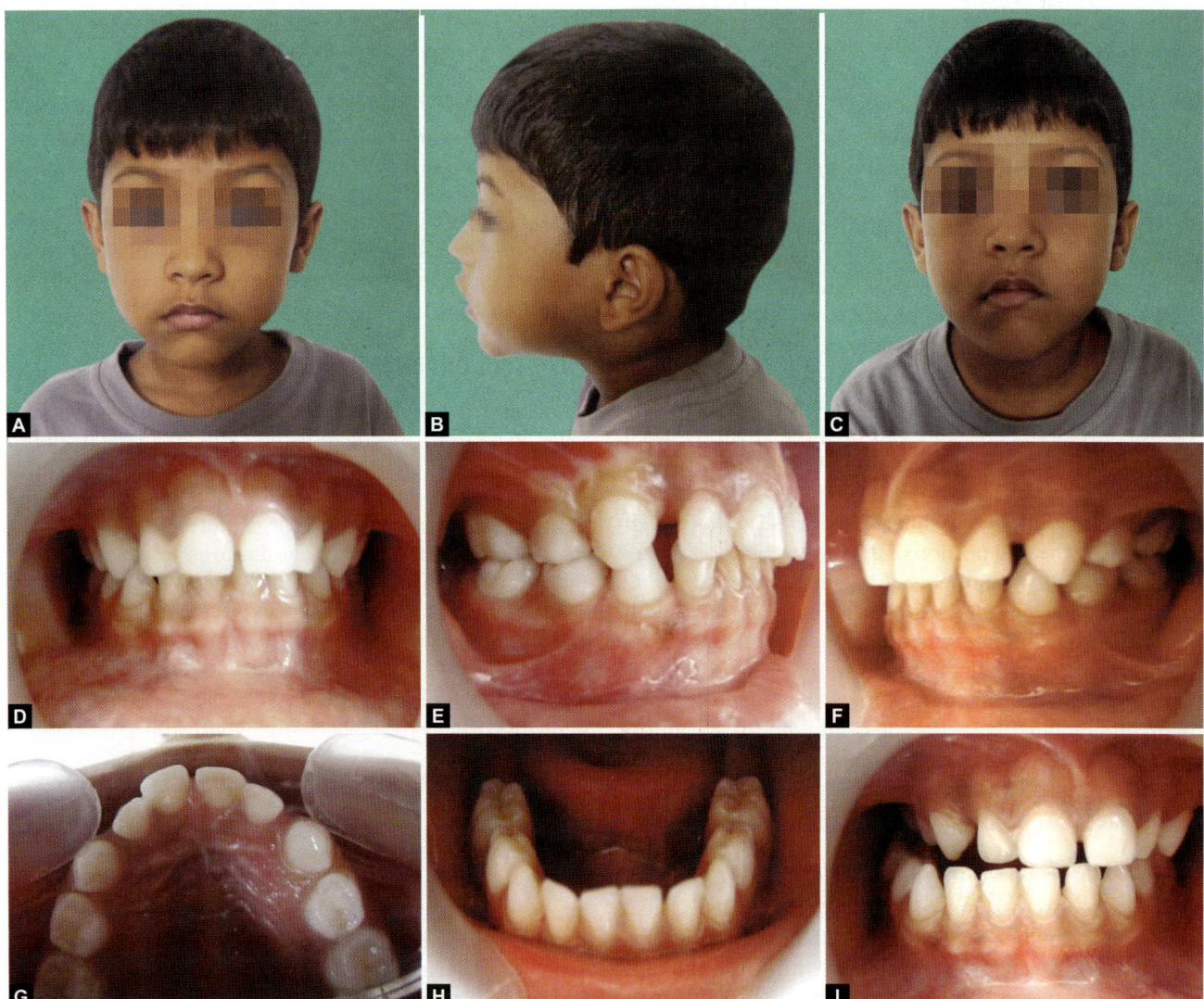

**Figs 20.3A to I:** Functional anterior crossbite. (A to H) Normal relationship of upper and lower arches, (I) Functional anterior crossbite

## CORRECTION OF OCCLUSAL INTERFERENCES

Occlusal interferences present during the development of occlusion can deflect the mandible anteriorly, laterally or posteriorly. Once occlusal prematurities are identified by using either occlusal wax or articulating paper, they are corrected by the reduction of crown height using pear-shaped stone in a center-angled handpiece. Occasionally, a lingually placed tooth particularly a maxillary lateral incisor or cuspid can deflect the mandible either anteriorly or posteriorly resulting in crossbite. In such situations, the interferences cannot be corrected by occlusal equilibration. Mechanotherapy will help in correcting the malocclusion by eliminating the interference.

## INTERCEPTION OF SKELETAL MALOCCLUSION

### Interception of Class II Malocclusion

- Class II malocclusion due to maxillary excessive growth can be intercepted by restricting the maxillary growth by the use of face bow with head gear
- Class II malocclusion due to mandible insufficiency can be intercepted by the use of myofunctional appliances such as Frankel II or orthopaedic appliance.

**Table 20.1:** Types of anterior crossbite and its treatment

| Type of anterior crossbite | Treatment |
|---|---|
| **Dentoalveolar Anterior Crossbite** | |
| • Developing anterior crossbite<br>• Existing anterior crossbite | • Tongue blade therapy<br>• Catlan's appliance<br>• Removable orthodontic appliance with finger springs and posterior bite plane for bite opening<br>• Fixed orthodontic appliance |
| **Skeletal Anterior Crossbite** | • Myofunctional appliances (FR-III appliance of Frankel) |
| • In growing patient<br>• In non-growing patient | • Orthopaedic appliances (Chin-cup appliance)<br>• Mandibular set back or maxillary advancement |
| **Functional Anterior Crossbite** | • Eliminating occlusal prematurities |

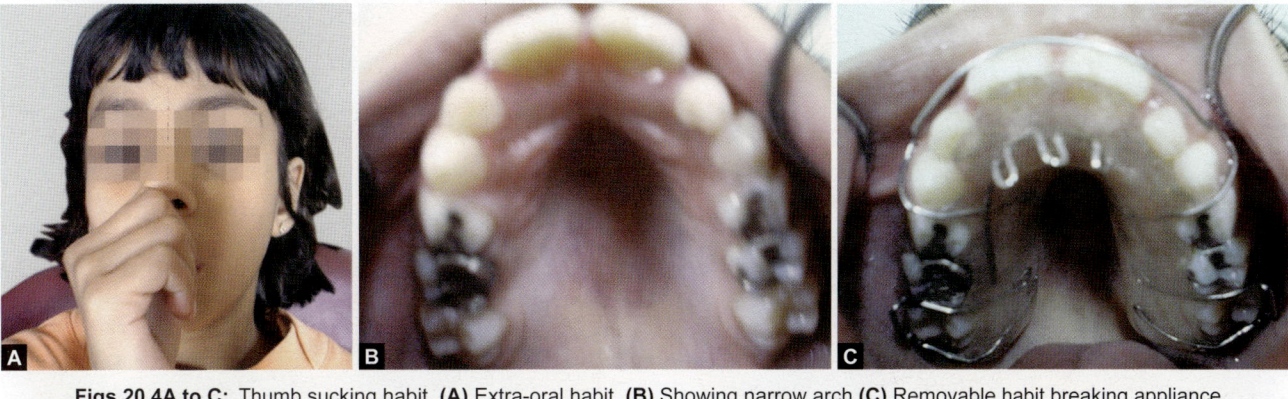

**Figs 20.4A to C:** Thumb sucking habit. **(A)** Extra-oral habit, **(B)** Showing narrow arch **(C)** Removable habit breaking appliance

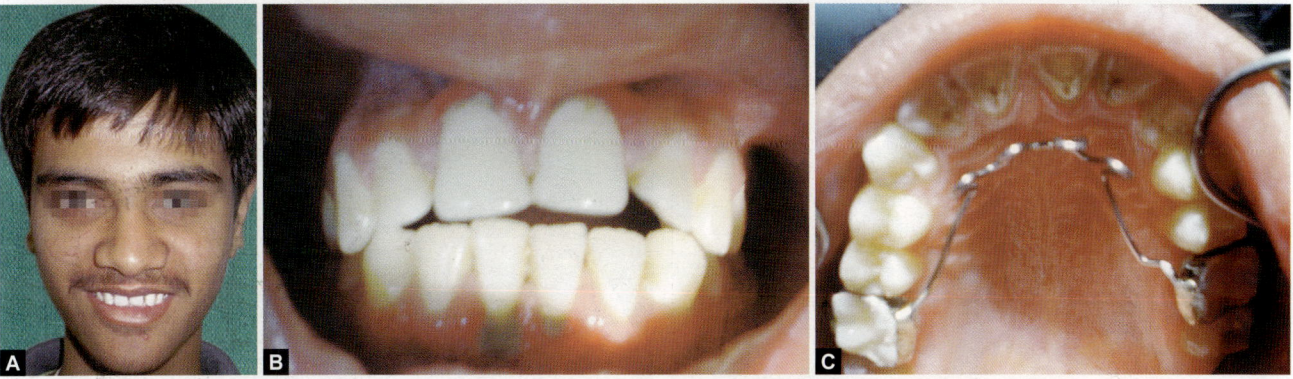

**Figs 20.5A to C:** **(A)** Tongue thrusting habit; **(B)** Open bite; **(C)** Fixed crib to curb the habit

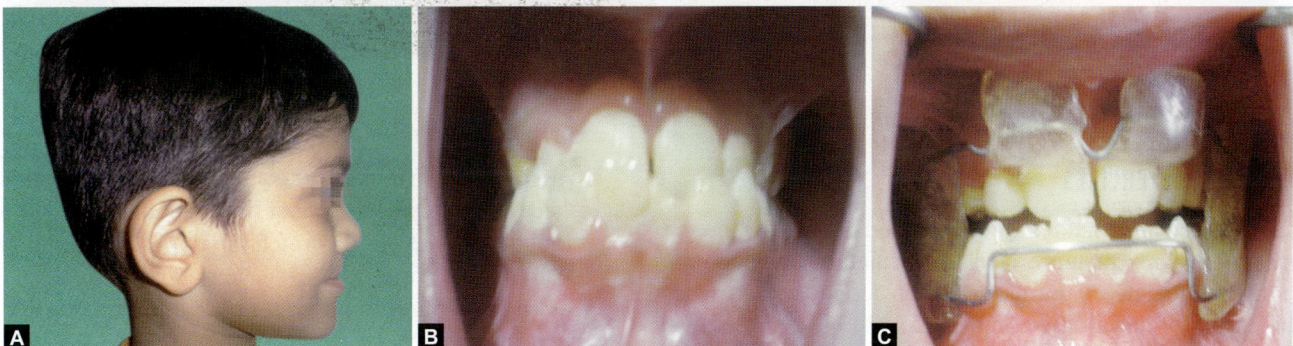

**Figs 20.6A to C:** Class III malocclusion due to maxillary deficiency can be intercepted by the use of Frankel III appliance

### Interception of Class III Malocclusion

- Class III malocclusion due to mandibular prognathism can be intercepted by restricting the mandibular growth by use of chin-cup with head gear
- Class III malocclusion due to maxillary deficiency can be intercepted by the use of myofunctional appliances such as Frankel II **(Figs 20.6A to C)** or orthopaedic appliance.

## SPACE REGAINING

### Space Regaining Using Cantilever Spring

Space lost by the mesial drifting of permanent molar and distal drifting of deciduous first molar, when second deciduous molar is lost prematurely, can be regained by the use of two finger springs, one on the mesial of first permanent molar and another on distal of first deciduous molar with retentive clasp (Adam's clasp) on incisors. The space is regained by the distalisation of molar by the use of removable orthodontic appliance with finger springs **(Fig. 20.7)**.

### Space Regaining Using Jack Screw

Space can also be regained by the use of removable orthodontic appliance that incorporates jack screw in such a way that an increase in arch length is obtained by the distalisation of the molar **(Fig. 20.8)**.

### Gerber Space Regainer

A seamless orthodontic molar band or stainless steel crown is selected for the tooth to be distalised. Gerber space regainer consists of a "U" shaped hollow tubing **(Figs 20.9A to D)**.

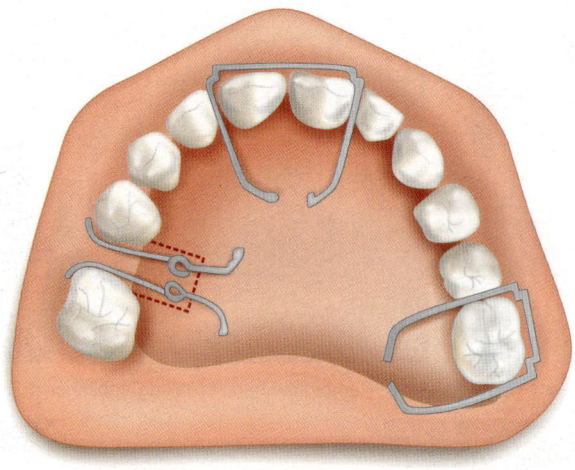

**Fig. 20.7:** The space regained by distalisation of molar

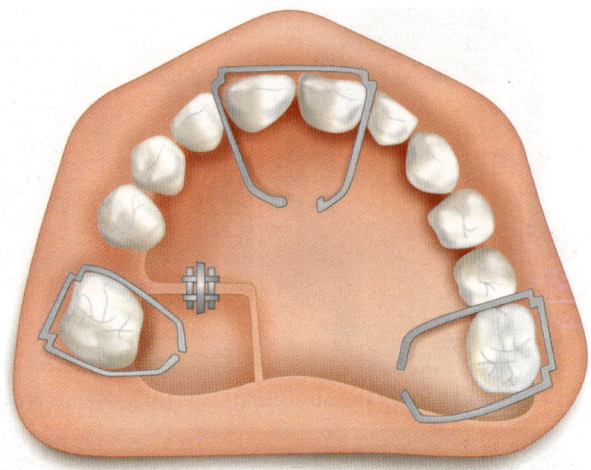

**Fig. 20.8:** Space regainer using Jack Screw

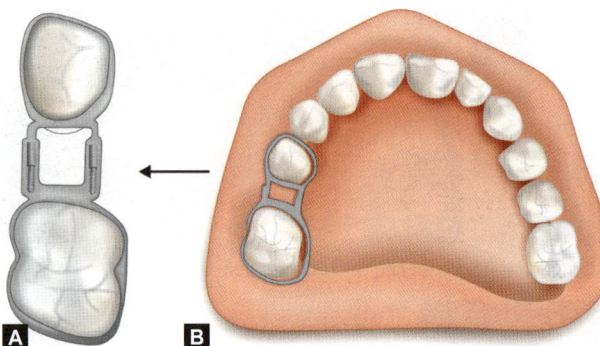

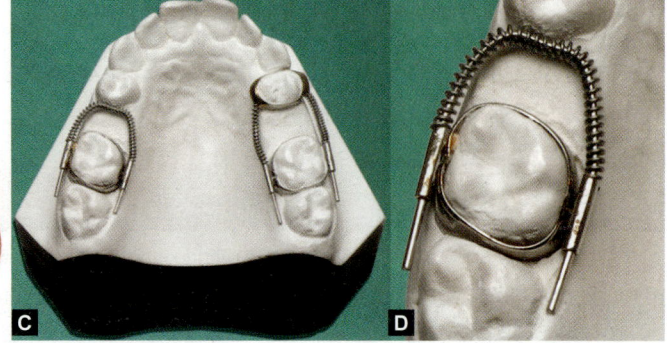

**Figs 20.9A to D:** Gerber's space regainer

## MUSCLE EXERCISES

Dentoalveolar structures are surrounded on sides by the soft tissue envelope made of orofacial musculature. Development and maintenance of normal occlusion depends on presence of normal orofacial muscular balance. Muscle exercises help in improving aberrant muscle activity.

### Exercise for the Masseter Muscle

Exercise of masseter muscle is done by asking the patient to clench teeth and to count from 1 to 10, and this is repeated for some duration of time.

### Exercises for Pterygoid Muscle

Exercises for pterygoid muscle are advised in patients with class II malocclusion where patient is asked to protrude the mandible as much as he can and then retract. The exercise should be repeated till the person is tired. Developing this habit helps in keeping the mandible in its correct position.

### Exercises for the Lips (Circumoral Musculatures)

A number of exercises have been advocated for the lips and circumoral musculature in patients with hypotonic lips and short upper lips:

- Stretching of the upper lip to maintain lip seal is an important therapeutic measure in patients having short hypotonic lips. To aid in the stretching, the patient is asked to hold a piece of paper between the lips
- Patient can be asked to stretch the upper lip inferiorly towards the chin
- Holding and pumping of water back and forth behind the lips
- Lip massaging.
- Button pull exercise
  - A button of one and half inch is taken and a thread passed through the button hole. Patient is asked to place the button behind the lips and pull the thread, while restricting it from being pulled out by using lip pressure.
- Tug of war exercise
  - This involves use of two buttons, with one kept behind the lips while the other button is held by another person to pull the thread.
- Playing a reed musical instrument
  - Playing a reed musical instrument produces fine lip tonicity.

### Exercise for Tongue

#### One Elastic Swallow

Use: Correction of positioning of the tongue.

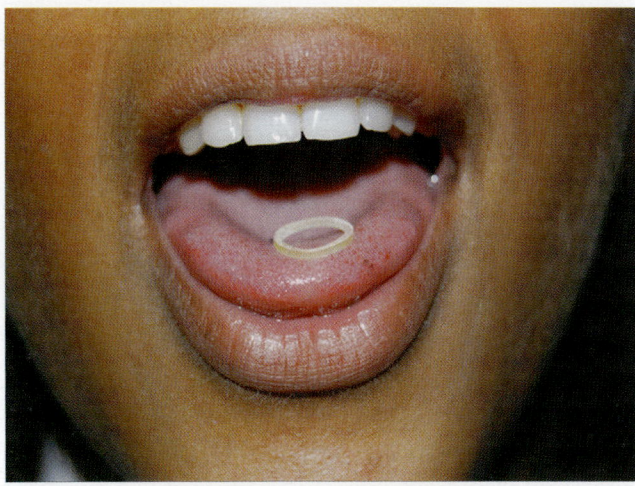

Fig. 20.10: One elastic swallow

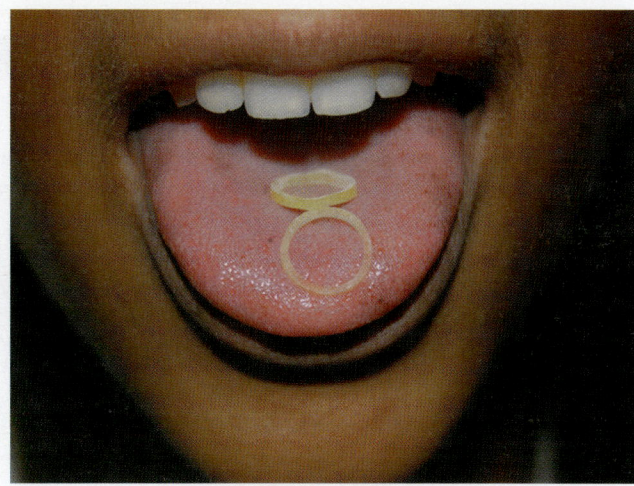

Fig. 20.11: Two elastic swallow

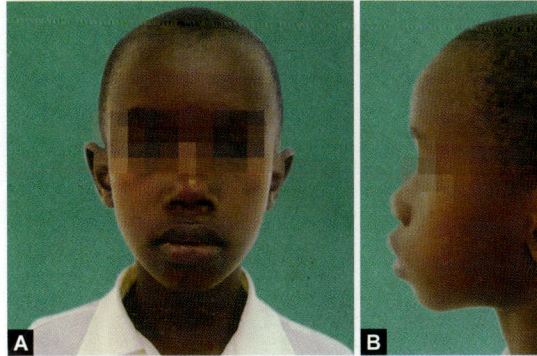
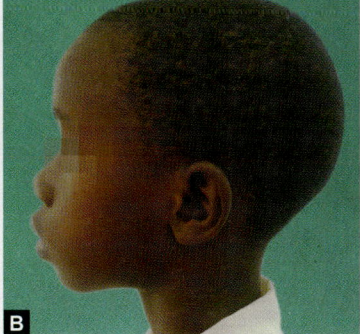
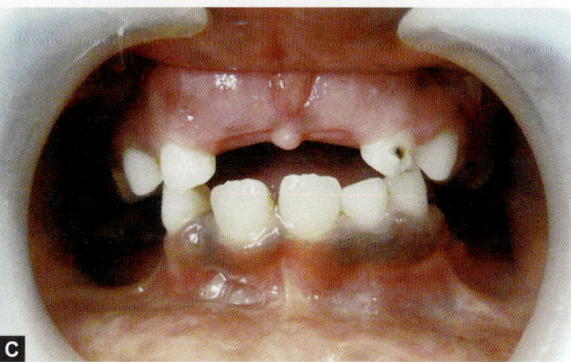

Figs 20.12A to C: A case indicated for surgical interceptive procedure involving incising the soft tissue over the alveolar ridge to facilitate the eruption of underlying permanent incisors

Procedure: Patient is asked to keep elastic of 5/16" on the tip of tongue and hold the tongue against the patient's rugae area and swallow **(Fig. 20.10)**.

### Two Elastic Swallow

Two elastics of 5/16", are replaced over the tongue, one in the midline and the other on the tip and the patient is asked to swallow with the elastic in position **(Fig. 20.11)**.

### The Tongue Holds Exercise

A 5/16" elastic is positioned over the tongue in a designated spot for a prescribed period of time with the lips closed. The patient is then asked to swallow with elastic in place and lips apart.

### The Hold Pulls Exercise

Use: The hold pull exercise helps in stretching the lingual frenum.
Procedure: The tip of the tongue and the midpoint are made to contact the palate and the mandible is gradually opened.

## REMOVAL OF SOFT AND BONY BARRIER

Removal of soft tissue and bony barrier is a surgical interceptive orthodontic procedure, which involves excision of the soft tissue **(Figs 20.12A to C)** and removal of bone, covering the crown of the unerupted tooth, to create the space so that the tooth can erupt without any hindrance. The extent of soft tissue and bone removal should be such that the greatest diameter of the crown of the tooth should be able to easily emerge. The surgical wound is given a cement dressing for a period of two weeks.

## BIBLIOGRAPHY

1. Ackerman JL, Proffit WR. Preventive and interceptive orthodontics: Strong theory work in practice. Angle Orthod 1980;50:75-86.
2. Dewel BF. A critical analysis of serial extraction in orthodontic treatment. Am J Orthod 1959;45:424-55.
3. Dewel BF. Serial extraction: its limitations and contraindications in orthodontic treatment. Am J Orthod 1967;53:904-21.
4. Dewel BF. Serial extraction in orthodontics: indications, objectives and treatment procedures. Am J Orthod 1954;40:906-26.
5. Norton A, Wickwire Na, Gellin ME. Space management in mixed dentition. J Dent Child 1975;42:0112-8.
6. Wright GZ, Kennedyt DB. Space control in the primary and mixed dentitions. Dent Clin North Am 1978;22:579-601.

## EXAM-ORIENTED QUESTIONS

### Long Essay or Long Questions

1. Interceptive orthodontics
2. Define and enumerate various interceptive orthodontic measures and write any two measures in detail.
3. Enumerate various interceptive orthodontic measures and describe serial extraction in detail.

### Short Essay or Long Notes

1. Interceptive orthodontics and describe serial extraction in detail
2. As an Interceptive orthodontic measure how to intercept developing crossbites
3. Grewe's method of serial extraction.

### Short Notes

1. Space regainer
2. Gerber's space regainer
3. Muscle exercise
4. Indication and contraindication of serial extraction
5. Interception of skeletal malocclusion.

# CHAPTER OVERVIEW

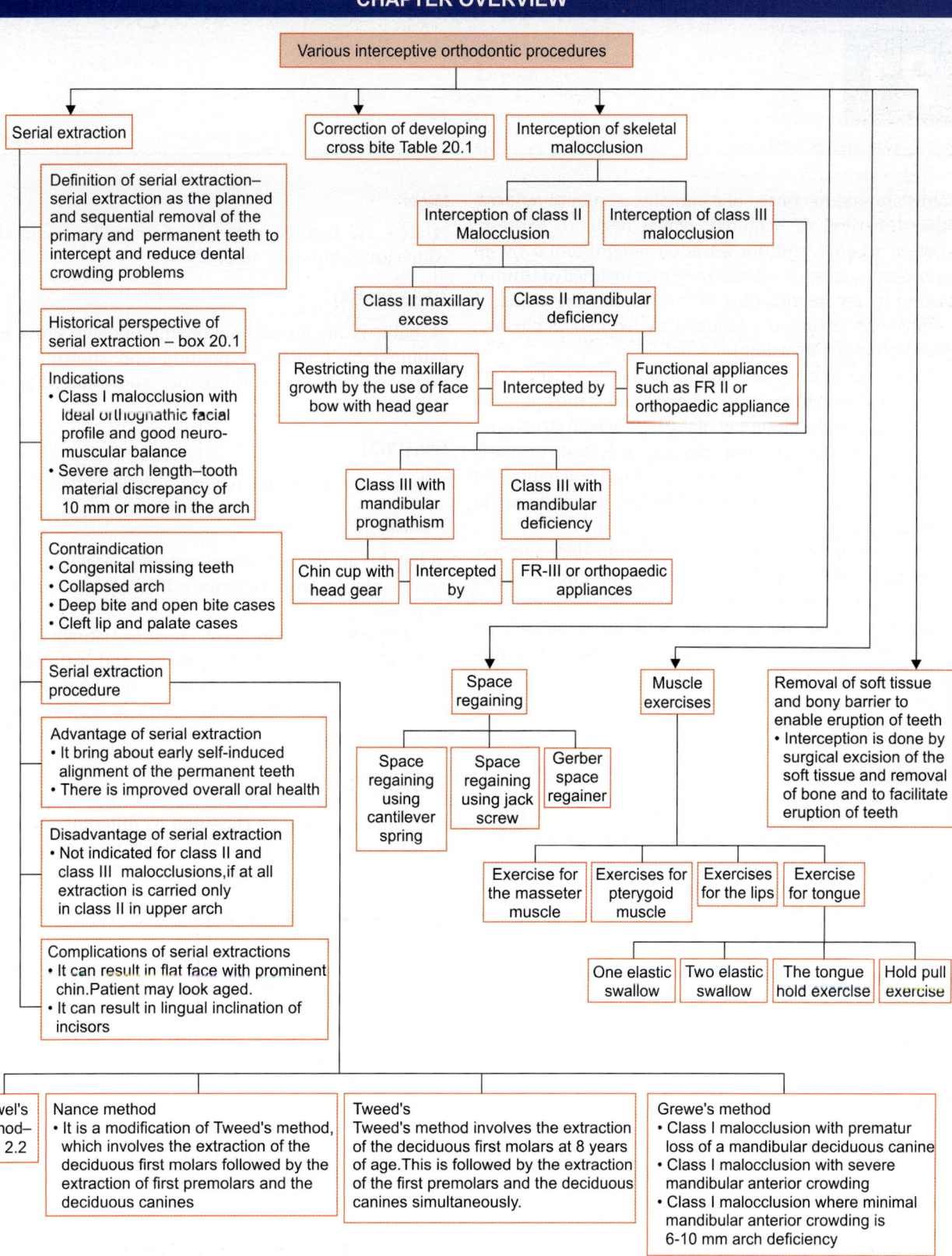

CHAPTER 20

Interceptive Orthodontics

205

# CHAPTER 21

# Oral Habits and their Management

*Phulari BS*

Habits are said to consist of a complex system of reflexes, either inherited or acquired, which begin to express/function when a child or an adult is confronted by an appropriate stimulus. Habits are either instinctive (thumb sucking in an infant), obstructive (mouth breathing in a child with enlarged adenoids) or learned behavioral patterns (tongue thrusting).

Most oral habits exert abnormal forces on the teeth and perioral structures, thus, adversely affect the optimum growth and the development of the dentofacial structures. The facial bones are not densely calcified in early childhood, so the abnormal pressures from oral habits can create abnormal developmental forces, which result in malocclusion.

Deleterious oral habits, such as thumb/digit sucking, lip sucking and biting, tongue thrusting, mouth breathing contribute directly or indirectly to the occurrence of different types of malocclusion and an imbalance of facial components, thus affecting esthetics, phonetics, mastication and swallowing. The consequences can be grave and immediate measures should be undertaken to break the deleterious habits.

## DEFINITIONS

A number of definitions are given by various authors. Some of the widely used definitions are given below.

### Dorland (1957)

"Habit can be defined as a fixed or constant practice established by frequent repetition."

### Buttersworth (1961)

"Habit can be defined as a frequent or constant practice or acquired tendency, which has been fixed by frequent repetition."

### Maslow (1949)

"Habit is a formed reaction that is resistant to change whether useful or harmful, depending to the degree to which it interferes with the child's physical, emotional and social functions."

### Mathewson (1982)

"Oral habits are learned patterns of muscular contractions."

### William James

"A new pathway of discharge formed in the brain by which certain incoming currents lead to escape."

### Moyer

"Habits are learned patterns of muscular contractions, which are complex in nature."

### Johnson (1938)

"A habit is an inclination or aptitude for some action acquired by frequent repetition and showing itself in increased facility to performance and reduced power of resistance."

### Finn (1972)

"A habit is an act, which is socially unacceptable."

### Stedman

"A habit is an act, behavioral response, practice or custom established in one's repertoire by frequent repetition of same act."

"Habit is an autonomic response to a situation acquired normally as the result of repetition and learning strictly applicable to only motor responses. At each repetition, the act becomes less conscious and can lead to an unconscious habit."

## CLASSIFICATION

Oral habits have been classified by different authors in a number of ways. Some of the widely used classifications are given below.

### Useful and Harmful Habits—William James (1923)

*Useful Habits*

These include habits that are essential for normal physiologic function.

For example, correct tongue posture, proper respiration and deglutition.

*Harmful Habits*

These include habits that have a harmful effect on the teeth and their supporting structures.

For example, thumb/digit sucking, tongue thrusting, mouth breathing, etc.

### Empty and Meaningful Habits—Klein (1971)

*Unintentional/Empty Habits*

These include habits that are not associated with any deep-rooted psychological problems.

For example, chin propping, abnormal pillowing, etc.

### Intentional/Meaningful Habits
These are habits that have a psychological basis.
For example, digit-sucking and lip-and nail-biting.

## Compulsive and Noncompulsive Habits–Finn

### Compulsive Habits
These are habits that have acquired a fixation in the child to the extent that he retreats to the practice of this habit whenever his security is threatened by events occurring around him. Compulsive habits express a deep-seated emotional need and attempts to correct them may increase the anxiety of the child.

### Non-compulsive Habits
These are the habits, which are easily learned and dropped from the child's behavioral pattern as he matures. Behavioral modification can replace the undesirable habits with the adaptation of new socially acceptable ones, without inducing anxiety in the child.

## Pressure, Nonpressure and Biting Habits

### Pressure Habits
These include habits that apply abnormal pressure on the teeth and their supporting structures.
For example, thumb/digit, lip and tongue sucking.

### Nonpressure Habits
These habits, although detrimental to the oral health, do not apply direct pressure/force on the teeth and their supporting structures.
For example, mouth breathing.

### Biting Habits
These include abnormal biting habits.
For example, lip, pencil and nail-biting.

## Kingsley (1956)
Kingsley classified the habits according to their nature as:
- Functional habits: Mouth breathing
- Muscular habits: Tongue-thrusting, cheek/lip-biting
- Combined muscular habits: Thumb- and finger-sucking
- Postural habits: Chin propping and abnormal pillowing

## Physiologic and Pathologic Habits

### Physiologic Habits
Habits that are required for normal physiologic functioning.
For example, nasal breathing and sucking during infancy.

### Pathologic Habits
Habits that are pursued due to pathologic reasons.
For example, mouth breathing developed secondary to deviated nasal septum (DNS)/enlarged adenoids.

## MECHANISM OF ACTION

An infant is born with some elementary reflexes whose pattern and order are inherited, e.g. sucking is an innate reflex in humans. On the other hand, a habit whose pattern and order are acquired, develops from constant repetition of the act, e.g. lateral tongue-thrusting habit developed due to extraction space in the posterior segment.

At the beginning, the infant makes an effort by frequent learning and practice, later on the muscles start responding more readily.

It has been observed that the unconscious pattern of a habit develops in response to five sources, namely—
  i. Instinct
  ii. Insufficient/incorrect outlet of energy
  iii. Pain or discomfort
  iv. Abnormal physical size of anatomic parts
  v. Imitation of/imposition by parents or others.

## THUMB SUCKING

Thumb/finger sucking collectively called as digit sucking **(Fig. 21.1A)** is one of the most commonly observed oral habits among children. Although presence of such a habit in first two years of life is considered as a part of normal development of the child, its persistence beyond preschool years would have profound deleterious effects on the developing dentofacial structures and occlusion and thus can lead to malocclusion.

The facial bones are not densely calcified in early childhood, so the sucking pressure between the maxillary and mandibular teeth creates an abnormal developmental force, which results in malocclusion **(Fig. 21.1B)**.

### Definition
- **Gellin (1978):** "Thumb sucking is defined as the placement of thumb or one or more fingers in varying depth into the mouth."
- **Moyer:** "Repeated and forceful sucking of thumb with associated strong buccal and lip contractions."

An understanding of the normal sucking reflex essential for survival of the infant is needed to appreciate the etiology and effects of abnormal sucking habits.

### Sucking Reflex

Sucking is the first coordinated muscular activity of the infant, which meets both nutritive, as well as psychological needs in the early years of life. Sucking is a reflex process, occurring in the oral stage of development and can be seen as early as 29th week of intrauterine life. It may disappear spontaneously during normal growth between the ages of 1 and 3½ years.

Apart from seeking nutritional satisfaction during breast/bottle feeding, infants also experience pleasurable stimuli from lips, tongue and oral mucosa and learn to associate these with enjoyable sensations, such as satisfaction of hunger, fondling and closeness of a parent. Babies who are restricted from sucking due to a disease or other factors become restless and irritable. This deprivation may motivate the infant to suck thumb/finger or the object which is most accessible for additional gratification.

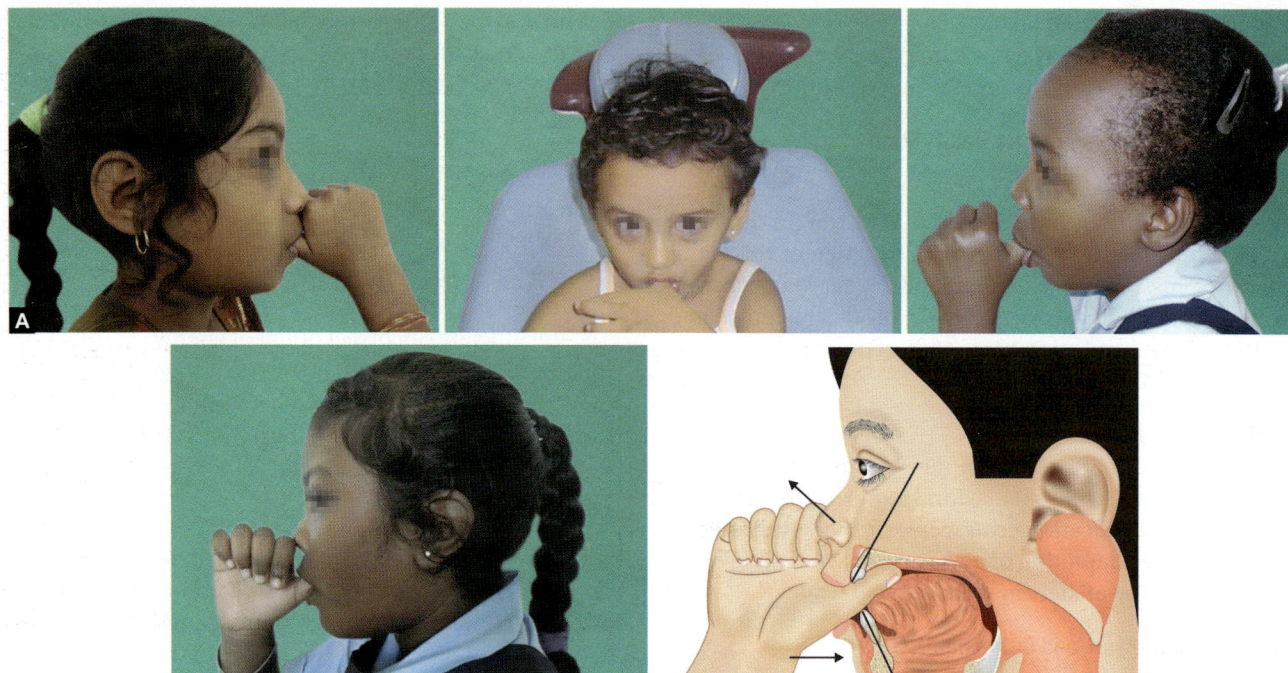

**Figs 21.1A and B:** Thumb-sucking habit

There are essentially two forms of sucking:
- Nutritive sucking
- Non-nutritive sucking.

### Nutritive Sucking

It is the sucking observed during breast/bottle feeding, which provides nutrition to the infant.

***During breastfeeding:*** Sucking by the infant stimulates the lactate glands and therein flow of milk. Breastfeeding stimulates circumoral musculature, tongue activity and protrusive mandibular movements, which are conductive to the normal development of teeth and jaws. The infant feels the warmth and security of being close to the mother.

In breastfeeding, the gum pads are apart, the tongue is placed in a plunger-like fashion so that the tongue and lower lip are in constant contact and the mandible moves up and down rhythmically and in forward and backward motion, while buccinator muscle alternatively contracts and relaxes.

***During bottle-feeding:*** Two forms of nipples are available for bottle-feeding. The physiologic nipple is preferred as it stimulates normal functional development and oral muscular activity.

### Conventional/Nonphysiologic Nipple

- Milk flow is continuous and, thus, does not allow muscles to work hard **(Fig. 21.2)**.
- Warmth associated with breastfeeding is lacking and the physiology of suckling is not duplicated.
- Mouth is held open more widely and lip seal is difficult with greater demand on buccinator.
- Pumping action of tongue and raising and lowering and rhythmic forward and backward movement of mandible are reduced.
- Suckling becomes sucking, with no stimulation of lower jaw exercise as seen in suckling.
- More air is gulped down during feeding.
- Milk is almost squirted into the throat, instead of being brought back by the peristaltic-like action of tongue and cheeks.
- Abnormal muscle pressures are exerted as a compensatory response to the excessive opening movement required.

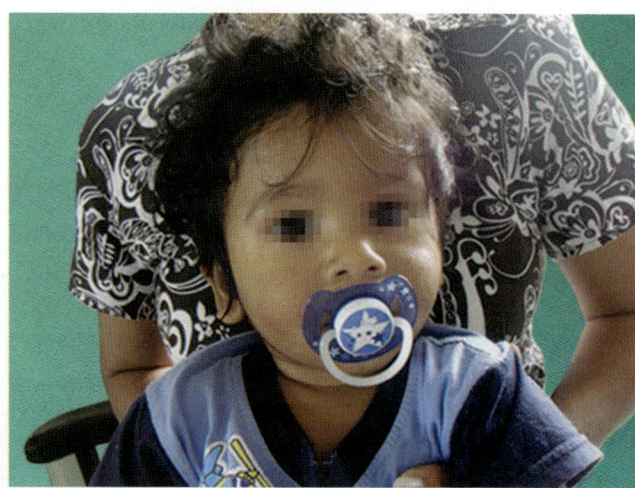

**Fig. 21.2:** Conventional/Nonphysiologic nipple

## Physiologic Nipple
- It closely simulates natural suckling activity.
- Lip seal is improved as the flat nipple base is flexible and adapts to the contour of the lips.
- Child has to exercise the tongue and lower jaw to squeeze milk.
- Milk flows down by peristaltic action of the tongue and cheeks.
- Example of physiologic nipple is Nuk sauger nipple.

## Non-nutritive Sucking (NNS)
As described by Johnson and Larson (1993), non-nutritive sucking habit (NNS) is the earliest sucking habit adopted by infants in response to frustration and to satisfy their need for contact. Children who are deprived of unrestricted breast-feeding and do not have an access to pacifier may develop digit/sucking habit in order to satisfy their emotional needs.

## Classification

### Cook (1958)
Cook classified thumb-sucking habit into following three patterns **(Flowchart 21.1)**:
a. Alpha group
b. Beta group
c. Gamma group.

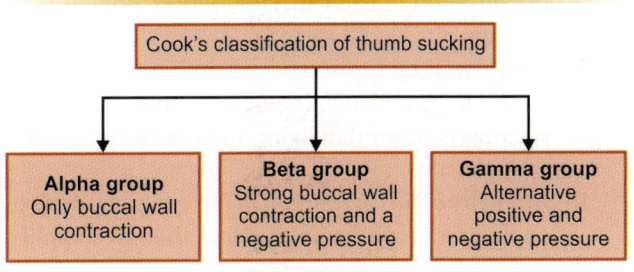
**Flowchart 21.1:** Cook's classification of thumb sucking

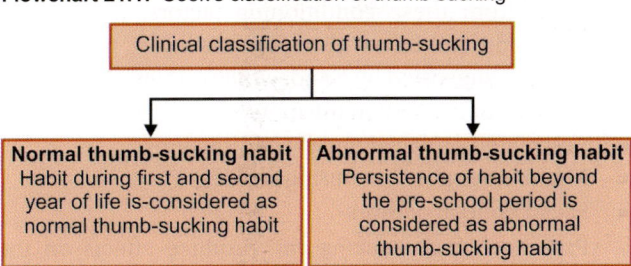
**Flowchart 21.2:** Clinical classification of thumb sucking

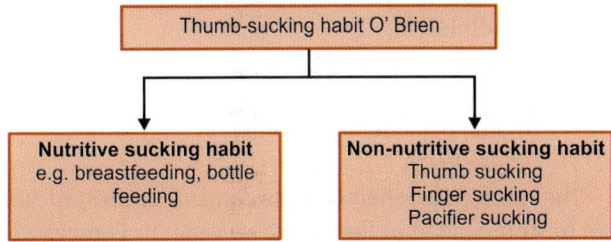
**Flowchart 21.3:** Thumb-sucking habit by O' Brien

## Clinical Classification of Thumb Sucking
Based on clinical observation, thumb sucking can be classified into following two types **(Flowchart 21.2)**:
1. Normal thumb sucking
2. Abnormal thumb sucking
   a. Physiological
   b. Habitual

Normal thumb-sucking habit is usually seen to disappear as the child matures. If not intercepted, this can cause deleterious effects on dentofacial structures.

Abnormal thumb-sucking habit is further classified into habitual and psychological habits.

### By O' Brien (1996)
O' Brien classified the habit into nutritive and non-nutritive **(Flowchart 21.3)**.

### Subtelny Classification (1973)
Subtelny has graded thumb sucking into four types depending on extent of the insertion of thumb into the mouth.

**Type A:** It includes the following features:
- This type is seen in 50% of children.
- In this type, whole digit is placed inside the mouth with the pad of the thumb pressing over the palate.
- Thumb is in contact with maxillary and mandibular anteriors.

**Type B:** It includes the following features:
- This type is seen in almost 13% to 24% of the children.
- In this type, the thumb is placed into the oral cavity without touching the vault of the palate.
- Contact of thumb with maxillary and mandibular anteriors is maintained.

**Type C:** It includes the following features:
- This type is seen in almost 18% of the children.
- In this type, thumb is placed into the mouth just beyond the first joint.
- Thumb is in contact with only maxillary incisors.
- There is no contact with mandibular anteriors.

**Type D**
- This type is seen in almost 6% of children.
- In this type only little portion of th*-umb is placed into the mouth.

### Johnson and Larson's Classification of Thumb Sucking (1993)
They classified non-nutritive sucking (NNS) habits and are given in **Table 21.1**.

## Pathophysiology of NNS Habits
Various theories have been proposed by psychologists to explain nonnutritive digit sucking habit. Some of the theories are given below:

### Psychoanalytical Theory: Sigmond Freud (1905)
- According to this classic theory by Freud, NNS develops from an inherent psychosexual drive, suggesting that all children possess an inherent biologic drive for sucking.

- Digit sucking is a pleasurable erotic stimulation of the lips and mouth, and an infant associates sucking with pleasurable feelings such as satisfaction of hunger, closeness to the parent and a sense of security.
- When subjected to deprivement of unrestrained feeding, feelings of insecurity, and internal conflicts, the child may find solace in sucking the most readily available object, i.e. thumb/finger.

*Oral Drive Theory: Sears and Wise (1982)*
- This theory suggests that the strength of the oral drive depends on how long a child continues to feed by sucking. In other words, prolongation of nursing strengthens the oral drive in the child and thus NNS is the result of prolongation of nursing and not the frustration of weaning.
- This theory agrees with Freud's theory that sucking increases the erotogenesis of the mouth.

*Benjamin's Theory (1962)*
He suggested that thumb sucking manifests from the rooting/placing reflex seen in all mammalian infants. Rooting reflex is the movement of infant's head and tongue towards an object touching his cheek. The object is usually the mother's breast while feeding, but may also be a finger or a pacifier. The rooting reflex usually disappears around 7–8 months of age.

*Oral Gratification Theory: Sheldon (1932)*
If the child is not satisfied with sucking during the feeding period, it will persist as a symptom of an emotional conflict/disturbance in the form of digit sucking.

*Learning Theory*
- Palermo (1956) suggested that thumb sucking arises out of a progressive stimulus-and-reward reaction and would spontaneously disappear unless it becomes an attention getting mechanism.
- Learning theorists believe that thumb sucking is a learned pattern with no underlying psychological basis.
- Recent studies indicate the thumb/finger sucking is a learned pattern in most patients although deeper emotional disturbance may be the cause in some cases.

### Effects of Prolonged Thumb Sucking

There is considerable controversy regarding the potential deleterious effects of thumb/finger sucking and their treatment modalities. However, most agree that if the habit is discontinued well before the permanent incisors erupt, no residual damage to the alignment or occlusion of the teeth is likely to result. In the first 3–4 years of life, the damage to the occlusion is largely confined to the anterior segment. This damage is usually temporary, provided the child starts with a normal occlusion.

Following cessation of the habit, there is generally some spontaneous correction in the form of reduction in open bite and maxillary incisor proclination. The extent to which malocclusion self-corrects varies and depends on the age of the patient at the time of habit cessation, as well as the severity of the malocclusion resulting from the habit. Due to emotional immaturity of the child under four years of age, in most cases, it is advisable to intercept the habit between the age of four years and eruption of permanent incisors (6–7 years).

**Table 21.1:** Classification of non-nutritive sucking (NNS) habits

| Levels | Descriptions |
|---|---|
| Level I (+/–) | Boys or girls of any chronological age with a habit that occurs during sleep |
| Level II (+/–) | Boys below age 8 with a habit that occurs at one setting during waking hours |
| Level III (+/–) | Boys under age 8 years with a habit that occurs at multiple setting during waking hours |
| Level IV (+/–) | Girls below age 8 or a boy over 8 years with a habit that occurs at one setting during waking hours |
| Level V (+/–) | Girls under age 8 years or a boy over age 8 years with a habit that occurs across multiple setting during waking hours |
| Level VI (+/–) | Girls over age 8 years with a habit during waking hours |

(+/–) designates willingness of the patients to participate in treatment

The severity of displacement of the teeth and investing tissues depends on the trident conditioning factors:

I. **Duration:** Amount of time spent on sucking: longer the duration of each sucking period, greater is the damage.
II. **Frequency of indulgence:** Number of times the habit is practiced: Frequent and continuous sucking is more damaging than occasional, short time practice.
III. **Intensity of force:** Amount of force exerted on teeth while practicing the habit: More the force applied, greater is the damage.

Apart from these conditioning factors, the type of malocclusion produced also depends on a number of variables as suggested by Nanda (1989). They include:
- Position of the digit in the mouth
- Associated orofacial muscle contractions
- Mandibular position during sucking
- Facial skeletal pattern.

Prolonged digit sucking can produce effects on the following:
I. Maxilla
II. Mandible
III. Inter-arch relationship
IV. Lip placement and function
V. Tongue placement and function
VI. Other effects.

The multitude effects of prolonged thumb sucking can be appreciated in the two cases given in **Figures 21.3 to 21.6.**

### Effects on Maxilla

- Proclination of upper anteriors **(Fig. 21.4)**: During the habit, finger is placed at an angle such that a labial and apical force is applied on the maxillary incisors, producing a pronounced labial flare of maxillary incisors.
- Increased maxillary arch length
- Anterior placement of maxillary apical base
- Increased SNA angle
- Increased clinical crown length of maxillary incisors **(Fig. 21.5A)**
- Counter-clockwise rotation of occlusal plane
- Decreased palatal arch width/constriction of maxillary arch: Lowering of the tongue and increased buccinator muscle activity during sucking creates an imbalance between the tongue and cheek pressures. This causes constriction of the maxilla with "V" shaped palate **(Fig. 21.5D, Fig. 21.7)**.
- Increased risk of trauma to the maxillary incisors due to their proclination.
- Atypical root resorption of primary central incisors.

### Effects on Mandible

- Retroclination of mandibular incisors: During finger sucking, lower incisors are often used for fulcrum/leverage applying a lingual and apical force on them and thus causing their retroclination **(Fig. 21.4C)**.
- Decreased SNB angle.

### Effects on Inter-arch Relationship

- Increased overjet **(Figs 21.3B and 21.4B)**: Flaring of upper incisors and retroclination of lower incisors increases the overjet.
- Decreased overbite **(Fig. 21.6B)**
- Anterior open bite **(Fig. 21.4A)**

Anterior open bite is caused by a combination of the following factors:
- Interference of normal incisor eruption by the interposed thumb
- Excessive eruption of the posterior teeth due to separation of the jaws opens up the bite further.

- Posterior crossbite **(Fig. 21.6A)**

It occurs as a consequence of maxillary arch constriction. Force exerted by the cheek muscles on

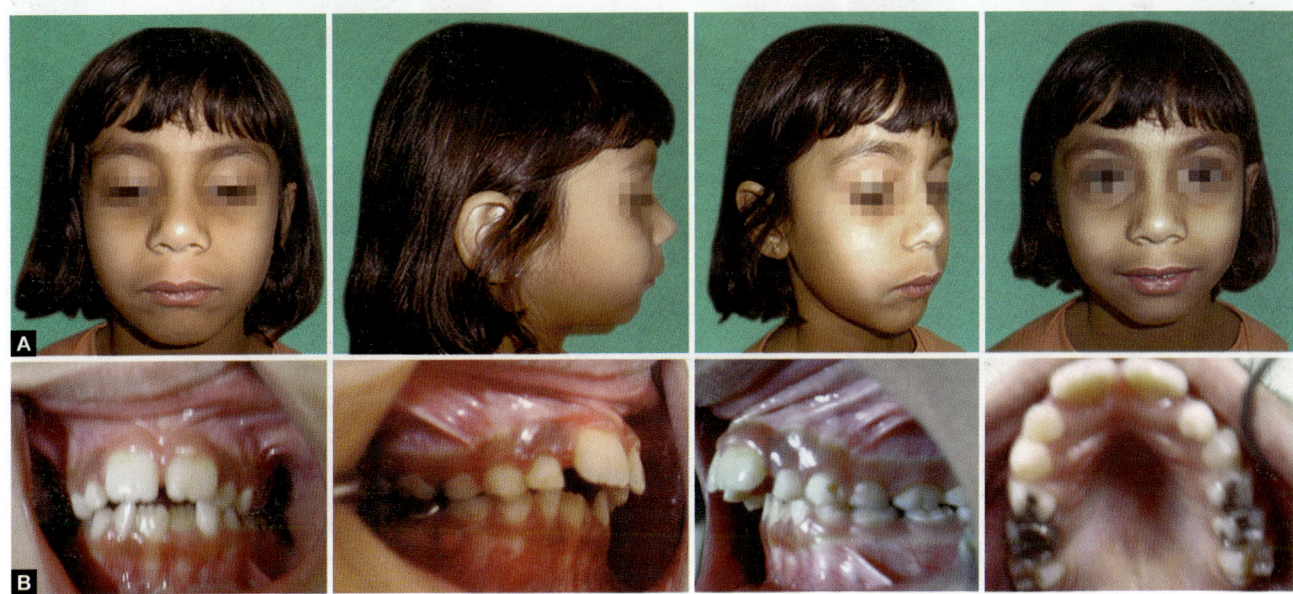

**Figs 21.3A and B:** The multitude effects of prolonged thumb sucking (A case of thumb sucking has resulted in skeletal class II division 1 malocclusion; (A) Extra-oral features: Convex facial profile, Decreased nasolabial angle, posterior facial divergence and incompetent lips; (B) Intra-oral features: Prognathic maxilla, retrognathic mandible, proclination of maxillary anteriors and "V" shaped maxillary arch)

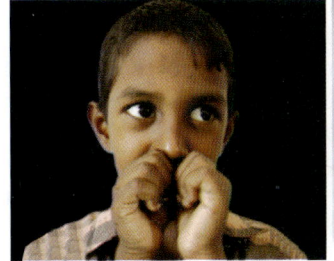 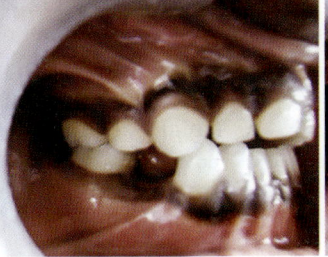 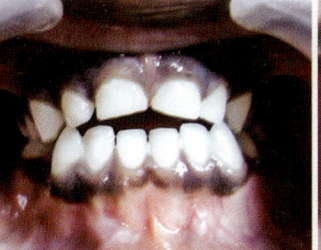 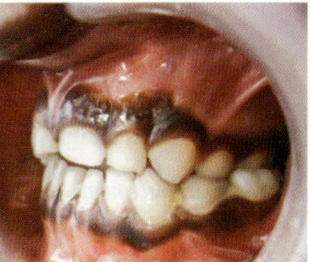

**Fig. 21.4:** Thumb sucking with thumb of both hands simultaneously
(Intra-oral features: Proclination of maxillary anteriors, prognathic premaxilla, retroclination of lower anteriors and anterior open bite)

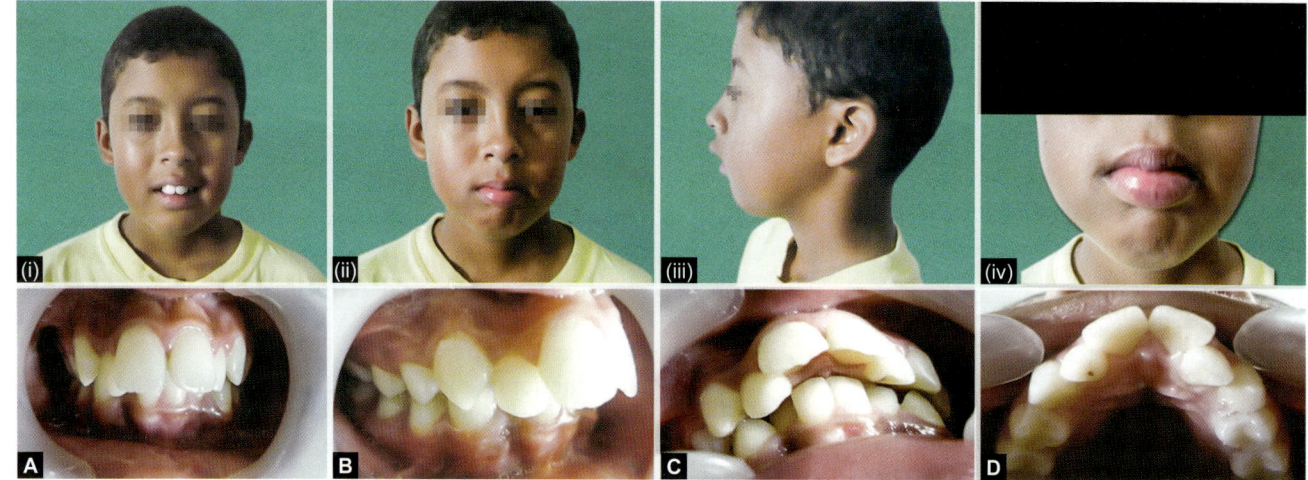

**Figs 21.5A to D:** Thumb sucking with lip sucking habit (Habit has resulted in skeletal class II division 1 malocclusion; Intra-oral features: Prognathic maxilla, retrognathic mandible, maxillary anterior proclination, crowding in the upper anteriors, increased overjet and overbite, "V" shaped maxillary arch. Extra-oral features: Convex facial profile, hypertonic lower lip, hyperactive mentalis, posterior facial divergence)

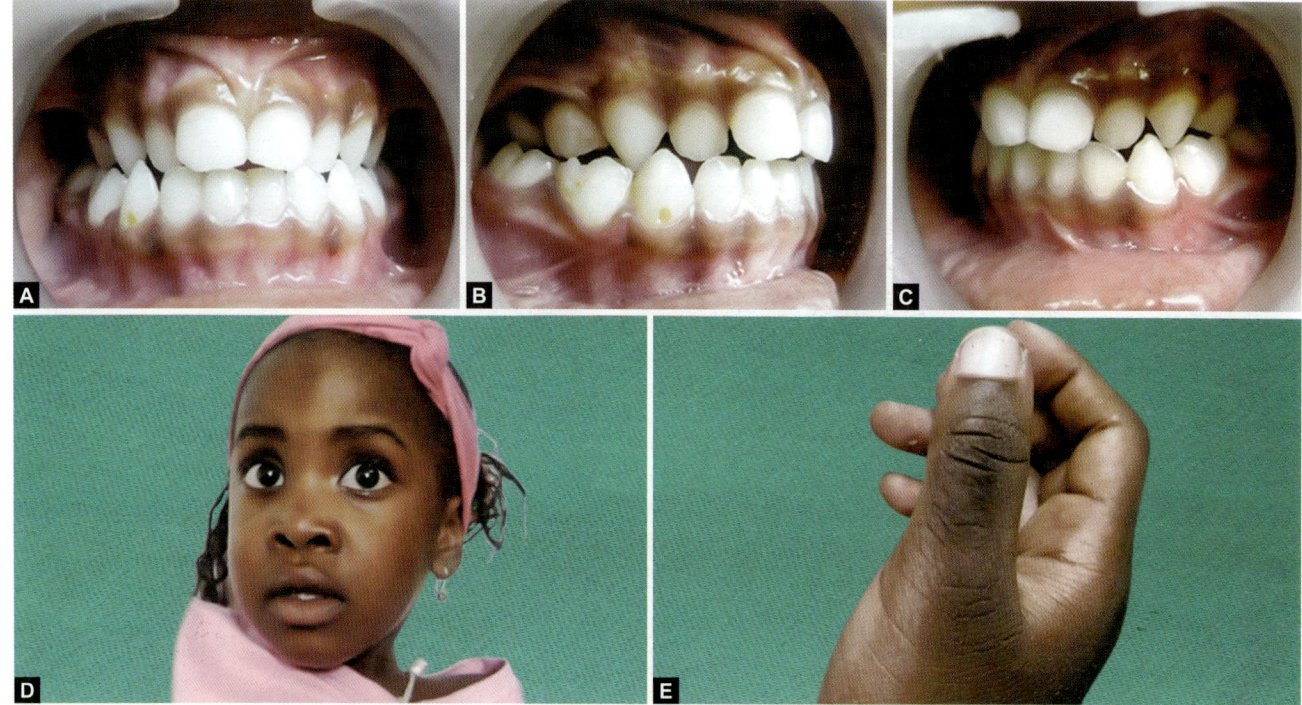

**Figs 21.6A to E:** Thumb sucking causing developing posterior crossbite.
Note: Fibrous roughened callus on the superior aspect of the offending finger

the maxilla is not balanced by the tongue musculature due to lowered tongue posture, while this results in maxillary constriction, there is no restriction of mandibular growth, eventually leading to bilateral posterior crossbite.
- Increased chances of developing class II molar and canine relationship.

### Effects on Lip Placement
- Lip is incompetence **(Fig. 21.5A)**
- Upper lip short and hypotonic **(Fig. 21.5D)**
  - Upper lip is passive during swallowing.
- Hyperactive lower lip
  - Lower lip is hyperactive due to hyperactive mentalis activity during swallowing. Puckering of the chin can be noted **(Fig. 21.5D)**.
- Lower lip placement lingual to upper anteriors:
  - Marked mentalis contraction causes sealing of lower lip lingual to upper anteriors rather than labially during swallowing.
  - Lower lip contacts the lingual surface of upper anteriors with some force accentuating the upper anterior proclination and overjet.

### Effects on Tongue Placement and Function
- Lowered posture of the tongue

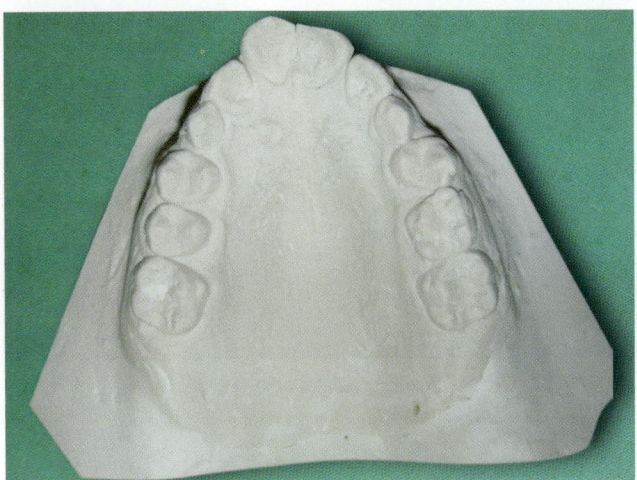

**Fig. 21.7:** Maxillary cast of a thumb-sucking patient showing "V"-shaped dental arch

- Increased chances of developing tongue thrust
  - Lack of lip seal and flaring of upper anteriors often leads to the development of compensatory tongue thrust so as to create a partial vacuum required during the swallowing act.

### Other Effects
- Risk to psychological health
- Deformation of the offending digit may occur
- Speech defects can develop (lisping) due to increase overjet and anterior open bite.

### Diagnosis of NNS Habit

#### History
Parents should be questioned about:
- Duration, frequency and intensity of sucking habit
- Feeding patterns and parental care of the child
- Presence of other secondary associated habits, such as hair pulling and twisting. Nose probing along with finger sucking should be determined. Cessation of secondary habit may stop the primary sucking habit.
- Any psychological stress should be assessed.

#### Extraoral Examination
Examination of digits may reveal the following:
- Offending digits is exceptionally clean and readily noted
- The digit can be reddened or sometimes deformed.
- Dishpan thumb with a short finger nail.
- Fibrous roughened callus may be present on the superior aspect of the offending finger **(Fig. 21.6E)**.

#### Intraoral Examination
Same as described in the effects of prolonged digit sucking.

### Management
A wide range of treatment modalities has been used in the management of NNS habits. Appropriate mode of treatment and timing of treatment should be decided upon keeping age and level of maturity of the child, severity of malocclusion, psychological status of the child and presence of any other habits, such as tongue thrusting, mouth breathing, etc.

#### Treatment Considerations
- No active intervention should be attempted before 3 years of age as due to emotional immaturity of the child.
- Most children discontinue the habit by 4–5 years of age.
- In most cases, it is advisable to initiate the treatment for a prolonged NNS habit between the age of 4–5 years and the eruption of the permanent incisors.
- Generally, malocclusion gets self-corrected, if the habit is stopped before eruption of permanent incisors.
- Before attempting treatment, the patient should express a desire to stop the habit. Without patient cooperation, treatment of a digit-sucking habit may not be successful.
- When indicated, habit-breaking appliances should act as reminders encouraging patient to stop the habit rather than punishing the child.
- Cooperation of the parents and an understanding of potential consequences of prolonged habit is also important.
- Parents should be advised not to rebuke or criticize the child, which will only aggravate the problem. Positive reinforcement and encouragement of the child is recommended.
- In presence of a psychological problem associated with digit-sucking habit, psychological consultation and necessary management are recommended before appliance therapy.

#### Psychological Approach and Behavior Modification
- Screening of patient for underlying psychological disturbances and referral to professionals for counseling.
- Parents should provide adequate emotional support and encouragement to the child.
- Positive behavior modification techniques, such as offering a small reward for dropping the habit can help.
- Dunlop's beta hypotheses: He suggested that forced purposeful repetition of a habit eventually associates it with unpleasant reactions and the habit is abandoned. The child is asked to repeat thumb sucking while sitting in front of a mirror, observing himself/herself as he/she indulges in the habit.

#### Reminder Therapy
This is for those children who wish to stop the habit but need assistance to do so.

***Mechanical methods:*** These include the following:
- Thermoplastic thumb post that covers the offending digit.
- Taping of the offending digit or tying it to the elbow.

***Chemical methods:*** These include the following:
- Hot tasting or bitter flavored preparations or distasteful agents are applied to the offending finger/thumb.

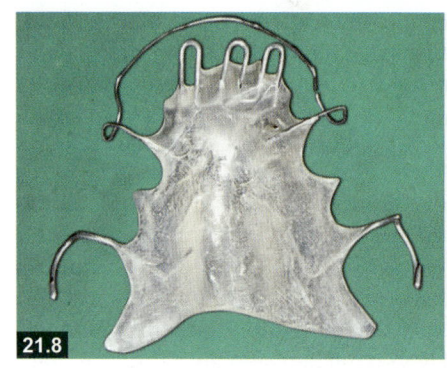 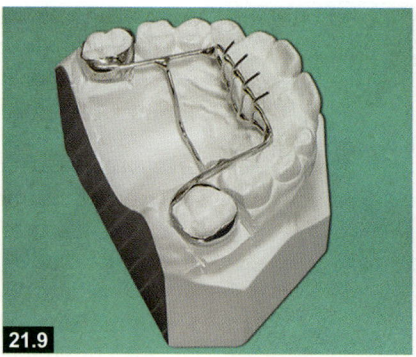 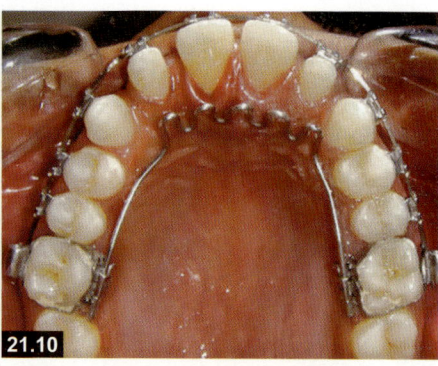

**Fig. 21.8:** Removable crib, **Fig. 21.9:** Fixed rake, **Fig. 21.10:** Removable maxillary palatal arch with crib

- In this method, agents, such as cayenne pepper, quinine, asafetida are used to paint the finger.

### Appliance Therapy

- Various removable and fixed orthodontic habit breaking/habit-retraining appliances are employed to discourage and eventually break the habit.
- The clinician should choose the most appropriate type of appliance after considering the child's age, malocclusion caused and oral habit pattern.
- Before giving the appliance, the child should understand the problem and express a desire to be helped in stopping the habit.
- The appliance should not be designed to "punish" the child by causing pain, but rather to serve as "reminders".
- These appliances generally consist of a palatal wire assembly placed palatal to maxillary incisors that pose a mechanical obstruction to the placement of a thumb.
- The appliances serve the purpose by—
  - Reminding the patient that he/she is indulging in the habit.
  - Rendering the finger habit meaningless by breaking the suction.
  - The feeling of satisfaction from the finger touching the palate is disrupted with the appliance. Patient stops the habit when he gets no real satisfaction from it.

The following appliances can be used for the purpose.

### Removable Habit-Breaking Appliances

Removable habit-retraining appliance consists of a palatal wire assembly embedded in the removable acrylic appliance. The appliance is retained by clasps on maxillary deciduous 2nd molars or 1st permanent molars.
  i. Cribs (**Fig. 21.8**)
  ii. Rakes/spurs (**Fig. 21.9**)

### Fixed Appliances

- Consist of maxillary lingual arch with cribs or rake soldered or inserted in lingual sheath (**Fig. 21.10**) in the anterior region.
- The lingual arch is soldered to the metal bands fabricated on maxillary deciduous 2nd molars or permanent 1st molars.

- Lingual arch with palatal crib
- Lingual arch with rakes/spurs
- Quad helix

### How Does Habit-breaking Appliance Work?

***Cribs:*** Incorporated in removable or fixed appliances, the palatal crib acts as follows:
- Renders the habit meaningless by breaking the suction.
- Makes the habit nonpleasurable as thumb cannot touch the palate.
- Breaks the thumb and tongue pressure applying on maxillary incisors.
- Appliance forces the tongue backward, distributes the pressure to posterior teeth as well.
- Acts as reminder not to indulge in the habit.

***Rakes/spurs:*** The blunt spurs projecting into palatal vault discourage not only thumb sucking but also tongue thrusting and improper swallowing habits as well.

***Quad helix:*** It includes the following:
- It is the ideal appliance for correction of posterior crossbite caused due to digit-sucking habit. Activation of Quad helix causes expansion of the dental arch.
- Its anterior portion with two helixes placed near the anterior palatal region acts as a reminder.

***Corrective mechanotherapy:*** After cessation of the habit any residual malocclusion present well after eruption of permanent incisors is treated by removable orthodontic appliances or fixed mechanotherapy (**Fig. 21.10**). It is also true for patients with continuation of the habit into adolescence and adulthood.

## TONGUE-THRUSTING HABIT

It is an abnormal tongue activity in which the tongue is thrust between the upper and lower teeth during swallowing (**Figs 21.11**). It often causes proclination of anteriors and an anterior open bite.

Tongue thrusting may be present in association with digit-sucking habit and should be considered in the diagnosis.

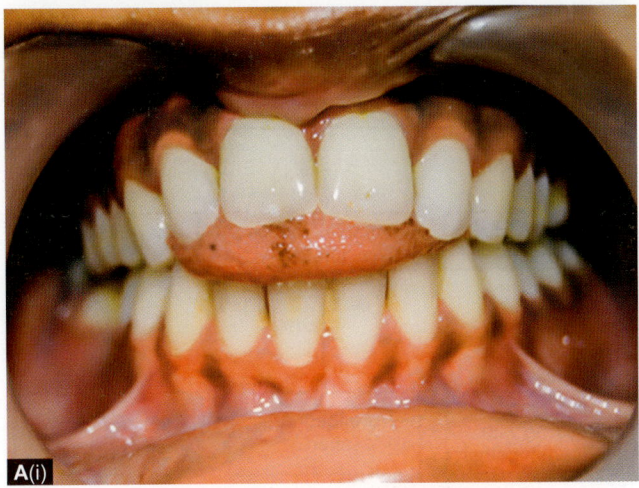
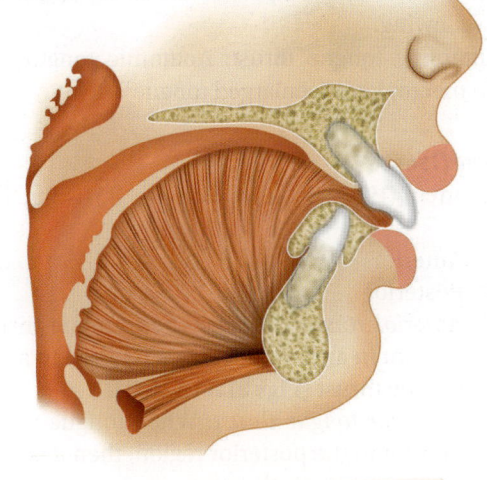
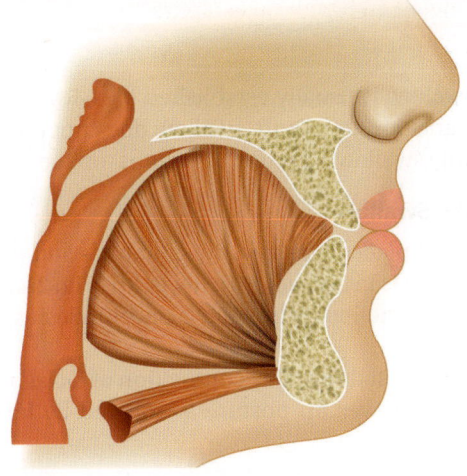
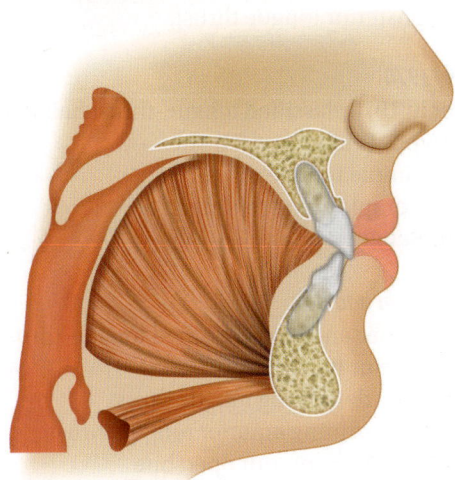

**Figs 21.11A to C:** A(i) and (ii) Tongue thrusting habit has resulted anterior open bite. (B) In infantile swallow: Tongue is placed between the gum pads and the tip of the tongue is in contact with lower lip (C) Mature swallow: Tip of the tongue is placed against anterior palate behind upper incisors; posterior teeth are in occlusion during swallowing; mandible is stabilized by contraction of muscles of mastication; downward and forward growth of mandible and vertical growth of alveolar bone increases intra-oral volume and assists in normal posture

## Definitions

### Brauer (1965)
A tongue thrust was said to be present, if the tongue was observed thrusting between and the teeth did not close in centric occlusion during deglutition.

### Tulley (1969)
Tongue thrust as the forward movement of the tongue tip between the teeth to meet the lower lip during deglutition and in sounds of speech, so that the tongue becomes interdentally.

### Barber (1975)
Tongue thrust is an oral habit pattern related to the persistence of an infantile swallow pattern during childhood and adolescence and thereby produces an open bite and protrusion of anterior tooth segments.

### Schneider (1982)
Tongue thrust is a forward placement of the tongue between the anterior teeth and against the lower lip during swallowing.

## Classification

### Etiologic Classification
Tongue thrust habit can be classified into following four types:
  I. Physiologic
  II. Habitual
  III. Functional
  IV. Anatomic

**Physiologic tongue thrust:** This comprises the normal tongue thrust swallow of infancy.

**Habitual tongue thrust:** The tongue thrust swallow is developed due to repeated placement of the tongue.

**Functional:** These include the following:
- When the tongue thrust mechanism is an adaptive behavior developed to achieve an oral seal, it is referred as functional tongue thrust.
- Swallowing requires the creation of an "oral seal" a partial vacuum. When there is no oral seal due to increased overjet, compensatory tongue thrust

develops in an attempt to establish the oral seal during swallowing.

Anatomic tongue thrust: Anatomic tongue thrust is due to macroglossia (enlarged tongue).

### Backland (1963)
Backland in 1963 classified tongue thrusting into two types:
I. Anterior
II. Posterior

I. *Anterior tongue thrust:* When tongue thrusting is present in anterior region, is referred to as anterior tongue thrust **(Figs 21.11A to C)**.
II. *Posterior tongue thrust:* When tongue thrusting is present in the posterior region, then it is termed as posterior tongue thrust.

### Moyer (1970)
Moyer in 1970 classified tongue-thrust habit into following three types **(Flowchart 21.4)**:
I. Simple tongue thrust
II. Complex tongue thrust
III. Retained infantile swallow.

### James Braner and Holt
James Braner and Holt classified tongue-thrust habits into following four types:

**Type I:** Nondeforming tongue thrust
**Type II:** Deforming anterior tongue thrust
a. Subgroup 1: anterior open bite
b. Subgroup 2: proclination of anteriors
c. Subgroup 3: posterior crossbite.
**Type III:** Deforming lateral tongue thrust
a. Subgroup 1: Posterior open bite
b. Subgroup 2: Posterior crossbite
c. Subgroup 3: Deep bite.
**Type IV:** Deforming anteriors and lateral tongue thrust
a. Subgroup 1: Anterior and posterior open bite
b. Subgroup 2: Proclination of anterior teeth
c. Subgroup 3: Posterior crossbite.

### Etiology
Tongue thrusting can be caused by various factors, which are as follows:

### Genetic Factors
- Inherited hyperactivity of orbicularis oris with specific anatomic configuration and neuromuscular activity may predispose to tongue thrusting.
- Genetically predetermined pattern of oral behavior.

### Persistence of Infantile Swallow Pattern
There is considerable evidence, which indicates that tongue thrust in many patients is merely retention of the infantile suckling mechanism. Infantile swallow normal in neonates, gradually disappears with eruption of teeth and

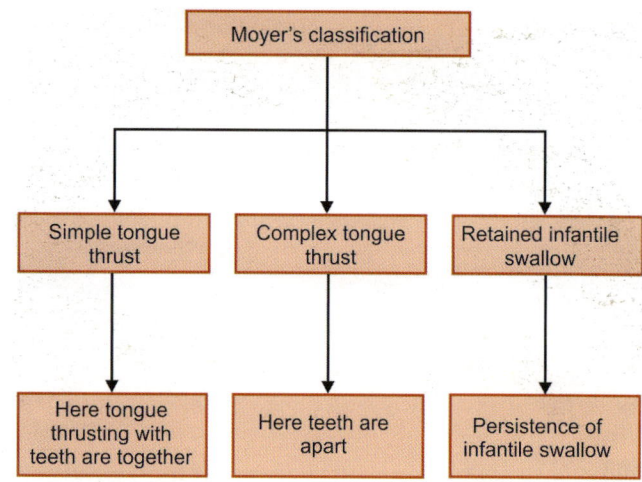

**Flowchart 21.4:** Moyer's classification

mature swallow is usually established by 4–5 years. If this natural transition to mature swallow does not take place, the infantile swallowing reflex persists as tongue thrusting.

### In Infantile Swallow
- Tongue is placed between the gum pads and the tip of the tongue is in contact with lower lip **(Fig. 21.11B)**
- Active contractions of lips and facial muscles, especially buccinator
- Mandible is stabilized by contraction of facial muscles
- Tongue-to-lower lip posture is adapted by infants at rest.

### Mature Swallow
- Cessation of lip activity with lips relaxed **(Fig. 21.11C)**
- Tip of the tongue is placed against anterior palate behind upper incisors
- Posterior teeth are in occlusion during swallowing
- Mandible is stabilized by contraction of muscles of mastication
- Downward and forward growth of mandible and vertical growth of alveolar bone increases intraoral volume and assists in normal posture.

### Adaptive Learned Behavior
- Improper bottle feeding.
- Prolonged tenderness of gums or teeth and thus the child learns to keep teeth apart during swallowing.
- Prolonged tonsillar/upper respiratory tract infection, which causes adaptive tongue patterns that are retained even after the infection subsides.
- Tongue held in open spaces during natural exfoliation of primary teeth or extractions.
- Prolonged thumb-sucking habit:
  - Prolonged thumb sucking has been observed to result in an increased tendency to develop tongue-thrusting habit.
  - When there is no oral seal due to increased overjet or open bite caused by thumb-sucking

habit, compensatory tongue thrust develops to establish oral seal and partial vacuum required for swallowing act.

### Mechanical Restriction

- *Macroglossia:* Large tongue limits the space in oral cavity and forces a forward thrust.
- *Enlarged tonsils and adenoids:* Reduces space available for tongue movement.
- Constricted dental arches.

### Neurological Disturbances

- Hyposensitive palate
- Moderate motor disability and loss of precision in oral function
- Disruption of tactile sensory control and coordination of swallowing.

### Psychogenic Factors

Children who are forced to discontinue other oral habits like thumb sucking may develop tongue thrusting habit.

## Effects of Tongue Thrusting

Depending on the duration, frequency and intensity of tongue-thrusting habit, some/all of the following features can be seen.

### Extraoral Features

- Lips: Incompetent lips **(Fig. 21.12A)**
- Anterior facial height: Increased **(Fig. 21.12B)**
- When tongue thrusts between anterior teeth, the posterior teeth are rendered out of occlusion. As a result, the posterior teeth may supraerupt and can gradually eliminate the interocclusal clearance between the upper and lower teeth. This increases the anterior facial and can also cause an open bite.
- Nasolabial angle is decreased **(Fig. 21.12C)**
- Hyperactive mentalis activity with puckering of chin (in case of anterior tongue thrust).

### Intraoral Features

Features pertaining to the maxillary arch **(Figs 21.13A to C)**: It includes the following:

- Maxillary anterior proclination
- Generalized spacing between the teeth
- Constricted arches near molar region—due to lowered posture of tongue.

**Mandible:** It includes the following **(Fig. 21.14)**:

- Retroclination of mandibular anteriors
- Proclination of mandibular anteriors
  - Degree of proclination or retroclination of mandibular incisors depends upon the type of tongue thrust present.

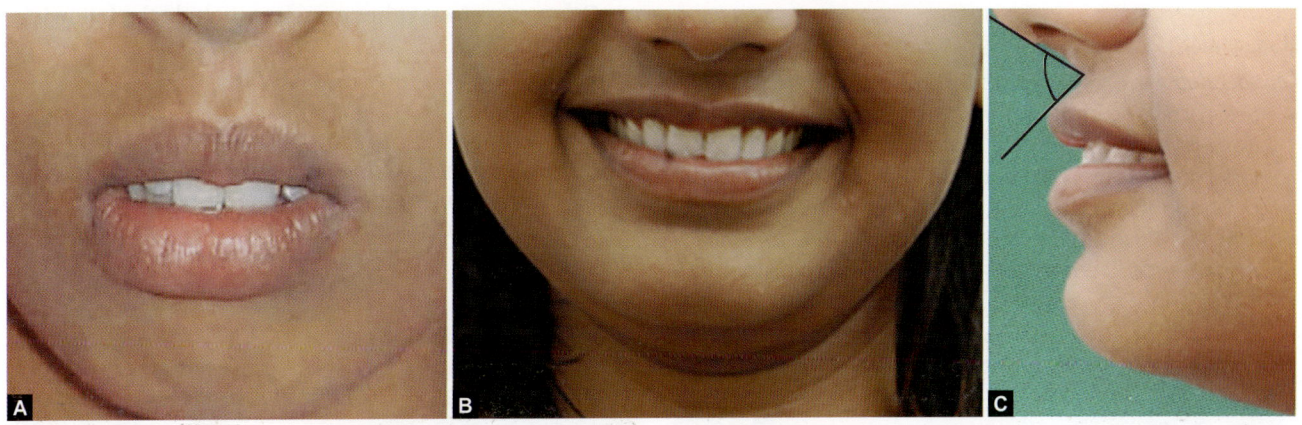

**Figs 21.12A to C:** Effects of tongue thrusting: (A) Incompetent lips. (B) Increased anterior facial height. (C) Decreased nasolabial angle

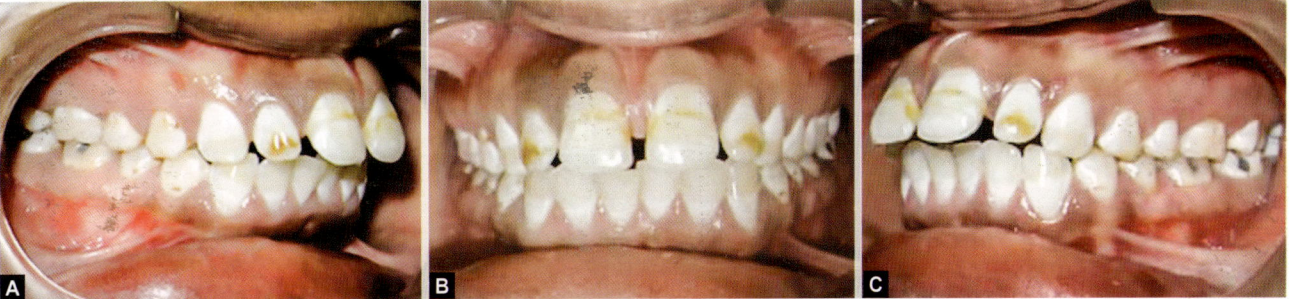

**Figs 21.13A to C:** A patient with tongue thrusting habit showing its effect on maxilla. Maxillary anterior proclination, spacing in the incisors region and constricted arches near molar region—due to lowered posture of tongue

## Intermaxillary relationships

It includes the following:
- Increased overjet **(Fig. 21.14)**
- Anterior open bite **(Fig. 21.15)**
- Posterior open bite—In case of lateral tongue thrust. It may be unilateral or bilateral
- Effect on speech: Hampered speech
- Tongue posture: The tongue tip at rest is observed to be at a lower level in the tongue thrust patients.
- Effects on mandible: Upward and backward movement of mandible with the tongue moving forward.

## Diagnosis

### History
- Any upper respiratory tract infections
- Digit-sucking habit
- Neuromuscular problems
- Swallow pattern in siblings and parents to check for hereditary factor.

### Tongue Examination
- *Tongue posture at rest:* It can be examined using lateral cephalogram or by seating the patient upright. In these patients, tongue usually assumes a lower posture at rest with the tip touching the cingulum/lingual fossae of lower anteriors, instead of resting behind upper incisors.
- *Tongue activity/function observed during swallowing:* Tongue activity is observed during swallowing act to know whether tongue thrust is simple/complex, anterior or lateral.

## Management

### Considerations
- *Self-correcting tongue thrusting:* Tongue thrust habit does not require any orthodontic treatment. It often self-corrects by 7–8 years of age by the time the permanent anterior teeth erupts completely.
- *Tongue thrusting without malocclusion or speech disturbance:* Treatment is generally not recommended when tongue thrust is present without any kind of malocclusion to any speech disturbances.
- *Tongue thrusting with malocclusion:* Orthodontic correction of the malocclusion caused by tongue thrusting will usually eliminate the tongue thrusting habit.
- *Associated with other oral habits:* If the patient has both thumb sucking and tongue thrusting, the thumb sucking should be treated first.

### Treatment

The treatment of tongue thrust can be divided into various steps:

### Training of correct swallow and posture of the tongue

a. **Myofunctional exercises:** The patient can be guided regarding the correct posture of the tongue during swallowing by various exercises. The child is asked to place the tip of the tongue in the rugae area for 5 min and is asked to swallow.

b. **Orthodontic elastics and sugarless fruits drop exercise:** This can be held by the tongue tip against the palate on the rugae area **(Fig. 21.16)**.

c. **4S exercise:** It includes identifying—
- Spot
- Salivating
- Squeezing the spot
- Swallowing

d. **2S exercise:** It includes identifying:
- Spot
- Squeeze

e. **Other exercises:** Other exercises include the following:
- Whistling
- Reciting the count from 60–69
- Gargling
- Yawning

All these exercises help in toning up respective muscles thereby eliminating tongue-thrust habit.

*Using appliance as a guide in the correct positioning of tongue*

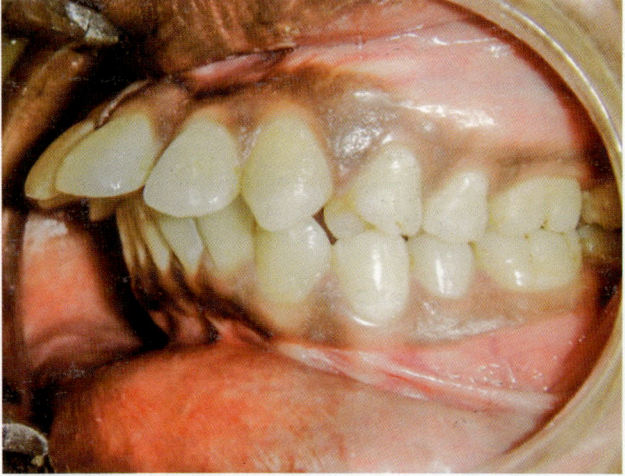

**Fig. 21.14:** Tongue-thrusting habit and mild anterior open bite

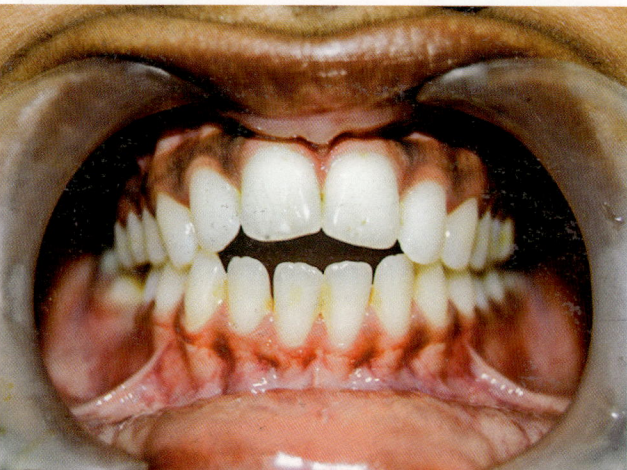

**Fig. 21.15:** Anterior open bite

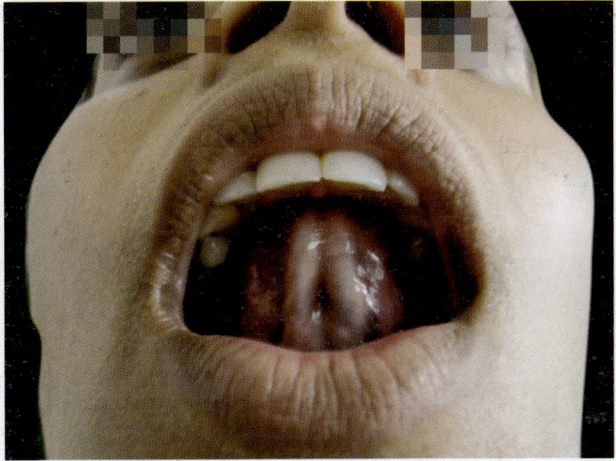

**Fig. 21.16:** Orthodontic elastics and sugarless fruits drop exercise where elastic is held by the tip of the tongue on the palatal rugae

An orthodontic appliance is given which acts as a guide in the correct positioning of tongue.
- Pre-orthodontic trainer for myofunctional training.
- Orthodontic trainer.

### Orthodontic Trainers (Fig. 21.17)

#### Tooth Guidance
Molded into the anterior section (similar to orthodontic arch wire).
1. Tooth channels
2. Labial bows

#### Myofunctional Training
1. *Tongue tag:* For the proprioceptive positioning of the tongue tip as in myofunctional and speech therapies.
2. *Tongue guard:* Stops tongue thrusting when in place and forces child to breathe through the nose.
3. *Lip bumpers:* Discourage overactive mentalis muscle activity.

#### Jaw Positioning
*Edge-to-edge class I jaw position:* It is produced when in place (same as most functional appliances). Combined with prevention of tongue thrusting and forcing the child to breathe through the nose.

#### Appliance Therapy

##### Using Removable Appliance
Various removable orthodontic appliances are used to break tongue-thrusting habit along with the correction of resultant malocclusion **(Fig. 21.18)**.
1. Habit-breaking appliance with tongue crib **(Fig. 21.19)**: This appliance is used to treat tongue-thrust habit.
   *Parts:* Tongue crib is comprised of the following parts:
   - Active component—bow
   - As a remainder—tongue crib
   - Retentive components
     ◆ Clasps—C clasp or Adam's clasp on maxillary 1st molars
     ◆ Plate—acrylic base plate.

2. *Nance palatal arch appliance:* In this appliance, acrylic button can be used as a guide to place the tongue in the correct position **(Fig. 21.20)**.
3. *Oral screen:* Another effective means of controlling abnormal muscle habits like tongue thrusting and at the same time utilizing the musculature to effect a correction of the developing malocclusion is vestibular/oral screen **(Fig. 21.21)**.

##### Using Fixed Orthodontic Appliances
Fixed orthodontic appliance with fixed rake or crib can be used to correct tongue thrust habit **(Figs 21.22A to E)**.

#### Surgery
- *Skeletal malocclusion:* The treatment of the retained infantile swallow behavior beyond adulthood is difficult and often consists of orthognathic surgical procedure to correct the skeletal malocclusion.
- *Tongue thrusting due to excessive lymphoid tissue:* Surgical reduction of lymphoid tissue will eliminate tongue thrusting.

## MOUTH-BREATHING HABIT

Mouth-breathing can cause malocclusion by disrupting the orofacial equilibrium of pressures on teeth and jaws. This is due to the altered posture of the mandible and tongue maintained during mouth breathing. If these postural changes are maintained, posterior teeth may supra-erupt increasing the facial height; mandible may rotate downward and backward opening up the bite and increasing the overjet.

### Definitions

#### Chopra RB (1951)
"Mouth breathing is defined as habitual respiration through the mouth instead of the nose."

#### Chacker FM (1961)
Mouth breathing as "a prolonged or continued exposure of the tissues of anterior areas of mouth to the drying effects of inspired air."

### Classification

#### Sim and Finn
Sim and Finn classified mouth breathers into the following three categories according to the etiology.
  I. Obstructive
  II. Habitual
  III. Anatomic.

#### Obstructive
Children with an increased resistance to or a complete obstruction of the normal flow of air through the nasal passage have difficulty in inspiring and expiring air

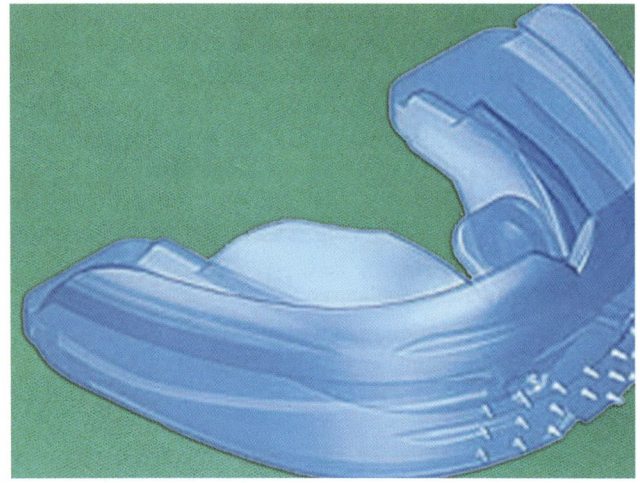

**Fig. 21.17:** Orthodontic trainer

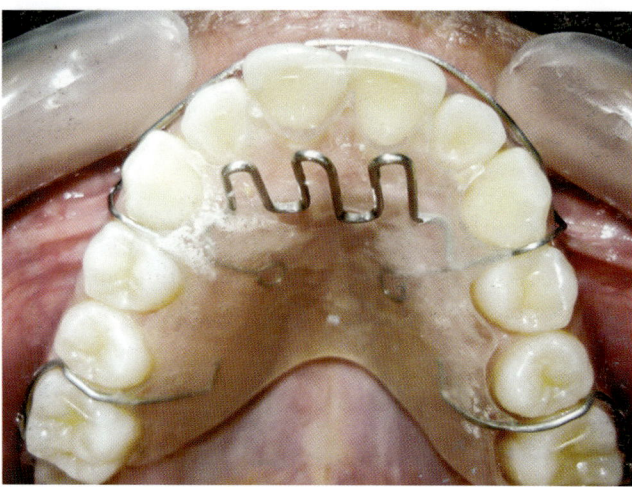

**Fig. 21.18:** Removable orthodontic appliance

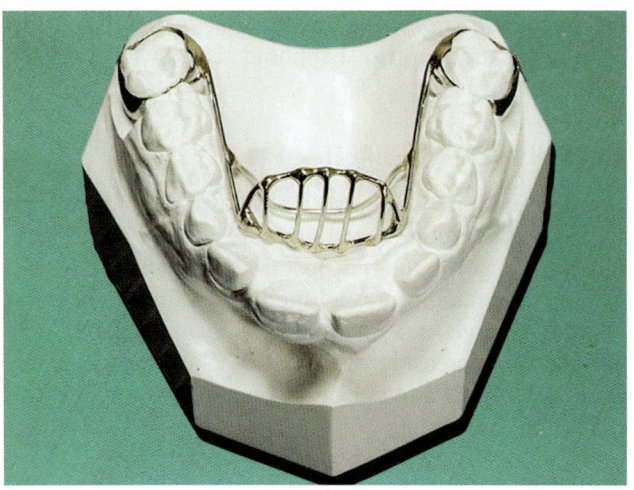

**Fig. 21.19:** Fixed habit breaking appliance with tongue crib

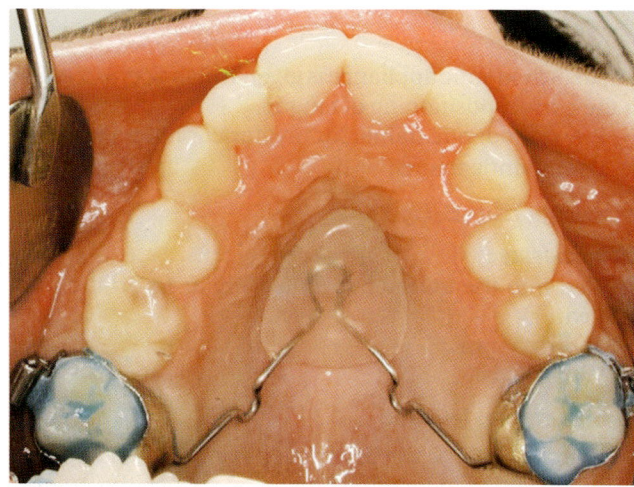

**Fig. 21.20:** Acrylic buttons of the Nance palatal arch appliance

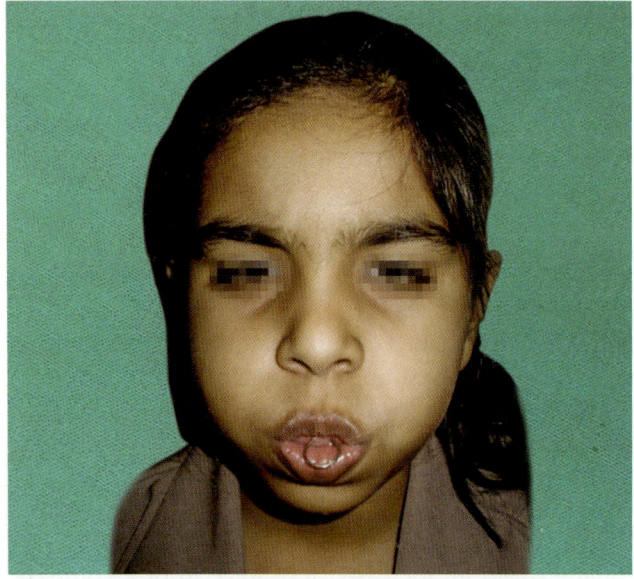

**Fig. 21.21:** Double oral screen can be used to treat tongue-thrusting habit

through nasal passages. These children are thus forced to breathe through the nose.

### Habitual

Habitual mouth breather is a child who continuously breathes through the mouth by force of habit, although the obstruction has been removed.

### Anatomic

The anatomic mouth breathing is seen in those, whose short upper lip does not permit complete closure without undue effort.

## Etiology

Common cause of mouth breathing is some form of obstruction to nasal airways. Nasal insufficiency can be due to facial form or other causes.

### *Facial Form: Genetic Predisposition*

Mouth breathing is typically seen in ectomorphic children with long, narrow faces and nasopharyngeal spaces.

Because of this genetic type of tapering face and nasopharynx, these children are more prone to have nasal obstruction than others (with wide facial form/brachycephalic).

### Nasal Obstruction

- *Hypertrophy of turbinate:* Can be caused by allergies, chronic infections of nasal mucosa, atrophic rhinitis, hot and dry climatic conditions or polluted air.
- Enlarged adenoids (pharyngeal tonsillar tissue):
  - Since adenoidal/lymphoid tissues are physiologically hyperplastic during childhood, mouth breathing from those causes are common in children.
  - In these cases mouth breathing may be self-correcting as the child grows older, the adenoid tissue would naturally shrink in size.

### Intranasal Defects

- Deviated nasal septum.
- Nasal polyps.
- Thick septum.

### Pathophysiology

Under normal conditions, pressure exerted by the tongue intraorally is balanced by the pressure of orofacial musculature. Nasal pattern of breathing does not disturb this equilibrium. In order to breathe through mouth, it is necessary to lower the mandible and the tongue and to extend the head. These postural changes disrupt the orofacial equilibrium of pressures on the jaws and teeth and thus can affect both the jaw growth and tooth position.

When these abnormal postural changes are maintained, malocclusion may be caused due to the following effects:

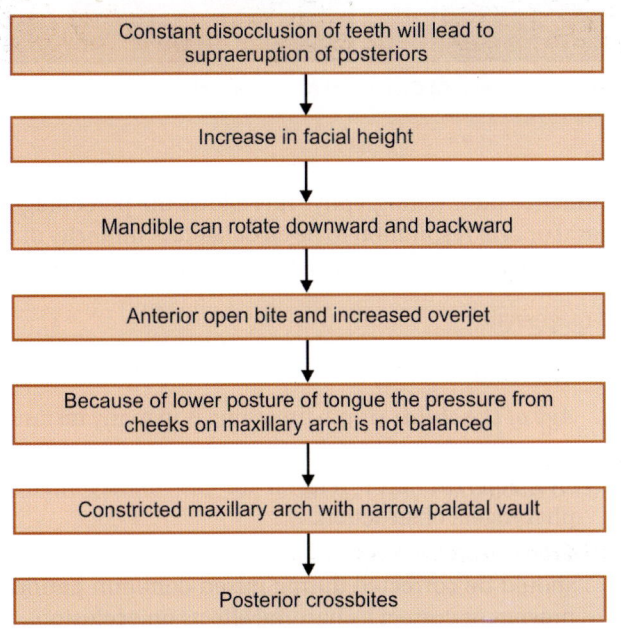

### Clinical Findings

#### Extraoral

- *Adenoid facies:* Patients typically exhibit "Adenoid facies" characterized by long, narrow face with narrow nose and nasal passages.
- *Dolichocephalic facial form:* With vertical skeletal growth pattern.
- Increased facial height.
- Short and flaccid upper lip with heavy and everted lower lip.
- *Incompetant lips:* Lips are apart at rest. Patient may have to close the lips with effort.
- Excessive appearance of maxillary anteriors due to long face.
- *Gummy smile:* On smiling, many patients reveal large amounts of gingiva.

#### Intraoral

- Proclination of maxillary anteriors.
- Increased overjet
- Constricted maxilla with narrow-shaped palate.
- Posterior crossbite.
- Mandibular incisors may be retroclined.
- Mandible is distal in relation to maxilla.
- *Gingiva:* Gingiva is hyperplastic, especially in relation to maxillary anterior teeth due to continuous exposure of the tissue to dry air. Marginal gingiva in this area is rolled out and inter-dental papilla is enlarged.

### Diagnosis

#### History

A good history should be recorded from the patient, as well as parents.

#### Clinical Examination

- *Mirror test:* In this test, a double-sided mirror is held between the nose and mouth **(Fig. 21.23A)**:
  - **Test is positive:** If fogging occurs on mirror facing oral cavity it indicates that patient is a mouth breather.
  - **Test is negative (nasal breathing):** If fogging is seen on nasal side of the mirror, then it indicates nasal breathing and test is negative.
- *Cotton test/Massler's butterfly test* **(Fig. 21.23B)**: Butterfly-shaped cotton strand is placed over the upper lip below nostrils. Patient observed as he/she breathes.
  - **Test is positive:** If cotton flutters down then test is positive, it indicates mouth breathing.
  - **Test is negative:** If cotton does not flutter down, then test is negative, it indicates nasal breathing.
- *Water test:* In this test the patient is asked to drink water and retain it for a period of time **(Fig. 21.23C)**.
  - **Test is positive:** If patient is unable to hold the water in the mouth, then test is positive, it indicates mouth breathing.
  - **Test is negative:** If the patient able to hold the water for sometime, then the test is negative, it indicates nasal breathing.

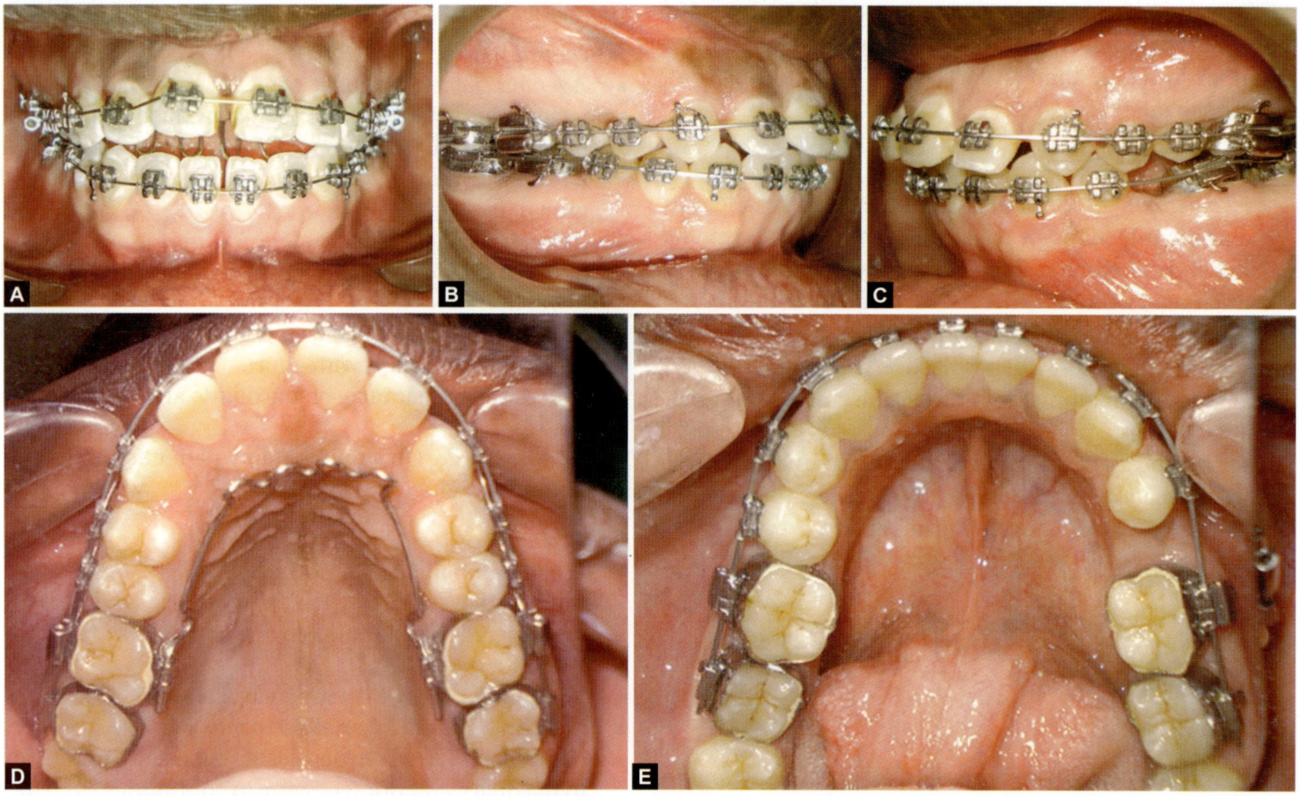

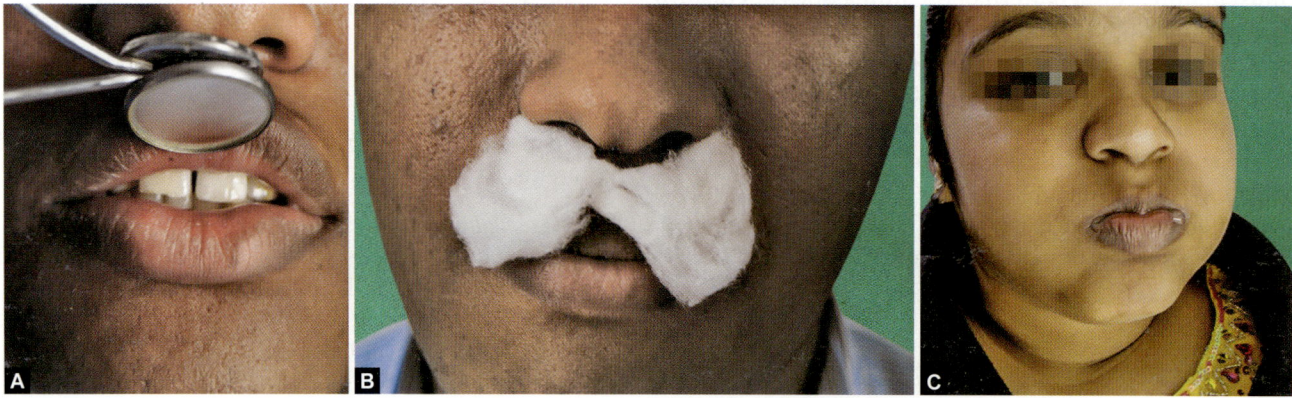

**Figs 21.22A to E:** Fixed orthodontic appliance with removable crib can be used to correct tongue-thrust habit

**Figs 21.23A to C:** Assessment of mouth breathing: (A) Mirror test (B) Cotton test (C) Water test

### Cephalometric Analysis

Cephalometric analysis of patient with mouth breathing reveals:
- A large face height
- Increased mandibular plane angle
- Vertical growth pattern
- Retrognathic maxilla
- Retrognathic mandible.

### Rhinomanometry

The only reliable way to quantify the extent of mouth breathing is to establish how much of the total air flow goes through the nose and how much through the mouth using inductive plethysmography. This allows the percentage of nasal or oral respiration to be calculated. A minority of the long faced children had less than 40% nasal breathing.

### Management

#### Considerations

1. *Age of the child:* Mouth breathing is in many instances self-correcting after puberty.
2. *ENT referral:* ENT referral for the management of pharyngeal obstruction.
3. *Correction of mouth breathing:* Mouth breathing should be corrected during mixed dentition period to prevent or correct its harmful effects on occlusion.

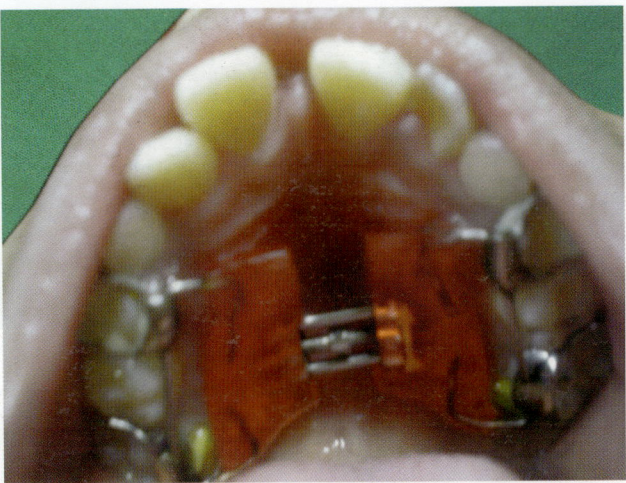

**Fig. 21.24:** Rapid maxillary expansion can widen the arch and increase nasal air flow

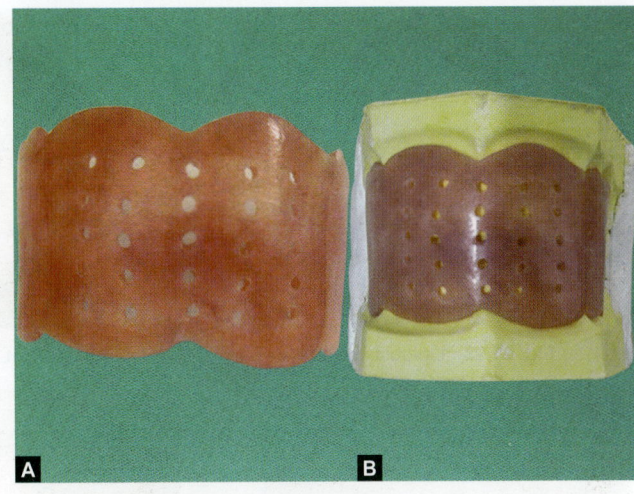

**Figs 21.25A and B:** Oral screen with holes can be used to treat mouth-breathing habit

4. ***Symptomatic treatment:*** Symptomatic treatment of gingival and periodontal tissue should be done.

### Treatment
1. ***Elimination of cause:*** Any nasal or pharyngeal obstruction should be removed by referring the patient to the ENT surgeon.
2. ***Interception of habit:*** If the habit continues even after the removal of the obstruction then it should be corrected.
   Correction can be done by the means of the following:
   a. ***Exercises:*** Breathing and lip exercises are instructed in patients with no physiologic cause.
   b. ***Physical exercises:*** This can be done in the morning and the night.
   c. ***Wind instrument:*** Playing a wind instrument may be a useful interceptive orthodontic procedure.
3. ***Rapid maxillary expansion:*** Rapid maxillary expansion, sing removable or fixed orthodontic appliances, helps in widening the constricted arches thereby increasing the nasal airflow and decreasing nasal resistance **(Fig. 21.24)**.
4. ***Oral screen:*** The most effective way to establish nasal breathing is to prevent air from entering the oral cavity. To do this either the lips or the mouth should be closed. For this purpose, oral screen can be used **(Figs 21.25A and B)**.

## LIP HABITS

### Definition
Habit that involves the manipulation of the lips and perioral structures are termed as lip habits.

### Classification
I. Lip habits are classified into:
   a. Wetting the lips with the tongue.
   b. Pulling the lips into the mouth between the teeth.

II. Lip habit can be of following three types:
   a. Lip sucking
   b. Lip wetting
   c. Lip biting.
   a. **Lip-sucking habit:** In lip sucking habit, the entire lip, including vermilion border is pulled into the mouth **(Fig. 21.26)**.
   b. **Lip-wetting habit:** In lip-wetting habit, tongue constantly wets the lips due to dryness/irritation, which later becomes a habit **(Fig. 21.27)**.
   c. **Lip-biting habit:** In lip-biting habit, either the upper or lower lips are bitten by incisal edges of upper and lower incisors **(Fig. 21.28)**.

### Clinical Features
- Malocclusion: Angle's class II division 1 malocclusion.
- Emotional stress
- Flabby cheeks

### Clinical Features of lip-sucking
1. In case of lower lip sucking **(Figs 21.29A to C)**:
   - Maxillary anterior proclination
   - Retroclination of mandibular anteriors.
2. In case of upper lip sucking:
   - Retroclination on maxillary anteriors
   - Proclination of mandibular anteriors
3. Vermilion border: Reddening of the vermillion border.
4. Cracking of lips
5. Hypertrophy of lips.

### Clinical Features of Lip Wetting
- Dryness of lips
- Irritation of lips

### Clinical Features of Lip Biting
- Abrasion on lips
- Indentation of incisors on lips
- Cuts on lips
- Proclination of maxillary anteriors
- Retroclination of mandibular anteriors.

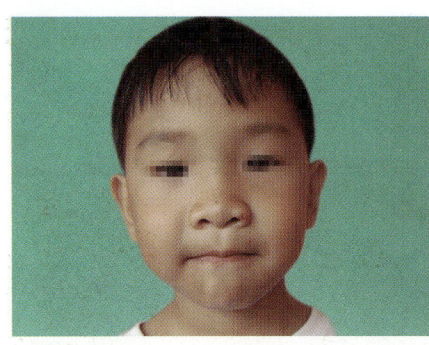
**Fig. 21.26:** Lip-sucking habit

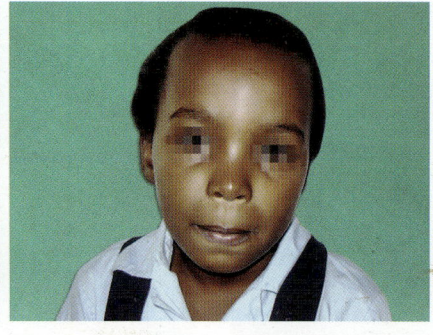
**Fig. 21.27:** Lip-wetting habit

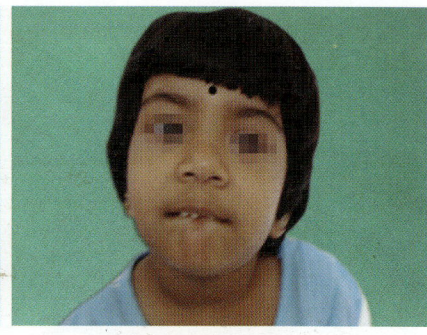
**Fig. 21.28:** Lip-biting habit

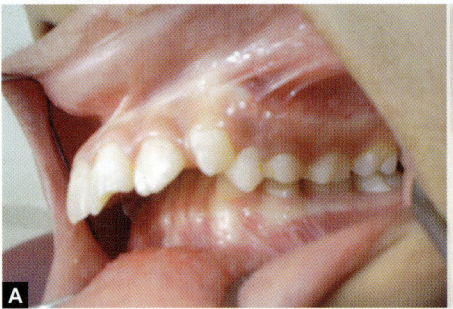
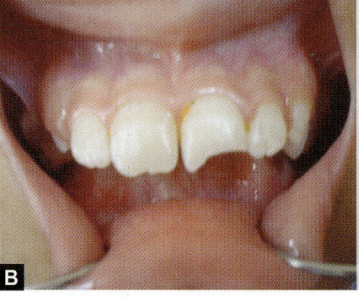
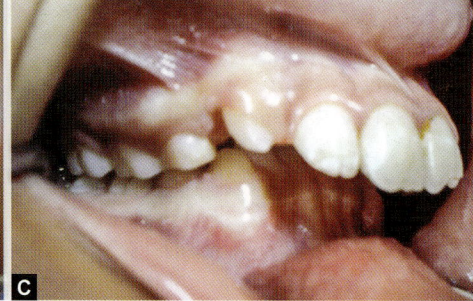

**Figs 21.29A to C:** A patient of lower lip-sucking habit showing proclination of maxillary anteriors and retroclination of lower anteriors, increased overjet and overbite

### Management

1. Elimination of cause
2. *Correction of malocclusion:* Removable or fixed orthodontic appliance can be used to correct malocclusion, which in turn, treats the habits.
3. *Appliance therapy:* It includes the following:
   - Oral screen which not only helps to stop the habit but also corrects the malocclusion.
   - Lip bumper appliance with fixed orthodontic appliance helps to stop the habit by keeping lips apart each other and even from teeth **(Fig. 21.30)**.

## CHEEK-BITING HABIT

Cheek-biting habit is an abnormal habit of keeping or biting the cheek muscles in between the upper or lower posterior teeth.

### Clinical Features

- Ulcer at the level of occlusion
- Open bite
- Individual tooth malposition.

### Treatment

- Removable orthodontic appliance with crib may be constructed to break the habit.
- A vestibular or oral screen may also be used to stop the habit.

## NAIL-BITING HABIT

Nail-biting habit is one of the most common habits in children **(Fig. 21.31A)** and adults **(Fig. 21.31B)**.

### Clinical Features

- Crowding
- Rotation
- Attrition of lower incisors or upper anteriors **(Fig. 21.31B)**
- Effect on nails: Inflammation of nailbeds and also nails.

### Management

- Mild cases—no treatment
- Avoid punitive methods, such as
  - Scolding

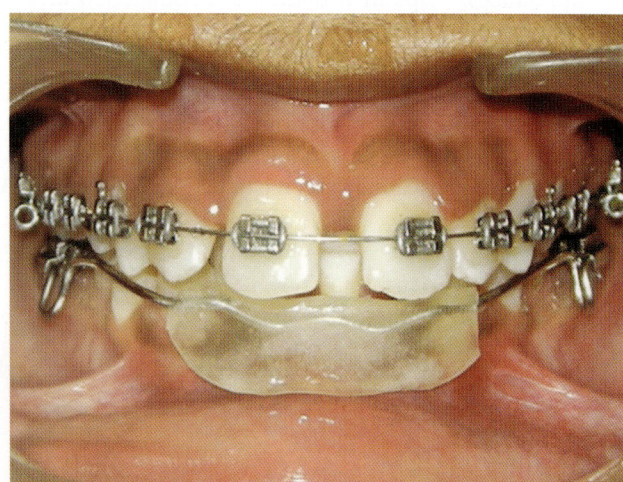

**Fig. 21.30:** Lip bumper appliances with fixed orthodontic appliance helps to stop the habit by keeping lips apart each other and even from teeth

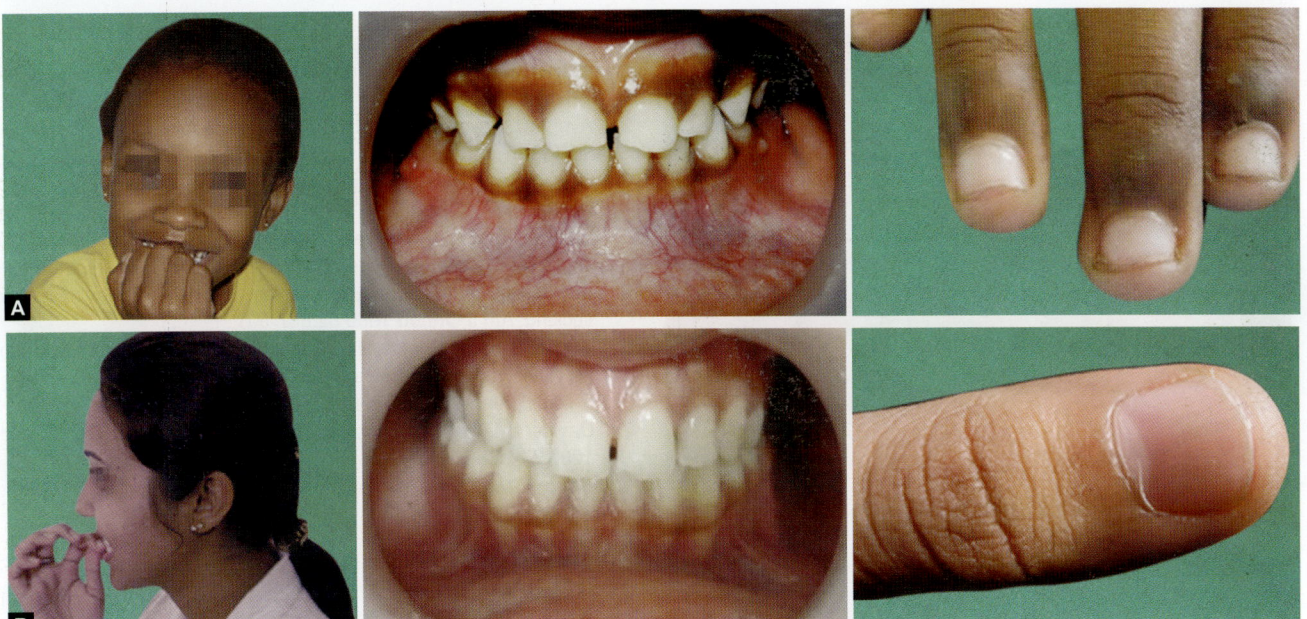

**Figs 21.31A and B:** Nail-biting habit: (A) A child with nail-biting habit. (B) An adult patient with nail biting habit; Note: Severe attrition of right maxillary central incisor and abrasion of the nail bed

- Nagging
- Threats
- Treat the basic emotional factors causing the habit
- Encourage outdoor activities, which may help in easing tension
- As a reminder, nail polish, tight cotton, mittens can be applied on nails.

## BRUXISM

### Definitions

#### Ramfjord (1966)
Bruxism is the habitual grinding of teeth when the individual is not chewing or swallowing.

#### Rubina (1986)
Bruxism is the term used to indicate nonfunctional contact of teeth, which may include clenching, smashing, grinding and tapping of teeth.

### Types

Bruxism is of two types:
1. Diurnal bruxism/day-time bruxism
2. Nocturnal bruxism/night-time bruxism.

Diurnal bruxism/day-time bruxism: It is conscious or subconscious grinding of teeth usually during the day.

Nocturnal bruxism/night-time bruxism: It is the subconscious grinding of teeth characterized by rhythmic pattern of masseter EMG activity.

### Etiology

- Psychological factors
  - Anxiety
  - Rage
  - Hate
  - Aggression
- Genetics
- Occlusal discrepancies
- Systemic factors
  - $Mg^{++}$ deficiency
  - Allergies
  - Enzymatic imbalance
- Occupational factors: Compulsive overachievers.

### Clinical Features

The signs and symptoms of bruxism depends on:
- Frequency
- Intensity
- Duration
- Occlusal trauma
  - Tooth mobility
  - Bone loss
- Tooth structure **(Fig. 21.32)**
  - Attrition of upper teeth
  - Attrition of lower teeth
- Muscular tenderness
  - Tenderness of jaw muscles
  - Muscular fatigue
  - Hypertrophy of masseter
- TMJ disorder
  - TMJ joint pain
- Headache
- Other signs and symptoms
  - Soft tissue trauma
  - Ulceration

### Treatment

- Occlusal adjustments: These include:
  - Correction of restoration
  - Coronoplasty

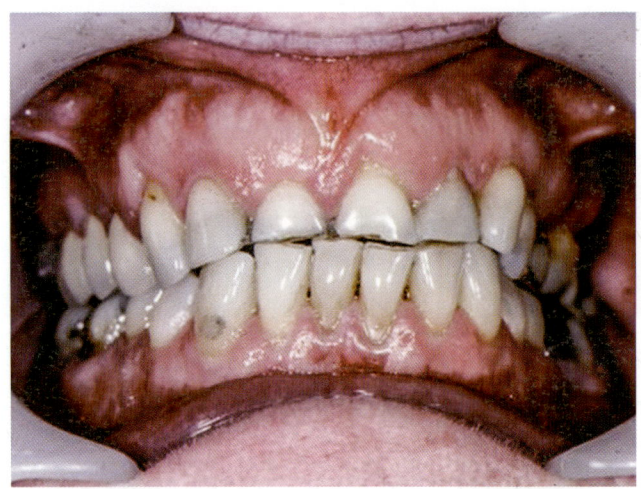

**Fig. 21.32:** An adult patient with bruxism has resulted in severe attrition

- **Occlusal splints:** Vulcanite splints have been recommended to cover the occlusal surface of all teeth as treatment of bruxism.
- **Restorative treatment:** Restorative treatment should be performed in case of abrasion.
- **Psychotherapy:** Counseling the patient can lead to decrease in tension and also create habit awareness.
- **Orthodontic correction:** Malocclusions such as class II and class III when associated with functional malocclusion may create a predisposition to bruxism, such malocclusions are corrected by removable or fixed orthodontic appliance.
- **Drugs**
  - Vapocoolants, such as ethyl chloride to relieve pain in the TMJ.
  - Diazepam: To induce sleep.
- **Electrical method:** Electrogalvanic stimulation for muscles relaxation is currently being utilized for the treatment of bruxism.
- **Acupuncture technique:** Acupuncture technique used for muscle relaxation.

## BIBLIOGRAPHY

1. Ardran GM, Kemp FH. A correlation between suckling pressures and the movements of the tongue. Acta Paediatr 1959; 48:261-72.
2. Ayer WJ. Psychology and thumbsucking. J Am Dent Assoc 1970; 80:1335-7.
3. Bakwin H. Persistent finger sucking in twins. Dev Med Child Neurol 1971;13:308-9.
4. Björk A. Timing of interceptive orthodontic measures based on stages of maturation. Eur Orthod Soc Trans 1972;61-74.
5. Bowden BD. A longitudinal study of the effects of digit and dummy sucking. Am J Orthod 1966;52:887-901.
6. Christensen JR, Fields HW, Adair SM. Oral habits. In: Pinkham AJ (Ed). Pediatric Dentistry: Infancy to Adolescence, 3rd edition. Philadelphia, WB Saunders; 1999.
7. Davidson DO. Thumbsucking, habit or symptom. J Dent Child 1967;34:252-9.
8. Good S. Mouth habits-mouth breathing. J India Dent Assoc 1966; 38:132-5.
9. Graber TM. Thumb and Finger sucking. Am J Orthod 1959; 45:258-64.
10. Hanson ML, Barnard L, Case JL. Tongue thrust in preschool children, 2nd edition. Dental Occlusal Patterns. Am J Orthod 1970;57:15-22.
11. Hanson ML, Barnard LW, Case JL. Tongue thrust in preschool children. Am J Orthod 1969;56:60-9.
12. Haryett RD, Hanson FC, Davidson PO, et al. Chronic thumb sucking: The psychologic effects and the relative effectiveness of various methods of treatment. Am J Orthod 1967;53:569.
13. Haryett RD, Hanson FC, Davidson PO. Chronic thumb sucking: A second report on treatment and its psychological effects. Am J Orthod 1970;57:167-78.
14. Klein J. Pressure habits, etiological factors in malocclusion. Am J Orthod 1952;38(8):569-87.
15. Massler M. Oral habits, origin, evolution and current concepts in management. Alpha Omegan 1963;56:127.
16. Norton LA. Management of digital sucking and tongue thrust in children. Dent Clin North Am 1968;363-82.
17. Popovich F. Prevalence of sucking habits and relation to malocclusion. Oral Health 1967;57:498-9.
18. Tewari A. Abnormal oral habits and malocclusion. J Indiana Dent Assoc 1970;42:81-4.
19. Whitman CL. Correction of oral habits. Dent Clin North Am 1969; 541.
20. Wright, Kennedy DB. Space control in primary and mixed dentition. Dent Clin North Am 1978;22(4):579-602.

## EXAM-ORIENTED QUESTIONS

### Long Questions
1. Define oral habits. Classify and discuss in detail about the features of Thumb sucking habit and its treatment modalities.
2. Classify tongue thrusting habit. Discuss its etiology, clinical features and management.

### Short Notes
1. Mouth breathing habit
2. Lip sucking & lip biting habit
3. Bruxism
4. Pernicious oral habits
5. Beta hypothesis.

# CHAPTER 22

# Orthodontic Treatment Planning

*Phulari BS*

Once the occlusal problem is diagnosed and the etiological factors contributing to the existing malocclusion assessed, the next step is to carefully plan the orthodontic treatment. Treatment planning is as important as the actual treatment itself for unless it is correctly planned, the treatment is unlikely to be successful. Treatment planning serves as a blueprint for the complete course of orthodontic treatment procedure and acts as a guide to achieve the desired results at the end of orthodontic therapy.

Treatment planning should be done systematically and the stages of assessment and planning may be considered as follows:

1. Summarizing the diagnostic findings and listing the orthodontic problems
2. Assessment of etiological factors and factors limiting the corrective treatment
3. Setting the goals for orthodontic treatment
4. Planning the actual treatment course:
   - Type and amount of tooth movement needed
   - Space needed for tooth movement
   - Anchorage sources
   - Selection and the type of appliances
   - Retention plan, which includes the following:
     ♦ Type of retention
     ♦ Duration of the retention.

## RECAPITULATING THE DIAGNOSTIC FINDINGS

Detailed procedure of diagnosis including case history, extraoral and intraoral examination and investigations are described in Chapter 13. Summarizing the diagnostic findings and listing the orthodontic problems would help in deciding the line of treatment appropriate in a given case.

### Recap of Diagnostic Findings

1. Chief concern
2. Medical history
3. Dental history
4. Facial form
5. Skeletal relationship
6. Dentition and occlusal findings:
   - Dental status: It includes the following:
     ♦ Teeth present, erupted, unerupted
     ♦ Teeth missing, supernumerary teeth
   - Restorative status: It includes:
     ♦ Caries, restorations, prosthesis
   - Periodontal status
   - Anteroposterior dental arch relationship:
     ♦ Angle's class
     ♦ Incisor overjet
   - Horizontal/lateral relationships
     ♦ Crossbites and scissors bites
     ♦ Midline shifts
   - Vertical relationship
     ♦ Incisor overbite
   - Individual tooth malpositions
   - Crowding/spacing
   - Functional shifts
7. Radiographic findings
8. Model analysis
9. Cephalometric analysis
10. Diagnosis
11. Treatment planning

> **Orthodontic Problem List**
> All the problems are listed, although each and every problem may not be treated. From the above diagnostic findings, a list of all the orthodontic problems present in given case should be made.

## ASSESSMENT OF ETIOLOGICAL AND LIMITING FACTORS

- Knowing the factors which have brought about the occlusal problems is important for understanding the problem and for planning the appropriate treatment.
- The main causative factors of most malocclusions are the skeletal relationship, the function of oral musculature and the size of the dentition in relation to the size of the jaw bones. Assessing the etiology of the occlusion is mainly important for deciding the treatment possibilities.
- Some etiological factors, can pose severe limitations to corrective treatment. For example, it may not be possible to overcome the effect of a severe skeletal discrepancy in anteroposterior relationship by orthodontic tooth movement alone. Such a condition may require orthognathic surgery along with orthodontic tooth movement.
- Age, growth and maturation of the patient are also important for assessing the potential changes occurring.

## TREATMENT OBJECTIVES

Having known what is wrong and why is wrong, it is necessary to outline the goals of orthodontic treatment. It must be borne in mind that, very few individuals show completely ideal occlusal characteristics and orthodontic treatment may only be needed when the degree of deviation is beyond a certain limit.

Furthermore, limitations to corrective treatment such as skeletal relationship and certain muscular anomalies

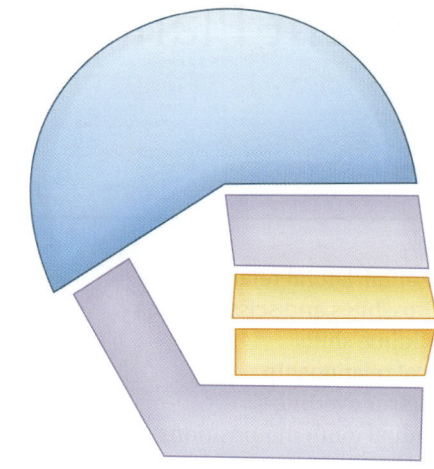 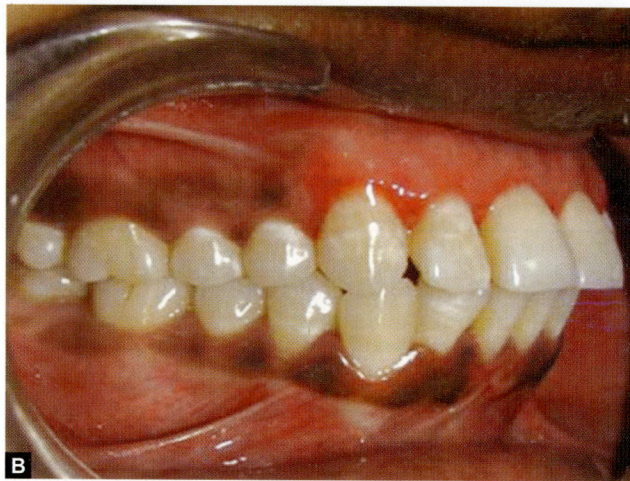

**Figs 22.1A and B:** Angle's class I malocclusion

must be considered. Thus, it may not be always necessary or possible to correct every deviation. Hence, it is necessary to outline objectives/goals of orthodontic treatment in a given case, which have to be achieved at the end of treatment phase.

Personal factors such as patient's ability for cooperation and patient's primary concern (e.g. esthetics) must also be considered while setting the goals of orthodontic treatment.

### Planning the Treatment Procedures

After deciding the goals of treatment, a detailed treatment plan should be formulated which depends on the following factors:

a. *The type of tooth movement needed:* The type of tooth movement needed will govern the amount of force required for movement and the type of appliance necessary. For example, tipping movement can be achieved by removable appliances while other types of movement usually need fixed appliances, which can apply forces over wide area of the tooth.
b. *The space needed for tooth movement:* Space is necessary for correction of crowding which is seen in the most of the cases of malocclusion and also for the correction of anteroposterior dental arch relationship. Accordingly, the required space can be gained by:
   - Arch expansion
   - Tooth extraction
   - Molar distalization
   - Proximal stripping, etc.

The amount and position of space required and the method of gaining this required space can be determined by model analysis. Patient's maturational age should also be considered.

### *Planning Extractions*

#### Angle's Class I Malocclusion Cases

In Angle's class I malocclusion where sagittal interarch relationship is normal, it is preferable to extract in both the arches in order to maintain the interarch relationship **(Figs 22.1A and B)**.

#### Angle's Class II Malocclusion Cases

- In most Angle's class II cases with upper anterior proclination and well-aligned lower arch, interarch relationship can be corrected by extraction only in the upper arch **(Figs 22.2A and B)**.
- However, in Angle's class II cases, where there is lower arch crowding or when molars are not in full class II occlusion, it may be necessary to extract in both the upper and lower arches to achieve proper sagittal interarch relation and to relieve crowding.

#### Angle's Class III Malocclusion Cases

- Angle's class III cases are preferably treated by extraction only in the lower arch **(Figs 22.3A and B)**. Extraction in upper arch is avoided as it may impair the forward development of the maxilla.

c. *Planning anchorage:* Planning the anchorage is very essential for successful orthodontic treatment. Anchorage sources, which can be used in a given case include headgear, transpalatal arches, interarch elastics, etc.
d. *Selecting the type of appliance:* Depending on the type and degree of tooth movement desired and other factors, the appropriate appliance is selected.
   - Removable, myofunctional, orthopedic appliances or fixed mechanotherapy may be needed.
   - Stages of the treatment procedures and approximate duration of the active treatment are also decided.
e. *Planning retention:* It includes the following:
   - It is usually necessary to apply passive mechanical retention at the end of successful active treatment, so as to prevent any relapse.
   - Retention phase is often overlooked by the patient and is the common cause of relapse. Thus, it is imperative to decide the type and duration of the

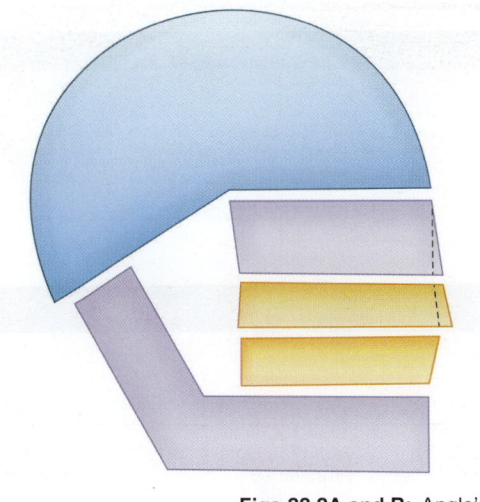 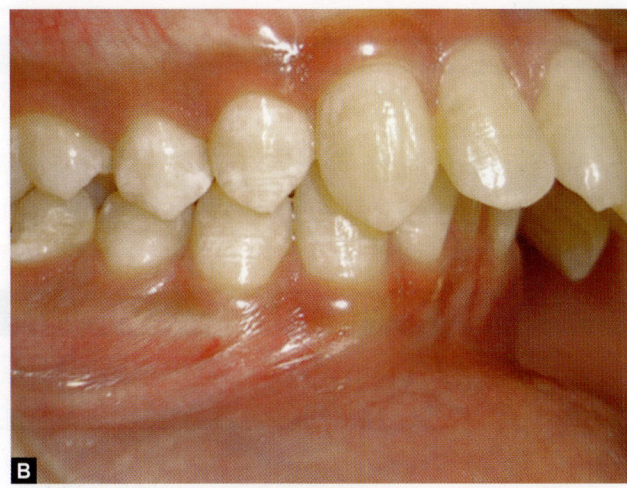

**Figs 22.2A and B:** Angle's class II division 1 malocclusion with well-aligned teeth

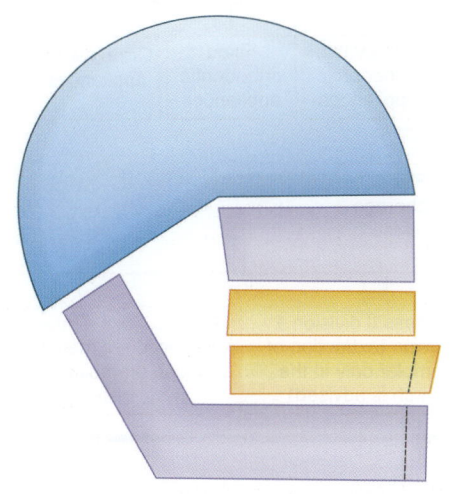 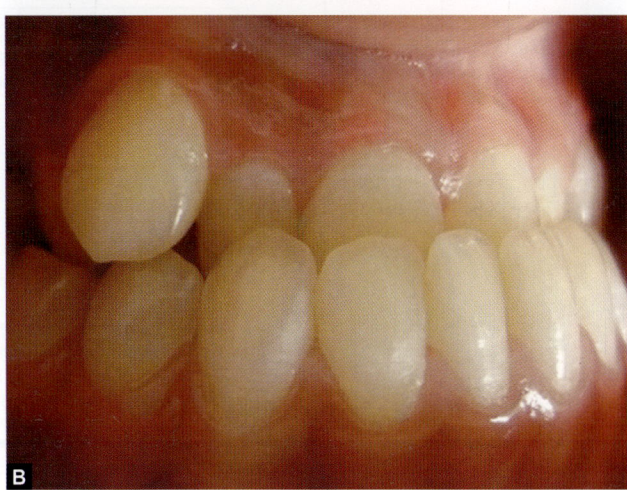

**Figs 22.3A and B:** Angle's class III malocclusion cases are preferably treated by extraction only in the lower arch

retention in a given case and the patient is educated about its importance.

- Type of retention and duration must be planned depending on the type of tooth movement achieved and patient's compliance. For example, rotation type of tooth movement requires longer period of retention. Fixed type of retainer should be opted in a case of an uncooperative patient.

## BIBLIOGRAPHY

1. Ackerman JL, Profitt WR. The characteristics of malocclusion: a modern approach to classification and diagnosis. Am J Orthod 1969;56:443-54.
2. Andrews LF. The six keys to normal occlusion. Am J Orthod 1972;62:296-309.
3. Begg PR. Begg orthodontic theory and technique, Philadelphia, WB Saunders, 1965.
4. Enlow DH, Moyers RE, Hunter WS, et al. A Procedure for the analysis of intrinsic factor form and growth. Am J Orthod 1969;56:6-14.
5. Graber TM, Vanarsdall RL. Orthodontics, Current Principles and Techniques. Mosby Year Book, Inc, 1994.
6. Graber TM. Orthodontics: Principles and Practice. WB Saunders, 1998.
7. Horowitz SI, Hixon EH. The number of orthodontic diagnosis. St. Louis: CV Mosby, 1966.
8. Koski K. The norm concept in dental orthopaedics. Angle Orthod 1955;25:113-7.
9. Profitt WR. Contemporary Orthodontics. St Louis: CV Mosby, 1986.
10. Schwanniner B, Shaye R. Management of cases with upper incisors missing. Am J Orthod 1980;100(5):710-2.
11. Thampson FG. Second premolar extraction in Begg technique. J Clin Orthod 1977;11:610-3.
12. Tung AW, Kiyak HA. Psychological influences on the timing of orthodontic treatment. Am J Orthod Dentofacial Orthop 1998;113:29-39.

# EXAM-ORIENTED QUESTIONS

## Long Essay or Long Question
1. Orthodontic treatment planning.

## Short Note
1. Planning of extraction in Angle's class I, II and III malocclusion cases.

## CHAPTER OVERVIEW

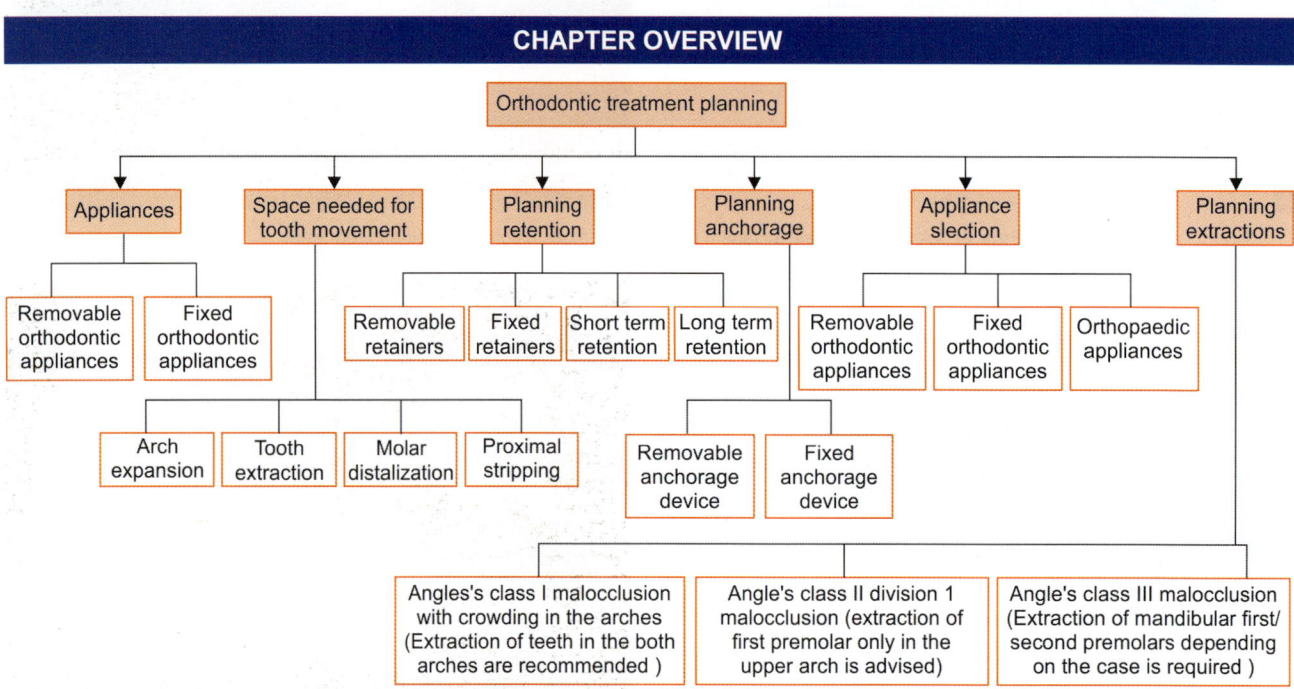

# CHAPTER 23
# Anchorage in Orthodontics

*Shah A, Phulari BS*

Teeth can be moved orthodontically by subjecting them to force. However, all teeth exhibit certain amount of resistance to tooth movement. Depending on their anatomy and position, different teeth have different resistance values to tooth movement. For example, multirooted, larger teeth like molars are more resistant to tooth movement than are the single-rooted anteriors.

Keeping this in mind, certain teeth can be used as anchor units in order to move other teeth into a more desirable position. For instance, proclined anterior teeth can be retracted distally by using the larger, multirooted posterior teeth as anchor units. Apart from teeth, other structures such as the palate, lingual alveolar supporting bone in the mandible, the occiput and the back of the neck can also be used as anchorage units. In recent years, mini implants are also being used for gaining anchorage in certain cases.

The resistance offered by other teeth not intended to be moved and other anatomic areas is used to apply force on the teeth to be moved. In simple terms, anchorage is the resistance offered by these anchor units to unwanted tooth movement.

To anchor is to hold or resist the movement of an object and anchorage is gaining of that hold. A sailboat anchored to the sea shore can serve as a suitable analogy to understand the concept of anchorage in orthodontics. The boat can be likened to the tooth to be moved, the rope to the arch wire or elastic and the anchor nail to the anchor unit (teeth or other anatomic areas) from which force is applied. Larger the boat, stronger should be the anchor.

Now, it can be appreciated that careful anchorage planning is essential for efficient tooth movement.

## DEFINITIONS

1. **Graber**
   Anchorage is defined as "the nature and degree of resistance to displacement offered by an anatomic unit when used for the purpose of affecting tooth movement".
2. **White and Gardner**
   Anchorage is defined as "the site of delivery from which a force is exerted".

## SOURCES OF ANCHORAGE

Anchorage can be obtained from several sources during orthodontic treatment, which can be either intraoral or extraoral sources **(Table 23.1)**.

## INTRAORAL SOURCES

### Teeth

Teeth by far are the most frequently used anchorage units in orthodontics. When certain teeth have to be moved; the remaining teeth can be used as anchorage units. Various factors can influence the anchorage potential of the teeth, such as:
   i. Root form
   ii. Size of the roots
   iii. Number of the roots
   iv. Anatomic position of the teeth
   v. Axial inclination of the teeth
   vi. Intercuspation of the teeth.

### Root Form

Root form has a definite bearing on the anchorage potential of a tooth. Cross-sections of roots of teeth may show any of the following three forms **(Figs 23.1A and B)**:
a. Round root form.
b. Flat (Mesiodistally) root form.
c. Triangular root form.

**Round:** In round root only about half of fibers of periodontal ligaments are stressed to resist force in any given direction. Thus, round root form of a tooth offers least anchorage **(Fig. 23.1A)**.

Round root form is seen in:
- Bicuspids
- Palatal root of maxillary permanent molar.

**Table 23.1:** Sources of anchorage

| |
|---|
| ***Intraoral sources*** |
| ▪ Teeth |
| ▪ Alveolar bone |
| ▪ Basal jaw bone |
| ▪ Musculature |
| ***Extraoral sources*** |
| ▪ Cranium |
|   • Occipital bone |
|   • Parietal bone |
| ▪ Facial bones |
|   • Frontal bone |
|   • Mandibular symphysis |
| ▪ Back of the neck (cervical bone) |

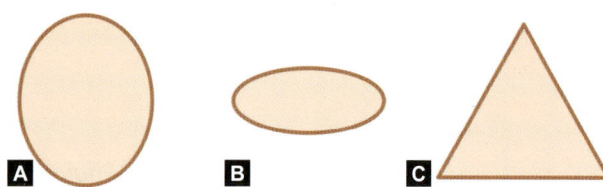

**Figs 23.1A to C:** Different forms of roots. (A) Round root form (B) Flat root form (C) Triangular root form

***Flat root form:*** Mesiodistally flat root can better resist tooth movement in a mesiodistal direction rather than in a labiolingual direction, as more number of periodontal ligament fibers is attached to the flatter surfaces as compared to narrow labiolingual surfaces **(Fig. 23.1B)**.

Examples of roots with flat form are:
a. Mandibular incisors
b. Mandibular molars
c. Buccal roots of maxillary molars.

***Triangular:*** When compared to round and flat roots, the triangular roots offer the maximum resistance **(Fig. 23.1C)**. Triangular form of root is seen in:
- Maxillary central incisors
- Canines.

In case of mandibular molars, the roots obtain an "I" form because of deep developmental depressions present on both mesial and distal root surfaces. This feature further enhances the anchorage due to larger surface area provided by such an arrangement.

The tripod arrangement of the roots as seen in maxillary molars also enhances the anchorage because of their arrangement in the alveolar bone.

### Size of the Roots

Larger and longer the roots, greater is the resistance they offer. Thus, maxillary canines provide good anchorage as they have long roots.

### Number of the Roots

Understandably, the multirooted teeth provide greater anchorage than that of the single rooted teeth, with comparable root lengths.

### Anatomic Position of the Tooth

The mandibular second premolars, due to their unique position between mylohyoid and external oblique ridges, offer an increased resistance to mesial movement.

### Axial Inclination of the Tooth

When the axial inclination of the tooth is in an opposite direction to that of the force applied, it can provide a greater resistance to movement.

### Proximal Contacts and Intercuspation between Teeth

Tight and broad contacts between adjacent teeth enhance anchorage potential of these teeth. A good intercuspation especially among posteriors augments anchorage since one tooth in the arch is related to two teeth in the opposing arch.

### Alveolar Bone

The investing alveolar bone around the roots offers resistance to tooth movement up to a certain amount of force, exceeding which there will be bone remodeling.

### Basal Bone

Certain areas of basal jaw bone such as hard palate and lingual surface of anterior mandible can be utilized in order to enhance the intraoral anchorage. "Nance palatal button" **(Fig. 23.2)** uses the anchorage provided by the hard palate to resist the mesial movement of maxillary molars.

### Musculature

Natural tonicity of the facial and masticatory muscles is conductive to the normal development of the dental arches. Hypotonic musculature can cause flaring of teeth

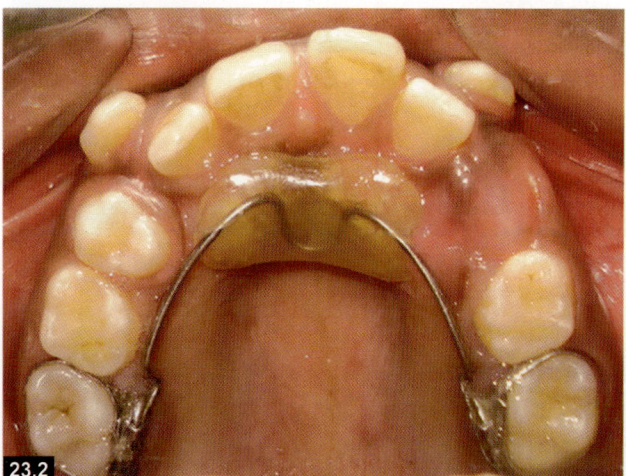
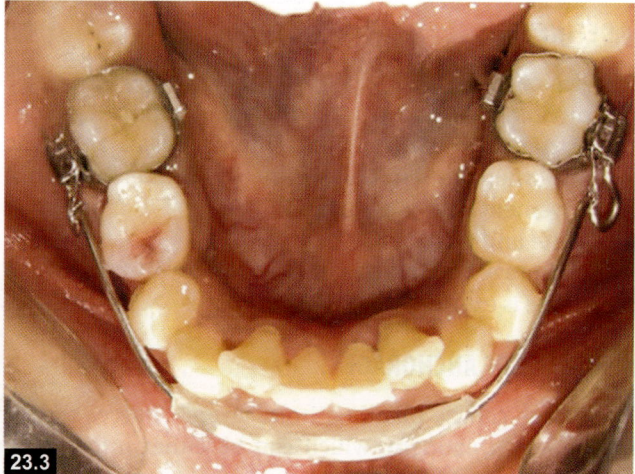

**Fig. 23.2:** Nance palatal button uses the anchorage by the hard palate; **Fig. 23.3:** Lip bumper

whereas, hypertonic musculature can force the teeth in a lingual direction.

The forces exerted by hypertonic labial musculature are utilized by the lip bumper appliance **(Fig. 23.3)** to augment the anchorage of mandibuar molars by preventing their mesial movement.

## EXTRAORAL SOURCES

Certain extraoral sites can be used as anchorage units to bring about orthodontic or orthopedic changes. They are used to reinforce anchorage when intraoral anchorage is insufficient.

Some of the most commonly used extraoral structures are the cranium, back of the neck, forehead and the chin. The main disadvantage however, is the lack of patient compliance as evidenced by bulky and extraorally noticeable anchorage assembly.

### Cranium (Occipital and Parietal Bones)

"Headgears" **(Fig. 23.4)** derive anchorage from occipital or parietal regions of the cranium. These are used along with a face bow to resist the growth of maxilla or to move the maxillary teeth distally.

### Back of the Neck (Cervical Region)

The "cervical headgears" derive anchorage from back of the neck or cervical region. They are also used to bring about changes in the maxilla or maxillary teeth.

### Facial Bones

The frontal bone (forehead region) and mandibular symphysis (chin area) are used as resistance units during face mask therapy so as to protract the maxilla. Such type of headgears which gain anchorage from forehead and chin regions are sometimes called the reverse headgears **(Fig. 23.5)**.

## CLASSIFICATION (MOYER'S)

Anchorage used in orthodontic treatment can be classified in a number of ways **(Table 23.2)**. However, one type of anchorage is not exclusive of that type. For instance, reciprocal anchorage used for closure of midline diastema is also an example of intramaxillary anchorage and intraoral anchorage.

**Table 23.2:** Moyer's classification

- According to the manner of force application
  - Simple anchorage
  - Stationary anchorage
  - Reciprocal anchorage
- According to jaws involved
  - Intramaxillary anchorage
  - Intermaxillary anchorage
- According to the site of anchorage
  - Intraoral anchorage
  - Extraoral anchorage
    - Cervical
    - Occipital
    - Cranial
    - Facial
  - Muscular anchorage
- According to the number of anchorage units:
  - Single or primary anchorage
  - Compound anchorage
  - Multiple or reinforced anchorage.

### According to the Manner of Force Application

#### Simple Anchorage

- Simple anchorage is the dental anchorage in which the manner and application of force is such that it tends to change the axial inclination of the anchor tooth or teeth in the plane of space in which the force is being applied.
- In other words, the resistance of the anchorage unit to tipping is utilized to move another tooth or teeth.

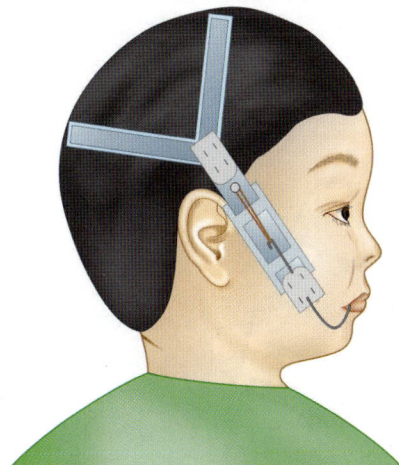
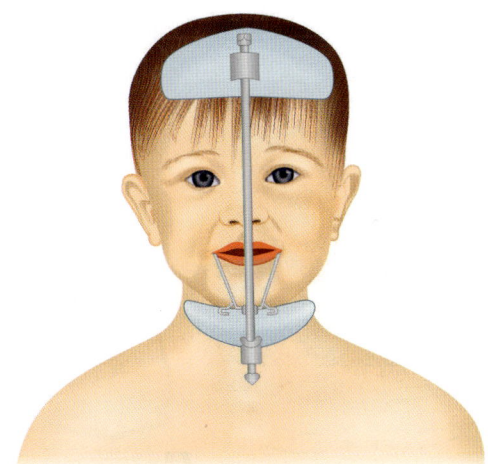

**Fig. 23.4:** Headgears derive anchorage from occipital or parietal regions of the cranium;
**Fig. 23.5:** Petit face mask derives the anchorage from forehead and chin

- In this type of anchorage, the appliance usually engages a greater number of teeth than are to be moved within the same dental arch. Ideally, the combined root surface area of the anchor teeth should be two times that of the teeth to be moved.
- The amount of force on each anchor tooth in simple anchorage is equal to the total moving force component of the appliance divided by the number of anchored teeth.

Amount of force on each anchor tooth

$$= \frac{\text{Total moving force component of appliance}}{\text{Number of anchor teeth}}$$

- Simple anchorage is frequently used and is satisfactory in many stages of orthodontic treatment.

### Stationary Anchorage

- Stationary anchorage is defined as dental anchorage in which the manner of application of force tends to displace the anchorage unit bodily in the plane of space in which this force is being applied.
- In this type of anchorage, the resistance of anchor teeth to bodily movement is utilized to move other teeth.
- Stationary anchorage provides greater resistance than simple anchorage to unwanted tooth movement.

### Reciprocal Anchorage

- The reciprocal anchorage refers to the resistance offered by two malposed units, when the dissipation of equal and opposite forces tends to move each unit towards a more normal occlusion.
- In some treatment procedures, it is desirable to move teeth or groups of teeth of equal anchorage potential in opposite directions. In such cases, it is possible to utilize their anchorage forces as moving forces to achieve the desirable changes.

### Examples

1. A frequently used form of reciprocal anchorage is known as intermaxillary traction in which the forces used to move the whole or part of one dental arch in one direction are anchored by equal forces by moving the opposite arch in opposite direction, thus, correcting discrepancies in both the dental arches.
2. Correction of midline diastema is another classic example of reciprocal anchorage (Fig. 23.6A).
3. Bilateral symmetrical expansion (Fig. 23.6B).
4. Correction of single tooth crossbite (Fig. 23.6C).

## According to the Jaws Involved

### Intramaxillary Anchorage

- Intramaxillary anchorage is the anchorage in which the resistance units are situated within the same jaw. If appliances are placed only in maxillary or mandibular dental arches, they are considered intramaxillary resistance units.
- For example, class I elastic stretched from first molar to canine teeth in either of the dental arches is an example (Fig. 23.7).

### Intermaxillary Anchorage

Intermaxillary anchorage is the anchorage in which the units situated in one jaw are used to effect tooth movement in the other jaw.

### Examples

a. Class II elastic stretched from upper canine to lower molar to effect correction of class II malocclusion (Fig. 23.8).
b. Class III elastic stretched from upper molar to lower canine to correct class III malocclusion (Fig. 23.9).

## According to the Site of Anchorage

### Intraoral Anchorage

When intraoral structures such as teeth, and other anatomic areas are used as anchor units it is called intraoral anchorage.

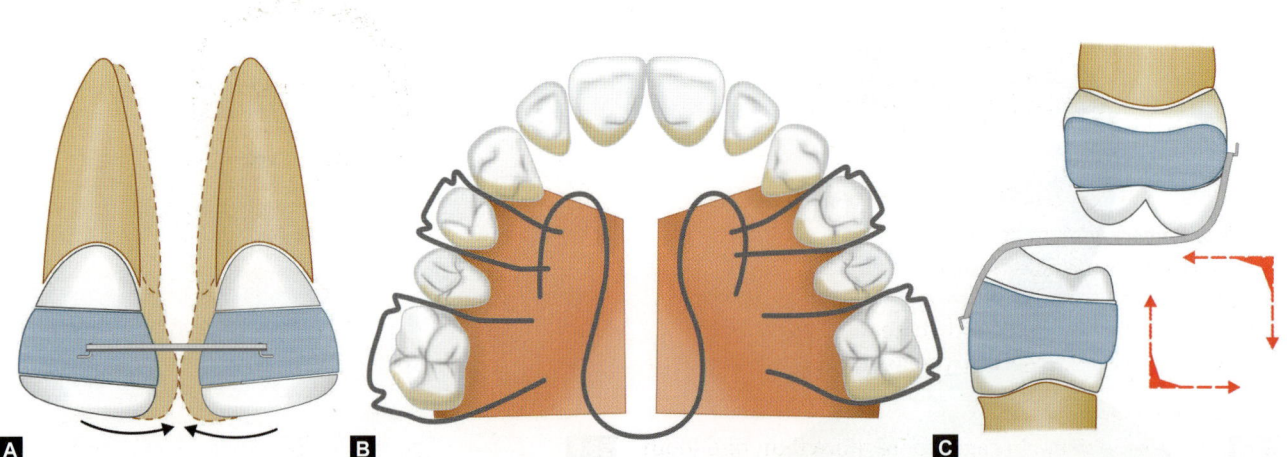

**Figs 23.6A to C:** Reciprocal anchorages: (A) Correction of midline diastema is another classic example of reciprocal anchorage. (B) Bilateral symmetrical expansion. (C) Correction of single tooth crossbite

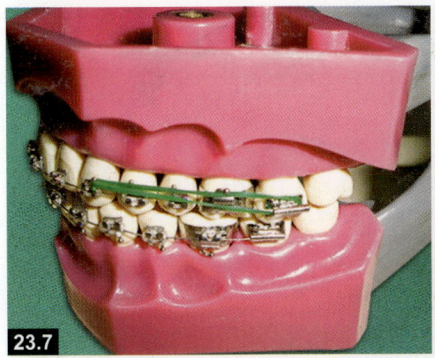 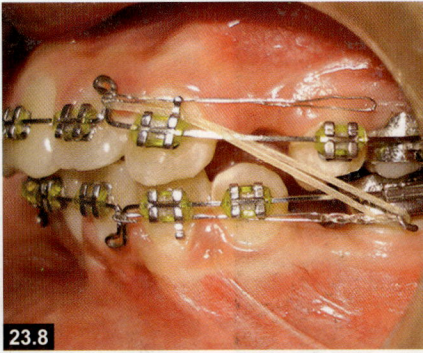 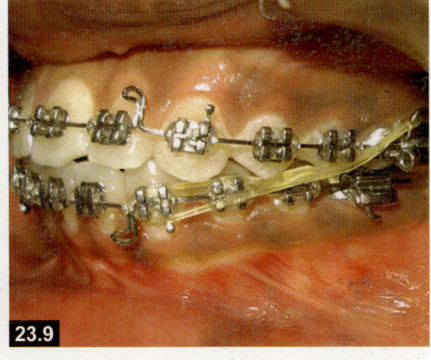

**Fig. 23.7:** Class I elastic/intramaxillary elastics; **Fig. 23.8:** Class II elastic stretched from upper canine to lower molar to effect correction of class II malocclusion; **Fig. 23.9:** Class III elastic stretched from upper molar to lower canine to correct class III malocclusion

### Extraoral Anchorage

Extraoral anchorage is the anchorage established from extraoral structures **(Figs 23.10A and B)**.

1. Cervical region: Use of cervical pull headgear.
2. Occipital region: Use of occipital pull headgear **(Fig. 23.10A)**.
3. Forehead and chin face mask **(Fig. 23.10B)**.

#### Advantages

- Anchorage established from extraoral anchorage source is much greater than intraoral anchorage source, since extraoral anchorage units are more stable.
- There is lesser risk of anchor loss.

#### Disadvantages

- When extraoral anchorage is employed, the success of the treatment lies entirely on patient compliance. Patient has to wear the extraoral appliance (headgear) for a minimum of 12–15 hours a day to achieve the desired effect.
- The metallic framework and noticeable gadgets of orthopedic orthodontic appliances (headgear or chin cup) may discourage the patient from wearing it.

### Muscular Anchorage

- Perioral musculature may be used as anchorage units in certain cases.
- For example, the lip bumper myofunctional orthodontic appliance utilizes the force exerted by lower lip musculature to bring about distalization of mandibular first molar **(Fig. 23.11)**.

### According to the Number of Anchorage Units

#### Single or Primary Anchorage

- Single or primary anchorage is defined as the resistance provided by a single tooth with greater alveolar support to move another tooth with lesser alveolar support.
- For example, retraction of a premolar using a molar tooth.

#### Compound Anchorage

- It is the type of anchorage where more than one tooth with greater anchorage potential are used to move a tooth/group of teeth with lesser support.
- For example, compound anchorage is routinely used in fixed mechanotherapy.

### Reinforced Anchorage/Multiple Anchorage

- It frequently happens that the teeth available for simple anchorage are not sufficient in number or in size to resist the forces necessary for orthodontic treatment and that reciprocal anchorage is not appropriate to the type of treatment to be carried out. In such circumstance, it is necessary to reinforce the anchorage to avoid unwanted movements of the anchor teeth.
- Anchorage is said to be reinforced when more than one type of resistance units are utilized.

### For example:

1. Transpalatal arch is often used to reinforce anchorage in fixed mechanotherapy **(Fig. 23.12)**.
2. Headgears can be used to augment intraoral anchorage.

## ANCHORAGE PLANNING

Success of orthodontic treatment depends on appropriate anchorage planning. One should consider the best possible resistant units in a given case to effectively move the malposed tooth/group of teeth.

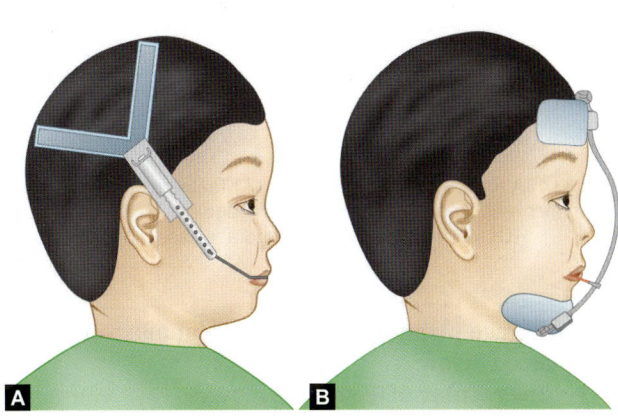

**Figs 23.10A and B:** Extraoral anchorage; (A) Occipital pull headgear (B) Face mask

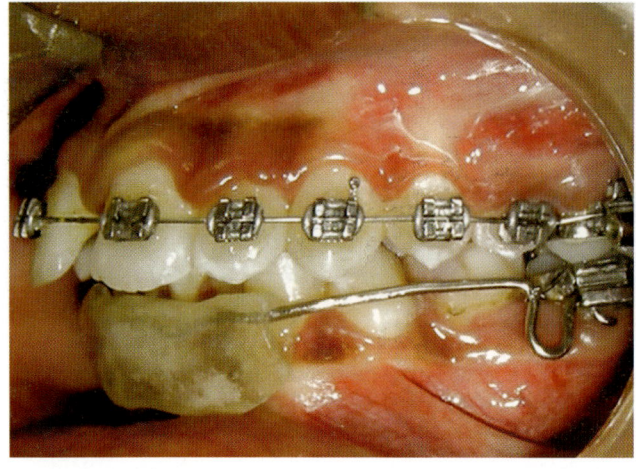

**Fig. 23.11:** "Lip bumper" myofunctional orthodontic appliance utilizes the force exerted by lower lip musculature to bring about distalization of mandibular first molar

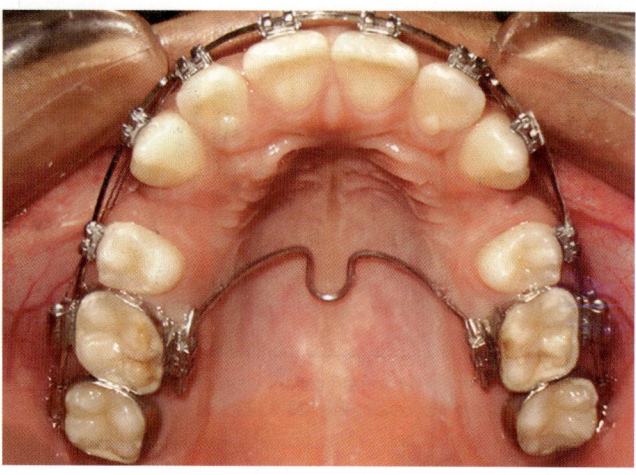

**Fig. 23.12:** Transpalatal arch is often used to reinforce anchorage in fixed mechanotherapy

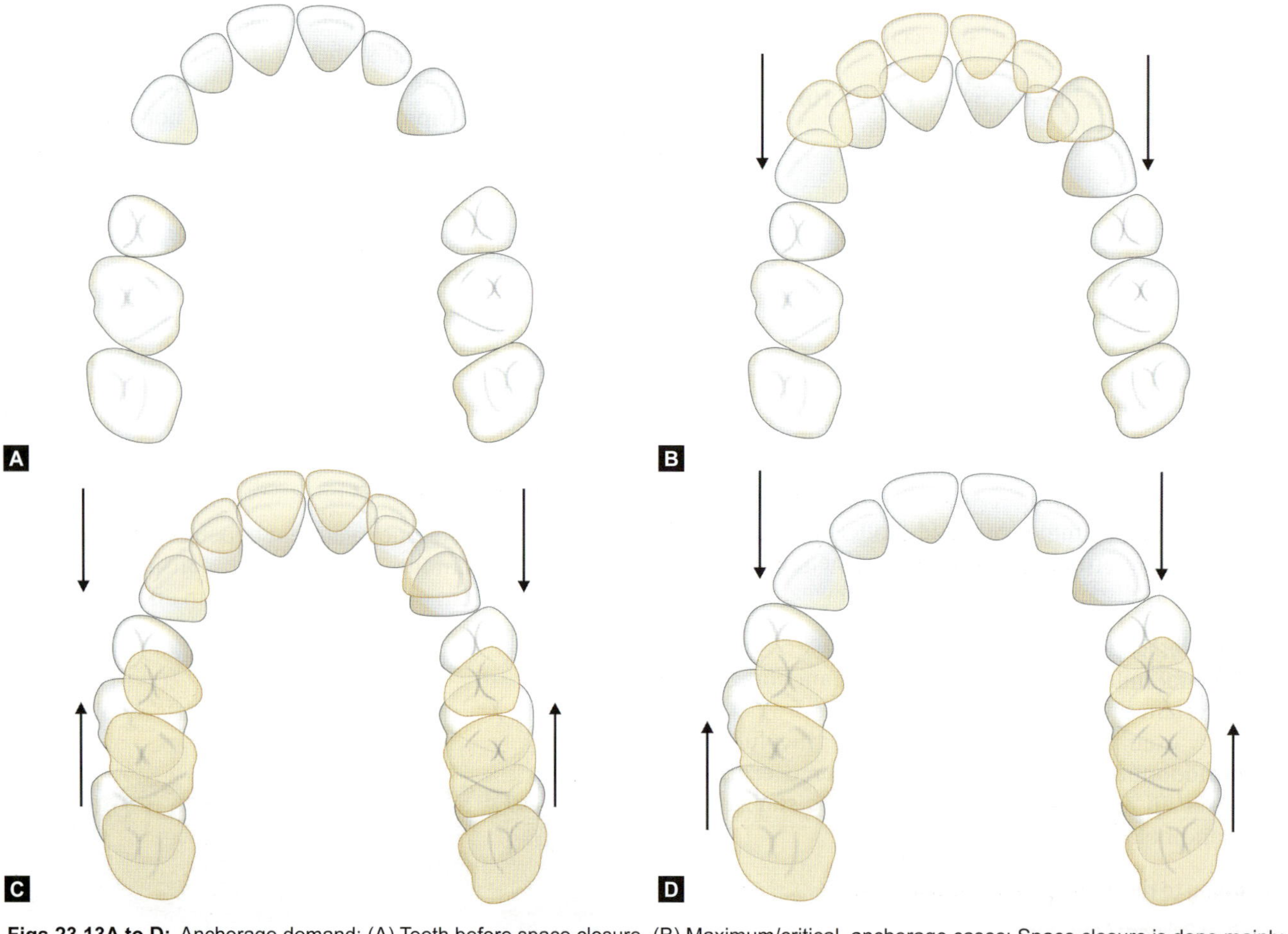

**Figs 23.13A to D:** Anchorage demand: (A) Teeth before space closure. (B) Maximum/critical anchorage cases: Space closure is done mainly by anterior retraction. (C) Moderate anchorage cases: Space closure is done by equal amounts of anterior retraction and posterior protraction. (D) Minimum/noncritical anchorage cases: Space closure is done by posterior protraction rather than anterior retraction

Anchorage planning depends on a number of factors as explained below:
   I. The number of teeth to be moved.
   II. The type of teeth to be moved
   III. Type of tooth movement.
   IV. Duration of tooth movement.

### I. The Number of Teeth to be Moved
Greater the number of teeth being moved, greater is the anchorage demand.

### II. The Type of Teeth to be Moved
Different types of teeth have different anchorage demand.

#### Examples
a. The movement of canine is tougher than incisors as it possesses a longer, larger and flatter root.
b. The movement of molars is more difficult than that of premolars as molars possess greater number of roots as compared to premolars.

### III. Type of Tooth Movement
Bodily movement of teeth requires more force as compared to tipping movement of same teeth.

### IV. Duration of Tooth Movement
Anchor teeth can withstand force for sometime as seen in short duration treatment. The anchor teeth might not be able to withstand the same force, if treatment is prolonged.

#### Anchorage Requirement
The term anchorage is only a relative one. Although ideally the anchorage teeth should not move, they also move to some extent along with the teeth against which the forces are primarily directed. Such unwanted movement of anchor teeth is called as "anchor loss". Some amount of anchor loss is inevitable during all orthodontic procedures and should be kept in mind while planning the treatment.

Depending on the amount of movement of posterior teeth permissible to close the extraction space, i.e. the amount of anchor loss permissible, the anchorage demand of an extraction case can be maximum, moderate or minimum **(Fig. 23.13A)**.

1. *Maximum/critical anchorage cases:* In maximum anchorage cases, no more than 25% of the extraction space should be lost by forward movement of the anchor teeth. In other words, 75% or more of the extraction space is needed for the retraction of the anteriors. In such cases anchorage should be reinforced to prevent undesirable movement of the posterior anchor teeth **(Fig. 23.13B)**.
2. *Moderate anchorage cases:* In cases where the anchorage demand is moderate, the anchor teeth can be allowed to move forward into the extraction space for about 50% of the total extraction space **(Fig. 23.13C)**. In other words, extraction space can be closed by equal movement of anterior and posterior teeth.
3. *Minimum anchorage cases:* In these cases, the anchorage demand is minimum or not critical. More than half the extraction space can be lost by the mesial movement of posterior teeth **(Fig. 23.13D)**. In these cases, distal movement of anteriors is not advised.

## BIBLIOGRAPHY

1. Block MS, Hoffman D. A new device for absolute anchorage for orthodontics. Am J Orthod Dentofacial Orthop 1995;107:251-8.
2. Block MS, Almerico B, Crawford C, et al. Bone response to functioning implants in dog mandibular alveolar ridges augmented with distraction osteogenesis. Int J Oral Maxillofac Implants 1998;12:342-51.
3. Branemark PI, Hansson BO, Adell R, et al. Osseointegrated implants in the treatment of edentulous jaw. Experience from a 10-year period. Scand J Plast Reconstr Surg 1977;16:1-132.
4. Costa A, Raffini M, Melsen B. Miniscrews as orthodontic anchorage: a preliminary report. Int J Adult Orthod Orthognath Surg 1998;13:201-9.
5. Creekmore TD, Eklund MK. The possibility of skeletal anchorage. J Clin Orthod 1983;17:266-9.
6. De Pauw GA, Dermaut L, De Bruyn H, et al. Stability of implants as anchorage for orthopedic traction. Angle Orthod 1999;69:401-7.
7. Douglass JB, Killiany DM. Dental implants used as orthodontic anchorage. J Oral Implantol 1987;13:28-38.
8. Erdmann L, Fernandez Valeron J, Fernandez Velazquez J. Implants in the orthodontic and prosthetic rehabilitation of an adult patient: a case report. Int J Oral Maxillofac Implants 1996;11:534-8.
9. Gainsforth BL, Higley LB. A study of orthodontic anchorage possibilities in basal bone. Am J Orthod Oral Surg 1945;31:406-17.

## EXAM-ORIENTED QUESTIONS

### Long Questions
1. Define anchorage. Explain in detail about different types of anchorage with examples.
2. Define anchorage. Classify orthodontic anchorage and explain with examples.
3. Define reinforced anchorage. Discuss methods of reinforcing anchorage.
4. Classify anchorage. Explain when, why and how would you like to reinforce it.
5. Define and discuss the various anchorage situations in removable and fixed appliances.

### Short Notes
1. Extraoral anchorage
2. Intermaxillary anchorage
3. Reciprocal anchorage
4. Anchorage planning
5. Stationary anchorage
6. Factors affecting anchorage
7. Cortical anchorage
8. Anchor loss.

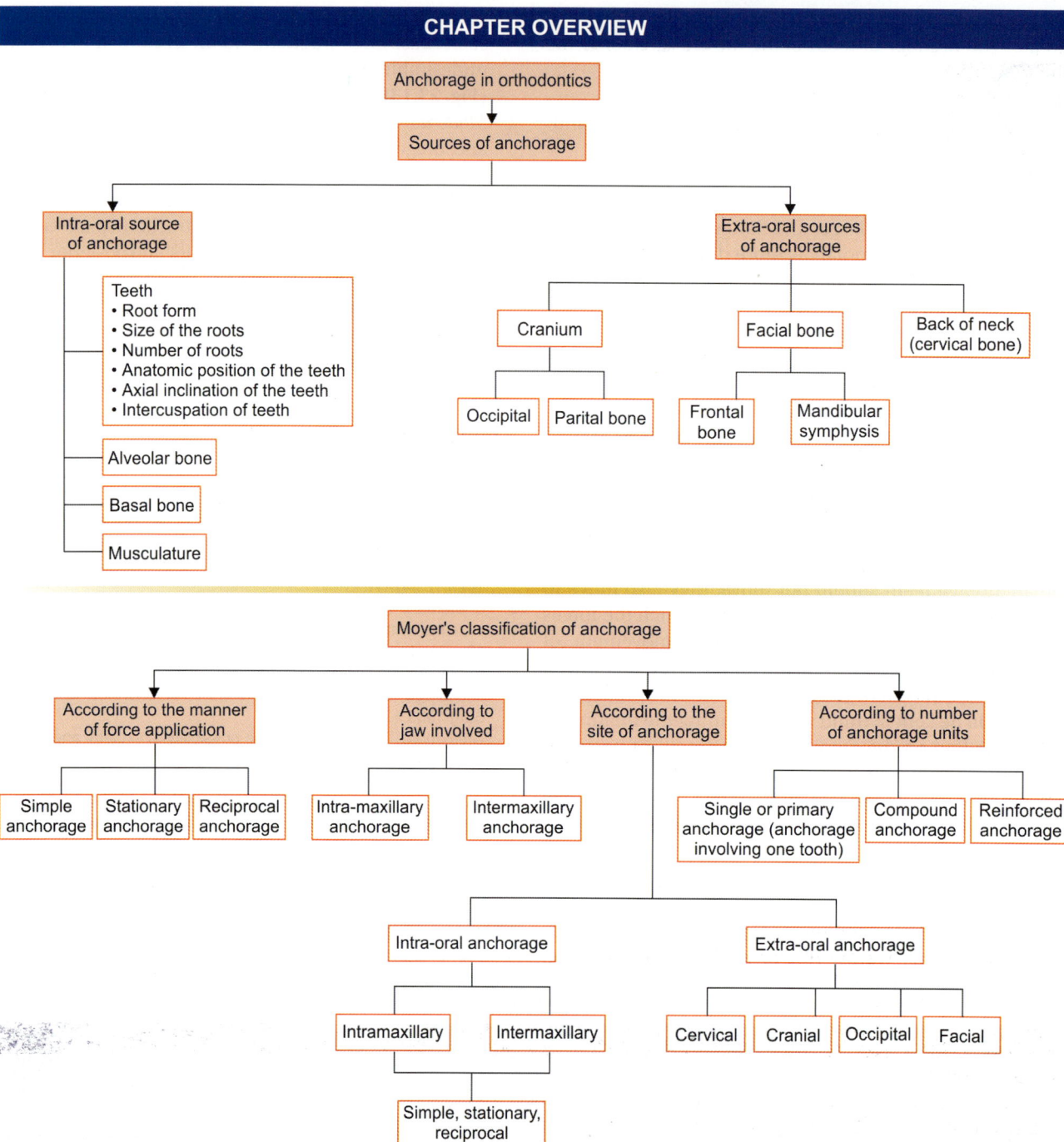

# CHAPTER 24

# Methods of Gaining Space

*Phulari BS*

Creation of space in the dental arch may be required to correct certain features of a malocclusion, such as crowding, overjet reduction, leveling of the curve of Spee or the correction of incisor inclination and angulations. The required space may be gained by a number of means including proximal stripping, arch expansion, extraction, etc. Appropriate means of obtaining the required space in a given case should be decided after careful examination and model analysis.

## METHODS OF GAINING SPACE

I. Proximal stripping
II. Expansion of the dental arches
III. Extraction of certain teeth
IV. Distalization of canines and molars
V. Uprighting of molars
VI. Derotation of posterior teeth
VII. Proclination of anterior teeth

## PROXIMAL STRIPPING

### Synonyms

- Proximal slicing of tooth
- Reproximation of tooth
- Proximal grinding of tooth
- Slendarization of tooth
- Proximal disking of tooth.

Proximal stripping is one of the routinely employed methods of gaining space when the space requirement is minimal up to 2.5 mm.

### Definition

Proximal stripping of a tooth is defined as a method by which the proximal surfaces of the tooth are stripped/sliced/disked in order to reduce the mesiodistal width of the tooth.

Proximal stripping can be opted as a method of gaining space in cases where mild crowding with minimal arch-length tooth material discrepancy of less than 2–3 mm is present. However, it should be carried out with caution so as to prevent dental caries and dentin hypersensitivity.

### Indications

- Proximal stripping is indicated to relieve mandibular anterior crowding most commonly and to some extent in maxillary anterior segment.
- If arch perimeter analysis and Nance Carey's analysis show discrepancy less than 2.5 mm, then proximal stripping is indicated.
- Proximal stripping is indicated if the Bolton's analysis shows discrepancy of mild tooth material excess.

### Contraindications

- Patients with high-risk of dental caries.
- In young patients with large pulp chambers.
- Presence of proximal caries in the teeth to be sliced.
- Patient with severely attrited teeth.

### Advantages

- It avoids extraction in borderline cases.
- It establishes favorable overjet and overbite relationship.
- It broadens the contact area thereby prevents rotation of teeth.

### Disadvantages

- Patient may experience sensitivity of teeth, which have undergone proximal stripping.
- Improper method of proximal stripping results in altered morphology of teeth.
- Proximally stripped teeth are more prone to dental caries.
- Food impaction may occur.

### Diagnosis

#### Model Analysis

Selection of proximal stripping as a method of gaining space depends on the amount of space required. Model analysis using orthodontic study models should be done to evaluate the usefulness of proximal stripping **(Flowchart 24.1)**.

- ***Arch perimeter analysis:*** Proximal stripping is indicated when discrepancy in the maxillary arch lies between 0–2.5 mm.
- ***Nance Carey's analysis:*** Proximal stripping is indicated when discrepancy in the mandibular arch lies between 0–2.5 mm.
- ***Peck and Peck analysis:*** If mesiodistal dimension of tooth is less than labiolingual dimension, then proximal stripping is indicated.
- ***Bolton's analysis:*** When there is an excess tooth material comparable to arch length in either of the arches, proximal stripping is indicated.

#### Intraoral Periapical Radiographs

IOPA of the teeth to be disked is advised to analyze the enamel thickness and pulp anatomy. It also gives an idea of how much enamel can be reduced without damaging the tooth.

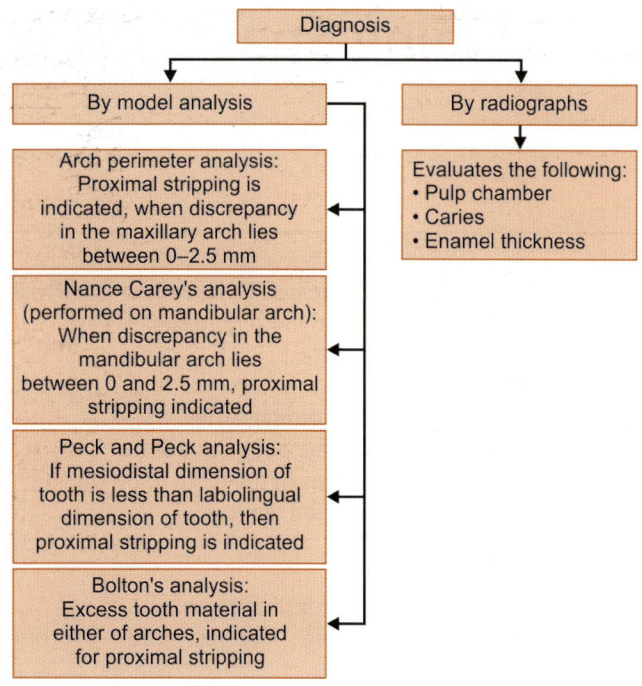

**Flowchart 24.1:** Diagnosis

**Figs 24.1A and B:** Metallic abrasive strips. (A) Single-sided metallic abrasive strip. (B) Double-sided metallic abrasive strip

## Procedure

Proximal stripping can be localized where stripping is performed for few teeth especially upper or lower anteriors or generalized where stripping is carried out for all the teeth. Care should be taken that not more than half the thickness of enamel is reduced from a side of the tooth.

Proximal stripping can be done using any of the following:
- Use of abrasive strips—single/double sided **(Figs 24.1A and B)**
- Use of long thin tapered fissure burs
- Use of safe-sided carborundum disk.

### Use

Abrasive strips used for proximal stripping can be of following two types:
1. Single-sided abrasive strip
2. Double-sided abrasive strip.

### Single-sided Abrasive Strip

This type of abrasive strip is used when reduction of one proximal surface either mesial or distal of a tooth.

### Double-sided Abrasive Strip

This type of abrasive strip is used when reduction of two teeth (distal surface of one tooth whereas mesial surface of another tooth).

Abrasive strip for stripping can be used with the following:
- Strip holder with strips **(Fig. 24.2A)**
- Needle holder or Mathew hemostat **(Fig. 24.2B)**
- Operator hands with strips **(Fig. 24.2C)**

### Methods of Proximal Stripping (Table 24.1)

| Table 24.1: Methods of proximal stripping |
|---|
| Use of abrasive strips **(Figs 24.2A to C)** |
| Use of long thin tapered fissure burs **(Fig. 24.2D)** |
| Use of safe-sided carborundum disk |

## ARCH EXPANSION

Arch expansion is a method of gaining space in a dental arch without extraction using a system of orthodontic appliances. There are various expansion appliances for this purpose and are described in detail in Chapter 25– Arch Expansion in Orthodontics.

## EXTRACTION

Teeth may have to be extracted to make more room in the crowded arch so as to allow proper alignment of the remaining teeth **(Figs 24.3A to C)** or because they are so badly positioned that alignment is impossible. First premolars are frequently extracted for gaining space during orthodontic management. This is so because the first premolars are situated at the center of each quadrant and thus the space gained by their removal can be used to relieve crowding in anterior or posterior segments of the arch.

## DISTALIZATION OF MOLARS

Distalization of molars is the procedure where molars are moved posteriorly by using removable or fixed intraoral orthodontic appliances or extraoral orthopedic appliances. The best time for molar distalization is during mixed dentition period before the eruption of second permanent molars.

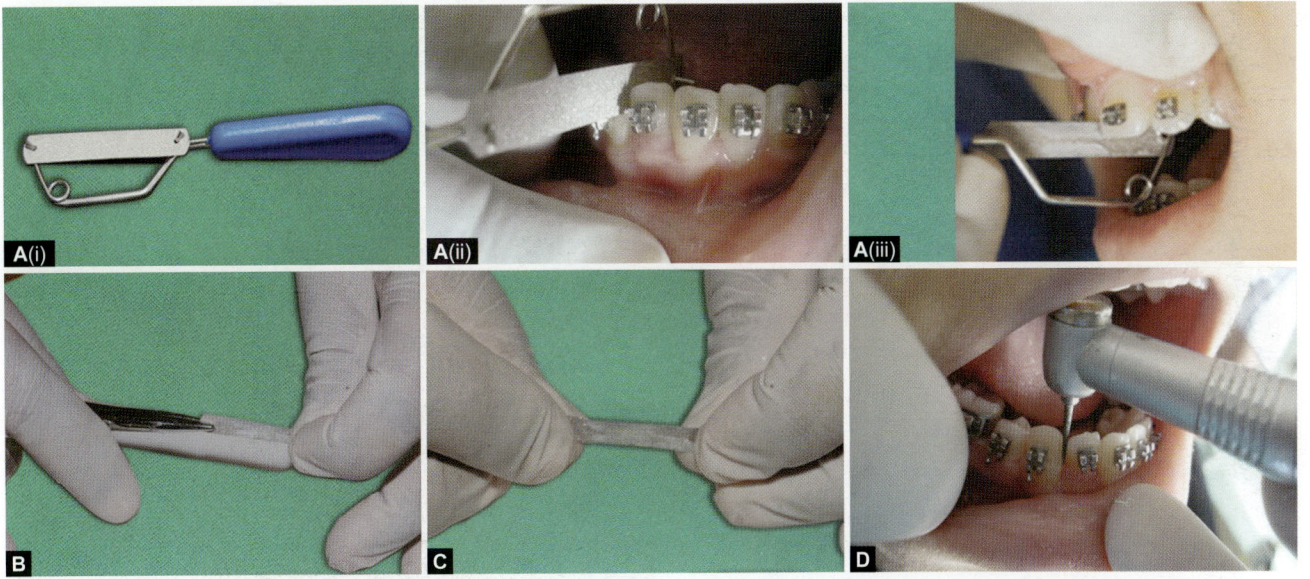

**Figs 24.2A to D:** Methods of proximal stripping. (A) Strip holder with strips. (B) Needle holder or Mathew hemostat and operator hands with strips. (C) Operator hand with strips. (D) Use of long thin tapered fissure burs

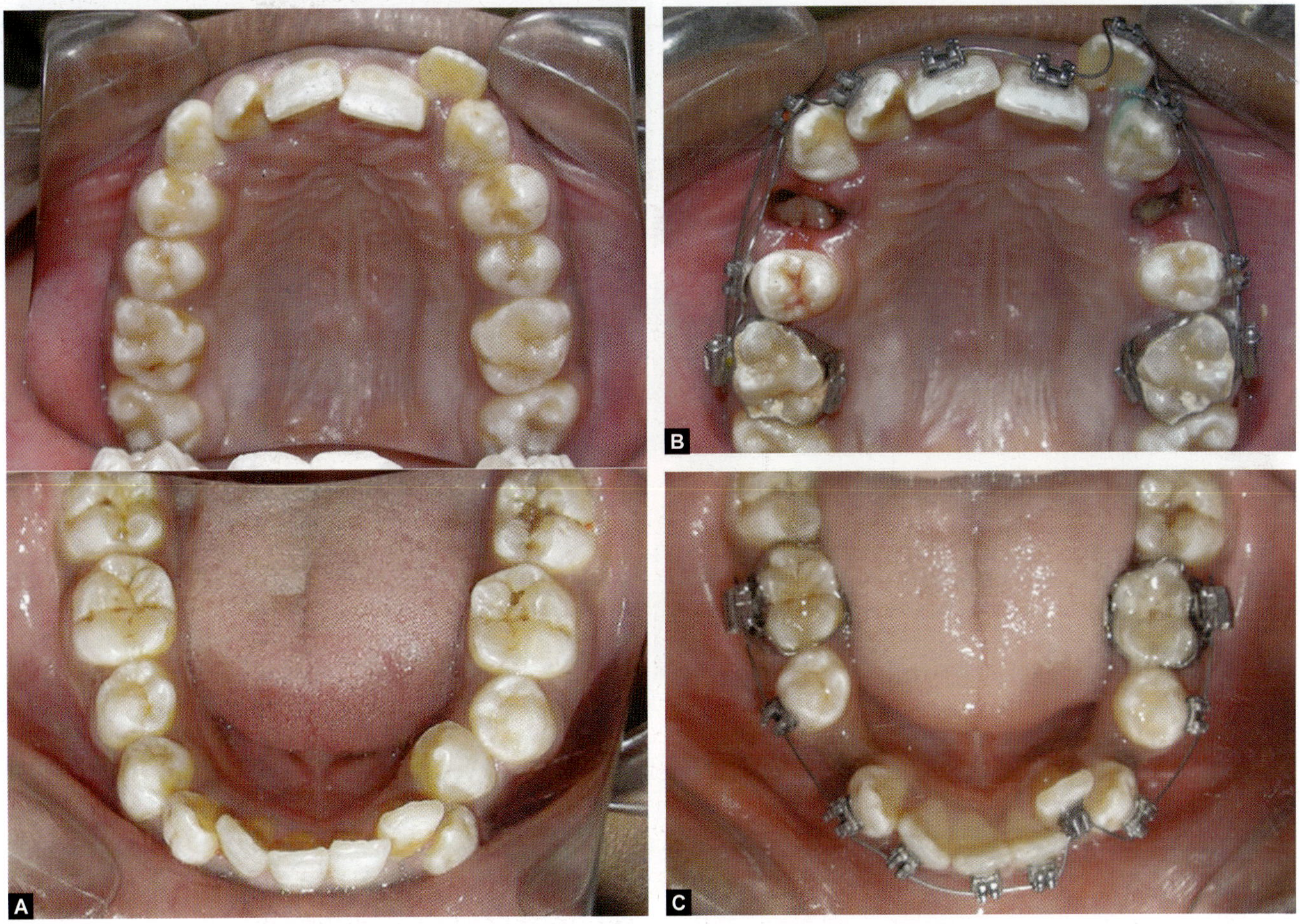

**Figs 24.3A to C:** Extraction of some teeth usually first permanent premolars is indicated to relieve the crowding

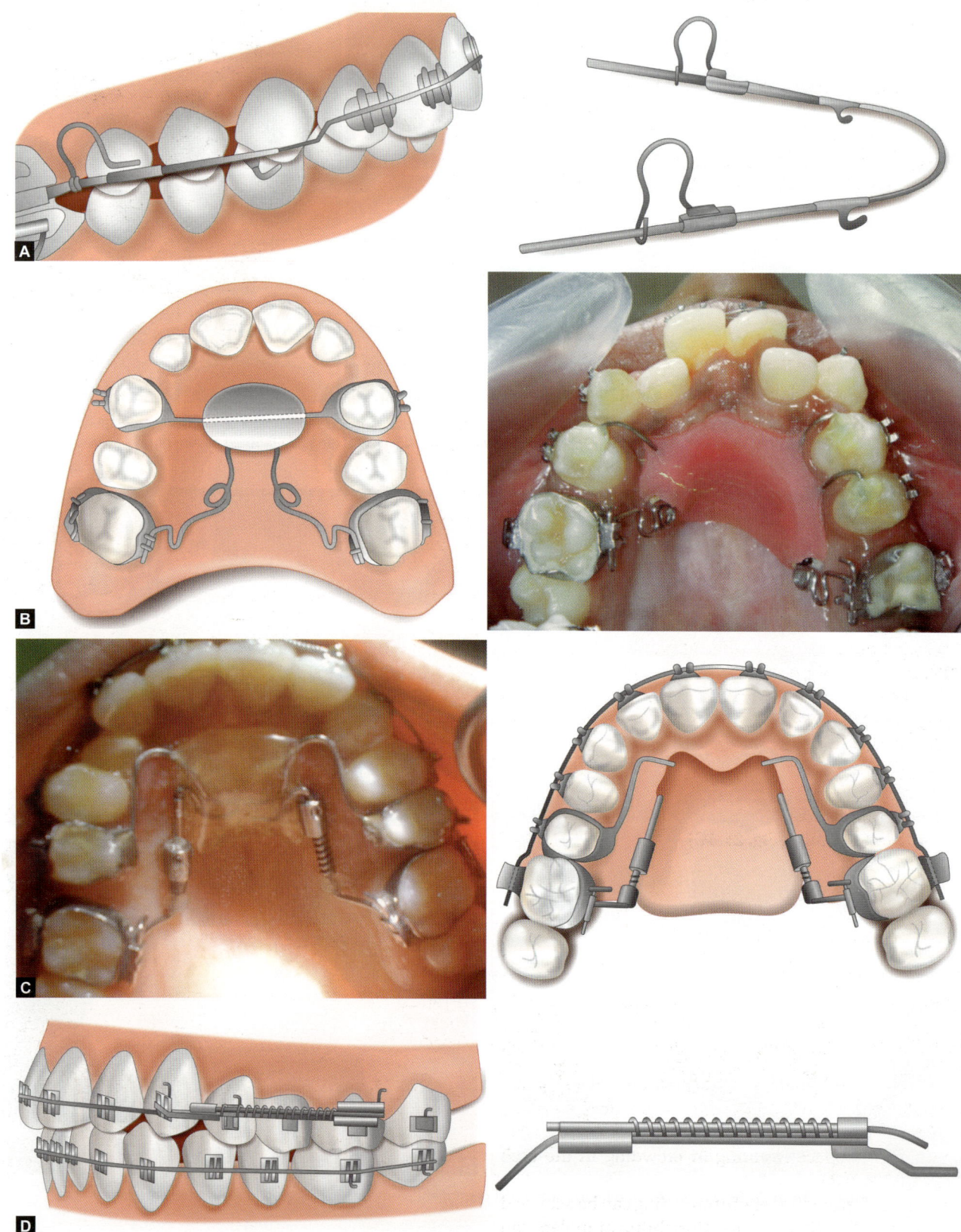

**Figs 24.4A to D:** Appliances used for molar distalization; (A) Wilson distalizing arch; (B) Pendulum appliances; (C) Distal jet appliance; (D) Lokar distalizing appliance

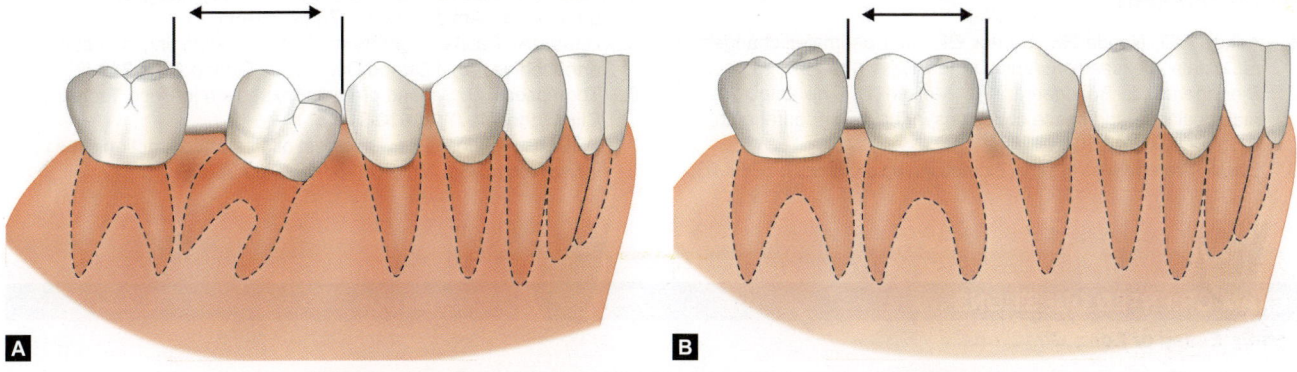

**Figs 24.5A and B:** Tilted molar occupies greater space than an upright one

### Advantages of Molar Distalization
- Distalization of molars helps in avoiding the extraction of teeth.
- It prevents arch collapse.

### Appliances Used for Molar Distalization
Following appliances are used for the distalization of molars:

*Intraoral Distalization Appliances*
- Schwartz appliance
- Sagittal appliance
- Wilson's distalizing arch **(Fig. 24.4A)**
- Pendulum appliance **(Fig. 24.4B)**
- Open coil spring appliance
- Veltri bilateral sagittal screws
- Monolateral sagittal screw
- First-class appliance
- Magnets
- Jones jig appliance
- Distal jet appliance **(Fig. 24.4C)**
- Fast appliance
- Jasper jumper
- Lip bumpers
- Lokar distalizing appliance **(Fig. 24.4D)**

*Extraoral Distalization Appliances*
- Headgears

## UPRIGHTING OF MOLARS

Extraction of permanent second premolar or early loss of deciduous second molar can cause mesial tilting of molars into the extraction site. Tilted molars occupy greater space resulting in crowding in the arch **(Figs 24.5A and B)**.

Gaining of space and relief of crowding can be achieved by uprighting the tilted molars. Uprighting of molars can be done using molar uprighting springs.

## DEROTATION OF POSTERIOR TEETH

A rotated posterior tooth occupies larger space and thus may cause crowding in the arch. Correction of rotated posterior teeth not only helps in relieving crowding but also aids in the prevention of dental caries and periodontal diseases. Correction of rotated posterior teeth is best done by fixed mechanotherapy using a force couple.

However, a rotated anterior tooth usually occupies less space in the arch and space has to be created in the arch for correction of anterior rotations **(Table 24.2)**.

## PROCLINATION OF ANTERIOR TEETH

Proclination of anterior teeth aids in gaining space thereby helps in relieving crowding in the arch. This method of gaining space is employed only in those patients where proclination of anterior teeth will not affect the basal bone relationship and soft tissue profile of the patient.

**Table 24.2:** Rotated posterior teeth vs rotated anterior teeth

| Difference | Rotated posterior teeth | Rotated anterior teeth |
|---|---|---|
| Space occupied by rotated teeth | More | Less |
| Time required for correction of rotated teeth | More | Less |
| Appliances used for the correction of rotated teeth | Mainly fixed orthodontic appliance | Removable orthodontic appliance (Z-spring, T-spring can be used) or fixed orthodontic appliances |
| Space | Space is gained by the derotation of rotated posterior teeth | Space required for the derotation of rotated anterior teeth |

## BIBLIOGRAPHY

1. Adkins MD, Nanda RS, Currier GF. Arch perimeter changes on rapid palatal expansion. Am J Orthod 1990;97:10-9.
2. Bjerregaard J, Bundgaard AM, Melsen B. The effect of the mandibular lip and space conditions in the lower dental arch. Eur J Orthod 1962;48:504-29.
3. Dewel. Prerequisites in serial extraction. Am J Orthod 1969;87-93.
4. Haas JA. Palatal expansion: Just the beginning of dentofacial orthopedics. Am J Orthod 1970;57:219-55.
5. Haas JA. Palatal expansion: Just the beginning of dentofacial orthopedics. Am J Orthod Dentofacial Orthop 1997;219-55.
6. Thompson FG. Second premolar extraction in Begg Technique. J Clin Orthod 1977;11:610-3.
7. Williams RT, Hosila FJ. The effect of different extraction sites upon incisor retraction. Am J Orthod 1976;69:388-410.

## EXAM-ORIENTED QUESTIONS

### Long Essay or Long Questions
1. Enumerate various methods of gaining space in orthodontics and write any three methods of gaining space in detail.
2. Distalization in orthodontic.

### Short Notes
1. Proximal stripping
2. Rotation posterior teeth vs rotated anterior teeth.

## CHAPTER OVERVIEW

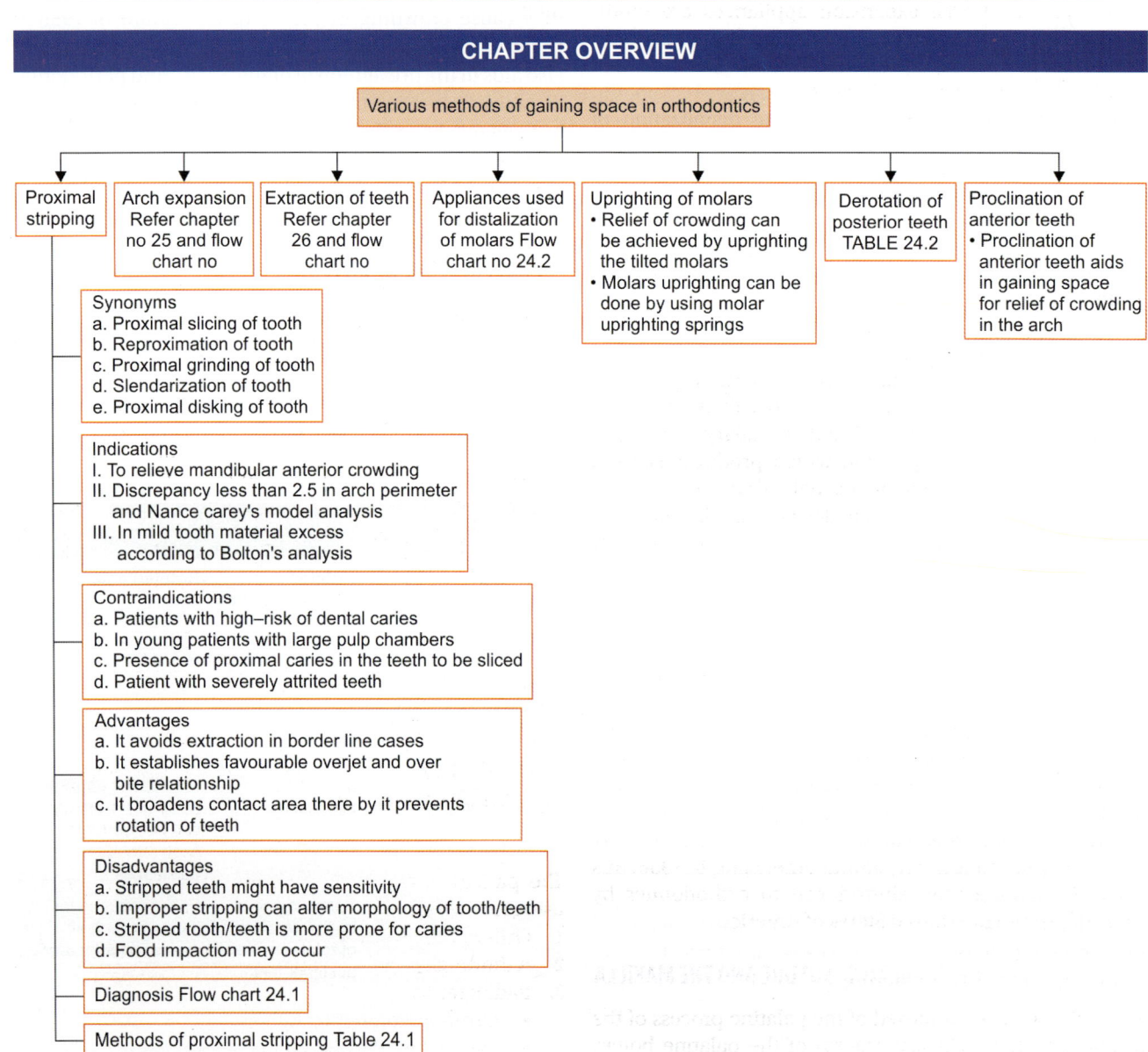

# CHAPTER 25

# Arch Expansion

*Tsipova V, Phulari BS*

Arch expansion is one of the methods of gaining space in orthodontics. The concept of arch expansion was explained for the first time by Emerson C Angel. Hence, he is considered as the Father of Expansion Appliances. Arch expansion can be slow or rapid, removable or fixed. Slow arch expansion brings about mainly dentoalveolar expansion whereas, rapid maxillary expansion brings about both skeletal as well as dentoalveolar expansion.

Removable expansion appliance may be a simple expansion appliance with incorporated jackscrew or coffin appliance. Fixed arch expansion appliances are tooth-borne expansion appliances (Hyrax, Isaacson) or tooth and tissue-borne expansion appliances (Derichsweiler Haas expansion appliance). How much and when to expand is evaluated by model analysis.

## RAPID MAXILLARY EXPANSION

Rapid maxillary expansion (RME) appliances are the best appliances for the orthopedic expansion; in that, the changes are produced mainly in the underlying skeletal structures rather than by the movement of teeth through the alveolar bone. Rapid maxillary expansion not only separates the mid-palatal suture but also affects the circumzygomatic and circum-maxillary sutural systems.

Rapid maxillary expansion is also called as palatal expansion or split palate. Rapid maxillary expansion is a skeletal type of expansion which produces skeletal changes by the separation of mid-palatal suture.

Rapid maxillary expansion device was first used by Emerson C Angel in the year 1860. He used a jack screw type of rapid maxillary expansion device between two premolars in maxillary arch on palatal side in a 14-year old girl and achieved arch expansion by ¼ inch in 14 days. For this significant valuable contribution to the expansion in orthodontics, he is considered as the Father of Rapid Maxillary Expansion.

Walter Coffin in 1877 developed a spring for the purpose of arch expansion, which has come to be known as coffin spring. This spring also produces arch expansion by the separation of mid-palatal suture, when used in young patients. This expansion device gained popularity by orthodontic community at that time. Later in 1956, this expansion device was reintroduced to orthodontics by Andrew Hass in the United States of America.

## ANATOMY OF THE MID-PALATINE SUTURE AND THE MAXILLA

The hard palate is composed of the palatine process of the maxilla and the maxillary process of the palatine bones. The palatine bones together with the maxilla also form the floor of the nose and a part of the lateral walls of the nasal cavity. The palatine bone articulates with the maxilla by a transverse palatal suture and up the lateral wall of the nasal cavity. Posteriorly, the palatine bone articulates with the pterygoid process of sphenoid. The maxillary bones are joined posteriorly and superiorly to various bones, including the frontal, ethmoid, nasal, lacrimal, zygomatic, etc. Thus, the anterior and inferior aspects are relatively free.

The interpalatine suture joins the paired palatine bones at their horizontal plates and is a continuation of the intermaxillary suture. Theoretically, it forms the junction of the three opposing pairs of bones—the premaxilla, the maxilla and the palatines. Practically, they are treated as a single entity—the mid-palatine suture (MPS).

Studies have indicated that the development of the mid-palatine suture passes through three distinct stages. Closure of palatine-suture shows a large individual variation, ranging from 15 to 19 years of age. A greater degree of obliteration occurs posteriorly than anteriorly with maximum obliteration in the third decade of life.

### Indications of RME

1. Posterior crossbite caused due to either maxillary deficiency or mandibular excess.
2. Class III malocclusion of dental or skeletal cause.
3. Along with face mask therapy, RME is used to loosen the maxillary sutural attachment in order to facilitate protraction of deficient maxilla.
4. The medical indications include:
    a. Allergic rhinitis
    b. Septal deformity
    c. Recurrent ear, nasal or sinus infections
    d. Poor nasal airway
    e. As a preliminary measure to septoplasty.
5. Cleft palate patients with collapsed maxillary arch.

### Contraindications

If more than half of the roots of deciduous teeth are resorbed, they cannot be used to provide retention in rapid maxillary expansion.

### Diagnosis

The patient is evaluated for rapid maxillary expansion using following diagnostic records:
1. Orthodontic study model
2. A thorough clinical history
3. Radiographs
    - Orthopantomogram OPG
    - Lateral and PA view cephalogram
    - Occlusal radiographs.

## EFFECTS OF RME

### Maxillary Skeletal Base

Effects of rapid maxillary expansion on maxillary skeletal base are as follows:

Triangular or fan-shaped opening of the mid-palatal suture with maximum opening in the maxillary incisors region and gradually diminishing towards the posterior part of the palate **(Figs 25.1A and B)**.

#### According to Korbs

- In sagittal plane, maxilla rotates in a downward and forward direction.
- In coronal plane, the two halves of the maxilla rotate away from each other.

### Maxillary Anterior Teeth

Activation of rapid maxillary expansion produces the separation of incisors in the midline resulting in midline diastema, which indicates that the expansion has been taken place. This midline diastema later will be closed as a result of the transseptal fiber traction in about 3–5 months **(Figs 25.2A and B)**.

### Maxillary Posterior Teeth

Effects of RME on maxillary posterior teeth are as follows:
- Buccal tilting of maxillary posterior teeth **(Fig. 25.3)**.
- Extrusion of maxillary posterior teeth to some extent.

### Mandible

Activation of rapid maxillary expansion results in a downward and backward rotation of the mandible due to extrusion of maxillary posterior teeth.

### Alveolar Bone

Alveolar bone bends buccally due to the compression of periodontal ligament fibers on activation of rapid maxillary expansion.

### Adjacent Cranial Bones and Sutures

Rapid maxillary expansion not only affects the maxilla, maxillary anterior and posterior teeth alveolar bone, but

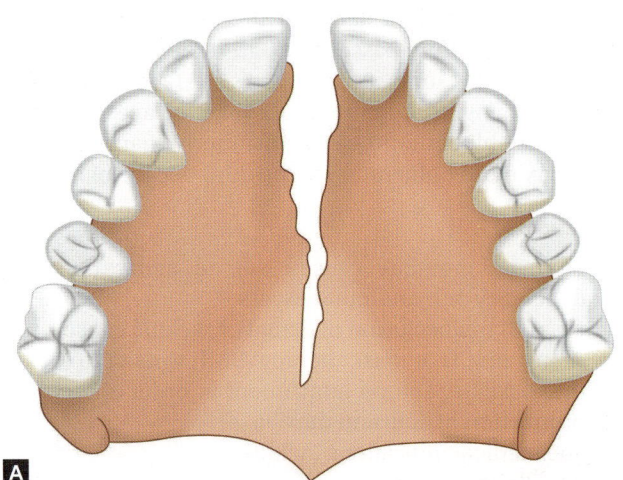
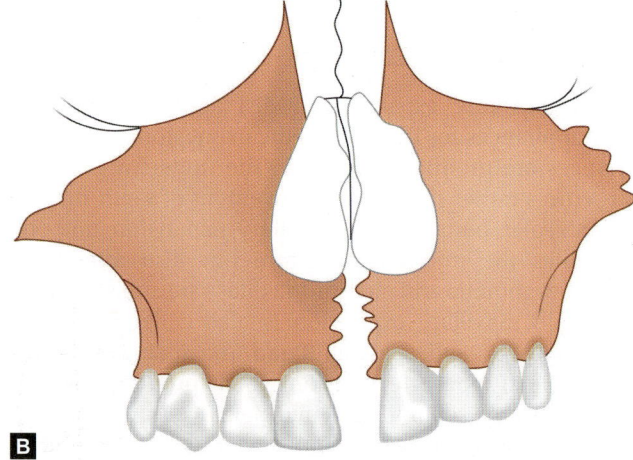

**Figs 25.1A and B:** RME causes triangular or fan-shaped opening of the mid-palatal suture with maximum opening in the maxillary incisors region and gradually diminishing towards the posterior part of the palate. (A) Transverse view. (B) Frontal view

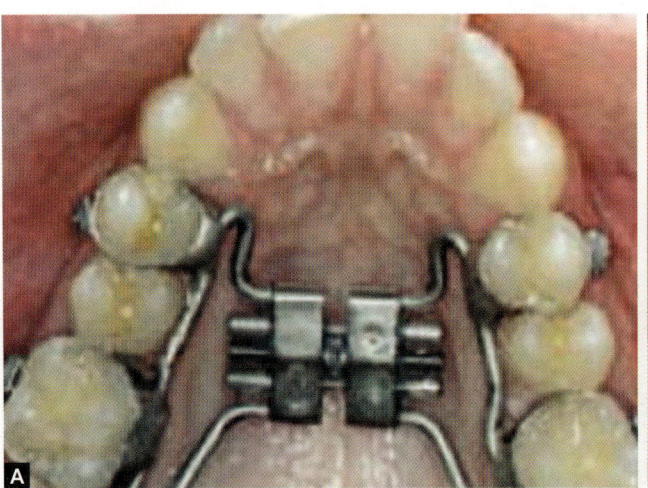
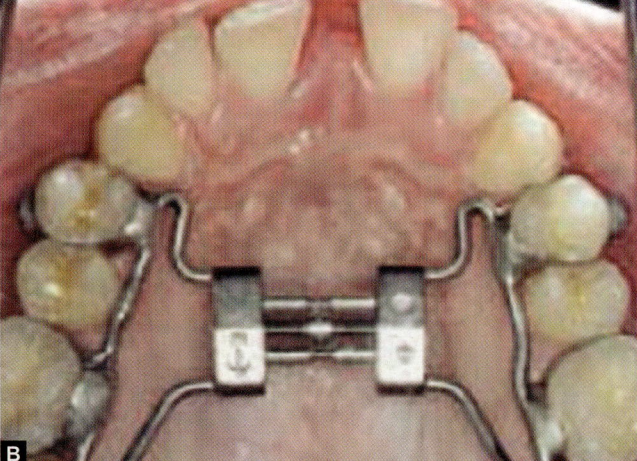

**Figs 25.2A and B:** Effect of RME on maxillary anterior teeth: (A) Before activation of RME. (B) After activation of RME. Note the appearance of midline diastema

also affects the adjacent cranial bones and sutures. The adjacent cranial bones, such as parietal and occipital bone are found to be displaced.

### Nasal Cavity

Activation of rapid maxillary expansion results in increased intranasal space due to separation of outer walls of the nasal cavity.

> **Expansion Achieved Followed by RME**
> With rapid maxillary expansion, expansion up to 10 mm can be achieved with the rate of 0.2–0.5 mm/day.

## TYPES OF RME APPLIANCES

1. Removable Appliances
2. Fixed Appliances
   - Tooth-borne
   - Tooth and tissue borne

### Removable Rapid Maxillary Expansion Appliances

Removable appliances produce skeletal expansion by the splitting of mid-palatal suture, when they are used in the deciduous or early mixed dentition. The reliability of these appliances in producing skeletal expansion is highly questionable when used in older adults.

Removable rapid maxillary expansion appliances consist of an expansion screw in the midline with split acrylic plate. It may also consist of retentive clasps ("C" or Adam's clasp) on the posterior teeth and a labial bow on the anterior teeth **(Figs 25.4A and B).**

Activation of screw is done by placing an expansion screw key in the central bossing of screw and turning the key up for 90º or 45º will produce split of mid-palatal suture and movement of the maxillary shelves away from each other.

### Fixed Rapid Maxillary Expansion Appliances

Fixed rapid maxillary expansion appliances are fixed expanders which cannot be removed by the patient. These fixed expanders can be classified into tooth and tooth tissue-borne appliances.

Most commonly used fixed expander of tooth and tissue-borne appliances are:
- Derichsweiler type
- Hass type.

Tooth-borne appliances are:
- Hyrax
- Isaacson type.

### Derichsweiler-type Expander

Derichsweiler expansion appliance consists of molar bands on right and left permanent first molars and first premolars with wire tags soldered into the palatal surface of all molar and premolar bands. The outer free ends of wire

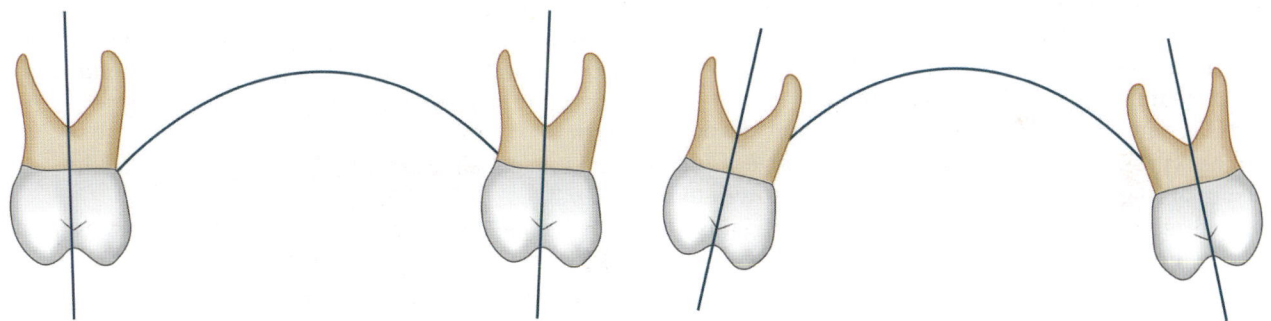

**Fig. 25.3:** Effect of RME on maxillary posterior teeth: Buccal tilting of maxillary posterior teeth

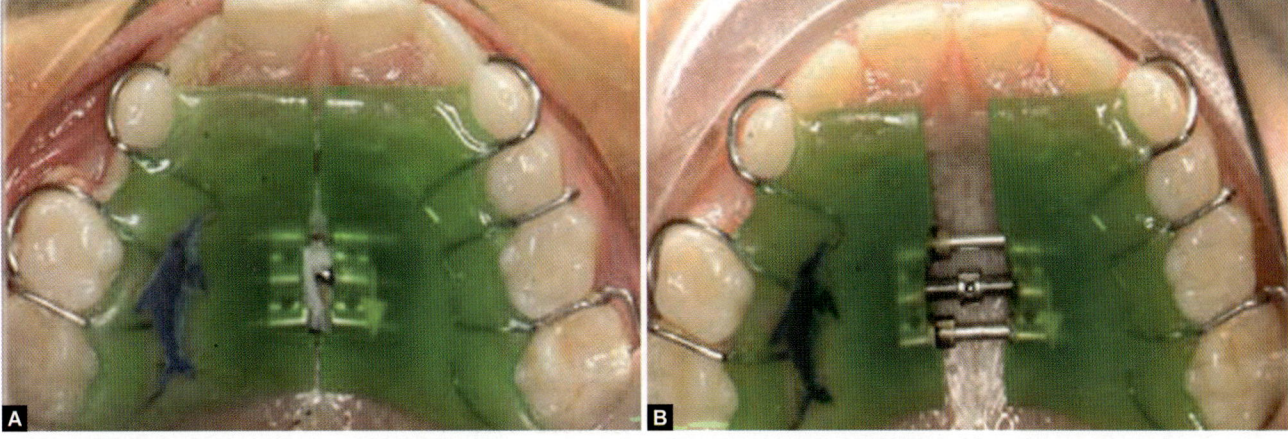

**Figs 25.4A and B:** Removable rapid maxillary expansion appliances, consisting of an expansion screw in the midline with split acrylic plate, Adam's clasp on the first molar and a labial bow on the anterior teeth

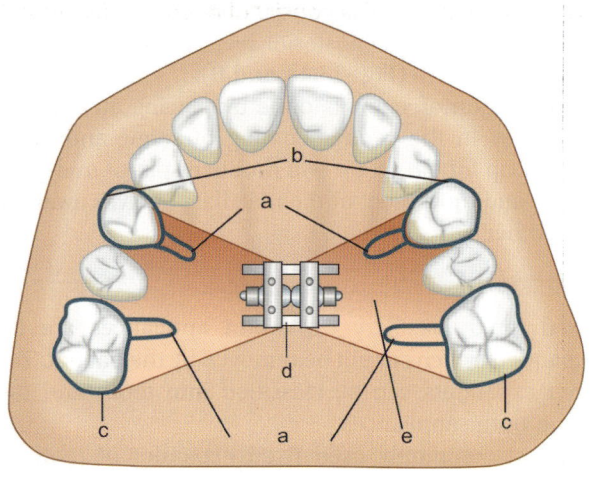

**Fig. 25.5:** Parts of Derichsweiler expansion appliance. (a) Wire tags, (b) Premolar bands, (c) Molar bands, (d) Expansion screw, (e) Acrylic plate

tags are inserted into split palatal acrylic, incorporating a jack expansion screw in its center **(Fig. 25.5)**.

### Haas-type Expander

Haas expander was designed and popularized by Andrew Hass in the year 1961. This appliance consists of molar bands on right and left permanent molars and premolars. A jack screw is incorporated in the midline into the two acrylic pads that closely contact the palatal mucosa. Support wires also extend anteriorly from the molars along the buccal and lingual surface of the posterior teeth to add rigidity to the appliance **(Figs 25.6A and B)**.

Haas states that more bodily movement and less dental tipping is produced when acrylic palatal coverage is added to support the appliance thus permitting the forces to be generalized not only against the teeth but also against the underlying soft and hard palatal tissues.

### Hyrax-type Expander

The more commonly used type of banded RME appliance is the Hyrax–type expander. This type of expander is made entirely from stainless steel. Bands are placed on the maxillary first molars and first premolars. The expansion screw is localized in the palate in close proximity to the palatal contour. Buccal and lingual wires may be added for rigidity **(Figs 25.7A and B)**.

### Isaacson Expansion Appliance

Isaacson expansion appliance is a fixed tooth-borne appliance without acrylic covering. This appliance consists of molar bands on first right and left permanent molars and premolar bands on right and left permanent premolars. Metal flanges are soldered into the molar and premolar bands on buccal and palatal sides **(Fig. 25.8)**.

A spring-loaded expansion screw (MINNE) expander, having a nut, which can compress the spring and is made to extend between palatal metal flanges.

*Activation:* It is activated by closing the nut so that the spring gets compressed.

### Bonded Rapid Maxillary Expansion

Bonded rapid maxillary expansion appliances consist of an acrylic splint, covering variable number of teeth on either side in the maxillary arch, to which a jack screw is attached. Splint can be either cast cap made of silver copper alloy or acrylic splint made of polymethyl methacrylate **(Fig. 25.9)**. A wire framework may be adapted around the teeth to reinforce the acrylic.

*Procedure of placement of bonded rapid maxillary expansion:* Procedure for the placement of bonded rapid maxillary expansion involves the following steps:

*Step 1*
Complete scaling and polishing of maxillary teeth.

*Step 2*
Teeth to be included in bonded rapid maxillary expansion are etched using 30% phosphoric acid.

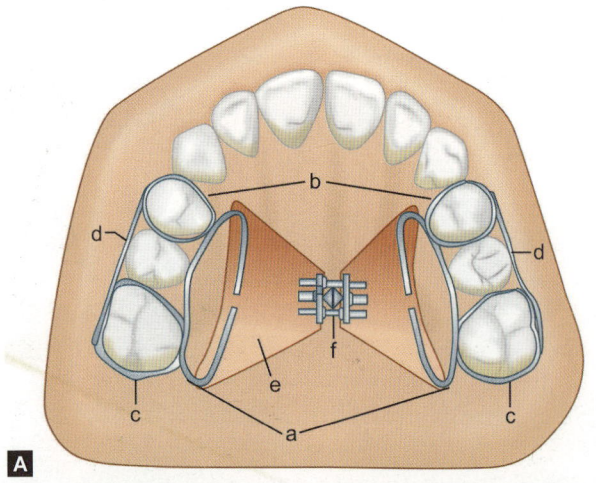
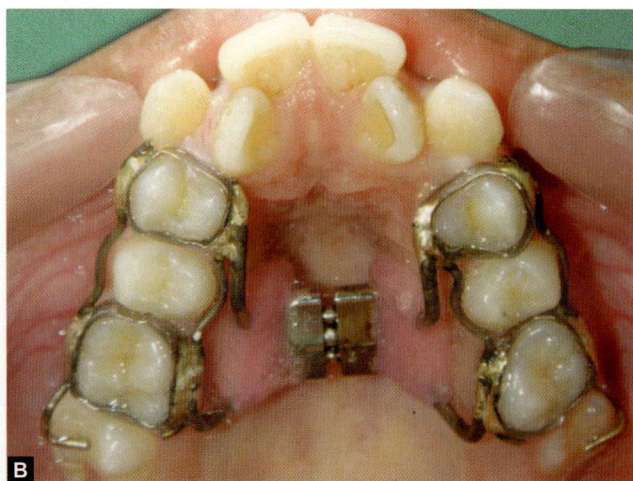

**Figs 25.6A and B:** (A) Hass type of expansion appliance. (a) Lingual support wire, (b) Premolar bands, (c) Molar band, (d) Buccal support wire, (e) Acrylic plate, (f) Expansion screw (B) A case treated with Haas Derichsweiler type of expansion appliance

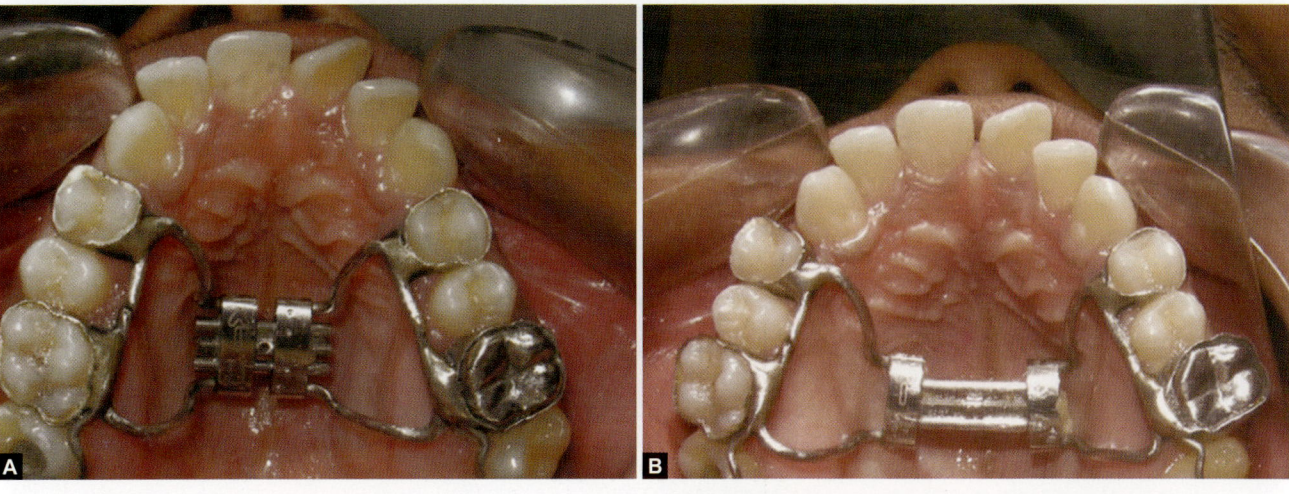

**Figs 25.7A and B:** Hyrax type of expansion appliance: (A) Pre-treatment. (B) Post-treatment of a patient treated with Hyrax rapid expander

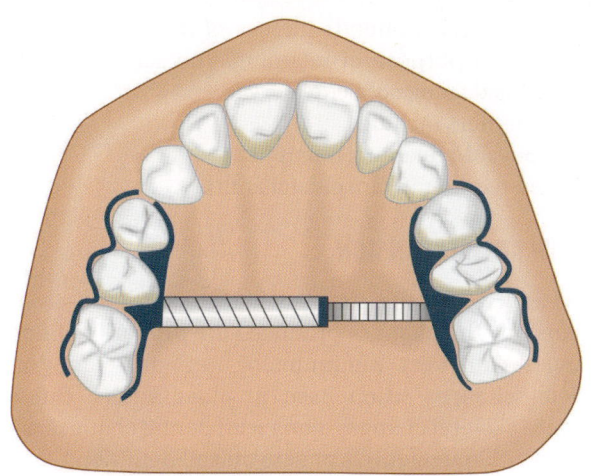

**Fig. 25.8:** Isaacson type of expansion appliance

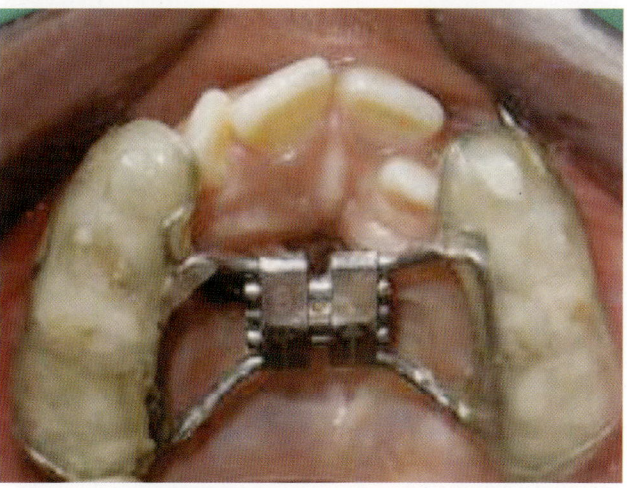

**Fig. 25.9:** Bonded rapid maxillary expansion appliances consist of an acrylic splint, covering variable number of teeth on either side in the maxillary arch to which a jackscrew is attached

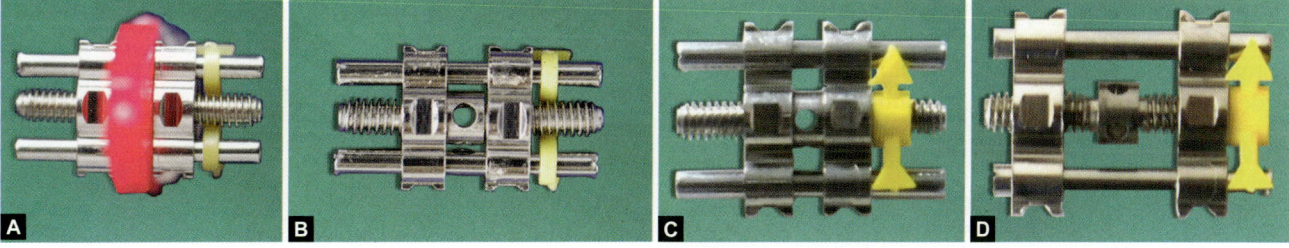

**Figs 25.10A to D:** A typical expansion screw. Note arrow mark. The key should be turned in the direction of the arrow given for activation

*Step 3*
Evaluation of etching.
*Step 4*
Bonded rapid maxillary expansion appliances are cemented onto the etched teeth using either glass ionomer cement or other bonding adhesives.

### Expansion Screw

A typical expansion screw (**Figs 25.10A to D**) consists of an oblong body divided into two halves. Each half has a threaded inner side that receives one end of a double-ended screw. The screw has central bossing with four holes. Theses holes receive a key called expansion screw key (**Figs 25.11A and B**), which is used to turn the screw.

Various types of expansion screws are available to carry out different types of expansion as enumerated in **Table 25.1**.
*Expansion screw activation schedule:* It includes:
*Timm's Schedule* (**Table 25.2**)

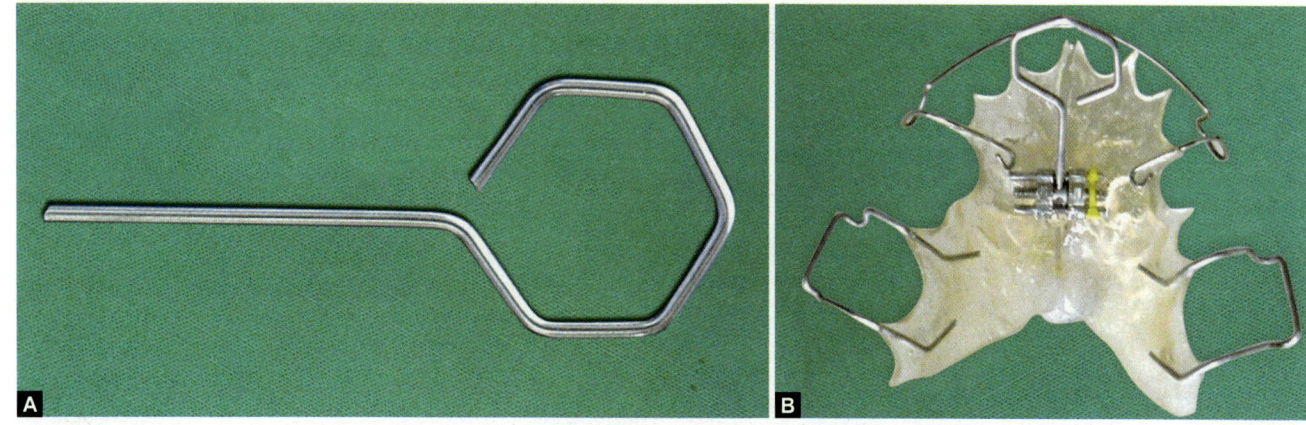

**Figs 25.11A and B:** Expansion screw key used for activating the expansion screw appliances: (A) Expansion screw key. (B) Showing how to activate the expansion appliance with the key. Usually for RME the key should be turned 90°

## TREATMENT EVALUATION DURING RME

Treatment evaluation of rapid maxillary expansion is done either clinically or radiographically.

Clinically the most noticeable feature during RME is the appearance of midline diastema. Studies by various authors show that the amount of incisors separation is roughly half of the amount of jackscrew separated. Hence, the amount of expansion achieved cannot be assessed on the amount of incisor separation (Midline diastema) alone.

Radiographically: Either maxillary occlusal view **(Figs 25.12A and B)** or PA (posteroanterior) cephalogram are used for the assessment of amount of expansion achieved. Radiographic assessment is considered to be the most reliable way in establishing the amount of rapid maxillary expansion.

### Retention Followed by RME

After the expansion is achieved by rapid maxillary expansion appliance, new bone deposition in the area of expansion occurs and the integrity of the midpalatal suture usually is re-established within 3–6 months. In order to prevent relapse, retainer should be given for the 3–6 months followed by RME.

| Table 25.1: Different types of expansion screws | |
|---|---|
| Expansion screw type | Use |
| Symmetrical bilateral expansion screw | Bilateral expansion |
| Traction screw | Closing spaces |
| Expansion screw with split activator | Separate expansion of maxilla or mandible |
| Three-dimensional screw | Anterior and bilateral expansion |

| Table 25.2: Timm's schedule of activation of expansion screw | | |
|---|---|---|
| Age of the patient | Degree of activation | Number of activation |
| Up to 15 years | 90° | 2 times in a day |
| More than 15 years | 45° | 4 times in a day |

Isaacson recommends the use of the RME appliance itself for the purpose of retaining. The screw should be immobilized using cold cure acrylic.

Other retainers include:
1. Removable retainer (Hawley's)
2. Fixed retainer (Transpalatal arch).

## SLOW ARCH EXPANSION

Slow arch expansion is also known as dento-alveolar expansion. The changes produced are primarily of dental changes with very minimum or negligible amount of skeletal changes when used in older adults. But can produce skeletal changes along with dental changes when used in either deciduous or early mixed dentition.

Slow arch expansion uses mild force of 2–4 pounds as compared to 10–20 pounds used in rapid maxillary expansion. The expansion produced with slow expansion is more physiologic with greater stability of having the least relapse tendency as compared to that of rapid maxillary expansion.

### Slow and Continuous Maxillary Expansion, Molar Rotation and Molar Distalization

An estimated 24–30% of all ortho patients can be benefitted from maximum expansion and 95% class II can be improved by molar rotation, distalization and expansion. Rapid palatal expanders such as Haas and Hyrax have traditionally been used for treating transverse maxillary discrepancies, but these appliances will not rotate or distalize molars.

Furthermore, rapid palatal expansion has been shown to produce forces ranging from 3 to more than 20 pounds. Studies have documented free-floating bone fragments, bleeding, microfractures, cyst formation, vascular disorganization and connective tissue inflammation in sutures sites during rapid expansion.

Stony and Ekstrom have suggested that slow expansion procedures allow physiologic adjustments and reconstitution of the sutural elements over a period

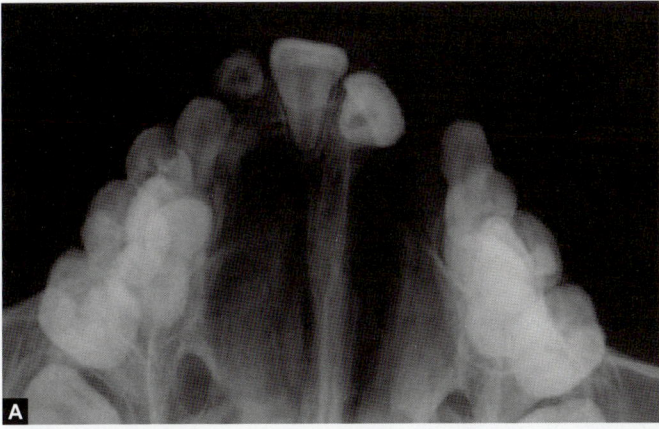 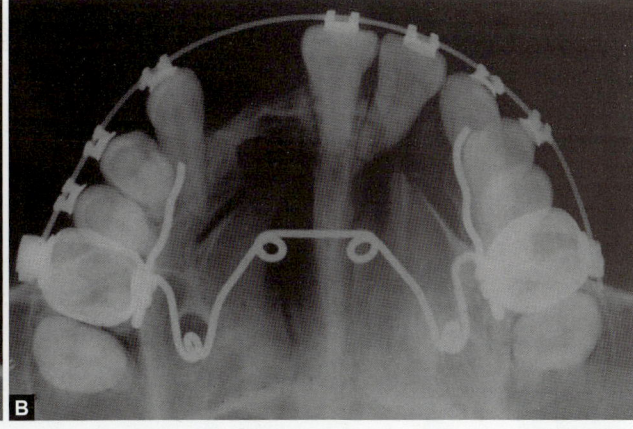

**Figs 25.12A and B:** Occlusal radiographs are used for assessing the progress of expansion: (A) Before expansion with Quad Helix appliance. (B) After expansion with Quad Helix appliance

of about of 30 days. McAndrews demonstrated that the application of light continuous forces in the areas of perisoteal growth allows normal arch dimensions to develop at any age without undue tipping of abutment teeth. Increased fibroblastic, osteoclastic and osteoblastic activity seems to occur when the maxilla is widened slowly.

Slower expansion has also been associated with more physiologic stability and less potential for relapse than rapid expansion. The neuromuscular adaptation of the mandible to the maxilla in slow expansion allows a normal vertical closure.

Differences between slow and rapid maxillary expansion can be seen in **Table 25.3**.

**Table 25.3:** Differences between slow and rapid maxillary expansion

| Features | Slow maxillary expansion | Rapid maxillary expansion |
|---|---|---|
| Rate of expansion | Slow | Rapid |
| Duration of treatment | Prolonged | Short |
| Force | Mild | Heavy |
| Tissue response | Physiologic | Pathologic |
| Frequency of activation | Less frequent | More frequent |
| Fabrication | Easy | Difficult |
| Type of appliance | Can be removable or fixed appliances | Mainly fixed appliance |
| Adjustment required | Minimal | More |
| Repair response | Greater | Less |
| Loss of attachment | Not seen | Seen to some extent |
| Post-expansion stability | Greater | Lesser |
| Trauma | Less | More |
| Relapse | Less chances | More chances |

## Appliances Used for Slow Arch Expansion

### Jackscrew
Various types of screws used for the rapid maxillary expansion can be used in slow arch expansion. Slow expansion using jackscrew can be used for expansion in both arches **(Figs 25.13A to C)**. Screws used in slow expansion are of smaller pitch and are less frequently activated as compared to screws used for the RME.

### Coffin Spring
Coffin spring was developed by Walter Coffin and is a type of removable orthodontic expansion appliance, which when used, brings about slow dentoalveolar expansion.

*Design of coffin spring:* The coffin spring consists of an omega-shaped wire, fabricated with 1.24 mm hard stainless steel wire and placed in the mid-palatal region. Only two outer free ends of omega wires are incorporated into the acrylic base material and the rest part of omega wire is kept free from acrylic **(Fig. 25.14)**.

The outer two free ends of omega wire are incorporated into acrylic base material covering the slopes of the palate.
**Indication:** The coffin spring is used to expand the arches in cases of unilateral crossbite.
**Activation:** The coffin spring is activated by the following two ways:
1. It can be activated by pulling the two sides apart manually.
2. It can also be activated by using three prong pliers by bending the omega wire at the center of the base.

### Quad Helix Appliance
It is believed that the Quad Helix is evolved from the coffin spring. As the name suggests, the appliance has four helices incorporated in its design. Quad helix can be used as a removable expansion appliance when its outer arms are placed in the lingual sheath and it can be made fixed orthodontic appliance when its outer arms are soldered to the palatal surface of molar bands **(Fig. 25.15)**.

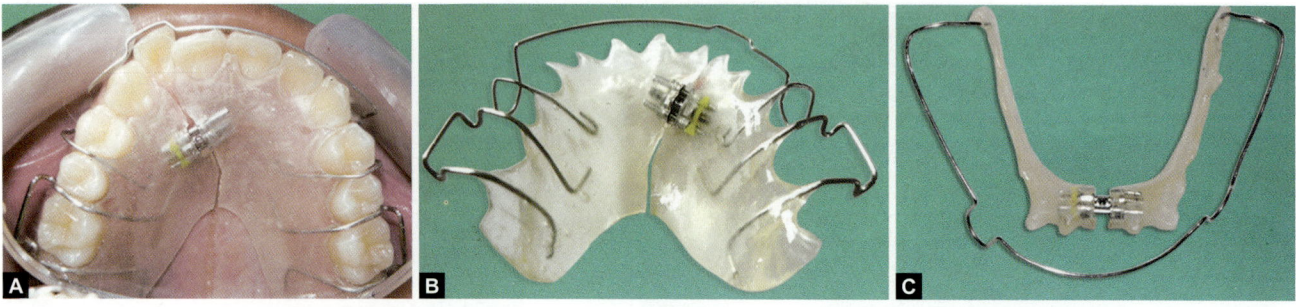

**Figs 25.13A to C:** Slow expansion using jackscrew can be used for expansion in both arches

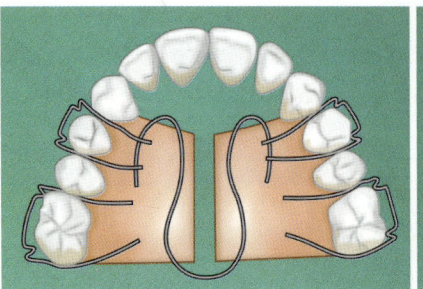

**Fig. 25.14:** Coffin spring

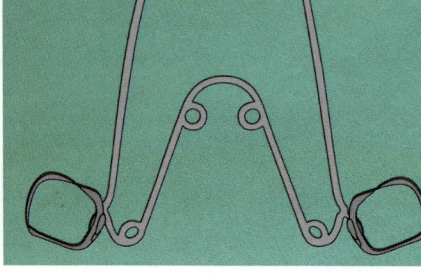

**Fig. 25.15:** Quad helix appliance

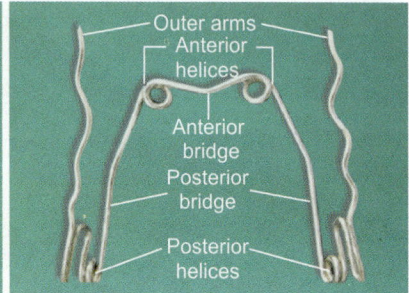

**Fig. 25.16:** Parts of quad helix appliance

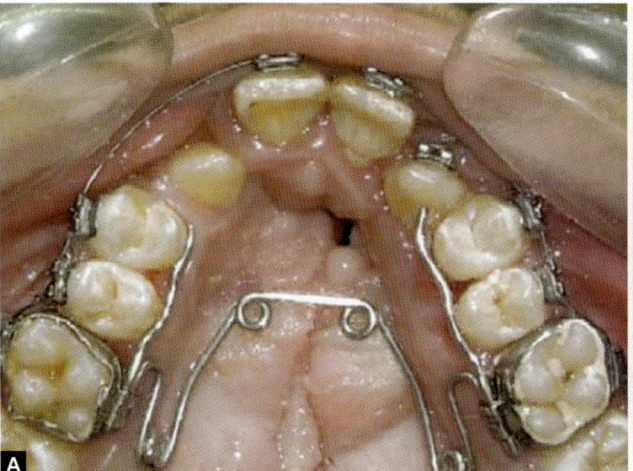

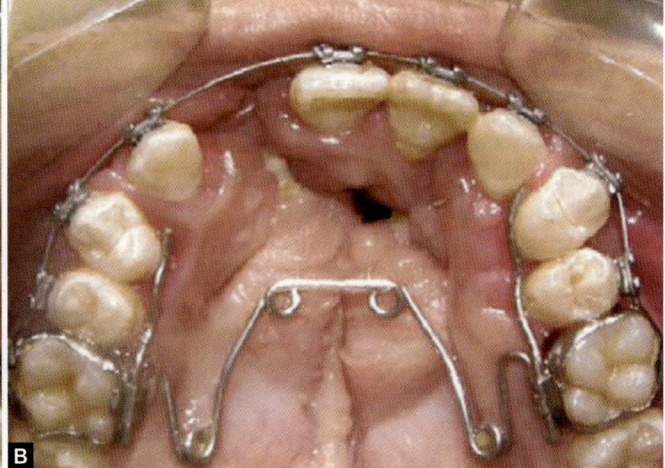

**Figs 25.17A and B:** Quad helix appliance used in a cleft palate case to expand constricted maxillary arch: (A) Before expansion. (B) After expansion

Design of quad helix: The parts of quad helix are as follows **(Fig. 25.16):**
1. Helices
   - The quad helix consists of four helices, two anterior and two posterior.
   - The diameter of each helix is about 3 mm.
2. *Anterior bridge:* Anterior bridge is the portion of wire between anterior helices and is one in number.
3. *Palatal bridge:* Palatal bridge is that portion of the wire that connects the anterior helix to posterior helices and are two in number.
4. Outer arms
   - There are two outer arms and are usually adapted close to the premolar teeth.
   - The outer arms are either soldered to molar bands or placed in lingual sheath (welded to palatal surface of band).

***Use:*** Quad helix appliance is used to expand constricted maxillary arch and also to bring about rotation of molars **(Figs 25.17A and B).**

***Activation:*** The quad helix can be activated by any one of the following ways:
a. By stretching the molar bands apart before the cementation of molar bands.
b. Three prong pliers can be used to activate quad helix appliance at two points, one at the center of anterior bridge and another at the center of palatal bridge.
c. Activating quad helix using three prong pliers at the center of anterior bridge produces bilateral expansion in the molar region **(Figs 25.18A and B).**

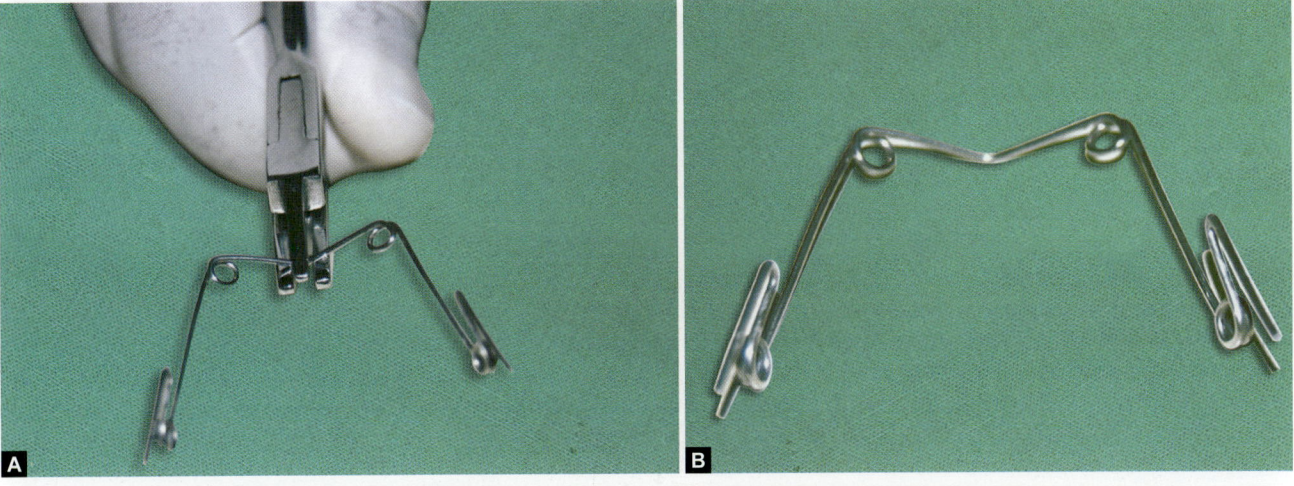

**Figs 25.18A and B:** Activating quad helix using three-prong pliers at the center of anterior bridge produces bilateral expansion in the molar region

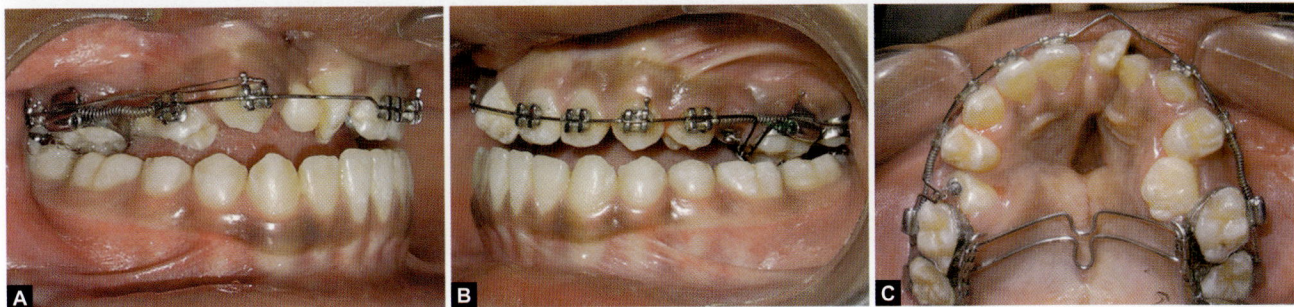

**Figs 25.19A to C:** Mild degree of arch expansion can be brought about by using expanded arch wires and appliances, such as transpalatal arch with fixed mechanotherapy

d. Activating quad helix using three-prong pliers at the center of palatal bridge brings about expansion in the premolar and molar region.
e. Activation of one side of palatal bridge of the quad helix brings about unilateral expansion in the premolar and molar region.
f. Activation of both sides of the palatal bridge of the quad helix produces bilateral expansion in the premolar and molar region.

### Arch Expansion Using Fixed Orthodontic Appliances

Mild degree of arch expansion can be brought about by using expanded arch wires with fixed mechanotherapy. Appliances such as quad helix or transpalatal arch can be used with fixed mechanotherapy **(Figs 25.19A to C)**.

### BIBLIOGRAPHY

1. Adkins MD, Nanda RS, Currier GF. Arch perimeter changes on rapid palatal expansion. Am J Orthod Dentofacial Orthop 1990;97:194-9.
2. Haas AJ. Palatal expansion: just the beginning of dentofacial orthopedics. Am J Orthod 1970;57:219-55.
3. Timms DJ, Moss JP. A histological investigation into the effects of rapid maxillary expansion on the teeth and their supporting tissues. Trans Europ Orthod Soc 1971;263-71.

## EXAM-ORIENTED QUESTIONS

### Long Essay or Long Questions
1. Define expansion and write different methods of expansion and discuss in detail about RME.
2. Rapid palatal expansion
3. Slow arch expansion
4. Effects of RME
5. Zimring and Timm's schedule of activation of expansion screw
6. Coffin spring.

### Short Notes
1. Expansion screw (jack screw)
2. Difference between slow and rapid maxillary expansion
3. Quad helix appliance
4. Hyrax appliance
5. Isaacson appliance
6. Indication and contra-indication of RME.

## CHAPTER OVERVIEW

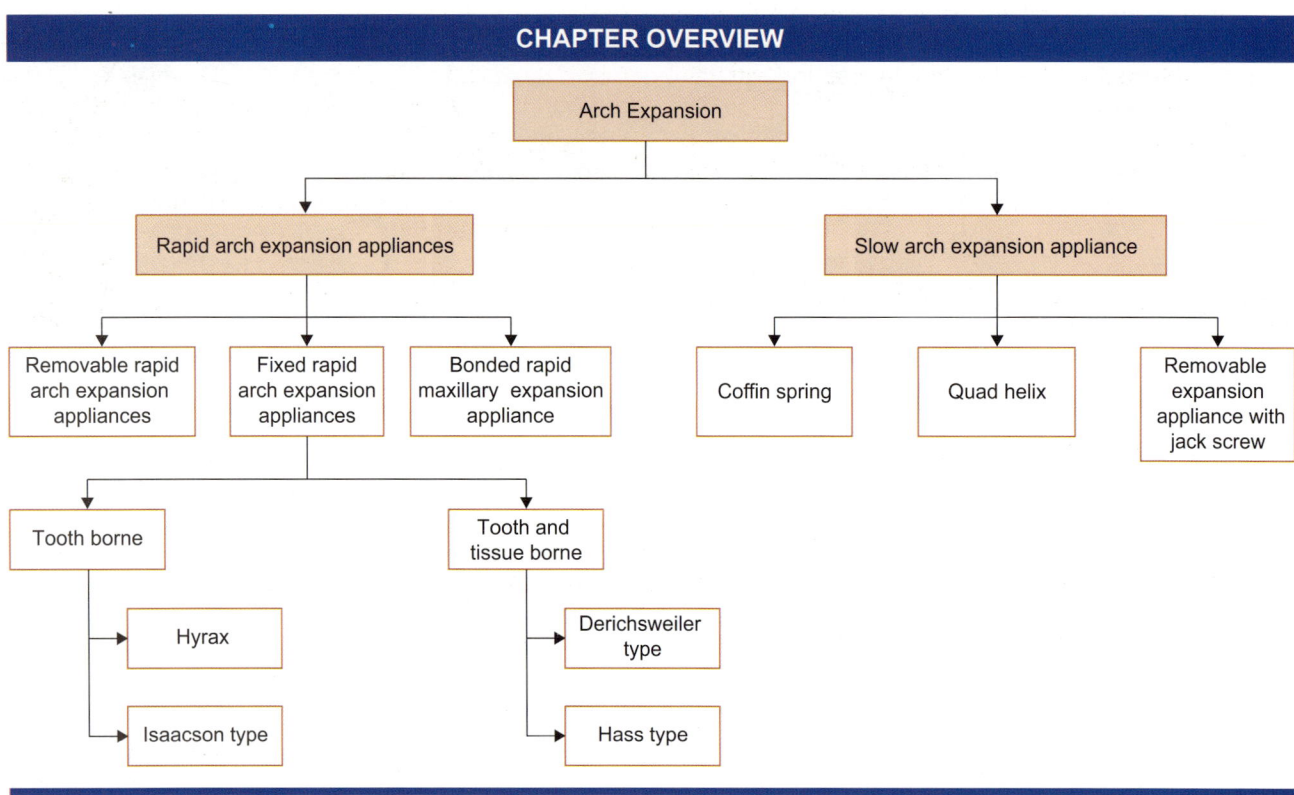

# CHAPTER 26

# Extraction in Orthodontics

*Phulari BS, Tsahannerr F*

Extraction of one or more teeth is sometimes necessary to establish normal functional occlusion, especially when the jaws are not large enough to accommodate all the teeth. Tooth extraction may also be needed to correct the anteroposterior dental arch relationships. The space gained by extraction is utilized to relieve crowding or to retract the proclined anteriors.

The decision of extraction should always be based on sound judgment taking patient's age, development and amount of space needed for tooth alignment into consideration. The decision to opt for extraction should only be made after careful clinical evaluation, cephalometric and model analysis to assess the need and outcome of such extraction. Injudicious extractions may lead to undesirable consequences, such as arch collapse, deep overbite, spacing and tissue damage. First premolars are most frequently extracted as a part of orthodontic treatment followed by the second premolars.

## EVOLUTION OF THE PHILOSOPHY OF EXTRACTION IN CONJUNCTION WITH ORTHODONTIC THERAPY

The role of extractions in orthodontic treatment has been a matter of controversy for years. Although **John Hunter** recognized the role of extraction as early as 1771 in his book Natural History of the Teeth, it was not until mid-20th century that extraction of teeth in conjunction with orthodontic therapy became more acceptable.

**Edward H Angle** (1907) was the major proponent of 'no extraction' philosophy. His theory was that "there shall be a full complement of teeth, and that each tooth shall be made to occupy its normal position." According to Angle, it was vital to maintain the full complement of teeth and to establish these teeth in ideal occlusion, if the results were to be considered successful. He advocated that if crowded teeth are aligned in correct relation to each other, the improved function of masticatory system will result in the growth of the jaws, which in turn, will create adequate space for the dentition. He thus advised expansion of arches in all orthodontic cases.

However, some orthodontists could not produce normal occlusion by means of expansion in all cases. In many instances, placing the teeth in the correct occlusal relationship to one another did not seem to develop normal bony support and the teeth would relapse to their original position of malocclusions or would collapse due to the lack of bony support as soon as the retention appliances were removed. Removal of one or two teeth in such cases seemed to permit the establishment of normal occlusions with great ease and post-treatment stability. Thus, the philosophy of extraction in conjunction with orthodontic treatment was introduced.

**Calvin Case**, a contemporary of Angle supported tooth extraction arguing that the jaw growth was not dependent on function and that if the jaws were too small to accommodate the teeth, then extraction of teeth will be necessary to relieve crowding and irregularity. Originally, Case was a genuine admirer of Angle. In fact, he gave up the general practice of dentistry because of Angle's influence. Case defended the discrete use of extraction as a practical procedure, while Angle believed in nonextraction. This led to the great extraction controversy between the two schools of thought. However, the unexpected result of this controversy was that it convinced general practitioners that they should not attempt orthodontic treatment but should refer the patients to a specialist.

The climax of the extraction controversy was a debate in 1911 at the annual meeting of the National Dental Association (former name of the ADA). Bitterness and animosity were rampant. It took many years after this episode for the problem to become a matter of calm and objective evaluation and respectful appreciation of various points of view, each of which has made its contribution to orthodontics.

By late 1940s, extraction was reintroduced as a part of orthodontic treatment by **Charles Tweed**, who found that post-treatment occlusion was more stable in patients treated with extractions. Tweed selected 100 failure cases among his previously treated patients without extraction and retreated them with extraction of four first premolars, for which he did not charge any fee. In 1940, he presented a paper on the need for extraction based on his 100 retreated cases with good post-treatment stability in a meeting of the Angle Society in Chicago. By early 1960s, extraction of teeth was fairly generally accepted in the orthodontic practice.

## NEED FOR EXTRACTION

Extraction of teeth in orthodontic treatment is necessary in two main circumstances:
1. For the relief of crowding caused by arch length-tooth material discrepancy
2. For the correction of anteroposterior sagittal dental arch relationship.

### Extraction for the Relief of Crowding

The size of dentition and the size of basal jaw bone are genetically determined. Crowding results from arch

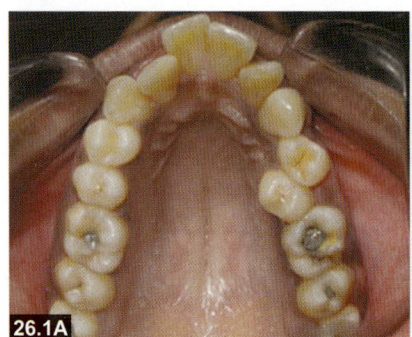
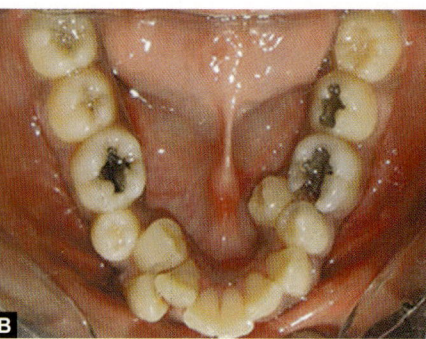
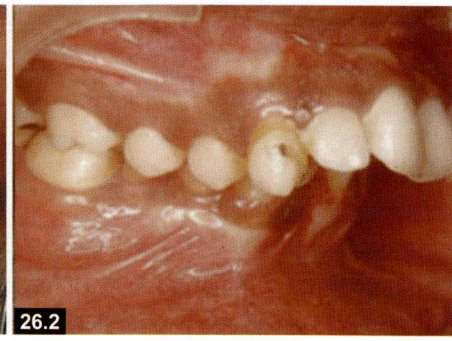

**Figs 26.1A and B:** Arch length-tooth material discrepancy where total tooth material is in excess of the arch length resulting in crowding. Extraction of some teeth (usually first or second premolars) is often needed to relieve crowding in such cases; **Fig. 26.2:** A patient's intraoral right lateral view showing severe skeletal class II division 1 malocclusion. Extraction of teeth may be required as a part of surgical correction of the jaws

length-tooth material discrepancy, where total tooth material is in excess of the arch length. Thus, when the dentition is too large to fit in the dental arch without irregularity, it is necessary to reduce the dentition size by extraction of certain teeth **(Figs 26.1A and B).**

Model analyses (Carey's analysis and Arch perimeter analysis) should be done to assess the amount of space needed for proper alignment and to select the teeth for extraction.

- Less than 4 mm discrepancy—extraction rarely advisable.
- 5-9 mm discrepancy—borderline cases, decision of extraction depends on other factors
- 10 mm or more—extraction almost always indicated.

### Extraction for the Correction of Sagittal Dental Arch Relationship

Apart from the relief of crowding, extraction of teeth is also needed for correction of discrepancies in the sagittal interarch relationship, such as Angle's class II and class III malocclusions.

Extraction of teeth impairs the forward development of dental arches and the alveolar process. Thus, extraction of teeth improves sagittal relationship not only by tooth movement, but also by selective forward growth impairment of the alveolar bone. In severe skeletal sagittal discrepancies, extraction of teeth may be required as part of surgical correction of the jaws **(Fig. 26.2)**.

### Angle's Class I Malocclusion Cases

In Angle's class I malocclusion where sagittal interarch relationship is normal, it is preferable to extract in both the arches in order to maintain the interarch relationship **(Figs 26.3A to H)**.

### Angle's Class II Malocclusion Cases

- In most Angle's class II cases with upper anterior proclination and well-aligned lower arch, interarch relationship can be corrected by extraction only in the upper arch **(Fig. 26.4)**.
- However, in Angle's class II cases, where there is lower arch crowding or when molars are not in full class II occlusion, it may be necessary to extract in both the upper and lower arches to achieve proper sagittal interarch relation and to relieve crowding.

### Angle's Class III Malocclusion Cases

Angle's class III cases are preferably treated by extraction only in the lower arch **(Figs 26.5A and B)**. Extraction in upper arch is avoided as it may impair the forward development of the maxilla.

## FACTORS TO BE CONSIDERED IN THE SELECTION OF TEETH FOR EXTRACTION

Whether teeth are extracted for the relief of crowding or for correction for interarch relationship, the following factors have to be considered before deciding which teeth are to be removed.

### Condition of the Teeth

- The condition of the teeth must be taken into account while planning extractions. Fractured teeth, hypoplastic teeth, grossly carious teeth and teeth with large restorations will be more favorable for extraction than sound healthy teeth.
- Long-term prognosis of tooth is given more importance than the appearance of the tooth while assessing the condition.

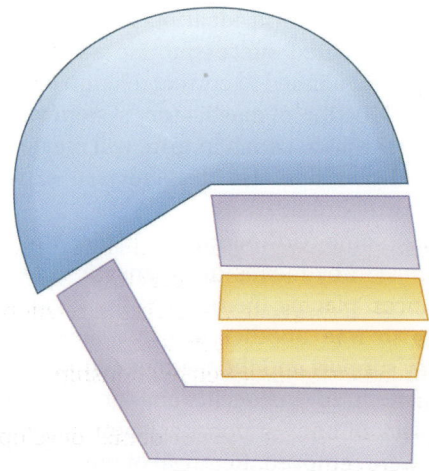

**Fig. 26.3A:** Angle's Class I Malocclusion Cases

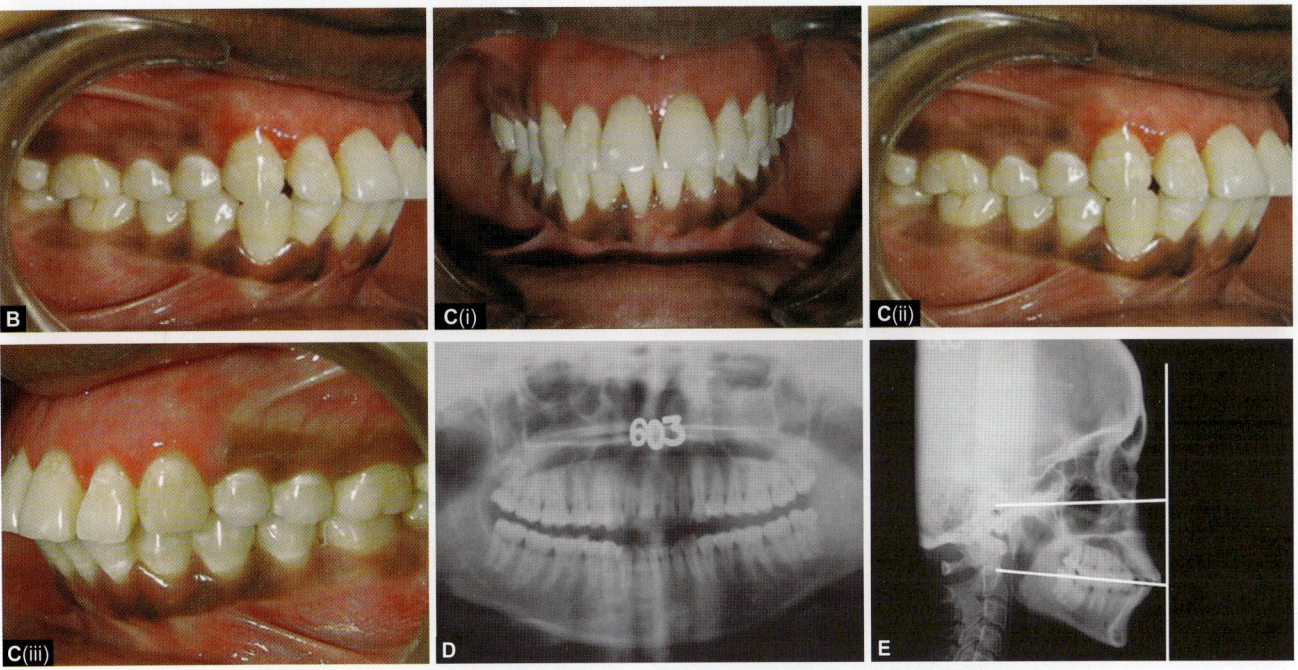

**Figs 26.3B to E:** Angle's Class I Malocclusion Cases

- It is important to consider the alveolar bone support of the teeth as well. Radiographic examination aids in scrutinizing the bone support.

### Position of the Crowding

The crowding can be readily corrected, if extractions are carried out in that part of the arch rather than in some remote uncrowded part. However, crowding of incisors is usually relieved by extraction of premolars as it gives a more esthetic appearance and occlusal balance than removal of incisors. First premolars are most commonly removed for relief of crowding as they are positioned in the center of each quadrant. Thus, the extraction space can be utilized for the relief of crowding in both anterior and posterior segments.

### Position of the Teeth

Teeth that are grossly malpositioned and which would be difficult to align are often the teeth of choice for extraction. Position of the apex of the teeth should be considered as it is usually more difficult to move the apex than to move the crown.

## CHOICE OF TEETH FOR EXTRACTION

The choice of teeth for extraction should be carefully made with consideration to the following factors:
- The amount of tooth material excess in relation to arch length, degree and site of crowding.
- The anteroposterior interarch relationship.
- Profile of the patient.
- Age of the patient and his/her dental developmental status.
- The direction of jaw growth.
- Carious status of the teeth.
- General health status of the dentition.

### Maxillary Central Incisors

Incisors are esthetically the most prominent teeth due to their position in the arches. Thus, extraction of incisors, especially that of upper centrals, is rarely undertaken unless their condition necessitates their extraction.

#### Indications

The following are some of the circumstances when upper central incisors are indicated for extraction:
- Unfavorably impacted maxillary central incisor, which cannot be aligned properly.
- Severely fractured maxillary central incisor.
- Grossly decayed tooth that cannot be conserved.
- Maxillary central incisor with severely dilacerated root, which cannot be moved orthodontically.

### Maxillary Lateral Incisors

Maxillary lateral incisors are the teeth that exhibit greatest variation, next to third molars in form, number and eruption pattern. Their extraction may be justified in some situations for the overall success of the orthodontic treatment.

#### Indications

The usual reasons for removal of maxillary lateral incisor are:
- Severe malposition of the tooth particularly when it is palatally blocked with good approximation of central incisor and the canine.
- When one maxillary lateral is congenitally missing, the lateral incisor on the other side of the arch may have to be extracted so as to balance the arch symmetry.

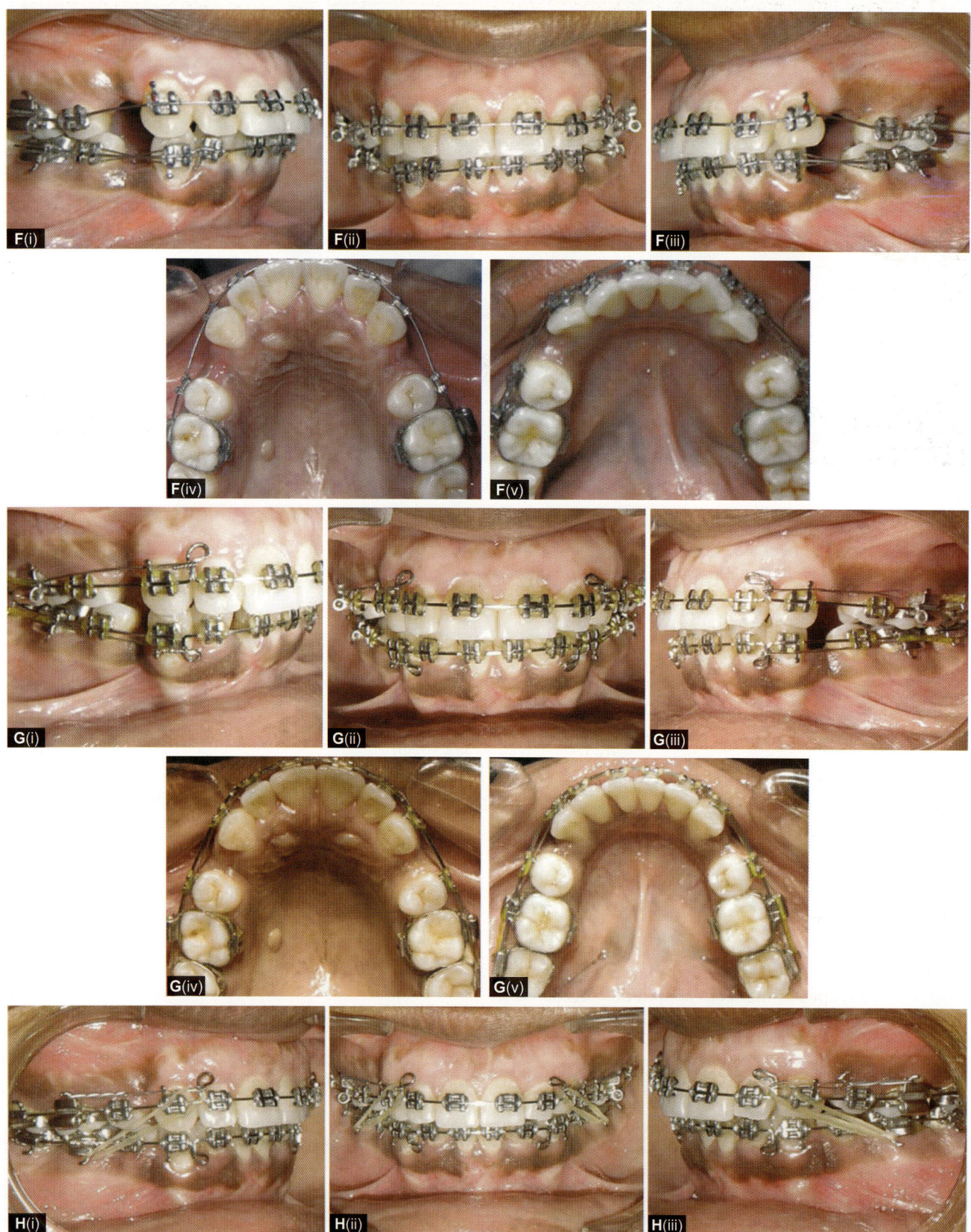

**Figs 26.3A to H:** A patient's intraoral photographs showing Angle's class I malocclusion with severe maxillary anterior proclination, increased overjet and overbite. Correction of such malocclusion may require extraction of first or second premolar in both the arches

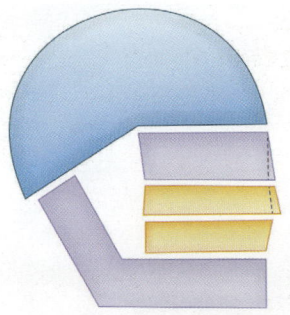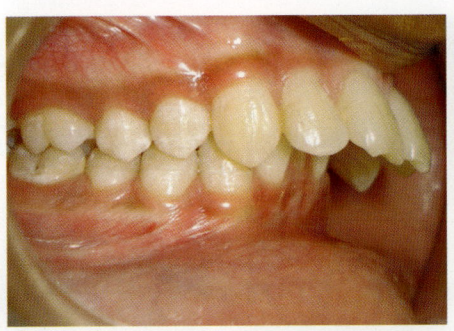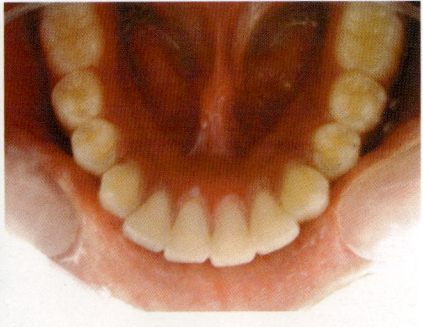

**Fig. 26.4:** A patient with Angle's class II division 1 malocclusion with well-aligned teeth in the lower arch can be corrected by the extraction of either first or second premolars only in the maxillary arch

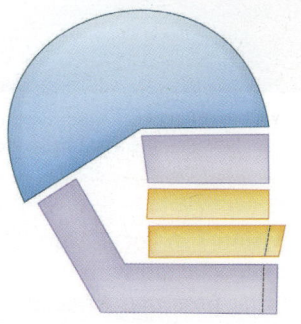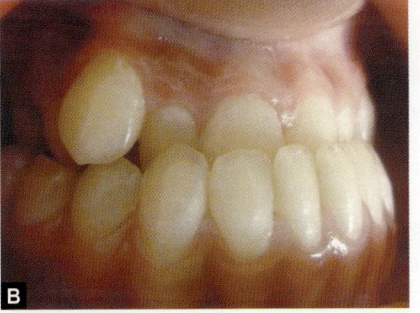

**Figs 26.5A and B:** Angle's class III malocclusion cases are preferably treated by extraction only in the lower arch

- Malformation of the tooth, the most common being the coniform crown.
- For the proper alignment of canines, sometimes lateral incisors may have to be compromised.
- When all the teeth in both the jaws are well-aligned except for maxillary lateral incisors, then in such cases lateral incisors may be extracted as a part of dental camouflage orthodontic therapy.

### Mandibular Incisors

Extraction of lower incisors should be avoided as far as possible although it can be tempting, particularly when crowding is confined to lower anterior segment. The result of lower incisor extraction is often disappointing except in certain special circumstances. This is because, lower incisor extraction is often followed by narrowing of intercanine width, lingual inclination of the remaining incisor teeth which results in deepening of the bite and eventually leads to collapse of the lower arch.

Consequently, the upper intercanine width may also be disturbed due to decreased lower intercanine width and may even cause reappearance of crowding. Thus, as a general rule, extraction of lower incisor should be avoided.

### Indications

Nevertheless, lower incisors may have to be removed in certain situations:
- When a lower incisor is completely excluded from the arch with good alignment of the remaining teeth **(Fig. 26.6)**.
- A lower incisor with poor periodontal support because of gingival recession and bone loss.
- In some cases of class III malocclusions with lower incisor crowding, a central incisor can be removed to obtain normal overjet, overbite and relief of crowding.

### Canines

Canines have the longest and strongest roots of all teeth that provide excellent anchorage in the alveolar bone. They help to establish normal facial expression at the corners of the mouth owing to their crucial position and prominence of canine eminence, and thus are of high esthetic value. The maxillary and mandibular canines also assist in guiding the teeth into intercuspal position by canine guidance. Furthermore, the contact established between lateral incisor and premolar is rarely satisfactory.

Due to all these reasons, extraction of canines should be guarded and only be attempted when it is absolutely necessary and completely justified.

### Indications

Extraction of canines may be considered in the following circumstances:
- Ectopically erupted or unfavorably impacted canines may need to be extracted **(Fig. 26.7)**. The maxillary canines have quite a long way to travel from their developmental position near the orbit to their final position in the arch. In addition, their sequence of eruption is after the eruption of one or both the maxillary premolars. Thus, maxillary canines are often observed to be impacted or deviated from their path of eruption.
- When maxillary and mandibular canine of one side is lost due to some reasons, extraction of the canine tooth on the other side of the arch may be considered

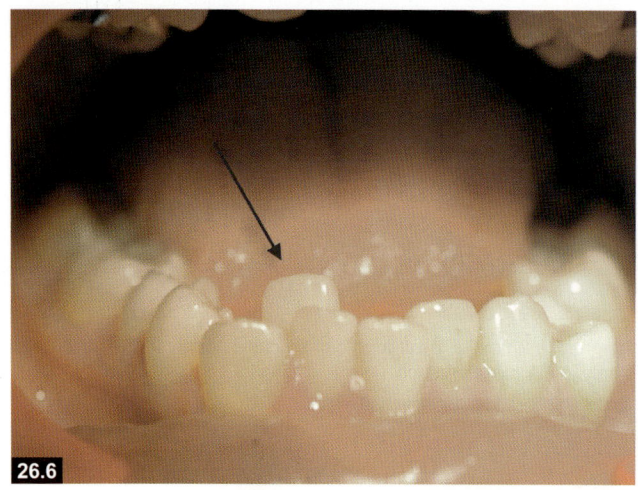 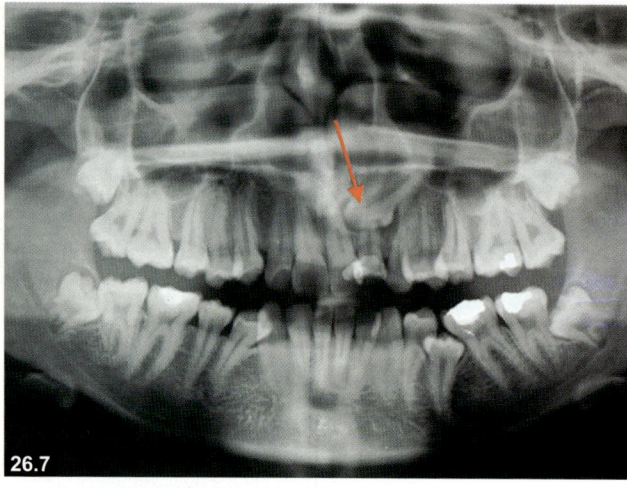

**Fig. 26.6:** Mandibular right permanent lateral incisor totally lingually blocked with the rest of the teeth well aligned. Lateral incisor may be extracted in such cases; **Fig. 26.7:** Unfavorably impacted canines may need to be extracted

to maintain the symmetry, provided the first premolar can be brought to the position of canine.
- When a canine is completely out of the arch with acceptable contact between lateral incisor and first premolar and its alignment is very difficult due to the unfavorable placement of its apex and then it may be sacrificed to improve the overall success of orthodontic treatment.

### First Premolars

First premolars are routinely extracted as a part of orthodontic treatment. The following are some of the reasons behind favoring their extraction:
- Since first premolars are positioned immediately next to the anterior segment, their extraction provides maximum space which can be utilized for the retraction of proclined anteriors and thus maximum lip retraction can be done.
- As they are positioned nearly at the center of each quadrant, the space created by first premolar extraction can be utilized for the correction of crowding in both anterior and posterior segments.

Extraction of first premolars leaves behind a posterior segment that has adequate anchorage potential for the retraction of the six anterior teeth; whereas, second premolar extraction leads to some anchorage loss as first molars have to retract eight teeth (six anteriors + two first premolars).
- The resultant contact between canine and second premolar is usually satisfactory.
- First premolar extraction is least likely to disturb molar intercuspation, which is especially important in case of class I malocclusion with bimaxillary protrusion.

### Indications
- First premolars are the teeth of choice for extraction to relieve moderate-to-severe anterior crowding where maximum space has to be gained **(Figs 26.8A to C)**.
- They are extracted for the correction of moderate-to-severe anterior proclination as in cases of class II division 1 malocclusion **(Figs 26.9A and B)** and class I malocclusion with bimaxillary protusion. Extraction of first premolar in such case often offers maximum space for retraction of the proclined anteriors.
- When anchorage demand is high, first premolar extraction is preferred over that of second premolars. The molars along with second premolars can offer sufficient anchorage in such cases.
- First premolars are also extracted as a part of serial extraction procedure undertaken in early mixed dentition period to intercept the development of crowding in the arches.

### Extraction of Second Premolars

Next to first premolars, the second premolars are the commonly extracted teeth during orthodontic treatment.

### Indications
- Extraction of second premolars is preferred when space required for the correction of malocclusion is minimum as in case of mild anterior crowding or mild anterior proclination. By extraction of second premolars in such cases, the soft tissue profile and facial esthetics can also be maintained.
- Second premolars are extracted when anchorage demand is minimum, i.e in cases where anchor loss is actually desirable. Here the extraction space is closed by the retraction of anteriors as well as by mesial movement of the molars.
- Premature loss of deciduous second molar may cause mesial migration of first permanent molar leaving inadequate space for second premolar eruption. In such cases, second premolar may erupt completely out of the arch and may be indicated for extraction **(Fig. 26.10)**.
- Unfavorably impacted second premolars may need to be extracted.
- Grossly carious or periodontally weakened second premolars may have to be sacrificed.

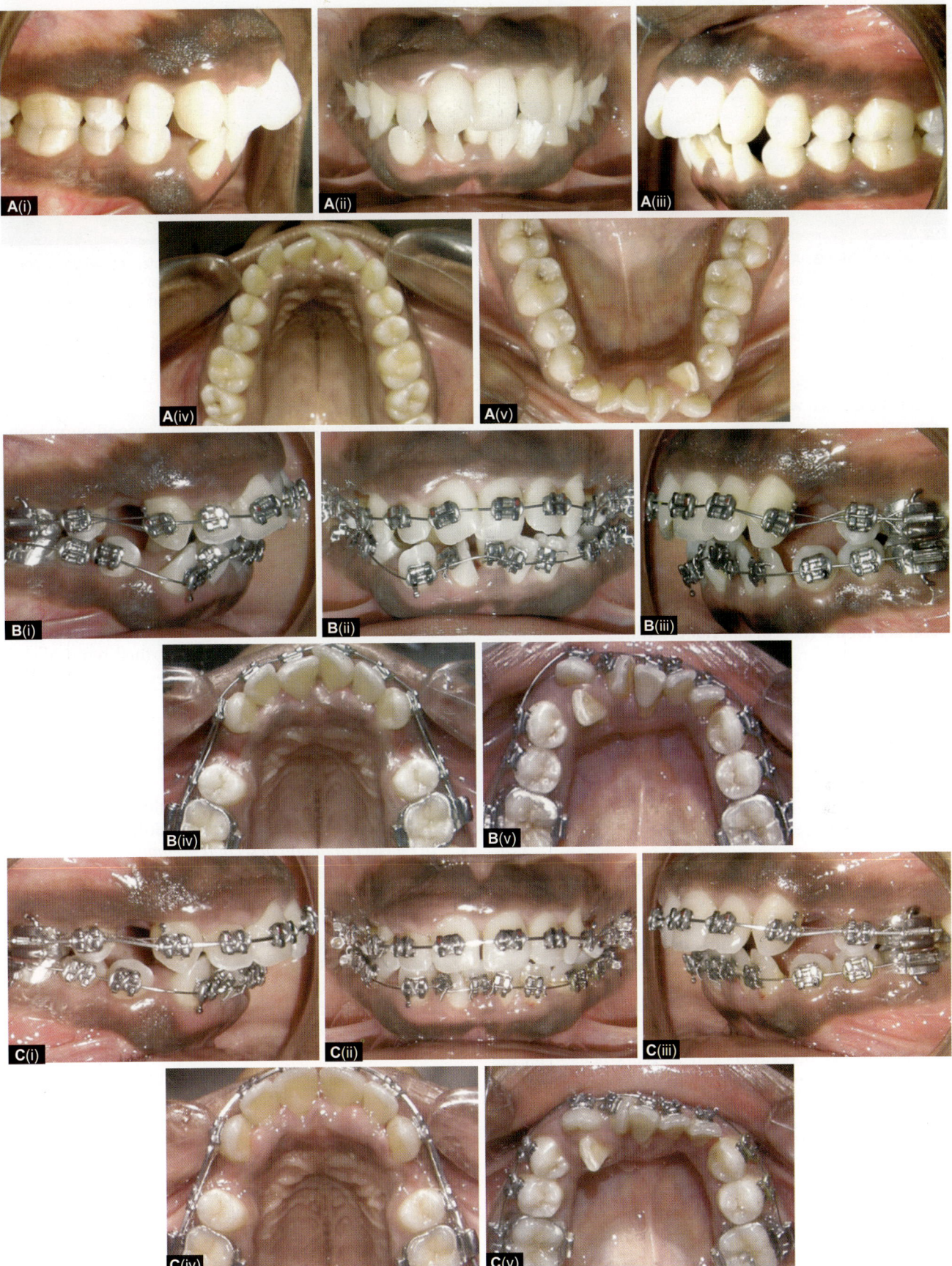

**Figs 26.8A to C:** First premolar extraction can be utilized for the correction of crowding in both anterior and posterior segments. (A) Pretreatment intraoral photographs of a patient with crowding in both arches. (B) During treatment with fixed orthodontic appliance by extraction of first premolars. (C) Nearing completion of treatment

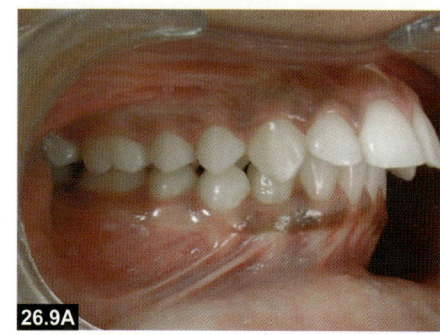 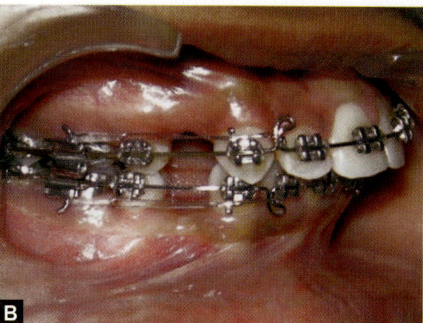 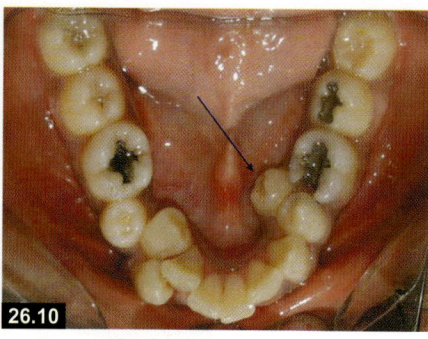

**Figs 26.9A and B:** A patient with class II division 1 malocclusion and extraction of first premolar in such case often offers maximum space for the retraction of the proclined anteriors. (A) Pretreatment intraoral right lateral view. (B) Intraoral right lateral view after extraction of first premolar with fixed orthodontic appliance; **Fig. 26.10:** Second premolar erupted completely out of the arch may be indicated for extraction

- Extraction of second premolars is preferred in open bite cases as it would encourage deepening of the bite.

### Extraction of First Molars

First molars are regarded as the cornerstones of dental arches and are considered to play a key role in the establishment of occlusion by Angle. They are usually not extracted unless otherwise indicated.

Extraction of first permanent molars is not advisable due to the following reasons:
- Extraction of first molars does not provide adequate space for the relief of anterior crowding.
- First molar extraction can lead to deepening of the bite, which may not be desirable in all cases.
- Following first molar extraction, the second premolar may tip into the extraction space.
- Masticatory function of the patient may get affected.

#### Indications
First molars may have to be compromised in certain conditions, such as the following:
- First molars are extracted when they are grossly decayed or heavily filled. First permanent molars are highly susceptible to dental caries, especially during childhood, immediately after their eruption.
- Extraction of first molars may be advantageous in open bite cases as this may lead to deepening of the bite.

### Wilkinson's Extraction

Wilkinson advocated extraction of entire first molars between the age of 8.5 years and 9.5 years. Reason for the extraction of first permanent molar by Wilkinson is that first permanent molars are highly prone for dental caries.

#### Benefits of Early First Permanent Molar Extraction According to Wilkinson
- Prevents impaction of third molars.
- It relieves crowding in the dental arch.
- It helps in decreasing the incidence and occurrence of dental caries.

#### Drawbacks of Wilkinson's Extraction
- It relieves crowding in the arches only to certain extent.

- Mesial drifting of second molar into the first permanent molar extraction space.
- Rotation of second premolars and second permanent molars.
- Extraction of permanent first molar results in lack of anchorage for orthodontic therapy.
- Extraction of first permanent molar will make it difficult to define the type of malocclusion according to Angle's classification.

### Extraction of Second Molars

Although second molars are not routinely extracted in conjunction with orthodontic therapy, their removal may be beneficial in certain situations as described below.

#### Indications
- *To prevent third molar impaction*
  Extraction of second molars may be considered in some cases for preventing third molar impaction. Removal of second molars prior to the eruption of third molars may result in satisfactory third molar position.
- *To relieve impaction of second premolar*
  Premature loss of second deciduous molars often results in forward drifting of first permanent molars and space required for the eruption of second premolar may become inadequate. Extraction of second molars in such a situation may create sufficient space for second premolar eruption by causing the distal movement of the first permanent molars.
- *To relieve lower incisor crowding*
  Mild crowding in the lower anterior region can be relieved by extracting the second molars.
- *For distalization of first molars*
  Extraction of second molars may be advantageous when distalization of first molars is planned.
- *In open bite cases*
  Removal of second molars may be beneficial in open bite cases, as this encourages deepening of bite.

### Extraction of Third Molars

Although extraction of third molars does not yield space for correction of crowding, it is undertaken for other reasons during orthodontic treatment.

### Indications

- Third molars are the most common teeth to be impacted in oral cavity.
- Impacted third molars, which are not likely to erupt into ideal position, are frequently extracted **(Fig. 26.11A)**.
- Pericoronitis development may also necessitate third molar extraction.
- Progressive crowding of lower anteriors is observed in adolescence and early adult life. This has often been blamed on the erupting lower third molar teeth although it is not proved. Some orthodontists advocate extraction of third molars to prevent such late crowding.
- Malformed third molars, which interfere with normal occlusion.
- Carious third molars which are difficult to restore **(Fig. 26.11B)**.

### DIFFERENT EXTRACTION PROCEDURES

- Balanced extraction
- Compensatory extraction
- Phased extraction
- Enforced extraction
- Therapeutic extraction
- Wilkinson's extraction
- Serial extraction.

#### Balanced Extraction

Balanced extraction is defined as the method of extraction, where removal of another tooth on the opposite side of the same arch is done. The teeth distal to the extraction space move into the space while the teeth mesial to the extraction space can also move distally into the space **(Fig. 26.12)**. Thus, the midline of the arch may shift to the side of the extraction space, creating asymmetry in the arch. To avoid unesthetic shifts of the dental arch, single side

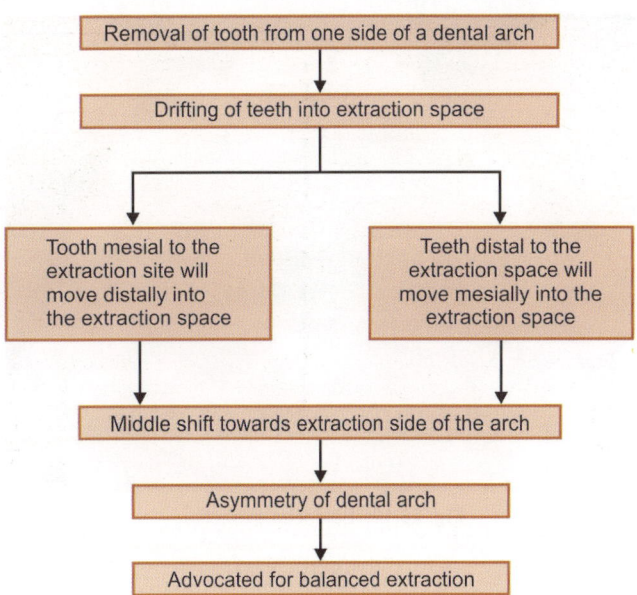

**Flowchart 26.1:** Balanced extraction

extraction is balanced by extraction of another tooth on the opposite side of the same dental arch **(Flowchart 26.1)**.

#### Compensatory Extraction

Compensating extraction refers to the extraction of a tooth in the opposite jaw of the same teeth group (antimere/antagonistic tooth). For example, if third molar is extracted in the right quadrant of the maxillary arch then the third molar in the right quadrant of the mandibular arch is also extracted. This type of extraction is called as compensatory extraction **(Flowchart 26.2)**.

When a tooth is removed in one arch, its antimere tooth (the opposing tooth of the other arch) may supraerupt leading to occlusal disharmony, compensatory extraction advocated in such cases.

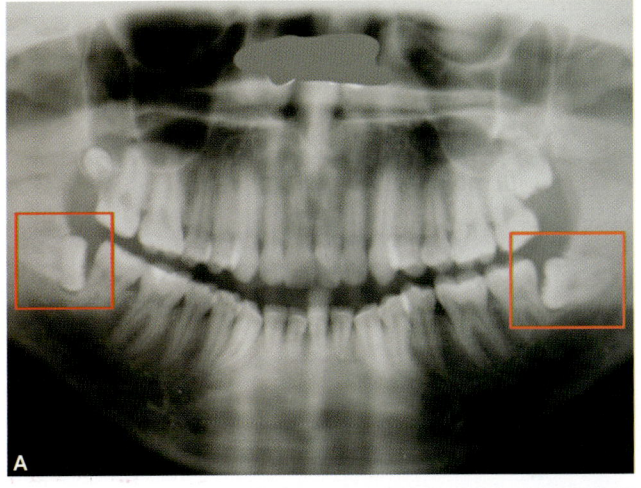
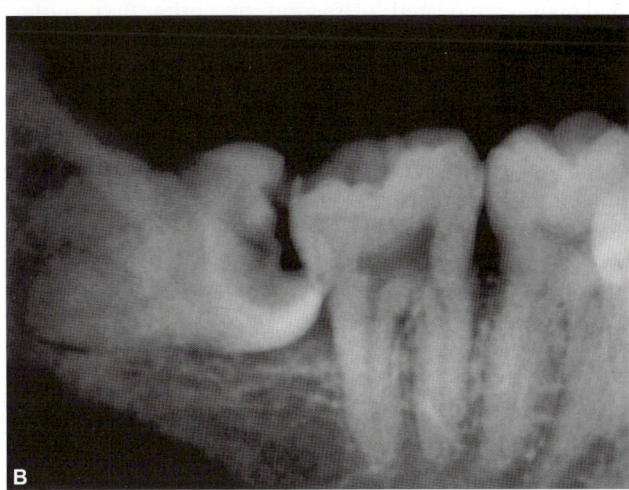

**Figs 26.11 A and B:** (A) Bilateral horizontally impacted third molars are frequently extracted; (B) Horizontally impacted carious 3rd molar

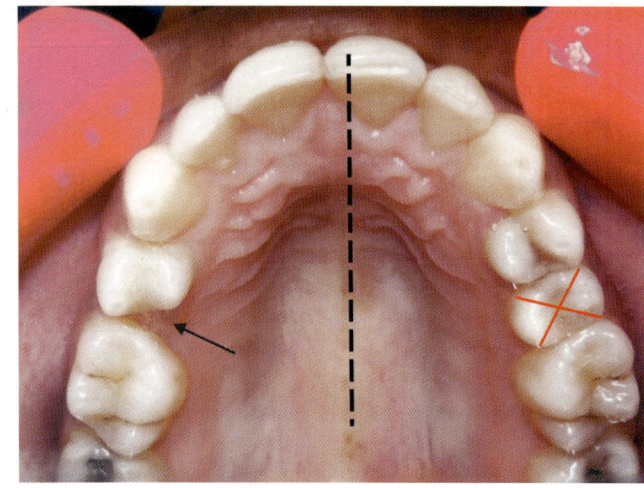

**Fig. 26.12:** Balanced extraction

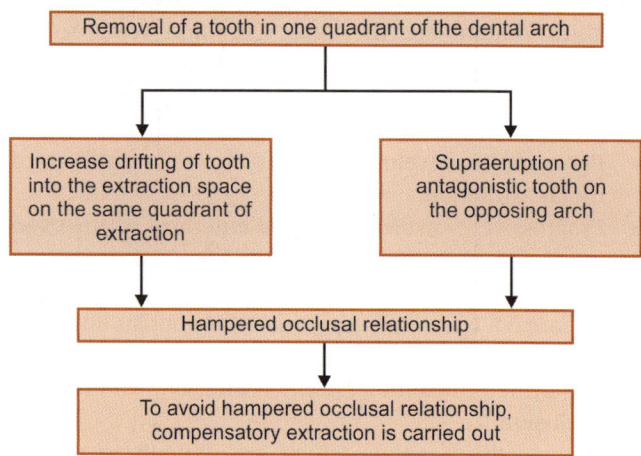

**Flowchart 26.2:** Compensatory method of extraction

### Phased Extraction

Sometimes, it may be advantageous to extract the indicated teeth in two phases, especially to effect a change in the molar occlusion. In this method, the tooth in one arch is extracted few months earlier than in the other arch.

### Enforced Extraction

Orthodontist is, sometimes, forced to extract the teeth in poor condition, e.g. grossly decayed, fractured, unfavorably impacted and periodontally compromised teeth. This is called enforced extraction.

### Therapeutic Extraction

Certain sound healthy teeth may have to be sacrificed to facilitate proper alignment of other teeth in cases of severe arch length-tooth material discrepancy. Such extraction of sound teeth or the purpose of orthodontic treatment is called as therapeutic extraction.

### Wilkinson's Extraction

Wilkinson advocated extraction of entire first molars between the age of 8.5 years and 9.5 years.

### Serial Extraction

Serial extraction refers to programmed removal of certain selected primary and permanent teeth during mixed dentition period so as to intercept the developing malocclusion with crowding in the arches (explained in detail in Chapter 20).

### BIBLIOGRAPHY

1. Barrer HG. Treatment timing of borderline cases. J Clin Orthod 1971;5:191-9.
2. Dewel BF. A question of terminology. Am J Orthod 1970;58:78-9.
3. Dewel BF. Precautions in serial extraction. Am J Orthod 1971;60:615-8.
4. Dewel BF. Serial extraction in orthodontics: indications, objectives and treatment procedures. Am J Orthod 1954; 40:906-26.
5. Dewel BF. Prerequisites in serial extraction. Am J Orthod 1969;55:633-9.
6. Dewel BF. Serial extraction: Its limitations and contraindications. Arizona Dent J 1968;14:14-30.
7. Fogel MS. Borderline malocclusions, differential diagnosis. Part one, J Clin Orthod 1971; 5:248-59. Part two, J Clin Orthod 1971;5:305-20.
8. Kjellgren B. Serial extraction as a corrective procedure in dental orthopedic therapy. Acta Odontol Scand 1948;8:17-43.
9. Klapper L, Navarro SF, Bowman D, et al. Effects of extraction and nonextraction treatment on growth patterns. Am J Orthod Dentofac Orthop 1992;101(5):425-30.
10. Mayne WR. Serial extraction: orthodontics at the crossroads. Dent Clin North Am 1968;341-62.
11. Nakai TT. The influence of serial extraction procedures on the soft tissues: profiles in class 2, division 1 malocclusions; a cephalometric study. Am J Orthod 1968;54:154.
12. Ringenberg QM. Serial extraction: stop, look, and be certain. Am J Orthod 1964;50:327-36.
13. Schwab DT. The borderline patient and tooth removal. Am J Orthod 1971;59:126-45.

# EXAM-ORIENTED QUESTIONS

## Long Questions

1. Describe in detail about extractions in orthodontics.
   Or
   What are the reasons for extraction in orthodontics? Discuss the choice of teeth for extractions.
   Or
   How will you plan extractions in orthodontic treatment?
2. Different tooth extraction procedures in orthodontics.

## Short Note

1. Wilkinson's extraction method
2. Dewel's method of serial extraction
3. Planning extractions in orthodontics
4. Impacted tooth and its orthodontic correction
5. Therapeutic extraction in Orthodontics.

# CHAPTER OVERVIEW

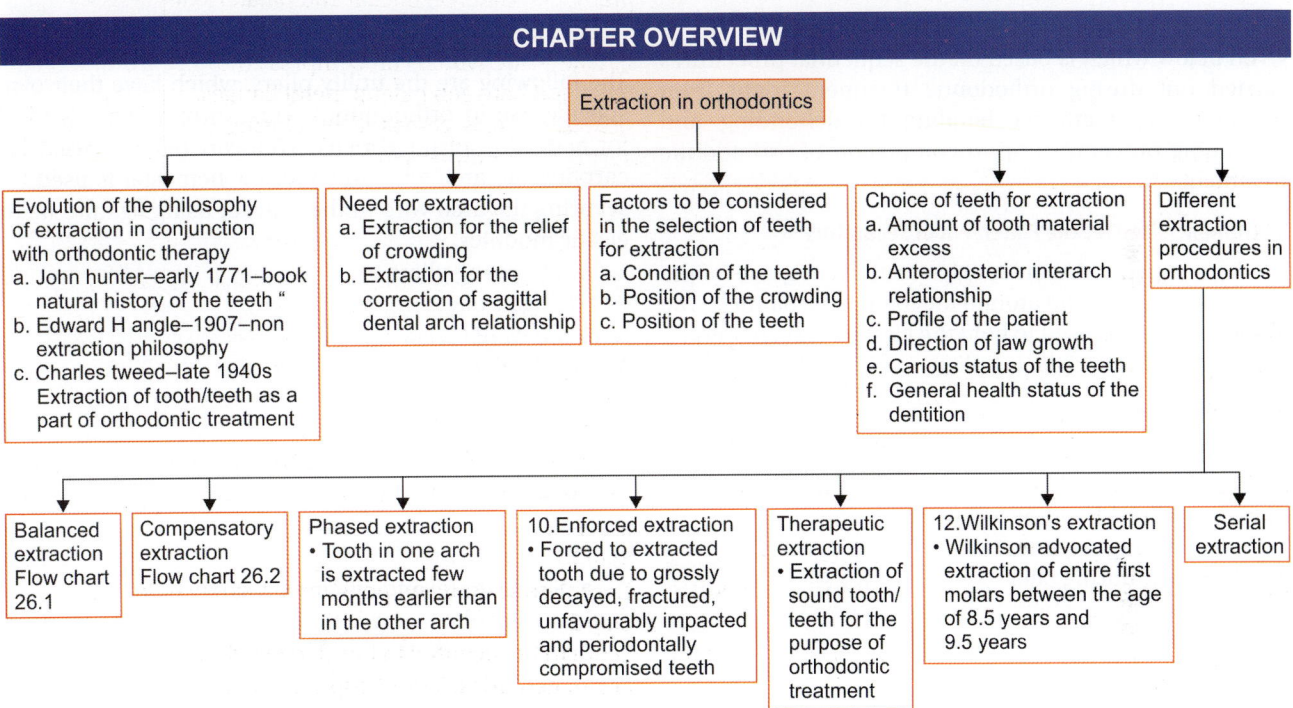

# CHAPTER 27

# Orthodontic Instruments

*Phulari BS*

Various instruments and pliers that are specially designed for orthodontic purposes are used in orthodontic practice. Basic set of orthodontic instruments along with newer advances in the filed such as 3D instruments are discussed in this chapter.

## CLASSIFICATION

A working classification of orthodontic instruments is given below which is based on the sequential procedures carried out during orthodontic treatment, right from separation of teeth for banding till debonding and debanding procedures up to completion of orthodontic treatment.

### Instruments Used for the Placement of Separators

Teeth are separated in order to have sufficient space for the placement of the band around the tooth to be banded. The following pliers is used to hold the elastic ring separator. Example: Separator placing pliers.

### Banding Instruments

Once the teeth are separated, the following sets of instruments are used for the fabrication of bands either by direct or indirect banding techniques.
1. Band-cutting scissors
2. Band-contouring plier
3. Band pinchable pliers
   a. Straight
   b. Curved
4. Band pusher
5. Band seater
6. Band crimping pliers.

### Bracket Positioning Instruments

After banding procedure, the brackets are bonded onto the remaining teeth. Boon's gauge and bracket positioning gauges are used for determining the appropriate position of the brackets on different teeth.
1. Boon's gauge
2. Bracket positioning height gauge
3. Direct bonding bracket holder.

### Wire-forming Pliers

The following set of instruments is used for the fabrication of arch wires.
1. Bird beak pliers (Light wire pliers)
   - With serrations
   - Without serrations
     - Short beak
     - Long beak
2. Clasp forming pliers
3. De La Rosa pliers
   - With grooves
   - Without grooves
4. Loop forming pliers
   - Tweeds style
   - Young style.

### Utility and Specialty Pliers

The following are the utility pliers, which have their own specific use in orthodontics. Three-prong pliers is used for activation of quad helix, Weingart pliers is used for carrying the arch wire and Mathew hemostat is used for securing the arch wire in the bracket using ligature tie or elastic modules.
1. Three-prong pliers
2. Weingart pliers
3. Mathew hemostat
4. Howe pliers.

### Wire-cutting Instruments

Following the placement of arch wire in the brackets slot, excess wire distal to the molar band is cut using distal end cutters.
1. Distal end cutter
   a. Microdistal end cutter with safety hold.
   b. Distal end cutter with safety hold.

Ligature wires are used to fasten the arch wire to the brackets on teeth. Excessive free ends of the ligature wires are cut using any of the ligature cutters.
2. Pin and ligature cutter
   a. Stein ligature cutter
   b. Mini ligature cutter
   c. Mini ligature cutter 15° angle
   d. Angled ligature cutter 30° angle
   e. Pin and ligature cutter 45° angle

### Debonding Pliers

Brackets are debonded using the following instruments:
a. Debonding pliers-anterior
b. Debonding pliers-posterior
c. Angulated bracket remover.

### Debanding Pliers

At the end of active orthodontic treatment, bands are removed using straight or curved band remover.
1. Band remover
   a. Straight band remover
   b. Curved band remover.

### 3D Modular Orthodontic Instruments

1. Howe pliers
2. Light wire pliers
3. Belzer wire cutter
4. Lingual arch forming pliers
5. Jaw pliers
6. Band director
7. Band pusher/Band seater
8. Angle wire bending pliers
9. Modular omega pliers.

### Pre-clinical Wire-bending Intruments

1. Universal pliers
2. Adam's pliers
3. 201 Three prong pliers/3 beak/3 jaw pliers
4. 53G Optical pliers
5. 139 Bird beak pliers
6. Hard wire cutter.

## INSTRUMENTS USED FOR THE PLACEMENT OF SEPARATORS

### Separator Placing Pliers

Separator placing pliers is used to place the elastic ring separator in the interproximal area between the tooth to be banded and the two adjacent teeth on either side of it **(Fig. 27.1)**.

Other separators such as brass wire separator and kesling metallic ring separators are placed using bird beak pliers/light wire pliers. The dumb-bell seaparator can be placed simply by pushing with fingers into the inter-dental area.

## BANDING INSTRUMENTS

### Band-cutting Scissors

Straight or curved band-cutting scissors are used for cutting the required length band material from the spool **(Fig. 27.2)**.

### Band-contouring Pliers

Band contouring pliers is used to contour the band material to follow the external contours of the tooth to be banded **(Figs 27.3A and B)**.

### Band Pinchable Pliers

The contoured band material is placed around the tooth to be banded and it is pinched near the lingual side of the tooth using band pinchable pliers **(Figs 27.4A and B)**.

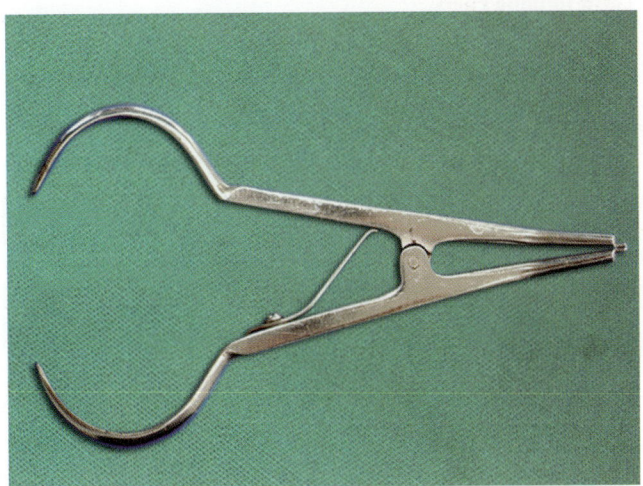

**Fig. 27.1:** Separator placing pliers

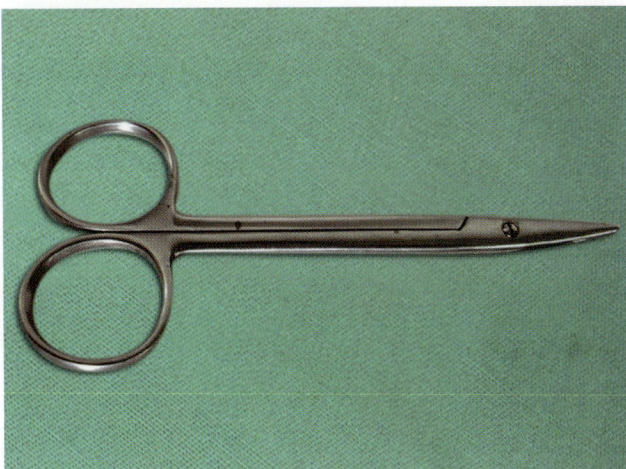

**Fig. 27.2:** Band cutting scissors

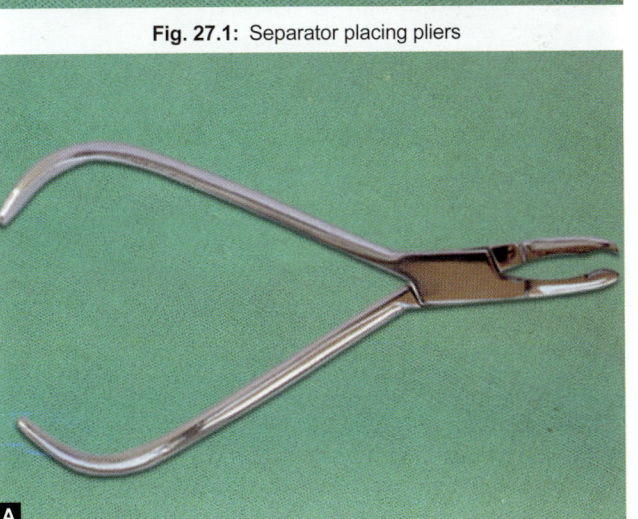

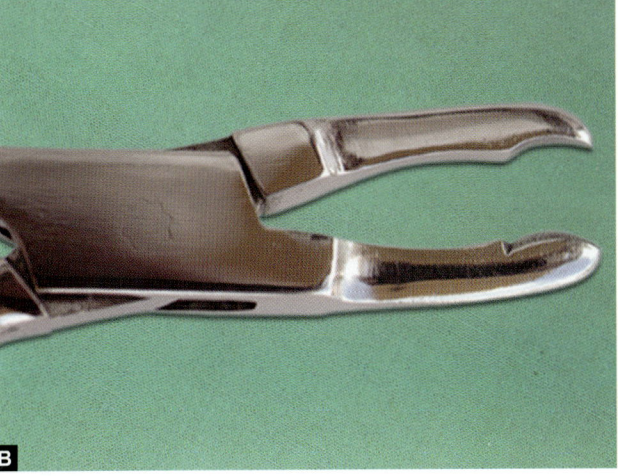

**Figs 27.3A and B:** Band contouring pliers

This helps in adjusting the diameter of the band according to the crown size of the tooth to be banded. This pliers is also used for recording the development grooves of the molars so that the band fits snugly around the tooth.

### Mershoon Band Pusher

Once the band is fabricated, Mershoon band pusher is used to push the band into its final position around the tooth to be banded **(Figs 27.5A to C)**.

### Band Seater

The band seater is used to seat and adapt the band around the tooth **(Figs 27.6A to C)**.

### Band Crimping Pliers

Band crimping pliers is used to modify the band according to the contours of the tooth to be banded so as to get a snug fit **(Fig. 27.7)**.

## BRACKET POSITIONING INSTRUMENTS

Precise bracket positioning is of utmost importance in fixed mechanotherapy. Boon's gauge and bracket positioning gauge did aid in proper positioning of brackets onto the tooth surfaces.

### Boon's Gauge

Boon's gauge is used to measure the bracket positioning heights of teeth and helps in proper positioning of the brackets **(Figs 27.8A to C)**. It has four measurements namely 3.5 mm, 4.0 mm, 4.5 mm and 5.0 mm to guide the brackets positioning on different teeth.

### Bracket Positioning Height Gauge

Bracket positioning height gauge also serves the same purpose as Boon's gauge, that is, determining the position of bracket placement **(Fig. 27.9)**. The markings are the same, nevertheless it has certain advantages over Boon's gauge because of its rectangular design. Along with the determination of height and placement of brackets it also helps in adjusting bracket into its final position.

### Direct Bonding Bracket Holder

Direct bonding bracket holder is used for holding, carrying and placing the bracket on the surface of the tooth at the desired position **(Figs 27.10A to C)**.

## WIRE-FORMING PLIERS

### Light Wire Pliers (Bird Beak Pliers)

Light wire, also known as bird beak pliers, and is used for adjusting and activating the 3D appliance **(Figs 27.11A to C)**. It can also be used for adjusting the 0.025 inch extenders on all 3D appliances.

### Clasp-forming Pliers

Arrow clasp-forming pliers, for wire up to 0.7 mm/.028" **(Fig. 27.12)**.

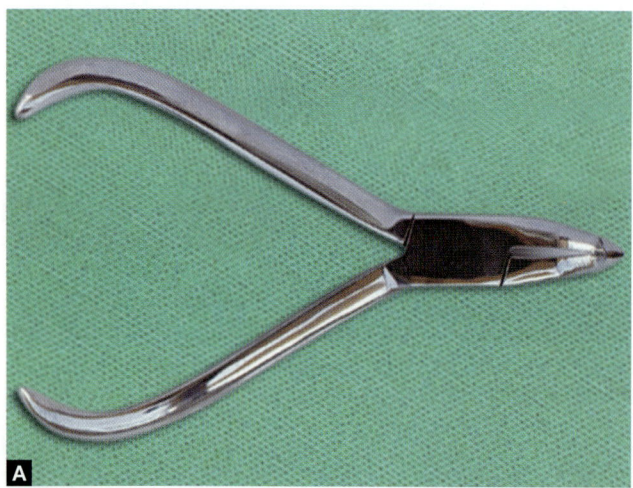
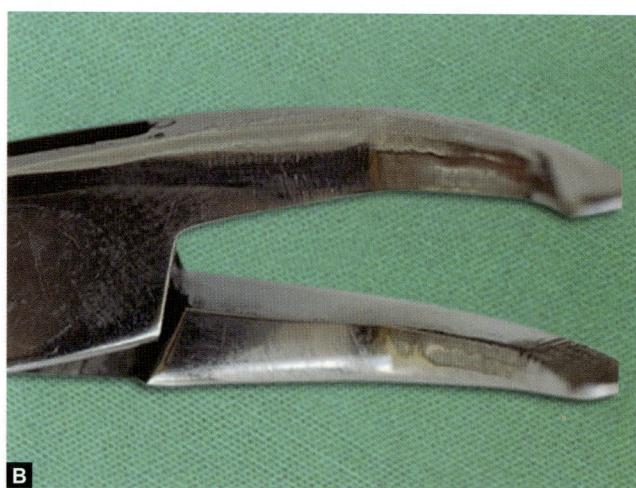

**Figs 27.4A and B:** Band pinchable pliers

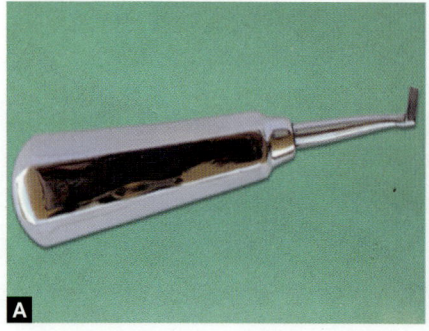
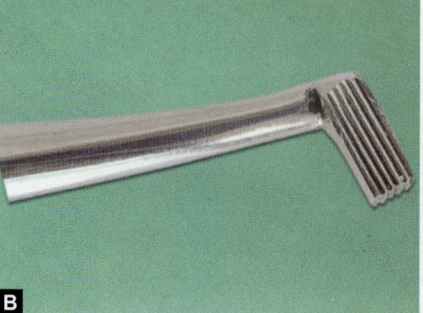
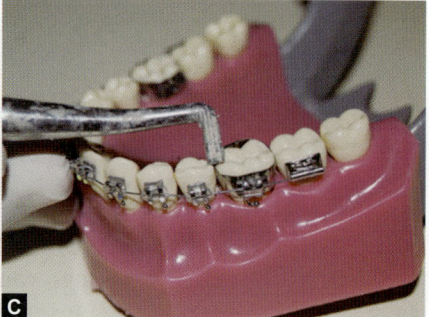

**Figs 27.5A to C:** (A and B) Mershoon band pushers. (C) Pushing the band into over the tooth to be banded using mershoon band pusher

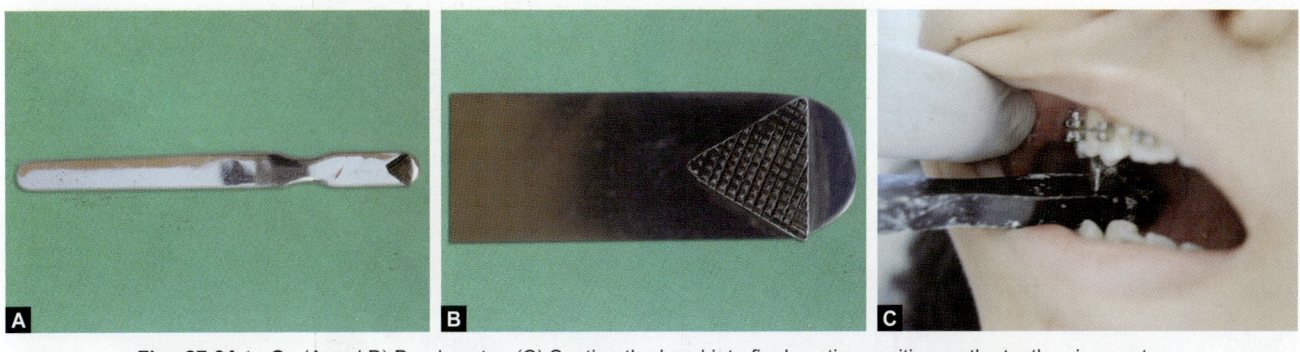

**Figs 27.6A to C:** (A and B) Band seater. (C) Seating the band into final seating position on the tooth using seater

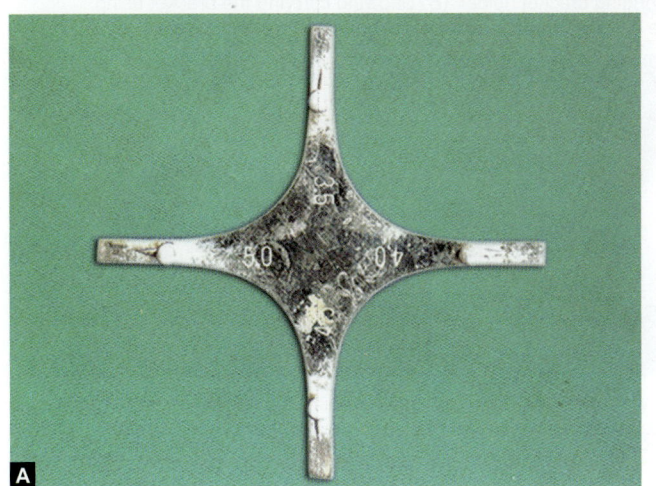
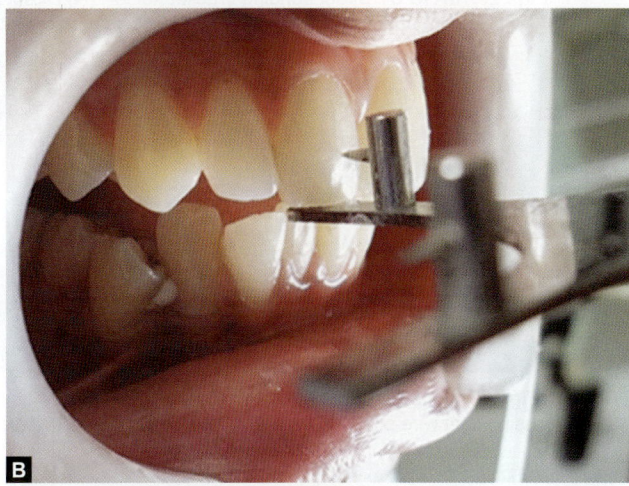

**Figs 27.8A and B:** (A) Boon's gauge. (B) B Measuring the bracket position on the tooth to be bracketed

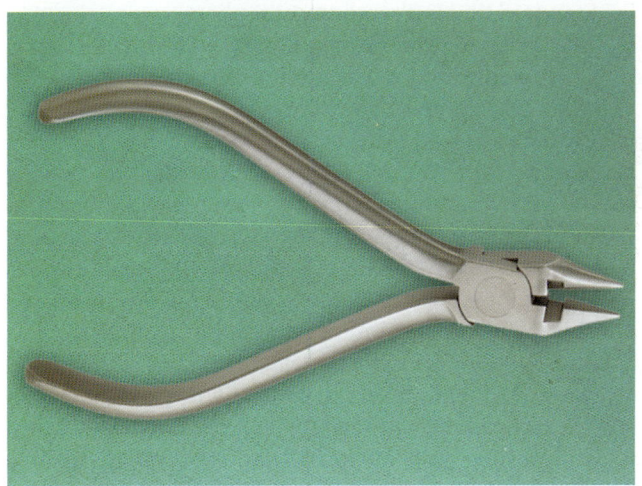

**Fig. 27.7:** Band crimping pliers

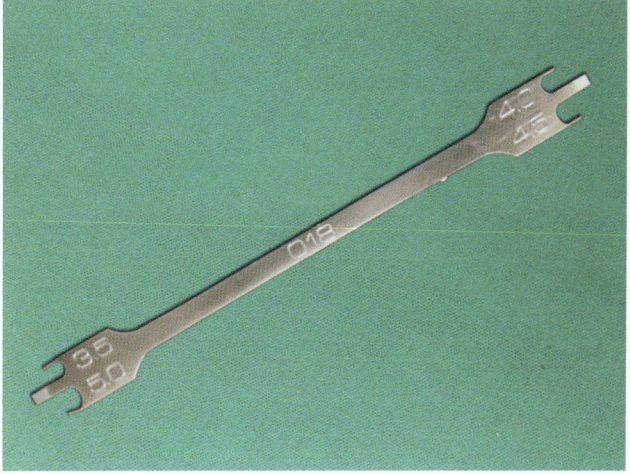

**Fig. 27.9:** Bracket positioning gauge

### De Le Rosa Pliers

It is used in fabrication of arch wire and helps to accentuate the curvature of the arch wire **(Figs 27.13A and B)**.

### Loop-forming Pliers

Various components of removable and fixed orthodontic appliances, such as bows, springs, canine retractors, etc. have loops of varying dimensions in their design. Loop-forming pliers are used to form such loops.

### Nance Loop-forming Pliers

The working end of Nance loop-forming pliers has four distinct step formations, which help in forming loops of varying sizes **(Figs 27.14A and B)**.

### Tweed Loop-forming Pliers

Tweed loop-forming pliers is an excellent pliers for making precise, consistent types of omega loops in round and rectangular wires **(Figs 27.15A and B)**.

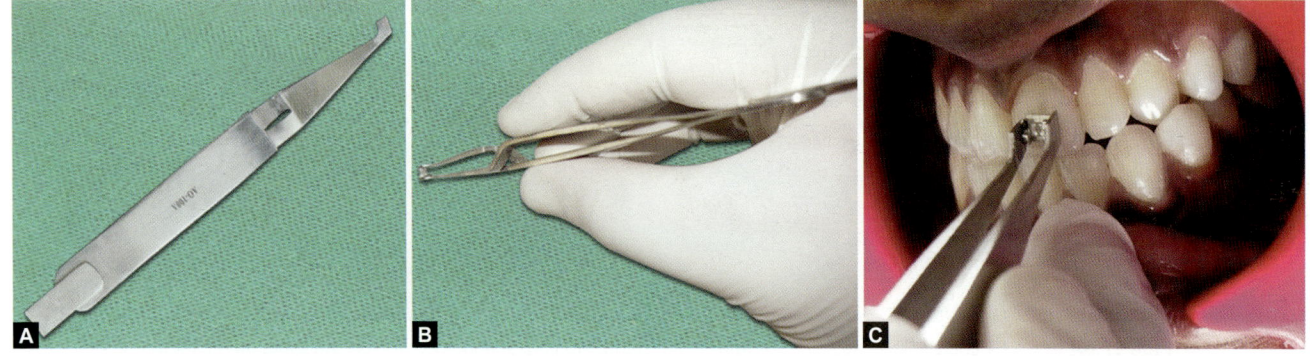

**Figs 27.10A to C:** Direct bonding bracket holder: (A) Direct bonding bracket holder. (B) Showing carrying the bracket using direct bonding bracket holder. (C) Showing placing the bracket on tooth using direct bonding bracket holder

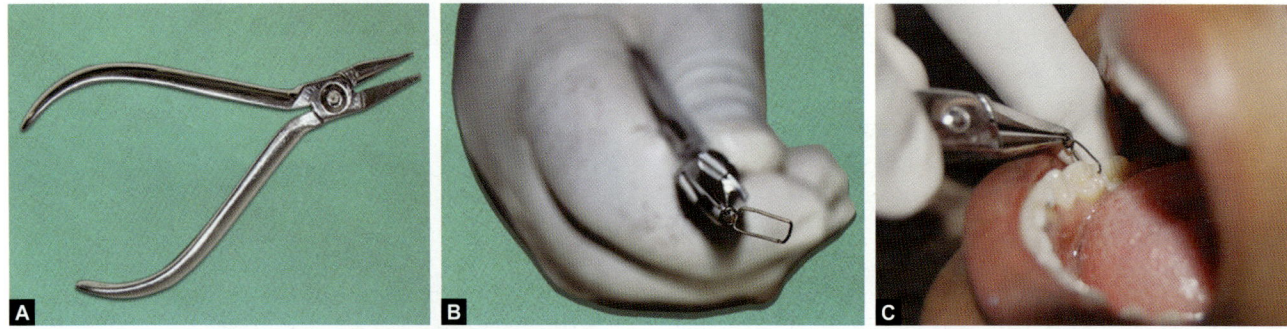

**Figs 27.11A to C:** Light wire pliers/Bird beak pliers: (A) Light wire pliers. (B) Showing how to secure the kesling separator using light wire pliers. (C) showing how to place the kesling separator on the tooth to be separated for banding procedure

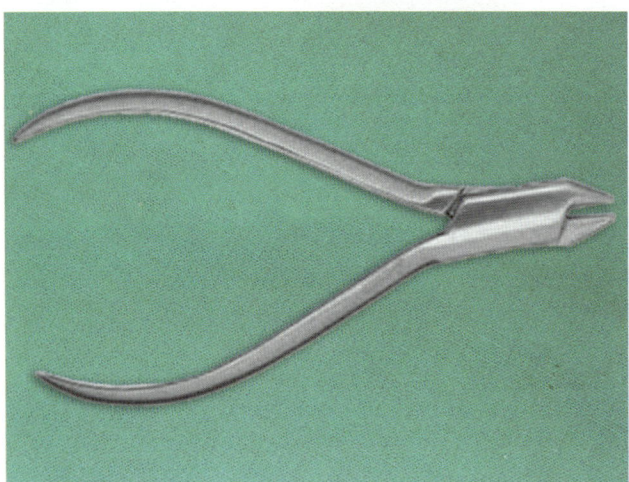

**Fig. 27.12:** Clasp-forming pliers

## UTILITY AND SPECIALTY PLIERS

### Three-prong Pliers

The working end of this instrument is used for the activation of quad helix appliance, which is often used for arch expansion **(Figs 27.16A and B)**.

### Matthew Pliers

There are a number of Matthew hemostats, which are mainly used for tieing ligature wires and fastening the elastic modules while securing the arch wires in the brackets slot.

a. Narrow tip Matthew hemostat.
b. Standard tip Matthew hemostat pliers.
c. Narrow tip Matthew (hollow form).
d. Crile needle holder hemostat.
e. Hook tip Matthew hemostat.
f. Carbide inserted Matthew hemostat.

a. *Narrow tips Matthew hemostat:* It is ideal for placing the elastic modules, although it can also be used for tieing ligatures **(Figs 27.17A to C)**.
b. *Standard tips Matthew:* Standard tip Matthew has slightly heavier construction with large tips. It is used for placing elastic modules and tieing ligatures.
c. *Narrow tips Matthew (hollow form):* The working end has a 0.20 inch groove at both the tips. Advantage of the grooved tip feature of this plier is that it allows firm and positive grip of elastic module without crushing the bracket during the procedure of placement modules.
d. *Crile needle holder:* Crile needle holder has a long handle and fine tips. It is also used for the holding and placing of elastic modules.
e. *Hook tip Matthew:* The working end has a small hook at its tip, which helps in securing elastic modules firmly. The hook also prevents slipping of modules out of the tip during the procedure.
f. *Carbide inserted Matthew:* It has carbide cross-cut serrations on its working end, which increases the longevity of this instrument. This is used for tying metal ligatures.

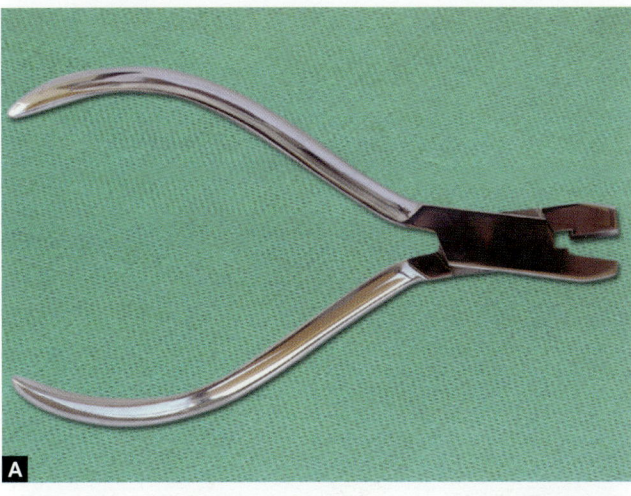 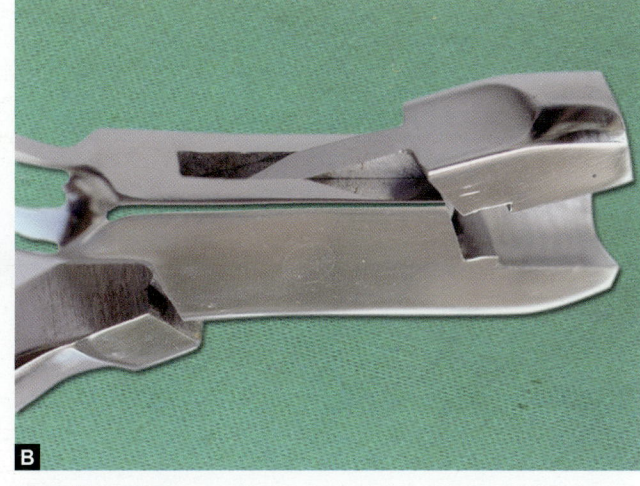

**Figs 27.13A and B:** De Le Rosa pliers

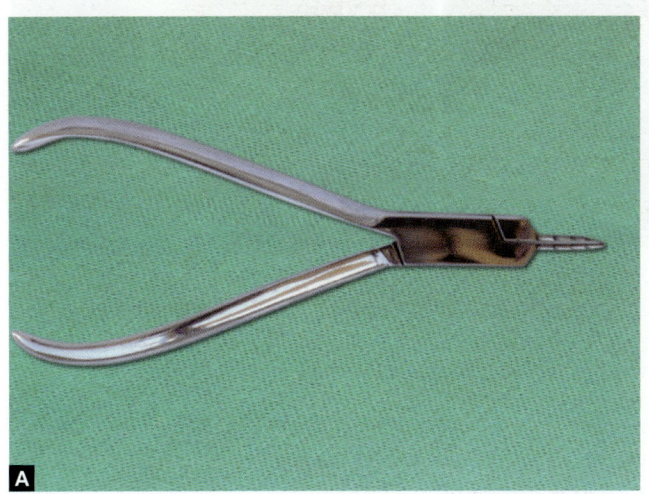 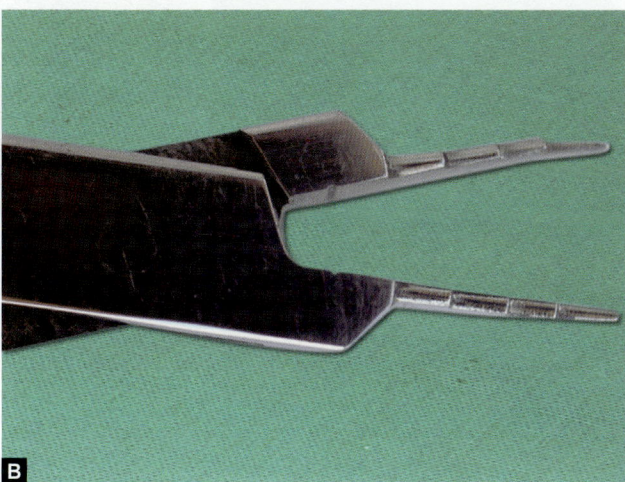

**Figs 27.14A and B:** Nance loop-forming pliers

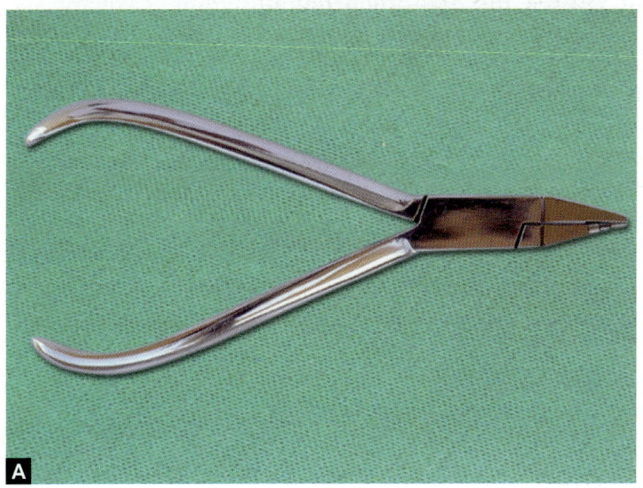 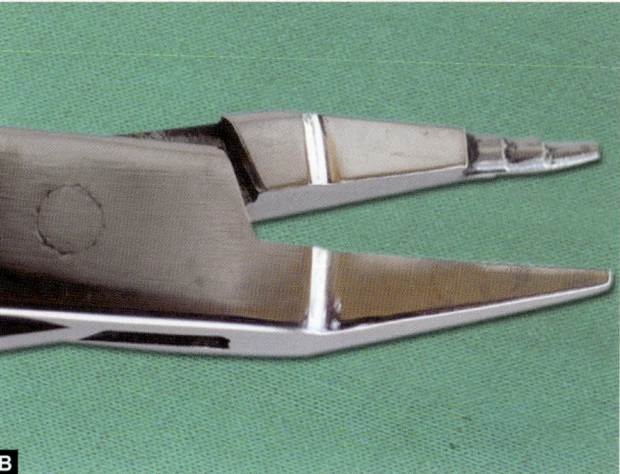

**Figs 27.15A and B:** Tweed loop-forming pliers

## Weingart Pliers

Weingart pliers are used for holding, carrying and placing the arch wires in the brackets slots **(Figs 27.18A to C)**.

There are various designs of Weingart pliers, such as:
a. Standard tip Weingart pliers.
b. Standard size Weingart pliers.
c. Heavy tip Weingart pliers.

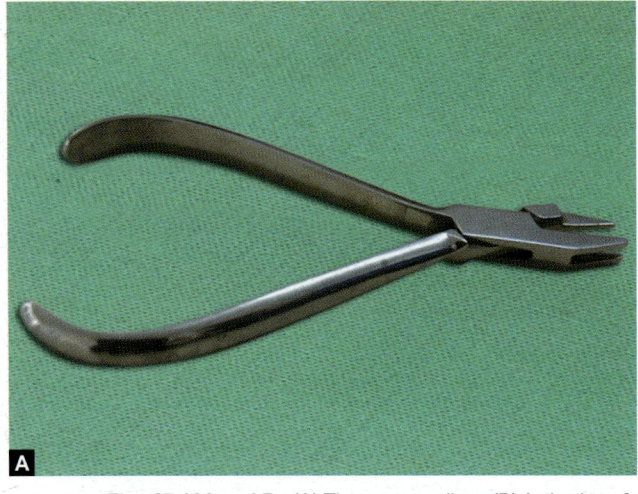
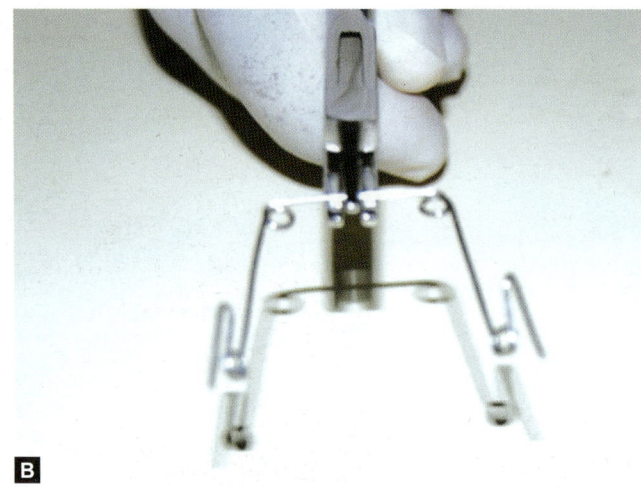

**Figs 27.16A and B:** (A) Three-prong pliers. (B) Activation of quad helix at the center of anterior bridge using three-prong pliers

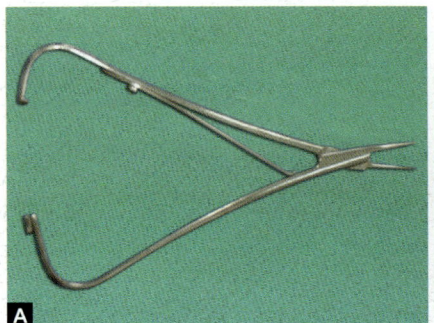
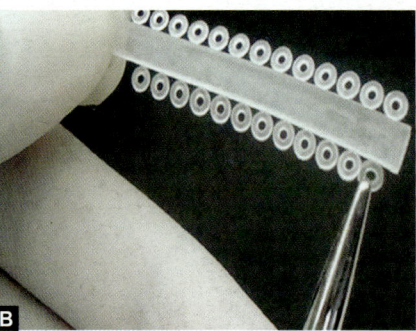
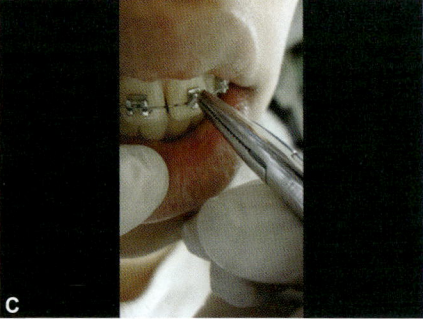

**Figs 27.17A to C:** (A) Mathew hemostat. (B) Showing dislodging the elastic module using Mathew hemostat (C) Placing elastic module on bracket to secure the arch wire into the slot of the bracket using Mathew hemostat

***Standard tip Weingart pliers:*** It has fully serrated cross-cut beaks and a convenient working angle to avoid injury to the soft tissue during arch wire placement.

***Standard size Weingart pliers:*** It has noninserted tips and is used to carry in the arch wire.

***Heavily tips Weingart pliers:*** This type of Weingart pliers has stubby inserted tips and is used to carry heavy arch wire.

## WIRE-CUTTING INSTRUMENTS

### Distal End Cutter

Distal end cutters are used to cut the excess arch wire distal to the molar band **(Figs 27.19A to C)**. The distal cutters are provided with safety hold mechanism. Due to this design of the pliers, the distal piece of wire after it is cut is held between the beaks of the cutter and thus prevents soft tissue injury and accidental swallowing.

#### Various Designs
- Micro distal end cutter with safety hold.
- Distal end cutter with safety hold.

### Pin and Ligature Cutter

Pin and ligature cutter is used to cut the terminal ends of lock pins in Begg's Technique and excessive ends of ligature wire **(Figs 27.20A to C)**.

## BRACKET DEBONDING PLIERS

### Debonding Pliers–Anterior

It is used for debonding brackets from maxillary and mandibular anteriors **(Figs 27.21A to C)**.

### Debonding Pliers–Posterior

It is used to debond the brackets from maxillary and mandibular posterior teeth. This can also be used to remove excess bonding material on the teeth **(Fig. 27.22)**.

### Angulated Bracket Remover–Wide

This bracket remover has an extra width of 6 mm and is angulated to increase accessibility in the posterior region.

## DEBANDING PLIERS

### Band Remover

During debanding procedure, the anterior and posterior band removers are used to remove the bands from anterior and posterior banded teeth, respectively **(Fig. 27.23A and B)**.

## 3D MODULAR ORTHODONTIC INSTRUMENTS

### Howe Pliers

Howe pliers is used for carrying all the 3D appliances to the arch, such as 3D lingual arch, 3D Wilson distalizing arch

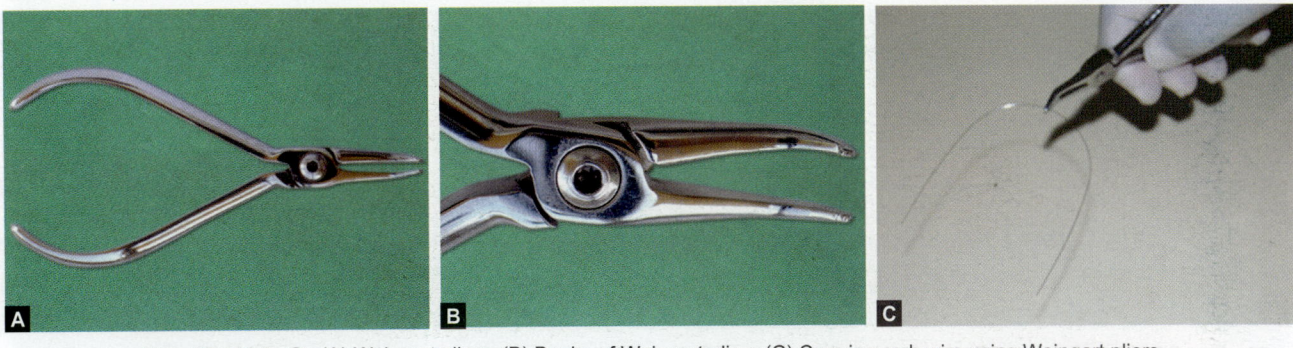

**Figs 27.18A to C:** (A) Weingart pliers. (B) Beaks of Weingart pliers (C) Carrying arch wire using Weingart pliers

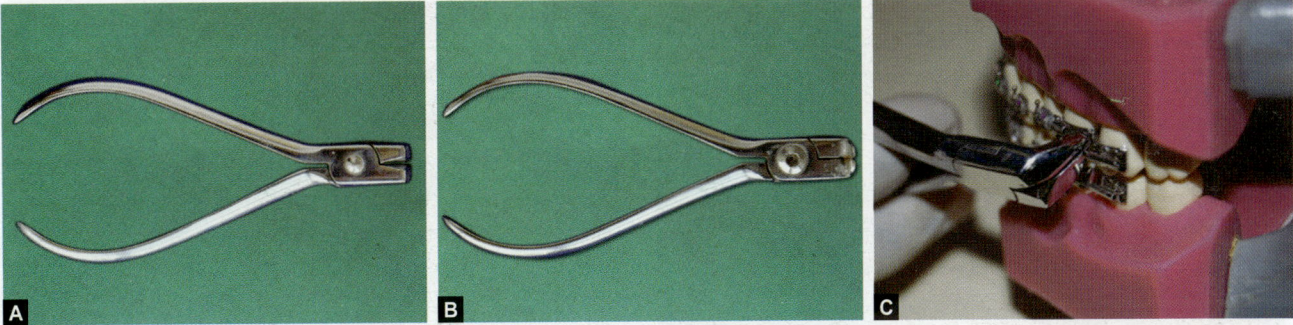

**Figs 27.19A to C:** (A and B) Distal end cutter. (C) Showing how excess wire distal to the molar buccal tube is cut using distal end cutter

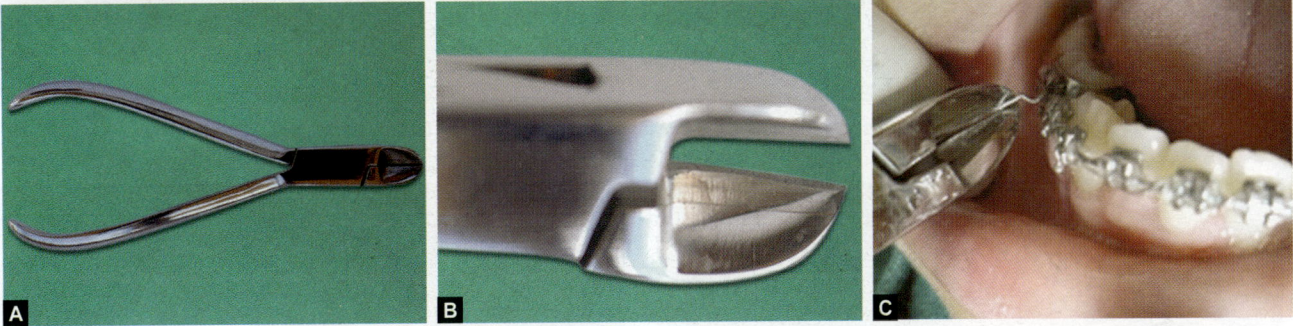

**Figs 27.20A to C:** (A and B) Pin and ligature cutters. (C) Cutting the excessive ends of ligature wire using pin and ligature cutter

and 3D quad helix appliances **(Fig. 27.24)**. It is also used for rotating, tipping and torquing of these 3D appliances.

### Light Wire Pliers (Bird Beak Pliers)

Light wire is also called as Bird Beak Pliers and is used for adjusting and activating the 3D appliance **(Fig. 27.25)**. It can also be used for adjusting the 0.025 inch extenders on all 3D appliances.

### Belzer Wire Cutter

Belzer wire cutter is used to crimp omega stop and tandem yoke onto arch. It can also be used for cutting excess wire from appliances.

### Lingual Arch-forming Pliers

It is used for holding the appliance with precision seated post during fabrication. It can also be used for rotation and torquing of 3D quad helix.

### Jaw Pliers

Jaw pliers are used for:

- Tightening wire formed 3D posts for any loose fit
- Adjusting quad helix appliance
- Adjusting 3D activators

### Band Director

Band director is used for seating of 3D posts in 3D lingual tubes.

### Band Scaler/Pusher

Band scaler/pusher is used for removing 3D appliance from 3D lingual tubes.

### Angle Wire Bending Pliers

Angle wire bending pliers is used for adjusting and activating 3D appliances.

### Modular Omega Pliers

It is used for adjusting the expansion or contraction of the omega loop on the 3D maxillary biometric distalizing arch.

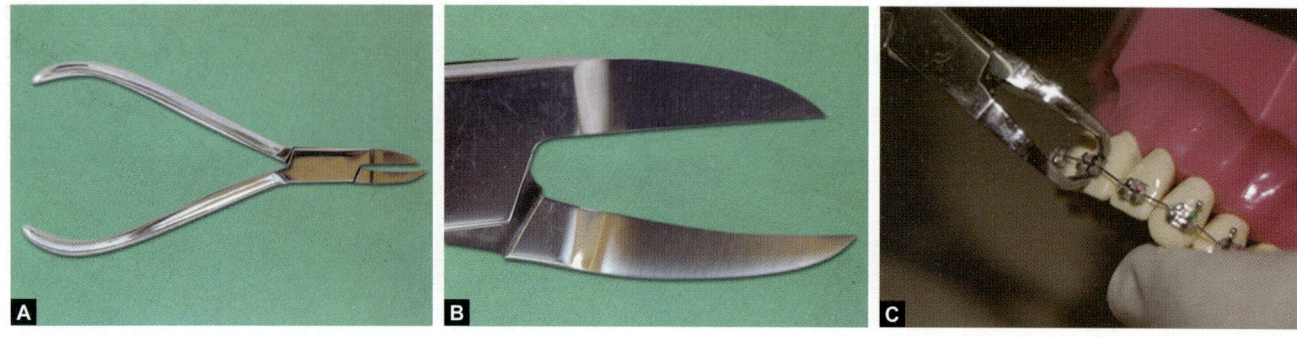

**Figs 27.21A to C:** (A and B) Anterior debonding pliers. (C) Showing debonding of anterior bracket using anterior debonding plier

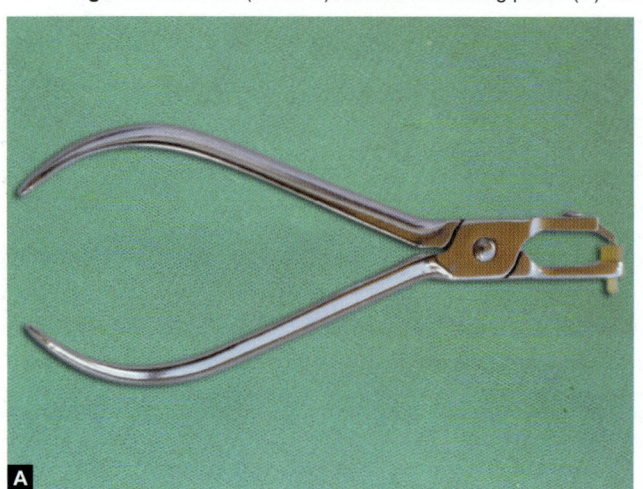 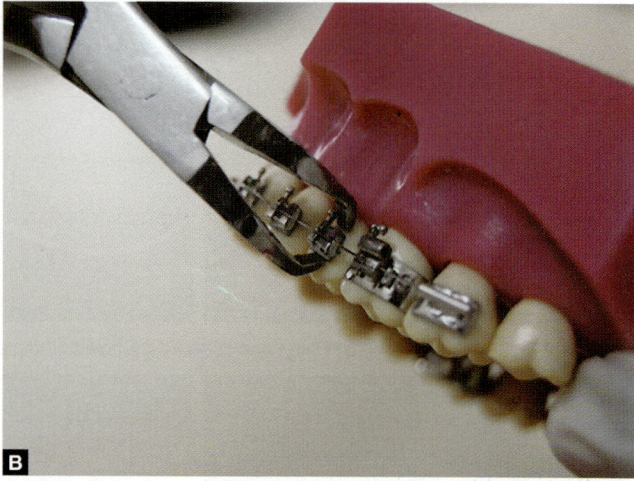

**Figs 27.22A and B:** Posterior debonding pliers: (A) Posterior debonding pliers. (B) Debonding the posterior bracket using the posterior debonding pliers

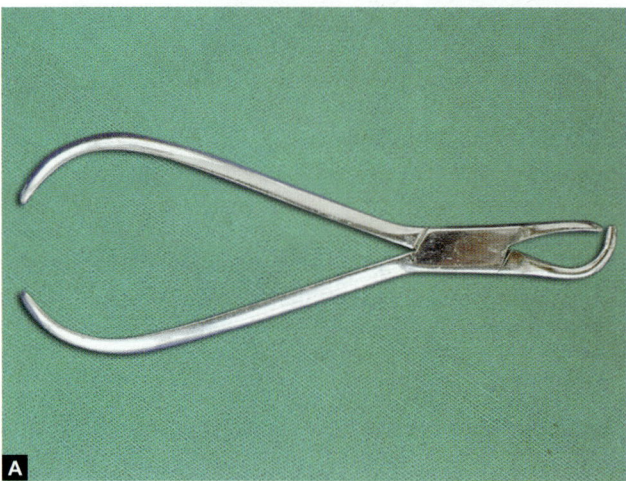 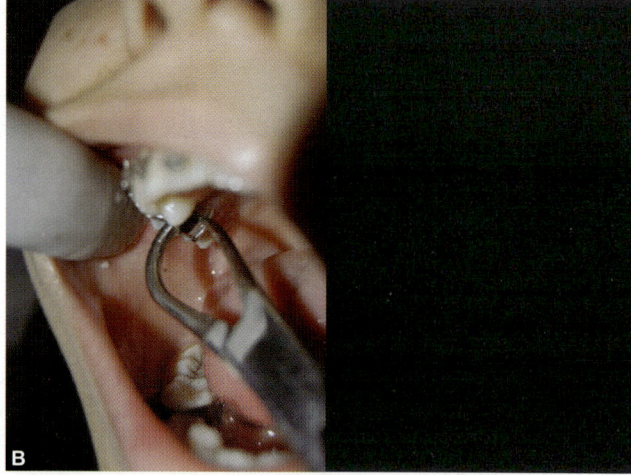

**Figs 27.23A and B:** (A) Band remover. (B) Removing the molar band using the band remover

## MAINTENANCE OF ORTHODONTIC INSTRUMENTS

### Rusted Pliers

- *Problem:* Pliers tips are rusted.
- *Reason:* Pliers were in touch with water.

*Solution:* Avoid use of soap and water to clean pliers.

### Discolored Plier

*Problem:* Black spots on the pliers.
*Reasons:* These include the following:

a. Pliers were in touch with water
b. Chemicals and minerals in the tap water are the reason for discoloration of the pliers.
  *Solution:* Avoid use of water to clean pliers.

### Dull Cutting Edges of Pliers

*Problem:* Dull cutting edge of pliers.
*Reasons:* These include the following:

- Pliers left too long in the ultrasonic cleaner
- Also check the bending and cutting specifications

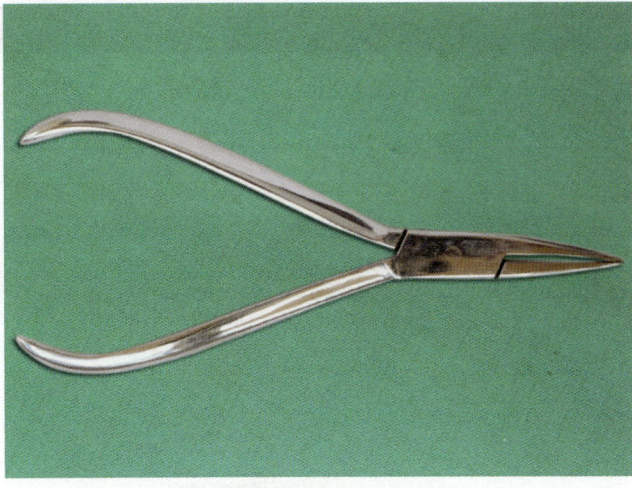

Fig. 27.24: Howe pliers

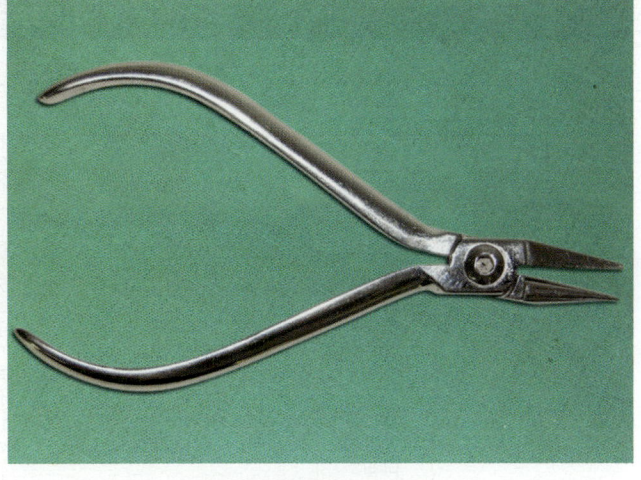

Fig. 27.25: Light wire pliers

- Pliers used to cut or bend a heavier wire than its standards.

**Solution:** Work with standards.

## STIFF AND SQUEAKY PLIERS

**Problem:** The joint and pliers are stiff and squeaky.
**Reasons:** These include the following:
a. Excessive sterilization causes the polish and the lubricant to disappear.
b. It might be the time to send them back for quality repair services.

**Solution:** Avoid excessive sterilization.

## DO's AND DON'Ts ABOUT STERILIZATION OF ORTHODONTIC INSTRUMENTS

### Do's

- Always use distilled water or surgical milk for precleaning.
- The pliers should be kept separately especially when they are in an ultrasonic cleaner.
- Check the wire sizes of pliers cutting and bending specifications.
- Clean pliers first with Y 10 surgical milk or distilled water solution.

### Don'ts

- One should never use soap and water to clean pliers. Distilled water cab is used in ultrasonic cleaner.
- Glutaraldehyde can also damage pliers. Do not put them in any glutaraldehyde solution.
- Do not brush pliers as hard brush might scratch pliers.
- Avoid excessive sterilization as it might damage the pliers polish.

## EXAM-ORIENTED QUESTIONS

### Long Essay or Long Questions

1. Classify orthodontic instruments and write any four orthodontics instruments in detail.
2. Classify orthodontic instruments and write about banding instruments in detail.
3. Banding orthodontic instruments.
4. Bracket positioning instruments.
5. Wire-forming pliers.
6. Orthodontic wire-cutting instruments.
7. Debonding orthodontic pliers.
8. 3D modular orthodontic instruments.
9. Pre-clinical wire bending orthodontic instruments.

### Short Notes

1. Debonding orthodontic pliers.
2. Maintenance of orthodontic instruments.
3. Do's and don'ts about sterilization of orthodontic instruments.

# CHAPTER OVERVIEW

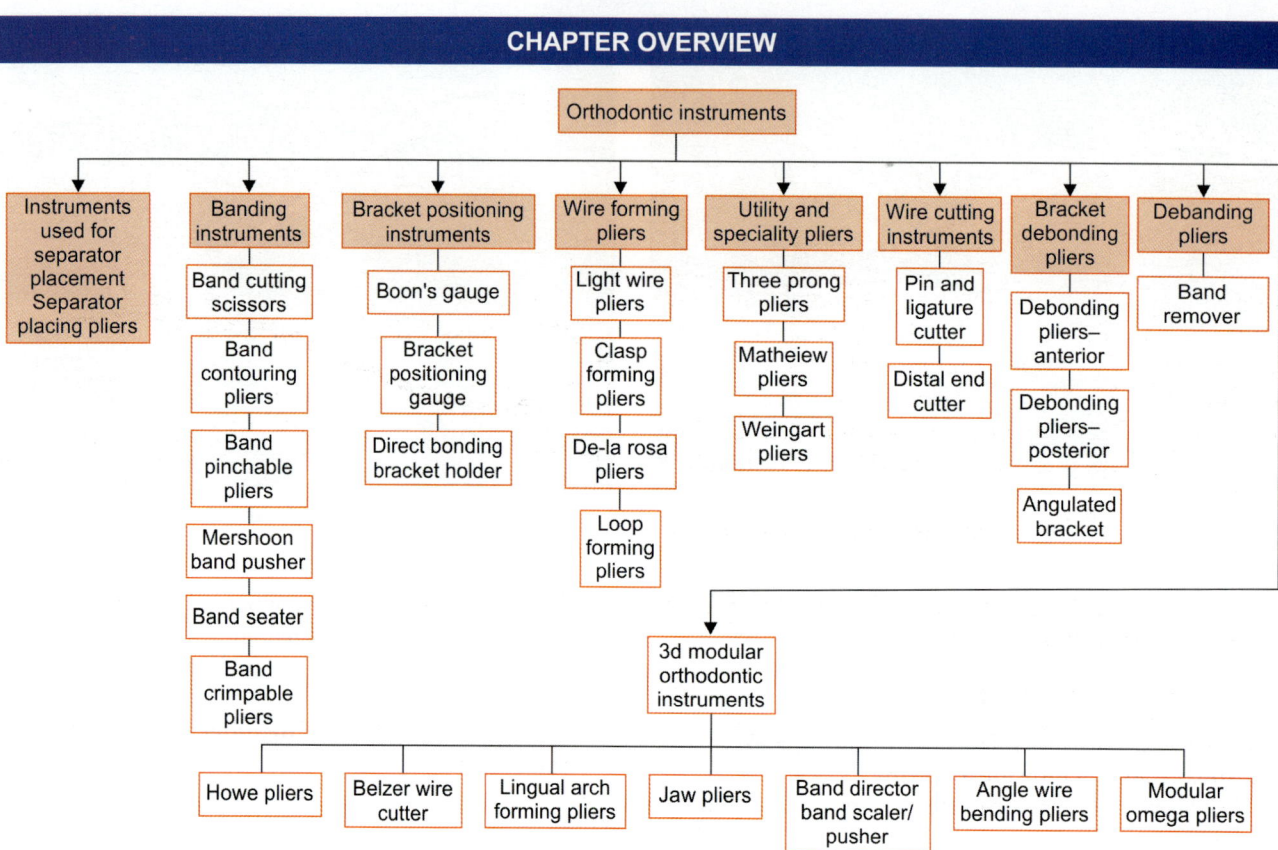

# CHAPTER 28

# Pre-clinical Orthodontics

*Phulari BS*

Wire bending is an integral part of orthodontic appliance fabrication. Various types of bends are given to stainless steel wire using pliers. The rationale of preclinical orthodontic exercise is to develop skills necessary to prepare various types of orthodontic components, which in turns, are used to fabricate various kinds of orthodontic appliance.

Basically, orthodontic wires used are for following two purposes:
1. To fabricate active components of orthodontic appliances, such as bows, springs and canine retractors that apply tooth moving forces.
2. To fabricate retentive components of orthodontic appliances such as clasps—that hold the appliance in contact with teeth.

In order to make active and retentive component of removable orthodontic appliance, the wire must be properly shaped in all three-dimension planes of space.

## BASIC BENDS

There are four basic types of bends that are used to fabricate orthodontic appliances. They are as follows:
   I. Right-angled bend.
  II. Loops and helices.
 III. Curves.
  IV. Control of plane in space.

### Right-angled Bend

To make right-angled bend, the thumb is placed as close to beaks as possible and wire is pushed over the round beak of the 139 pliers **(Figs 28.1A to D)**.

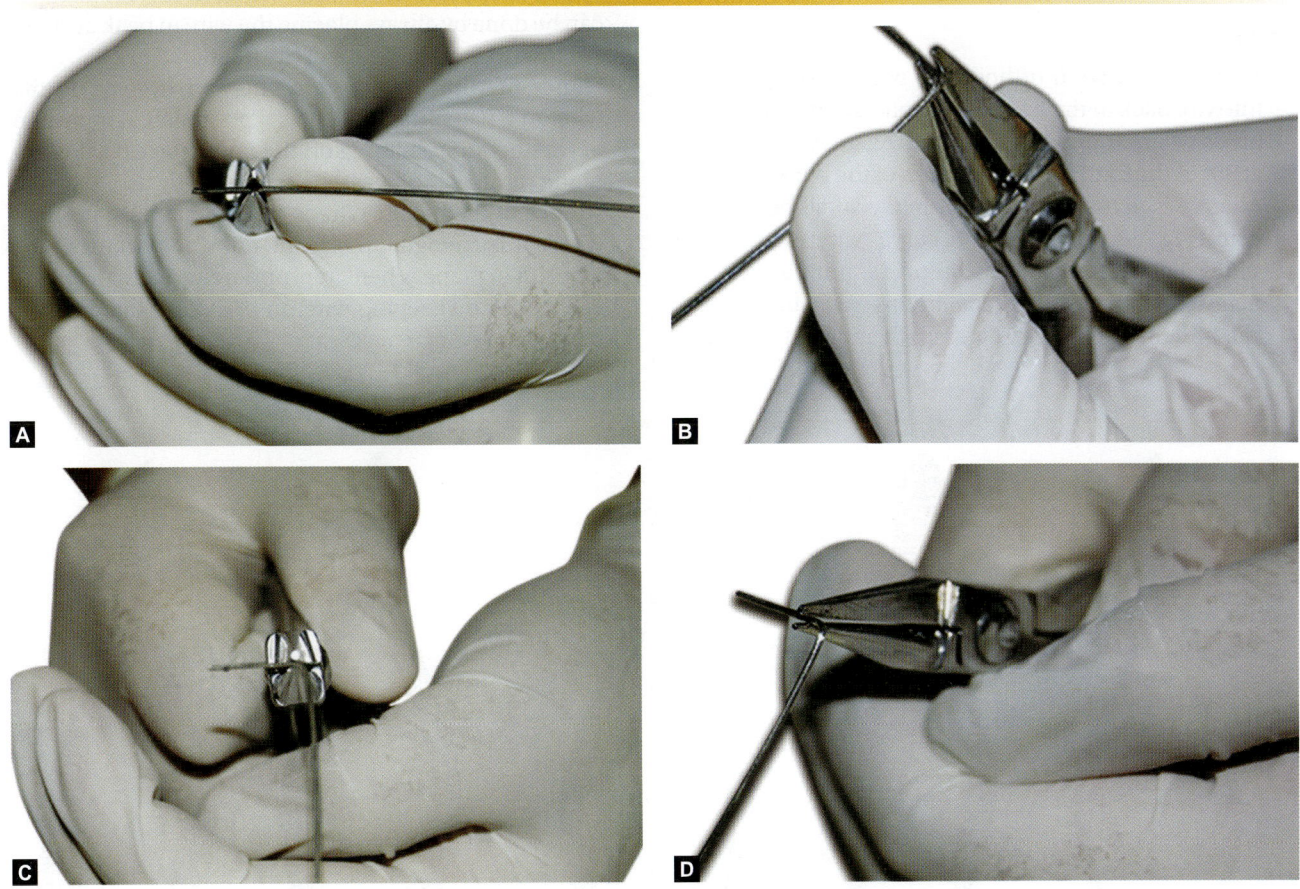

**Figs 28.1A to D:** To make right-angled bend, the thumb is placed as close to beaks as possible and wire is pushed over the round beak of the 139 bird beak pliers

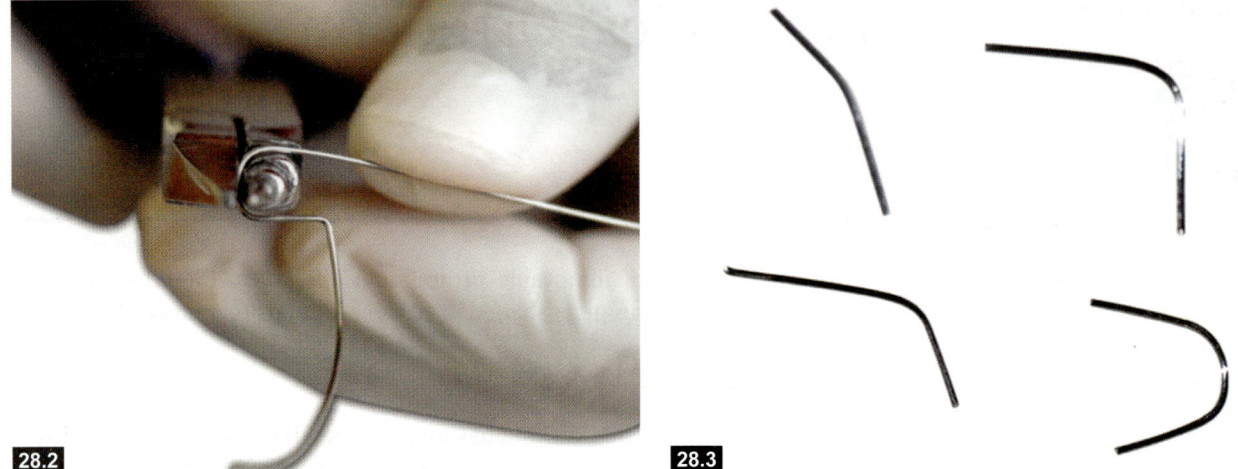

Fig. 28.2: Round beaks of the pliers can be used to make a loop by placing the wire half way back in the beaks and again at 90 degree to the long axis of the pliers, with the thumb, the wire is pushed at around the round beak of the pliers,

Fig. 28.3: A curve is a series of many small bends in a wire

### Loops and Helices

Place the wire half way back in the beaks and again at 90° to the long axis of the pliers, with the thumb the wire is pushed at around the round beak of the pliers. Then a smooth loop is formed just to the shape of the round beak of the pliers **(Fig. 28.2)**.

### Curve Bend

- To bend a curve in orthodontic wire, start by placing the wire back in the beaks of the pliers, a portion of the pliers where round beak is larger. Again wire is placed at 90° to the long axis of the beaks of the pliers.
- A curve is actually a series of many small bends in a wire **(Fig. 28.3)**. To make a curve, wire is bent and slides along the beaks of the pliers, until a series of many small bends are made. In this way a bend curve can be achieved and that is smooth and continuous.
- The flat portion of the beak of the pliers can be used to open up the overly curved (sharp bend) portions of the wire, keeping wire in beaks and squeezing it.

### Control of Plane in Space

- Orthodontic wire must be formed accurately in all planes of space. The wire should be in correct plane. It can be done by always placing the wire in beak at 90° to the long axis of the beaks of the pliers.
- Planes of wire bending are checked by placing the wire on a flat surface, such as a glass slab. If a portion of wire bending is lifting off the flat surface (that is not in the same plane) it can be corrected by using the flat surface of the beaks. Wire is held in flat base portion, where it is changing the plane and the portion of the wire not in plane is bent appropriately. Again the plane is checked by keeping wire on the glass slab and any bends are given, if necessary.

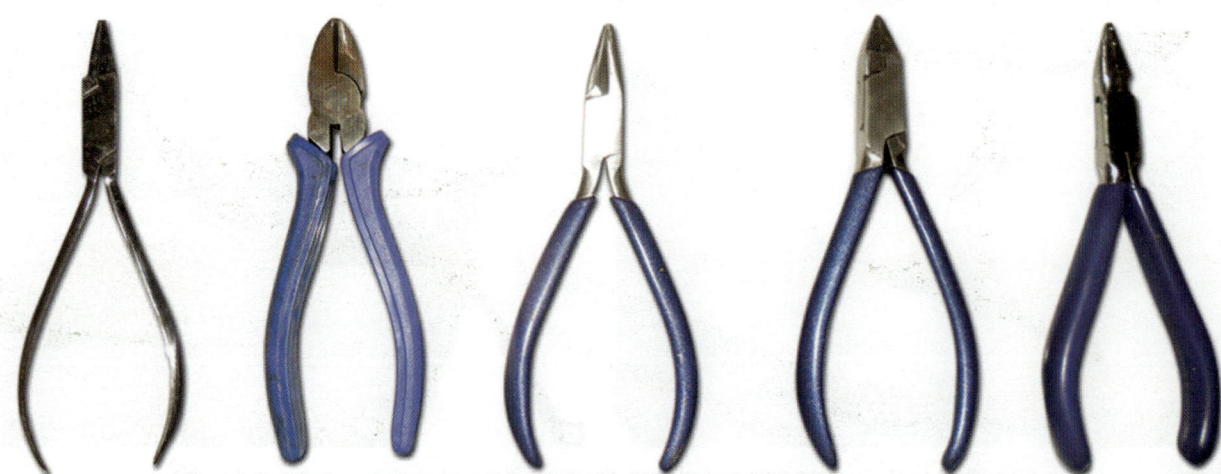

Fig. 28.4: Armamentarium to perform wire bending

## ARMAMENTARIUM

Armamentarium required to perform preclinical wire bending procedures are as follows **(Fig. 28.4)**:
1. Pliers
   - Universal pliers
   - Adam's pliers
   - 201 Three-prong pliers/3 beak/3 jaw plierd
   - 53G Optical pliers
   - 139 Bird beak pliers
   - Hard wire cutter
2. Laminated graph paper
3. Metallic scale with markings in centimeter and inch scale
4. Lead pencils
5. Glass slab
6. Sponge
7. Cotton or gauze rolls
8. Box to store the fabricated wire components.

## UNIVERSAL PLIERS

Universal pliers **(Fig. 28.5)** is so called, because it can be used for fabricating many of the wire components, such as bows, clasps, springs and wire components of myofunctional orthodontic appliance.

### Parts

Universal pliers consists of the following parts **(Fig. 28.6)**:
1. Working end
   a. Looped beak portion
   b. Non-looped beak portion
2. Hinge
3. Handle.

### Working End

The working end of the universal pliers has two beaks or two halves:

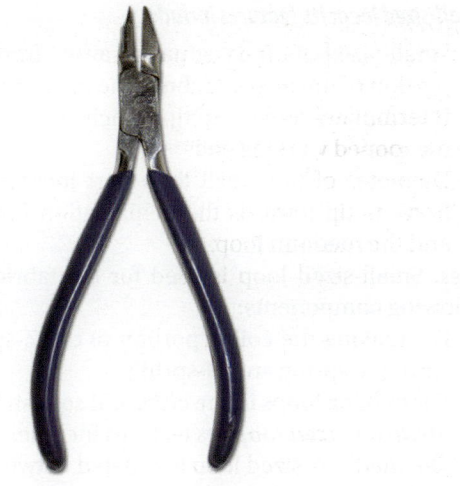

**Fig. 28.5:** Universal pliers

a. Looped beak portion
b. Non-looped portion.

#### Looped Beak Portion

- The looped beak portion is also called as the looped half of the working end.
- Looped portion is so called because it consists of three loops of varying diameter:
   - Small-sized loop
   - Medium-sized loop
   - Large-sized loop
- The three different sized loops are distinctly demarcated.
- Each loop has progressively increasing diameter throughout its length.
- Each loop in the looped beak portion has its own significance.

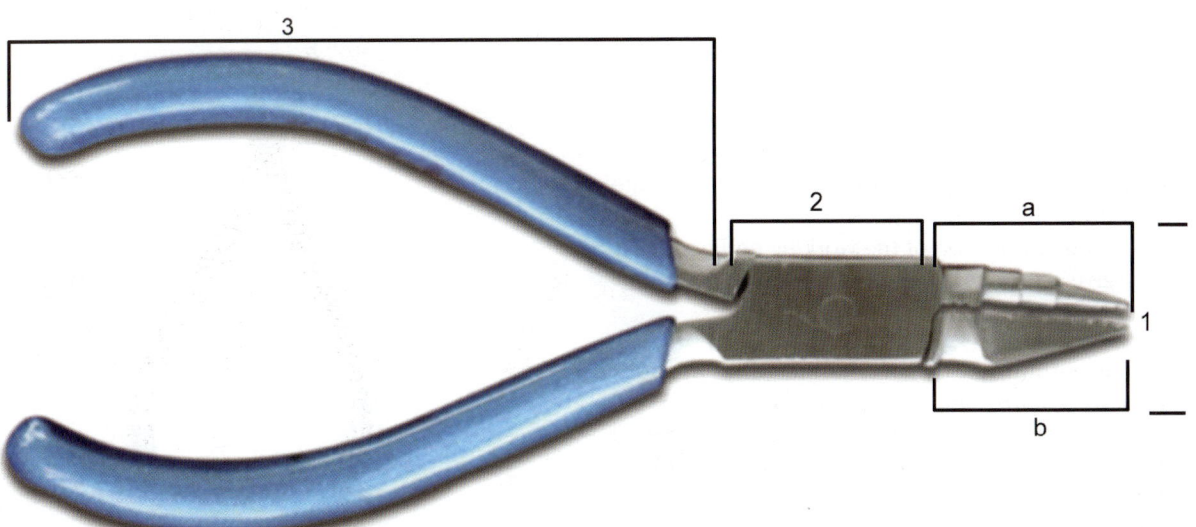

**Fig. 28.6:** Parts of Universal pliers: (1) Working end, a—Looped beak portion, b—Non-looped beak portion, (2) Hinge, (3) Handle

*Small-sized loop: Its features include:*
- Small-sized loop is situated away from the hinge portion of the pliers or above the medium-sized loop.
- It terminates as a sharp tip, which also forms the tip of the looped working end.
- Diameter of the small loop part increases gradually from its tip towards the demarcation line between it and the medium loop.

*Uses:* Small-sized loop is used for the fabrication of the following components:
- For making the coiled portion of the Z-spring, Finger spring, T-spring and M-spring.
- For making loops in the cribs and squash loop.

***Medium-sized loop:*** Its features include:
- The medium-sized loop is situated between the small- and large-sized loops.
- Diameter of this loop is greater than the small-sized loop but smaller than the large-sized loop.
- The medium-sized loop also exhibits progressively increase in diameter from the demarcation line and separates it from the small-sized loop to the second demarcation line separating it from the large-sized loop.

Medium-sized loop is used for the fabrication of the following components:

The medium-sized loop part of the working end is used in fabrication of the bows and canine retractors to incorporate coils and U loops.

***Large-sized loop:*** Its features include:
- This loop is present near the hinge of the pliers.
- Even this loop like the other two loops has progressively increasing diameter throughout its length.

***Uses:*** Large-sized loop is used to fabricate Mills retractor.

*Non-Looped Portion*
- Non-looped portion is devoid of any loops.
- It is smooth in all the sides of its design, except one side, which is grooved.
- Non-looped beak converges towards the tip, as does the looped portion to form the tip of the plier.
- Horizontal grooves/indentations are present on the inner surface of the non-looped portions, usually 3–4 in number.
- The grooves in the non-looped beak portion helps in holding the wire to be cut firmly against the uneven looped beak while cutting, test the wire may slip.
- Continuous use of the pliers over the time, may create some more shallow indentations.
- The non-looped portion of the working end generally used to give acute sharp bends in the wire.

### Hinge
- The hinge portion, like that of any other pliers provides hinge-like opening and closing mechanism to the pliers. The two beaks of the working end are opened and closed through the use of the hinge during wire bending.
- Hinge movement should be smooth and unrestrained for carrying out wire-bending procedures properly.

### Handle
- Handle part of the pliers is greater in length as compared to the other two parts.
- The handle consists of mesial and distal halves.
- Each half of the handle has convexity outer surfaces and concave inner surfaces, which aid in better stabilization of the plier in the operator's hand.
- Each half of the handle may be wrapped with colored rubber material, which again facilitates better grip.
- The pliers is held firmly in the palm of the right hand (left hand for left-handed person) with one part of the handle held near the thumb, while the other half is supported by the rest of the fingers. The index finger is placed between the inner surfaces of the two halves of the handle to facilitate opening and closing movements of the pliers.

## ADAM'S PLIERS

Adam's pliers was developed by Philip C Adam. He also designed one of the most versatile clasps used in orthodontic appliance, the Adam's clasp.

### Parts (Fig. 28.7)
1. Working end.
   a. Right half/right beak
   b. Left half/left beak
2. Hinge
3. Handle

### Working End
- The working end of Adam's pliers consists of two halves or two beaks both of which are non-looped.
- Both the halves are smooth, shiny and similar in shape and design.
- Generally, there are no serrations on both of the beaks.
- Both the halves of the working end are symmetrical and converge gradually from the base near the hinge towards their tips.

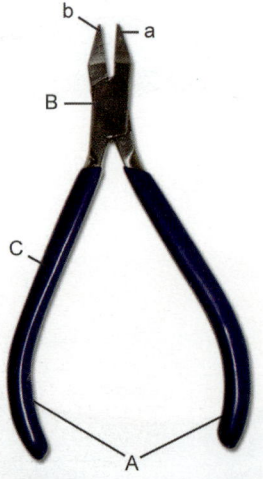

**Fig. 28.7:** Parts of Adam's pliers: (A) Working end: a—Right half/right beak, b—Left half/left beak, (B) Hinge, (C) Handle

- Thus, both the beaks acquire the shape of a wedge with the base at the hinge and their ends forming the tip of the pliers.

### Hinge
Hinge portion of the Adam's pliers is similar to that of the universal pliers. It should allow smooth, non-restrictive hinge movement of the pliers.

### Handle
- Handle portion, like that of the Universal plierforms the major length of the pliers.
- Handle consists of mesial and distal halves.
- Both halves of the handle have a convex outer and concave inner surface/sides that provide better stabilization of the pliers in the palm of the hand.
- They may be wrapped in colored rubber material to enhance the grip.

### Uses
Adam's pliers is mainly used for the fabrication of Adam's clasp and all its modifications.

## 201 THREE-PRONG PLIERS/3 BEAK/3 JAW PLIERS

201 Three prong pliers/3 beak/3 jaw pliers **(Fig. 28.8)** has three beaks. The wire is placed between the three beaks, which are perpendicular to the long axis of the pliers beaks. Simply by squeezing the wire, the bend is made using this pliers.

## 53 G OPTICAL PLIERS

Optical pliers has one round beak and one beak that is concave. The round beak fits into the concave opposite beak of the pliers. Optical pliers also will bend by simply squeezing the wire **(Fig. 28.9)**.

## 139 BIRD BEAK PLIERS

Most of orthodontic wire bending can be made with 139 pliers. It has one round beak and is opposed by a flat surface beak. The base portions of both beaks are flat. To bend a wire with 139 pliers hold the pliers with right hand with round beak away from the chest. Place the wire in beaks of pliers at 90º to the long axis of the beaks of the pliers **(Fig. 28.10)**.

## HARD WIRE CUTTER

Hard wire cutter is an essential tool in the armamentarium required for wire bending exercises. Orthodontic wires of different gauges are generally supplied in the form of spools. The required length of the wire is cut from the spool for fabrication of a given wire component using a hard wire cutter. It is also necessary to cut the excess wire (after fabricating a wire component) at the end of a wire bending exercise.

### Parts
1. Working end
2. Hinge
3. Handle **(Fig. 28.11)**

### Working End
- The working end of hard wire cutter has two halves.
- Both the halves are symmetrical in shapes and design.
- Each has a wide base that joins with the hinge and a sharp tip at the end.
- Each half of the working end exhibits a sharp, linear, wedge-shaped cutting edge.
- When the two halves are joined as while cutting, a triangular (or pyramid shaped) depression can be noted on one side of the working end and a flat surface on the other side.

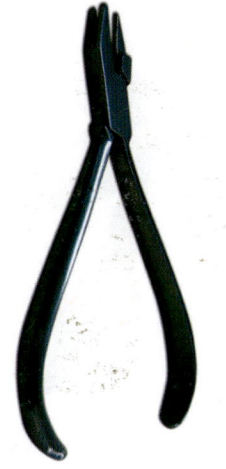
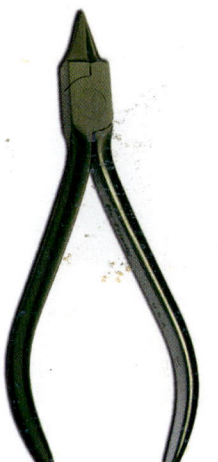
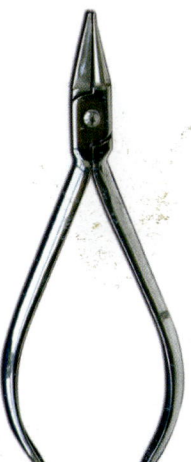

**Fig. 28.8:** 201 Three-prong pliers/3 beak/3 jaw pliers, **Fig. 28.9:** 53G Optical pliers, **Fig. 28.10:** 139 Bird beak pliers

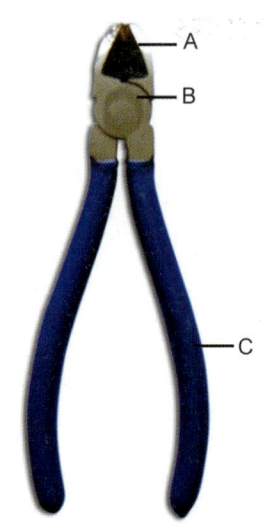

**Fig. 28.11:** Parts of hard wire cutter: (A) Working end, (B) Hinge, (C) Handle

- The triangular depression (that forms on closing the cutter) has less convergence on the sides of the triangular and the greatest depth at the base of the triangle.

### Hinge

Hinge portion is similar to that of the other pliers. It should be smooth, neither too tight nor too loose to allow proper cutting.

### Handle

The handle of hard wire cutter is similar to that of the other pliers. It has two halves, which exhibit convex outer and concave inner surfaces. Metal handle may be covered with colored rubber material to facilitate firm grip in the handle.

### Uses

Hard wire cutter is used to cut hard stainless steel wires.

### Precautions during Use of Hard Wire Cutter

Considerable force is generated when a wire is cut using the hard stainless steel wire with discarding piece of the wire moving at a high speed. Improper handling of the hard wire cutter may sometimes cause injury to the operator or the person in vicinity. Thus, the following precautions should be exercised/observed while using the cutter.

- Always hold the cutter away from the face while cutting).
- Always incline the cutter towards a rough surface of the floor **(Fig. 28.12)**.
- Do not face the discarding part of the wire towards glass floor/or any polished surface because the discarded piece of wire may get reflected and may cause injury.
- Do not direct the cut end of the wire towards any operator.
- After cutting, the wire piece to be discarded is carefully picked and placed in a container meant for waste wire disposal.
- It is a good practice to use a thick slab of sponge during cutting procedure. While cutting, the cutter is held slanted near the sponge, such that the triangular depression side of the working end with the discarding part of the wire faces the sponge **(Fig. 28.13)**.
- By doing this, the cut piece of the wire not be reflected and lost and lies in the sponge. Thus, preventing possible injury and saving time.
- The cutter should be sharp in good condition to be effective. Bunt cutting edges and tight hinge make cutting procedure more tedious, time-consuming and risky as well.

### Steps in Cutting Procedure

The operator should hold the cutter firmly in the palm of his/her right hand (left hand for left-handed person) such that, one half of the handle is at the thumb portion of the palm/ while the other half of the handle is supported by rest of the fingers.

- The index finger is usually placed between the two handles to aid in opening and closing movement.

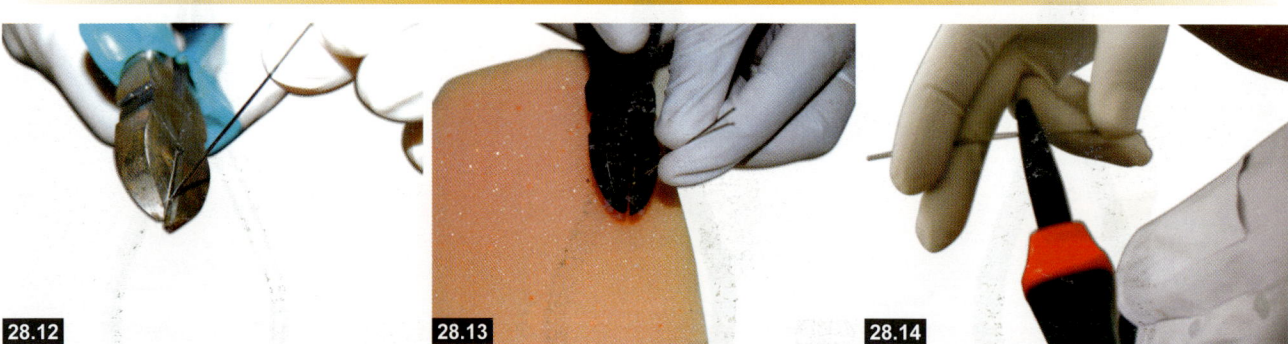

**Fig. 28.12:** Always incline the cutter towards a rough surface of the floor while cutting a wire, **Fig. 28.13:** It is a good practice; use a thick slab of sponge during cutting procedure. While cutting, the cutter is held slanted near the sponge such that the triangular depression side of the working end with the discarding part of the wire faces the sponge, **Fig. 28.14:** When a wire is being cut, the left hand (non-operating hand) is used to hold the non-discarding part of the wire

- When a wire is being cut, the left hand (non-operating hand) is used to hold the non-discarding part of the wire **(Fig. 28.14)**.
- When the required length of wire has to be cut from a spool **(Fig. 28.15)**, it is advisable to hold both the parts of the wire on either side of the cutter, using sides of index and middle fingers and pads of thumb and with finger of the nonworking hand.
- Make sure which type of wire (diameter) and where it has to be cut. Point at which the wire is to be cut can be marked with a glass marker for precision.
- The operator should hold the nondiscarding part of the wire in left hand (non-operating hand) while the cutter firmly in the right hand.
- Wire should be placed between the cutting edges of the working end in such a way that the non-discarding part should be towards the flat side of the working end and the part of wire to be discarded is towards the triangular depression side of working end **(Fig. 28.16)**.
- It is advantageous to engage the wire to be cut nearer to the hinge towards the tip to more force while cutting.
- Incline the hand wire cutter with triangular depression side of working end, facing the rough surfaced floor or sponge.
- After the wire is cut, piece of the wire not required is discarded properly.
- Sometimes cut end of the wire may be irregular, sharp or have unsupported edges **(Fig. 28.17)**. Those irregular edges have to be smoothened with a file sand paper to avoid soft tissue injury to the patient on placing the appliance with the fabricated wire component in mouth.

### Straightening of Wire

#### Step 1
- A piece of wire 6" in dimension is cut from the spool to make a straight wire of 4" dimension **(Fig. 28.18A)**.
- The 2-excess provides working space for the pliers.
- The 2 inches will be removed once the wire has been straightened (1 inch from each side) **(Fig. 28.18B)**.

#### Step 2
- Adam's or Universal pliers are used for the straightening of the round hard stainless steel wire.
- For a right-handed individual, the pliers are held in the left hand and vice versa.
- For a left-handed person, the pliers should be held in the palm of the hand with the beak facing away from the body.
- Any end of the wire is placed into the beak of the Adam's/universal pliers.
- Three fingers are used of the operating hand that is the pad of the middle finger, the index finger and the thumb.
- The fingers are positioned in such a way; the pad of the middle finger should rest on the beak of the pliers with the pad of the finger touching the wire **(Fig. 28.18C)**.
- The pad of the index finger should touch the wire on the same side as the middle finger at a slightly highest level.
- The pad of the thumb should contact the wire on the opposite side of the index finger.

#### Step 3
- The position of the pliers and the fingers should be as shown in the figure **(Fig. 28.18D)**.
- The wire should be positioned in the pliers in such a way that the convexity faces towards the operator **(Fig. 28.18E)** so that the force applied by the pad of the thumb will facilitate/assist in the straightening of the wire.
- The straightening force of the wire is applied by the pad of the thumb, while the pad of the index and the middle finger will guide the straightening of the wire. The straightening force should begin at wire near the beak of the pliers and go throughout the length of the wire **(Fig. 28.18F)**.
- Consecutive forces in a similar manner are applied until the wire becomes straight **(Fig. 28.18G)**.
- The excess wire can be cut 1 inch at both ends **(Fig. 28.18H)**.

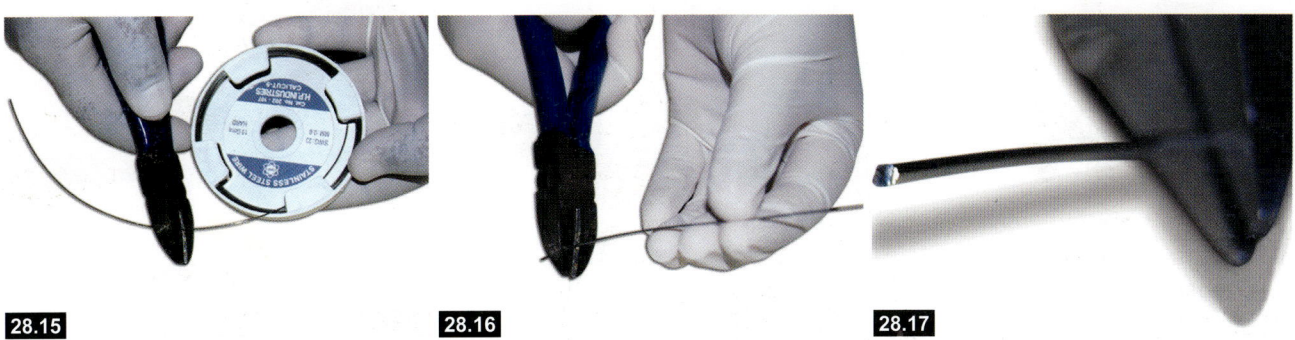

**Fig. 28.15:** When the required length of wire has to be cut from a spool, it is advisable to hold both the parts of the wire on either side of the cutter, **Fig. 28.16:** Wire should be placed between the cutting edges of the working end in such a way that the non-discarding part should be towards the flat side of the working end, **Fig. 28.17:** Sometimes cut end of the wire may be irregular, sharp or have unsupported edge. Those irregular edges have to be smoothened with a file/sand paper to avoid soft tissue injury

## Step 4

Evaluation of straightened wire. There are three methods of evaluation:

### Method 1: Inspection with the "Naked Eye"

The wire should be held in the pliers, in the palm of the hand at a lower level than the chest.

With one eye closed, try to observe the straightened wire from the one tip end **(Fig. 28.18I)**, if only the tip is visible that indicates the wire is straight, on the other hand, if the tip along with some other portions of the wire is visible, it then indicates that the wire is not straight throughout the length.

### Method 2: Graph paper method

In this method, the wire is placed on the graph paper and is matched with the drawn straight line **(Fig. 28.18J)**. If the wire coincides with the straight line, it denotes that the wire is straight.

### Method 3: Glass slab method

In this method, the glass slab **(Fig. 28.18K)** is used to evaluate the straightened wire. The glass slab should be—
  i. Clean
  ii. Moist free
  iii. Transparent glass is preferable.

- The straightened wire should be placed on the glass slab and held at eye level and checked that the wire lies flat on the glass plane **(Fig. 28.18L)**.
- If the wire is flat with no gaps visible, it indicates that it is straight.
- If the gap exists at a particular point, it indicates that the wire is not straight.

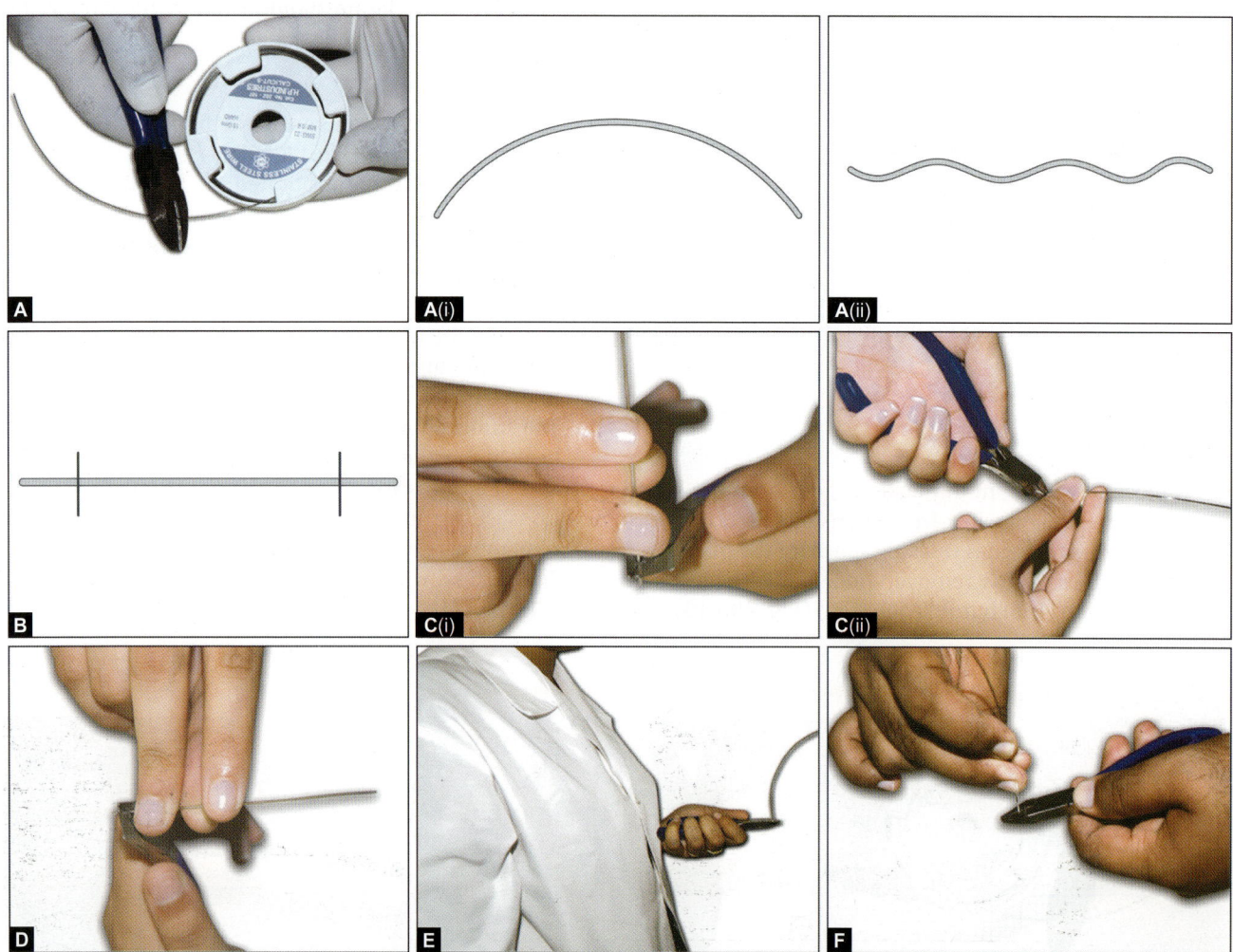

**Figs 28.18A to F:** (A) A piece of wire 6" in dimension is cut from the spool, to make a straight wire of 4" dimension. (B) The 2 inches will be removed once the wire has been straightened (1 inch from each side). (C) The fingers are positioned in such a way; the pad of the middle finger should rest on the beak of the pliers with the pad of the finger touching the wire. (D) The position of the pliers and the fingers. (E) The wire should be positioned in the pliers in such a way that the convexity faces towards the operator, so that the force applied by the pad of the thumb will facilitate / assist in the straightening of the wire. (F) The straightening force of the wire is applied by the pad of the thumb, while the pad of the index and the middle finger will guide the straightening of the wire. The straightening force should begin at wire near the beak of the pliers and go throughout the length of the wire.

## Significance of Straightening of Wire

- For any orthodontic wire bending, the wire has to be straight prior in order to obtain an accurate design wire bending [A clasp, bow, spring **(Fig. 28.19)**, canine retractors] this, when used clinically, helps in achieving the desired results.
- Unstraightened wire used for fabrication of any wire bending would result in inaccurate wire bending which, when later clinically used, will result in undesired tooth movement.

### Fabrication of One "U"

#### Step 1

The wire should be straightened following the wire straightening procedure.

The "U" should be drawn on the graph paper **(Fig. 28.20A)**.

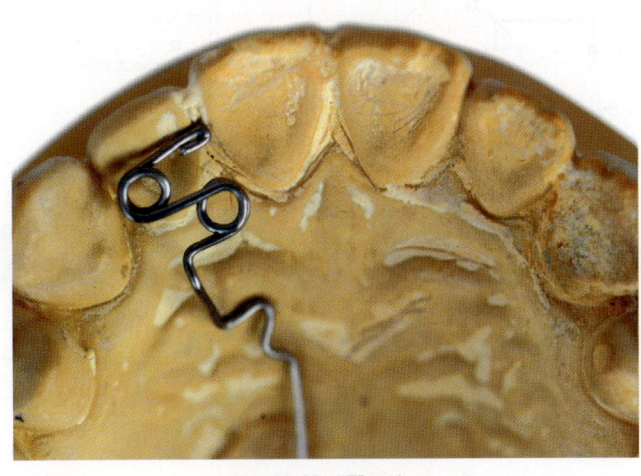

**Fig. 28.19:** "Z" spring

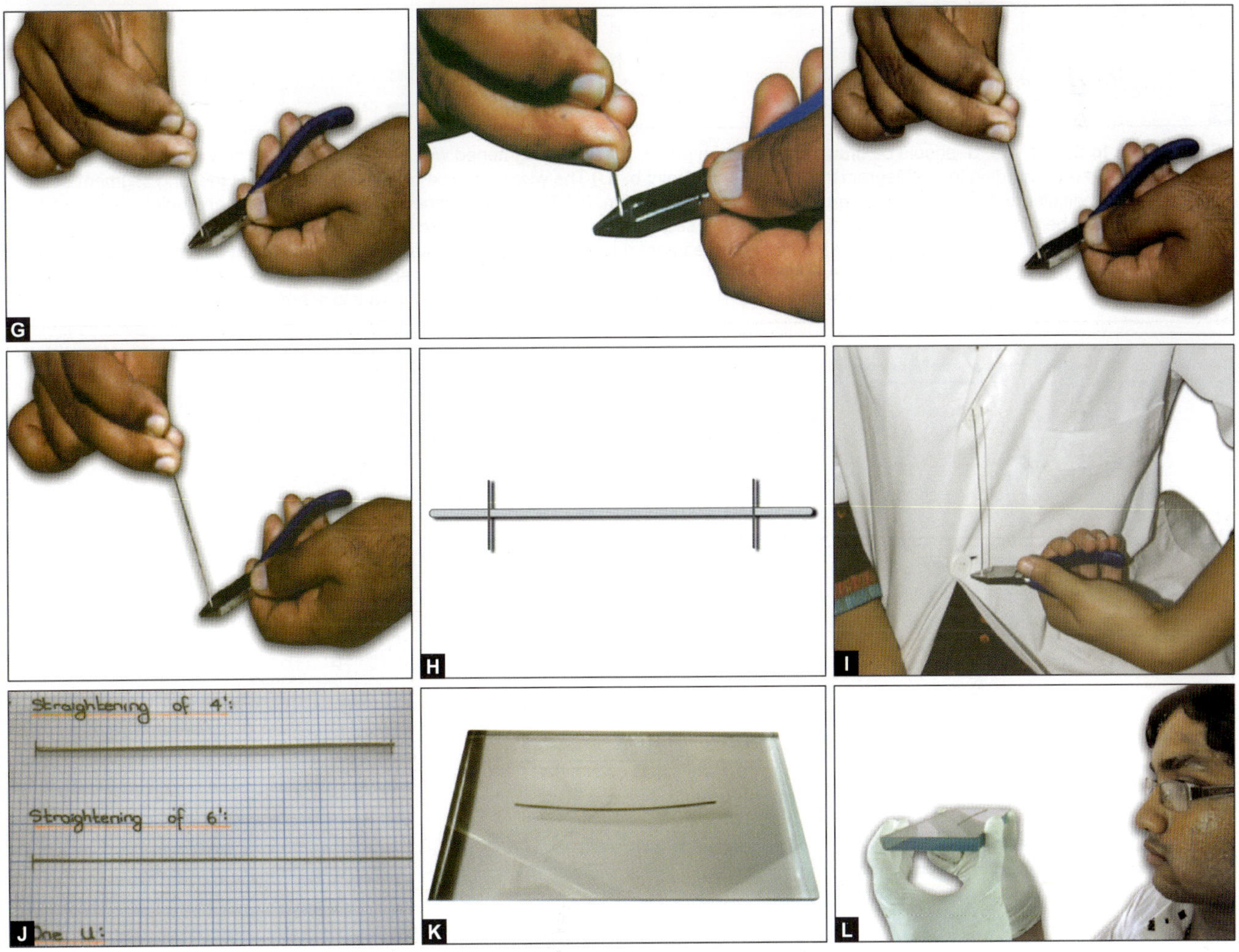

**Figs 28.18G to L:** (G) Consecutive forces in a similar manner are applied until the wire becomes straight. (H) The excess wire can be cut 1 inch at both ends. (I) The wire should be held in the pliers, in the palm of the hand at a lower level than the chest. With one eye closed, try to observe the straightened wire from the one tip end. (J) In this method, the wire is placed on the graph paper and is matched with the drawn straight line. (K) In this method, the glass slab is used to evaluate the straightened wire. The glass slab should be clean, moist free and transparent glass is preferable. (L) The straightened wire should be placed on the glass slab and held at eye level and checked that the wire lies flat on the glass plane

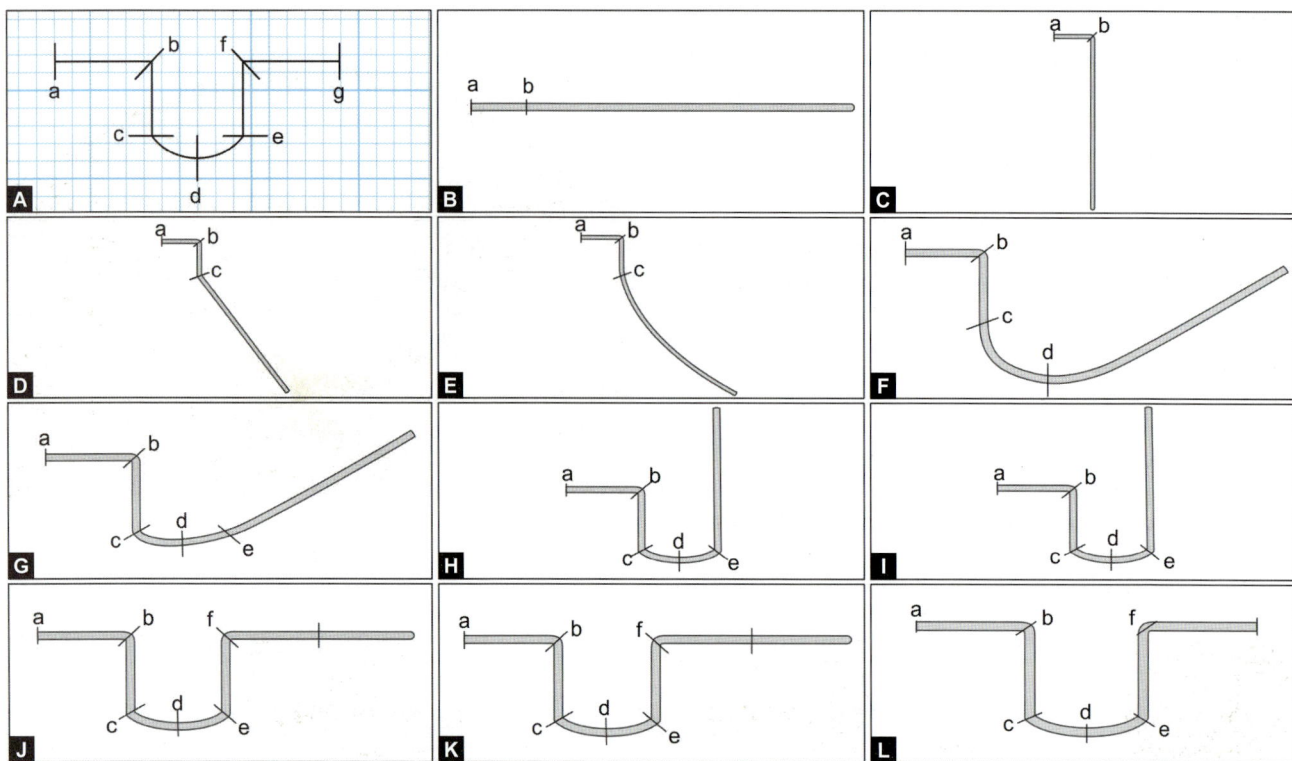

**Figs 28.20A to L:** (A) The "U" should be drawn on the graph paper. (B) The straightened wire is placed on the U drawn on the graph paper, the wire is marked according to the diagram from point a and point b. (C) The wire has to be bent at point b so that the long segment of the wire is perpendicular to the short portion (a-b) in a downward direction. (D) The wire is placed on the graph paper and point c is marked. (E) The wire is bent at point c towards point d, forming the segment c-d (one half of the arc of the U). (F) The wire is marked at point d. (G) The wire is bent at point d towards point e, forming the segment d-e (another half of the arc of U). (H) The point e is marked on the wire. (I) From point e, the wire is bent to form the segment e-f. (J) The point f should be marked as shown in the figure. (K) At point f, the wire is bent to form the segment f-g. (L) Point g is marked and the excess wire is discarded

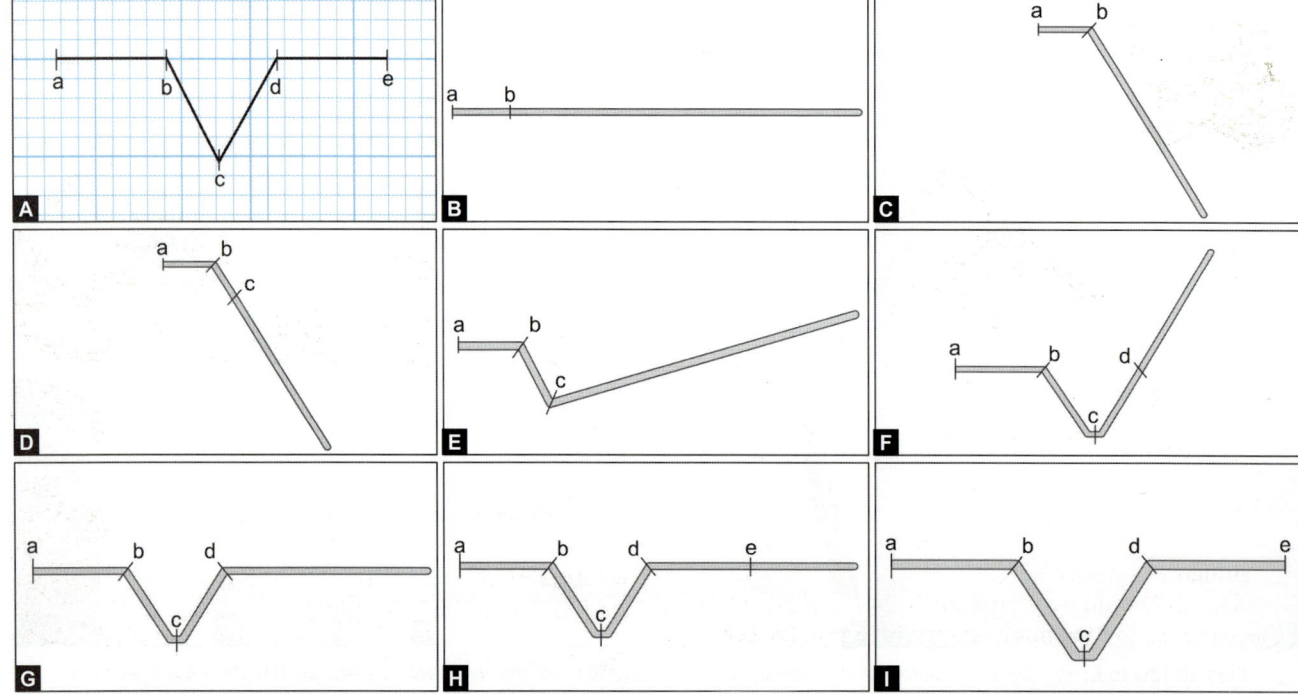

**Figs 28.21A to I:** (A) The "V" should be drawn on the graph paper. (B) The wire is marked according to the diagram from point a and point b. (C) The wire has to be bent at point b so that the long segment of the wire is perpendicular to the short portion (a-b) in a downward direction. (D) The wire is placed on the graph paper and point c is marked. (E) The wire is bent at point c towards point d, forming the segment c-d. (F) The wire is marked at point d. (G) At point d, the wire is bent to form the segment d-e, which should be same length as portion a-b. (H) The point e is marked on the wire. (I) The excess wire is removed by cutting the wire at point e

### Step 2

The straightened wire is placed on the U drawn on the graph paper. The wire is marked according to the diagram from point a and point b **(Fig. 28.20B)**.

### Step 3

The wire has to be bent at point b so that the long segment of the wire is perpendicular to the short portion (a-b) in a downward direction as shown in **Figure 28.20C**.

### Step 4

The wire is placed on the graph paper and point c is marked as shown in the **Figure 28.20D**.

### Step 5

- The wire is bent at point c towards point d, forming the segment c-d (one half of the arc of the U) **(Fig. 28.20E)**.
- The wire is marked at point d as shown in **Figure 28.20F**.

### Step 6

- The wire is bent at point d towards point E, forming the segment d-e (another half of the arc of U) **(Fig. 28.20G)**.
- The point e is marked on the wire as shown **Figure 28.20H**.

### Step 7

- From point e, the wire is bent to form the segment e-f, as shown in **Figure 28.20I**.
- The segment e-f should be parallel to segment b-c.
- The point f should be marked as shown in **Figure 28.20J**.

### Step 8

- At point f, the wire is bent to form the segment f-g **(Fig. 28.20K)**.
- f-g should be same as a-b
- f-g should be perpendicular to e-f.

### Step 9

Point g is marked and the excess wire is discarded **(Fig. 28.20L)**.

## Fabrication of One "V"

### Step 1

- The wire should be straightened following the wire straightening procedure.
- The "V" should be drawn on the graph paper with the following dimensions as shown in **Figure 28.21A**.

### Step 2

- The straightened wire is placed on the "V" drawn on the graph paper.
- The wire is marked according to the diagram from point a and point b **(Fig. 28.21B)**.

### Step 3

The wire has to be bent at point b so that the long segment of the wire is perpendicular to the short portion (a-b) in a downward direction as shown in **Figure 28.21C**.

### Step 4

- The longer segment of the wire is bent at point b, so that the segment b-c is formed.
- The wire is placed on the graph paper and point c is marked as shown in **Figure 28.21D**.

### Step 5

- The wire is bent at point c towards point d, forming the segment c-d **(Fig. 28.21E)**.
- c-d must be equal to b-c.
- The wire is marked at point d as shown in **Figure 28.21F**.

### Step 6

- At point d, the wire is bent to form the segment d-e, which should be of same length as portion a-b **(Fig. 28.21G)**.
- The point e is marked on the wire as shown in **Fig. 28.21H**.

### Step 7

- The point e is marked on the wire.
- The excess wire is removed by cutting the wire at point **(Fig. 28.21I)**.

## Fabrication of an Equilateral Triangle of 1 Inch from All Sides

### Step 1

- The wire should be straightened following the wire straightening procedure.
- The equilateral triangle should be drawn on the graph paper **(Fig. 28.22A)**.

### Step 2

The wire is placed on the equilateral triangle on the graph paper and segment a-b is marked as shown **(Fig. 28.22B)**

### Step 3

At point b, the wire is bent perpendicular in an upward direction as shown **(Fig. 28.22C)**.

### Step 4

- The long portion of the wire should be held in the back of the Adam's pliers.
- At point b, the long portion of the wire is bent to form segment b-c **(Fig. 28.22D)**.

### Step 5

Point c is marked as shown **(Fig. 28.22E)**.

### Step 6

At point c, the wire is bent towards the direction of c-d as shown **(Fig. 28.22F)**.

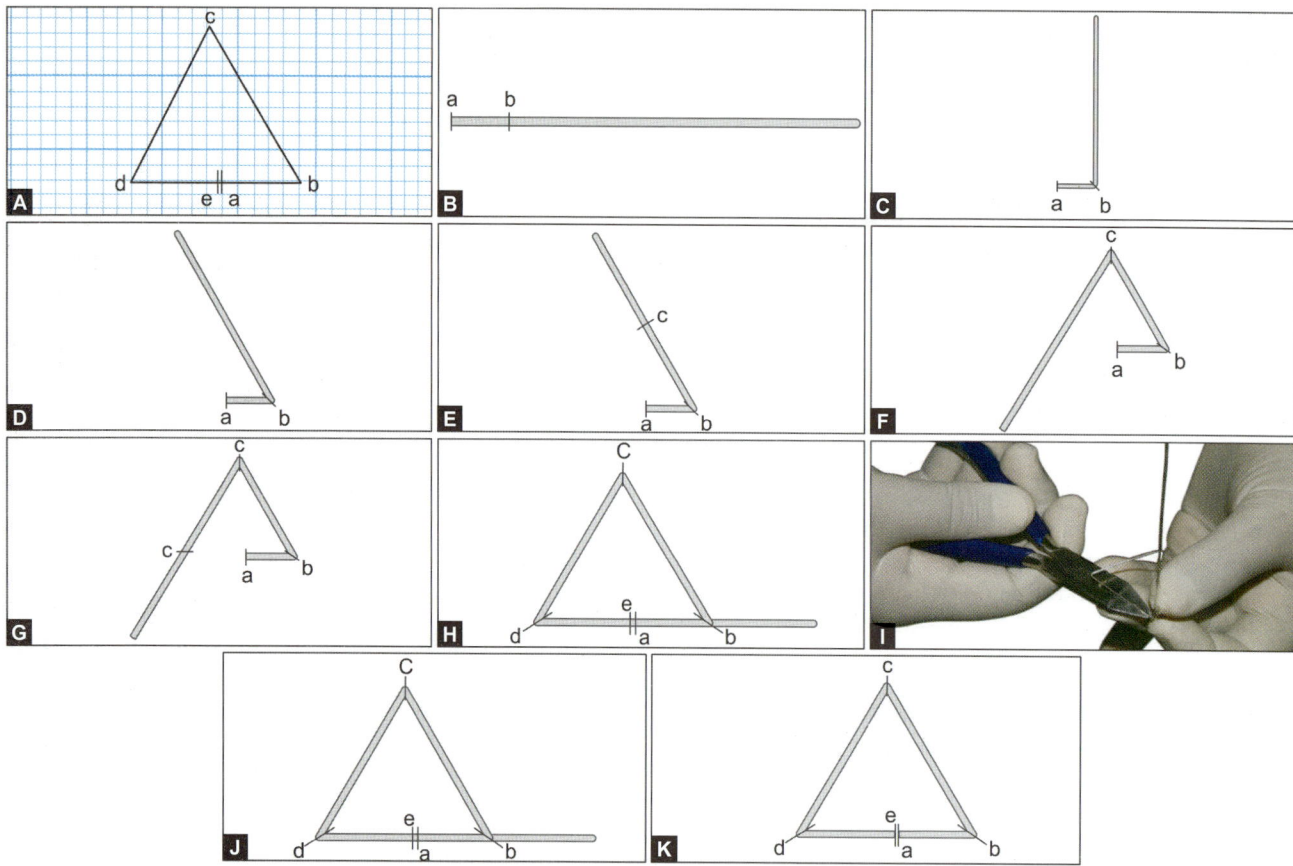

**Figs 28.22A to K:** (A) The "Equilateral triangle" should be drawn on the graph paper. (B) The wire is placed on the equilateral triangle on the graph paper and segment a-b is marked. (C) At point b, the wire is bent perpendicular in an upward direction. (D) At point b, the long portion of the wire is bent at 45° to form segment b-c. (E) Point c is marked. (F) At point c, the wire is bent towards the direction of c-d. (G) Point d is marked. (H) Wire is bent at 45° near point d. (I) To achieve the segment d-e, the wire is held in the beak of Adam's pliers. (J) The wire is bent to form d-e. (K) Point e is marked. At point e, excess wire is cut

### Step 7
The wire is bent to form c-d as shown **(Fig. 28.22G)**.

### Step 8
Point d is marked as shown **(Fig. 28.22G)**.

### Step 9
Wire is bent at point d as shown **(Fig. 28.22H)**.

### Step 10
To achieve the segment d-e, the wire is held in the beak of Adam's pliers as shown **(Fig. 28.22I)**.

### Step 11
The wire is bent to form d-e, as shown **(Fig. 28.22H)**.

### Step 12
- Point e is marked **(Fig. 28.22J)**.
- d-e should be equal to a-b.

### Step 13
At point e, excess wire is cut **(Fig. 28.22K)**.

## Fabrication of Square of All Sides 1 Inch

### Step 1
- The wire should be straightened following the wire straightening procedure.
- The square of all sides 1 inch should be drawn on the graph paper **(Fig. 28.23A)**.

### Step 2
The wire is placed on the square of all sides 1 inch on the graph paper and segment a-b is marked as shown in the **(Fig. 28.23B)**.

### Step 3
At point b, the wire is bent to form b-c, as shown in the **(Fig. 28.23C)**.

### Step 4
Point c is marked using marking pencil as shown in the **(Fig. 28.23D)**.

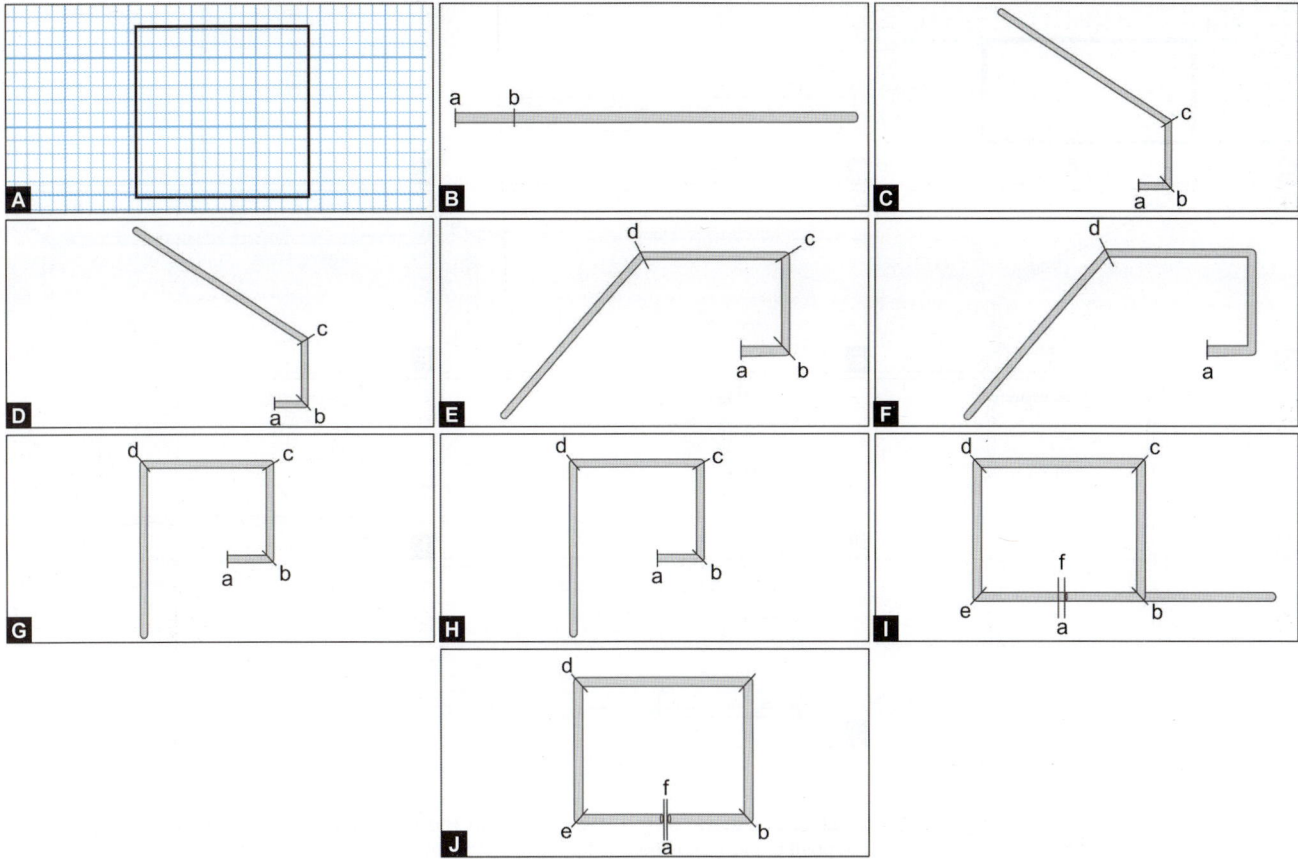

**Figs 28.23A to J:** (A) The "Square of all sides 1 inch" should be drawn on the graph paper. (B) The wire is placed on the square of all sides 1 inch on the graph paper and segment a-b is marked. (C) At point b, the wire is bent to form b-c. (D) Point c is marked using marking pencil. (E) At point c, the wire is bent towards the direction of point d. (F) At point d, the wire is bent towards the direction of point e. (G) The wire is bent to form the segment d-e. (H) Point e is marked. (I) The wire is bent to form e-f. (J) At point f, the excess wire is removed

### Step 5
At point c the wire is bent towards the direction of point d as shown in **Figure 28.23E**.

### Step 6
The wire is bent to form c-d (**Fig. 28.23E**).

### Step 7
Point d is marked as shown in **Figure 28.23E**.

### Step 8
At point d, the wire is bent towards the direction of point E, as shown in **Figure 28.23F**.

### Step 9
The wire is bent to form the segment d-e (**Fig. 28.23G**).

### Step 10
Point e is marked as shown in **Figure 28.23H**.

### Step 11
At point e, the wire is bent towards the direction of point f.

### Step 12
The wire is bent to form e-f as shown in **Figure 28.23I**.

### Step 13
- At point f, the wire is marked (**Fig. 28.23I**).
- e-f should be equal to a-b.
- At point f, the excess wire is removed (**Fig. 28.23J**).

## Fabrication of Rectangle 2/1 Inch

### Step 1
The wire should be straightened following the wire straightening procedure.

The rectangle of 2/1 inch should be drawn on the graph paper (**Fig. 28.24A**).

### Step 2
The wire is placed on the rectangle of 2/1 inch on the graph paper and segment a-b is marked as shown in **Figure 28.24B**.

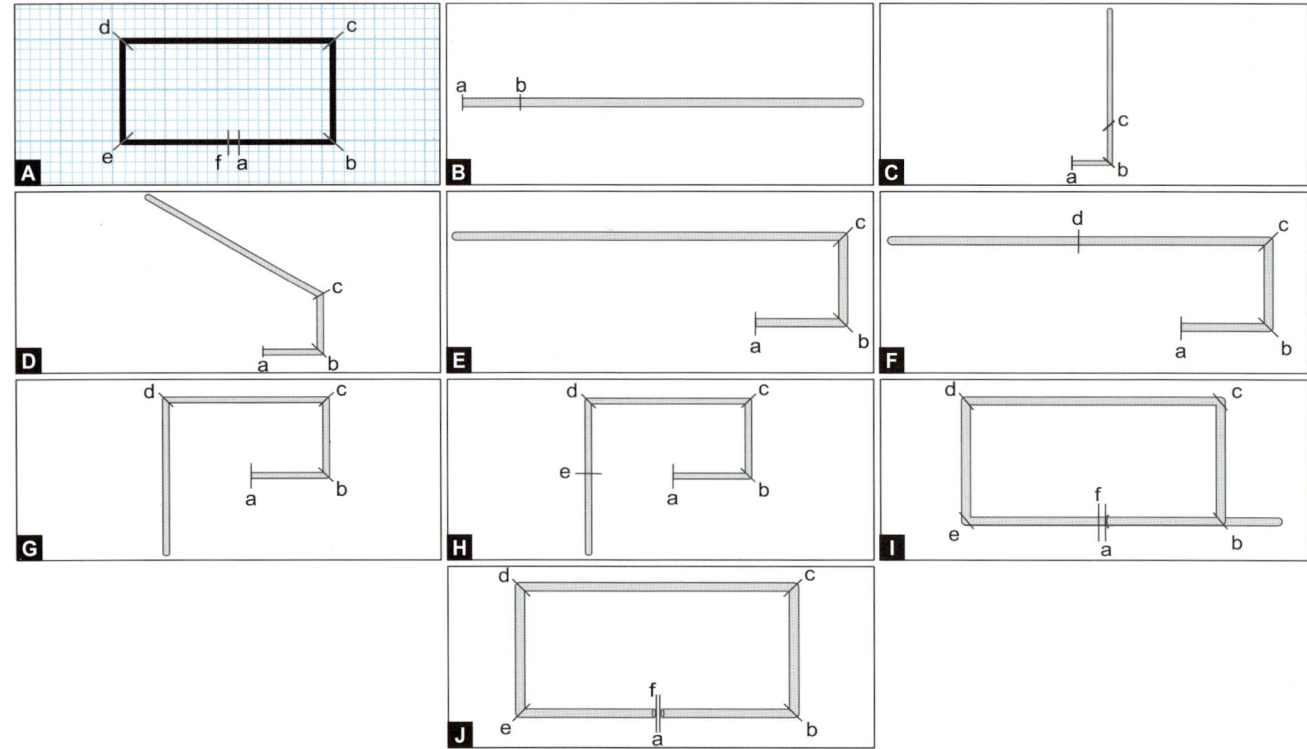

**Figs 28.24A to J:** (A) The "Rectangle of 2/1 inch" should be drawn on the graph paper. (B) The wire is placed on the rectangle of 2/1 inch on the graph paper and segment a-b is marked. (C) At point b, the wire is bent to form b-c. (D) Point c is marked using marking pencil. (E) At point c, the wire is bent towards the direction of point d. (F) The wire is bent to form c-d. (G) At point d, the wire is bent towards the direction of point e. (H) Point e is marked. (I) The wire is bent to form e-f. (J) At point f the excess wire is removed.

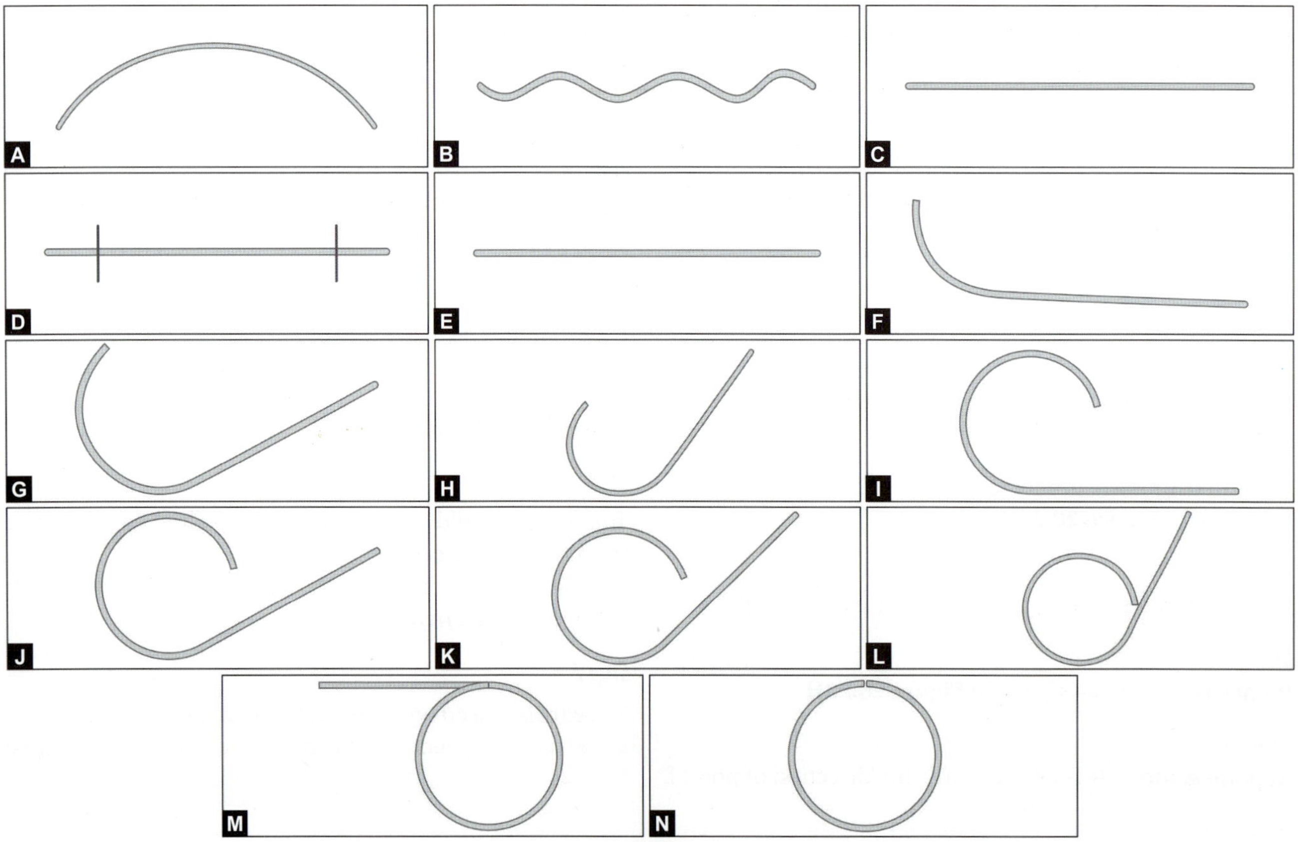

**Figs 28.25A to N:** Fabrication of circle

### Step 3
At point b, the wire is bent to form b-c, as shown in the **Figure 28.24C**.

### Step 4
Point c is marked using marking pencil as shown in **Figure 28.24D**.

### Step 5
At point c, the wire is bent towards the direction of point d as shown in **Figure 28.24E**.

### Step 6
The wire is bent to form c-d **(Fig. 28.24F)**.

### Step 7
Point d is marked as shown in **Figure 28.24F**.

### Step 8
At point d, the wire is bent towards the direction of point e, as shown in **Figure 28.24G**.

### Step 9
The wire is bent to form the segment d-e, as shown in **Figure 28.24G**. The side d-e should be equal to side b-c.

### Step 10
Point e is marked as shown in **Figure 28.24H**.

### Step 11
At point e, the wire is bent towards the direction of point f, as shown in **Figure 28.24H**.

### Step 12
- The wire is bent to form e-f as shown in **Figure 28.24I**.
- d-c is equal to the addition of e-f and a-b.

### Step 13
- At point f, the wire is marked **(Fig. 28.24I)**.
- e-f should be equal to a-b.
- At point f, the excess wire is removed **(Fig. 28.24J)**.

## FABRICATION OF CIRCLE

Fabrication of circle is also one among the important pre-clinical exercise. Universal pliers is need for the fabrication of circle. Circle is formed by giving a series of small curves as shown in the **Figures 28.25A to J**.

---

### EXAM-ORIENTED QUESTIONS

**Long Essay or Long Questions**

1. Preclinical orthodontics.
2. Write in detail about straightening of orthodontic wire in preclinical orthodontics.
3. Write in detail about fabrication U-shape using orthodontic wire in preclinical orthodontics.
4. Write in detail about fabrication V-shape using orthodontic wire in preclinical orthodontics.
5. Write in detail about fabrication *-shape using orthodontic wire in preclinical orthodontics.
6. Write in detail about fabrication rectangle-shape using orthodontic wire in preclinical orthodontics.
7. Write in detail about fabrication square-shape using orthodontic wire in preclinical orthodontics.
8. Write in detail about fabrication circle-shape using orthodontic wire in preclinical orthodontics.

**Short Note**

1. Basic orthodontic bends in preclinical orthodontics.

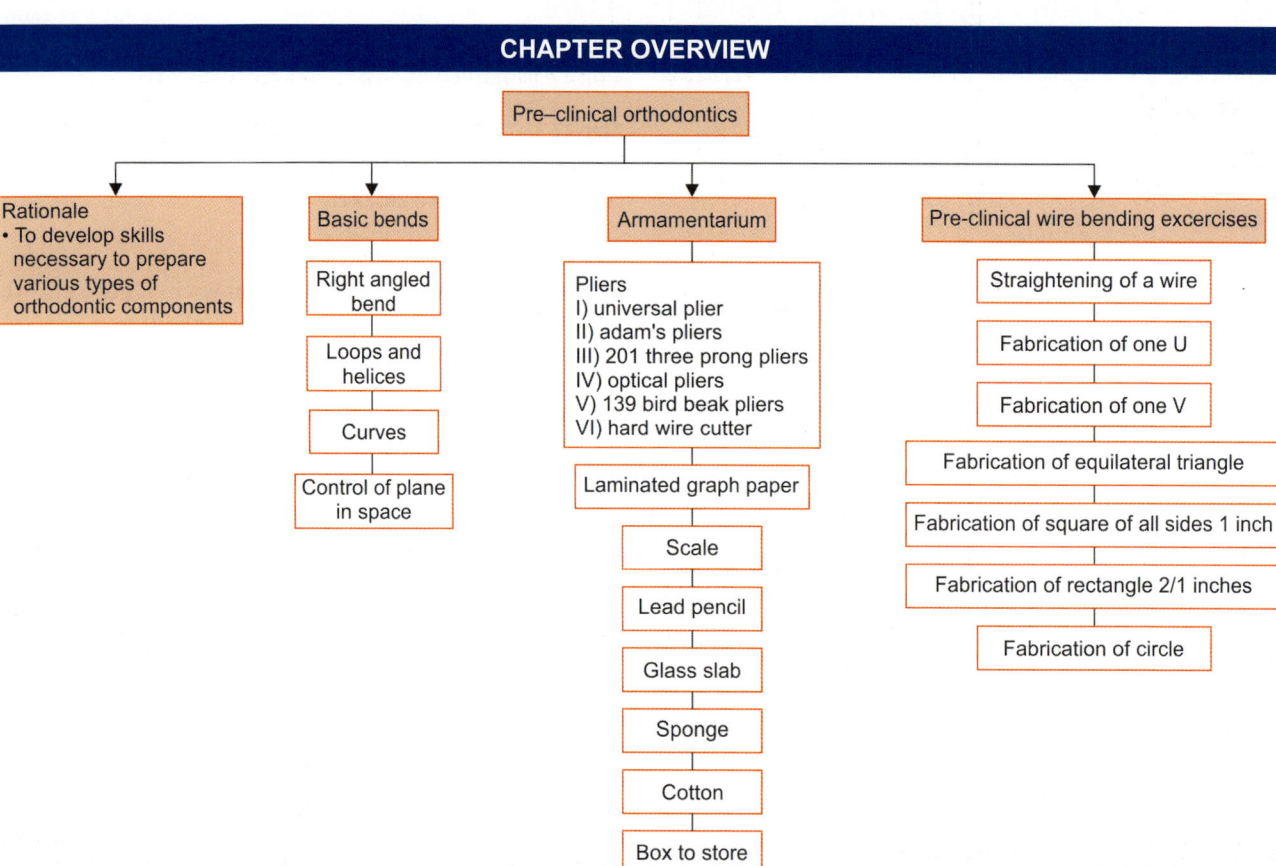

# CHAPTER 29

# General Principles of Orthodontic Appliances

*Naik P, Phulari BS*

Orthodontic treatment is based on application of force to the teeth or to the jaw bones to bring about desirable tooth movement or jaw growth modification. Orthodontic appliances are the means of applying force to the teeth and/or the jaw bones to effect dental and/or skeletal changes that are aimed at correcting malocclusions.

Orthodontic appliances can be defined as "devices, which create and/or transmit forces to individual teeth/a group of teeth and/or maxillofacial skeletal units so as to bring about changes within the bone with/without tooth movement, which will help to achieve the treatment goals of functional efficiency, structural balance and esthetic harmony".

Orthodontist today is equipped with a wide array of orthodontic appliances from which the appliance, that is most appropriate in a particular clinical situation, is selected. The design of various orthodontic appliances is continuously being refined to increase the efficiency, patient comfort and esthetics during the treatment period. Careful selection of the appliance and its skillful management is the key to the success of orthodontic treatment. This chapter gives an overview of various orthodontic appliances in use today.

## CLASSIFICATION

Orthodontic appliances can be classified in a number of ways. The most common and practical way of classifying orthodontic appliances is based on patient's ability to remove the appliance from the mouth.

### Based on Whether it is Active or Passive

#### Active Orthodontic Appliances

Active appliances are those which bring about movement of the teeth. These may either incorporate active forces within the appliance or transmit forces from another source, usually the muscles of mastication or the circumoral musculature.

For example, all removable (**Fig. 29.1**) and fixed appliances that bring about active tooth movement.

#### Passive Orthodontic Appliances

Passive appliances are those that maintain the position of the teeth. These are commonly used for space maintenance after premature loss of deciduous teeth or for the maintenance of tooth position at the completion of active mechanotherapy.

For example, space maintainers (**Fig. 29.2A**) and retainers (**Fig. 29.2B**).

### Based on Patient's Ability to Remove Appliance from Oral Cavity

#### Removable Orthodontic Appliances

Removable orthodontic appliances are so called because they are designed to be fitted and removed by the patient. They can be active or passive.

- *Active removable orthodontic appliances:* These are designed to achieve tooth movement by means of active components, such as springs, bows and expansion screws, etc. (**Fig. 29.1**).
- *Passive removable orthodontic appliances:* These are designed to maintain the teeth in their current/present position.

For example, removable retainers given at the end of active orthodontic therapy to enhance stability of the orthodontic correction (**Fig. 29.2B**).

#### Fixed Orthodontic Appliances

Orthodontic devices in which attachments are fixed to the teeth (by cementation/direct bonding) and forces are applied by arch wires or auxiliaries via these attachments to the teeth are called as fixed orthodontic appliances. Like removable orthodontic appliances, these can also be active or passive.

- *Active fixed appliances:* Most of the corrective orthodontic procedures are best carried out with fixed active mechanotherapy, which allows multiple tooth movements. They apply forces to the teeth by arch wire or auxiliaries (elastic bands, open and closed coiled springs, etc.) thereby effecting active tooth movement. For example, fixed mechanotherapy to correct malocclusions using various techniques, such as Begg's technique, edge-wise technique, straight wire technique (**Fig. 29.3**), etc.
- *Passive fixed appliances:* Fixed orthodontic appliances may also be used for the passive maintenance of teeth in their current position after active mechanotherapy. For example, fixed lingual bonded retainers given at the retention phase of treatment (**Fig. 29.4**), fixed type of space maintainer, such as distal shoe, band and spur, etc.

#### Semi-fixed/Fixed Removable Combination Appliance

It is sometimes beneficial to combine the properties of fixed and removable appliances to achieve the advantages of both. Generally, such combined appliances are used to achieve a type of tooth movement which cannot be achieved with removable appliance alone, but the use of a removable component facilitates oral hygiene maintenance and makes the construction of the appliance simpler.

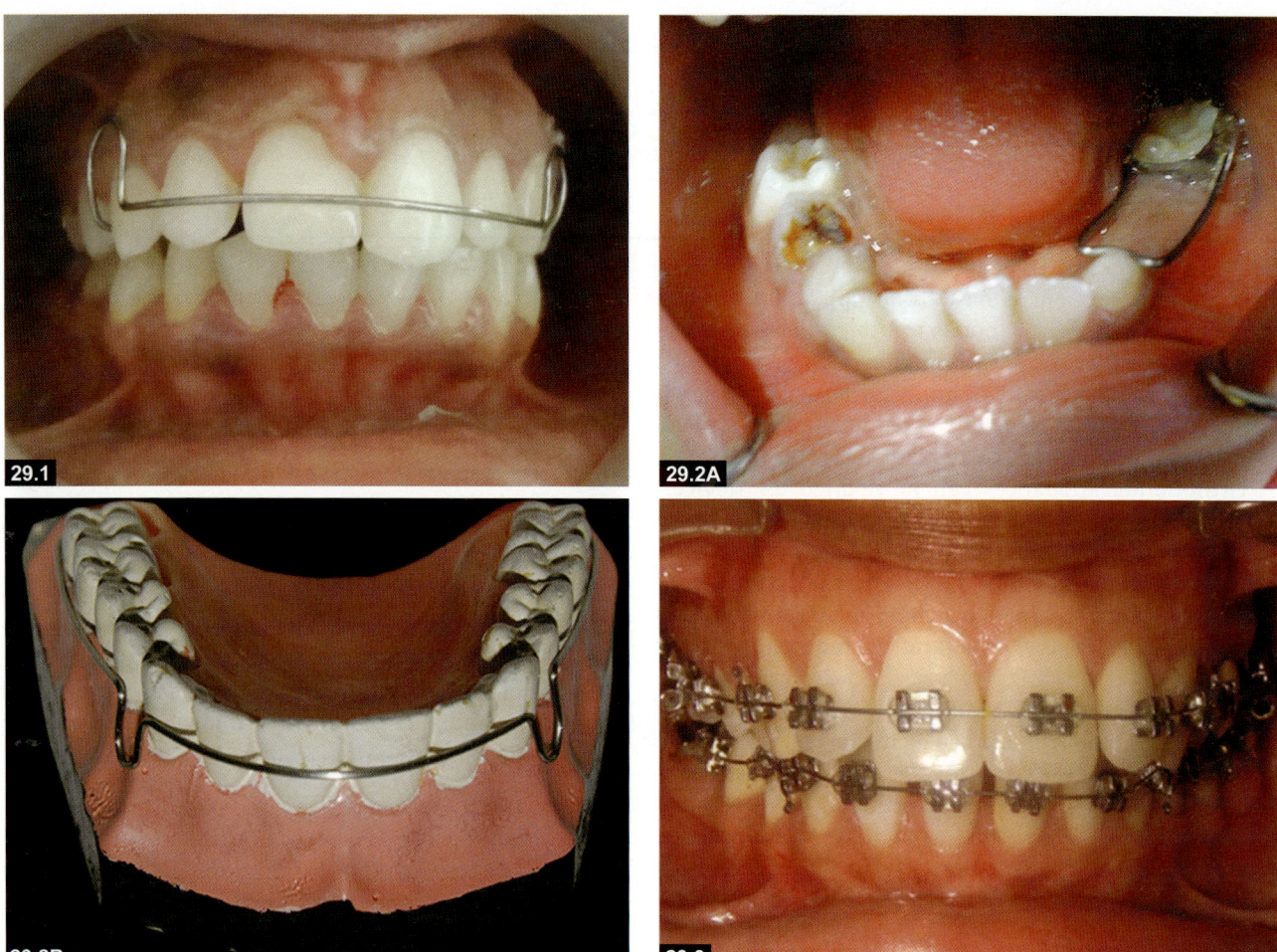

**Fig. 29.1:** Active removable orthodontic appliance consisting of short active labial bow as an active component to bring about overjet reduction by retraction of upper anteriors; **Figs 29.2A and B:** Passive orthodontic appliances: (A) Band and loop space maintainer. (B) Begg's retainer is a passive removable orthodontic appliance used to hold teeth in their corrected positions after active orthodontic treatment; **Fig. 29.3:** Fixed orthodontic appliance (Straight wire technique)

For example, lip bumber appliance **(Fig. 29.5)**. The appliance is attached to the buccal tubes on the molar bands and can be removed for cleaning.

### Depending on the Mode of Action

#### Mechanical Appliances

Most orthodontic appliances act by applying mechanical forces to the teeth to move them and are called as mechanical appliances. They possess active components such as springs, screws arch wires, elastics, etc. that generate mechanical forces. Mechanical appliances include removable orthodontic appliances and fixed orthodontic appliances **(Fig 29.6)**. Extraoral force appliances (orthopedic appliances) that apply heavy orthodontic forces to bring about skeletal changes also come under this category.

#### Functional (Myofunctional Appliances)

In contrast to mechanical appliances that generate and apply mechanical forces to the teeth, the functional appliances utilize natural forces of the orofacial and masticatory musculature for their action. Instead of applying active forces, they harness and transmit the natural forces of the circumoral musculature to the teeth and/or jaw bones. Functional appliances generally cause a change in the surrounding soft tissue envelop of the teeth (functional matrix) thereby leading to a more harmonious relationship of the jaws to each other and to the other bones of the facial skeleton.

For example, Frankel's functional regulator and oral screen **(Figs 29.7A and B)**.

### Working Classification

1. Removable orthodontic appliances
2. Fixed orthodontic appliances
3. Functional orthodontic appliances
4. Orthopedic orthodontic appliances.

## IDEAL REQUIREMENTS OF ORTHODONTIC APPLIANCES

All appliances should be comfortable to wear and readily acceptable by the patient. Ideal requirements of orthodontic appliances are as follows:

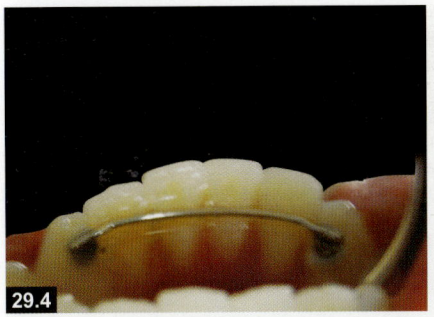 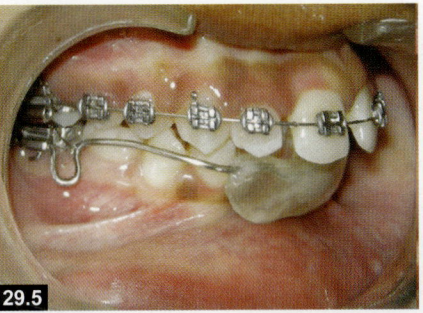 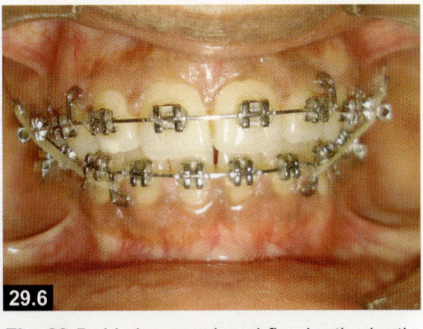

**Fig. 29.4:** Fixed lingual bonded canine to canine retainer given at retention phase of treatment; **Fig. 29.5:** Lip bumper (semi-fixed orthodontic appliance); **Fig. 29.6:** Fixed orthodontic appliance is a type of mechanical appliance, which acts by applying forces to teeth

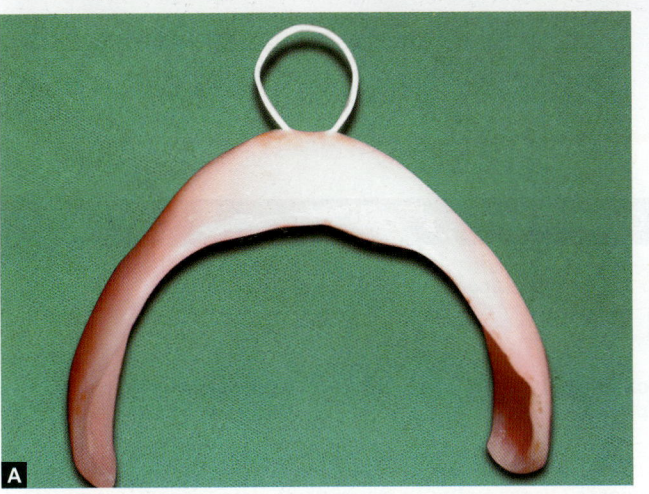 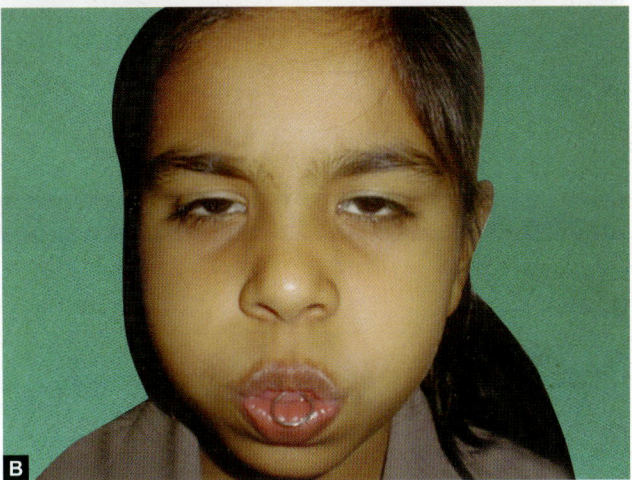

**Figs 29.7A and B:** Oral screen: (A) Hotz type of oral screen. (B) Patient with oral screen in mouth used to eliminate mouth breathing habit

- Biologic requirements
- Mechanical requirements
- Esthetic requirements

### Biologic Requirements

- The appliance should bring about the desired tooth movements efficiently.
- It should be well tolerated by the oral tissues, i.e. should be biocompatible without causing any allergic or toxic reactions.
- While inducing the desired tooth movement, it should not produce any detrimental effects on teeth such as root resorption, periodontal ligament damage or tooth nonvitality.
- The appliance should not interfere with normal growth.
- It should not interfere with normal functions, i.e. mastication, deglutition and phonetics.
- It should not move other teeth, which are not intended to be moved, i.e. should not move the anchor teeth.
- The appliances should not hinder oral hygiene maintenance. The design of the appliance should allow the patient to carry out routine oral hygiene measures throughout the treatment.

### Mechanical Requirements

- The appliance should be able to deliver controlled forces of desired intensity, for a desired duration and in the desired direction.
- It should be sufficiently strong to withstand the stresses of oral functions.
- It should not be overly bulky and uncomfortable for the patient to wear.
- It should be comfortable to wear and readily acceptable by the patient.
- The appliance should be versatile, i.e. should be able to correct various types of malocclusions and should be able to bring out different types of tooth movement.
- The appliance should be simple to fabricate and should allow repair in case of any damage.
- It should be easy to activate the appliance.

### Esthetic Requirements

The appliance should be esthetically acceptable to the patient. It should not draw attention and must be as inconspicuous as possible. The duration of orthodontic treatment is long when compared to other dental procedures. Thus the appliance, because of its appearance should not interfere in patient's professional and social lives during the orthodontic treatment.

It is almost impossible for a single appliance to fulfill all these requirements. The clinician should select appliance, keeping specific treatment needs and level of cooperation of the patient in mind.

## BIBLIOGRAPHY

1. Badcock JH. The screw expansion plate. Trans Brit Soc Orthod 1911;3-8.
2. Graber TM, Neumann B. Removable Orthodontic Appliances. Philadelphia: WB Saunders, 1977.
3. McNamara JA. Jr. Utility arches. J Clin Orthod 1986;20:4526.
4. Ricketts RM, Bench R, Gugino CF, et al. Bioprogressive Therapy. Denver: Rocky Mountain Orthodontics, 1979;25.
5. Roth RH. Treatment mechanics for the straight wire appliance. In: Graber TM, Swin BF (Eds). Orthodontics: Current principles and Techniques. St. Louis: Mosby 1966.
6. Schwarz AM, Gratzinger M. Removable Orthodontic Appliances. Philadelphia: WB Saunders, 1966.
7. Tulley WJ, Campbell AC. A Manual of Practical Orthodontics. Bristol: J Wright and Sons, 1960.
8. Tweed CH. Clinical Orthodontics. St. Louis: Mosby, 1966.
9. Zachrisson BU. Bonding in orthodontics. In: Graber TM, Vanarsdall RL (Eds). Jr. Orthodontics: Current Principles and Techniques, 3rd edition. St. Louis: Mosby, 2000.

## EXAM-ORIENTED QUESTIONS

### Long Question

Define classify orthodontic appliances and discuss in detail about ideal requirements, mechanical requirements and esthetic requirements of orthodontic appliances.

## CHAPTER OVERVIEW

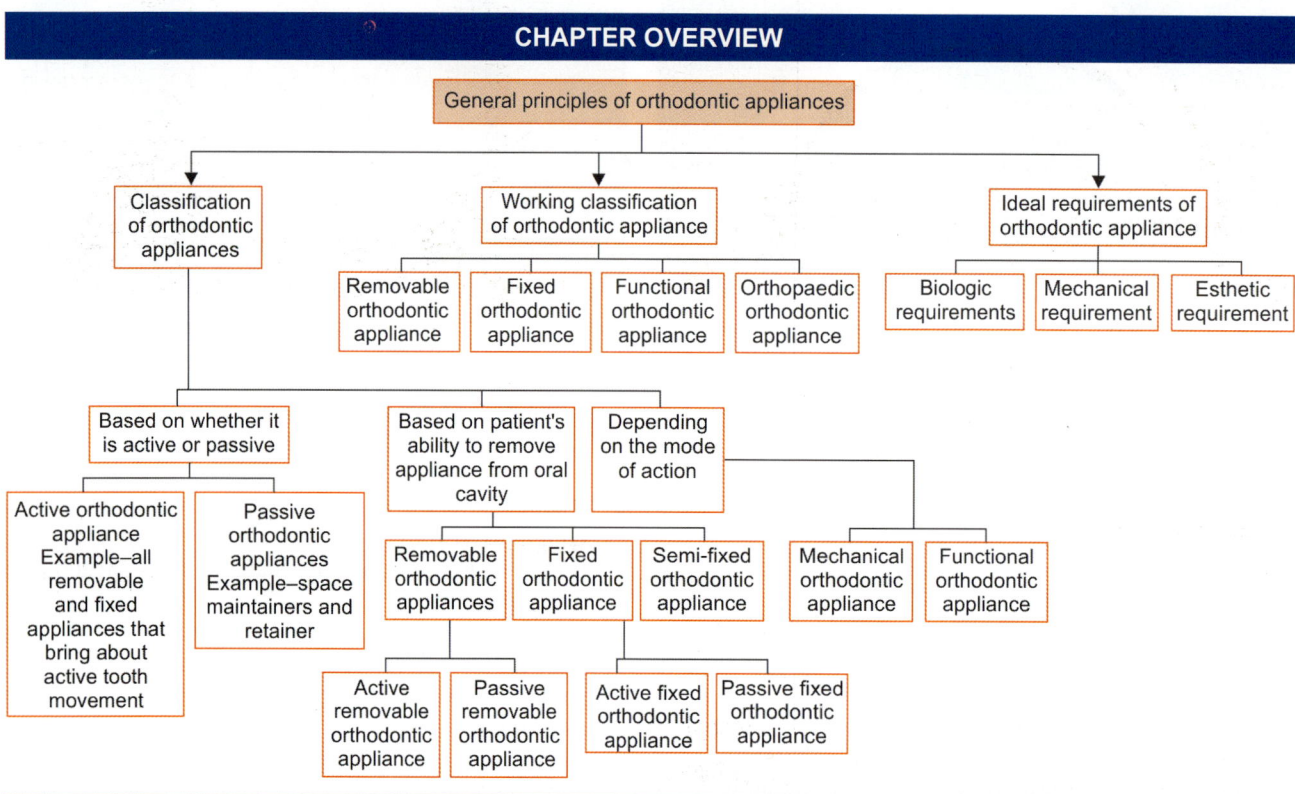

# CHAPTER 30

# Removable Appliances

*Rashmi GS*

Removable orthodontic appliances are so called because they are designed to be fitted and removed by the patient. Removable orthodontic appliances are limited to tipping and simple rotatory movements of teeth, which are sufficient for many orthodontic treatments. They depend on cooperation and a certain degree of skill on the part of the patient. Removable orthodontic appliances may be active or passive.

Use of removable appliances requires careful case selection for the success of the treatment. They are ideally used when simple tipping movement of teeth is sufficient to correct a certain type of malocclusion. The range of malocclusions that can be treated with removable appliance alone is limited. They can also be used as passive appliances to maintain teeth in their corrected positions after active phases of orthodontic therapy, e.g. retainers. Removable orthodontic appliance is often used in conjunction with fixed mechanotherapy.

## INDICATIONS

Use of removable orthodontic appliances requires careful selection. They should not be used in circumstances where fixed orthodontic appliance therapy would be more appropriate. May be used as an adjunct to fixed orthodontic appliance treatment.

## CONTRAINDICATIONS

Removable orthodontic appliances are contraindicated in case where bodily movements of the teeth are required.

## ADVANTAGES

Advantages of removable orthodontic appliances are listed here:
1. Removable appliances permit easy cleaning.
2. They need less chairside time.
3. They are good for overbite reduction.
4. They can tip the teeth efficiently.
5. They eliminate occlusal interferences.

## DISADVANTAGES

Disadvantages of removable orthodontic appliances are listed below:
1. Removable orthodontic appliances can bring about only a limited type of tooth movement.
2. Anchorage of tooth movement is sometimes difficult, since anchor teeth cannot be prevented from tilting.
3. Retention of removable orthodontic appliance is more difficult than with fixed appliances.
4. A high degree of cooperation and a certain amount of skill is required from the patient, who has to remove, clean and replace the appliance at frequent interval.
5. Limited scope on lower arch.
6. Removable orthodontic appliance can hamper the phonation.

## COMPONENTS

Removable orthodontic appliance consists of the following three components **(Flowchart 30.1)**:

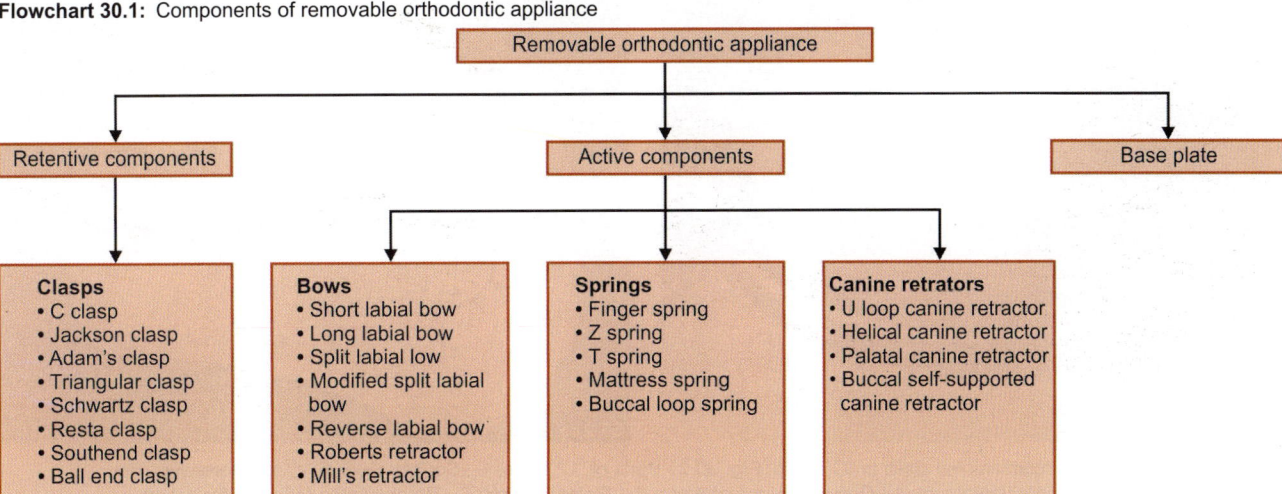

**Flowchart 30.1:** Components of removable orthodontic appliance

1. Retentive components
2. Active components
3. Base plate.

### Retentive Components

The success of a removable orthodontic appliance mainly depends upon good retention of the appliance. Adequate retention of a removable orthodontic appliance is achieved by incorporating certain wire components that get engaged into the undercuts on the teeth. These wire components that help in retention of a removable appliance are called clasps.

### Clasps

Clasps are the essential retentive components of removable orthodontic appliances. Various designs of clasps can be used depending on the clinical need. The clasps utilize mesiodistal or buccolingual undercuts for retention. Some of the commonly used clasps are described below. Other clasps include occlusal rest clasp, duyzing clasp, lingual extention clasp, eyelet clasp, delta clasp, arrow-pin clasp, Visick clasp and wrought Roach clasp.

### 'C' Clasp

Circumferential clasp, also known as "three-quarter clasp" or 'C' clasp, is fabricated from round, hard stainless steel wire of 0.7 mm.

#### Design

'C' clasp has a simple design and utilizes buccocervical undercut of the teeth. The wire is extended circumferentially from one proximal undercut along the cervical margin, to reach the other proximal side and is then brought occlusally over the embrasure to end lingually as retentive arm and tag **(Fig. 30.1)**. The retentive arm and tag later get embedded in the acrylic base material. Incorporation of a squash loop at the beginning of 'C' prevents soft tissue trauma and injury while cleaning the appliance.

#### Parts of 'C' Clasp

Parts of circumferential clasp are listed below **(Fig. 30.2)**:
1. Squash loop: Prevents soft tissue injury.
2. Circumferential arm: Follows the buccal circumference of the tooth to be clasped.
3. Buccal interdental arm: Extends from buccal proximal undercut to the level of occlusion interdentally.
4. Occlusal interdental arm: Runs occlusally between the tooth to be clasped and its adjacent tooth.
5. Retentive arm: Gets embedded in acrylic base material.
6. Retentive tag: The terminal end of retentive arm is bent to form a tag, which increases the amount of wire embedded in acrylic base material.

Wire used for construction: Hard stainless steel wire of 0.7 mm is used for the fabrication of this clasp.

#### Advantages

Advantages of circumferential clasp are as follows:
1. Simplicity in design.
2. Easy to fabricate.
3. Less occlusal interference.
4. Provides adequate retention.
5. Having squash loop in the clasp helps in preventing soft tissue trauma and injury while cleaning the appliance.

#### Disadvantages

Disadvantages of the circumferential clasp are as follows:
1. It does not provide adequate retention when used for an active removable orthodontic appliance.
2. It should be considered only as a supporting clasp.
3. It is not comparable to Adam's clasp in retention ability, as it engages only one undercut area of the clasped tooth.
4. It cannot be used in teeth that are partially erupted, as the cervical undercut cannot be seen.
5. It cannot be fabricated on deciduous molar.
6. It can be easily distorted during insertion or removal of the appliance by the patient.

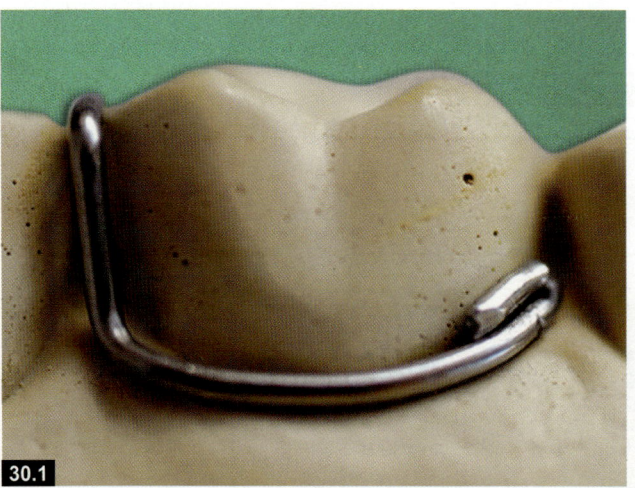
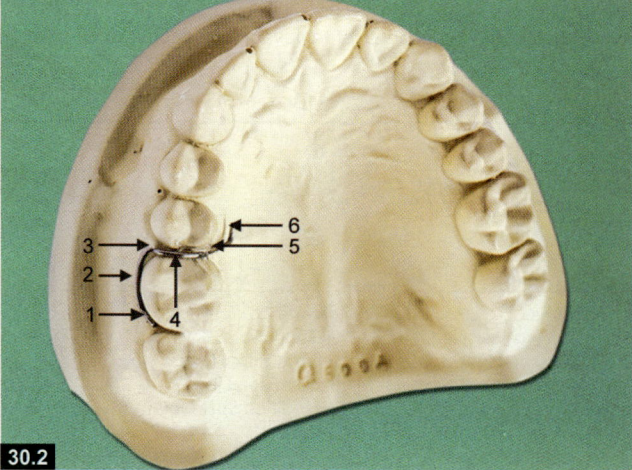

**Fig. 30.1:** Circumferential clasp or "C" clasp; **Fig. 30.2:** Parts of "C" clasp. 1—Squash loop; 2—Circumferential arm; 3—Buccal interdental arm; 4—Occlusal interdental arm; 5—Retentive arm; 6—Retentive tag (see text for detail);

## Uses

1. Circumferential clasp is often used on first permanent molar or second permanent molars.
2. Circumferential clasp is occasionally used on permanent canines.

A variation of this clasp is incorporated into many wrap around labial bow designs.

### Jackson Clasp/Full Clasp

Jackson clasp is also called as "full clasp" or "U" clasp. It was introduced by Jackson in the year 1906. It is fabricated with 0.7 mm hard round stainless steel wire. This clasp is adapted along the buccal cervical margin and extends along the mesial and distal undercuts over the occlusal embrasure to end in two retentive arms on either side of the teeth **(Figs 30.3A and B)**.

### Adam's Clasp

Adam's clasp is the most useful and versatile clasp for contemporary removable appliances. It provides excellent retention and accepts a number of modifications to suit various clinical situations. This clasp was introduced by C Phillips Adams and hence, the name Adam's clasp, it is also called by the name universal clasp, Liverpool clasp and modified arrowhead clasp.

### Design

Adam's clasp has two arrowheads, which engage the mesiobuccal and distobuccal proximal undercuts of the tooth to be clasped and are connected by a bridge. The bridge should be such that it is at the level of middle third of the crown and at an angulation of 45° to the long axis of the tooth **(Figs 30.4A and B)**.

The outer ends of both the arrowheads continue occlusally over the mesial and distal embrasures to end lingually as two retentive arms that get embedded in acrylic base material.

***Thickness of wire used:*** Hard stainless steel wire of 0.7 mm or 21 gauges is used for the fabrication of the clasp.

### Parts

Following are the parts of the Adam's clasp **(Fig. 30.5)**:
1. Two arrowheads
   - Mesiobuccal arrowhead
   - Distobuccal arrowhead.

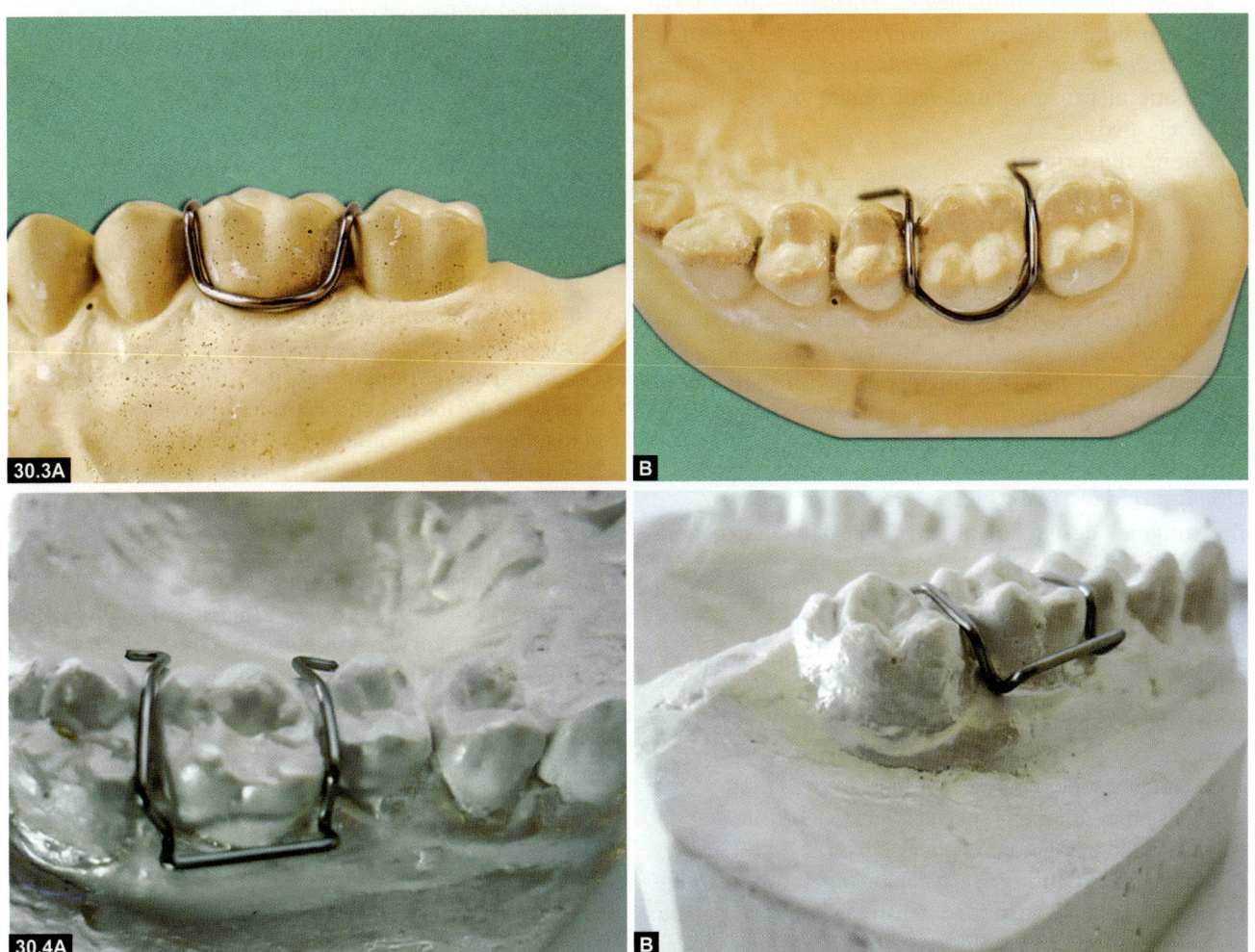

**Figs 30.3A and B:** Jackson clasp; **Figs 30.4A and B:** Adam's clasp

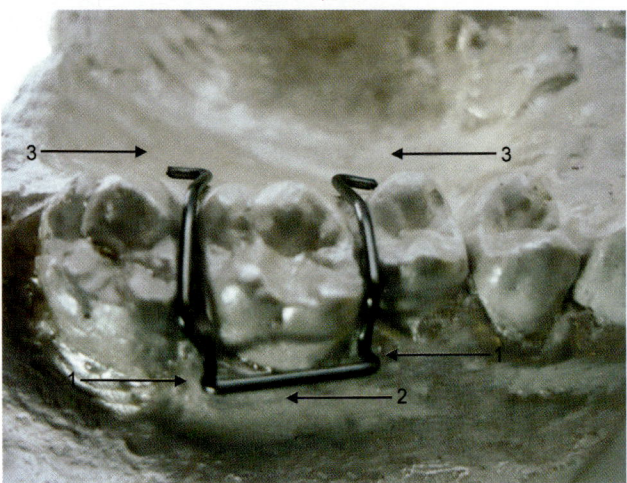

**Fig. 30.5:** Parts of Adam's clasp

2. Connecting bridge.
3. Two retentive arms with two retentive tags.

1. Arrowheads of Adam's Clasp
   Adam's clasp is composed of two arrowheads, which are:
   - *Mesiobuccal arrowhead:* Engages on mesial proximal undercut region of tooth to be clasped.
   - *Distobuccal arrowhead:* It engages on distal buccal proximal undercut region of tooth to be clasped.
2. Connecting bridge
   - Connecting bridge, so called because it connects mesiobuccal proximal undercut arrowhead to distobuccal proximal undercut arrowhead of clasp.
   - It should be in middle third area of crown of clasped tooth.
   - It should have 45° angulations with long axis of clasped tooth.
   - It should be parallel with buccal cusps.

### Advantages of Adam's Clasp

The unique design of Adam's clasp offers general advantages as listed below:
- It has excellent retentive properties as it engages both the proximal undercuts of the clasped tooth.
- It can be fabricated on both deciduous and permanent teeth.
- It can be constructed on any tooth in the arch, i.e. incisors, canines, premolars and molars.
- It can be used on partially or fully erupted tooth.
- Does not require any special pliers to fabricate it and is fabricated using Adam's pliers.
- If it is broken during use, it can be repair by soldering.
- The clasp has an added advantage that it permits modifications in its design to meet various clinical needs.

### Disadvantages of Adam's Clasp
- This is difficult to fabricate.
- It possesses greater occlusal interference than that of a circumferential clasp.

### Modifications of Adam's Clasp and their Uses

Adam's clasp offers a unique feature that its design can be modified in a number of ways to suit various clinical requirements. The following are some of the modifications of Adam's clasp **(Figs 30.6A to H)**:
1. Adam's clasp with incorporated helix **(Fig. 30.6A)**
   *Use:* For the attachment of elastics
2. Adam's clasp with soldered hook **(Fig. 30.6B)**
   *Use:* For the attachment of elastics
3. Adam's clasp with traction hook **(Fig. 30.6C)**
   *Use:* For the attachment of elastics
4. Adam's clasp with additional arrowhead **(Fig. 30.6D)**
   *Use:* For additional retention.
5. Adam's clasp with single arrowhead **(Fig. 30.6E)**
   *Use:* For partially erupted teeth
6. Adam's clasp with soldered buccal tube **(Fig. 30.6F)**
   *Use:* For the attachment of face bow
7. Double Adam's clasp on maxillary central incisor **(Fig. 30.6G)**
   *Use:* For additional retention
8. Adam's clasp with distal extension **(Fig. 30.6H)**
   *Use:* For the attachment of elastic and additional retention.

### Points to be Checked in Adam's Clasp
1. Arrowhead should be pointed at the bucco-proximal undercut.
2. The bridge should be placed parallel to the buccal surface at the middle third of the tooth.
3. The bridge should be placed at about 2 mm away from the buccal surface of the tooth.
4. When viewed from the side, the bridge should be at an angle of 45° to the buccal surface of tooth.
5. Retentive arms should not interfere with occlusion.
6. Retentive tags should be placed at the end of the retentive arms for retaining the clasp securely in the acrylic base.

### Clinical Adjustment of an Adam's Clasp
- Tightening the clasp by bending it gingivally at the point where the wire emerges from the base plate.
- Adjustment of the clasp by bending the retentive arms inward.
- Usually adjustment of the clasp is done after repeated insertion and removal of the appliance.
- If it is broken during use, it can be repaired by soldering.
- This clasp permits modifications in its design, as per the requirement.

### Triangular Clasp

Triangular clasp is so called because it acquires the shape of a triangle **(Fig. 30.7)**.

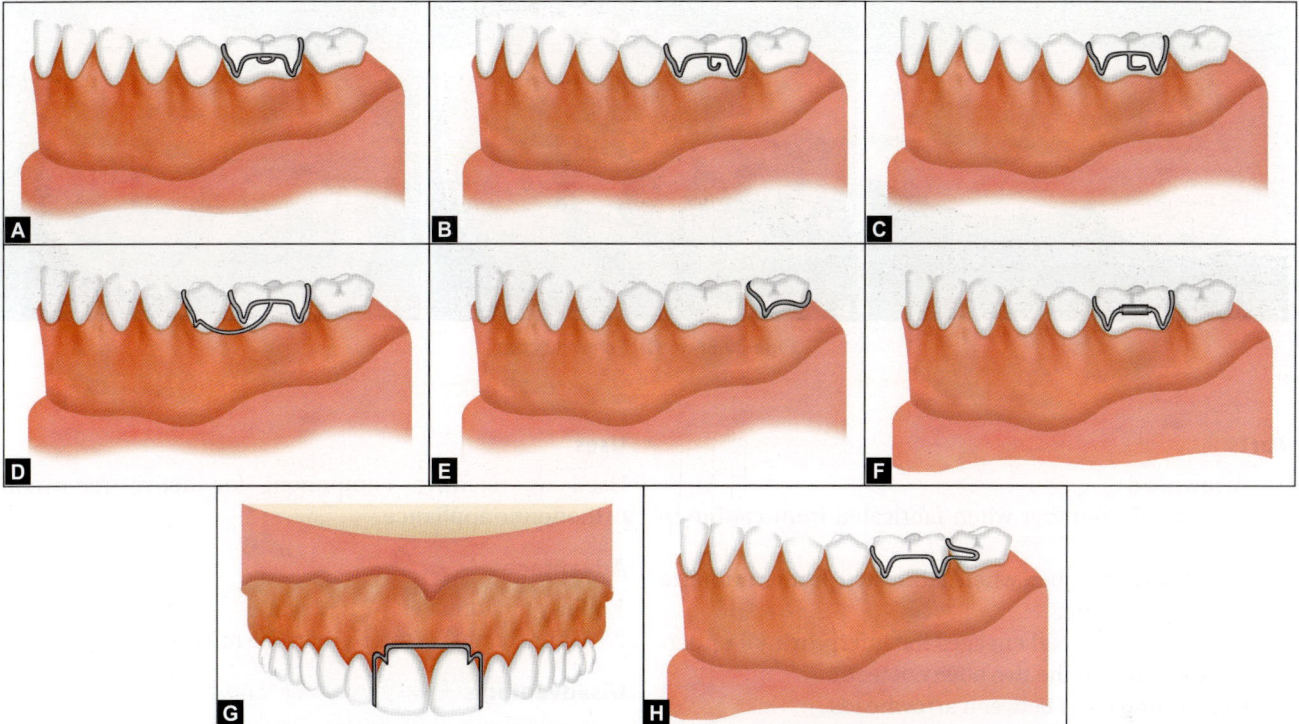

**Figs 30.6A to H:** Modifications of Adam's clasp. **(A)** Adam's clasp with incorporated helix. **(B)** Adam's clasp with soldered hook. **(C)** Adam's clasp with traction hook. **(D)** Adam's clasp with additional arrowhead. **(E)** Adam's clasp with single arrowhead. **(F)** Adam's clasp with soldered buccal tube. **(G)** Double Adam's clasps on maxillary central incisor. **(H)** Adam's clasp with distal extension

## Parts

Parts of triangular clasp are:
1. Base of triangle: Away from embrasure
2. Apex of triangle: Faces embrasure
3. Retentive arm: Long
4. Retentive tag.

## Uses

1. Triangular clasps are used as accessory clasps.
2. They are used to provide additional retention.

## Advantages

1. They are small-sized clasps thus do not interfere with the maintenance of oral hygiene.
2. Easy to fabricate.
3. They can be fabricated between two adjacent teeth, mainly between two adjacent posterior teeth.
4. They engage proximal undercuts between two adjacent teeth.

## Disadvantages

Triangular clasp cannot provide adequate retention when used alone.

## Wire Used

Hard stainless steel wire of 21 gauge or (0.7 mm) is used to fabricate this clasp.

## Pliers Used

Adam's pliers are used to construct this clasp.

### Schwartz Clasp

Schwartz clasp is also called as "arrowhead clasp" as it is made up of a number of arrowheads **(Figs 30.8A to C)**. The design of an Adam's clasp is, in fact, a modification of Schwartz clasp.

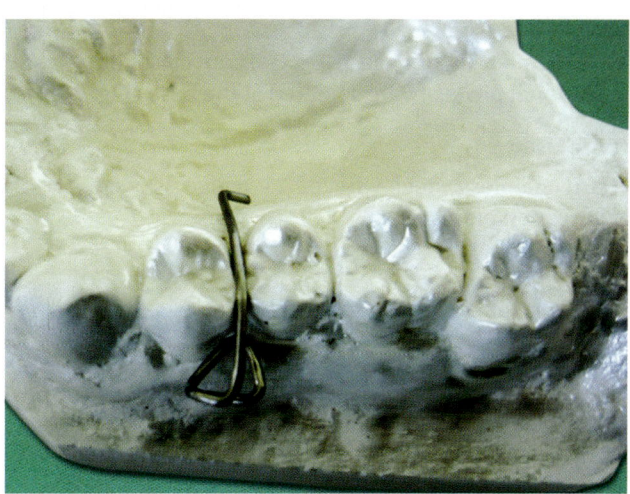

**Fig. 30.7:** Triangular clasp

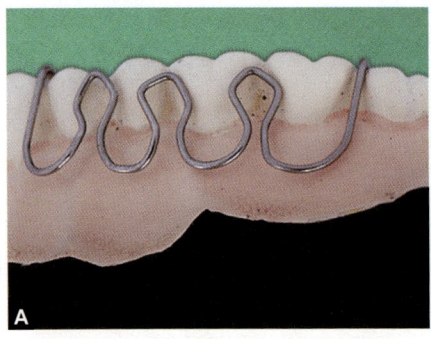 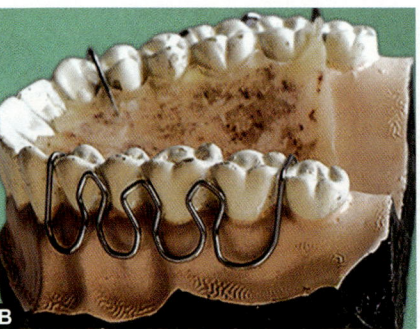 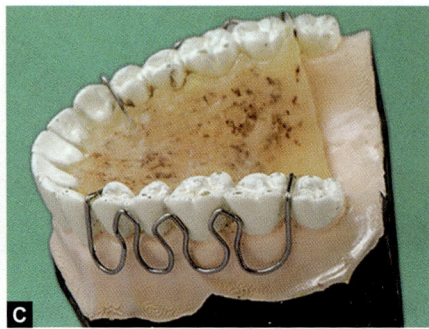

**Figs 30.8A to C:** Schwartz clasp

### Parts

1. Arrowhead
   - Three in number when fabricated from canine to first molar.
   - Four in number when fabricated from canine to second molar.
   - Each arrowhead engages the interproximal undercut between the two adjacent teeth.
2. Connecting parts between arrowheads.
3. Two retentive arms and retentive tags.

### Advantages

Schwartz clasp provides better retention than triangular clasp.

### Disadvantages

This clasp is not routinely used due to a number of disadvantages:
a. It is a bulky clasp and occupies a large amount of space in the buccal vestibule.
b. The arrowheads may cause injury to interdental soft tissues.
c. Needs special arrowhead forming pliers for its fabrication.
d. Fabrication is tedious and time consuming.

### Crozat Clasp

It is similar to full clasp or Jackson clasp but has an additional piece of wire soldered at the base **(Fig. 30.9)**.

### Wire Used

Hard stainless steel wire of 21 gauge is used for the fabrication of this clasp.

### Pliers Used

Universal plier can be used to fabricate this clasp.

### Parts

Parts of Crozat clasp are listed below:
1. *Circumferential arm*: Follows buccal contours of the tooth to be clasped.
2. *Additional piece of wire*: Soldered to circumferential arm at the base.
3. *Retentive arm and tags*: Mesial and distal.

### Uses

Used as retentive component for active removable orthodontic appliance.

### Advantages

1. Easy to fabricate.
2. Offers better retention than the full clasp.

### Disadvantage

It requires soldering machine for soldering the additional piece of wire at the base of circumferential arm of Crozat clasp.

### Resta Clasp

The Resta clasp is a modified version of Adam's clasp.

### Design

- It uses the arrowhead retentive point from the Adam's clasp and ball from ball end clasp to engage two undercut areas on the buccal surface of the anchor tooth.
- The clasp wire passes over the occlusal surface of the clasped tooth either on its mesial or distal side **(Figs 30.10A and B)**.

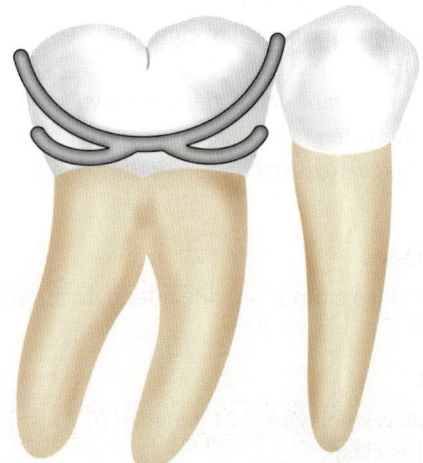

**Fig. 30.9:** Crozat clasp

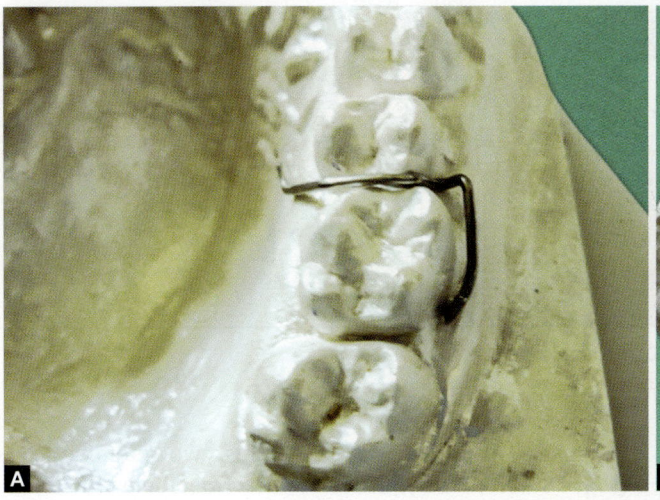 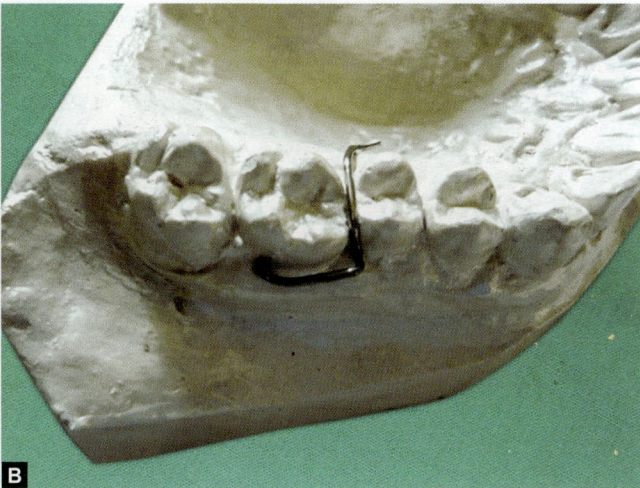

Figs 30.10A and B: Resta clasp

### Wire Used

The hard round stainless steel wire of 22 gauge (0.7 mm) is used for its fabrication.

### Pliers Used

- Pliers: Adam's pliers or universal pliers
- Cutter: Hard wire cutter.

### Parts

Parts of Resta clasp are as follows
1. Squash loop
2. Arrowhead
3. Retentive arm
4. Retentive tag.

### Uses

The clasp is useful when interocclusal clearance or space is available on only the mesial or distal side of the tooth to be clasped.

### Advantages

1. Making of this clasp is easier and quicker than the forming of an Adam's clasp.
2. It can be modified to be part of wraparound retainer design.

### Disadvantages

Retentive ability of this clasp is less than that of an Adam's clasp.

### *Southend Clasp*

Southend clasp is used when retention is required in the anterior segment of the arch.

### Design

The wire is adapted along the cervical margins of both the central incisors. The distal ends are carried over occlusal embrasures and to end as retentive arms and tags on the lingual side **(Figs 30.11A to C)**.

### Wire Used

Hard stainless steel wire of 21 gauge.
- Pliers used: Universal pliers
- Cutter used: Hard cutter wire

### Parts

Parts of southend clasp are as follows:
1. Circumferential arm: Two in number.
2. Interdental embrasure arm: Two in number
3. Retentive arm and tags.

### Advantages

This clasp can be used when upper incisors are not proclined and where there is limited undercut.

### Disadvantages

In case of proclined incisors, the clasp is flexed unnecessarily during the placement and removal of the appliance and can fracture frequently.

### *Ball End Clasp*

Ball end clasp is used as an accessory clasp when additional retention is required.

### Design

The clasp is made of stainless steel wire with a knob/ball-like structure at one end of the wire. The ball end is formed by using a silver solder. The thickened ball end engages the proximal undercut between the two adjacent posterior teeth. The distal end of the wire passes over the occlusal embrasure to end as retentive arm and tag lingually **(Fig. 30.12)**.

## ACTIVE COMPONENTS

### Bows

Bows also form the active components of removable orthodontic appliance. They are usually used for overjet reduction. They can also be used for space closure in the

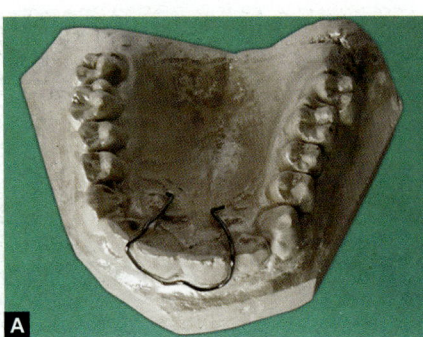 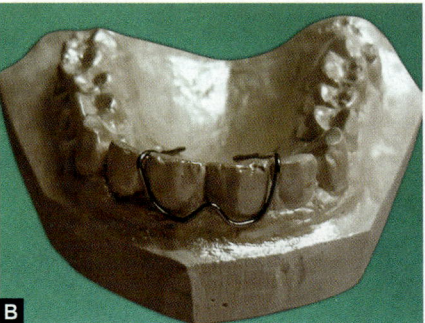 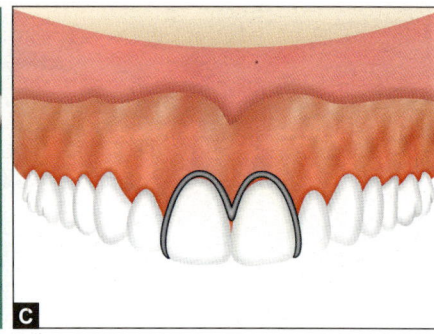

**Figs 30.11A to C:** Southend clasp

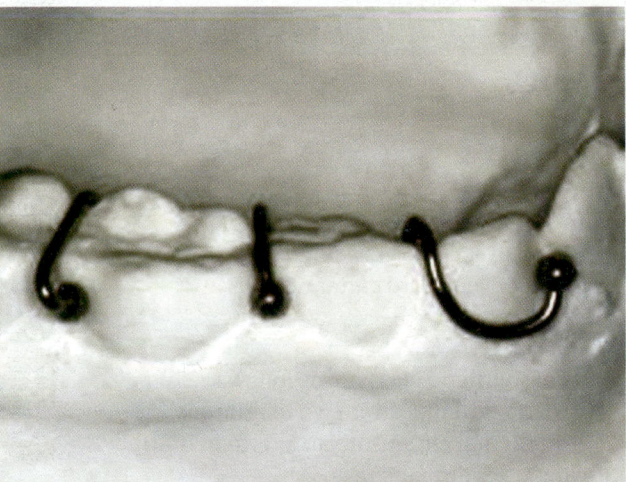

**Fig. 30.12:** Ball end clasp

anterior segment as well as space distal to canines. The following are some of the routinely used designs of labial bows:
1. Short labial bow
2. Long labial bow
3. Split labial bow
4. Modified split labial bow
5. Reverse labial bow
6. Robert's retractor
7. Mill's retractor
8. Fitted labial bow
9. High labial bow with apron spring.

The amount of overjet reduction possible depends on the length of the wire used in fabrication of bow. Longer the wire used, greater is the flexibility. For example, short labial bow allows overjet reduction up to 4 mm, whereas Mill's retractor incorporating long wire can be used to achieve overjet reduction up to 7 mm.

Labial bows are also used in the retention phase after active orthodontic therapy and are referred to as passive labial bows (e.g. short labial bow in the design of Hawley's retainer).

### Short Labial Bow
The short labial bow is constructed from canine to canine region in both the maxillary and mandibular arches. It consists of a bow, two "U" loops, two retentive arms (**Figs 30.13A and B**), which are described below.

### Bow
1. It contacts with the most prominent labial surface of the anterior teeth.
2. Bow should be exactly in the center of the crown on labial surface of the anterior teeth.
3. There should not be any bends in the bow.

### "U" Loops
1. There are two U-shaped loops, one on right canine another one on left canine.
2. The bow terminates just mesial to labial ridges of canines on either side, where the wire is bent to form "U" loops.
3. The distal leg of "U" loop passes interdentally between canine and first premolar to end lingually as retentive arm.

### Retentive Arms
1. Short labial bow has two retentive arms—mesial and distal.
2. The retentive arms should follow the anatomy of palate and lingual mandibular area in respective jaws.
3. A clearance of 0.5 mm between the tissue surface and retentive arm is needed for acrylization.

### Indications
1. Minor overjet reduction.
2. Anterior space closure.
3. For the purpose of retention at the termination of active orthodontic therapy.

### Activation
It is activated by compressing the "U" loop by 1 to 2 mm.

### Long Labial Bow
Long labial bow is a modification of short labial bow where in the bow extends from left first premolar to right first premolar (**Figs 30.14A and B**). Thus, greater length of the wire used allows greater anterior retraction as compared to short.

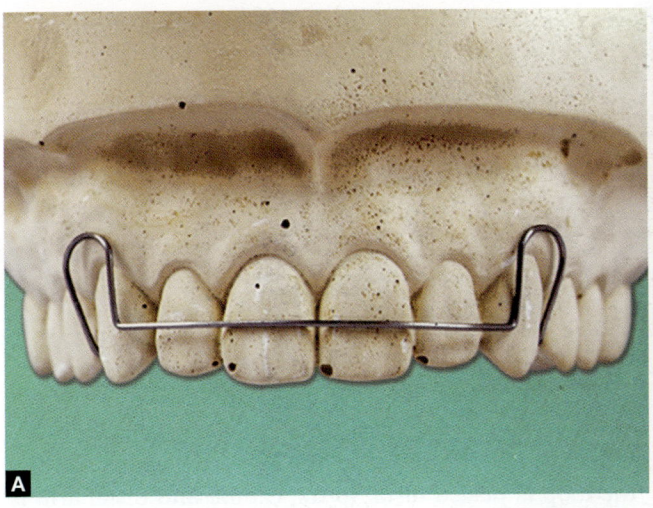
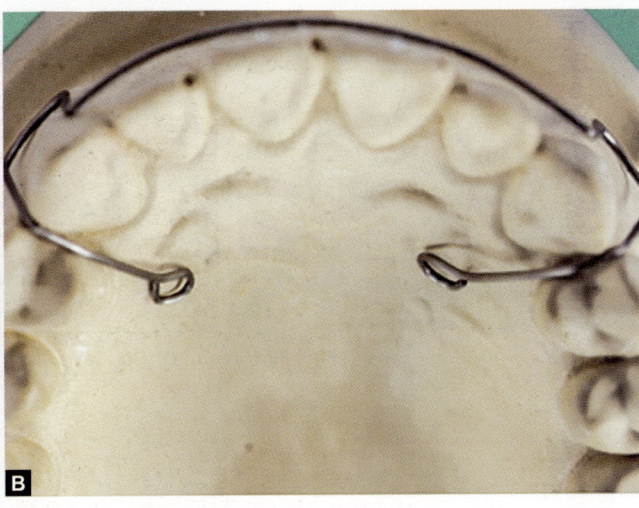

**Figs 30.13A and B:** Short active labial bow

### Bow

1. The bow extends from right first premolar to left first premolar.
2. It contacts with the most prominent labial surface of the anterior teeth.
3. Bow should be exactly in the center of the crown of labial surface of the anterior teeth.
4. There should not be any bends in the bow.

### "U" Loops

1. There are two U-shaped loops, one on right first permanent premolar and another one on left first permanent premolar.
2. U-loop should be (2–3 mm) below the gingival margin of the premolar.
3. U-loops end as the retentive arms.

### Retentive Arms

Long labial bow has two retentive arms—mesial and distal.

### Indications

1. Anterior space closure.
2. Closure of space distal to the canine.
3. Guidance of canine during canine retraction.

### Activation

It is activated by compressing the loops by 1–2 mm.

#### Split Labial Bows

Split labial bow is a modification of the conventional short labial bow in that it is split in the midline; this results in two separate buccal arms, having a "U" loop each **(Figs 30.15A and B)**. This type of bow is not routinely used as the bow lacks enough rigidity and stability and the degree cut ends may cause soft tissue injury. Although more flexible, this clasp has least clinical applicability.
Parts of split labial bow are as follows:

This bow is formed from 0.7 mm hard round stainless steel wire.

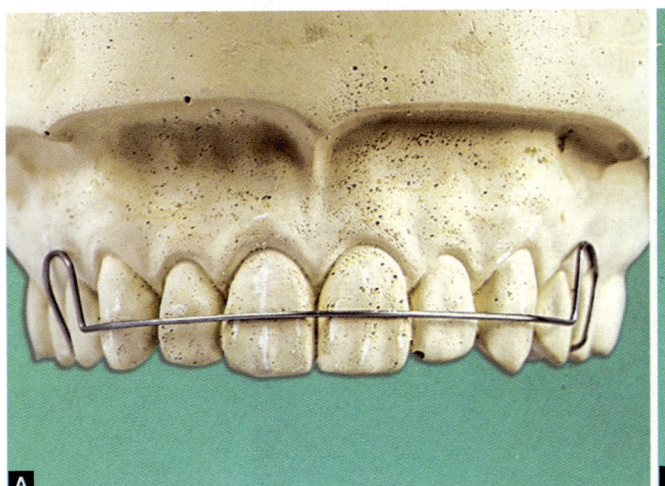
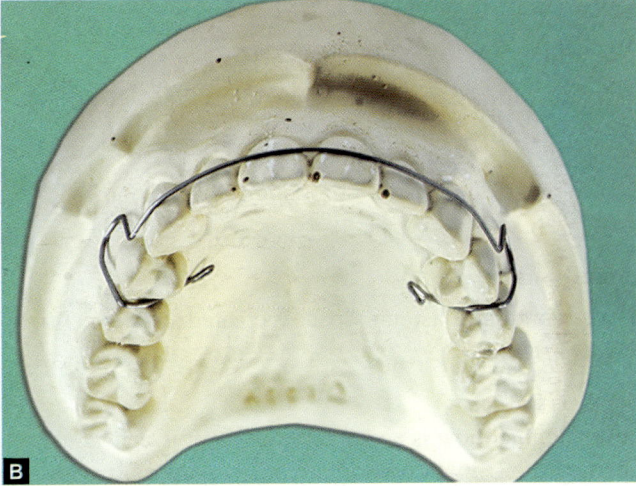

**Figs 30.14A and B:** Long active labial bow

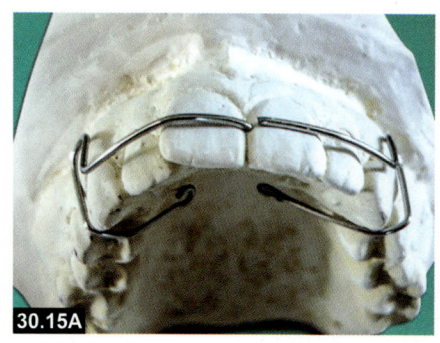 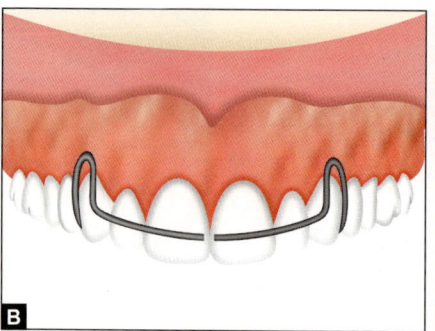 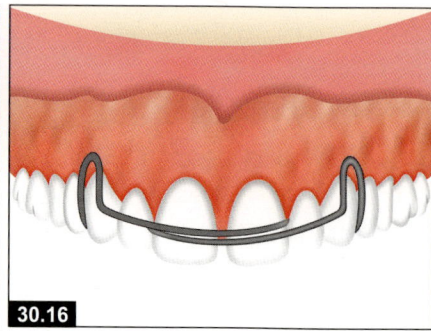

Figs 30.15A and B: Split labial bow; Fig. 30.16: Modified split labial bow

1. Bow
2. U-loops
3. Two retentive arms

### Indications
Used for retraction of anteriors especially incisors.

### Activation
It is done by compressing the U-loops of the bow by 1 to 2 mm.

### Modified Split Labial Bow
Modified split labial bow is a modification of the split labial bow; wherein the free ends of the buccal arms of labial bow are made to hook onto the distal surface of the opposite to central incisors **(Fig. 30.16)**.

### Wire Used
It is fabricated using 0.7 mm hard round stainless steel wire.

### Parts of Modified Split Labial Bow
1. Bow to engage opposite central incisors: The free ends of left and right buccal segments of the bow cross each other in the midline to engage the distal surface opposite to central incisors.
2. Two U-loops
3. Two retentive arms.

### Indications
Used in closure of midline diastema.

### Activation
Activation is done by compressing the "U" loop by 1–2 mm.

### Limitations
It closes midline diastema; space is created distal to central incisors.

### Reverse Labial Bow
Reverse labial bow is so called because it is activated by opening the U-loop, instead of compressing as is seen in the other conventional bows.

### Design
The loop is placed distal to the canine and distal arm is bent at right angle to extend anteriorly as the labial parts of the bow and mesial arm is bent to pass between canine and first premolar and thereafter it ends as retentive arm and tag and gets incorporated into the acrylic base plate **(Figs 30.17A and B)**.

### Activation
It is activated by opening the loops make the lowering of the labial bow in the incisor region. For maintaining the proper level of the bow a compensatory bend is then given at the base of the loop.

### Robert's Retractor
Robert's retractor **(Fig. 30.18)** has two helices instead of U loops in its design. This type of bow is fabricated from thin gauge stainless steel wire of 0.5 mm smaller diameter of wire and incorporation of helices renders the bow highly flexible and thus can bring about greater anterior retraction.

However, it lacks adequacy and needs support in vertical plane. The distal part of the retractor is supported by a stainless steel tubing of 0.5 mm internal diameter.

### Mill's Retractor
Mill's retractor has a complexly designed labial bow. The bow has extensive looping of the wire designed to increase the flexibility and range of action. It is called as extensive labial bow **(Fig. 30.19)**.

### Uses
It is indicated in patient with large overjet.

### Drawback
a. Difficulty in fabrication.
b. Poor patient compliance due to its complex design.

### Fitted Labial Bow
This type of labial bow is so called, as it is adapted to the contours of the labial surface of anteriors **(Fig. 30.20)**.

### Use
Mainly for retention after completion of fixed orthodontic treatment.

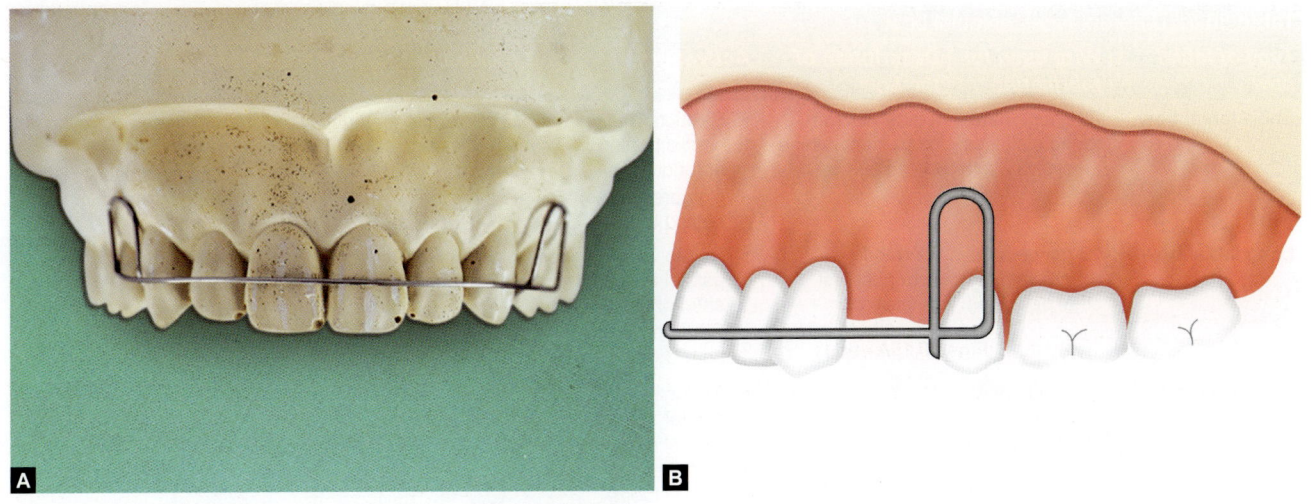

**Figs 30.17A and B:** Reverse labial bow

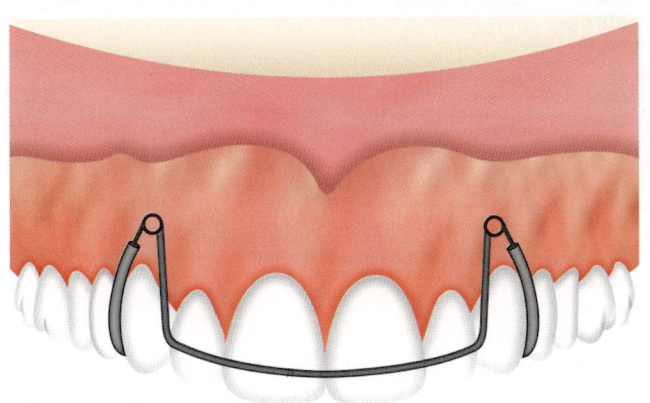

**Fig. 30.18:** Robert's reatractor

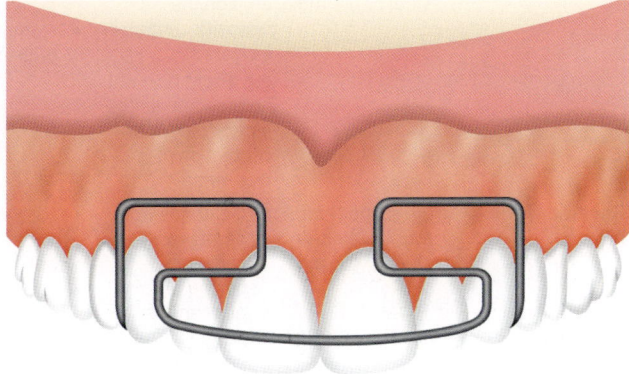

**Fig. 30.19:** Mill's retractor

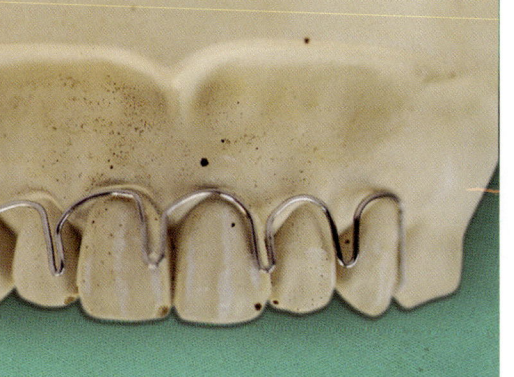

**Fig. 30.20:** Fitted labial bow

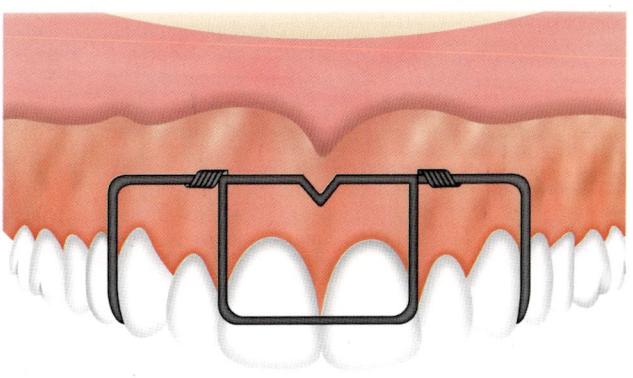

**Fig. 30.21:** High labial bow with apron spring

**Table 30.1:** Different types of labial bow

| Type of labial bow | Wire used for fabrication | Description of the bow | Activation | Flexibility | Indications |
|---|---|---|---|---|---|
| Short labial bow | 23 gauge hard round stainless steel or 0.7 mm | It extends from permanent canine to canine | • Reduction of palatal acrylic behind anteriors<br>• Compression of both U loops | Less flexible than any other type of labial bows | • Minor overjet reduction (upto 3.5 mm)<br>• Mild space closure in the anterior segment |
| Long labial bow | 23 gauge hard round stainless steel or 0.7 mm | It extends from right first permanent premolar to left first premolar | • Reduction of lingual palatal acrylic of anterior<br>• Compression of both U loops | More flexible than short labial bow | • Minor overjet reduction<br>• Minor anterior space closure<br>• Closure of space distal to canine |
| Split labial bow | 23 gauge hard round stainless steel or 0.7 mm | The bow is split in midline | • Reduction of lingual palatal acrylic behind anteriors<br>• Compression of both U loops | More flexible than short labial bow | Anterior retraction |
| Modified split labial bow | 23 gauge hard round stainless steel or 0.7 mm | The bow is modified to engage the opposite central incisors, e.g: Right bow will engage left central incisor below the contact point and vice versa | • Reduction of lingual palatal acrylic behind anteriors<br>• Compression of both U loops | More flexible than short, long and split labial bow | Mainly used for closure of midline diastema |
| Reverse labial bow | 23 gauge hard round stainless steel or 0.7 mm | • It extends from permanent canine to canine or permanent premolar to premolar<br>• The bow is reversed | • Reduction of lingual palatal acrylic behind anteriors<br>• Opening the loop resulting in lowering the bow incisally and compensatory bend is given to maintain proper level of bow | More flexible than short, long, split, modified split labial bow | Overjet reduction (5 to 7 mm) |
| Robert's retractor | 23 gauge hard round stainless steel or 0.5 mm | • It extends from permanent canine to canine<br>• It incorporates an helix on either side<br>• The diameter of both helix should be 3 mm | • Reduction of lingual palatal acrylic behind anteriors<br>• Closing both the helices | More than short, long, split, modified split and reverse labial bow | Increased overjet (7 to 9 mm) |
| Mill's retractor | 23 gauge hard round stainless steel or 0.7 mm | Bow having extensive looping | • Reduction of lingual palatal acrylic behind anteriors<br>• Compression of looping | More than short, long, split, modi-fied split, reverse labial bow and Robert's retractor | Large overjet (more than 9 mm) |
| High labial bow with apron spring | • 21 gauge hard round stainless steel or 0.9 mm<br>• Apron spring fabricated with 0.4 mm | • Extends in buccal vestibule<br>• Apron springs are made to rest on incisors | • Activated only by apron spring<br>• Apron spring is activated by bending it toward the teeth | Apron spring is highly flexible because it is fabricated with thinner gauge wire | Proclined incisors |
| Fitted labial bow | 23 gauge hard round stainless steel or 0.7 mm or 21 gauge hard round stainless steel or 0.9 mm | It is made to be fitted in the contour of all anteriors | It is not activated | Least as compared to all other types of bows | Mainly used or retentive after completion of fixed orthodontic therapy |

### High Labial Bow with Apron Spring

This type of labial bow extends high into the labial vestibule. It is made up of a thicker gauge stainless steel wire (0.9–1 mm). The labial bow acts as a support onto which apron springs (made from 0.4 mm wire) are attached. Apron springs help in retraction of one or more upper anteriors **(Fig. 30.21)**. This type of bow is highly flexible because of the springs and is, therefore, used for retraction in cases with large overjet.

Apron spring is activated by bending it towards the teeth, up to 3 mm at a time. Since it generates light forces, it is also useful in adult patients. However, it is difficult to construct and can cause soft tissue injury. It may also lack patient compliance as too much of wire is visible.

Different types of labial bows are given in **Table 30.1**.

## SPRINGS

Springs are active components of removable orthodontic appliances, which are used to bring about tooth movement. There are different types of springs, which can be used according to the need. The basic principle behind using springs is that when a wire is deflected, it tries to regain its prefabricated original shape and while trying to do so the springs move the teeth along their path **(Table 30.2)**.

### Classification

Springs can be classified in a number of ways.

1. Depending on Presence/Absence of Helix in their design
   a. Simple spring: No helix
   b. Compound spring: With helix incorporated.
2. Depending on whether helix or loop is present
   a. Helical springs: With helix in their design
   b. Looped springs: Helix, loop is incorporated in their design.
3. According to nature and stability of the spring
   a. *Self-supported springs:* These springs are fabricated from wires of thicker gauge and thus are self-supporting.
   b. *Supported springs:* These springs lack stability as they are made of thinner gauge wires. They are supported by encasing a section in metallic tubes or acrylic.

### Principles of Designing Springs

Several factors are considered while designing of spring. Ideally, orthodontic forces should be of low magnitude and longer duration.

Spring should exert adequate amount of force and at the same time they should also be flexible as to remain for a longer period. Force exerted by the spring is related to diameter and length of the wire used as follows:

$F = D^4/L^3$: where  F = Force
D = Diameter of the wire
L = Length of the wire

**Table 30.2:** Different types of springs and their activation and indications

| Types of springs | Wire used for fabrication | Description of the spring | Activation | Indication |
|---|---|---|---|---|
| Finger spring | 0.5 mm or 0.6 mm stainless steel | • Consist of active arm, helix and retentive arm<br>• Helix is of 3 mm in diameter and should rest on the long axis of root of the tooth to be moved<br>• Retentive arm is of 4–5 mm in length and is made to get embedded in acrylic base | Opening the helix and moving active arm towards the tooth to be moved | For closure of minor anterior space<br>For closure of midline diastema |
| Z-spring | 0.5 mm or 0.6 mm stainless steel | Consists of two helices arranged in pattern of Z that's why also known as double cantilever spring | • Activation depends on its indication<br>• For correction of minor rotation, then only one upper helix is activated by opening the helix<br>• For labial movement of incisors the spring is activated by opening both the helices | • Correction of minor rotation<br>• Labial movement of incisors<br>• Labial movement of tooth in case of single or segmental crossbite |
| T-spring | 0.5 mm or 0.6 mm stainless steel | It consists of T-shaped arm | Pulling the free end of T towards the intended direction of tooth movement | Buccal movement of premolars |
| Mattress spring | 0.6 mm round stainless steel wire | It is shaped like a mattress with "U" loops extending up to the retentive arm | — | Labial movement of upper teeth in cross-bite |
| Helical coil spring | 0.6 mm round stainless steel wire | Free-ended spring with two helices formed on different arms | — | To regain the lost space |

***Diameter of wire:*** Force is directly proportional to the diameter of the wire by using a thicker wire, the force can be increased but flexibility of the spring decreases. By doubling the diameter of the wire, force increases by almost 16 times.

***Length of wire:*** Flexibility is an important desirable quality of a spring. By increasing the length of the wire, force decreases but flexibility increases. Springs that are made of longer wire are more flexible and remain active for a longer duration of time. By doubling the length of the wire, force can be reduced up to 8 times. Helices and loops are incorporated in the design to render springs more flexible and long acting.

***Force to be applied:*** The amount of force that should be generated by the spring depends on the number of teeth to be moved, root surface area and patient comfort. In general, an average force of 20 gm/cm of root area is recommended for tooth movements.

The other factors that have to be considered while designing a spring are:

***Direction of tooth movement:*** The spring should be designed, keeping in mind the direct direction of tooth movement. The direction of tooth movement is determined by the point of contact between the spring and the tooth.

For example, lingual movement of tooth is brought about by buccally placed springs while palatally positioned springs effect labial tooth movement.

***Patient comfort:*** Spring should be such that it does not cause discomfort to the patient by way of its design, size or the force it exerts.

### Finger Spring

Finger spring, also called as single cantilever spring, has a simple design and is useful for mesiodistal tooth movement **(Fig. 30.22)**.

Parts of Spring **(Fig. 30.23)**
- ***One helix:*** Diameter 3 mm
- ***Active arm:*** It is of about 12 to 15 mm long
- ***Retentive arm:*** It is of about 4 to 5 mm long
- Retentive tag.

***Helix of finger spring:*** Finger spring has a single helix of 3 mm internal diameter (the helix is placed near the point of attachment of the spring to the acrylic base).

***Active arm:*** The free end of the spring is the active arm, which contacts the tooth to be moved. The active arm is about 12 to 15 mm long and circumscribe one-third of the crown surface of the tooth to be moved.

***Retentive arm:*** Retentive arm of finger spring is 4–5 mm long and is kept away from the tissue in the acrylic.

***Retentive tag:*** Retentive arm ends as a small retentive tag, which later gets embedded in acrylic base material.

### Fabrication of Finger Spring

1. Wire used: 0.5 or 0.6 mm or 23 gauge hard stainless steel wire is used for the fabrication of finger spring.
2. Fabrication of finger spring.
3. Finger spring should be constructed such that the helix lies along the long axis of the tooth to be moved and it should be perpendicular to the direction of movements prior to the acrylization. Helix and active arm of finger spring are boxed in the wax to support the thin wire. The direction of the coil should be opposite to that of the intended direction of tooth movement.

### Activation

The finger spring is activated either by moving the active arm towards the tooth to be moved or by opening the helix. Activation of up to 3 mm is considered optimum when spring is made of 0.5 mm wire and up to 1.5 mm when 0.6 mm wire is used for fabrication of the spring.

### Indications

The finger spring is used to effect mesiodistal movement of teeth, such as closure of anterior diastemas. It can be used only on those teeth, which are in proper alignment buccolingually along the arch.

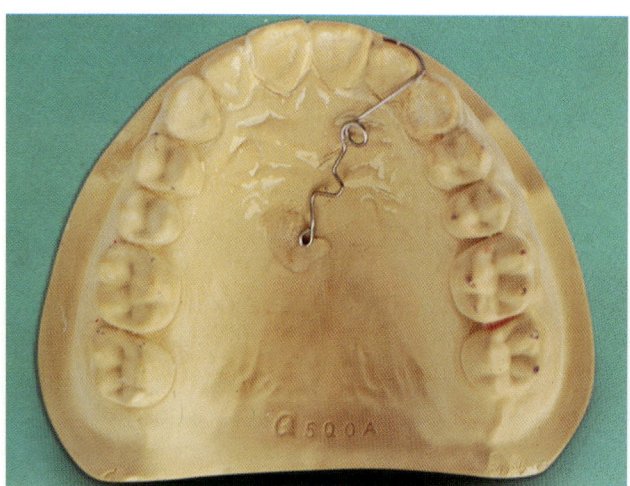

**Fig. 30.22:** Finger spring

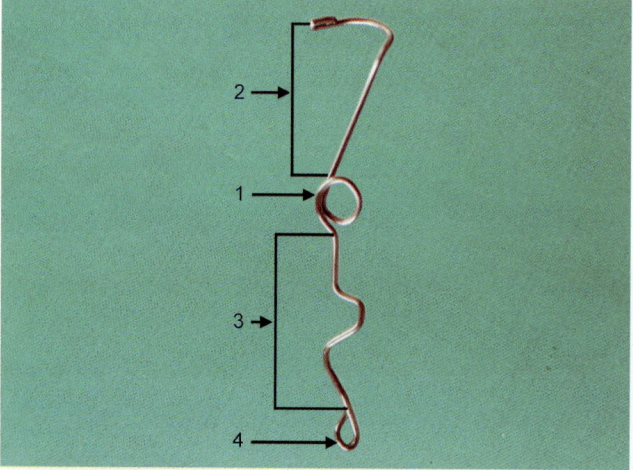

**Fig. 30.23:** Parts of finger spring: 1—Helix—3 mm in diameter; 2—Active arm; 3—Retentive arm; 4—Retentive tag

## Z-Spring

Double cantilever/Z-spring can be used for the labial movement of palatally locked incisors and also for correcting minor rotations of these teeth **(Fig. 30.24)**.

### Parts of Z-Spring
a. Square loop
b. Two helices
c. Retentive arm
d. Retentive tag. **(Fig. 30.25)**

### Helices of Z-spring
There are two helices of small internal diameter.

***Squarsh loop:*** Active arm with squarsh loop is incorporated at the free end of active arm and it helps in preventing soft tissue damage.

***Retentive arm:*** It has a long retentive arm of about 10 to 12 mm length, which gets embedded in acrylic base material.

***Retentive tag:*** Retentive tag of Z-spring is perpendicular to the retentive arm and is of 2 to 3 mm in length.

### Fabrication
- Stainless steel wire of 0.5 mm or 23 gauge is used for the fabrication of Z-spring.
- Pliers used: Universal pliers can be used for the fabrication of Z-spring.
- Z-spring can be designed to more one or two incisor in a labial direction over equal distances.
- The spring is constructed such that it is perpendicular to the palatal surface of the teeth to be moved.
- Z-spring is a supported spring and needs boxing in the wax prior to acrylization. However, the helices are kept free from acrylic so that they can be activated.

### Activation of Z-Spring
- For labial movement of incisors, the Z-spring is activated by simultaneously opening both helices by 2 to 3 mm.
- For correction of minor rotations, activation is done by opening only upper helix by 2 to 3 mm.

### Uses
Z-spring is used for:
a. Labial movement of one or two incisors. It is often used for correction of anterior crossbite occurring due to palatally locked upper incisors.
b. It can also be used for the correction of mild rotation of incisors.

## T-Spring

T-spring (having a T-shaped active arm) can be used to effect the buccal movement of premolars and sometimes that of canines **(Fig. 30.26)**.

### Parts of T-Spring
a. T-shaped active arm that contacts the tooth to be moved.
b. Loops incorporated in the arms.
c. Retentive arms, which get embedded in acrylic.
d. Retentive tag **(Fig. 30.27)**.

### Construction
- The spring should be perpendicular to palatal surface of the tooth to be moved.
- The head of the "T" is slightly curved to follow the palatal contour of the tooth.
- As the tooth moves buccally, the head, the "T" can still be made to remain in contact with the crown by opening up the loops incorporated in the arms.

### Uses
1. T-spring is used for the buccal movement of premolar.
2. It can also be used in some cases for the buccal movement of canines.

### Activation
The spring is activated by pulling the free end of the "T" towards the intended direction of tooth movement.

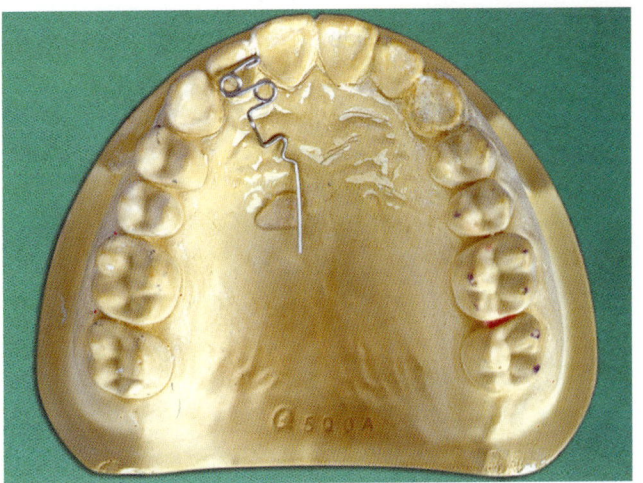

**Fig. 30.24:** Z-spring

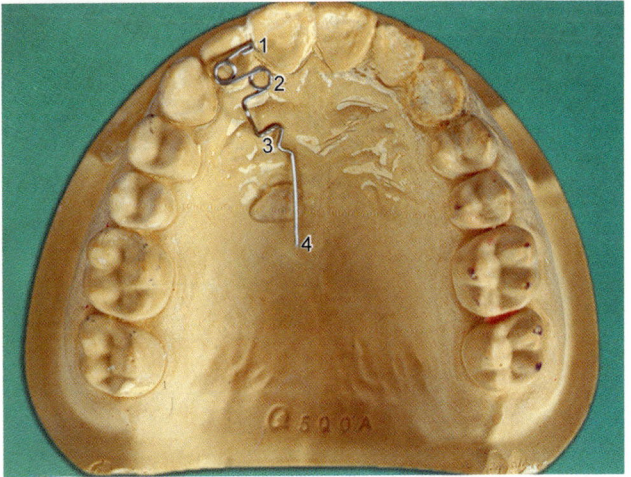

**Fig. 30.25:** Parts of Z-spring: 1—Square loop; 2—Two helices; 3—Retentive arm; 4—Retentive tag

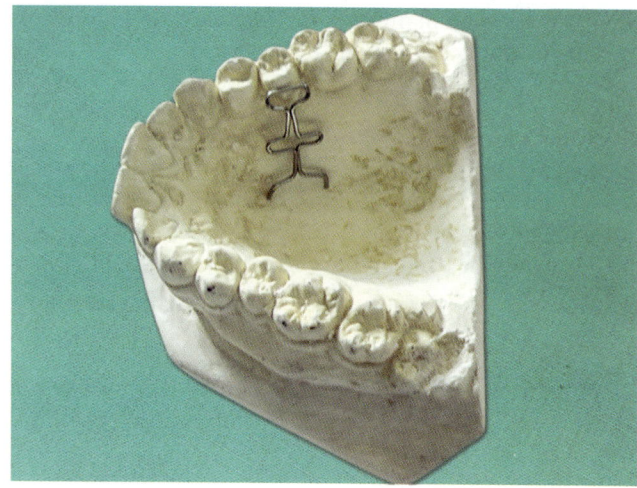

**Fig 30.26:** T-spring

### Mattress Spring

A mattress spring can be used for the labial movement of upper teeth in crossbite, when there is sufficient space for tooth movement **(Fig. 30.28)**.

#### Construction

Mattress spring is fabricated from stainless steel wire of 0.6 mm diameter. It is shaped like a mattress with "U" loops, extending up to the retentive. The free end engages the tooth to be moved, close to gingival margin.

### Helical Coil Spring

Following extraction of a tooth, the adjacent teeth tend to migrate towards the extraction space. Helical coil spring can be used to regain the lost space **(Fig. 30.29)**.

#### Construction

Helical coil spring is a free-ended spring with two helices formed on different arms. The two free ends act as active arms and engage the teeth on either side of the extraction space. It is constructed from a stainless steel wire of 0.6 mm diameter. The connecting arm between the two helices acts partly as a retentive arm.

#### Activation

Activation is done by opening the helices. Depending upon the amount of tooth movement requires the two sides can be activated to different degrees.

## CANINE RETRACTORS

Canine retractors are springs that are used to move canines in a distal direction.

They can be classified in a number of ways as shown in **Table 30.3**.

Usefulness of canine retractors depends on the angulations of the canine to be retracted. The removable orthodontic appliance with canine retractor can be efficiently used only when the canine is mesially angulated. When used on up righted or canines, the removable canine retractors can worsen the situation. Thus, fixed orthodontic appliances have greater control over tooth movement and are preferred over removable canine retractors.

### "U" Loop Canine Retractor

*Wire used:* 0.6 or 0.7 mm hard stainless steel wire is used for the fabrication of this type of canine retractors.

Parts of "U" loop canine retractor **(Fig. 30.30 A and B)**:
a. Active arm
b. "U" loop
c. Retentive arm
d. Retentive tag.

a. Active arm: It includes:
   - Active arm is bent at right angles from the mesial leg of the loop.
   - Active arm is adapted around the canines.
b. U-loop: It includes:
   - The base of the "U" loop is placed 2–3 mm below the cervical margin.

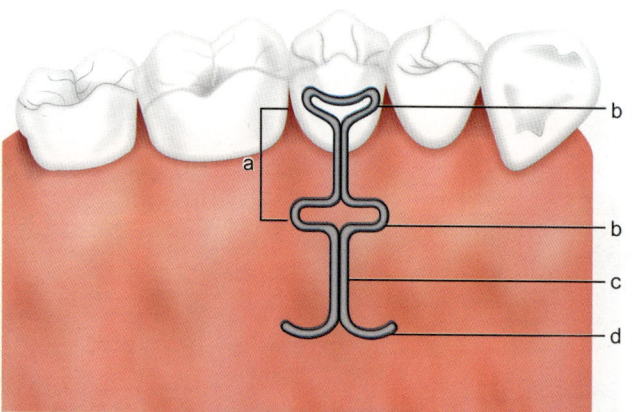

**Fig. 30.27:** Parts of T-spring. a–T-shaped active arm; b–Loops; c–Retentive arms; d–Retentive tags

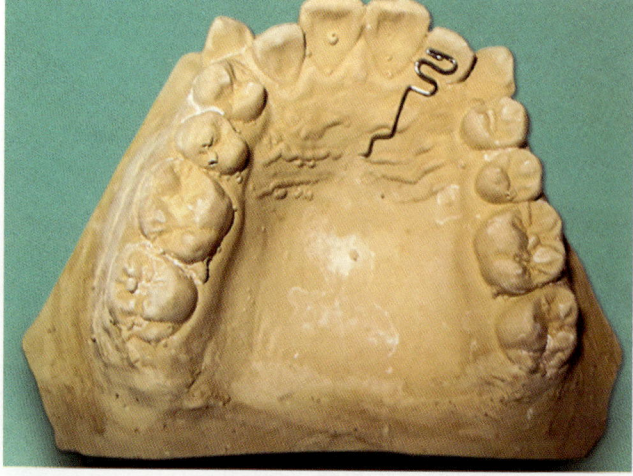

**Fig. 30.28:** Mattress spring

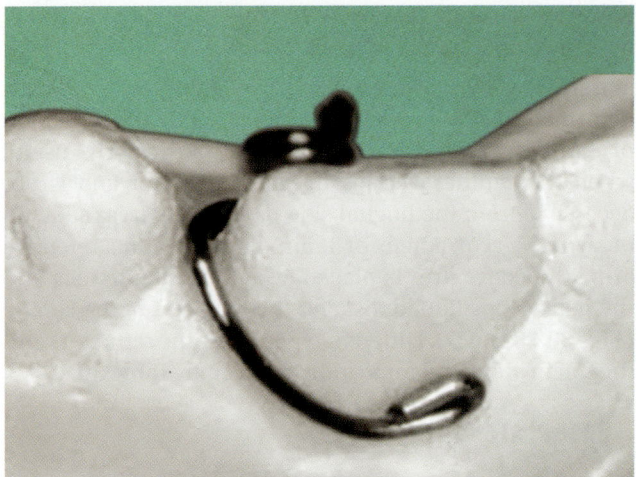

**Fig. 30.29:** Helical spring

| Table 30.3: Classification of canine retractors | |
|---|---|
| **According to their location, canine retractors can be classified as:** | |
| Buccal | Placed buccally |
| Palatal | Placed palatally |
| **According to the presence of helix or loop** | |
| a. Helical canine retractor | |
| b. Looped canine retractor | |
| **According to their mode of action** | |
| a. Push type | |
| b. Pull type | |
| **The following are some of the commonly used canine retractors** | |
| 1. "U" loop canine retractor | |
| 2. Helical canine retractor | |
| 3. Palatal canine retractor | |
| 4. Buccal self-supported retractor | |

- "U" loop consists of the two legs:
  1. Mesial leg
  2. Distal leg
c. Retentive arm:
  - The distal leg of the loop extends as the retentive arms.

### Activation of "U" Loop Canine Retractor
This retractor is activated by compressing the loop or by cutting the free end of the active arm by 2 mm and readapting it.

### Indication
This type of canine retractor is indicated when the minimal canine retraction of 1 to 2 mm is required.

### Helical Canine Retractor
*Wire used:* 0.6 or 0.7 mm hard stainless steel wire is used for the fabrication of this type of canine retractors **(Figs 30.31A and B)**.

### Parts of Helical Canine Retractor
a. Active arm
b. Helix
c. Retentive arm
a. Active arm: It includes:
  - The distal arm is bent at right angles to form this arm.
  - Active arm engages the canine.
b. Helix
  - Diameter of the helix should be of 3 mm.
  - Helix is placed 3 to 4 mm below the gingival margin.

### Indication
This type of canine retractor is indicated when the minimal canine retraction is required.

### Activation
This type of canine retractor is activated by opening of helix or by cutting of 2 mm from the end of the active arm and readapting it around the canine.

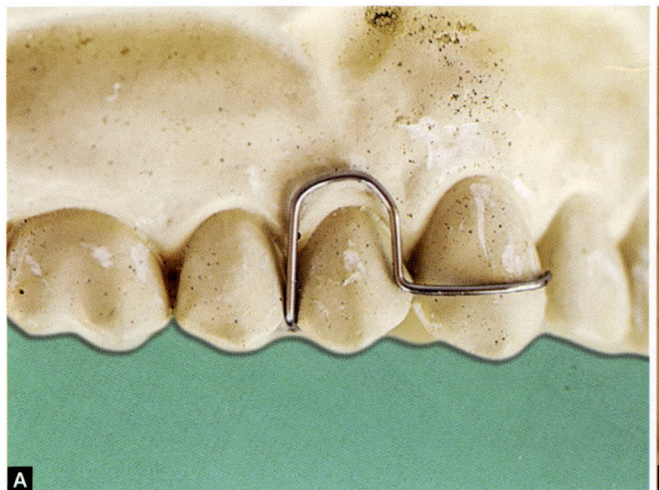 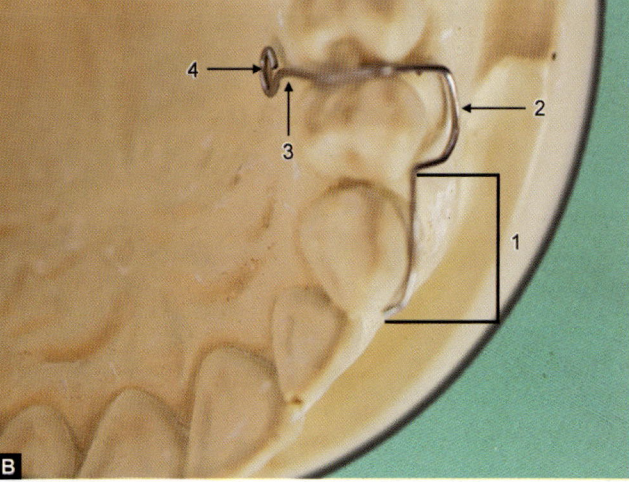

**Figs 30.30A and B:** (A) "U" loop canine retractor; (B) Parts of "U" loop canine retractor. 1— Active arm; 2—U-loop; 3—Retentive arm; 4— Retentive tag

### Palatal Canine Retractor

*Wire used:* 0.6 or 0.7 mm hard stainless steel wire is used for the fabrication of this type of canine retractors **(Figs 30.32A and B)**.

Parts of palatal canine retractor:
a. Active arm
b. Helix
c. Guide arm

a. *Active arm:* Placed mesial to the canine
b. *Helix:* It includes–
   • Helix of 3 mm diameter
   • Placed along the long axis of the canine.

#### Indication

This type of canine retractor is indicated for retraction of palatally placed positioned canines.

#### Activation

This type of canine retractor is activated by opening of helix by 2 mm.

### Buccal Self-supported Canine Retractor

As the name suggests, this canine retractor is made from a thicker gauge wire (0.7 mm), which helps to resist deformation of the spring. It is indicated for the retraction of buccally placed canine and is particularly useful when the canine overlaps the lateral incisor and is not accessible from the lingual side of the arch. It is made up of an active arm, a helix of 3 mm diameter and a retentive arm. The active arm is placed away from the tissues and the helix is positioned distal to the long axis of the canine **(Figs 30.33A to D)**. Different types of canine retractors and their activation and indications is given in **Table 30.4**.

## BASE PLATE

Base plate has a greater percentage of bulk in removable orthodontic appliance than other components. The design of base plate varies with the type of removable orthodontic appliance. Self-cure or autopolymerizing acrylic resins are used for the fabrication of base plate. It joins all other (active and retentive) components of removable

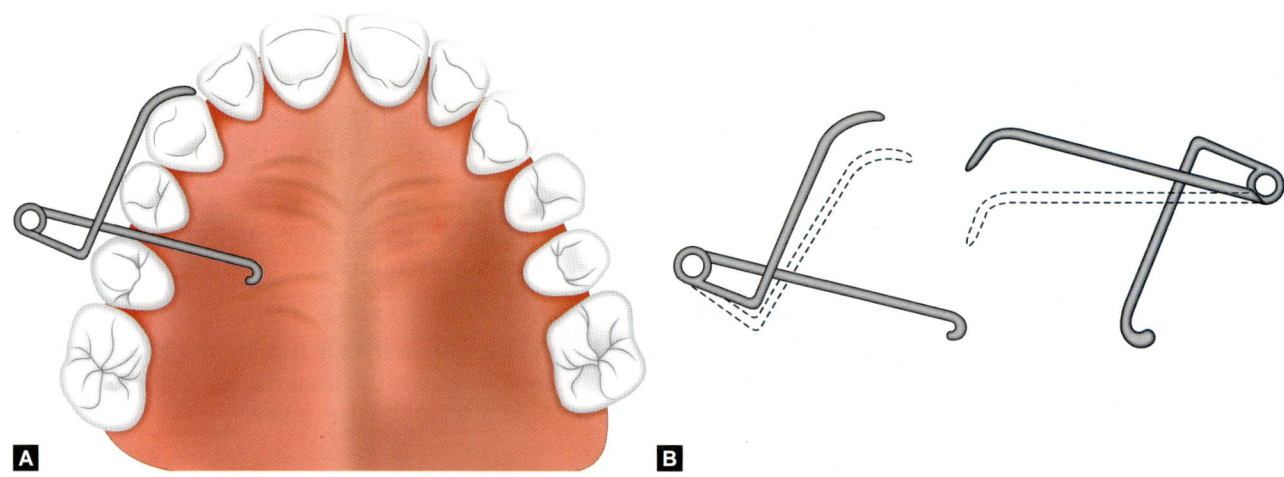

**Figs 30.31A and B:** Helical canine retractors

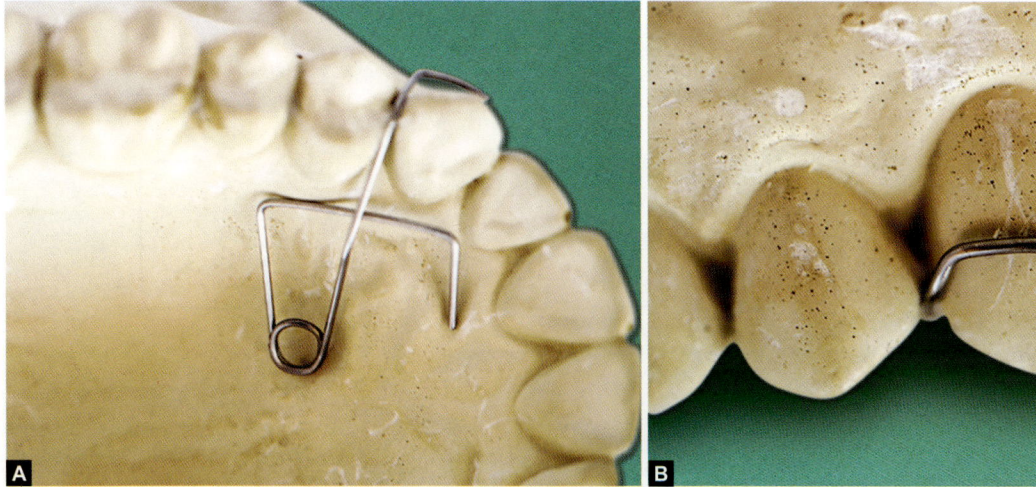

**Figs 30.32A and B:** Palatal canine retractor

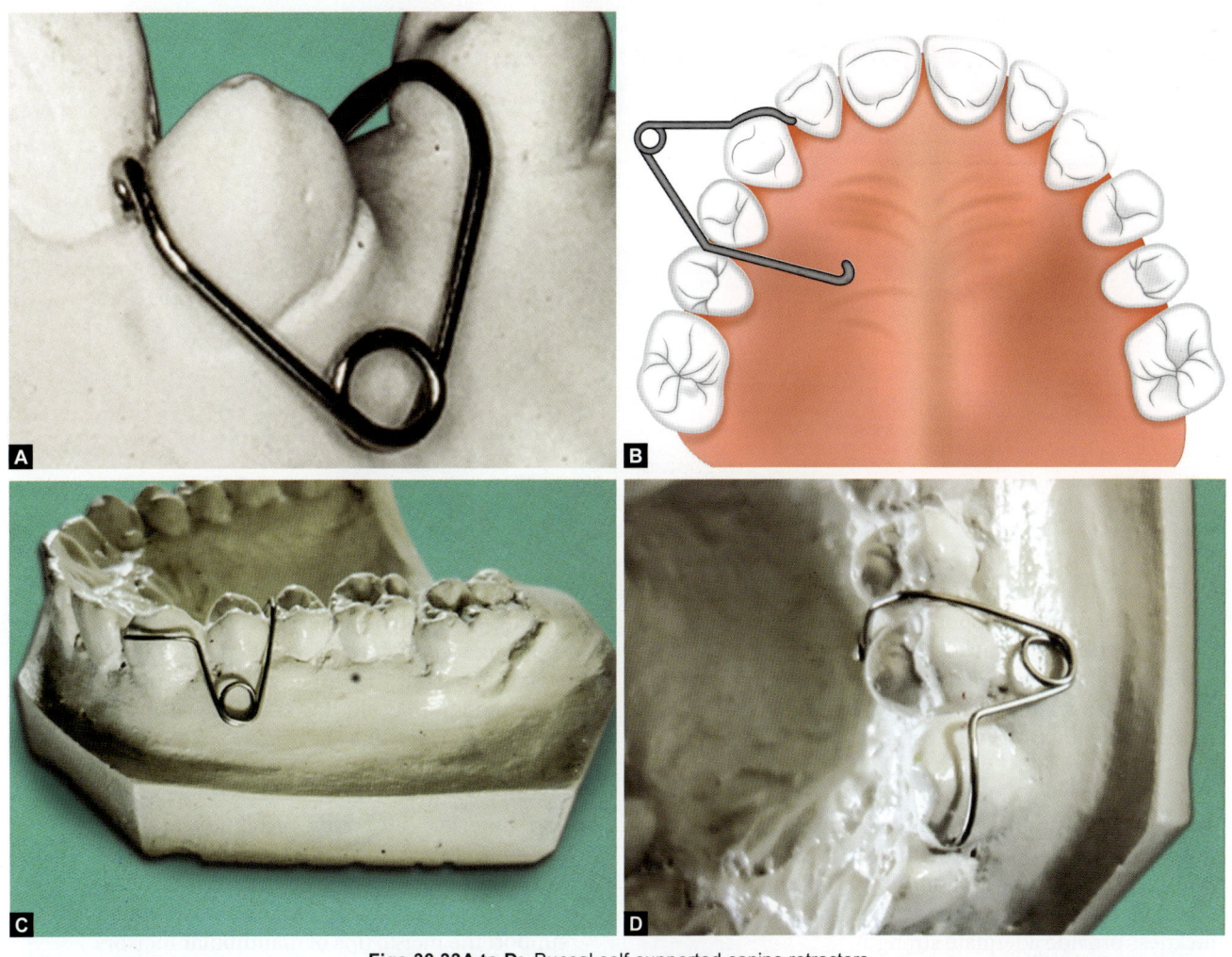

**Figs 30.33A to D:** Buccal self-supported canine retractors

| Types of canine retractor | Wire used for fabrication | Description of canine retractor | Activation | Indication |
|---|---|---|---|---|
| "U" loop canine retractor | 0.6 or 0.7 mm | It consists of "U" loop, active arm and retentive arm | Compressing the loops 1 to 2 mm or cutting the free ends of active arm by 2 mm and re-adapting it | For canine retraction |
| Helical canine retractor | 0.6 or 0.7 mm | It consists of a coil of 3 mm diameter and active arm and retentive arm | Opening the helix by 1 mm or by cutting 1 mm of free ends and re-adapting it | Retraction of canine |
| Palatal canine retractor | 0.6 or 0.7 mm | It consists of coil of 3 mm diameter, active arm and guidearm | Opening the helix 2 mm at a time | For retraction of palatally placed canine |
| Buccal self-supported canine retractor | 0.6 or 0.7 mm | It consists of coil of 3 mm diameter, active arm and retentive arm | Activation is done by closing helix 1 mm at a time | For retraction of buccally placed canine |

**Table 30.4:** Different types of canine retractors and their activation and indications

orthodontic appliance together into a single functional unit.

## Uses of Base Plate

The following are the uses of base plates in removable orthodontic appliance:

1. Base plate carries and unites all the components of removable orthodontic appliance into a single functional unit.
2. It helps in the retention of removable orthodontic appliance.
3. It also provides anchorage by preventing unwanted drift of teeth.

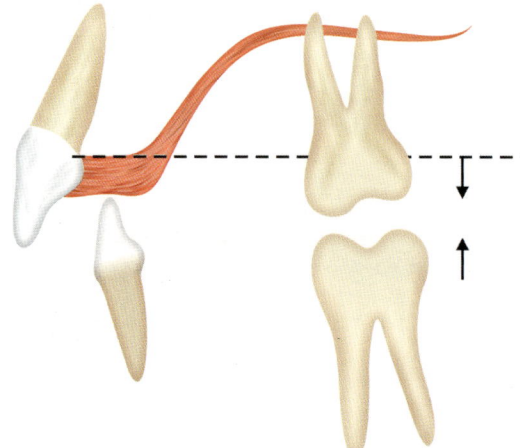

**Fig. 30.34:** Anterior bite planes are used to correct deep bite by facilitating extrusion of posterior teeth

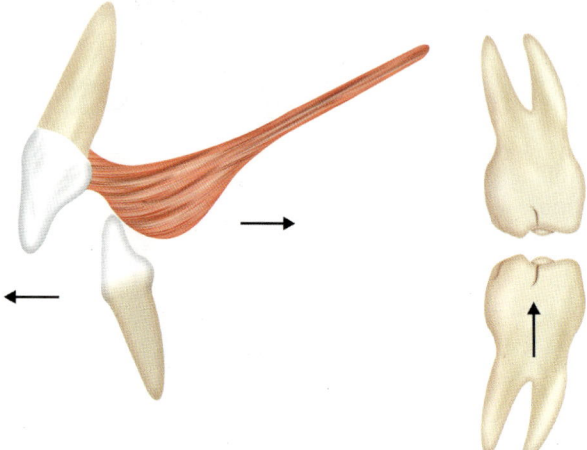

**Fig. 30.35:** Anterior inclined bite plane is flat, inclining downward and inferiorly at an angle of 60° to the occlusal plane

4. It transmits forces uniformly throughout the area.
5. It can be used to support the springs made of smaller gauge wire, which lack strength.
6. Base plate can be extended to form various types of bite planes that are used to treat different types of malocclusions.

### Design of Base Plate

The base plate is routinely fabricated from cold cure (self-polymerizing) acrylic resin although it can be fabricated from heat cure resin. It should be of minimal thickness to be tolerated by the patients. Base plates of 1.5 to 2 mm thickness provide adequate strength.

Maxillary base plate is usually extended up to distal end of first molar covering the entire palate such wide area coverage enhances its strength. Less bulky, narrow horse-shoe shaped maxillary base plate can also be used but are less stable and may get dislodged during tongue movements.

The mandibular base plates are usually shallow to avoid soft tissue irritation at the lingual sulcus and are extended posteriorly up to the first molars.

### Bite Planes–"Modification" of Base Plate

Base plates are extended to form various kinds of bite planes as listed below:
1. Anterior bite plane (for upper arch)
2. Anterior inclined bite plane (for upper arch)
3. Sed bite plane
4. Mandibular anterior inclined bite plane (Catlan's appliance)
5. Posterior bite planes:
   a. For upper arch
   b. For lower arch

### Anterior Bite Plane (for Upper Arch)

Anterior bite plane is fabricated by extending the acrylic base plate behind the maxillary incisors on palatal rugae from right canine to left canine.

Anterior bite planes are used to correct deep bite by facilitating extrusion of posterior teeth. Lower facial height can be increased in such cases. By placing bite planes in the anterior region, the upper and lower posterior teeth are prevented from occluding each other, thus stimulating their extrusion **(Fig. 30.34)**.

**Important Points to be Remembered**

- The anterior bite planes should be flat and not inclined. This is to prevent proclining forces on the lower incisors.
- Grooves can be provided in the anterior bite planes to support the incisal tips of mandibular incisors.
- Anterior bite plane should have labial bow, which prevents protrusion of maxillary anterior.
- Upper incisors can also be capped to prevent supraeruption or flaring of incisors.
- The thickness of the bite plane should be sufficient to open the bite by about 4 to 5 mm in the premolar region.
- Anterior bite plane is indicated in low FMA angle cases.

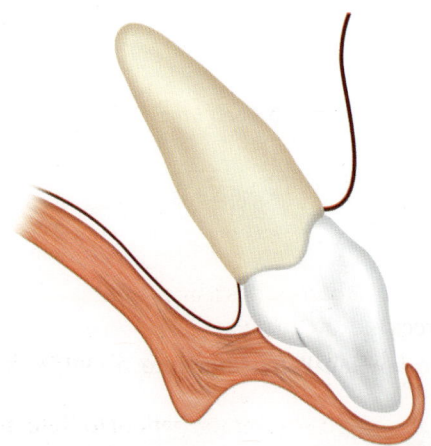

**Fig. 30.36:** Sved bite plane is a modified form of anterior inclined bite plane where the bite plane extends over the incisal edges of the maxillary anteriors. Sved bite plane also reinforces the anchorage

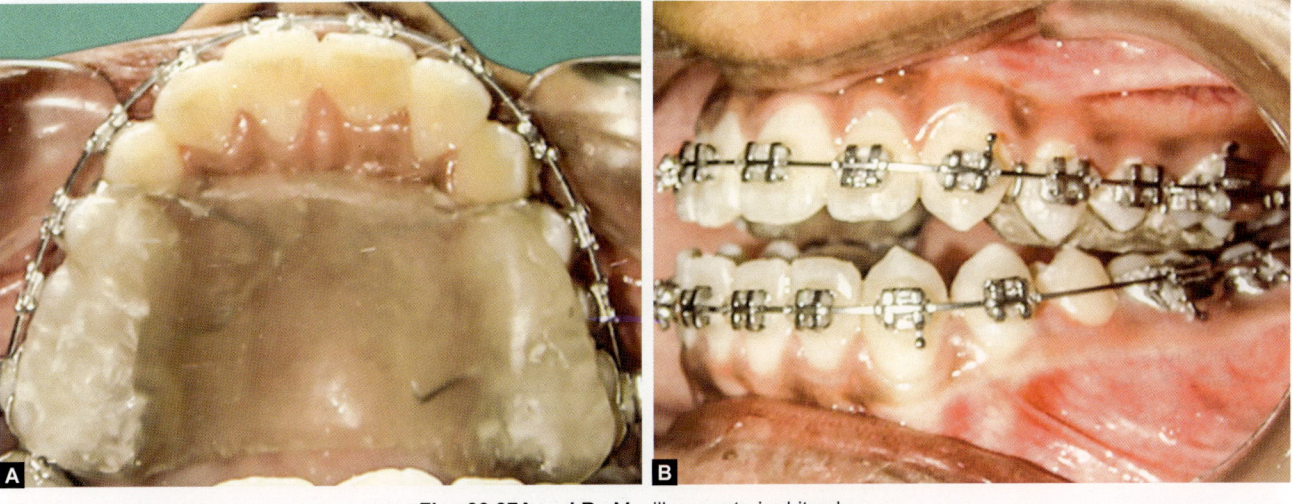

**Figs 30.37A and B:** Maxillary posterior bite plane

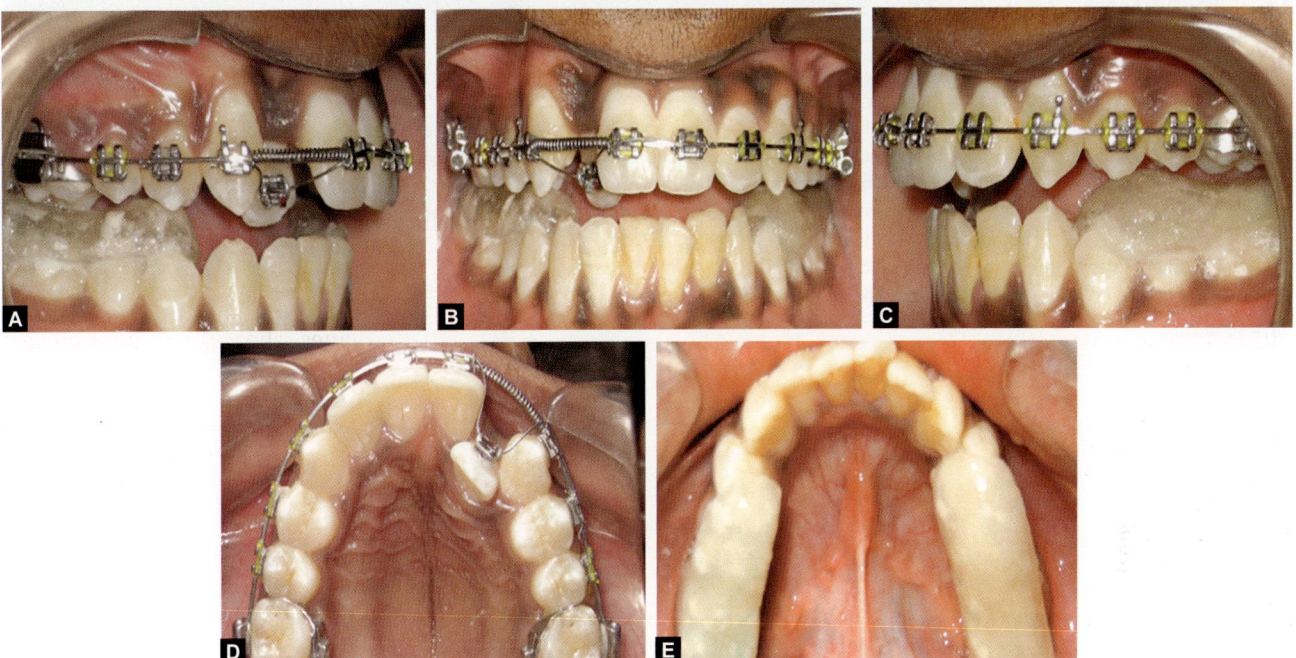

**Figs 30.38A to E:** Mandibular posterior bite plane

### Anterior Inclined Bite Plane

Anterior inclined bite plane is a modification of the anterior bite plane. Anterior inclined bite plane is flat, inclining downward and inferiorly at an angle of 60° to the occlusal plane **(Fig. 30.35)**.

### Uses

1. Correction of anterior deep bite.
2. Reinforces the anchorage.
3. Can be used when mandibular anterior teeth are proclined.
4. The inclined plane causes the patient to "bite" in a more forward position and thus may guide the mandible to grow forward.

### Sved Bite Plane

Sved bite plane is a modified form of anterior inclined bite plane where the bite plane extends over the incisal edges of the maxillary anteriors **(Fig. 30.36)**. Sved bite plane also reinforces the anchorage.

### Posterior Bite Plane

Posterior bite plane is modification of base plate, in which there is extension of acrylic base plate over the occlusal surface of posterior teeth. Posterior bite plane can be fabricated on maxillary and mandibular arches of jaw called maxillary posterior bite plane **(Figs 30.37A and B)** and mandibular posterior bite plane **(Figs 30.38A to E)**, respectively. The thickness of the bite plane should be sufficient enough to free the teeth to be moved from occlusal interference.

### Indications

a. While correcting a lingually placed maxillary anterior tooth.
b. Used in the correction of posterior crossbite either unilateral or bilateral.
c. Used to eliminate occlusal interferences in patient with TMJ pain dysfunctions.

### BIBLIOGRAPHY

1. Adams CP. Removable appliances yesterday and today. Am J Orthod 1969; 55(6):202-18.
2. Adams CP. The modified arrowhead clasps. Dental Record 1950; 70:143-4.
3. Adams CP. The modified arrowhead clasp—some further considerations. Dent Record 1953; 73:332-3.
4. Badcock JH. The screw expansion plate. Trans Brit Soc Orthod 1911; 3-8.
5. Graber TM, Neumann B. Removable Orthodontic Appliances. Philadelphia: WB Saunders, 1984.
6. Graber TM, Neumann B. Removable Orthodontic Appliances. Philadelphia: WB Saunders, 1977.
7. Profitt WR. Contemporary Orthodontics. St Louis: CV Mosby, 1986.
8. Schwartz AM, Gratzinger M. Removable Orthodontic Appliances. Philadelphia: WB Saunders, 1966.
9. Tulley WJ, AC Campbell. A Manual of Practical Orthodontics. J Wright and Sons, Bristol, 1960.
10. Zachrisson BU. Bonding in orthodontics. In: Graber TM, Vanarsdall RL (Eds). Jr. Orthodontics: current principles and techniques, 3rd edition. St. Louis: Mosby, 2000.

### EXAM-ORIENTED QUESTIONS

#### Long Essay or Long Questions

1. What are bows in orthodontics; enumerate various/different types of bows and discuss in detail about wire used for fabrication, description, activation and indication of specific types of bow.
2. Define clasps in orthodontics, enumerate different types of clasps and write down in detail about additional clasps used in retention.
3. What are clasps used in orthodontics retention appliances and discuss in detail about Adam's clasp and its modifications.
4. What are springs and discussion detail on different types of springs and their description activation and indications?
5. What are canine retractors and classify them and discuss in detail about helical canine retractor?
6. Base plate in removable orthodontic appliance.
7. Active components of removable orthodontic appliance.
8. Passive component of removable orthodontic appliance.

#### Short Notes

1. Clasps
2. Bows
3. Springs
4. Canine retractors
5. Z-spring
6. Finger spring
7. Mattress spring
8. Adam's clasp
9. Helical canine retractor
10. Addition clasps for retention
11. Activation of different types of springs
12. Activation of different types of bows
13. Activation of different types of canine retractors
14. Bite planes.

# CHAPTER 31

# Fixed Appliances and Techniques

*Naik P*

Fixed orthodontic appliances are called so because they are fixed to the teeth and cannot be removed by the patient. Fixed orthodontic therapy involves the fixation of attachments (brackets) to the teeth and application of forces by arch wires or auxiliaries via these attachments. Fixed appliances are indicated when multiple tooth movements are required for correction of malocclusion such as rotations, bodily movement of teeth. Fixed mechanotherapy allows fine finishing and settling of occlusion.

## Indications

Fixed orthodontic appliances are indicated where multiple tooth movements are required, e.g. derotation, bodily movement of teeth and controlled space closure.

## Contraindications

- Poorly motivated patients.
- In patients with poor dental health.
- In patients with poor periodontal health.

## Advantages

Advantages of fixed orthodontic appliances are listed below:
- Retention presents no problem, since the appliance is cemented to the teeth.
- Less skill is required from the patient in the management of the appliance.
- Multiple tooth movements are possible with fixed orthodontic appliances.

## Disadvantages

- Difficult to maintain good oral hygiene during fixed orthodontic treatment.
- Excessive force damages the supporting structures of the teeth.
- The potential disadvantage of fixed orthodontic appliance is the possibility of producing adverse tooth movements.
- They can hamper esthetics.

## Components

The components, which form any fixed orthodontic appliance system can be of the following two types depending upon their ability to generate forces:
1. Active components **(Flowchart 31.1)**.
2. Passive components **(Flowchart 31.2)**.

## ACTIVE COMPONENTS

Active components of fixed appliances are those, when used to generate force for bringing about tooth movement. Various active components are described below.

### Separators

Separators are used to create space between two adjacent teeth for banding procedures.

There are four types of separators, which are the following:
I. Elastic ring separator
II. Dumb-bell separator
III. Brass wire separator
IV. Kesling metallic ring separator

### Elastic Ring Separator

Elastic ring separators are small elastic rings **(Fig. 31.1A)**.

**Flowchart 31.1:** Active components of fixed orthodontic appliances

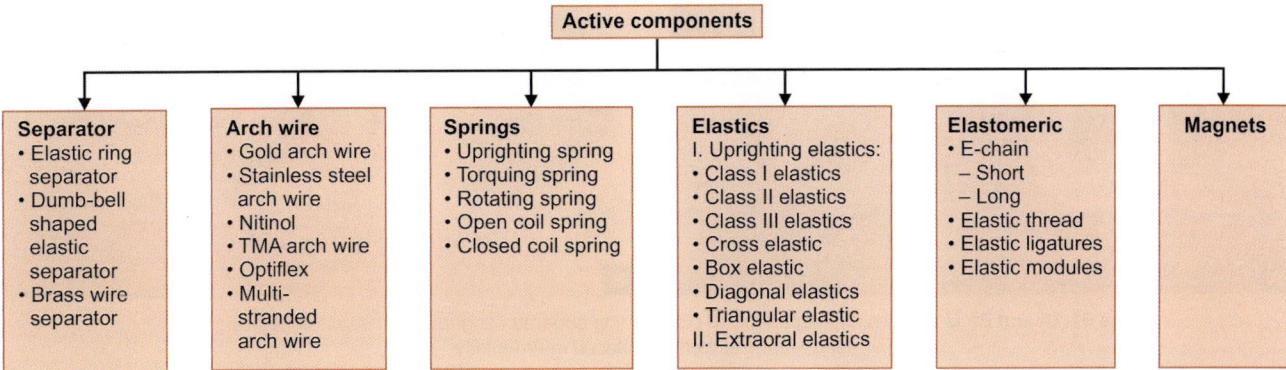

Flowchart 31.2: Passive components of fixed orthodontic appliances

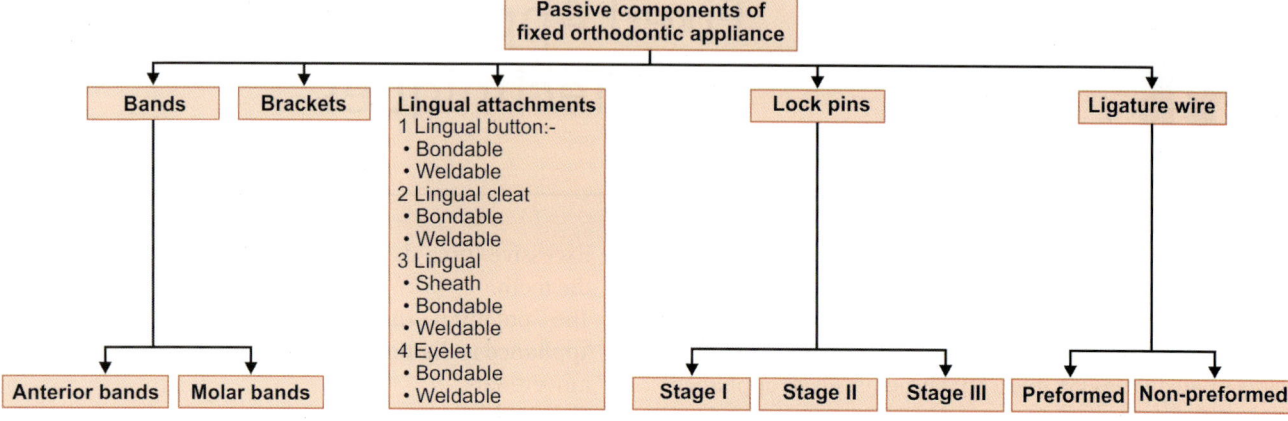

## Use

They are used to create space between two adjacent teeth for banding procedure.

***Application procedure***: Elastic ring separator is grasped in separator placing pliers and then stretched and placed interdentally **(Fig. 31.1B)**.

## Types

Elastic ring separator may be:
a. Round
b. With edges.

## Time Required for Separation

When elastic ring separator is used, separation of teeth takes place in about seven days.

## Advantages

- Elastic ring separators are the most comfortable for the patient.
- Elastic ring separators fit snugly in the interdentally region.

### *Dumb-bell Shaped Elastic Separator (Fig. 31.2A)*

As the name itself specifies, this type of separator is dumb-bell shaped.

## Use

They are used to create space between two adjacent teeth for banding procedure.

## Application Procedure

Dumb-bell shaped elastic separator is stretched and passed through the contacts between adjacent teeth **(Fig. 31.2B)**.

## Time Required for Separation

When dumb-bell shaped elastic separator is used, separation of teeth takes place in about 4 days.

## Advantage

Special pliers are not required for the placement.

### *Brass Wire Separator*

Soft brass wire of 0.5 or 0.6 mm is used for the separation of teeth.

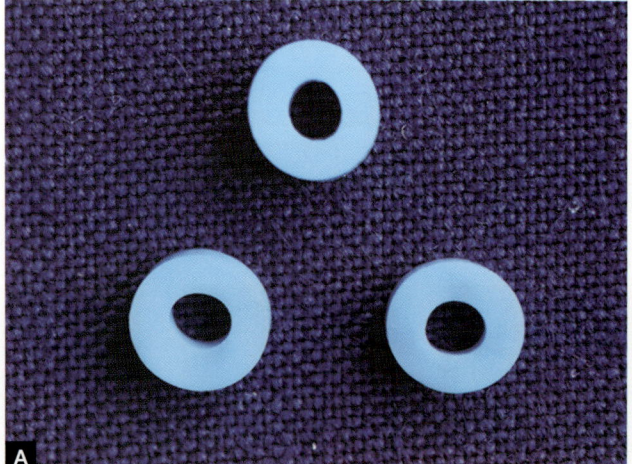
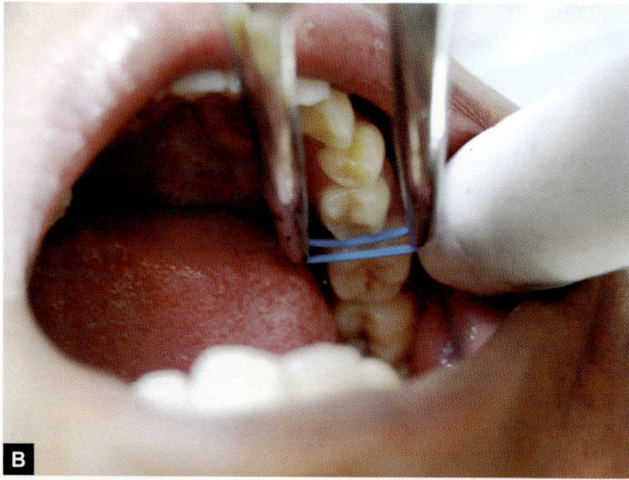

**Figs 31.1A and B:** (A) Elastic ring separator; (B) Elastic ring separator is grasped in separator placing pliers and then stretched and placed interdentally

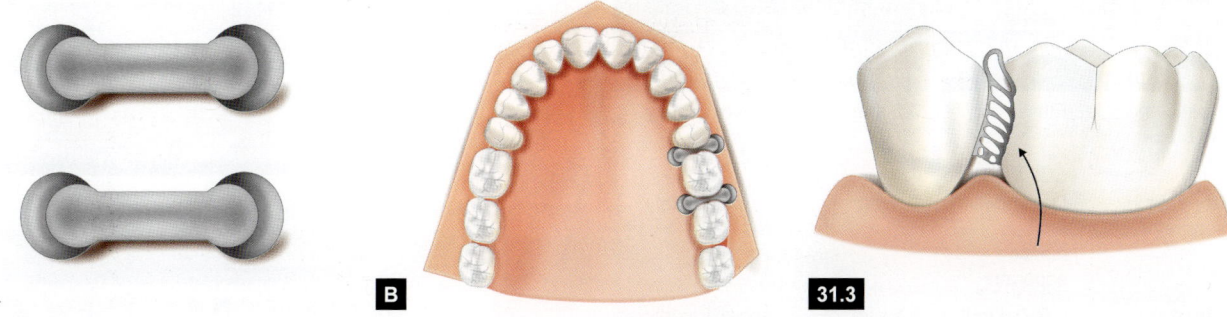

**Figs 31.2A and B:** (A) Dumb-bell shaped separator; (B) Dumb-bell shaped separator placed interdentally on mesial and distal of 1st molar for separation for banding procedure; **Fig. 31.3:** Brass wire separator is twisted and tucked between two adjacent teeth for tooth separation

### Use

They are used to create space between the two adjacent teeth for banding procedure.

### Application Procedure

A soft brass wire of 0.5 to 0.6 mm is passed around the contact and the ends are twisted tightly together. The end is made short and then tucked between the teeth (Fig. 31.3).

### Advantage

Ease in application.

### Disadvantages

Disadvantages of brass wire separators are as follows:
a. Soft tissue damage can occur
b. Poor patient acceptance.

### Kesling Metallic Ring Separator

Kesling metallic ring separator is a spring separator.

#### Parts of Kesling Metallic Ring Separator (Fig. 31.4A)

Following are the parts of Kesling metallic ring separator:
- Coil/helix
- Occlusal arm
- Gingival arm
- Retentive arm.

### Use

Kesling metallic ring separators are used to create space interdentally for banding procedure.

*Wire used:* Australian austenitic arch wire of 0.016 round wires.
*Plier used:* Light wire pliers or bird beak pliers or Weingart pliers are used **(Fig. 31.4B)**.
*Placement:* Kesling metallic ring separator is grasped in tight wire pliers and then placed in such a way that coils part of separator should be on buccal side of the teeth **(Fig. 31.4C)**.

### Time Required for Separation

Kesling metallic ring separator brings about separation for banding in about two days.

### Advantage

Space created interdentally is faster as compared to other types of separator.

### Disadvantage

It can be dislodged and can cause tissue damage.
Different types of separators are given in **Table 31.1**.

## ARCH WIRES

Arch wire is one of the active components of fixed orthodontic appliances, which when used, brings about various tooth movements (tipping, bodily, torque, rotational and vertical movements) through the medium of brackets and welded buccal tube on the palatal aspect of the molar bands.

The classification of arch wires is given in **Table 31.2**.

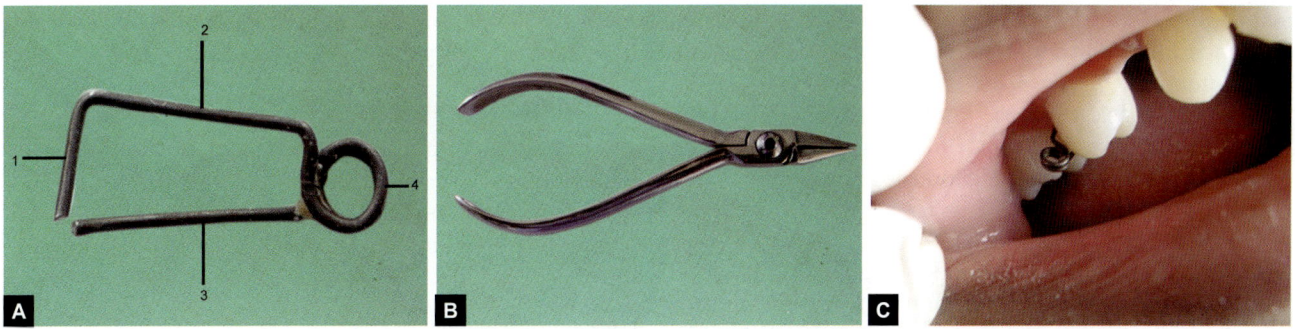

**Figs 31.4A to C:** (A) Parts of Kesling metallic ring separator: 1–Coil/helix, 2–Occlusal arm, 3–Gingival arm, 4–Retentive arm; (B) Light wire pliers; (C) Kesling metallic ring separator is grasped in light wire pliers and then placed in such a way that coils part of separator should be on buccal side of teeth

Table 31.1: Different types of separators

| Types of separators | Wire used | Amount of separations | Time required for separation |
|---|---|---|---|
| Elastic ring separator | Elastic ring | 0.5 mm | Approximately 7 days |
| Dumb-bell separator | Dumb-bell shaped elastic separator | 0.5 mm | Approximately 2–4 days |
| Brass wire separator | 0.5–0.6 mm soft brass wire | 0.5 mm | Approximately 4–5 days |
| Kesling metallic ring separator | 0.016 Australian austenitic arch wire | 0.5 mm | Approximately 2 days |

Table 31.2: Classification of arch wires

| I. Based on material used |
|---|
| 1. Gold and gold alloys |
| 2. Stainless steel |
| 3. Nickel-titanium alloys |
| 4. Beta-titanium |
| 5. Cobalt–Chromium-Nickel alloys |
| 6. Optiflex arch wires |
| II. Based on cross-section (Figs 31.5A to D). |
| 1. Round |
| 2. Square |
| 3. Rectangular |
| 4. Multistranded |

## Gold

Gold alloy were used in the manufacture of orthodontic arch wire. It was intensively used before 1940. Gold and gold alloy arch wire exhibit excellent formability, environmental stability and biocompatibility. The main drawbacks of these arch wires include high-cost, low-spring back and low-yield strength.

## Stainless Steel

Stainless steel was introduced by Wilkinson in 1929. Stainless steel arch wire exhibits adequate strength, high resilience, formability, high stiffness, biocompatibility and are economical.

The drawback of these arch wires includes high modulus of elasticity; more frequent activations are required to maintain the same force level.

## Nickel Titanium Alloys

Nickel titanium alloy, also known by nitinol (Nickel Titanium Naval Ordinance Laboratory) was invented by William R Buchler at Naval Ordinance Laboratory. The main advantage of this alloy over others is the high elasticity and shape-back memory. However, the drawback of these

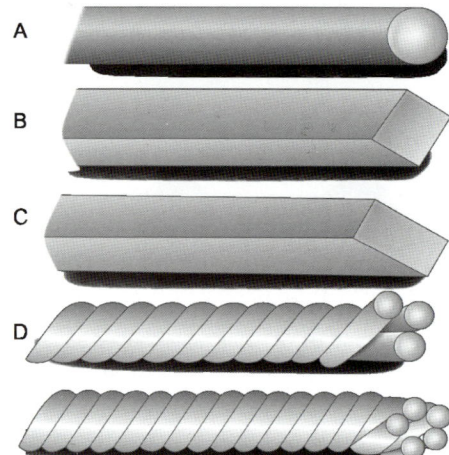

Figs 31.5A to D: Classification of arch wire based on cross-section into: (A) Round; (B) Square; (C) Rectangular; (D) Multistranded

arch wires is that they cannot be welded or soldered and cannot receive bends or loops or helices.

## Beta Titanium or TMA or CAN Wire

Goldberg and CJ Burrstone invented beta titanium and they are also known by TMA or CAN wires. The main advantages of these arch wires include high range of action, high spring back, receive bends, loops and helices and they can be welded or soldered.

## Cobalt-Chromium-Nickel Alloy

Cobalt-Chromium-Nickel alloy is also known as elgiloy. These wires exhibit excellent formability, jointability, spring back and biocompatibility.

## Optiflex Arch Wire

Optiflex arch wire was invented by MF Talass in 1992. Optiflex arch wires are composed of clear optical fibers and are, therefore, highly esthetic. The drawback of these arch wire is that they cannot receive sharp bends.

## Multistrand Arch Wires

Multistranded arch wires are made up of a number of thin wires. They can be round or rectangular and braided or twisted and may have three strands or six strands. The main advantage of these arch wires is that they exhibit increased flexibility.

## Physical Properties of Wires

The first group of properties is concerned with the elastic behavior, which represents the internal stress/strain in the wire. This is produced by an external force deflecting the wire, the stress being the internal load and the strain, the internal distortion.

### Stiffness/Springiness

i. **Pseudoelastic effect:** When an austenitic wire is placed in the mouth and deformed by forcing it into the misaligned brackets, the pseudoelastic effect is induced. This transforms the austenitic alloy into a martensitic state, which as the teeth align, gradually reverses to the austenitic state.

ii. *Thermoelastic effect:* Martensitic active alloys are stable at room temperature, but when raised to mouth temperature, the material changes into an austenitic state, which exhibits shape memory.

- *Martensitic stabilized alloy (e.g. Unitek's Original Nitinol):* The alloy, introduced in 1970 by Andreasen, is stabilized by introducing a certain amount of work hardening during processing and does not show true memory shape properties.
- *Austenitic active alloy:* "Active" means that it exhibits the shape memory, in this case of the pseudoelastic type, the shape memory effect being induced by stress distorting the arch wire in malaligned teeth. Examples of superelastic NiTi are Titanol from Forestadent and Nitinol SE from Unitek.
- *Martensitic active alloy:* Again this exhibits shape memory, but of the thermally activated variety. This alloy is stable at low temperatures but when is placed in the mouth and the temperature increased to mouth temperature, it exhibits the shape memory effect. Examples of thermally activated NiTi are Noe-Sentalloy from GAC and Nitinol XL from Unitek.

### Range of Deflection–Spring Back

The range of wire is the distance it will bend elastically before permanent deformation occurs. If the wire is deflected beyond its yield point, it will not return to its original shape.

### Strength of the Wire

The strength of a wire is important because it determines the maximum force it can deliver.

The above three properties are related by the formula:
Strength = Stiffness × Range.

### Formability

This is the amount of permanent deformation a wire can withstand before it breaks.

### Solubility and Weldability

Stainless steel can be soldered and welded but NiTi cannot. Miura recently reported a method of soldering nickel titanium wires. TMA is weldable as described by Burrstone.

### Friction

The laboratory understanding of friction is not relevant to the clinical situation because every time the patient bites together, the tooth is liable to move a small distance in all three planes of space. More important is the concept that the two components, bracket and wire, may damage each other as they moved across their surfaces. This is evident by the fact that it is difficult to slide teeth with ceramic brackets along a wire, as the abrasiveness of the ceramic notches the surface of the metal.

### Environmental Stability

Any material used for the construction of the wire must be stable in the oral environment. This has been one of the limitations of the esthetics.

### Shape Memory Effect

The shape-memory effect, exhibited by the more recent nickel titanium wires, has revolutionized the selection of wires for appropriate tooth movement. The wires manufactured for orthodontic purposes are composed of an alloy of nearly equal parts of nickel and titanium. The shape memory effect is brought about by a change in the internal crystal formation from the martensitic phase with a hexagonal crystal structure to or from the austenitic phase with a cuboid crystal structure (Kusy, AJO Sep 1991).

The shape in crystalline structure can be brought about by either:

a. Stress, as in the **pseudoelastic effect** in the austenitic active alloy.
b. Heat, as in the **thermoelastic effect** in the Martensitic active alloy where the transition temperature is between room and mouth temperatures.

## SPRINGS

Springs are one of the active components of fixed orthodontic appliance.

### Types of Springs

Followings are the different types of springs:
  I. Uprighting spring
 II. Torquing spring
III. Rotating spring
 IV. Open coil spring
  V. Closed coil spring **(Table 31.3)**.

### Uprighting Springs

Uprighting springs are fabricated from 0.012 or 0.014 inch. Australian austenitic wire using light wire pliers **(Figs 31.6A and B)**. They are used to move the tooth roots in a mesial direction in order to upright the tooth.

They are of two types:

i. Standard design, which can be used with Begg or Tip-edge technique.
ii. Sidewings design, which can be used with only Tip-edge technique.

### Torquing Spring

Torquing springs as the name suggests, bring about torquing movement of the tooth root that is they move root in a labial or lingual direction. They are fabricated from Australian austenitic wire of 0.012 or 0.014 inch using light wire pliers **(Figs 31.7A** and **B)**. Torquing springs are generally used in Begg technique at the finishing phase of the treatment.

**Table 31.3:** Different types of springs and their use

| Types of spring | Use |
|---|---|
| Uprighting spring | For uprighting tooth |
| Torquing spring | For torquing roots of teeth |
| Rotation spring | For derotation of rotated teeth |
| Open coil spring | To open the space between teeth |
| Closed coil spring | To close the space between the teeth |

### Rotating Spring

Rotating springs are used to affect derotation of the rotated teeth. They are often used in conjunction with Begg and Tip-edge techniques. They are made of either stainless steel or nickel titanium alloy (**Figs 31.8A** and **B**). Depending on their design, these springs can bring about clockwise/counterclockwise movement of the teeth.

### Open Coil Spring

Open coil springs, made of stainless steel or nickel titanium alloy, are often used to open up space between the teeth (**Figs 31.9A** to **C**). When an appropriate length of open coil spring is compressed between two/more teeth, space is created between its points of attachment as the coil tries to spring back to its original length. Force applied depends on the length of the spring used, as well as the diameter of the spring.

### Closed Coil Spring

Closed coil springs are also made up of stainless steel or nickel titanium alloy and are used to close spaces between the teeth (**Fig. 31.10**). To effect the closures of space between the two teeth, the closed coil spring of appropriate length is stretched between two teeth. The teeth are moved towards each other as the spring tries to gain its original length.

## ELASTICS

wElastics of latex and nonlatex materials are often used to effect different types of tooth movement in conjunction with fixed mechanotherapy. They are available in various dimensions and strengths and are color coded for easy identification.

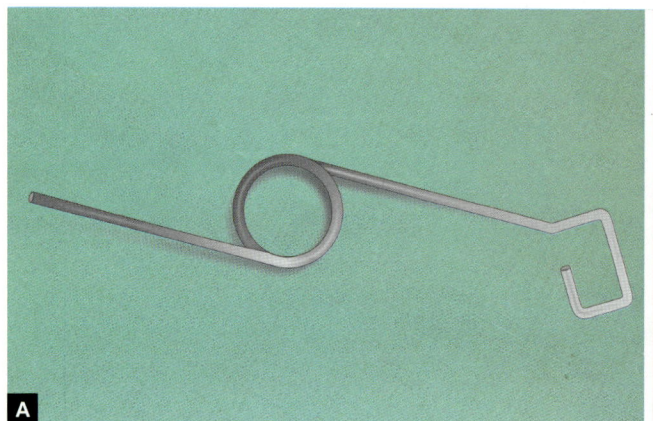
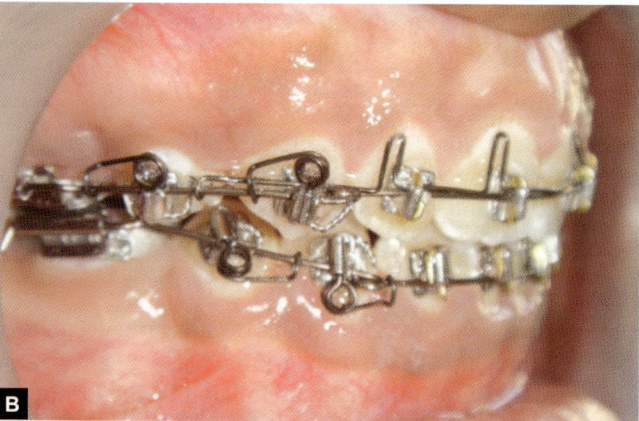

**Figs 31.6A and B:** Uprighting springs are used to move the tooth roots in a mesial direction in order to upright the tooth
[*Courtesy:* Dr Nikunj Patel MDS (Ortho)]

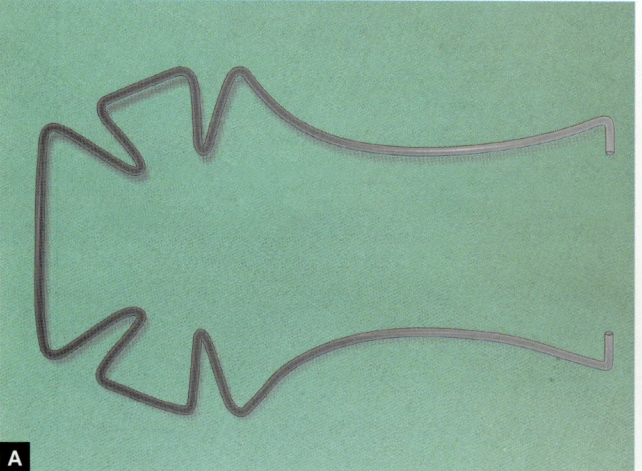
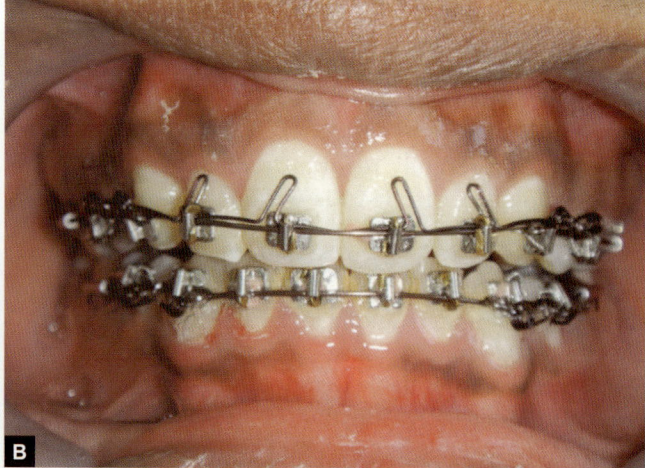

**Figs 31.7A and B:** Torque springs bring about torquing movement of the tooth root, i.e. they move root in a labial or lingual direction
[*Courtesy:* Dr Nikunj Patel MDS (Ortho)]

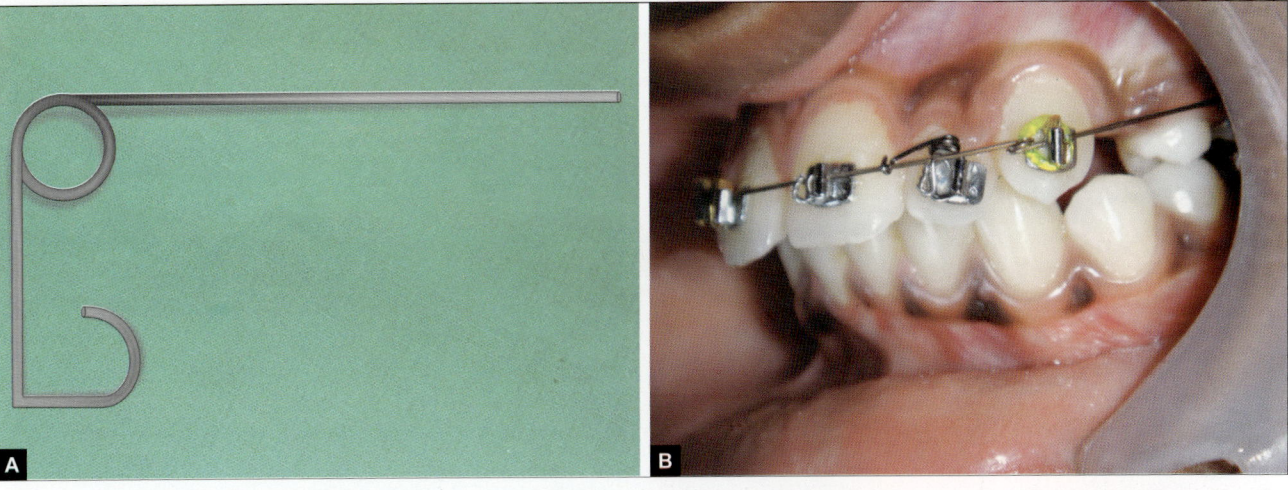

**Figs 31.8A and B:** Rotating springs are used to affect derotation of the rotated teeth. They are often used in conjunction with Begg and tip-edge techniques [*Courtesy:* Dr Nikunj Patel MDS (Ortho)]

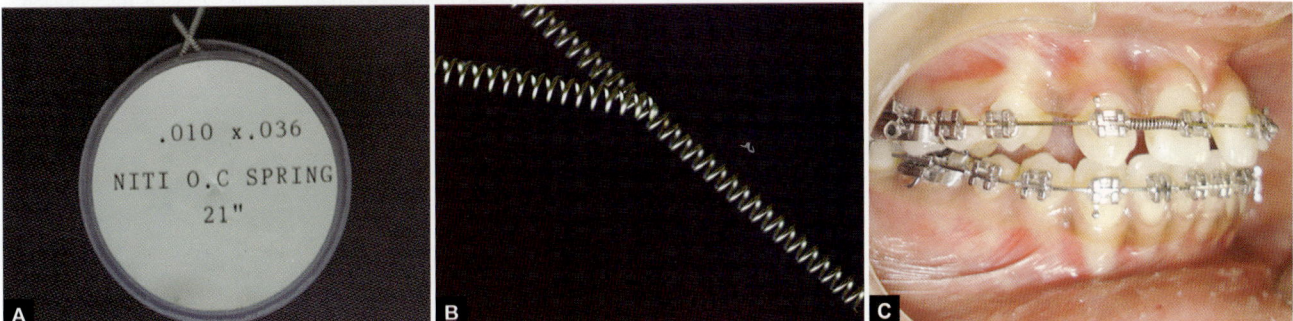

**Figs 31.9A to C:** Open coil springs made of stainless steel or nickel titanium alloy are often used to open up space between the teeth

Various kinds of tooth movements are possible with elastics, such as:
- Closure of spaces,
- Correction of open bites,
- Correction of crossbites, and
- Correction of interarch molar relationship.

Elastics are generally named, depending on the purpose they serve as desired below.

### Class I Elastic
Class I elastics/intra-arch elastics are stretched between molars and anterior of the same arch. They are generally used for closure of spaces and retraction of anterior teeth **(Fig. 31.11)**.

### Class II Elastic
Class II elastics are inter-arch/inter-maxillary elastics placed between the mandibular molars and maxillary anterior. They are generally used in the management of Angle's class II malocclusion. They bring about a reduction in overjet by retracting the maxillary anterior **(Fig. 31.12)**.

### Class III Elastic
These are also intermaxillary elastics, but their attachment between maxillary molars and mandibular anteriors. Class III elastics are generally used in the treatment of Angle's class III malocclusion. They bring about retrusion of mandibular anteriors and protrusion of maxillary anteriors **(Fig. 31.13)**.

### Crossbite Elastic
These intermaxillary elastics are used for the correction of crossbites in posterior region. The tooth in crossbite and its antagonistic tooth, in the opposing arch are engaged with crossbite elastic through the bite **(Figs 31.14A and B)**.

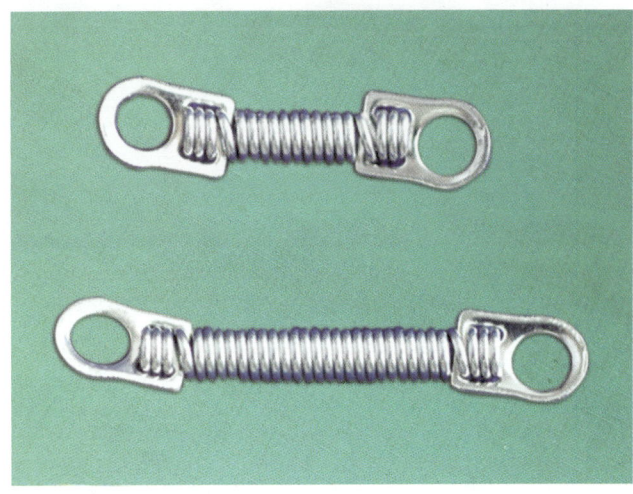

**Fig. 31.10:** Closed coil springs are also made up of stainless steel or nickel titanium alloy and are used to close spaces between the teeth

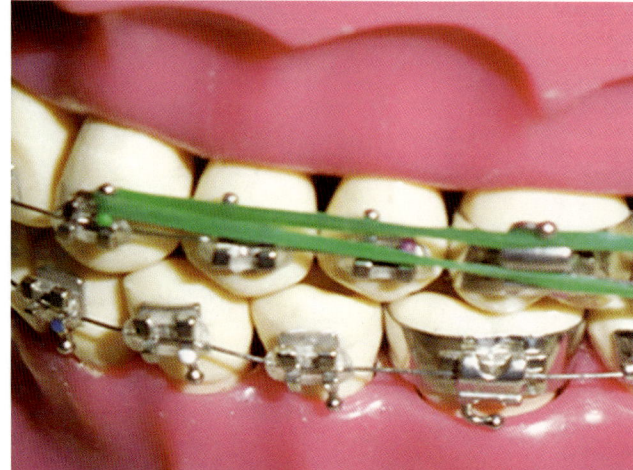

**Fig. 31.11:** Class I elastic/Intra-arch elastic are stretched between molars and anterior of the same arch. They are used in Angle's class I malocclusion

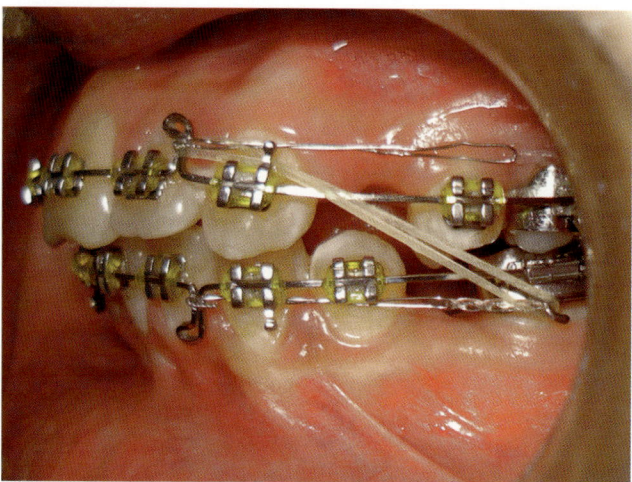

**Fig. 31.12:** Class II elastics are interarch/intermaxillary elastics placed between the mandibular molars and maxillary anterior. They are generally used in the management of Angle's class II malocclusion

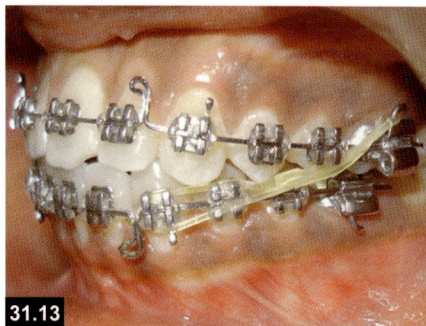
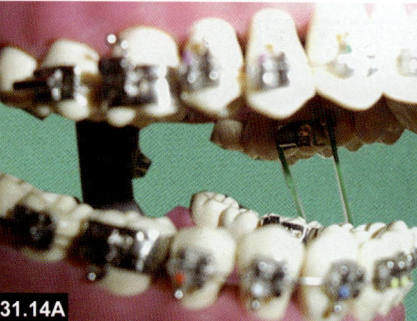
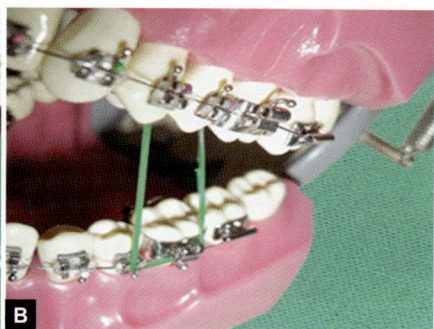

**Fig. 31.13:** Class III elastics, generally used in the treatment of Angle's class III malocclusion; **Figs 31.14A and B:** Crossbite elastics are extended between palatal surfaces of maxillary molars/premolars and buccal surfaces of mandibular molars/premolars or vice versa. They are used for correction of crossbites; (A) Showing placement of elastics; (B) For correction of multiple tooth crossbites

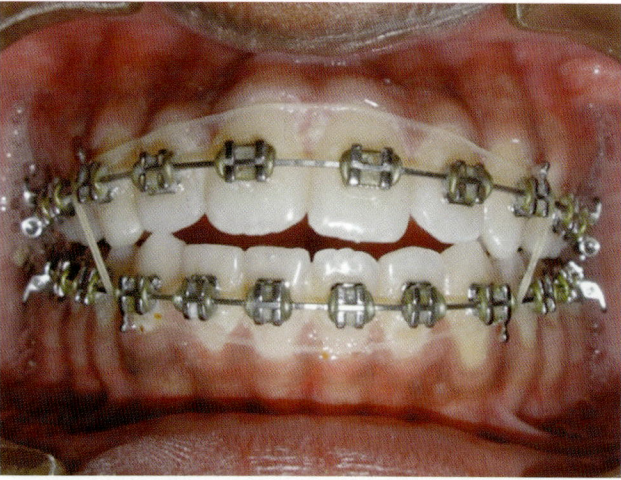

**Fig. 31.15:** Box elastic engages maxillary and mandibular anteriors in a box-like fashion. These elastics are used for correction of anterior open bite cases

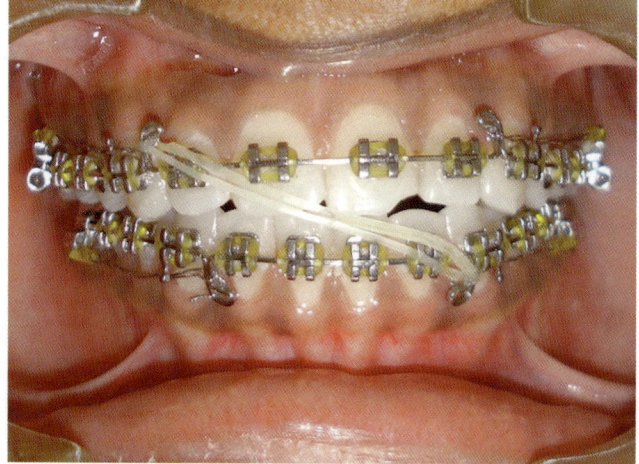

**Fig. 31.16A:** Diagonal elastics are worn diagonally across the maxillary and mandibular anteriors for correction of midline deviations

Depending on the types of crossbite, the elastics are extended between palatal surfaces of maxillary molars/premolars and buccal surfaces of mandibular molars/premolars or vice versa.

## Box Elastics (Fig. 31.15)

These elastics are used for the correction of anterior open bite cases. The elastic engages maxillary and mandibular anteriors in a box-like fashion and brings about the closure

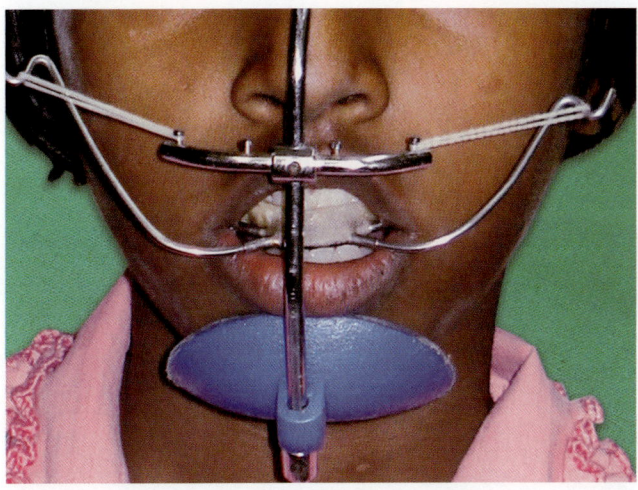

**Fig. 31.17:** The extraoral elastics are sometimes used in conjunction with orthopedic appliance, such as face mask

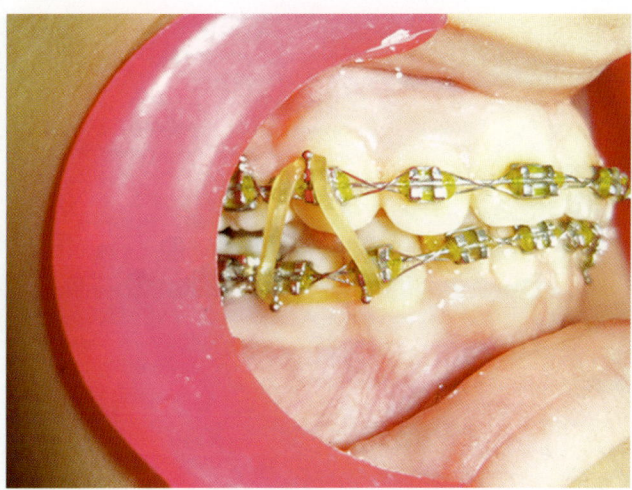

**Fig. 31.16B:** Triangular elastic

| Table 31.4: Elastic chains also known as E-chains are often used for space closure in fixed mechanotherapy. | | | | |
|---|---|---|---|---|
| **Types of elastics** | **Figures** | **Description of the elastics** | **Action of elastics** | **Used in** |
| Class I elastic | Fig. 31.11 | Stretched from molar to canine in the same arch | Brings about space closure | Angle's class I malocclusion |
| Class II elastic | Fig. 31.12 | Stretched from upper canine to lower molar | Brings about retraction of upper anteriors and protrusion of lower anteriors | Angle's class II malocclusion |
| Class III elastic | Fig. 31.13 | Stretched from upper molar to lower canine | Brings about retraction of lower anteriors and protrusion of upper anteriors | Angle's class III malocclusion |
| Crossbite elastic | Figs 31.14A and B | Elastics are extended between the palatal surfaces of maxillary molars/premolars and buccal surfaces of mandibular molars/premolars or vice versa | Buccal movement of upper molar and lingual movement of lower molar | Crossbite in the posterior region |
| Box elastic | Fig. 31.15 | The elastic engages maxillary and mandibular anteriors in a box like fashion | Brings about closure of the bite by effecting forced eruption of maxillary and mandibular anteriors | Open bite cases |
| Diagonal elastic | Fig. 31.16A | Worn diagonally across the maxillary and mandibular anteriors | Mesial movement of one incisors and distal movement of another incisor | Closure of midline diastema |
| Triangular elastic | Fig. 31.16B | Worn in the form of triangle involving three teeth | Brings about mild extrusion of upper and lower teeth | Cuspal interdigitation |
| Extraoral elastic | Fig. 31.17 | | Brings about extrusion and distal movement of molars | Used in conjunction with extraoral appliance, such as face mask, headgear |

of the bite by effecting the forced eruption of maxillary and mandibular anteriors.

### Diagonal Elastic (Fig. 31.16A)

These are worn diagonally across the maxillary and mandibular anteriors for the correction of midline deviations.

### Triangular Elastics (Fig. 31.16B)

These are worn in the form of triangle involving three teeth, for example, involving one tooth in maxillary arch and two teeth in the mandibular arch or one tooth in mandibular form and two teeth in the maxillary arch. These types of elastics are used for cuspal interdigitation and are used with fixed mechanotherapy in finishing phase of fixed orthodontic treatment.

### Extra-oral Elastics (Fig. 31.17)

The extraoral elastics are sometimes used in conjunction with extraoral appliance, such as face mask. These exert forces ranging from 8 Oz to 14 Oz.

Different types of elastics and their uses are given in **Table 31.4**.

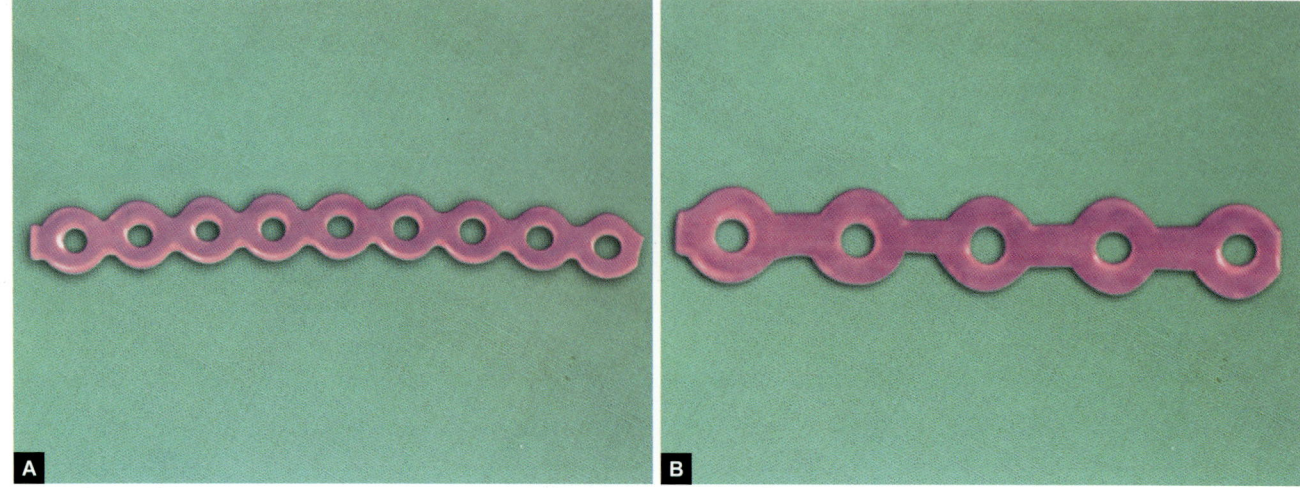

**Figs 31.18A and B:** Elastomerics in orthodontics are made up of synthetic polyurethane material are often used with fixed orthodontic appliances for space closure; (A) Short E-chain; (B) Long E-chain

## ELASTOMERICS

Elastomerics in orthodontics are made up of synthetic polyurethane material, are often used with fixed orthodontic appliances. The various forms of elastomerics are as follows:
1. Elastic chain/E-chain
2. Elastic thread
3. Elastic ligature
4. Elastic modules

### Elastic Chain/E-Chain

Elastic chains also known as E-chains are often used for space closure in fixed mechanotherapy.

They are available in various strengths, depending on the distance between the adjacent rings:
1. Continuous E-chain: Distance between the rings is conti-nuous.
2. Short E-chain: Distance between the rings is short **(Fig. 31.18A)**.
3. Long E-chain: Distance between the rings is long **(Fig. 31.18B)**.

### Elastic Thread

Elastic thread made of special elasticized cotton is sometimes used along with fixed orthodontic appliances for consolidation of anterior spacing **(Fig. 31.19)**.

### Elastic Ligature

These are elastic rings, which are used to secure the arch wire in the brackets **(Figs 31.20A to C)**. They are available in different colors.

### Elastic Module/Elastomeric Links

Elastic modules or elastomeric links are two elastic rings separated by a variable distance.

They are generally used for space closure and derotation of teeth.

## MAGNETS

Magnets can be used in conjunction with fixed orthodontic appliances in their attraction mode to effect space closure and in repulsion mode for regaining lost space between the teeth. Magnets commonly used are:
- Samarium cobalt magnet
- Neodymium-iron-boron magnet.

### Passive Components

Passive components are those components of fixed orthodontic appliances, which by themselves, are not capable of generating tooth moving forces but help providing attachment for other auxiliaries to the tooth.

### Bands

Bands are passive components that provide space for fixing various attachments onto the teeth **(Fig. 31.21A)**. They are generally made of soft stainless steel. Weldable brackets

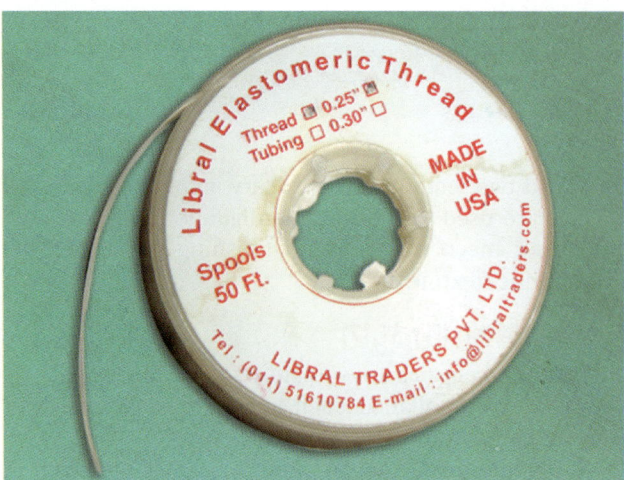

**Fig. 31.19:** Elastic thread

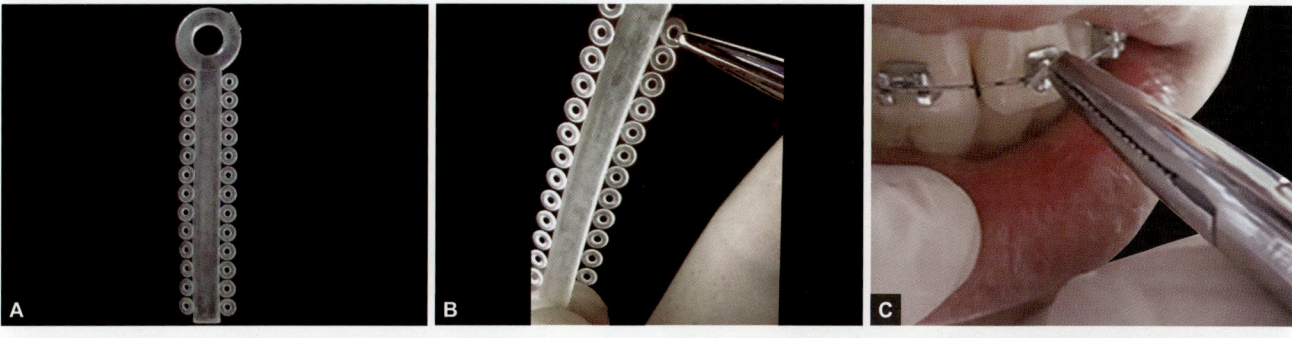

**Figs 31.20A to C:** Elastic ligatures are elastic rings, which are used to secure the arch wire in the brackets. (A) Elastic modules in a key; (B) Deattaching the module from the key using Weingart pliers; (C) Placing module on the bracket using Weingart pliers

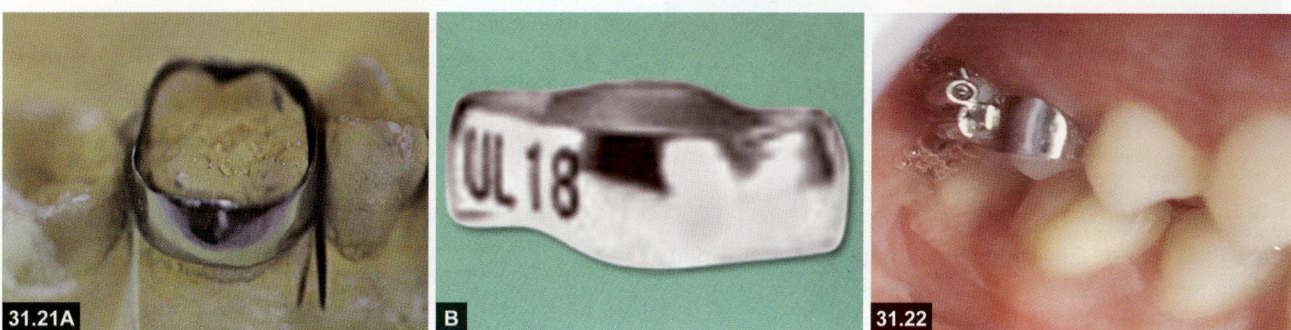

**Figs 31.21A and B:** (A) Custom-made band; (B) Preformed band; **Fig. 31.22:** Direct banding procedure: Where bands are fabricated as a chair-side procedure, in presence of the patient

buccal tubes and other auxiliary attachments are soldered or welded over the bands, which are then cemented around the intended teeth.

### Availability

1. Custom-made bands are fabricated using band materials, which are available in the form of spools **(Fig. 31.21A)**.
2. Preformed seamless bands are available in different sizes, which can be directly cemented around the tooth **(Fig. 31.21B)**. Preformed bands are increasingly being used in recent years.

Different width and thickness of stainless steel strips are given in **Table 31.5**.

### Banding Procedures

Bands are fabricated by the following any of the two ways:

### Direct Banding Procedure

Where bands are fabricated as a chair side procedure, with presence of the patient **(Fig. 31.22)**.

### Indirect Banding Procedure

In this procedure, bands are fabricated on the diagnostic cast of the patient in the laboratory **(Fig. 31.23)**.

### Steps in Banding (Figs 31.24A to Q)

### Step 1: Separation of Teeth

Teeth have to be separated so as to create adequate space for the placement of the band. Any of the different separators described earlier can be used for the purpose and may take 24 hours or more to effect the separation of interdental contact depending on type of separator used.

### Step 2: Selection of Band Material

Band material of appropriate width and thickness is selected depending on the type of tooth to be banded.

### Step 3: Pinching of the Band

Band material of adequate length is taken and two ends are assembled and then welded together using a spot welder. The band is then passed through separated interdental contacts of the tooth to be banded. Using band pinch able pliers, the band is tightly drawn around the tooth to form a ring and pinched. The pinched band is removed from the tooth and welded close to the pinched ends. The excess band material is then cut off and the ends are adapted close to the band and the bent portion is spot welded. The margins are smoothened and gingival contouring is done on the material and distal gingival margins.

**Table 31.5:** The stainless steel strips are available in different widths and thickness to suit different teeth

| Teeth | Band thickness (inches) | Band width |
|---|---|---|
| Incisor | 0.003 | 0.125 |
| Canine | 0.003 | 0.150 |
| Premolar | 0.003 | 0.150 |
| Molar | 0.005 | 0.018 |
| | 0.006 | 0.018 |

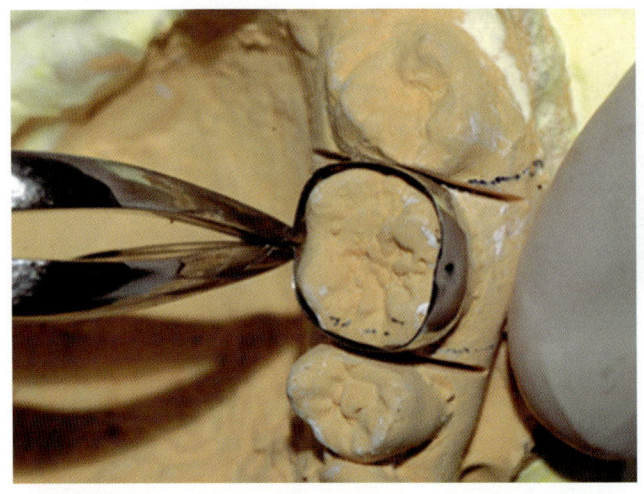

**Fig. 31.23:** Indirect banding procedure: In this procedure, bands are fabricated on the diagnostic cast of the patient

### Step 4: Fixing the Attachments

Once the band fabrication is complete, appropriate attachments are selected and welded on the buccal/palatal surface of the band according to the need.
Attachments include:
1. A bracket of weldable type
2. Buccal tubes often used on a molar band
3. Lingual attachments
   a. Lingual buttons
   b. Lingual sheath
   c. Lingual cleats
   d. Lingual eyelets
   e. Lingual ball and hooks
   f. Seating lugs.

From buccal or labial aspect, seated band should allow visualization of cusps of the tooth to be banded and it should be in the middle third of the tooth.

### Step 5: Cementation of the Band

#### Lingual Attachments

Brackets and buccal tubes are usually placed on buccal aspect of the teeth. Sometimes, attachments may also be needed on the lingual surface of the tooth for example, for engaging the elastics. Their attachments can be weldable or bondable. Classification of various forms of lingual attachments are available and are described below.
a. Lingual buttons
b. Lingual sheath
c. Lingual cleats
d. Lingual eyelets
e. Lingual ball and hooks
f. Lingual seating lugs

a. Lingual Buttons **(Flowchart 31.3) (Figs 31.25A and B)**
   - Buttons with different base shapes are available for attachment of elastics/elastomerics can be weldable bond.
   - Flat based ones are for centering on molars.
   - Curved ones for mesial/distal placement on molars and extra-curved ones are used on premolars.

b. Lingual sheaths **(Flowchart 31.4) (Fig. 31.26)**

Lingual sheaths may be weldable/bondable and are used for attaching accessories, such as transpalatal arches, Quad helix, NITI molar rotators and expanders.

c. Lingual Cleats **(Flowchart 31.5) (Figs 31.27A and B)**

These are available in weldable/bondable forms, are welded/bonded in the center with the ends being open. They are also used for engaging elastics/elastomerics.

d. Lingual Eyelets **(Fig. 31.28)**

They are hollow in the center and their two sides are welded. These are used for tying elastic threads/ligature wires.

e. Lingual Ball End Hooks **(Fig. 31.29)**

There are small balls attached to weldable flat arm. They are used to engage elastic/elastomerics from lingual aspect.

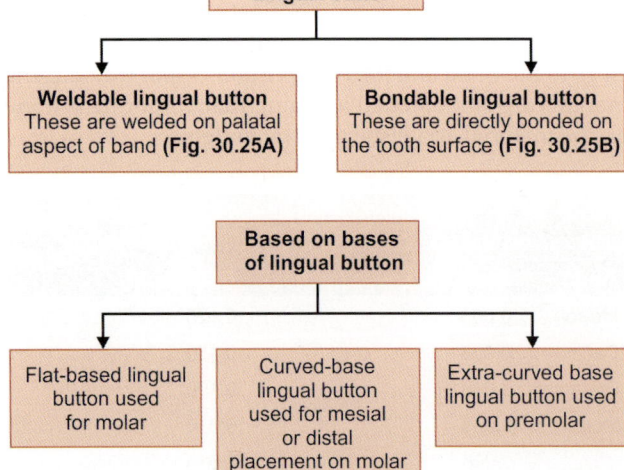

**Flowchart 31.3:** Classification of lingual button

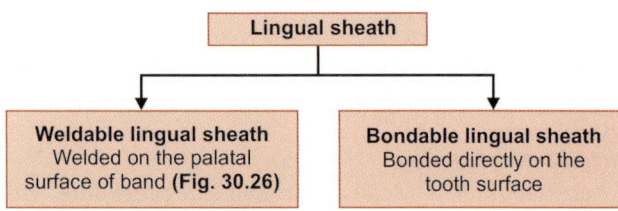

**Flowchart 31.4:** Types of lingual sheath

**Flowchart 31.5:** Types of lingual cleat

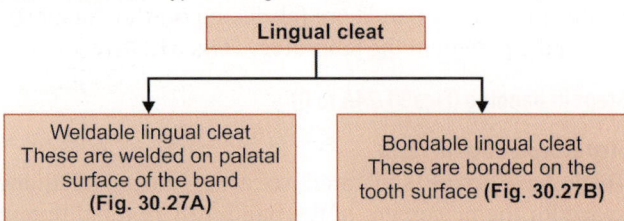

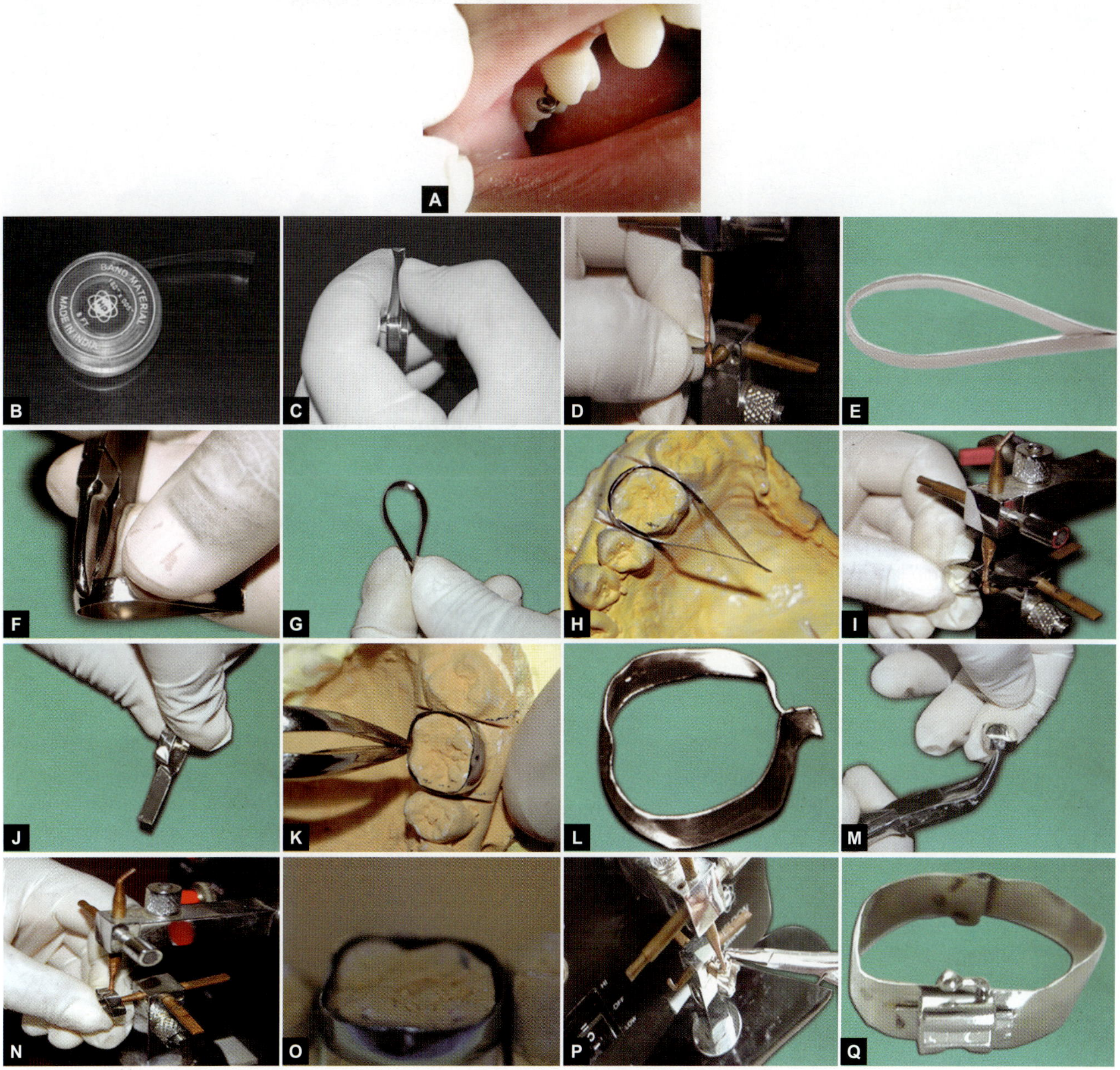

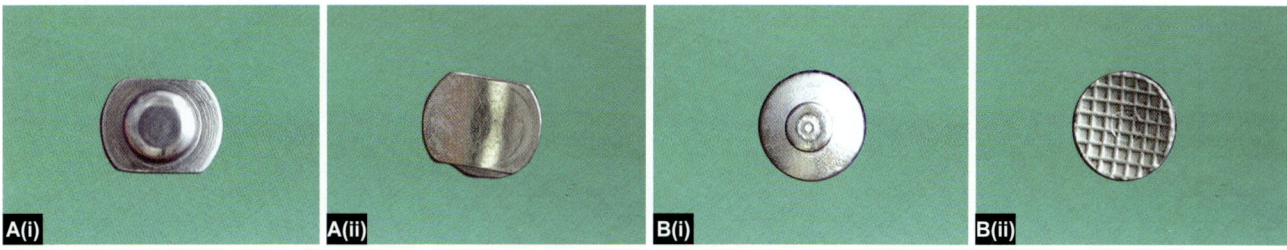

**Figs 31.24A to Q:** (A) Kesling metallic ring separator is placed interdentally; (B) Molar band material; (C) Band material of adequate length is taken and then assembled; (D and E) Assembled ends of band are welded using spot-welder; (F) Contoured the band material; (G) Appearance of band material after complete contouring using band contouring plains; (H) Contoured band material placed on the tooth to be bounded; (I) Pinching the band using band pinchable plier; (J) Pinched band is removed from the tooth and welded close to the pinched ends; (K) Excess band material is then cut off using band cutting scissors; (L) Ends of band are adapted close to the band; (M and N) The bent portions is again welded using spot-welder; (O) Completed band; (P) Welding buccal tube to the band; (Q) Appearance of band after welding buccal tube

**Figs 31.25A and B:** (A) Weldable lingual button; (B) Bondable lingual button

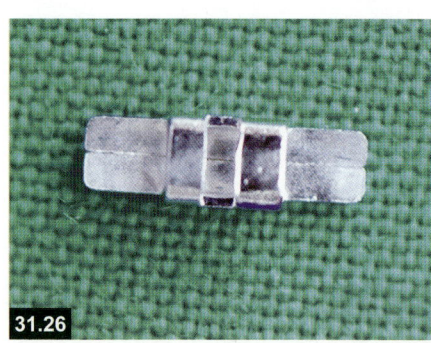
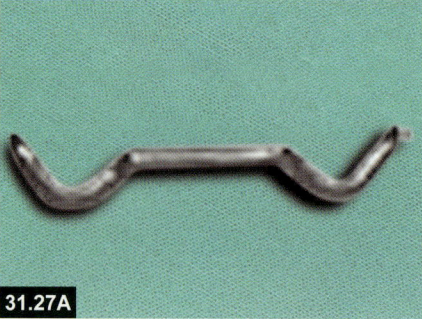
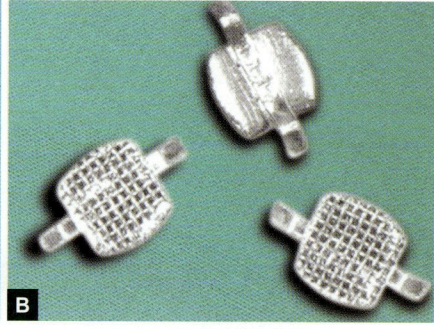

**Fig. 31.26:** Weldable lingual sheath; **Figs 31.27A and B:** (A) Weldable lingual cleat; (B) Bondable lingual cleat

f. Lingual Seating Lugs **(Fig. 31.30)**

Lingual seating lugs are helpful in the placement of the bands.

Based on the base: Lingual seating lugs, based on its base, are of two types:
1. *Flat:* Used for anteriors and molars
2. *Curved:* Used for cuspids and bicuspids.
   *Use:* These help in seating of the bands.

## BRACKETS

Brackets are passive components, which provide a means of transferring tooth moving forces from arch wires, elastics and other active components of fixed orthodontic appliances.

They can be welded to the bands, which are then cemented onto the teeth (weldable brackets). Bondable brackets being increasingly used in recent years, although weldable ones have to be opted in some cases.

Brackets manufactured from a variety of materials are available and they can be of various designs suitable for different orthodontic techniques.

Brackets can be classified in a number of ways as listed below:

I. **Depending on material used for manufacture**
   1. Metal brackets
      i. Gold
      ii. Stainless steel
      iii. Titanium
   2. Plastic brackets
   3. Ceramic brackets
II. **Depending on mode of attachment**
   1. Weldable brackets
   2. Bondable brackets
III. **Depending on technique for which they are used**
   1. Ribbon arch brackets
   2. Begg's modified ribbon arch brackets
   3. Tip-edge brackets
   4. Edgewise brackets
   5. Preadjusted Edgewise brackets
   6. Lingual brackets

### I.1. Metal brackets

- Metal brackets are routinely used in orthodontic practice of which steel brackets are the most frequently used. Although biocompatible, gold brackets are expensive **(Fig 31.31)**.
- Titanium brackets are recently introduced and have high biocompatibility and low friction.

*Advantages of metal brackets:*

These include–
a. They can be sterilized.
b. They can be recycled.
c. They resist deformation and fracture.
d. Exhibit less friction with the arch wire.
e. They are comparatively less expensive (cost-effective).

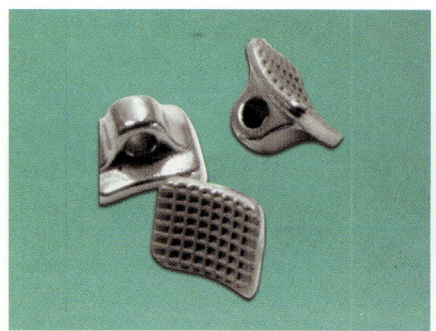
**Fig. 31.28:** Lingual eyelet

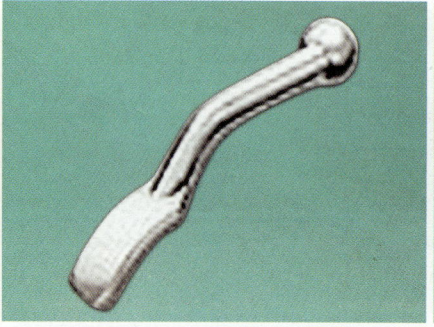
**Fig. 31.29:** Lingual ball-end hook

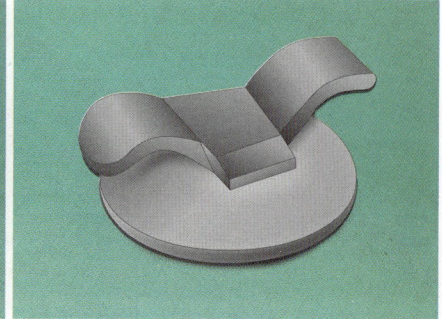
**Fig. 31.30:** Lingual seating lugs

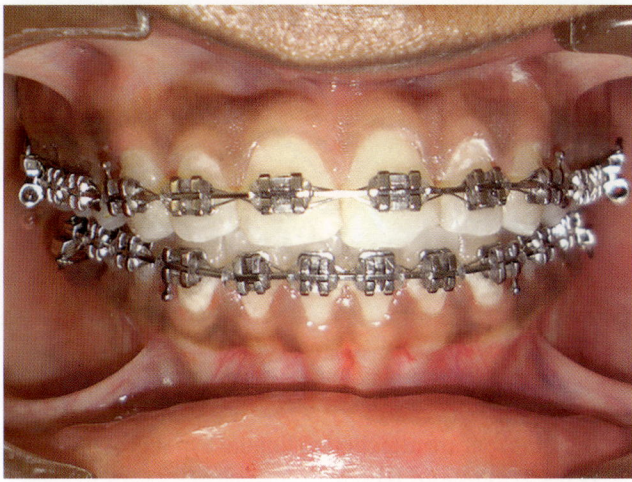

Fig. 31.31: Metal brackets

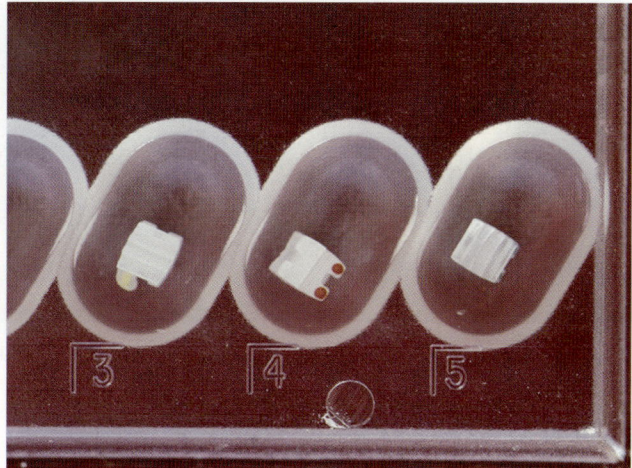

Fig. 31.32: Plastic brackets

***Disadvantages:***
These include–
   a. Easily noticeable, metallic brackets are esthetically not pleasant
   b. They may corrode and cause staining of the teeth.

### I.2. Plastic brackets
Plastic brackets made of polycarbonate and other related materials were introduced to improve esthetics (**Fig. 31.32**). However, they are not preferred as they have a number of disadvantages, such as:
1. They tend to get discolored easily, especially in patients who smoke or drink coffee, tea, etc.
2. They have poor dimensional stability
3. Their slots tend to distort
4. There is a high amount of friction between plastic bracket and metal archwire.

### I.3. Ceramic brackets
Ceramic brackets were introduced in 1987 and offer a good alternative when esthetics is a major concern while undergoing orthodontic treatment. Transparent and opaque tooth colored ceramic brackets are available and are generally made of alumina or zirconium-based products (**Figs 31.33A** and **B**).

***Advantages of ceramic brackets are:***
1. They are highly esthetic and not easily noticeable
2. Resist discoloration unlike plastic brackets
3. Dimensionally stable, do not distort in oral cavity

***Disadvantages***
These include:
1. They are very brittle and thus tend to fracture easily during active treatment and also while debonding.
2. Exhibit greater friction at wire/bracket interface than metallic brackets.
3. High cost of material, and are highly expensive.

### II.1. Weldable brackets
- They are either welded or soldered to the band, which is then cemented over the teeth (**Fig. 31.34**).

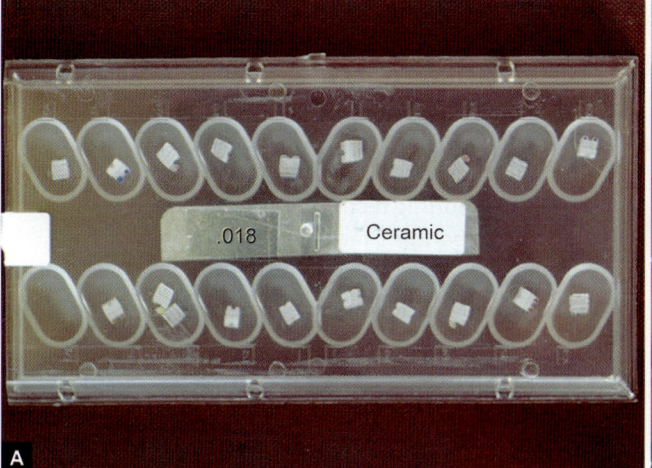

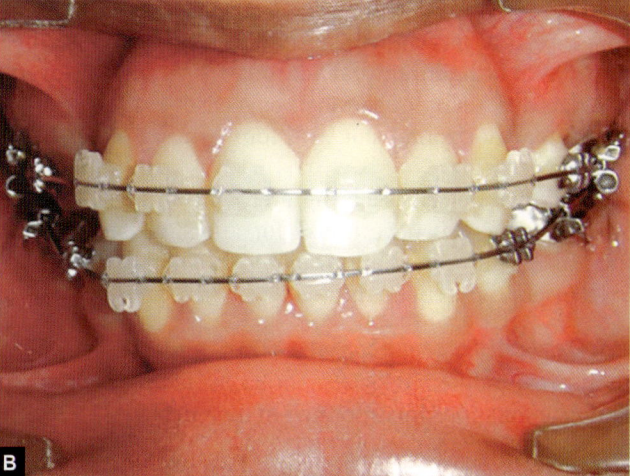

Figs 31.33A and B: Ceramic brackets

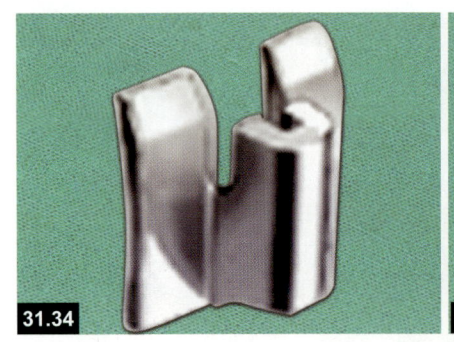 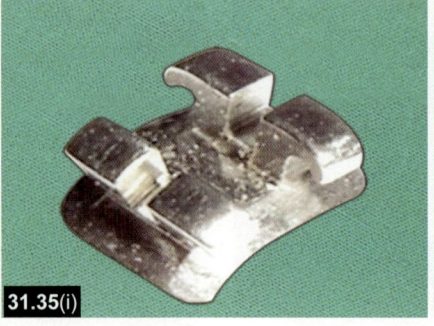 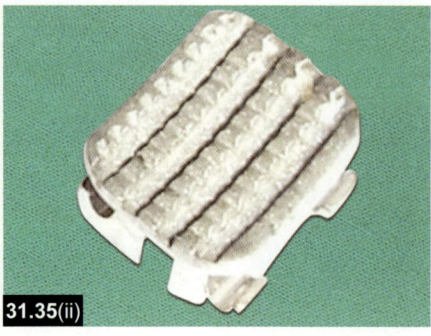

**Fig. 31.34:** Weldable brackets; **Figs 31.35(i and ii):** Bondable brackets

- Weldable brackets have metal flanges on the base to facilitate welding.

### II.2. Bondable brackets

- They are directly bonded onto the teeth using bonding adhesives **(Fig. 31.35)**.
- Base of these brackets generally exhibit meshwork or indentations to facilitate bonding with the adhesive material.

### III.1. Ribbon arch brackets

- Ribbon arch brackets had a simple design with occlusally facing vertical slot in it.
- They were used in ribbon arch technique.

### III.2. Modified ribbon arch/Brackets in Begg technique

- Begg technique uses modified ribbon arch brackets in which the vertical slot is facing gingivally rather than occlusally.
- This modification allowed easy tipping of the teeth.

### III.3. Tip-edge brackets

They are used in the tip-edge technique. The bracket design is a modification of the conventional edgewise bracket where two diagonally opposite corners of the conventional edgewise bracket slot are removed and a vertical rectangular slot is also added.

### III.4. Edgewise brackets

Edgewise brackets and their modifications become the mainstay in orthodontic practice today. They are employed in Edgewise technique. Most edgewise brackets have rectangular horizontal slot with four wings, two gingival and two occlusal.

The rings help in securing arch wire in the slot and brackets may also have hooks for attaching auxiliaries, such as elastics. They are available as a set of different brackets for different teeth.

### III.5. Preadjusted edgewise brackets

They are modified edgewise brackets with inbuilt tip, torque angulations incorporated in their design.

### III.6. Lingual brackets

- They are used in lingual orthodontic technique where the brackets are attached to lingual aspects of the teeth **(Figs 31.36A and B)**.
- Indirect bonding procedure is preferred for attaching these onto the teeth, due to inadequate visibility of lingual aspects.

### Buccal Tubes

Buccal tubes are also referred as molar tubes.
I. Buccal tubes can be classified into the following two types based on the mode of attachment.
   1. Weldable buccal tubes: Weldable buccal tubes have a flat contoured metal flange base and are welded to the bands that are cemented on the molars.
   2. Bondable buccal tubes: The bondable buccal tube has a mesh base and is bonded directly to the tooth surface.

Buccal tubes can be welded to the bands or directly bonded to the tooth surface **(Flowchart 31.6)**.
II. Based on number of tubes, they can be classified as
   1. Single buccal tube
   2. Double buccal tube
   3. Triple buccal tube.
III. Buccal tubes are of two types based on their shape in the cross-section:
   1. Round
   2. Flat-oval.

### Orthodontic Bonding

***The basic mechanism of bonding teeth:*** The term bonding in dentistry is used to describe the attachment of the bracket using bonding resins to the enamel surfaces.

***Classification of orthodontic bonding:*** Orthodontic bonding can be classified into the following two types:
   i. Direct bonding technique
   ii. Indirect bonding technique

No matter which technique is used, the basic mechanism of bonding has remained the same and involves prophylaxis, enamel surface preparation—enamel etching and bonding the bracket to the enamel surface.

***Prophylaxis:*** Enamel prophylaxis before etching has been shown to result in maximum bond strength. This procedure removes oral debris, pellicle, and accentuates the irregularities present in the natural enamel and enhances

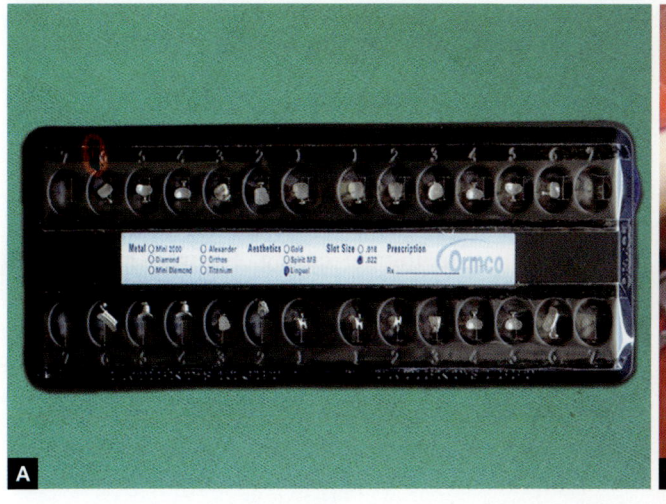 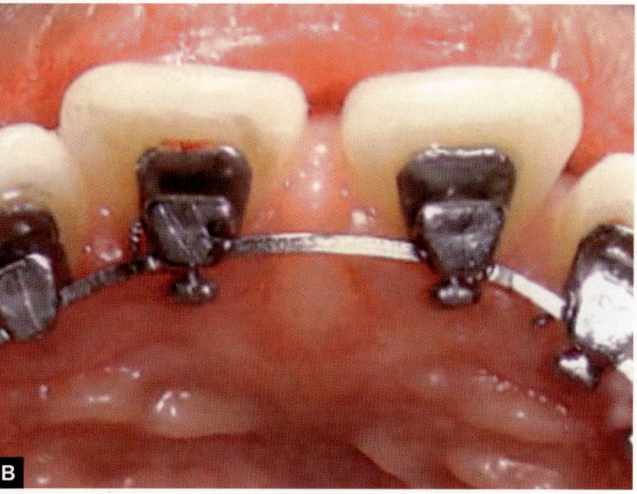

**Figs 31.36A and B:** Lingual brackets

the wetting of the enamel surface by the acid. Scaling is done to remove any calculus on teeth surface **(Fig. 31.37)**. Later, polishing is carried out using a polishing brushes **(Fig. 31.38A)** or rubber cup **(Fig. 31.38B)**, and thin slurry of medium of grain pumice powder, or prophylactic paste **(Figs 31.39A and B)** and water on slow-speed handpiece. Teeth after prophylaxis enhance bond strength **(Fig. 30.40)**.

### Isolation and Moisture Control

The prepared enamel surface requires proper isolation and moisture control for successful bonding. Isolation of moisture control is done by using chick retractors and a plastic bite block to open the bite and saliva ejectors.

### Enamel Etching

Following proper isolation and moisture control, the tooth or segment of teeth to be etched are dried using an oil and moisture-free air source. This procedure is carried out with 35% unruffled phosphoric acid and the etching time should be between 15 and 31 minutes **(Fig. 31.41)**. The etched surface should have a highly frosted, matte, dull or whitish appearance **(Figs 31.42A and B)**.

### Bracket Positioning

Preadjusted appliances have built-in adjustments in the bracket slot required to facilitate achieving the proper position of the individual teeth. These adjustments include mesiodistal tip, labiolingual torque and in-out horizontal movement. However, these brackets work properly when they are positioned accurately on the individual teeth. Individual bracket on the tooth should be positioned in such a way that they are at center of the clinical crown mesiodistally.

### Bonding Material

There are three types of filled acrylic–(BIS-GMA) based composite resins available for orthodontic bonding depending on the mode of polymerization curing (chemically cured, light-cured and a combination of thermal and chemically cured).

### (i) Direct Bonding

The direct bonding technique refers to the direct attachment of orthodontic appliances to etched teeth using chemically and light-cured adhesives. The initial steps with the direct bonding technique involves prophylaxis, isolation of the arches to be bonded, cheek retraction with tongue restraint and enamel etching.

Steps of direct bonding technique are as follows:

1. Enamel surface preparation is performed **(Figs 31.42 and 31.43)**.
2. Unfilled liquid sealant is applied to the bracket base and the etched tooth surface.

**Flowchart 31.6:** Classification of buccal tubes

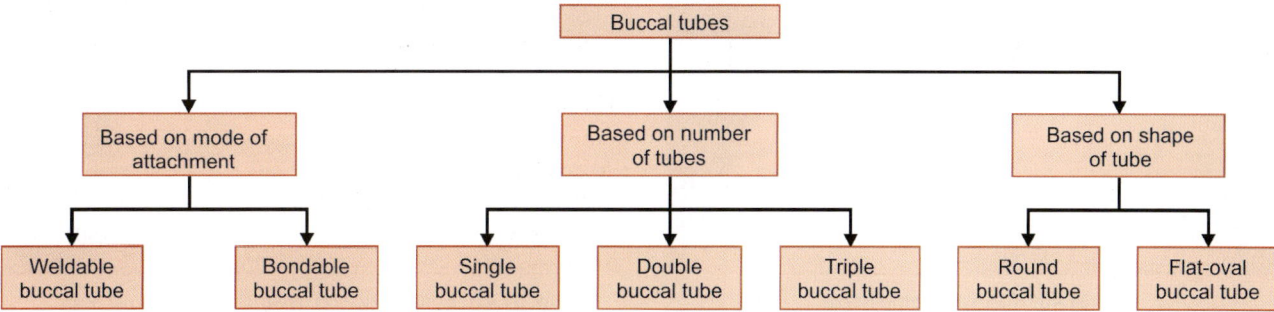

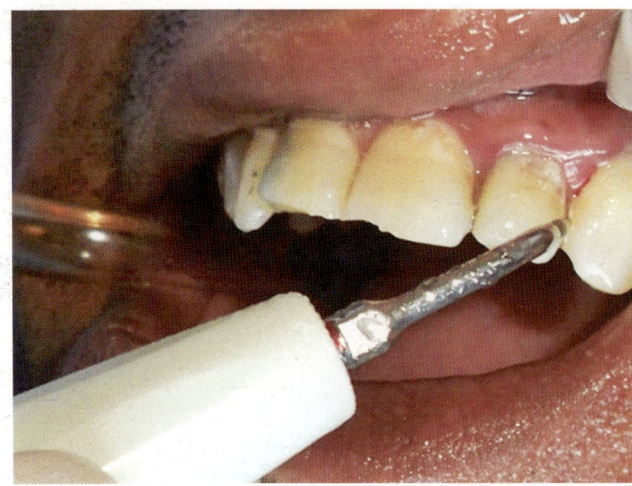

Fig. 31.37: Scaling using ultrasonic scaler

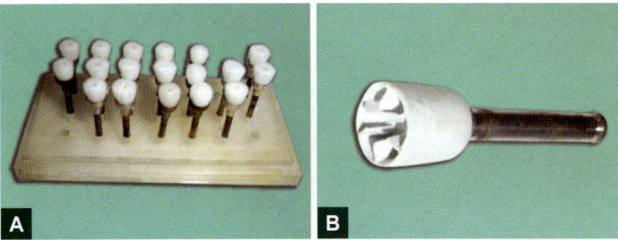

Figs 31.38A and B: (A) Prophylactic brushes; (B) Rubber cup

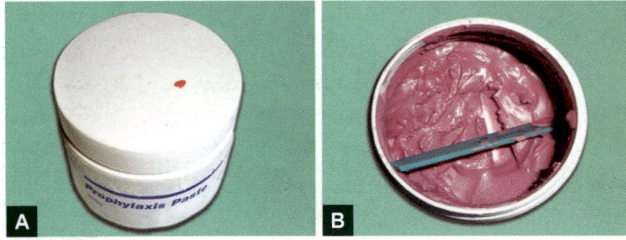

Figs 31.39A and B: Prophylactic paste

3. Filled resin paste is applied on the base of the bracket and carried to tooth surface using bracket holder **(Fig. 31.43A)**.
4. The resin-loaded bracket is placed on the tooth surface **(Fig. 31.43B)** and the excess resin is removed before setting the material. The desired bracket position is confirmed and the bracket slot height is verified using a gauge. Light–cured resin requires a light source to initiate curing. **Figure 31.44** shows bonding and brackets completed and arch wires are secured.

### (ii) Indirect Bonding

In this procedure precise positioning of brackets is done on the sutdy models rather than directly on patients' teeth. Impression of study models is taken with brackets. Brackets are then transferred onto the teeth and cured. This method is usually used for lingual ortho appliances.

### Ligature Wires

- Ligature wires are soft stainless steel wires of 0.008 to 0.010 inch in diameter **(Fig. 31.45)**. These may be used to secure the arch wire in the slot of bracket or to tie the segment of teeth together.
- Ligature wire can also be placed in the fashion of figure of eight around the bracket to prevent opening of space between.

## LOCK PINS

Lock pins **(Fig. 31.46)** are mainly used in Begg's technique for securing arch wire in the ribbon arch/bracket. Lock pins are made up of brass or soft stainless steel.

Lock pins are of the following types based on their use in the stages of Begg's technique:
1. Stage I
2. Stage II
3. Stage III.

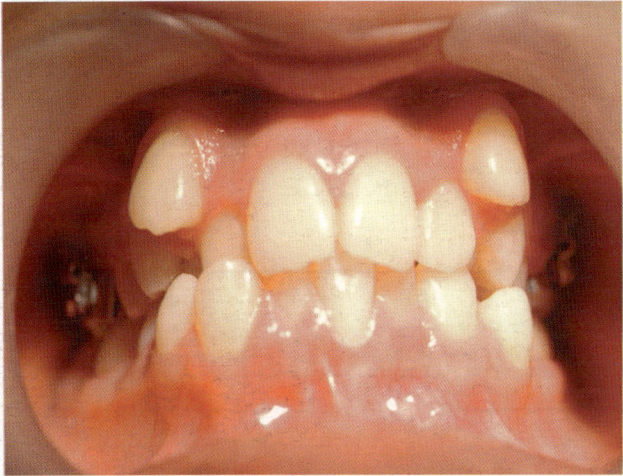

Fig. 31.40: Teeth after prophylaxis

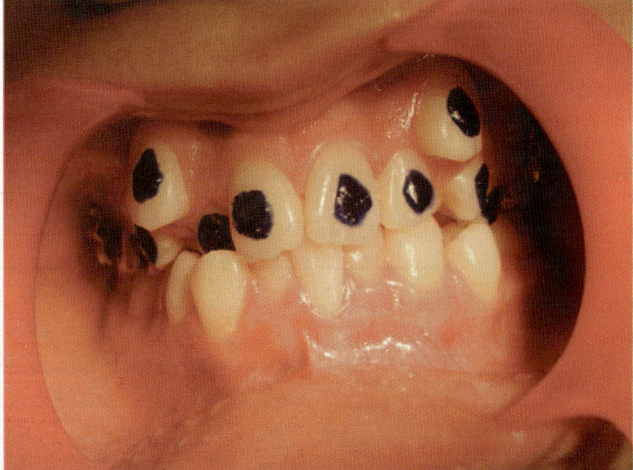

Fig. 31.41: Enamel etching using 35% phosphoric acid

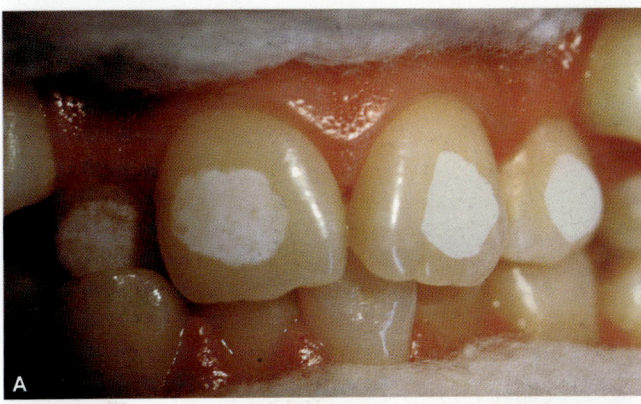 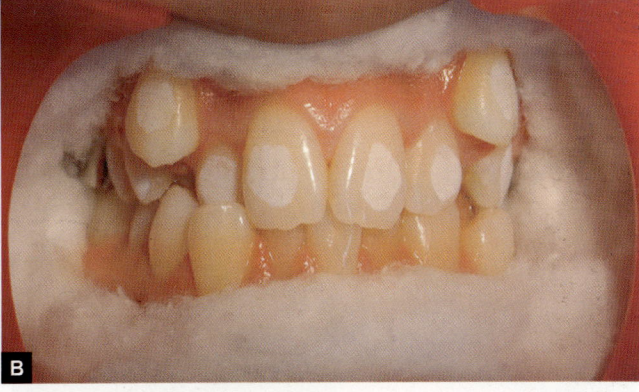

**Figs 31.42A and B:** Frosted, matte, dull or whitish appearance after electing

## FIXED ORTHODONTIC APPLIANCE TECHNIQUES

### E-Arch Appliance

E-arch appliance was developed by Angle in early 1900. It is also referred to as Edward Angle's E-arch. It was the first Angle's orthodontic appliance developed to treat malocclusions. E-arch appliance consists of bands, which are placed on molar teeth on either side of the arch of a heavy labial arch wire extended around the arch. The ends of labial extended arch wire threaded to the buccal aspect of the molar bands allowed the arch wire to be advanced so that the arch perimeter increased. Individual teeth were ligated with the heavy labial extended arch wire with the ligature wire of 0.010 inch.

*Advantage:* It is simple in design.
*Disadvantages:* These include:
1. Poor oral hygiene maintenance.
2. Poor patient compliance/acceptance.

*Force:* The E-arch appliance can deliver only heavy-interrupted force.

*Tooth movement:* The E-arch appliance brings about the tippling movement of the malposed teeth to the line of occlusion.

### Pin and Tube Appliance

Pin and tube appliance was also developed by Edward H Angle. In this pin and tube appliance, all teeth are banded. Vertical tubes were welded to the bands on the labial surface in the center of the crown for all teeth in the arch. Arch wires were secured with soldered pins that inserted into the vertical tubes. Tooth movement was achieved by altering the placement of these pins. Pin and tube appliance is also used for treating malocclusions.

*Advantage:* This appliance brings about bodily movement of teeth.

*Disadvantages:* These include:
1. This appliance is complex in design. Tedious to fabricate.
2. Poor oral hygiene maintenance as all the teeth in the arch are banded.
3. Time-consuming procedure.
4. It requires frequent appointments for activation.

*Force:* This appliance can deliver heavy force.

*Tooth movement:* This appliance brings about bodily tooth movement.

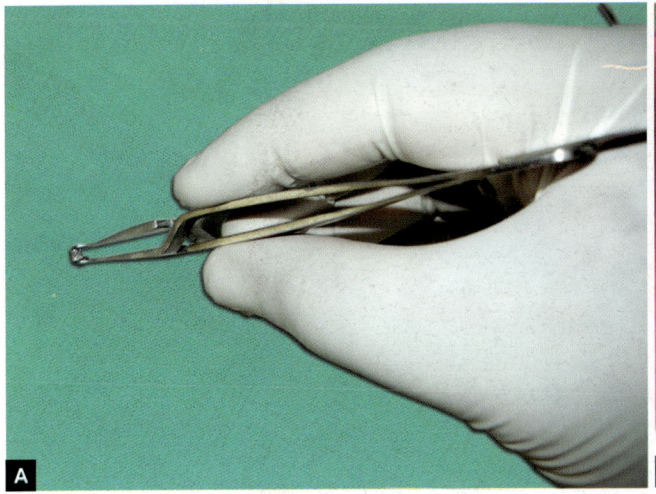 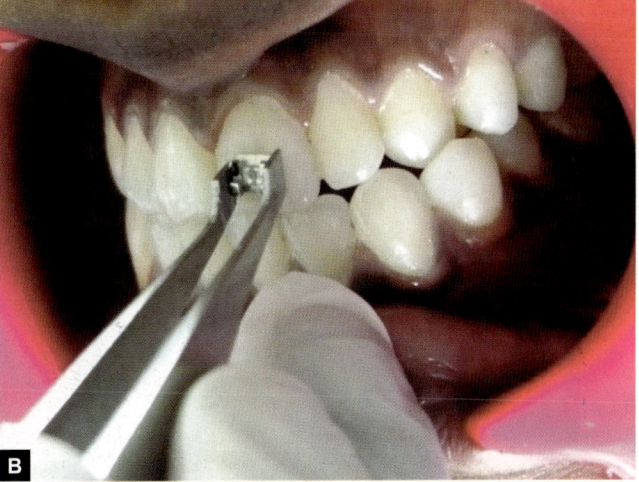

**Figs 31.43A and B:** (A) Holding the bracket with bracket holder after applying filled resin onto base of the bracket; (B) Showing placement of bracket on a tooth

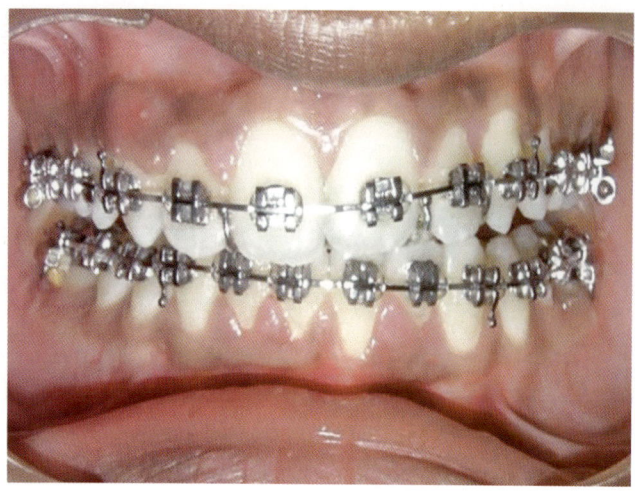

Fig. 31.44: After completion of bracket bonding and archwire insertion

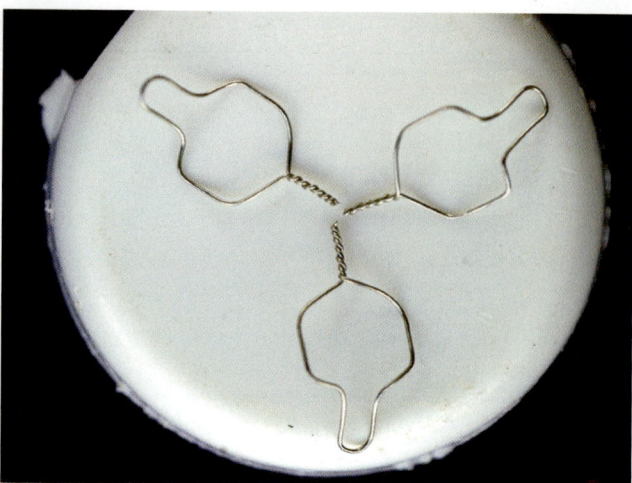

Fig. 31.45: Ligature wire of 0.010 inch in diameter used to secure arch wire in bracket

## Ribbon Arch Appliance

Ribbon arch appliance was also developed by Edward H Angle and it is the modification of pin and tube appliance. This appliance was introduced in 1910. Ribbon arch was the first appliance to use a true bracket. The bracket has a vertical slot facing occlusally. The brackets were attached to the bands at the center of labial surface of teeth.

*Arch wire used:* Angle used gold arch wire in this technique, as gold wire is flexible, biocompatible, and resilient and formable.

*Pins:* Pins were used to secure gold arch wire in the ribbon arch vertical rectangular slot.

*Advantage:* This appliance was quite efficient in aligning malposed teeth.

*Disadvantages:* This appliance provides relatively poor control of root position.

## Edgewise Appliance

In order to overcome the deficiencies encountered with his previous techniques, Angle devised a metal bracket that could give a better control over individual tooth movement. The Edgewise bracket has a rectangular slot facing labially, rather than occlusally or gingivally, which receives a rectangular arch wire. This unique feature of rectangular arch wire in a rectangular slot enabled control of tooth movement in all the three planes of space. Furthermore, the bracket has four wings, two occlusal and two gingival, which increase the surface of arch wire with the bracket slot and thus, give accurate control over the tooth movement **(Figs 31.47A and B)**. The term Edgewise refers to the method by which rectangular arch wire is inserted into the horizontal slotted bracket. The Edgewise appliance was developed and introduced to Orthodontics by Edward H Angle in the year 1925.

### Edgewise Bracket

- The Edgewise bracket has a bracket slot measuring 0.022 × 0.028 inch with single or double to the wings.
- The Edgewise bracket has a horizontally projected slot.
- The Edgewise brackets are available in 2 forms:
  1. *Weldable:* Welded to band.
  2. *Bondable:* Bonded directly to tooth surface.

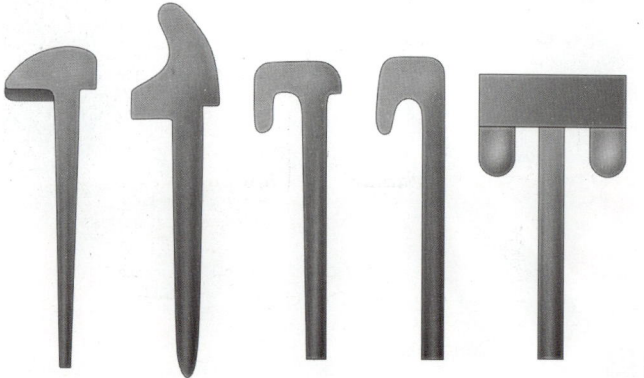

Fig. 31.46: Lock pins

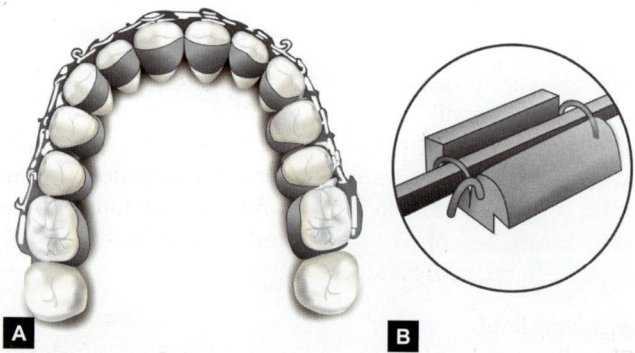

Figs 31.47A and B: Edgewise appliance also was introduced by Edward H Angle

**Table 31.6:** Occlusogingival positioning of the brackets assisted by predetermined measurement

|    |    |    | 3.5 | 3.5 | 4.5 | 3.0 | 3.5 | 3.5 | 3.0 | 4.5 | 3.5 | 3.5 |    |    |    |
|----|----|----|-----|-----|-----|-----|-----|-----|-----|-----|-----|-----|----|----|----|
| 28 | 27 | 26 | 25  | 24  | 23  | 22  | 21  | 11  | 12  | 13  | 14  | 15  | 16 | 17 | 18 |
| 48 | 47 | 46 | 45  | 44  | 43  | 42  | 41  | 31  | 32  | 33  | 34  | 35  | 36 | 37 | 38 |
|    |    |    | 3.0 | 3.0 | 3.5 | 2.5 | 2.5 | 2.5 | 2.5 | 3.5 | 3.0 | 3.0 |    |    |    |

Boons gauge/bracket positioning height gauge is used to measure the accurate height of bracket placement on different types of teeth.

## Bracket Placement

Proper bracket positioning is of the utmost importance for achieving the desired tooth movement.

Accurate placement of the brackets on tooth surfaces is an important prerequisite for achieving the desired tooth movement. The brackets should be placed in the center of the tooth crown mesiodistally and along the long axis of the tooth. Occlusogingival positioning of the brackets assisted by predetermined measurement given different tooth types as listed in the **Table 31.6**.

### Maxillary Arch

Central incisor – 3.5 mm from incisal edge
Lateral incisor – 3.0 mm from incisal edge
Canine – 4.5 mm from cusp tip
First premolar – 3.5 mm from buccal cusp tip
Second premolar – 3.5 mm from buccal cusp tip.

### Mandibular Arch

Central incisor – 2.5 mm from incisal edge
Lateral incisor – 2.5 mm from incisal edge
Canine – 3.5 mm from cusp tip
First premolar – 3.0 mm from buccal cusp tip
Second premolar – 3.0 mm from buccal cusp tip

All brackets are bonded in the center of the crown along the axis of the tooth.

### Molar Bands

Molar bands are fabricated in such a way that some portion of a cusp should be visible and the band should be cemented in the middle third of the crown.

### Bondable Buccal Tubes

These tubes are directly bonded to the buccal surface of crown of molars in the middle third of crown.

### Arch Wire Fabrication

The basic arch wire is formed on an Edgewise arch former using the Bonwill Hawlay chart. The width of the arch wire is primarily dictated by the inner cuspid and the inner buccal segment width in the regional malocclusion. After the arch wire width and symmetry are found to be satisfactory, the first order, second order and third order bends can be incorporated.

### First Order Bends

The first order bends or in-out bends are placed to compensate for differences in the buccolingual prominence of the teeth. They comprise of the lateral inset, the canine offset and the molar offset **(Figs 31.48)**.

### Second Order Bends

The second order bends are placed to achieve correct mesiodistal axial inclination of teeth. They comprise the tip back bends placed in the posterior segments **(Figs 31.49)**.

### Third Order Bends

The third order bends or torque are placed to get correct buccolingual position by moving the roots. They are placed by twisting the arch wire **(Figs 31.50)**.

Over the years, a number of modifications of Edgewise technique have come. Some of the routinely used current techniques are preadjusted Edgewise appliance and tip-edge appliance (straight wire appliance). In preadjusted technique, the brackets are designed such that they have in-built tip, torque and angulations for each tooth type.

### Begg's Appliance

The Begg's appliance was introduced by Dr PR Begg in the year 1930. Begg studied in Angle's School of Orthodontics and later began practicing in Australia. After a couple of years of practicing neither his patients nor himself were satisfied with the treatment using appliances available then, namely ribbon arch and pin and tube appliance. The treatment period was too long, oral hygiene a prime issue and soft tissue irritation and oral ulcers due to extensive metallic design were common. These problems led him to think of solution and he came up with the light wire differential force technique, now popular by the name

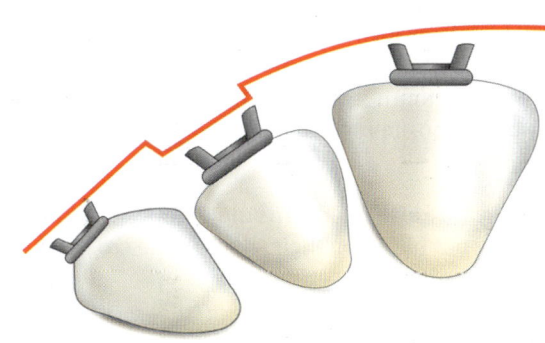

**Fig. 31.48:** First order bend

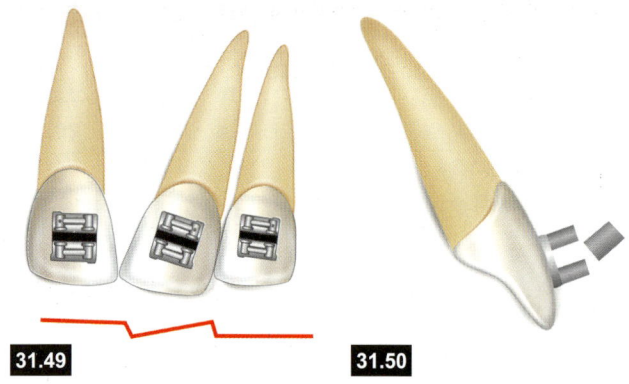

**Fig. 31.49:** Second order bend; **Fig. 31.50:** Third order bends

Begg's technique. He modified the ribbon arch bracket and with a vertical slot facing gingivally.

Although biocompatible, the gold arch wire was expensive and the forces were insufficient. In such of an alternative, Begg approached his friend AJ Willcock, who was a metallurgist. Willcock developed Australian austenitic arch wires, which were biocompatible, flexible, formable, malleable, resilient and also inexpensive. Begg's technique advocates the use of differential force and tipping of teeth crowns rather than bodily movement. Roots are torqued at the end of the treatment.

Although a number of other advanced fixed techniques have been developed lately. Begg's technique is still used in many parts of the world. Begg's appliance/technique uses stainless steel arch wires along with a number of auxiliaries and springs to achieve the desired tooth movement.

### Components Used in the Begg's Technique

#### Bracket

Modified ribbon arch bracket is used in the Begg's technique. Modified ribbon arch bracket has a single vertical slot, with opening gingivally.

The bases of the brackets can be of following two types:
a. Flat
b. Curved

Modified ribbon arch brackets are of two types, based on their mode of attachment to the tooth surface. The brackets can be either weldable/bondable.

***Weldable bracket:*** These brackets are welded to the bands which later on are cemented to the tooth surface.

***Bondable brackets:*** These brackets are directly bonded to the tooth surface with either using surface or light cure composite resins.

#### Buccal Tubes

Buccal tubes are also referred as molar tubes. Buccal tubes are of two types based on their shape in the cross-section:
a. Round
b. Flat-oval

Buccal tubes can be welded to the bands or directly bonded to the tooth surface.

***Weldable buccal tubes:*** Weldable buccal tubes have a flat contoured metal flange base and are welded to the bands that are cemented on the molars.

***Bondable buccal tubes:*** The bondable buccal tube has a mesh base and is bonded directly to the tooth surface.

#### Lock Pins

Lock pins are used to secure the arch wire into the vertical slot of modified ribbon arch bracket in Begg's technique. Lock pins are made of brass or stainless steel.

***Types:*** Various types of lock pins are:
- One-point safety pin
- High hot safety pin
- Double safety pin
- Hook pin
- Universal T-pin

#### Arch Wire

AJ Wilcock Australian austenitic arch wire is used in the Begg's technique, which are available in various diameters.

#### Elastics

Latex or nonlatex elastics of different diameters are used to apply the forces of different magnitude depending upon the stage of treatment in the Begg's technique.

#### Springs

The following springs are used in the Begg's technique:
i. Rotating spring
ii. Uprightening springs
iii. Torque springs
iv. Reverse torque springs

i. ***Rotating springs (see Fig. 31.8):*** Rotating springs in the Begg technique are used for the derotation of spring.
ii. ***Uprighting springs (see Fig. 31.6):*** Uprightening springs in the Begg technique are used for uprighting the teeth.
iii. ***Torque springs (see Fig. 31.7):*** Torque springs bring about torque of tooth, i.e. movement of root in one direction and crown in another direction. These springs are used at the end stage of this technique to achieve normal axial inclination of the teeth.

### Stages of Begg's Technique

In Begg's technique, malocclusion is treated in three stages:
1. Stage I: Alignment of teeth is achieved.
2. Stage II: It is concerned with space closure.
3. Stage III: Torquing of the roots is done.

### Stage I

The objectives of stage I of Begg's technique are:
- Open (or close) the anterior overbite.
- Eliminate anterior crowding or spacing.
- Overcrowding of rotated cuspids and bicuspids.
- Correct any posterior crossbite.
- Overcorrect any mesiodistal relationship of the buccal segment.

***Arch wire used in stage I:*** Plain or looped initial arch wire of diameter 0.012 and 0.014 inch are used.

### Elastics of stage I
- Elastic of 2 to 2.5 oz force is used.
- *Pattern:* Class II elastic.

### Stage II
The objectives of stage II is to maintain all corrections achieved at stage I and closing remaining spaces.

***Arch wire used in stage II:*** Plain 0.018 inch arch wire with premolar offset and slight decrease in anchor bends.

### Elastics of stage I
- Elastic of 2 to 2.5 oz force is used.
- *Pattern:*
  - Class I elastic
  - Class II elastic.

### Stage III
All corrections achieved during stage I and stage II are maintained and mechanics are undertaken to achieve desired axial inclination of all teeth.

***Arch wire used:*** The 0.020 inch Australian austenitic arch wire is used with molar offsets.

***Springs used:*** Torque, reverse torque and uprightening springs are used in stage III of Begg technique to correct axial inclination of individual teeth.

### Elastics of Class III:
- Elastics of 2 to 2.5 oz are used.
- *Pattern:* Class II or class III elastics depending on the conditions.

## Straight Wire Appliance

Straight wire appliance/technique is a modification of Edgewise appliance and it was developed by Lawrence F Andrew in the year 1970, based on his six keys to normal occlusion. Brackets used in this technique are having pre-built tip, angulation and torque.

### Advantages
- Minimal wire bending required in this technique.
- This technique enables good finishing of the cases.

### Disadvantages
Since tip, angulation and torque are in built in the brackets, accurate bracket placement is important to have desired tooth movements.

### Stages of Straight Wire Technique
1. Leveling and aligning.
2. Overbite reduction.
3. Overjet reduction and space closure.
4. Finishing and occlusal detailing.

1. **Leveling and aligning:** Leveling and aligning signifies placement of bracket in both vertical and horizontal planes of space. It is the major treatment objective in the early stage of the treatment. Achievement of objective during this stage would help in future movement and adjustment.

   The initial leveling and aligning can be done with a light round arch wires such as nickel, titanium or braided stainless steel arch wire as they apply gentle forces. Progressively larger diameter wires are placed to achieve the objectives of leveling and alignment (**Figs 31.51A to C**).

2. **Overbite reduction:** Overbite reduction should be undertaken soon after the leveling and aligning phase. Deep bite can be corrected by intrusion of upper and lower anteriors and extrusion of upper and lower posteriors (**Fig. 31.52**). There are a number of ways to achieve this. Correction of deep bite is explained in detail in the chapter "Management of deep bites". Intrusion of anteriors can be done by using intrusion arches, which includes utility arches (**Fig. 31.53**) and reverse curve of Spee wires and extrusion of posteriors can be achieved by bite planes and headgear.

3. **Overjet reduction and space closure:** Overjet reduction should be followed by overbite reduction in order to have smooth movement of teeth in the horizontal plane. One of the major objectives of fixed orthodontic appliance is to achieve a normal overjet relationship between the maxillary and mandibular arches and to obtain class I canine relationship. In addition to this, there is another objective of closing any remaining space (**Figs 31.54A and B**), especially in cases where some teeth have been extracted for orthodontic treatment.

Anterior retraction is done using—
a. Friction mechanics
b. Frictionless mechanics

a. **Friction mechanics:** Friction mechanics is also called as sliding mechanics. In this mechanics, anterior retraction can be done by using steel wires, such as 0.018 inch × 0.025 inch or 0.019 inch × 0.025 inches. Hooks are soldered onto the arch wire either mesial or distal to the canine and elastics or NiTi coil springs are applied from this post to the hooks present on the molar bands. These results in retraction of the anterior teeth by the arch wire sliding through the slots of the posterior brackets. Care should be taken to adequately reinforce the posterior anchorage.

b. **Frictionless mechanics:** Frictionless or loop mechanics relies on springs and loops design aimed at producing a controlled force system that can be modulated for anterior retraction or posterior protraction depending upon the anchorage need of the patient. Various designs of loop are available, such as T-loop, omega loop, key whole loop and tear drop loop.

   *Anterior retraction can be done by either friction or loop mechanics:*
   i. *Enmass retraction:* Here the entire anterior segment is retracted. This kind of retraction demands maximum anchorage.

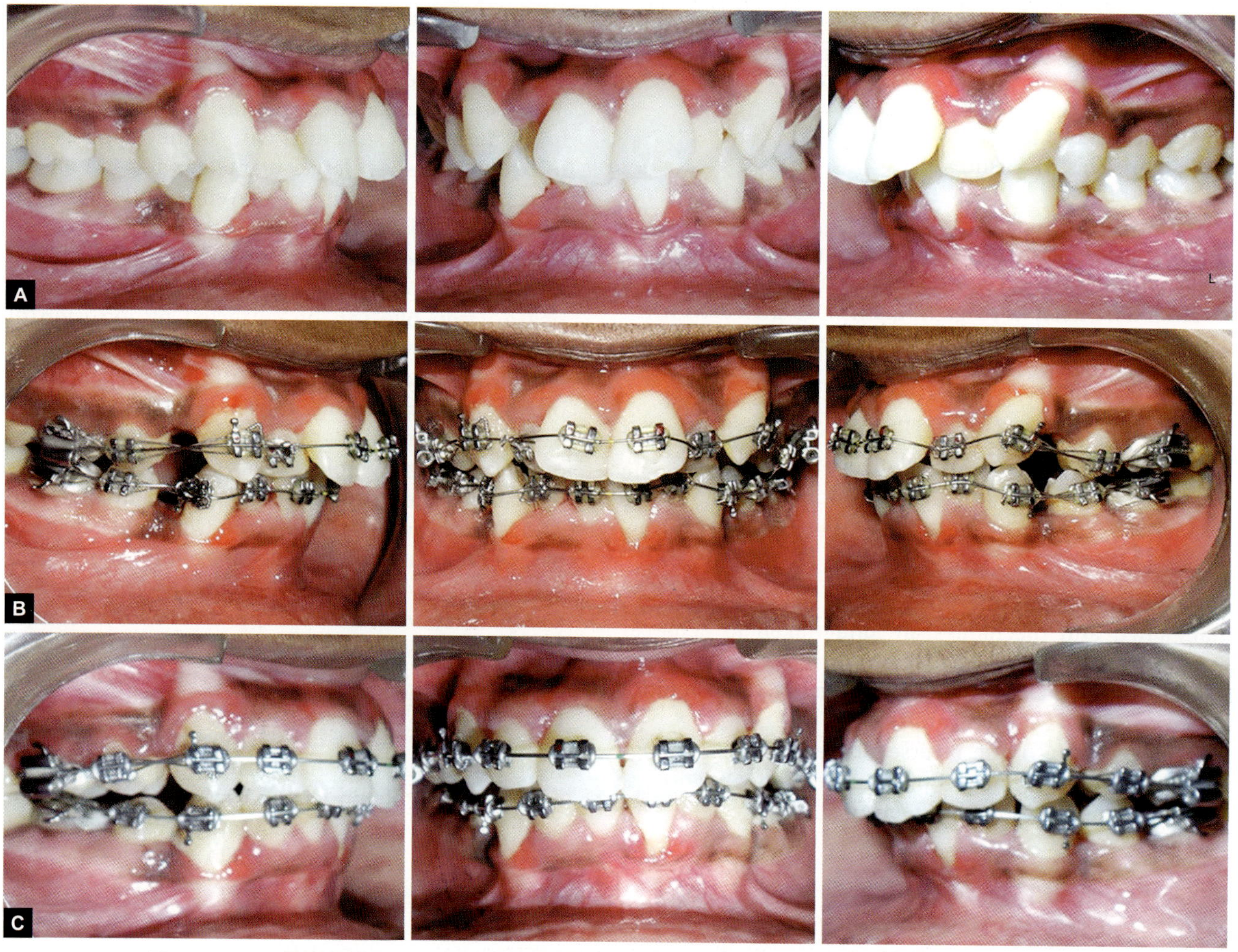

**Figs 31.51A to C:** The initial leveling and aligning can be done with a light round arch wires, such as nickel, titanium or braided stainless steel arch wire as they apply gentle forces

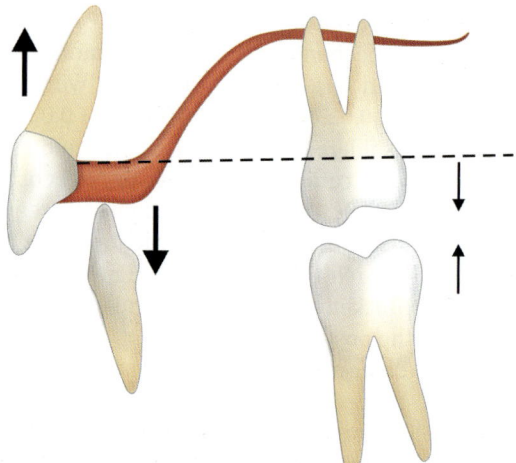

**Fig. 31.52:** Deep bite can be corrected by intrusion of upper and lower anteriors and extrusion of upper and lower posteriors

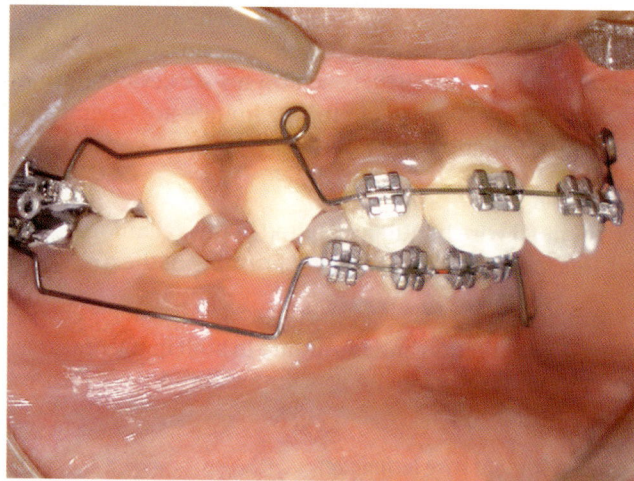

**Fig. 31.53:** Intrusion of anteriors can be done by using intrusion arches, which include utility arches

ii. *Canine retraction followed by incisors retraction:* Here only canine is retracted first and then later incisors are retracted. This enhances the posterior anchorage control during space closure.

4. **Finishing and detailing of occlusion:** This phase of treatment is aimed at finishing and occlusal detailing. This is thus a fine tuning of the tooth position in terms of axial inclination and angulations to optimize the occlusion.

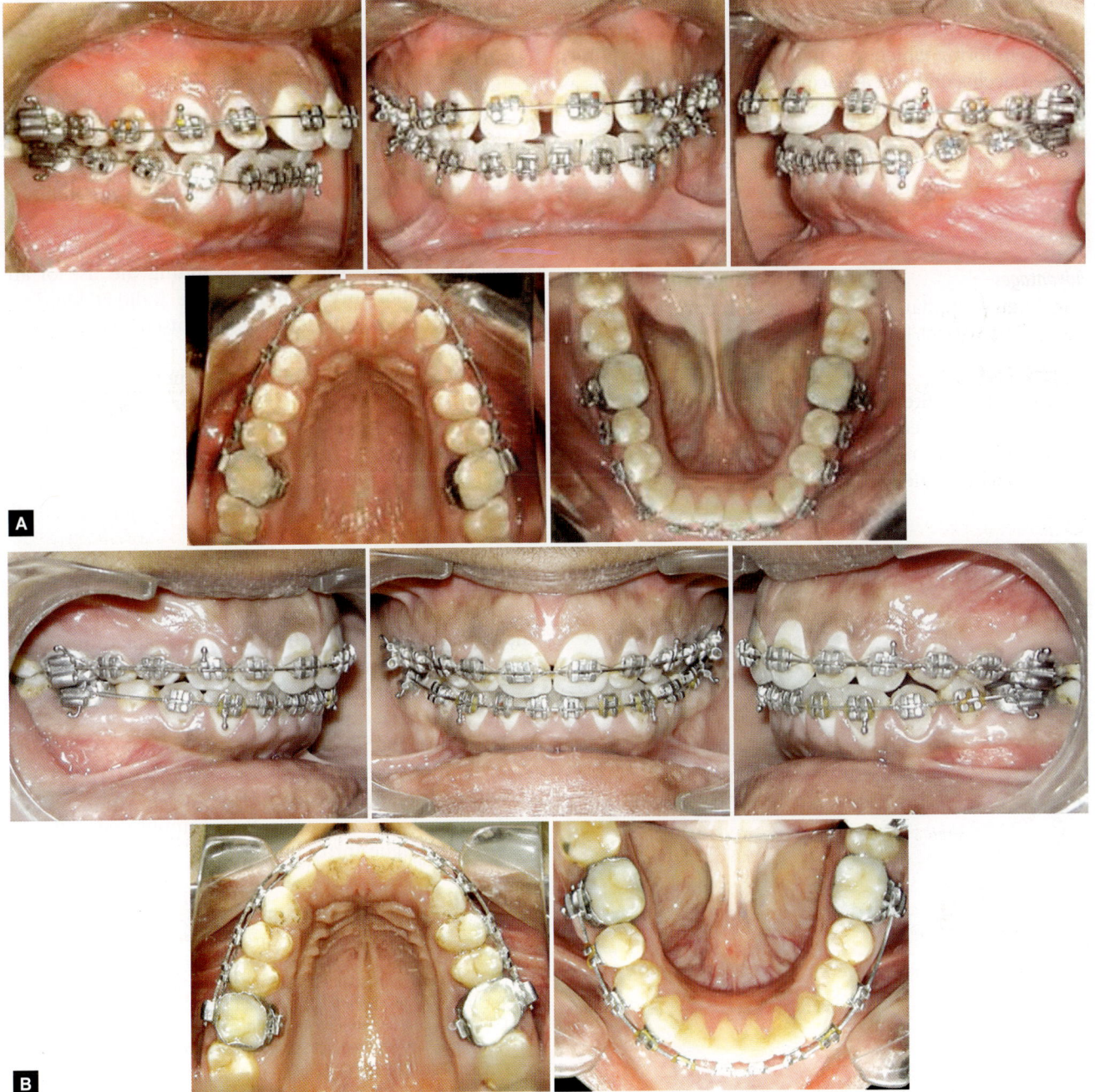

**Figs 31.54A and B:** Fixed orthodontic appliance main objective is closing any remaining space using elastomerics (E-chain)

Finishing and occlusal detailing can be done with smaller diameter wires, such as 0.016 inch stainless steel wire or rectangular beta titanium as they are more flexible and allow precise finishing. Minor arch wire bends in first, second or third order may be required for detailing of tooth position. Finishing elastics ("M" elastics or "W" elastics) are used for the settling of elastics. Triangular elastic is also used to achieve cuspal interdigitation.

### Lingual Technique

The lingual technique was introduced by Craven Kurz in 1976. Dr Craven Kurz, an assistant professor at UCLA School of Dentistry, realized that many of his patients were adults.

This led to the development of the concept of the lingually bonded appliance, consisting of plastic lee fisher brackets bonded to the lingual aspect of the anterior dentition and metal brackets bonded to the lingual aspect of the posterior dentition. The plastic brackets were used for the inherent ease of recontouring and reshaping them to avoid direct contact with the opposing teeth.

Dr Fujita of Japan published cases treated with his modification of the Begg's light wire appliance. He had bonded the Begg's brackets lingually or palatally and used the same AJ Wilcock Australian austenitic arch wires contoured to the lingual aspect of the teeth. He explained the arch form, which resembled a mushroom (when viewed occlusally) and advocated the same basic steps as in the conventional Begg's technique to be used with the Begg's brackets with a modified base.

In this appliance, the brackets are placed on the palatal surface of the upper teeth and lingual surface of the lower teeth **(Figs 31.55A and B)**. This technique is a combination of Edgewise and Begg's Technique.

### Advantages

The lingual appliances are highly esthetic as they are bonded on palatal/lingual surface of the teeth.

### Disadvantages

1. Difficulty of direct viewing and access, particularly of retroclined anterior teeth.
2. Variations in morphology of the lingual surfaces, especially on the maxillary anterior teeth.
3. Wide range of labiolingual thickness of the teeth—from 4.6 mm for lateral incisors to 9.2 mm for canines-necessitating numerous in-out bends.
4. Critical relationship between the vertical height of lingual brackets and the labial surface torque, due to the distance of the lingual brackets from the labial surface.
5. Much smaller-inter bracket distances in the anterior region, making compulsory bends difficult.
6. They are time-consuming and require specialized technical skills, sometimes including the use of an outside laboratory to prepare the indirect bonding trays. If an outside laboratory is used, the clinician can only verify the correct bracket positions after the brackets have been bonded in the mouth.
7. Many measurements and the other steps are needed before the brackets can be bonded to the cast and the final transfer tray prepared, increasing the possibility of errors.
8. Changing a bracket position requires an additional laboratory procedure of expense.

### Indications of Lingual Appliance

Following are the five distinct conditions where lingual appliance may be more effective than labial appliance because of their unique mechanical characteristics:

1. Intrusion of anterior teeth
2. Maxillary arch expansion
3. Combing mandibular repositioning therapy with orthodontic movement
4. Distalization of maxillary molar
5. Treatment of cases with case complicated with an existing tongue-thrust habit.

## BIBLIOGRAPHY

1. Graber TM. Orthodontics: Principles and Practice. WB Saunders, 1998.
2. Graber TM, Vanarsdall RL. Orthodontics, Current Principles and Techniques. In: Sarver DM, Proffit WR, Ackerman JL, (Eds). Diagnosis and Treatment Planning in Orthodontics, Mosby, 2000.
3. Harradine NW. Self-ligating brackets and treatment efficiency. Clin Orthod Res. 2001;4(4):220-7.
4. Harradine NW. Self-ligating brackets: Where are we now? J Orthod. 2003;30:262-73.
5. Miles PG. Self-ligating brackets in orthodontics: do they deliver what they claim? Aust Dent. J 2009;54:9-11.
6. Profitt WR. Contemporary Orthodontics. St Louis, CV Mosby, 1986.
7. Rinchuse DJ, Miles PG. Self-ligating brackets: Present and future. Am J Orthod Dentofacial Orthod. 2007;132:216-22.
8. Roth RH. Treatment mechanics for the straight wire appliance: In: Graber TM, Swain BF (Eds). Orthodontics: Current Principles and Techniques. The CV Mosby Company, St Louis, 1966.
9. Tweed CH. Clinical Orthodontics. The CV Mosby Company, St Louis, 1966.
10. Zachrisson BU. Bonding in orthodontics. In: Graber TM, Vanarsdall RL (Eds). Orthodontics: Current Principles and Techniques, Ed 3, St Louis, Mosby, 2000;557.

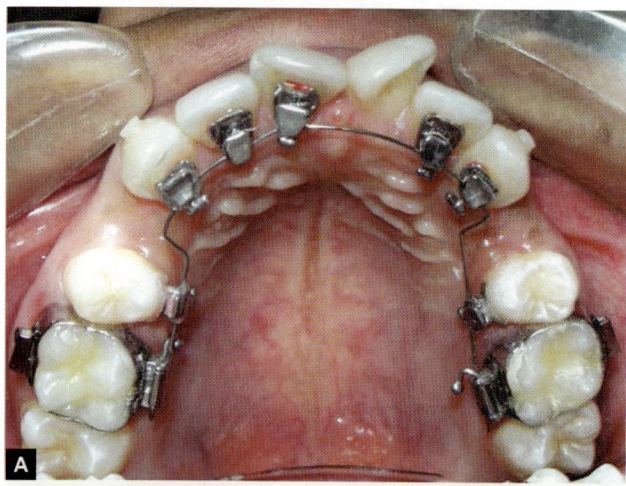
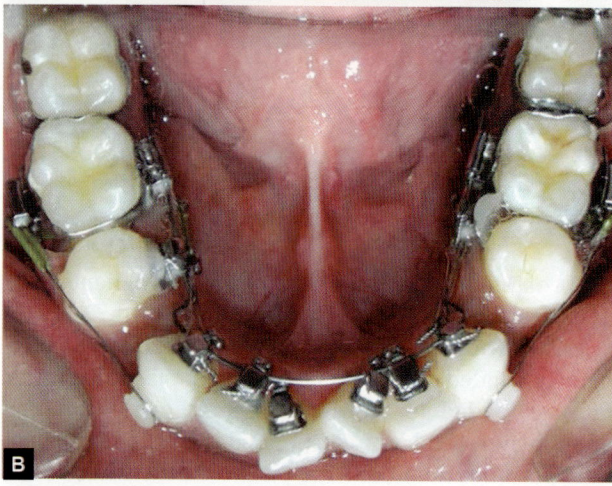

**Figs 31.55A and B:** In lingual appliance, the brackets are placed on the palatal surface of the upper teeth and lingual surface of the lower teeth

## EXAM-ORIENTED QUESTIONS

### Long Essay or Long Questions

1. What are the components of fixed orthodontic appliances?
   - Write about different bracket systems used in fixed mechanotherapy.
2. What are the active components of fixed orthodontic appliances?
   - Write about different arch wires used in fixed mechanotherapy.
3. Explain various fixed orthodontic appliance techniques.

### Short Notes

1. Elastics in fixed orthodontics
2. Lingual attachments
3. Buccal tubes
4. Lingual orthodontics
5. Straight wire technique
6. Different types of separators
7. Different types of springs used in fixed mechanotherapy
8. Magnets
9. Banding procedure
10. Brackets
11. Bonding procedure
12. Pin and tube appliance
13. Lock pins
14. Begg's appliance.

# CHAPTER 32

# Functional Appliances

*Shah A, Phulari BS*

Functional/myofunctional appliances are devices that alter patient's functional environment in an attempt to influence and permanently change the surrounding hard tissue.

Most of the functional appliances are mainly designed to correct skeletal class II relationship by positioning the mandible downward and forward to theoretically enhance mandibular growth. All functional appliances are intraoral devices. Functional appliances may be removable or fixed.

## DEFINITION

- By Moyer: "Functional appliances are loose removable appliances designed to alter the neuromauscular environment of the orofacial region to improve occlusal development and/or craniofacial skeletal growth."
- By Proffit: "Functional appliances are appliances which alter the posture of the mandible, holding it open or closed and forward or backward."
- Functional appliances are appliances which act by either harnessing the muscular forces or by preventing aberrant muscular forces.

## CLASSIFICATION

Functional appliances are classified in a number of ways; a simple easily understandable classification is described below.

Functional appliances can be divided into removable functional appliances or fixed functional appliances. Removable functional appliances can further be classified into removable tooth-borne functional and removable tissue-borne functional appliances **(Flowchart 32.1)**. The fixed functional appliances are tooth borne.

### Removable Functional Appliances

Removable functional appliances include removable tooth-borne and removable tissue-borne functional appliances.

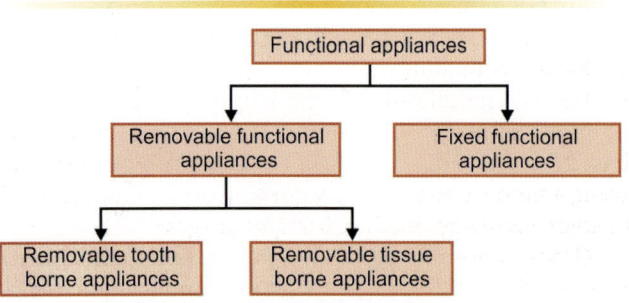

**Flowchart 32.1:** Classification of functional appliances

### Removable Tooth-Borne Appliances

These appliances depend on the stretch of the soft tissues caused by the mandible being positioned downward and forward, as well as by the muscle activity generated by the mandible attempting to return to its original position.
*Examples*:
- Activator
- Bionator
- Twin block appliance.

### Removable Tissue-Borne Functional Appliances

These appliances are used to minimize unwanted tooth movement and to recontour the facial soft tissue adjacent to the teeth as well as posture of mandible downward and forward.
*Example*: Functional regulator/functional corrector/Frankel appliance.

### Fixed Tooth-Borne Functional Appliances

The fixed tooth borne functional appliances are fitted on the teeth and cannot be removed by the patient at will.
*Example*: Herbst appliances.

Other classifications of functional appliances are listed in **Table 32.1**.

## MODE OF ACTION

Most of the functional appliances act by utilizing one or more of the following:
- A forced mandibular posture, which transmits forces to the teeth and jaws.
- Bite planes, which produce differential eruption.

## ADVANTAGES

Advantages of functional appliances are as follows:
- Functional appliances are effective in vertical control of increased overbite.
- Functional appliances can be used in the mixed dentition.
- Functional appliances require minimal chairside adjustment.

## DISADVANTAGES

Disadvantages of functional appliances are listed below:
- The success of functional appliances therapy solely depends on patient cooperation.
- Precise tooth movement is not possible with functional appliances.
- Treatment duration of functional appliances is often prolonged.

**Table 32.1:** Classification of functional appliances

*Tom Graber classification when functional appliances were removable*
- Group A: Teeth-supported appliances, e.g. catlans appliance, inclined planes, etc.
- Group B: Teeth/tissue supported, e.g. activator, bionator, etc.
- Group C: Vestibular-positioned appliances with isolated support from tooth/tissue, e.g. Frankel appliance, lip bumpers.

*With advent of fixed functional appliances*
- Removable functional appliances, e.g. activator, bionator, Frankel, etc.
- Semi-fixed functional appliances, e.g. Den Holtz, Boss appliances, etc.
- Fixed functional appliances, e.g. Herbst, Jasper jumper, Churro jumper, Saif springs, and Adjustable corrector.

*With concept of hybridization by Peter Vig, functional appliances were classified as:*
- Classification functional appliances, e.g. activator, Frankel's appliance, etc.
- Hybrid appliances, e.g. propulsor, double oral screen, hybrid bionators, bass bionators.

*Classification by Proffit:*
- Teeth-borne passive appliances: myotonic appliances, e.g. Andresen/Haüpl activator, Herren activator, Woodside activator, Balter's bionator, etc.
- Tooth-borne active appliances: myodynamic appliances, e.g. elastic open activator, Bimler's appliance, modified bionator, stockfish appliance, etc.
- Tissue-borne passive appliance, e.g. oral screen, lip bumpers, etc.
- Tissue-borne active appliances, e.g. Frankel appliances.
- Functional orthopedic magnetic appliances (FOMA)

- Functional appliances often need two-phases treatment to complete the treatment. Functional appliances may be used for definitive treatment or as phase-1 of two-phase treatment. Phase-1 treatment is aimed at reducing the overjet, overbite and to correct sagittal jaw relationship, while phase-2 treatment is aimed at completing the final alignment using fixed mechanotherapy.

## EFFECTS

Effects of functional appliances include effects on the dentition and skeletal structures.

### Effects on Dentition

Functional appliances typically cause some intrusion of maxillary incisors. This is caused by a lingual force transmitted from the labial bow or torquing springs against these teeth when the mandible attempts to reposition back to its normal position. This natural repositioning attempt by the mandible causes protrusion of mandibular incisors caused by a labial force transmitted from the portion of the appliance lingual to these teeth.

### Effect on Skeletal Structures

Functional appliances are designed to stimulate the growth in the condylar region and can also produce change in the direction of growth of the jaws. Functional appliances can also bring about downward and forward remodeling of the glenoid fossa. Functional appliances are also capable of restricting the growth of the jaws.

### Muscular Effect

Functional appliances are designed to improve the tonicity of orofacial musculature.

## ACTIVATOR

Norman Kingsley, an early influential American orthodontist, has been credited with the development of the first appliance to position the mandible forward as early as 1879. However, most consider Pierre Robin to have developed the earliest removable functional appliance, in France in 1902.

Hotz devised a "Vorbissplatte," which was a modified form of Kingsley's vulcanite palatal plate. This was used to treat retrognathism associated with deep bite.

**Pierre Robin** devised an appliance called 'Monobloc', made up of a single block of vulcanite. He used it to position the mandible forward in patients with glossoptosis and severe mandibular retrognathism. By positioning the mandible forward, it reduced the risk of airway obstruction.

**Viggo Andresen,** in 1908 in Denmark, designed a loose fitting appliance, which he first used on his daughter. He made a modified Hawley type of retainer on the maxillary arch to which he added a lower lingual horse-shoe shaped flange, which helped in positioning the mandible forward. He used this appliance on his daughter who was going on a three-month vacation. On her return three months later, he found a marked sagittal correction and improvement of the facial profile.

Although it was developed more than 70 years ago, the Andresen appliance, which is also known as an activator or monobloc, has been successfully used by many generations of orthodontists. The activator is generally used for the treatment of Class II division I malocclusion.

During the time of Viggo Andresen and Haupl, the appliances were made of vulcanized rubber, but this gave way to acrylic in the 1950s. Over the years, various modifications have been made to the original design of Andresen's appliance, such as:
- The bow activator of AM Schwartz
- Wanderer's modification
- The propulsor
- Cut out or palate free activator
- The reduced activator or cybernator of Schmuth
- Kawetzky modification
- Herren's modification of the activator.

Most of the modifications of Andresen appliance were based on Andresen's concepts. There can be advantages to using a simple design in terms of patient cooperation, ease of adjustment and freedom from breakages.

Graber observed that numerous modifications have been made to the Andresen Haupl monobloc and have been described in texts and periodical contributions by

Petrik, Escher, Hafler, Grossman and others. These are surprisingly effective at times but generally a simpler design of appliance is preferred.

Effects produced by activator are categorized into following two categories:
1. The dental changes produced by activator
   a. The incisor changes
   b. The vertical molar changes
   c. Upper molar expansion.
2. The skeletal changes produced by activator
   a. Mandibular growth changes
   b. Changes on growth of the maxilla
   c. Changes in lower facial height.

## Dental Changes Produced by Activator

### Incisor Changes
The activator helps in successful overjet and overbite reduction by retroclination of upper incisors and proclination of lower incisors **(Fig. 32.1)**.

### Vertical Molar Changes
The design of the activator permits removal of occlusal acrylic above the lower molar and premolars. This facilitates upward and forward eruption of the lower molars and makes the activator a logical choice for low angle class II division 1, where there is a need for the molars to be free to erupt into the freeway space **(Fig. 32.2)**. Lower molar eruption of this kind is assumed to be a favorable factor in correcting the class II molar relationship and reducing the deep incisor overbite.

### Upper Molars Expansion
The activator with an incorporated expansion screw produces expansion in the upper molar region.

### Changes In Lower Facial Height
The activator produces an increase in lower facial height by encouraging eruption of lower molars when acrylic is trimmed above the lower molars **(Fig. 32.3)**.

## Skeletal Changes Produced by the Activator

### Changes on Mandibular Growth of the Mandible
The activator produces a downward and forward growth of the mandible **(Fig. 32.4)**.

### Changes on Growth of the Maxilla
Upper anteriors retrocline during Andresen wear and point "A" can move distally with the incisor roots. This indicates an apparent maxillary skeletal change in studies where point "A" is used to assess the position of maxilla.

### Indications
- Class I malocclusion with deep bite
- Class II malocclusion with open bite
- Class II division 1 malocclusion
- Class II division 2 malocclusion after aligning the incisors
- Class III malocclusion (reverse activator)
- Serves as space regainer in mixed dentition where acrylic is extended into the space of missing tooth
- Used for treating patients who snore during sleep.

### Contraindications
- Crowded arch
- Increase lower facial height
- Extreme vertical mandibular growth
- Severe proclined lower incisors
- Retroclined upper incisors
- Crossbite tendency
- Gross intra-arch irregularities.

### Advantages
- Treating mixed and deciduous dentition is possible
- Appointments can be delayed over 2 months
- Tissues not injured
- Worn at night time only
- Helps to eliminate abnormal habits
- Oral hygiene is maintained.

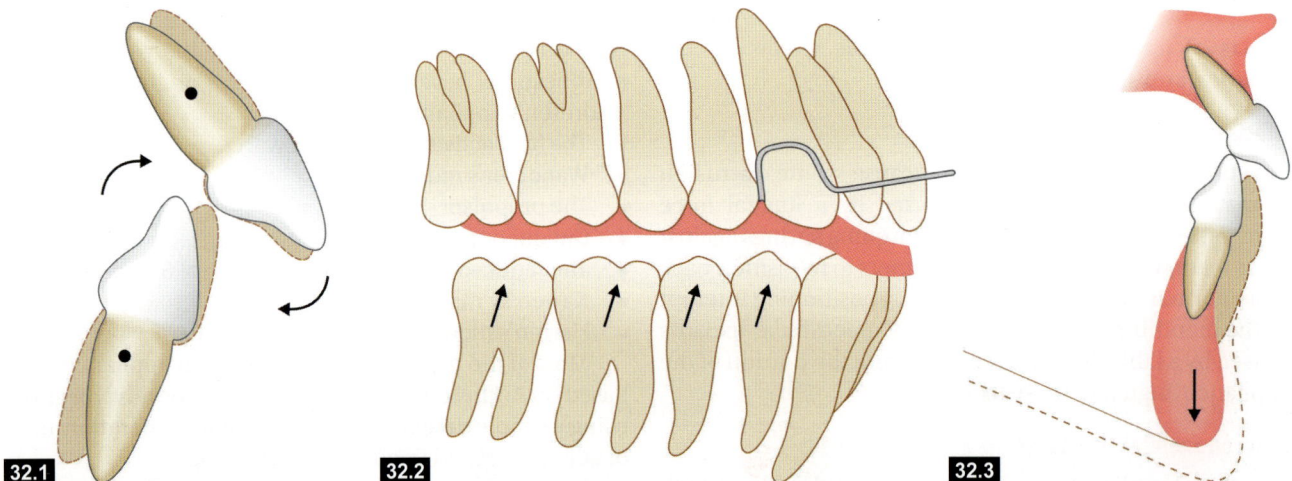

**Fig. 32.1:** The activator helps in successful overjet and over-bite reduction by the retroclination of upper incisors and proclination of lower incisors; **Fig. 32.2:** Activator is the appliance of choice in low angle class II division 1 cases, where there is a need for free eruption of molars; **Fig. 32.3:** The activator produces increase in lower facial height when acrylic is trimmed above the lower molars into free way space

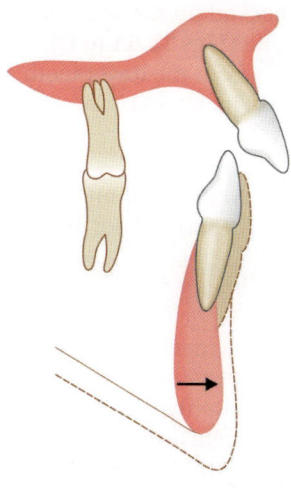

**Fig. 32.4:** The activator produces the downward and forward growth of the mandible

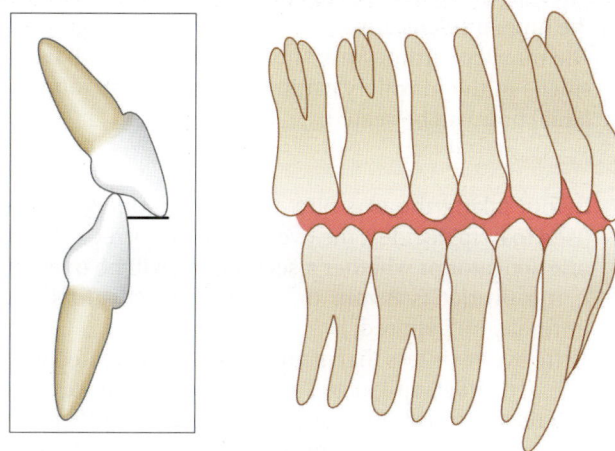

**Fig. 32.5:** If the overjet is less than 8 mm it can be corrected with one activator appliance

## Disadvantages

- Fully rely on patient cooperation
- Little value in cases with crowding
- Force on individual tooth can not be controlled
- Little or no response in older patients
- Bulky and uncomfortable.

## Impressions for Activator

- High quality impressions are needed and perforated trays or similar are preferred, with some soft wax build up in the lower molar lingual sulcus.
- The alginate mix should not be too liquid, as firmer material carries better into the important lingual sulcus area.
- After placing lower tray loaded with alginate impression material partly into position the patient is asked to put his/her tongue over the top with a gesture from the orthodontist, so that they gently protrude the tongue on the instruction, 'now relax your tongue,' the tongue drops back to a relaxed position and then the

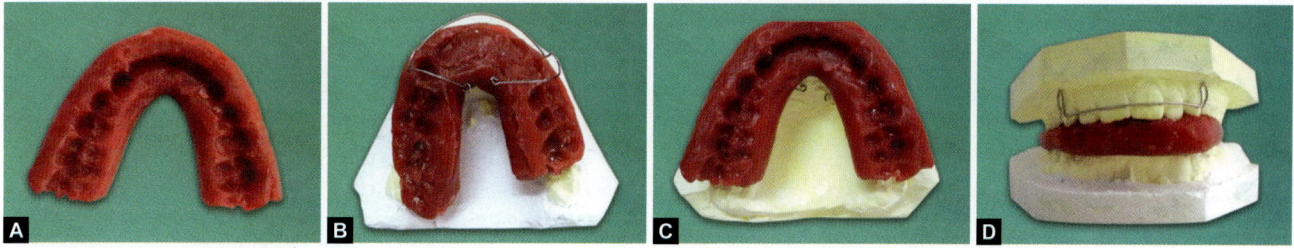

**Figs 32.6A to D:** The softened wax is pressed onto the upper teeth and then the lower jaw protruded, then the wax bite is cooled and if necessary, trimmed with a sharp knife. It should be checked on the study models

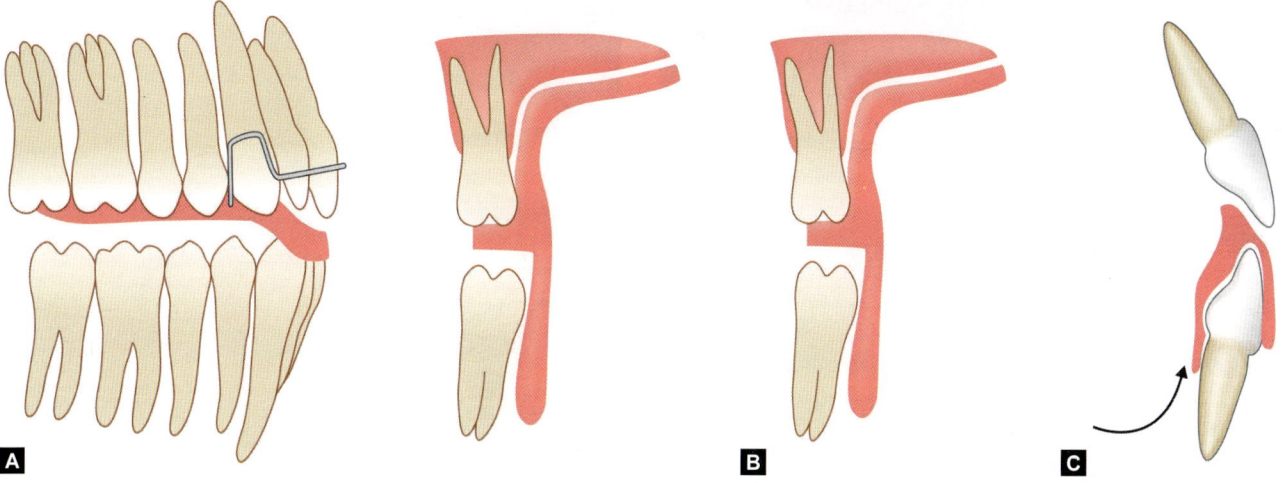

**Figs 32.7A to C:** Grind away the acrylic in the lingual sulcus areas, partially adjacent to the molar and lower anteriors

tray may be fully seated to ensure a good impression in the lingual sulcus area.
- The maxillary impression should include the full labial sulcus in the maxillary canine regions, where loops of labial bow will be seated.

### The Wax Bite

- Before taking the wax bite, the study models can be used to help decide if the overjet can be corrected with one activator or whether a second one will be needed. If the overjet is 8 mm or more, two activators will normally be required
- If the overjet is less than 8 mm, it can be corrected with one activator appliance. For these cases, the wax bite can be taken with the mandible protruded sufficiently to bring the incisors almost edge-to edge **(Fig. 32.5)**.
- A piece of good quality pink wax of approximately 6 × 8 cm dimensions is warmed in hot water and folded over two or three turns to make a soft sausage of wax. A slightly more bulky sausage will be needed for deep bite low angle cases
- The softened wax is pressed onto the upper teeth and then the lower jaw protruded. Then the wax bite is cooled and if necessary, trimmed with a sharp knife.

It should be checked on the study models and in the mouth, if possible **(Figs 32.6A to D)**.
- The indentations from the lower teeth should be only 2 or 3 mm deep **(Fig. 32.6A)**.

### Casting the Impressions

The impressions are poured in dental stone and carefully mounted on a plane line articulator ensuring that the bite is correct.

### Fitting the Appliance

There are three main mechanical requirements when fitting the activator.
1. It is necessary to ease the acrylic in the lingual sulcus areas, partially adjacent to the molar and lower anteriors by grinding away a little acrylic **(Fig. 32.7A to C)**.
2. The labial bow must be passive; otherwise the appliance will not be worn. The bow should be about half way up the labial surface of the upper incisors and resting passively on the enamel surface or functionally away from it **(Figs 32.8A and B)**.
3. During appliance construction, acrylic needs to be trimmed to allow unimpeded eruption of lower molars and premolars **(Fig. 32.9)**.

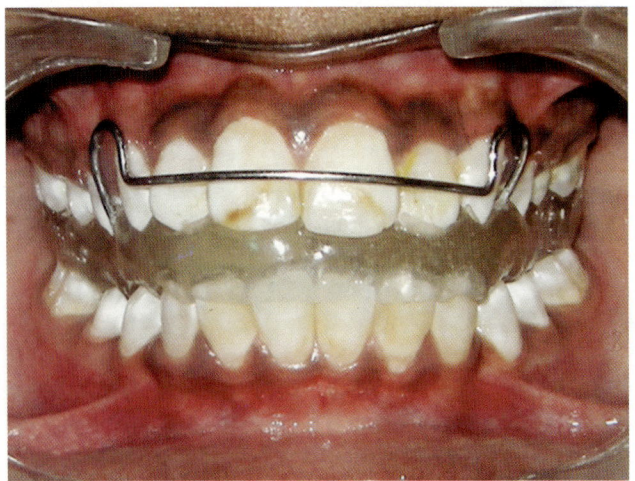
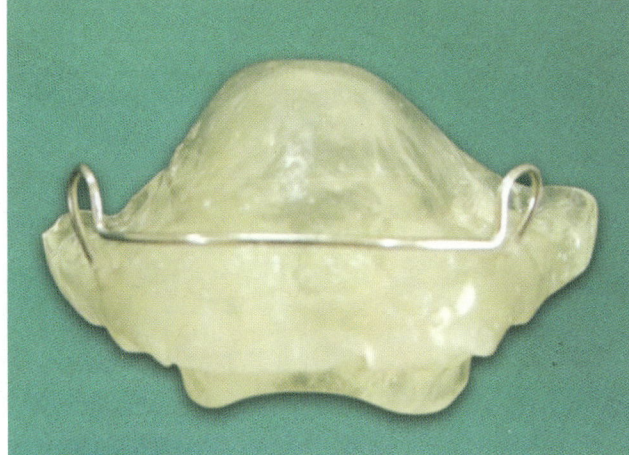
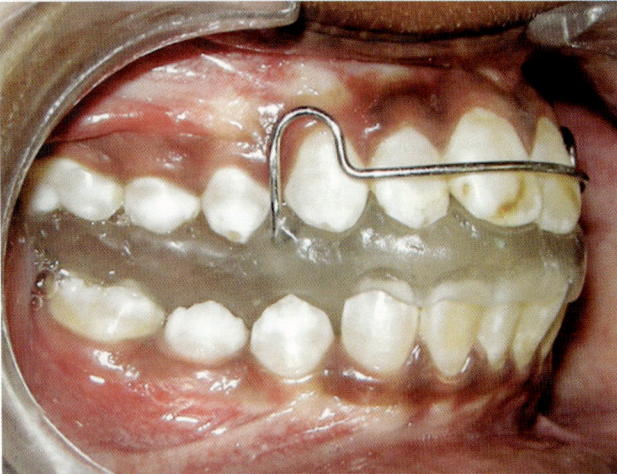
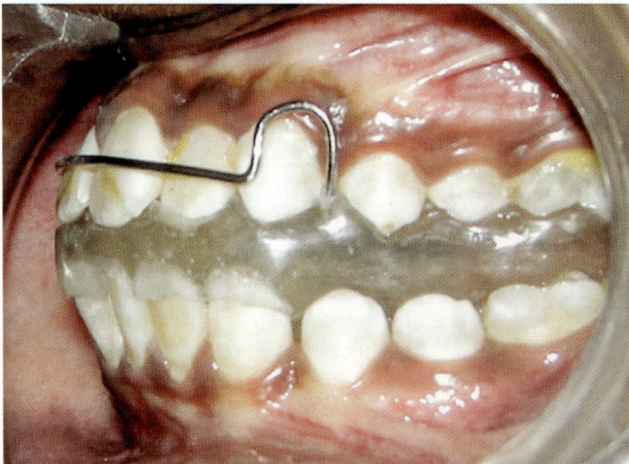

**Fig. 32.8A:** The labial bow must be passive; otherwise the appliance will not be worn. The bow should be about half way up the labial surface of the upper incisors and resting passively on the enamel surface or functionally away from it

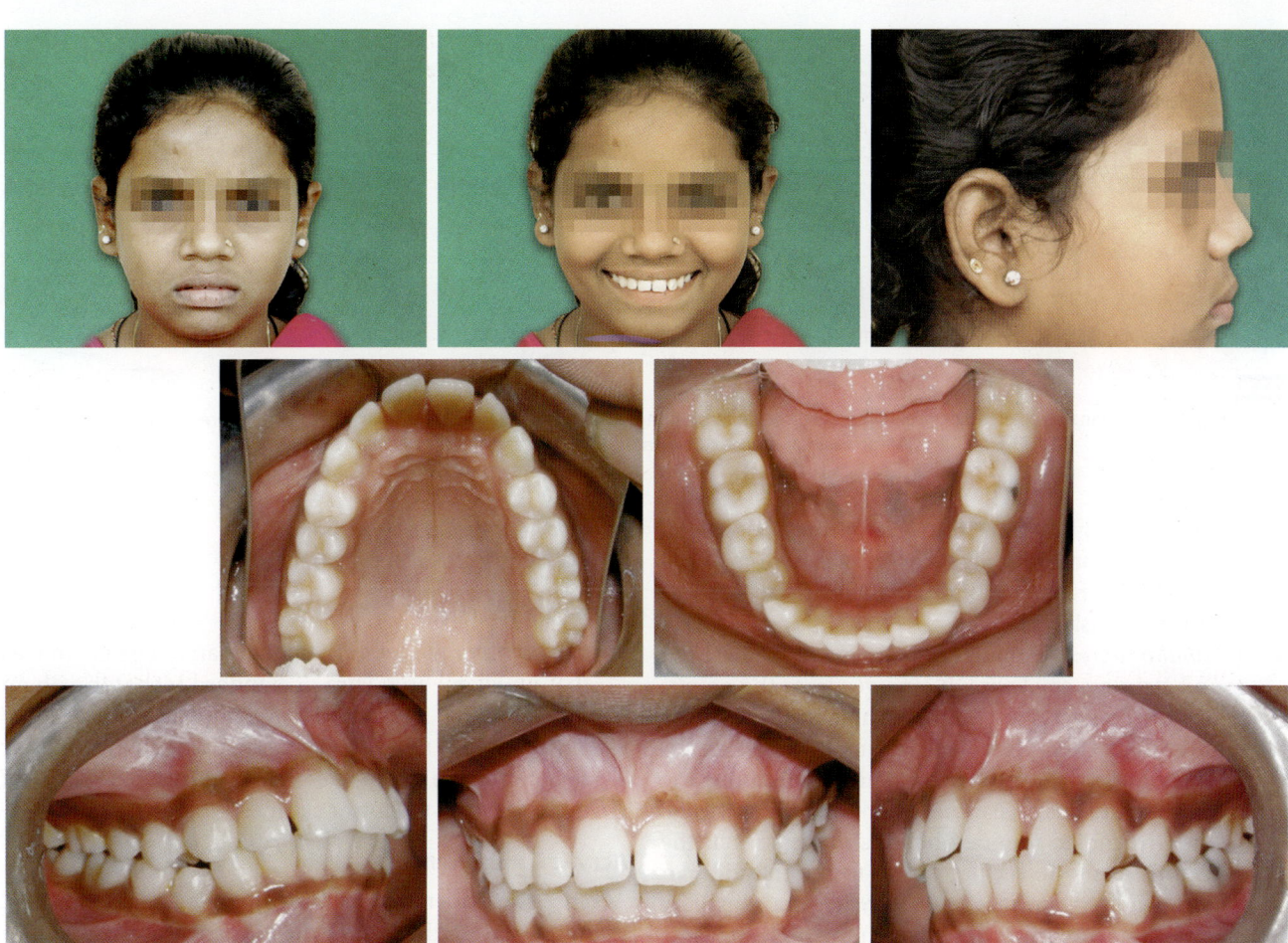

**Fig. 32.8B:** A case report—11-year-old girl with class II division 1 malocclusion treated with activator [*Courtesy*: Dr Dharm Pal hada, MDS (Ortho)]

## Patient Instructions after Delivering the Activator

- The patient is asked to wear the activator at least 10–12 hours in a day at the beginning, and few hours in a day when patient is used to the appliance and then instructed to be worn at night also.
- Patient is asked to keep the appliance in the mouth or in the box not elsewhere.
- Patient is instructed to clean the appliance with a little toothpaste and a toothbrush using cold water.
- Patient is also instructed to keep the appliance away from pets.
- Patient is asked not to keep the appliance in hot water.
- As soon as the overjet and overbite are close to normal levels, the hours of wear can be reduced from evening and nights to one hour in the evening and sleeping or sleeping only.

The activator is normally checked every six weeks. The aim is to achieve an overjet reduction of 1 or 2 mm every visit. At each visit, it is necessary to check that the activator appliance is still active as the overjet reduces.

## BIONATOR

The bionator was developed in Germany by Wilhelm Balter in the early 1950s to increase patient's comfort and facilitate daytime wear to increase the functional use of the appliance. Balter accomplished this by drastically reducing acrylic bulk of the appliance.

### Standard Bionator

Standard bionator is used for the treatment of class II division 1 malocclusion and Angle's class I malocclusion having constricted dental arch.

### Components of Standard Bionator

- Wire components
  - Palatal arch
  - Vestibular wire.
- Acrylic components
  - Maxillary acrylic part
  - Mandibular acrylic part
  - Interocclusal acrylic part. **(Figs 32.10 and 32.11)**

### Wire components

- *Palatal arch*: The palatal arch is made up of 1.2 diameter stainless steel wire. It emerges opposite the middle of the first premolars on the palatal side, follow the contour of the palate joining a curve that extends till the distal surface of the first permanent molar. The

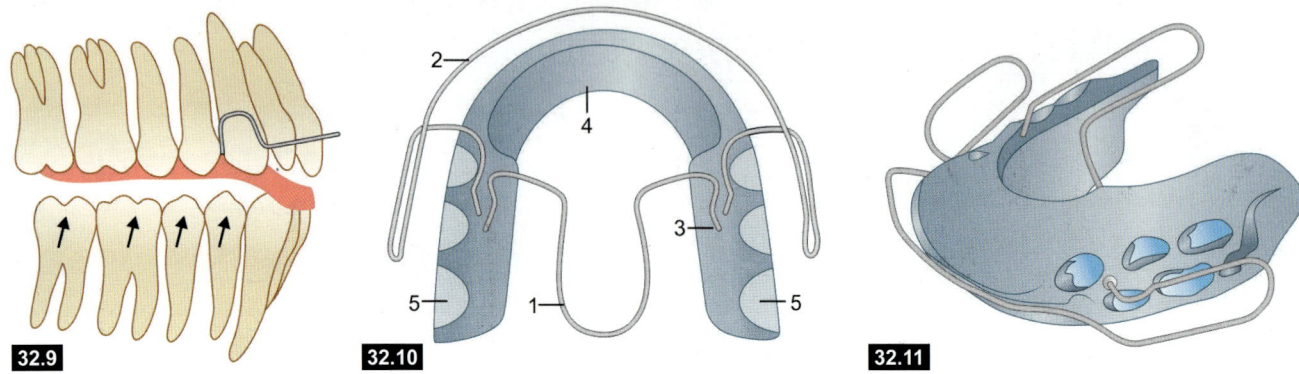

**Fig. 32.9:** During appliance construction acrylic needs to be trimmed to allow unimpeded eruption of lower molars and premolars; **Fig. 32.10:** Components of standard bionator; **Fig. 32.11:** Standar bionator-side view

palatal arch is placed 1 mm away from the palatal mucosa. The palatal arch helps in orientation of the tongue and directing mandible anteriorly to achieve class I relationship.

- *Vestibular wire*: Vestibular wire is made of 0.9 hard round stainless steel wire. It emerges from the acrylic below the contact point between the maxillary canine and maxillary first premolars. It runs vertically and is bent at right angles and made to run distally along the middle of the maxillary premolars crowding mesial to the first molar, rounded bend is made so that the wire runs at the lower papilla up to the mandibular canine where again it is bent to reach the maxillary canines. It forms a mirror image on the opposite side. The vestibular wire is kept free from the surface of the incisor teeth anteriorly and is kept sufficiently away from buccal surface of posterior teeth on either side of the arch to allow lateral expansion.

### Acrylic component

- *Maxillary acrylic part*: In the maxillary arch acrylic covers only the molars and the premolars with the anterior region remaining uncovered.
- *Mandibular acrylic part*: The standard bionator consists of a mandibular horseshoe-shaped acrylic lingual plate extending from the distal of the last erupted molar to the corresponding point on the other side.
- *Interocclusal acrylic*: The interocclusal space of some of the buccal teeth is filled with acrylic extending arch half of the occlusal surface of the teeth to stabilize the appliance.

### Class III or Reverse Bionator

Class III bionator is also known as reverse bionator and is used for the treatment of Angle's Class III malocclusion caused due to mandibular prognathism.

### Components of Class III or Reverse Bionator

- Wire components
  - Palatal arch wire
  - Vestibular wire.
- Acrylic components
  - Maxillary acrylic part
  - Mandibular acrylic part
  - Interocclusal acrylic part.

### Wire components

- *The palatal arch wire*: The palatal arch wire is same as that of palatal arch wire of standard bionator with an exception that it is placed in the opposite direction.
- *The vestibular wire*: The vestibular wire in the anterior region is made to run over the lower incisors instead of terminating at the lower canines.

### Acrylic Components

Acrylic components, including acrylic in the maxilla, mandible and in the interocclusal space is exactly similar to that of acrylic components of standard bionator.

### Openbite Appliance

This type of bionator is used in open bite cases.

### Components of Open Bite Appliances

Like standard and class III bionator, even open bite appliances also consist of the following components (**Fig. 32.12**):

- Wire components
  - Palatal arch wire
  - Vestibular wire.
- Acrylic components
  - Maxillary acrylic
  - Mandibular acrylic
  - Interocclusal space.

### Wire Components

The palatal arch wires and vestibular wires are same as that of palatal arch wire and vestibular wires of standard bionator.

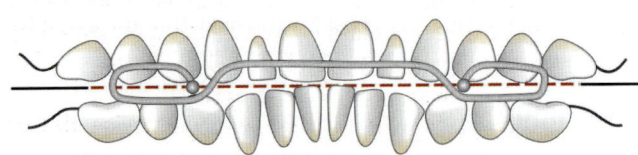

**Fig. 32.12:** Open bite bionator

### Acrylic Components

The maxillary acrylic portion is modified so that even the anterior area is covered to prevent tongue thrusting. Other two acrylic components are same as standard bionator.

### Uses of Bionator

- Class II malocclusion.
- Class III malocclusion.
- Deep bite cases.
- Open bite cases.

## FRANKEL APPLIANCE

The function regulator (FR) appliances are developed by "Rolf Frankel". The function regulators (FR) are orthopedic exercise devices that aid in the maturation, training and reprograming of orofacial neuromuscular system. Function regulators have been designed to overcome functional disorders and re-establish physiologic conditions within the orofacial complex.

### Types of Frankel Appliance

There are five types of Frankel's appliances:
1. FR-I is further divided into three types:
    a. FR-I a
    b. FR-I b
    c. FR-I c
2. FR-II
3. FR-III
4. FR-IV
5. FR-V.

### Indications of Various Types of Frankel Appliances

- *FR-I a appliance of Frankel*: Treating Angle's class I malocclusion with deep bite.
- *FR-I b appliance of Frankel*: Indicated for treating the cases of Angle's class II division 1 malocclusion where the overjet does not exceed 5 mm.
- *FR-I c appliance of Frankel*: Indicated for treating the cases of the Angle's class II division 1 malocclusion where the overjet is more than 7 mm.
- *FR-II appliance of Frankel*: Indicated for treating cases of Angle's class II division 1 malocclusion and class II division 2 malocclusion.
- *FR-III appliance of Frankel*: Indicated for Angle's class III malocclusion.
- *FR-IV appliance of Frankel*: Indicated for treating bimaxillary protrusion and open bite.
- *FR-V appliance of Frankel*: It is used with headgear.

### FR-II Appliances of Frankel

FR-II appliances of Frankel are the appliance of choice in patients with severe class II malocclusion classified by not only mandibular skeletal relations but also significant neuromuscular imbalance **(32.13A to D)**.

The FR-II appliance is used as an exercise device in retaining the associated musculature and indirectly producing changes in the skeletal and dentoalveolar relationship by reprogramming the central nervous system. Frankel II appliance is used for the treatment of Angle's class II Division 1 and Division 2 malocclusion.

### Wire Components of Frankel II Appliances

Wire components of the Frankel II appliances are as follows:
- Labial bow
- Canine extensions
- Palatal bow
- Upper lingual wire
- Lingual crossover wire
- Lower lingual springs
- Support wire of lip pads.

The Acrylic components of Frankel II appliance are as follows:
- Buccal shield
- Lip pads
- Lower lingual pad.

### Wire Components

Wire component of the Frankel II appliances are as follows:
- *Labial bow:* The labial bow, used for Frankel II appliance, is a passive type and it runs in the middle third of the labial surface of the maxillary incisors. The labial bow turns gingivally at the right angle from the distal margin of the lateral incisor. The labial bow should be bent in an ideal contour and not in the contour of malaligned teeth, and then it ends in the vestibular shield on either side.
- *Canine extensions:*
    - Canine extensions are also called as canine guards.
    - Loop of the canine extensions hook to the distal surface of the canine and extends distally about 2-3 mm away from the buccal surface of canine and ends in the vestibular shield.
    - They are two in number, one on right permanent canine and another on left permanent canine.
    - They help in the elimination of restrictive muscle function and in transverse development in the canine region.
- *Palatal bow:* It should follow the curvature of the palate and should have a clearance of 2-3 mm between the bow and the palatal tissue. Lateral extensions of the bow cross interdentally between mesial to first permanent molar and distal to the second permanent premolar and enter the acrylic buccal shield. The recurved ends of the bow terminate as occlusal rest on the occlusal surface between the mesiobuccal and distobuccal cusp of first permanent molar. Similarly, palatal bow transverses on another side of the same arch.
- *Upper lingual wire:* It is also called as lingual stabilizing wire or protrusion bow. The wire prevents tilting of maxillary incisors. It is a sort of labial bow fabricated on palatal surface of maxillary anterior teeth. It originates from vestibular shield and reaches palatal surface by passing distal to canine. The loop is fabricated on

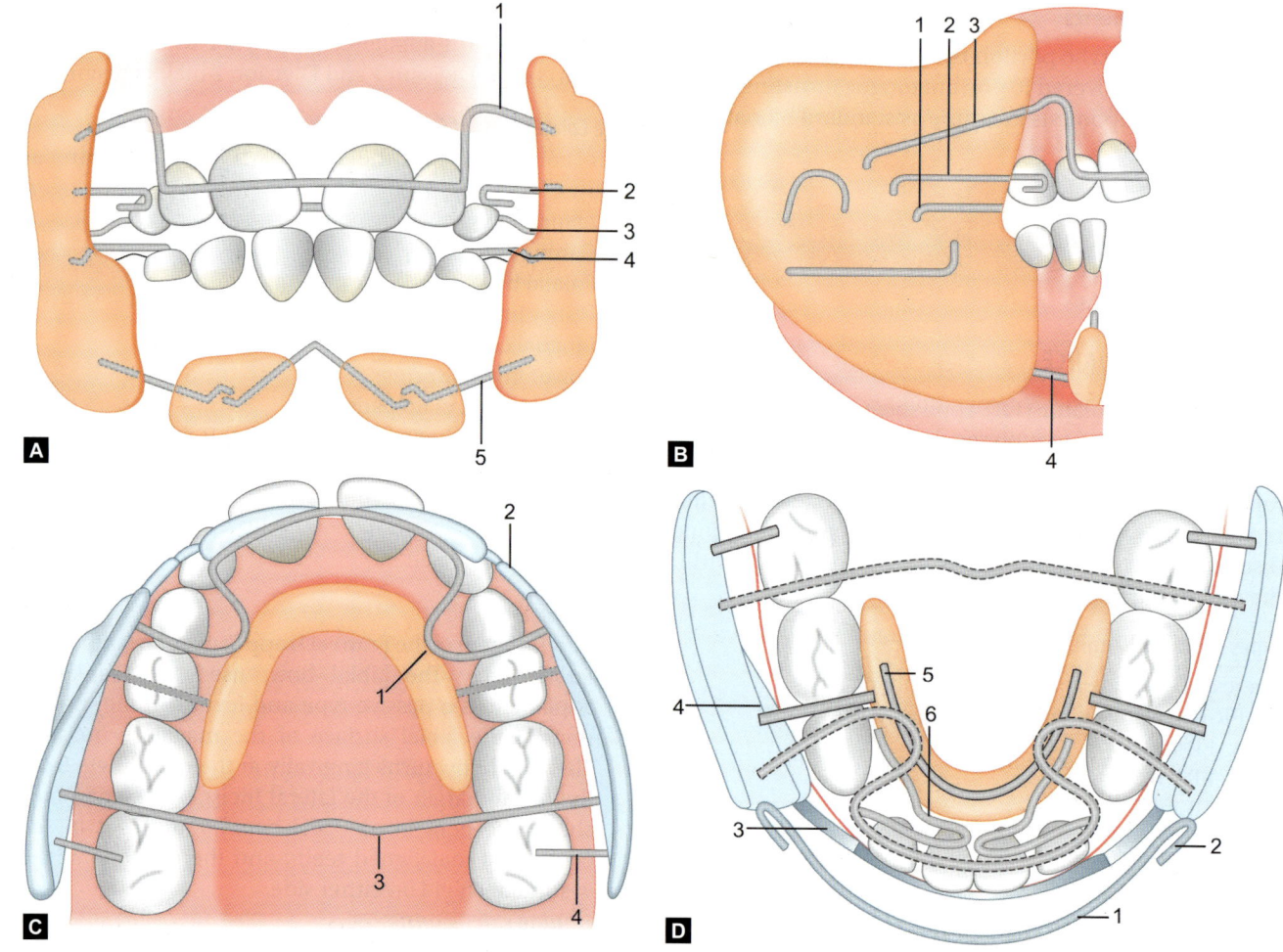

**Figs 32.13A to D:** (A) FR-II appliance of Frankel: 1—Upper labial wire, 2—Canine extension wire, 3—Maxillary lingual wire, 4—Crossover wire, 5—Lower labial wire. (B) Lateral view FR-II appliance of Frankel: 1—Upper labial wire, 2—Canine extension wire, 3—Maxillary lingual wire, 4—Lower labial wire. (C) Maxillary occlusal view FR-II appliance of Frankel: 1—Upper labial wire, 2—Canine extension wire, 3—Palatal wire with occlusal rest. 4—Crossover wire (D) Mandibular occlusal view FR-II appliance of Frankel: 1—Upper labial wire, 2—Canine extension wire, 3—Lower labial wire, 4—Crossover wire, 5—Support wire within the lower lingual shield, 6—Lower lingual spring

canine, then passes on the palatal surface of anterior teeth at the level of the cingulum till it reaches distal marginal ridge of other side lateral incisor and then another loop is fabricated. The distal arm of the loop enters the vestibular shield by passing through the distal surface of another canine.

- *Lingual crossover wire:* Lingual crossover wire follows the contour of the lingual mucosa 3-4 mm below the lingual margin of the mandibular incisors.
- *Lower lingual springs:* They are also called so because they are made to rest on the lingual surface of the mandibular anterior teeth and they are used to prevent the supra-eruption of lower incisor and also to procline the lower anteriors, when the lower anteriors are retroclined.
- Support wire of lip pads.

### Acrylic Components

- *Buccal shield:* Buccal shields are also called the vestibular shields. Buccal shields are composed of acrylic and extends in the buccal vestibule. All the wire components are embedded in this buccal shield.

- *Lip pads:* Lower labial lip pads are also called as pellots. The lip pad helps in elimination of abnormal perioral activity for example, hyperactive mentalis muscle activity.

### Treatment Effects Produced by the FR-II of Frankel Appliance

Treatment effects produced by the FR-II of Frankel appliance can be arbitrarily divided into following two types:

1. Effects on dentoalveolar development: Treatment effects produced by FR-II of Frankel appliance on dentoalveolar development have three effects onto the dentition, they are:
- The cheek is held away from the dentition by the vestibular shield.
- The tongue becomes relatively more of a force because the counter balancing force of cheek musculature is shielded.
- This effect of the Frankel appliance is a result of the vertical extension of the vestibular shields.

*Frankel hypothesizes* that

Verical extension of the shields
↓
Stretch on the alveolar mucosa
↓
Subsequent tension produced on the periosteum
↓
New bone deposition occurring on the lateral borders of the alveolus

Frankel theorizes that the appliance system is especially valuable when treatment begins in early mixed dentition period.

The appliances can utilize the ability of an erupting tooth to act as a "matrix" for alveolar growth. Arch expansion can be best achieved with this appliance, when used before and during the eruption of the canines and premolars.

2. *Effects on skeletal growth:* In the treatment of a class II division 1 malocclusion, the appliance prompts a forward position of the mandible.
- Correction of the malocclusion.
- Increase in the mandibular length by 18.9 mm.
- Posterior facial height (ramus length) increases.
- Facial axis angle is closed.
- A more horizontal vector of facial growth.
- Increase in lower anterior facial height.
- Dental-arch expansion.

### Duration of Treatment with FR-II of Frankel
- Middle or late mixed dentition.
- Duration of treatment is usually 18–24 months of full time appliance wear.

### Clinical Evaluation of Appliance Wear
- Soft tissue: It features
  - Irritation of soft tissue.
  - Hyperemia of the tissue, particularly in the lower labial region.
  - Ulceration or fibrous tissue building.
- The pterygoid response: It includes
  - After 3–4 months of appliance wear, a clinical sign of adaptation is the occurrence of the so called: "pterygoid response".
  - The pterygoid response is indicated by the patient by the inability of the patient to reposition the mandible in a more posterior direction following full-time appliance wear.
  - The "pterygoid response" is mainly because of the lateral pterygoid muscles which are the only orofacial muscles that take part in determining the mandibular posture and translation.
  - Absence of "pterygoid response" clearly indicates that the patient is not wearing the appliance as expected.

### Home Care Instructions
- Appliance should be worn 20–22 hours/day.
- Appliance should be removed in only following situations:
  - Eating
  - Brushing the teeth
  - Practicing a foreign language
  - Playing contact sports
  - Swimming in lake or river.
- Frequent appointments must be given to the patient so as to evaluate the following:
  - Sore spots
  - Patient cooperation
  - Working on patient motivation.
- Parents and siblings should be told to avoid teasing the patient about wearing the appliance and avoid making comments on changes in facial appearance.

### Lip Seal Exercises
- The establishment of a competent oral seal is a major goal of Frankel therapy.
- Patient is instructed to keep the lips together at all times.
- Patient often are given reminders, which are useful in encouraging lip closure.
- During lip seal exercises, the mentalis muscle is relaxed by the lower labial lip pads.
- The patient can be instructed to press on the muscles with his or her fingers, by doing so, increased activity of the orbicularis oris muscle is encouraged.
- Dierkes (1992) instructs the patient to drink with a straw, which strengthens the lip musculature.

### Function Regulator (FR-III) of Frankel
1. The FR-III version of the function regulator of Frankel has been used during **(Fig. 32.14)**
   - Deciduous dentition
   - Mixed dentition
   - Early permanent dentition.
2. Used to correct class III malocclusions primarily characterized by maxillary skeletal retrusions.
3. According to Frankel, the vestibular shields and upper labial pads function to counteract the forces of the surrounding musculature that restricts forward maxillary skeletal development and cause a retrusion in maxillary tooth position.
4. Frankel (1983) also has stated that vestibular shields should stand away from the alveolar process of maxilla but fit closely to the tissue of the mandible, thus, stimulating maxillary alveolar development and restricting mandibular alveolar development.

### Parts of FR-III of Frankel
Acrylic Components of FR-III of Frankel
- Buccal shields.
- Upper lip pads.

Wire Components of FR-III of Frankel
- Upper labial wires (three wire designs).

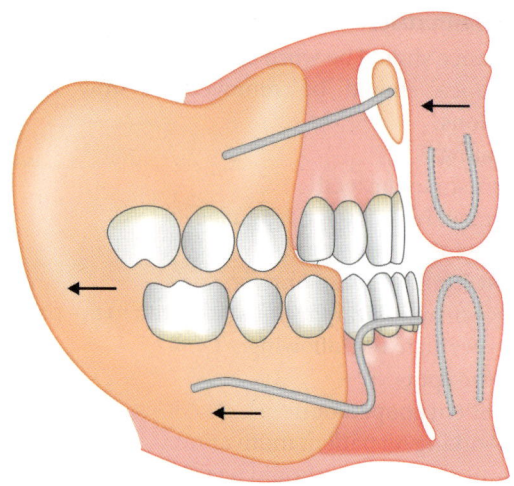

**Fig. 32.14:** FR-III appliance of Frankel

- Lower labial supporting wire.
- Upper lingual wire.
- Upper occlusal rest.
- Palatal wire.
- Lower occlusal rest.

### Acrylic Components of FR-III of Frankel

- *Vestibular shields:* The vestibular shields extend from the depth of the mandibular vestibule to the height of maxillary vestibule. These shields act to remove the restrictive forces created by the buccinators and associated facial muscles against the lateral surface of the alveoli and buccal dentition.
- *Labial pads:* Labial pads lie above the upper incisors and anterior to the maxillary mucosa. The upper labial pads are larger and more extended than the corresponding lower pads of the FR-II.

### Upper Lip Pads

**Shape:** The upper labial lip pads of the FR-III are fabricated in an inverted tear drop shape in sagittal view.
**Location:** They should lie in the height of vestibular sulcus with a contour similar to that of alveolus.

### Wire Components of Frankel III Appliance

- *Upper labial wire:* The upper labial pads are connected to the vestibular shields by a series of three adjacent wires called upper labial wires.
- *Lower labial wire:* Lower aspect of the vestibular shields is connected by a lower labial wire that rests against the labial surface of the lower incisors.
- *Upper lingual wire:* On the lingual surface, an upper lingual wire originates in the vestibular shields, transverses the interocclusal space and rests against the cingula of the upper incisors.
- *Upper occlusal rest:* The upper occlusal rest originates in the posterior aspect of the vestibular shield, traverses the central groove of the upper first molars and then recurves back on itself. Upper occlusal rest is designed in this manner so as not to restrict the forward movement of the maxilla during functional appliance therapy. The upper occlusal rests are necessary only in the cases of anterior crossbite.
- *Palatal wire:* This wire originates in the vestibular shields and traverses the palate. The palatal wire crosses the palate behind the last molar present, thus the maxillary dentition is not restricted in its forward movement by the wires of the appliance.
- *Lower occlusal rests:* All FR-III appliances have lower occlusal rest that originates in the vestibular shield, make a gentle right angle bend along the central groove of the lower first molar and then extend again back into the vestibular shield posterior. The purpose of this type of occlusal rest is to prevent the eruption of the lower first molar.

### Treatment Effects Produced by the Fr-III Appliance

- FR-III of Frankel produces both
  - Skeletal
  - Dentoalveolar changes.
- Treatment effects of FR-III of Frankel, includes more forward movement of maxillary skeletal and dental landmarks, as well as a backward rotation or repositioning of the mandible combined with an increase in lower facial height.
- FR-III of Frankel can also be used as a retainer following orthopedic facial mask therapy.
- Eirew and coworkers stated that FR-III is an excellent retraining device and an aid to musculature reeducation following the surgical correction of Angle's class III malocclusion.
- Petite use of heavy orthopedic forces generated by the facial mask to achieve initial correction of the malocclusion.

## ORAL SCREEN (VESTIBULAR SCREEN)

Newell in 1912 introduced oral screen. It is composed of acrylic base material, which fits in the buccal/labial vestibule of the mouth.

### Indications

Indications for oral screen include:
- Oral habits, such as:
  - Thumb sucking **(Fig. 32.15A)**
  - Mouth breathing
  - Tongue thrusting **(Fig. 32.15B)**
  - Lip biting **(Fig. 32.15C)**.
- In the cases of mild proclination of maxillary anterior teeth **(Fig. 32.16)**.

### Mechanism of Action

- Oral screen **(Fig. 32.17A)** acts like a mechanical barrier between teeth and lips, tongue, thumb and thereby help in correcting the oral habits, such as mouth breathing, thumb sucking, lip biting and tongue thrusting.

- Oral screen is made to contact the proclined teeth when it is used to retrocline the incisors. It transmits the forces of peri-oral musculature to the teeth and thereby retroclining the proclined anterior teeth.
- It is also used as a muscle exerciser to stimulate the hypotonic perioral muscles.

### Modifications of Oral Screen

Oral screen is modified in many ways:

- For the treatment of mouth breathing habit, the oral screen is modified with a number of holes and they are closed gradually in a phased manner **(Fig. 32.17B)**.
- For the treatment of tongue thrusting, oral screen is modified in such a way that there is an additional screen, which is attached to the regular oral screen by means of a thick wire that runs through the bite in the lateral incisor region **(Fig. 32.17C)**.

### Hotz Modifications

- The oral screen can be fabricated with a metal ring projecting between the upper and lower lips **(Fig. 32.17D)**.

## LIP BUMPER

The lip bumper is a fixed functional orthodontic appliance that works by altering the equilibrium between cheeks, lips and tongue and by transmitting forces from perioral muscles to the molars where it is applied **(Fig. 32.18)**.

### Uses

Uses of lip bumper include **(Fig. 32.19)**:

a. Lip bumper is used to treat lip suckling habit.
b. Lip bumper is used to treat lip biting habit.
c. Lip bumper is used as a molar anchorage.
d. Lip bumper is used for space gaining in the lower arch.

### Characteristics of the Lip Bumper

- The lip bumper has a removable part and a fixed part. The removable part is composed of a 0.045 inch stainless steel wire that runs in the lower vestibule from molar to molar between teeth, lip and cheeks. Fixed part of lip bumper is composed of two molar bands

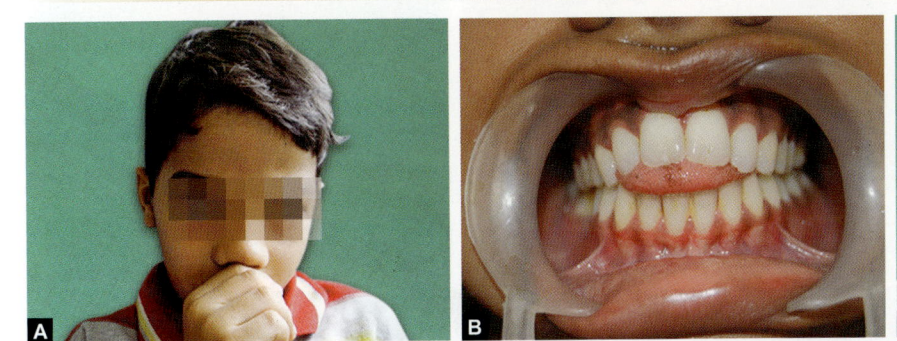
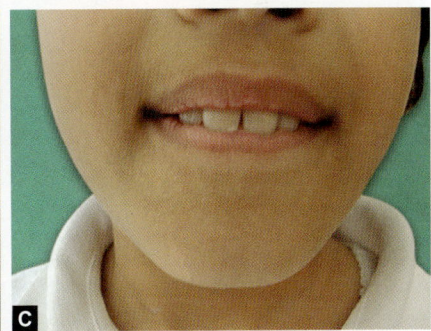

**Figs 32.15A to C:** **(A)** Thumb sucking habit. **(B)** Tongue thrusting habit. **(C)** Lip biting habit

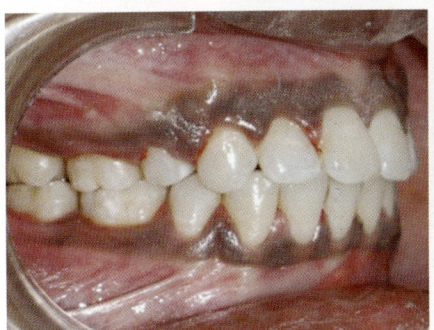
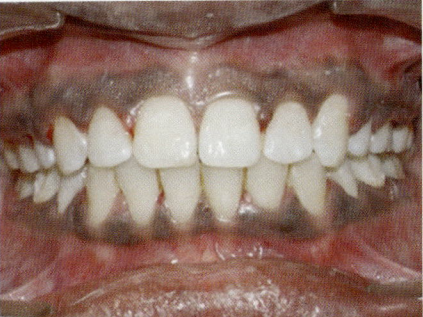
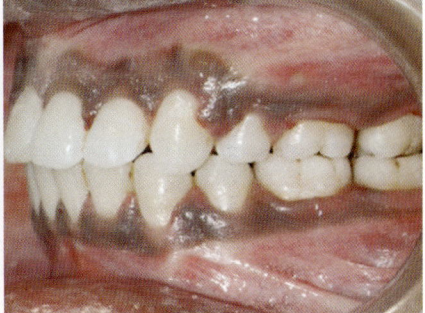

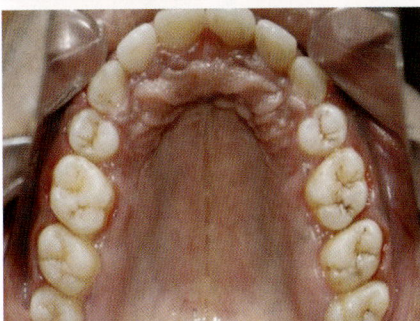
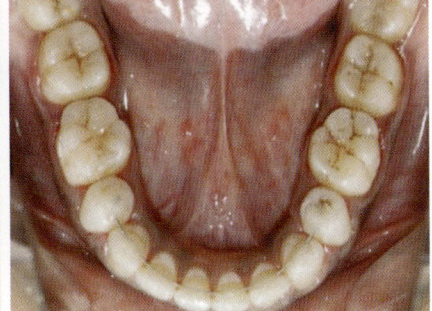

**Fig. 32.16:** A patient of Angle I malocclusion with proclination of teeth, such a malocclusion can be treated by using an oral screen

cemented to first or if possible second molar with 0.045 inch tubes **(Figs 32.20)**.
- The lip bumper may be preformed lip bumper or custom made lip bumper.
- Performed lip bumper is having four loops, two adjustment loops mesial to each molar and two in the canine area. It can be used for class III elastics in more severe cases.
- The custom made lip bumper has only two loops and is located mesial to each molar.
- The appliance must be worn 24 hours a day and should be removed only for meal and hygiene.

### Fitting the Lip Bumper

The lip bumper must keep cheeks and lips away from the lower dentoalveolar area and it should be wider

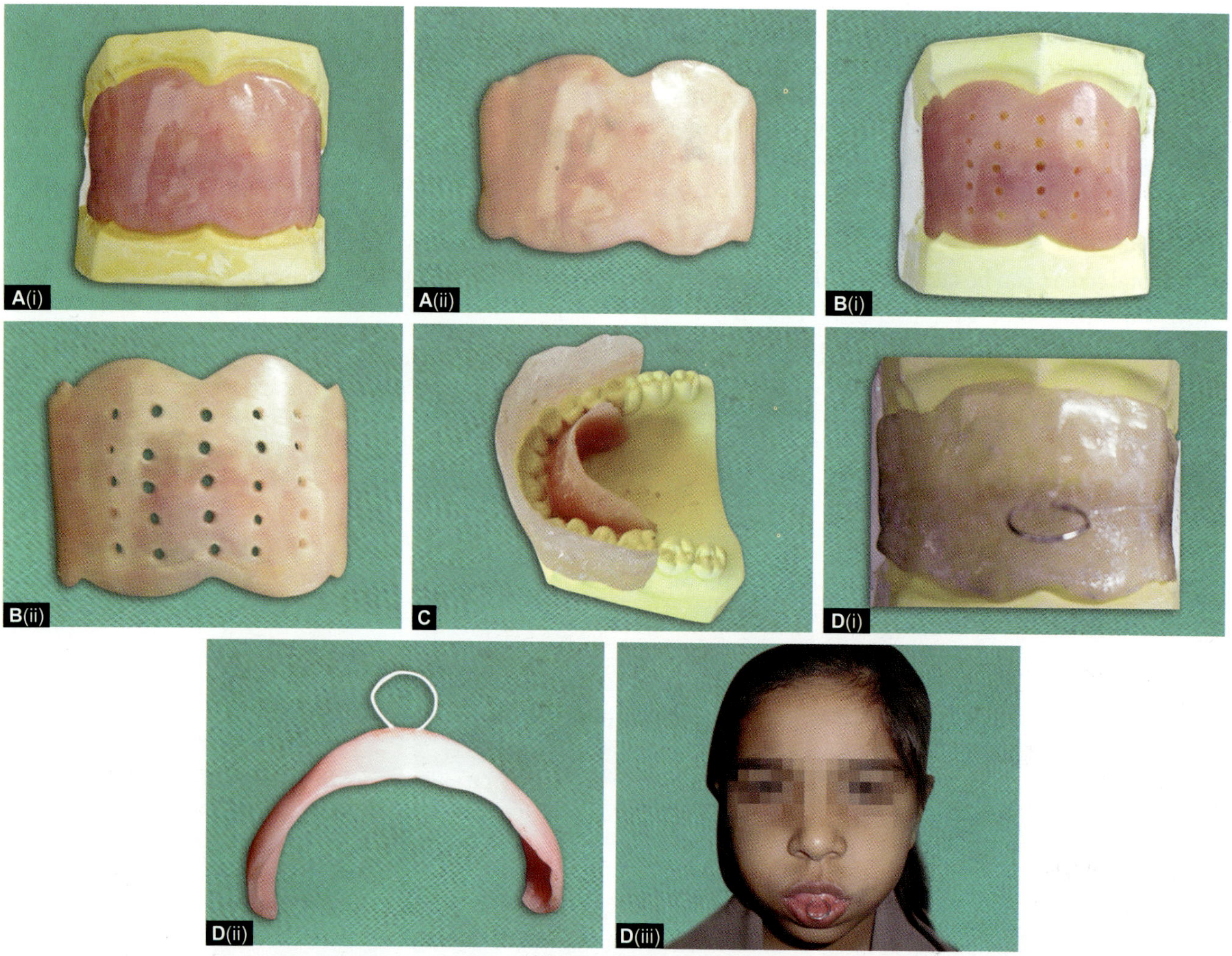

**Figs 32.17A to D:** (Ai and ii) Oral screen, (B i and ii) Oral screen with wholes used to treat mouth breathing habit, (C) Double oral screen, (Di, ii and iii) Hotz type of oral screen used to treat mild proclination of upper anterior teeth sucking habit and digit sucking

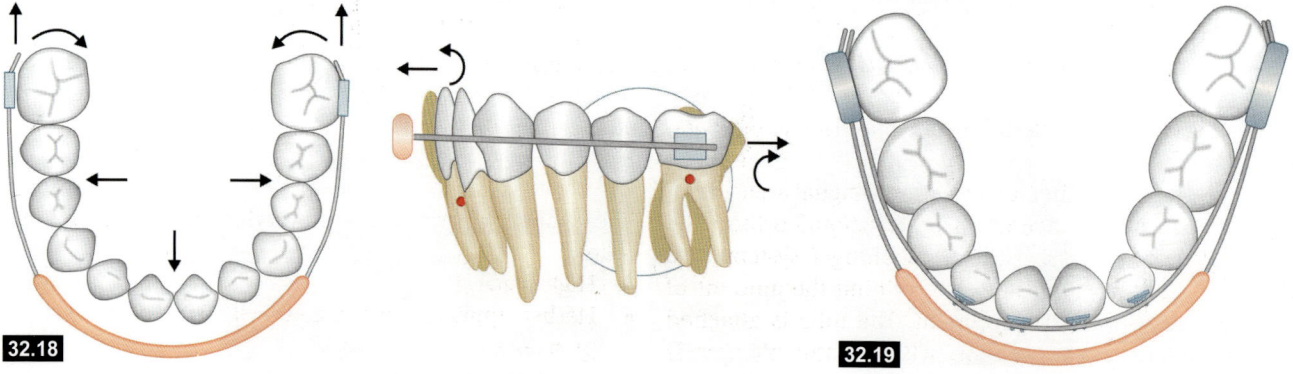

**Fig. 32.18:** Lip bumper; **Fig. 32.19:** Lip bumper in conjunction with fixed orthodontic appliance

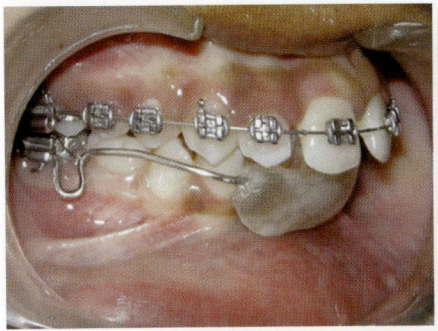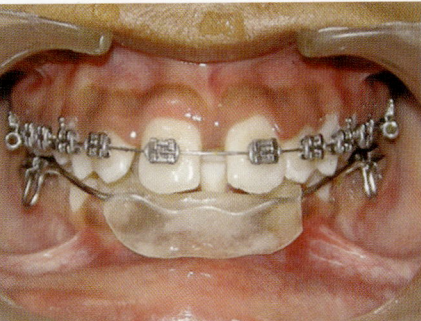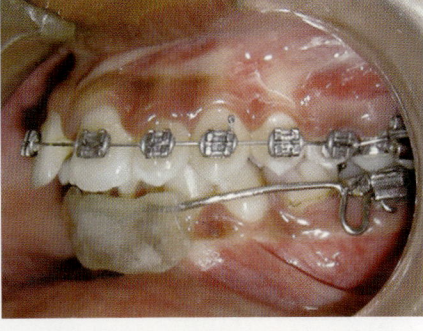

**Fig. 32.20:** Fixed part of lip bumper is composed of two bands on first molars with 0.045 inch tubes

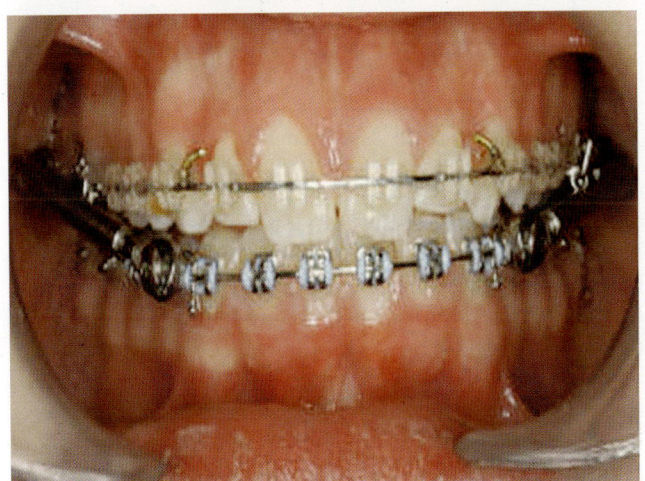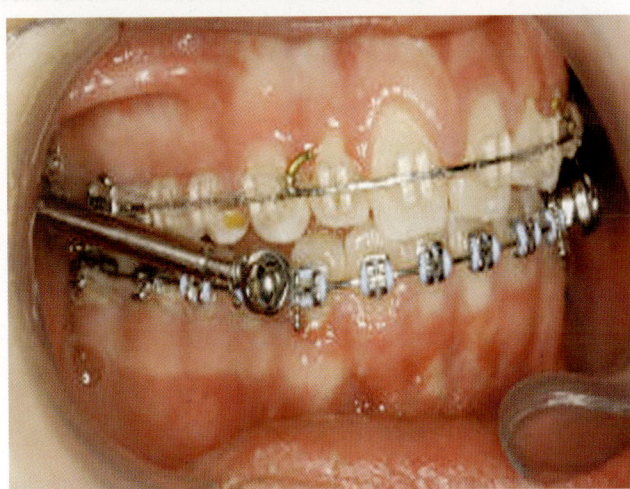

**Fig. 32.21:** Herbst appliance

buccally and flatter anteriorly. It should not exert any expansion or contraction on the molar and must be easy for the clinician and the patient to insert and remove.

## HERBST APPLIANCE

The Herbst bite jumping mechanism was developed by Emil Herbst in the early 1900s. The original banded design of this appliance was introduced at the International Dental Congress in Berlin (Germany) by Herbst in 1905. It was introduced by Pancherz. Pancherz used a banded Herbst design that involved the following:
- Maxilla
  - Placement of bands on molar and premolar
  - Bands are connected by copper lingual wire.
- Mandible
  - Bands on lower right first molar and lower right first premolar
  - Bands are connected by a lower lingual arch wire.

The Herbst appliance is a fixed functional orthopedic appliance having passive tube and plunger system with the exact length of the tube determining the amount of anterior mandibular development. The tube is attached to a maxillary posterior root, whereas the plunger is fixed anteriorly to the mandibular dentition and slides through the tube during opening and closing movements **(Fig. 32.21)**.

### Indications
Herbst appliance is indicated in the following conditions:
- Dental class II malocclusion.
- Deep bite with retroclined mandibular incisors.
- Skeletal class II mandibular deficiency.

### Contraindications
Herbst appliance is contraindicated in the following conditions:
- Dental and skeletal open bites.
- Cases prone to root resorption.

### Advantages
The advantage of Herbst appliance includes abundant documentation availability and variety of modifications to suit the need of individual clinician.

### Disadvantages
The major disadvantages of Herbst appliance are as follows:
- High cost.
- Herbst appliance associated with more chances of breakage.
- Less patient acceptance.

## JASPER JUMPER

An American orthodontist James Jasper replaced the rigid telescopic mechanism used in Herbst appliance with a flexible plastic cover open coil spring that can be attached directly to auxiliary wires with a complete partial or fixed appliance in place **(Fig. 32.22)**. It is the most successful and widely used interarch force delivery system used with fixed mechanotherapy. It is used with push force rather than the more common pull force of class II elastics and other extension springs.

The Jasper jumper is essentially a heavy coil spring encased in plastic that uses pivoting attachments at both ends. To permit a greater range of opening, an auxiliary is frequently used.

### Advantages

- Ease of insertion of activation
- It generates intrusive forces on molars and incisors.

### Disadvantages

- It is more prone for breakage
- Lack of force when the mouth is held open slightly, such as in sleeping mouth breather.

## TWIN-BLOCK APPLIANCE

Twin-block appliance is a functional jaw orthopedic appliance developed by Scottish orthodontist William Clark in the year 1977.

The Twin-block appliance is composed of maxillary and mandibular retainers that fit tightly against the teeth, alveolus and adjacent supporting structures. Delta clasps are used bilaterally to anchor the maxillary

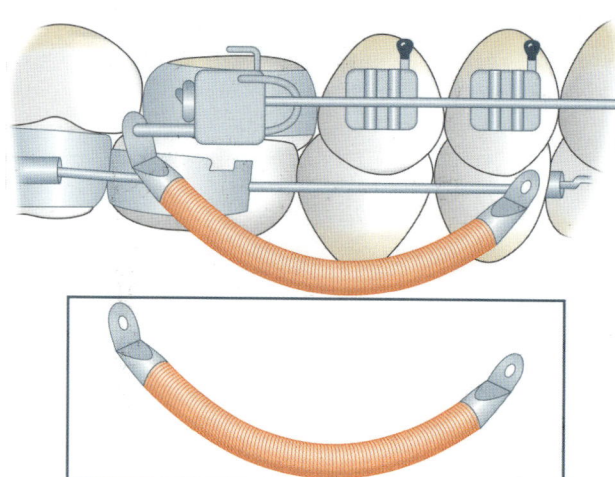

**Fig. 32.22:** Jasper jumper appliance

appliance to the first permanent molars and 0.030 inch ball clasps are placed in the interproximal areas anteriorly **(Figs 32.23)**. The precise clasp configuration depends on the type of deciduous or permanent teeth and number of teeth present at the time of appliance construction.

Various designs are available for the lower part of the twin block appliance. The original design advocated by Clark consists of a horseshoe of acrylic that extends anteriorly from the mesial of the first permanent molars.

The acrylic covers the lingual aspect of the premolar/deciduous molars and the canines and incisors. In this design, delta clasps are used to anchor the appliance to the first premolar/first deciduous molar and ball clasp are present between the canines and lateral incisors, additional ball clasps can be placed between the incisors,

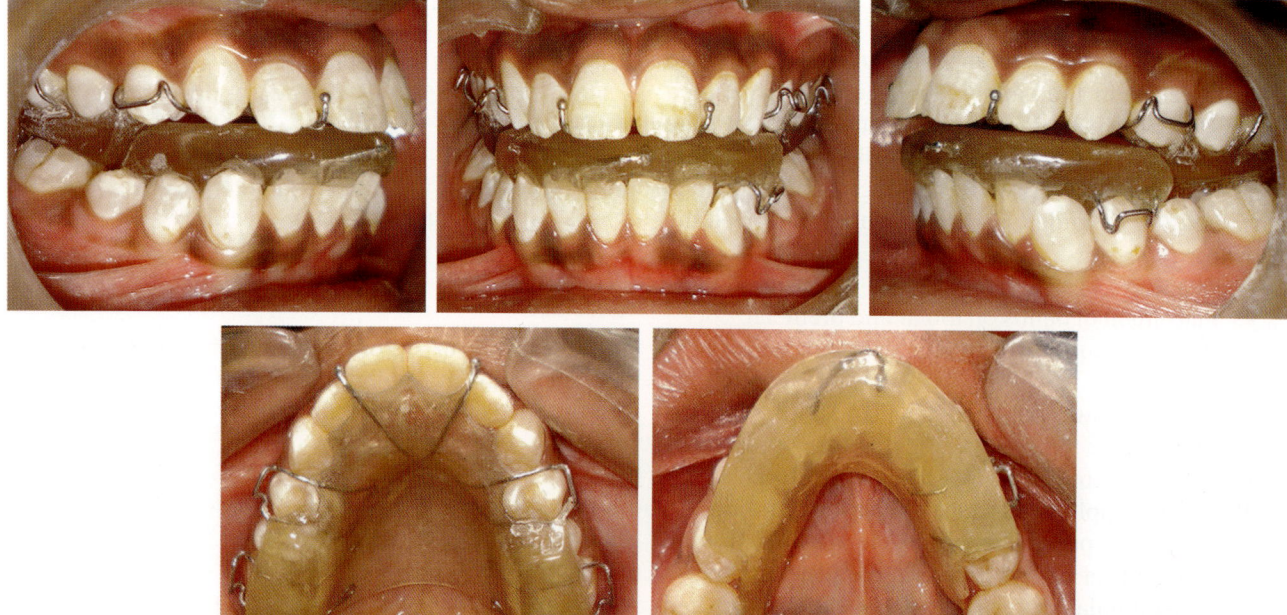

**Fig. 32.23:** Twin-block appliances

if appliance retention is thought to be a problem. There should not be any acrylic material touching the lower molars, this allows the lower molar to erupt vertically, if the acrylic on the maxillary block is trimmed to increase the vertical dimension.

The twin block appliance has been shown to produce increase in mandibular length, incisor proclination and variations in lower anterior facial height.

The posterior bite blocks of the twin block appliance can be trimmed to facilitate the eruption of the lower posterior teeth in patient with a deep bite and an accentuated curve of Spee. The blocks also can be left untouched to prevent the eruption of the posterior teeth in patients with a tendency toward an anterior open bite.

### Indications

Twin-block appliance is most commonly used in the treatment of class II malocclusions.

A case report on class III malocclusion has been illustrated to give the full insight of the case.

### Duration of Treatment

Full time wearing of twin block appliance is advised including while eating and the duration of treatment usually is about (9–12) months.

## BIBLIOGRAPHY

1. Bishara SE, Ziaja RR. Functional appliances: a review. Am J Orthod Dentofacial Orthop 1989;95(3):250-8.
2. Clark WJ. The twin block technique. A functional orthopedic appliance system. Am J Orthod Dentofacial Orthop 1988;93(1):1-18.
3. Falck F, Frankel R. Clinical relevance of step-by-step mandibular advancement in the treatment of mandibular retrusion using the Fränkel appliance. Am J Orthod 1989; 96(4):333-41.
4. Frankel R. A functional approach to orofacial orthopedics. Br J Orthod 1980;7:41-51.
5. Logan WR. The clinical management of the Fränkel appliance, F.R.1. Dent Pract Dent Rec 1971;21(6):205-11.
6. McNamara JA Jr, Huge SA. The functional regulator (FR-3) of Fränkel. Am J Orthod 1985;88(5):409-24.
7. McNamara JA, Howe RP. Clinical management of the acrylic splint Herbst appliance. Am J Orthod Dentofacial Orthop 1988;94(2):142.
8. Pancherz H, Anehus-Pancherz M. The headgear effect of the Herbst appliance: a cephalometric long-term study. Am J Orthod Dentofacial Orthop 1993;103(6):510-20.
9. Pancherz H. The effects, limitations and long-term dentofacial adaptations to treatment with the Herbst appliance. Semin Orthod 1997;3(4):232-43.
10. Sessle BJ, Woodside DG, Bourque P, et al. Effect of functional appliances on jaw muscle activity. Am J Orthod Dentofacial Orthop 1990;98(3):222-30.
11. Stucki N, Ingervall B. The use of the Jasper Jumper for the correction of Class II malocclusion in the young permanent dentition. Eur J Orthod 1998;20(3):271-81.
12. Wieslander L. Long-term effect of treatment with the headgear-Herbst appliance in the early mixed dentition. Am J Orthod Dentofacial Orthop 1993;104(4):319-29.

---

### EXAM-ORIENTED QUESTIONS

#### Long Questions

1. Principle and mode of action of functional appliances. Discuss Frankel appliance in detail.
2. Define and classify functional appliance. Discuss principles and mode of action of functional appliance and also advantages, disadvantages and effects of functional appliance.
3. Write down indications, contra-indications, advantages, fabrication and effects of activator.
4. Write in detail about bionator.
5. Write in detail about Frankel's appliance.
6. Discuss about twin-block appliance in detail.

#### Short Notes

1. Lip bumper
2. Herbst appliance
3. Jasper jumper appliance
4. FR III appliance
5. Differences between FR-I and FR-II APPLIANCE.

# CHAPTER 33

# Orthopedic Appliances

*Phulari BS*

There are essentially three alternatives for treating any skeletal malocclusions—growth modification, dental camouflage and orthognathic surgery. While all three may be possible in growing patients, only the latter two options can be used in adults.

Ideally, growth modification should be opted wherever applicable because this precludes the need for tooth extractions and surgery. The goal of growth modification is to alter the unacceptable skeletal relationships by modifying the patient's remaining facial growth to favorably change the size or position of the jaws.

Basically, there are three types of orthodontic appliances that can be used for modifying the growth of maxilla and/or mandible; orthopedic appliances, functional appliances and inter-arch elastic traction. This chapter discusses the essential aspects of orthopedic appliances.

## ORTHODONTIC FORCE VS ORTHOPEDIC FORCE

There are two types of forces used in orthodontics. One is "orthodontic force," which when applied brings about dental change; the other is "orthopedic force," that brings about skeletal change. Unlike orthodontic forces which are light forces (50–100 gm) bringing about tooth movement, orthopedic forces are heavy forces, generally in the range of 300–500 gm (over 400 gm) per side, that bring about changes in the magnitude and direction of bone growth. The appliances that produce skeletal changes by applying orthopedic forces are known as "orthopedic appliances." Since they employ heavy forces, adequate anchorage required is gained by extraoral means using occipital, parietal, frontal cranial bones and cervical vertebrae. The most widely used orthopedic appliances are headgear, protraction face mask (reverse pull headgear) and chin cup.

## RATIONALE ORTHOPEDIC APPLIANCE THERAPY

Orthopedic appliances generally use teeth as "handles" to transmit forces to the underlying skeletal structures. Basis of orthopedic appliance therapy resides in the use of intermittent forces of very high magnitude. Such heavy forces when directed to the basal bones via teeth, tend to alter the magnitude and direction of the jaws by modifying the pattern of bone apposition at periosteal sutures and growth sites.

Immediate tooth movement does not occur since hyalinized zones in periodontal ligament caused by heavy forces prevent direct frontal resorption of the socket wall. Orthopedic appliances are worn intermittently for only about 10–12 hours a day. Tooth movement is also reduced significantly by replenishment of normal circulation when the appliance is not worn.

Thus, skeletal changes rather than tooth movement occur during orthopedic appliance therapy, although some tooth movement is inevitable.

## PRINCIPLES OF USING ORTHOPEDIC APPLIANCES

The following are the basic principles of using orthopedic appliances effectively:

### Magnitude of Force

- Light orthodontic forces used for tooth movement (50 to 100 gm per tooth) are not sufficient for orthopedic purposes to modify skeletal growth.
- Extraoral forces of much greater magnitude, in excess of 400 gm per side, is required to bring about skeletal changes. Most orthopedic appliances employ forces in the range of 400 to 600 gm per side for a total of two to three pounds to maximize skeletal change and to minimize dental change. Such heavy forces compress the periodontal ligament on the pressure side and cause hyalinization, which prevent tooth movement.

### Duration of Force

- In contrast to continuous light forces that are effective in producing orthodontic tooth movement, orthopedic changes are best produced by employing intermittent heavy forces. Intermittent forces of 12–14 hours duration per day appear to be effective in producing orthopedic changes.
- Since most orthopedic appliances are tooth-borne an increase in the duration of appliance wearing more than 16 hours/day and decrease in the magnitude below 400 gm will produce dental changes rather than skeletal changes.
- Thus intermittent forces employed in dentofacial orthopedics minimize tooth movement while still providing for skeletal changes. An intermittent heavy force is also less damaging to the teeth and periodontium than a continuous heavy force.

### Direction of Force

- Orthopedic force should be applied in the appropriate direction to have a maximum skeletal effect.
- The desired changes are best achieved when the line of force passes through the center of resistance of the skeletal structures to be moved.

- The force direction or force vector should be decided depending on the clinical needs. For example, while treating class II malocclusion with headgear therapy, the selection of cervical attachment produces a force vector that is below the center of resistance of maxillary molars resulting in distalization as well as the extrusion of the molars; while an occipital attachment produces the intrusion of molar
- An appropriate site of anchorage should be selected based on what type of skeletal and tooth movement would be beneficial in a given case.

### Age of the Patient
- It is advisable to begin orthopedic appliance therapy while patient is still in the mixed dentition period, to make most of the active growth occurring during prepubertal growth spurt.
- Treatment may have to be continued until the completion of adolescent growth, so as to prevent relapse caused by the re-expression of patient's fundamental growth pattern after the cessation of orthopedic therapy.

### Timing of Force Application
- Optimum timing of extraoral force application is considered to be during evening and night. This is because, an increased release of growth hormone and other growth-promoting endocrine factors has been observed to occur during the evening and night rather than during the day.
- Evidence suggests that skeletal growth is associated with sleep onset and follows a circadian pattern. Thus patients are advised to wear the appliance in the evening after school hours and throughout the night, which is also advantageous in the terms of patient compliance.

## APPLIANCES

The following are the commonly used orthopedic appliances:
I. Headgear
II. Protraction face mask
III. Chin cup appliance

### Headgear

Headgears are the most widely used extraoral orthopedic appliances. They are mainly used in the management of skeletal class II malocclusion by growth modification. They are also used for the distalization of maxillary molars, as well as for reinforcing intraoral anchorage.

A typical headgear is attached to the teeth via a face bow and is anchored from the back of the head/neck by means of head cap/neck strap **(Fig. 33.1A)**.

### Components
1. **Force-delivering Unit**
   - Face bow **(Fig. 33.1B)**
   - 'J' hook.
2. **Force generating unit (Fig. 33.1C)**
3. **Anchor unit**
   - Head cap or
   - Neck strap **(Fig. 33.1D)**
1. **Force Delivering Unit**

Headgears employ either a face bow or a 'J' hook for delivering extraoral forces to the maxillary posterior teeth.

#### Face Bow
Face bow is a metallic framework made of large gauge wire. It is more versatile than the 'J' hook as it can be attached to teeth either via brackets (fixed orthodontic appliance) or removable appliance.

#### Parts
Face bow consists of **(Fig. 33.2)**:
i. Outer bow/Whisker bow
ii. Inner bow
iii. Junction.

i. **Outer bow:** It includes the following features:
   - The outer bow is made of a round stainless steel wire of 0.051" or 0.062" that is contoured to fit around the face.
   - The length of the outer bow can be adjusted to produce the desired force vector/line of force.
     a. *Short-outer bow:* Outer bow is shorter than the inner bow.
     b. *Medium-outer bow:* Outer bow is as long as the inner bow.
     c. *Long-outer bow:* Outer bow is longer than the inner bow.

   Outer bow on both sides at the distal end is curved to form a hook that gives attachment to the force generating unit.

ii. **Inner bow:** It includes the following features:
   - The inner bow is made of 0.045" or 0.052" (1.25 mm) round stainless steel wire and is contoured to follow the shape of the dental arch.
   - The inner bow is inserted into the round buccal face bow tube, which is welded to the buccal surface of maxillary first permanent molar band.
   - The inner bow is well-adapted according to the shape of the arch.
   - Stops in the form of U-loops, bayonet bends and friction stops are placed in the bow mesial to the buccal tube of first permanent molar to prevent the inner bow from sliding too far distally through the buccal tube.

iii. **Junction:** It includes the following features:
   - It is the point of attachment of the inner and outer bow, which may be soldered or welded.
   - The junction is usually situated in the midline of the bows, although it can be shifted either right or left side depending upon asymmetrical force needed.
     *Face bow fitting:* Points to remember while fitting face bow are:
   - Preformed face bows are available and are modified to fit the arch form of the patient.
   - Inner bow should fit closely to the arch.

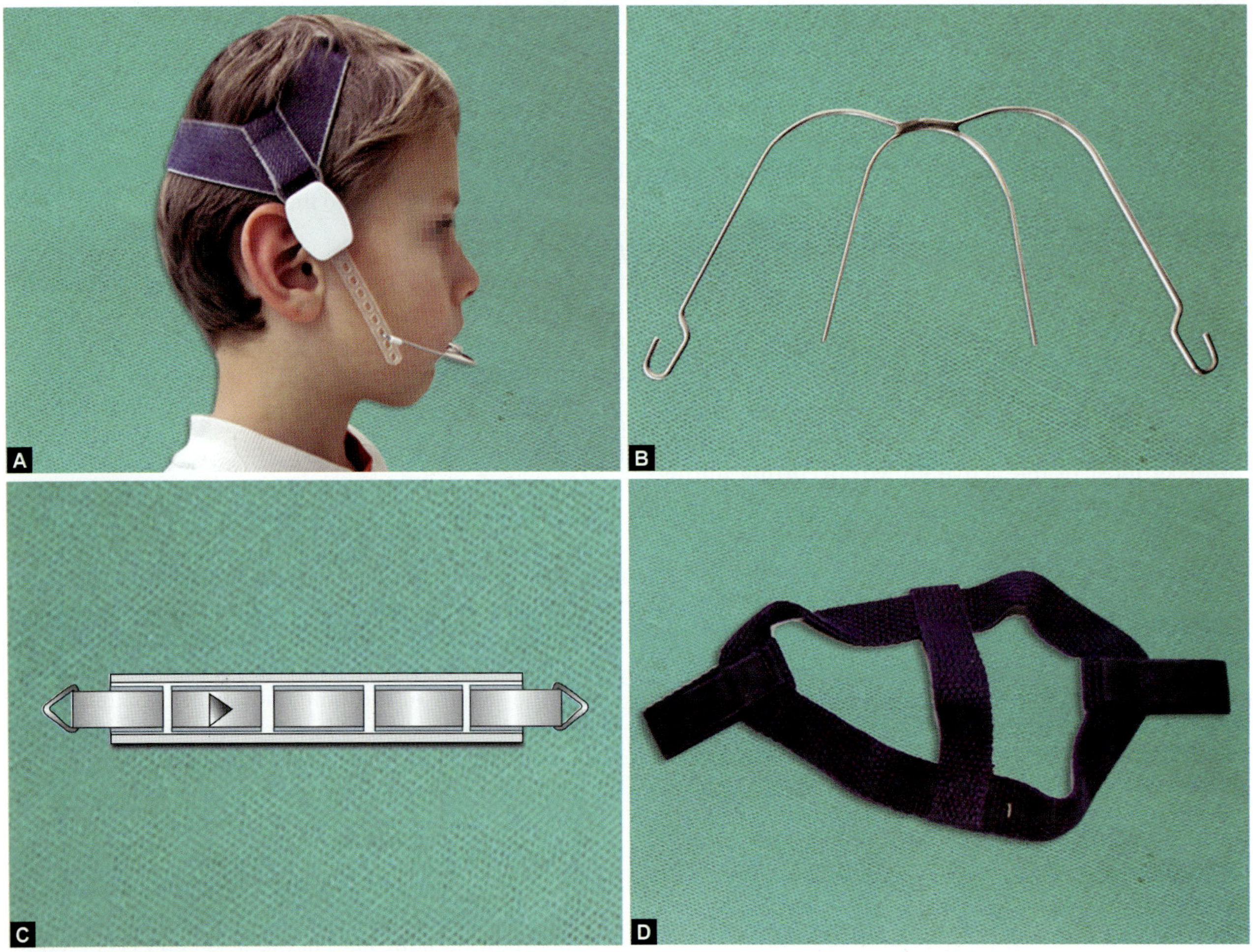

**Figs 33.1A to D:** (A) Patient with headgear appliance; Components; (B) Face bow; (C) Force-generating unit; (D) Strap

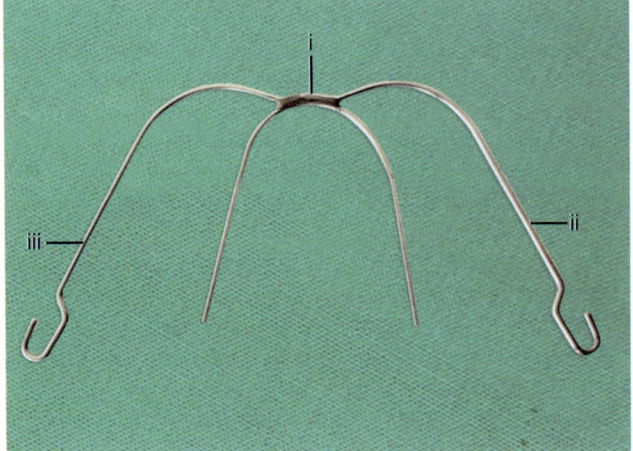

**Fig. 33.2:** Parts of face bow: i-Junction, ii-Inner bow and iii-Outer bow

- Stops provided in the inner bow should allow the anterior portion of the bow to be placed about 4–5 mm away from the maxillary incisors.
- Anterior portion of the bow should fit comfortably between the lips at rest.
- The outer bow is adjusted to confirm the cheeks, and should rest several mm away from the cheeks.

2. **Force-generating Unit**
   - It is the force-generating element of the assembly, which produces heavy forces to effect skeletal changes.
   - Force-generating unit also connects the face bow to the anchor unit (head cap or neck strap).
   - Force-generating unit may be in the form of:
     - springs
     - elastics, or
     - other stretchable material
   - Force thus produced is delivered to the teeth through the face bow and then to the underlying skeletal structures via teeth.
   - Springs are preferred as they provide a constant force whereas elastics tend to undergo force decay.

3. **Anchor Unit**
   - Headgear appliance derives anchorage from extraoral sites using the rigid bones of skull and/or the back of the neck.
   - There are two basic types of extraoral attachments that provide anchorage for headgear:
     a. Cervical attachment/neck strap
     b. Occipital attachment/head cap
   - A combination of cervical and occipital attachments may also be used to distribute the external forces over a wide surface area.

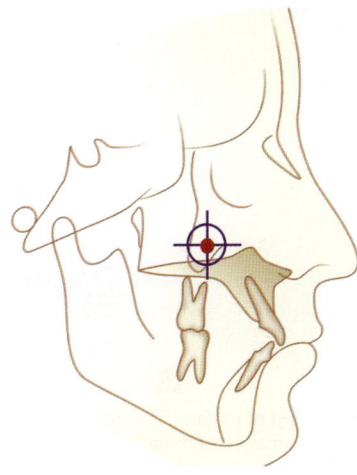

Fig. 33.3: Center of resistance of maxilla is usually located between the roots of the premolar teeth

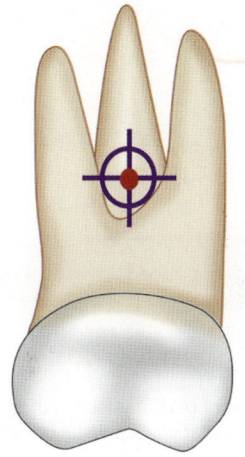

Fig. 33.4: Center of resistance of maxillary molar

## Mode of Action

- A headgear when used for growth modification is designed to deliver heavy extraoral orthopedic forces to the sutures of maxilla. Such heavier forces compress the maxillary sutures and thus modify the pattern of bone apposition at these sites. This, in turn-changes the magnitude and direction of growth of the maxilla.
- The goal of the treatment in the management of skeletal class II malocclusion is to restrict the maxillary growth, while the mandible continues to grow forward an adequate amount to "catch up" with the maxilla, thus correcting the anteroposterior jaw relationship.
- The forces need to be of sufficient magnitude, applied in an appropriate direction, and delivered for an adequate length of time, during a period of active mandibular growth for there to be a positive treatment prognosis.

## Indications of Headgear Therapy

1. *Growth modification:* Headgears can be used to treat a variety of skeletal class II problems. However, ideal circumstances to use the extraoral orthopedic effect of headgears is when skeletal class II malocclusion is caused by maxillary protrusion (anteroposterior excess of maxilla) with normal mandibular skeletal and dental morphology, and when there is continued active mandibular growth in a forward direction.
2. For distalization of maxillary molars.
3. To reinforce intraoral anchorage.

## Biomechanical Principles of Headgear Therapy

The clinician must follow the biomechanical principles so as to control the direction and magnitude of the forces produced by different headgear designs and to determine the type of clinical changes that can be expected.

## Center of Resistance

A force passing through the center of resistance causes pure translation in the direction of the line of force. Any other force not acting through the center of resistance produces translation as well as rotation.

*Center of resistance of maxilla:* Center of resistance of maxilla is usually located between the roots of the premolar teeth **(Fig. 33.3)**. The forces must be directed perfectly through this point to effectively restrain maxilla without tipping it.

*Center of resistance of maxillary first molar:* Because the intraoral point of attachment of force is localized to the bands on the maxillary first permanent molars, it is usually the molar center of resistance that is considered when determining the direction or vector of force of the headgear.

- The center of resistance of maxillary first molar lies at the trifurcation area **(Fig. 33.4)**. Forces acting through the center of resistance of the molar tend to translate it **(Fig. 33.5A)**, while any other forces tend to tip the tooth.
- If the force is applied below the center of resistance, it causes a distal crown tipping **(Fig. 33.5B)**, while force acting above the center of resistance will cause a mesial crown tipping **(Fig. 33.5C)**.

## Line of Force Action

Extraoral orthopedic force must be applied in the appropriate direction to have a maximum skeletal effect. Although superior and posterior force through the center of resistance appears to be the most appropriate direction to affect the maxillary sutures, some modification of the angle of that force vector may be necessary in specific situation.

According to the specific clinical needs, the force direction or vector can be altered by the following means:

a. Selection of the appropriate extraoral anchorage site (type of attachment):
- The cervical or occipital extraoral attachment can be selected to establish a low- or high-angle force vector, respectively.
- By using the cervical attachment/neck strap, the extraoral force is directed inferiorly as well as posteriorly, with the force vector acting below the center of the resistance of maxillary molars **(Fig. 33.6)**.

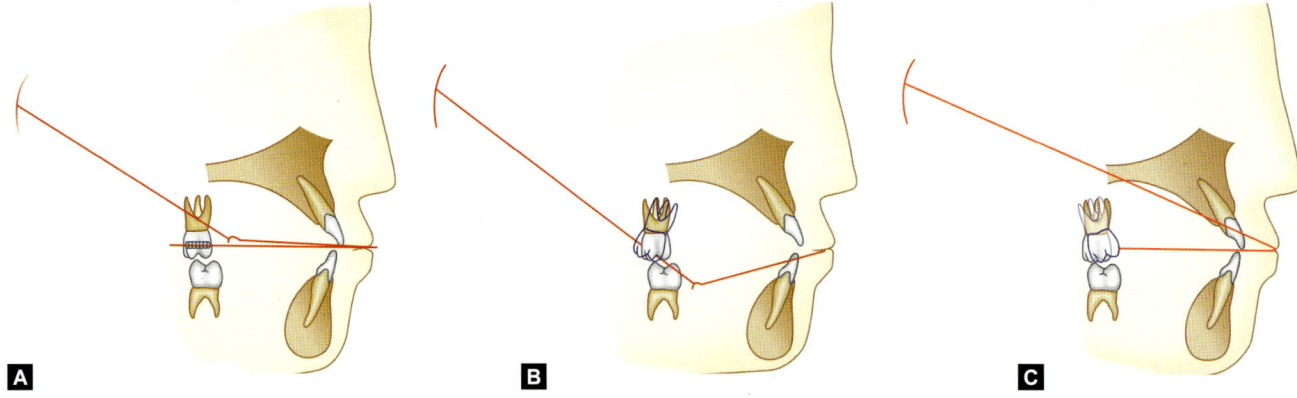

**Figs 33.5A to C:** Line of (A) Force acting through the center of resistance causes bodily movement of molar; (B) Force passing below the center of resistance of molar causes distal crown tipping; (C) Force passing above the center of resistance of molar causes distal root tipping

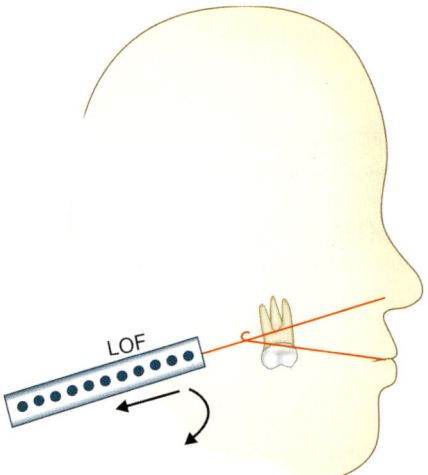

**Fig. 33.6:** Line of force in headgear with cervical attachment is directed inferiorly as well as posteriorly, and acts below the center of resistance of maxillary molars

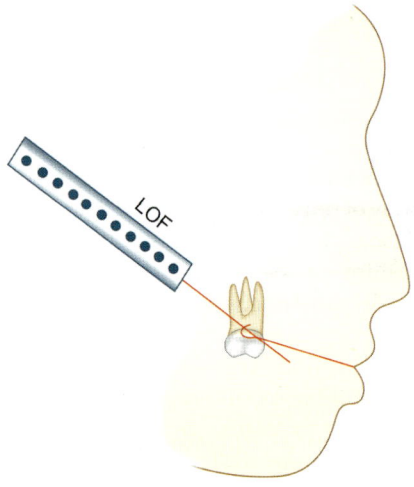

**Fig. 33.7:** Line of force occipital headgear acts vertically and posteriorly through the center of resistance of maxillary molars, resulting in intrusion and retraction of the molar

Such a force vector results in distalization as well as extrusion of the molars, while distalization of molars is favorable in class II corrections, extrusion is not.
- Use of occipital attachment results in a line of force that acts vertically and posteriorly through the center of the resistance of maxillary molars. This line of force acts to intrude and retract the molar, which is favorable in class II management **(Fig. 33.7)**.
b. By altering the length and height of the outer bow:
   Force vector can also be altered suitably by varying the length of the outer bow or by changing its vertical height **(Figs 33.8A and B)**.

### Amount, Duration and Timing of Force
- Headgears should apply extraoral forces in the magnitude of 400–600 gm per side, intermittently for a duration of 12 to 16 hours a day to bring about the desired skeletal effects.
- Headgear therapy is initiated in the mixed dentition period and maintained until the cessation of maxillary growth.
- Patients are advised to wear the appliance in the evening and throughout the night. Headgear treatment is usually given at 8.5 to 10.5 years in females and 9.5 to 11.5 years in males.
- Excessive force greater than 1,000 gm will result in trauma to the teeth periodontium, while force of lesser magnitude may produce dental changes rather than skeletal changes.

### Types of Headgears
There are several types of headgears that can be used to bring about a desired effect. The type of headgear and the appropriate force level should be selected according to the specific treatment objectives in a given patient.

According to location of anchor unit, headgear can be of the following types:
a. Cervical pull headgear
b. Occipital pull headgear
c. High pull headgear
d. Combination pull headgear

### Cervical Headgear (Figs 33.9A and B)
- Cervical headgear derives anchorage from the back of the neck using a neck strap.

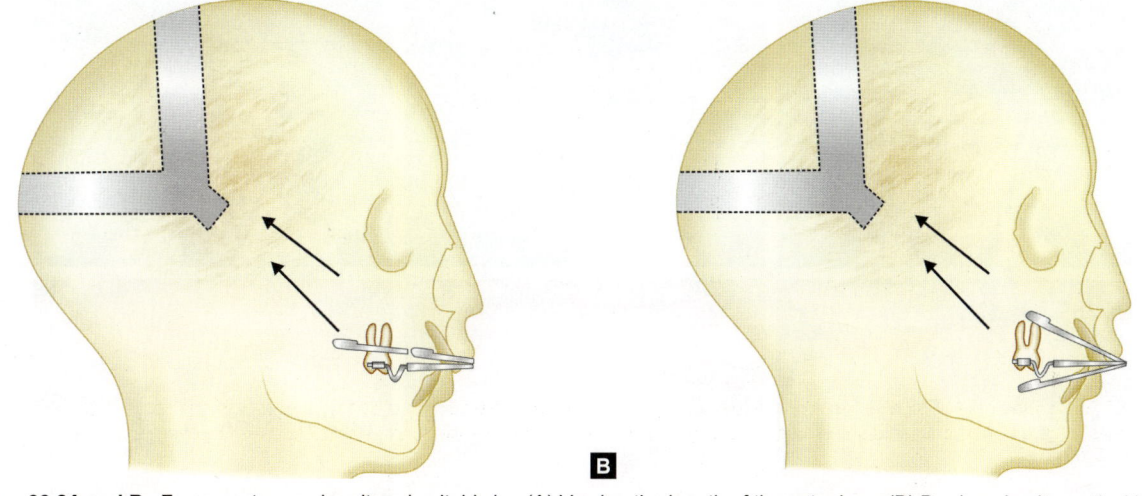

**Figs 33.8A and B:** Force vector can be altered suitably by: (A) Varying the length of the outer bow; (B) By changing its vertical height

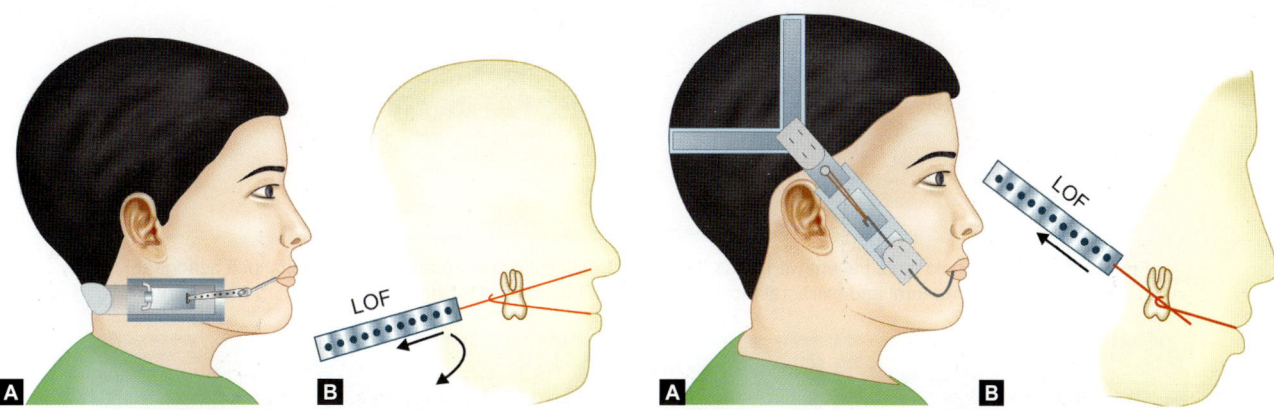

**Figs 33.9A and B:** Cervical headgear

**Figs 33.10A and B:** Occipital headgear

- Cervical headgear produces a distal and inferior line of force resulting in distal movement of maxilla and maxillary molars as well as the extrusion of the molars.
- Extrusion of maxillary molars results in the backward rotation of mandible with a tendency to open the bite.
- Thus cervical headgear should be used only in patients with flat mandibular and occlusal planes in which an increase in facial height is desired.

***Contraindications:*** Cervical headgears is contraindicated in:
- Patient with open bite
- High mandibular plane angle
- Long face with lower facial height.

***Advantage:*** Better patient compliance due to its simple design of the assembly having only one strap.

***Disadvantage:*** It produces extrusion of maxillary molars, which is not favorable in class II correction because it opens the bite by rotating the mandible downward and backward.

### Occipital Pull Headgear (Figs 33.10 and 33.11)

- Occipital headgear derives anchorage from occipital region of the head. An occipital headgear is usually constructed with the outer bow cut short at a position adjacent to the first molar. This results in a line of force that acts vertically and posteriorly through the center of resistance.
- This high angle of the force vector created results in a distal and intrusive force on the maxillary molars.
- Occipital headgear is effective not only in the correction of anteroposterior maxillary excess, but also in the correction of vertical maxillary excess.

### High Vertical-Pull Headgear (Fig. 33.12A)

- High-pull headgear derives anchorage from the parietal region.
- It produces intrusion and distalization maxillary molars.
- It is used when vertical maxillary excess is also to be addressed.

### Combination Pull Headgear (Fig. 33.12B)

- It uses a combination of the cervical and occipital attachments to distribute the external force over more surfaces
- It provides a convenient means of modifying the direction of the force vector. Magnitude of force can be distributed equally or unequally between the two attachments to alter the direction of force vector.

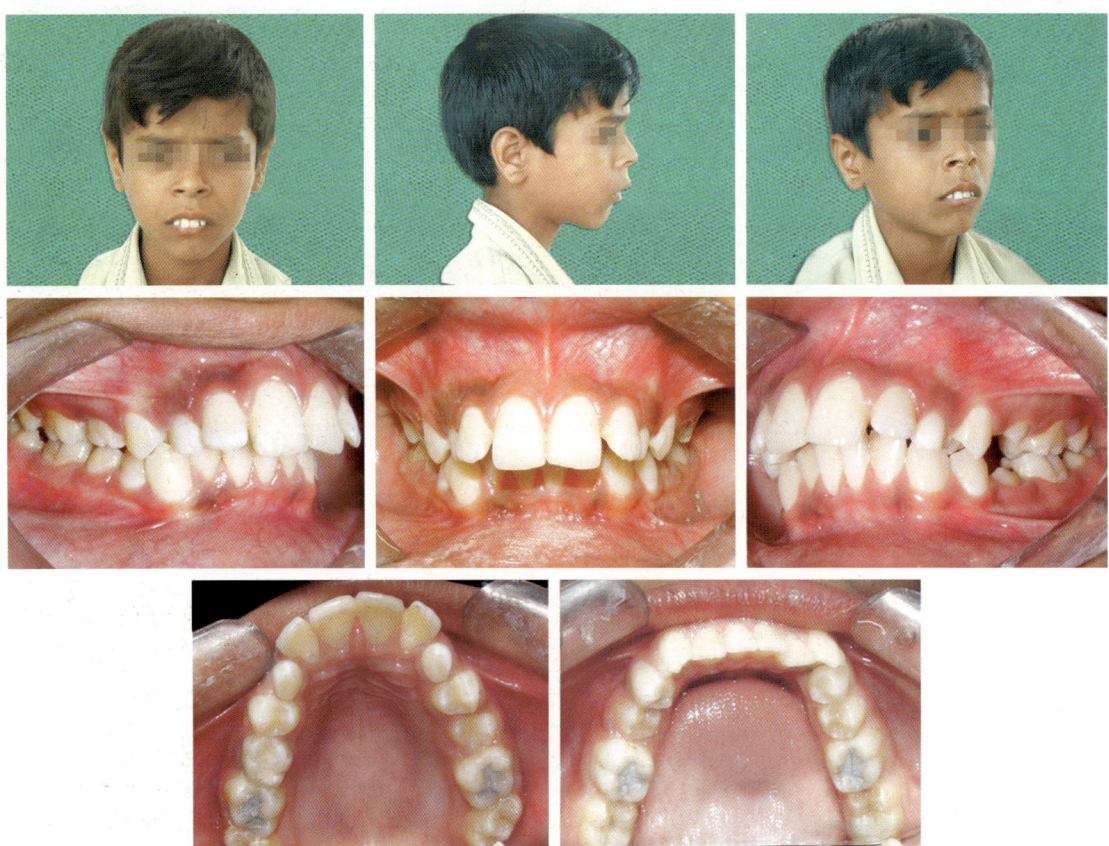

**Fig. 33.11A:** 11-year-old male patient with class II division 1 malocclusions treated using occipital pull headgear. (A) Pre-treatment intraoral and extraoral facial photographs [*Courtesy:* Dr Dharmpal Hada, MDS (ORTHO)]

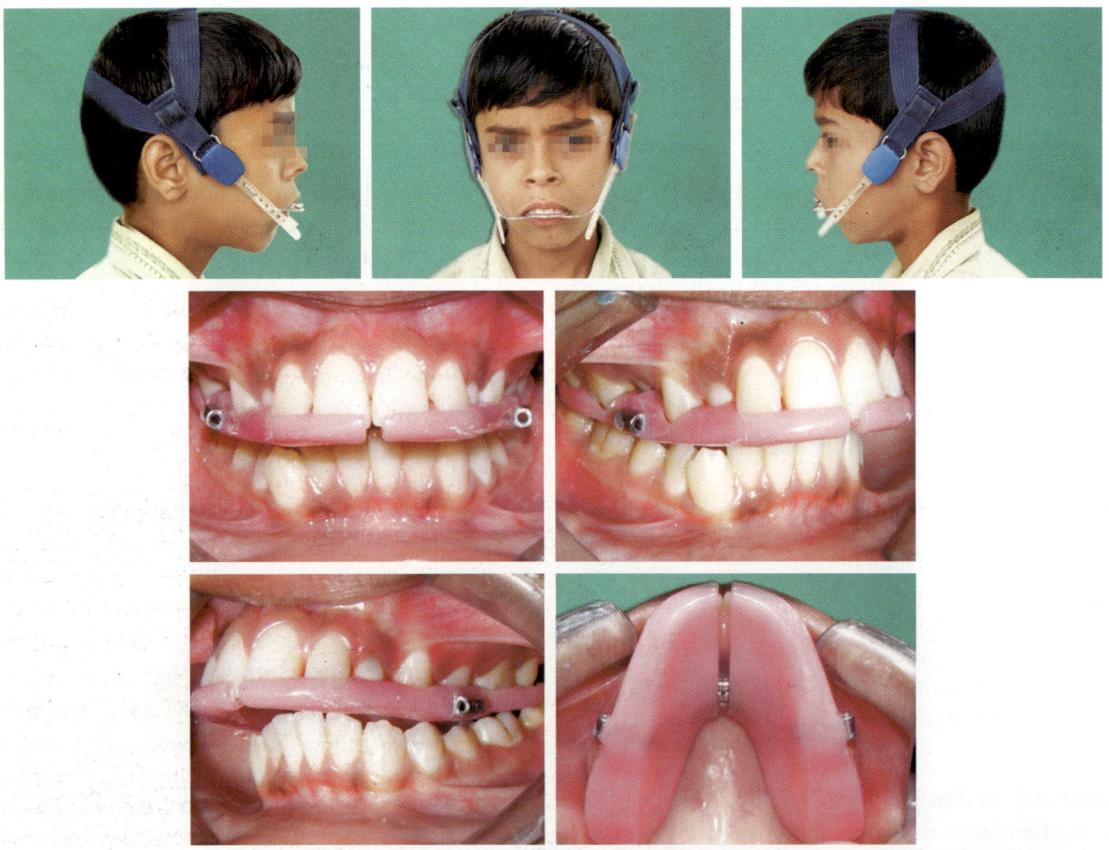

**Fig. 33.11B:** During treatment with occipital pull headgear [*Courtesy:* Dr Dharmpal Hada, MDS (ORTHO)]

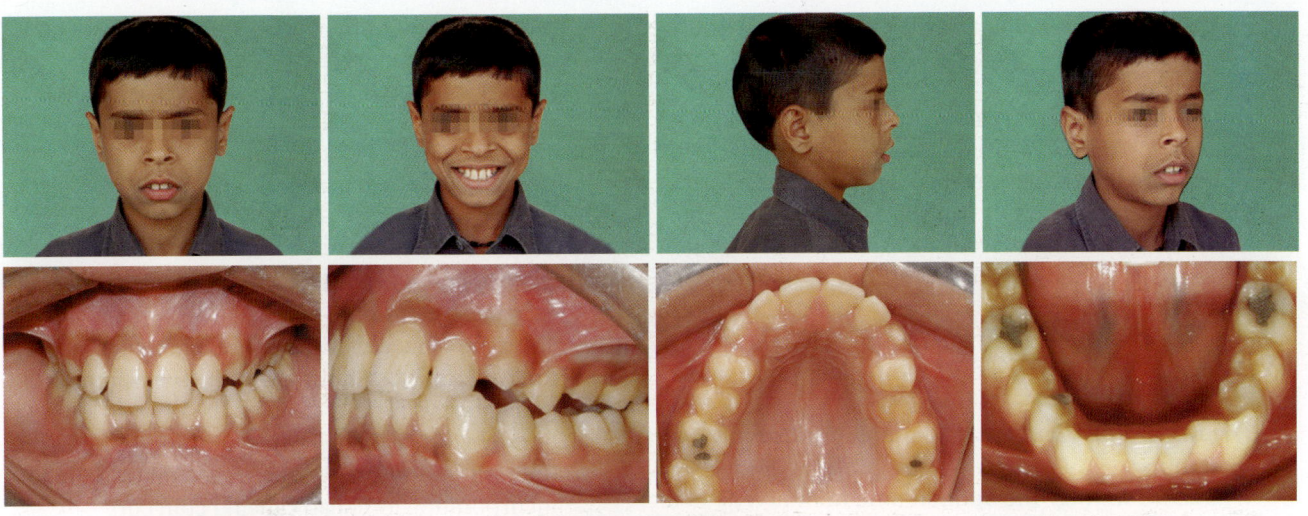

**Fig. 33.11C:** After 1½ year of treatment with occipital pull headgear [*Courtesy:* Dr Dharmpal Hada, MDS (ORTHO)]

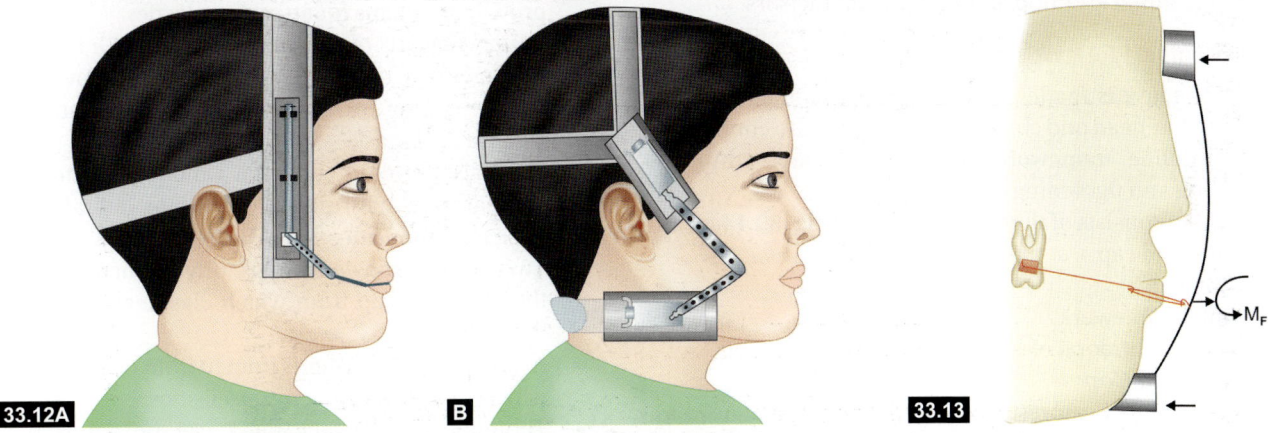

**Figs 33.12A and B:** (A) High pull headgear; (B) Combination headgear; **Fig. 33.13:** Face mask/reverse-pull headgear produces forward movement of maxilla by exerting a mesial force on maxilla with an equal and opposite force on the chin and forehead. It is used to treat class III malocclusion due to maxillary deficiency

- The combination attachment creates a force vector that is between the one created by either attachment alone.

  ***Advantages:*** The ease with which the force vector can be modified and it also provides patient comfort due to the increased force distribution.

  ***Disadvantage:*** Patient compliance/cooperation becomes more challenging because of the increased number of parts that the patient has to wear.

## FACE MASK (PROTRACTION FACE MASK)

Face mask is also called as "reverse pull headgear" or "protraction headgear." Face mask has been used in the treatment of patients with class III malocclusion and a maxillary deficiency. It exerts a mesial force on the maxilla with an equal and opposite force on the chin and forehead, thereby causing a forward movement of maxilla **(Fig. 33.13)**.

### Indications

- The face mask can be used in the treatment of mild to moderate skeletal class III malocclusions with a retrusive maxilla and a hypodivergent growth pattern.

- It can even be used for the selective rearrangement of the palatal shelves in cleft patients.

### Mode of Action

Development of the nasomaxillary complex is influenced by changes occurring at circummaxillary sutures (e.g. frontomaxillary, nasomaxillary, zygomaticotemporal, zygomaticomaxillary, pterygopalatine, etc.). Face mask produces forward displacement of the maxillary complex by effecting significant changes in the circummaxillary sutures and in the maxillary tuberosity.

### Principles of Face Mask Therapy

Clinically, the maxilla can be advanced 2–4 mm over an 8–12 month period. The amount of forward maxillary movement is influenced by a number of factors such as:

a. Age of the patient
b. Design of anchorage system (with or without expansion appliances)
c. The force level
d. Direction of force
e. Treatment duration
f. Treatment timing.

a. ***Age of the patient:*** Some studies suggested that face mask may be most effective in the primary or early mixed dentition.
b. ***Design of anchorage systems:*** The design of anchorage systems for maxillary protraction varies from palatal arches to rapid maxillary expansion appliances.
c. ***Force level:*** Successful maxillary protraction has been reported using a force of 300–500 gm/side in the primary and mixed dentitions.
d. ***Direction of force:*** Hata et al. suggested that an effective forward displacement of the maxilla can be obtained clinically from a force applied 5 mm above the palatal plane.
e. ***Treatment duration:*** Treatment time varies from 3 to 16 months.
f. ***Treatment timing:*** The optimal time to intervene in a patient with early class III malocclusions is at the time of the initial eruption of upper central incisors.

### Components of Face Mask

The face mask is made of two pads that contact the soft tissue in forehead and chin region. The pads are connected by a midline framework and are adjustable through loosening and tightening of a set screw.

Face mask consists of the following parts **(Fig. 33.14)**:
a. Forehead cap
b. Chin cup
c. Metal framework
d. Slots for intraoral elastics.

***a. Forehead Cap***
- Forehead cap rests on frontal bone and is used to derive anchorage from forehead.

***b. Chin Cup***
- Chin cup is used to derive anchorage from chin. It can be prefabricated or can be custom made. It is attached to the metal framework of the face mask.

***c. Metallic Framework***
- The metallic framework connects all parts of the face mask
- It contributes major percentage as compared to other parts and this extensive metal framework hampers patient esthetics and thus less patient acceptance.

***d. Intraoral Appliances***
- Intraoral appliance may consist of metallic-banded palatal expansion appliance (bands fitted on molars are joined by soldering heavy wire to the palatal plate, incorporated hyrax-type screw in the midline) or an acrylic bonded palatal expansion appliance with incorporated hyrax-type screw into a wire framework or multibanded appliances with rigid wire.

***e. Elastics***
- Elastics are used to apply forward pulling force on the upper arch.
- Elastics are stretched from the buccal tube hook, which is welded on the molar band, or soldered hook on the arch wire to the slots on the anterior part of the framework, which brings about downward and forward pull of the maxilla.

### Types of Face Mask

Following are the types of face mask:
1. Delaire type of face mask
2. Tübinger type of face mask
3. Petit type of face mask.

*Delaire type of face mask* **(Fig. 33.15)**: Features of Delaire type of face mask include:
- This type of face mask was developed by Delaire in the 1960s and is squarish with rigid metal framework.
- Metal framework of Delaire face mask consists of two vertical metal wires running parallelly in the front of the ears on the either sides of the face incorporating forehead cap and chin cup.
- A horizontal metal wire in front of the mouth provides a means for attaching elastics.

*Tübinger type of face mask* **(Fig. 33.16)**: Features of Tübinger type of face mask include the following:
- Tübinger type of face mask is a modification of Delaire face mask.
- It consists of chin cup from which originates two vertical rods that run in the midline, lateral to the nose on either side.
- Two vertical rods end superiorly by incorporating the forehead cap from which elastic encircles the head.
- A horizontal bar extends from in front of the mouth, which can be used to engage elastics.
- Tübinger type of face mask can be adjusted at forehead cap and horizontal bar to suit individual patients.

*Petit type of face mask* **(Figs 33.17A to C)**: Features of Petit type of face mask include the following:
- Even this type of face mask is also a modification of Delaire face mask.
- It consists of chin cup and forehead cap with a single vertical rod running in the midline from chin to the forehead cap.
- A horizontal bar extends from vertical rod in the front of mouth and is used to attach elastics. It can be adjusted at forehead cap, chin cup and horizontal bar to suit individual patients.

## CHIN CUP

Chin cup is an extraoral orthopedic orthodontic appliance used to treat skeletal class III malocclusions caused due to mandibular prognathism. It covers the chin and is connected to a headgear.

Chip cup appliance is aimed at restraining the forward growth of the mandible.

### Chin Cup Assembly

Chin cup assembly consists of:
i. Chin cup—covers chin

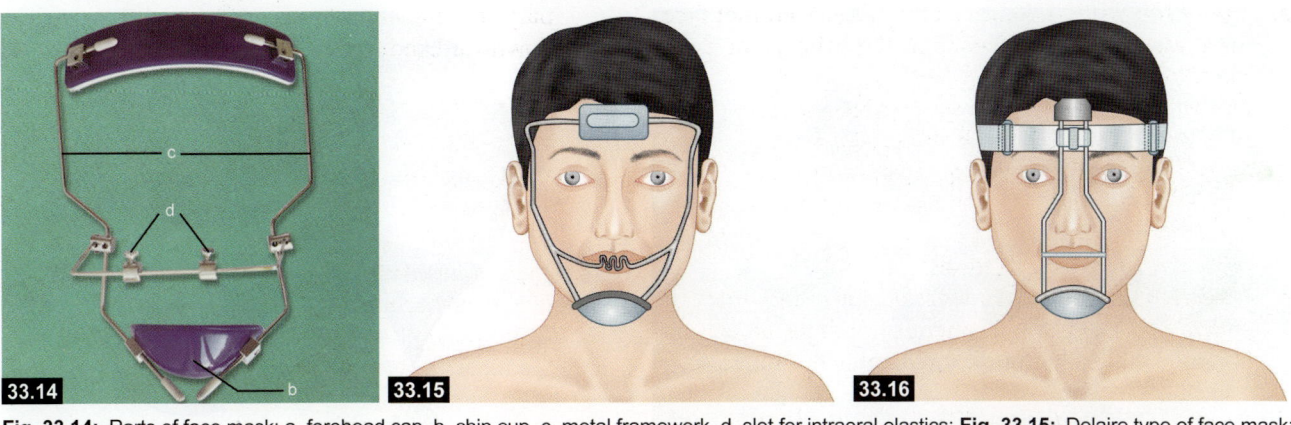

**Fig. 33.14:** Parts of face mask: a. forehead cap, b. chin cup, c. metal framework, d. slot for intraoral elastics; **Fig. 33.15:** Delaire type of face mask; **Fig. 33.16:** Tübinger type of face mask

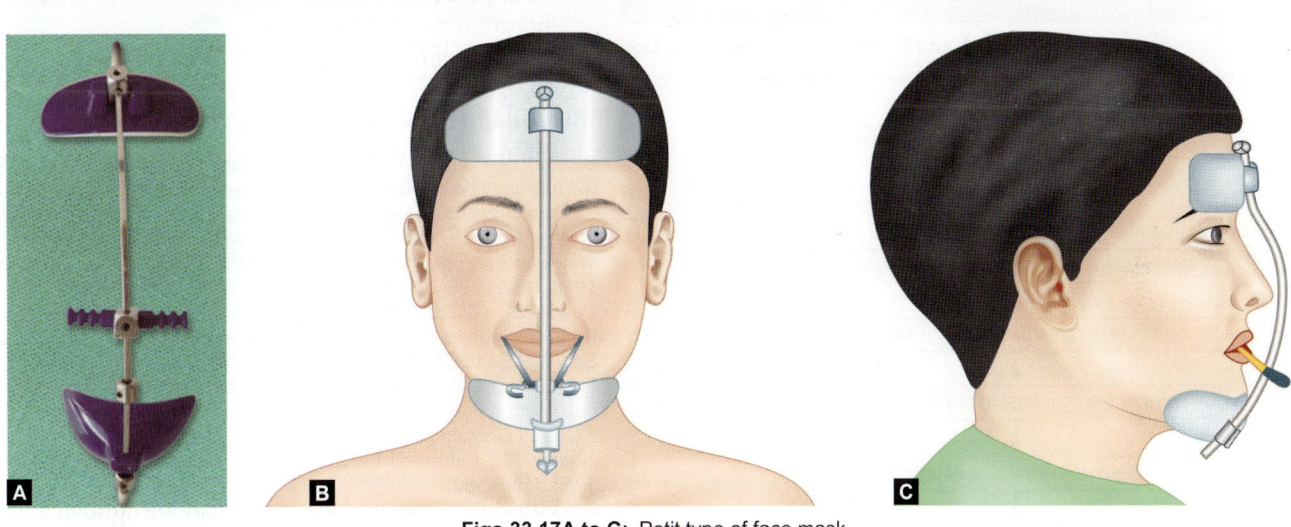

**Figs 33.17A to C:** Petit type of face mask

ii. Head cap—covers the head
iii. Elastic strap—connects the chin cup with the head cap.

## Types of Chin Cup

Chin cups are available in following types:
1. Occipital pull chin cup
2. Vertical pull chin cup.

*Occipital pull chin cup (Fig. 33.18A):* Features of occipital pull chin cup includes the following:
- Occipital pull chin cup is called so because in this type of chin cup the anchorage is derived from the occipital region of the head.
- Occipital pull chin cup is one of the most commonly used chin cups.

*Uses:* Various uses of occipital pull chin cup include:
- It is used in class III malocclusion or mild-to-moderate mandibular prognathism.
- Moderately proclined mandibular incisors.

Vertical pull chin cup **(Fig. 33.18B)**: Features of vertical pull chin cup include:

Anchorage is derived from the parietal region of the head in this type of chin cup.

*Use:* It is indicated in patient with open bite.

## Fabrication of Chin Cup

Chin cups are either custom made (fabricated for a patient) or preformed which are commercially available.

Custom fabrication of chin cup is shown in **Flowchart 33.1.**

***Force used:*** A force of 150–300 grams is used at the time of the appliance delivery and over the next two months, the force is gradually increased to 450–700 grams per side.

***Duration of wear:*** The patient is asked to wear the chin cup appliance for 12–16 hours/day to have the desired results.

## Effects of Chin Cup Appliance

- Redirection of mandibular growth in a downward or backward direction.
- Remodeling of the mandible and a decrease in mandibular plane angle or gonial angle.
- Lingual tipping of lower incisors.
- Improvement in skeletal and soft tissue profile.

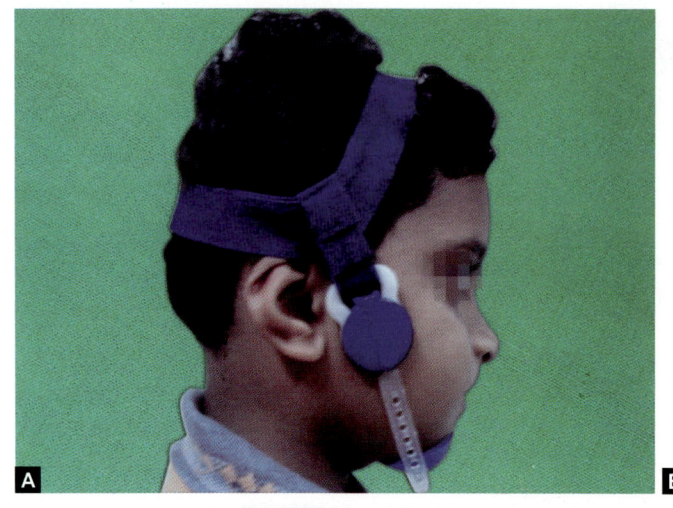 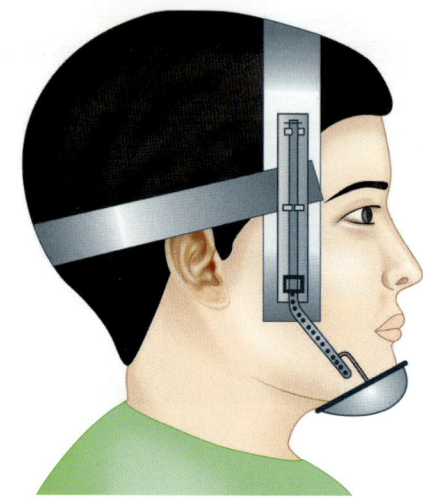

**Figs 33.18A and B:** Chin cup appliance. (A) Occipital pull chin cup; (B) Vertical pull chin cup

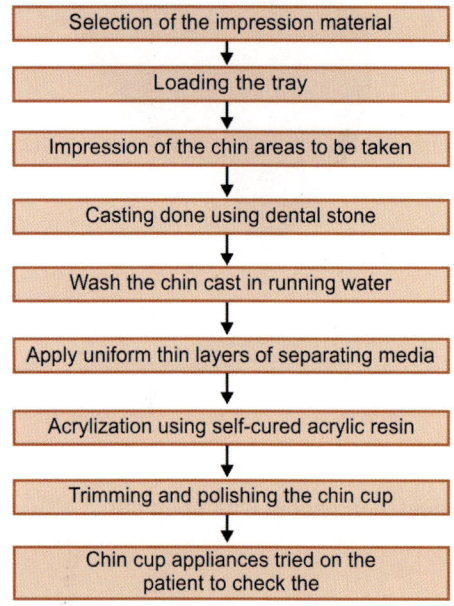

**Flowchart 33.1:** Custom fabrication of chin cup

### Indications

Chin cup appliances are indicated in:
  i. Patients with a mild skeletal prognathism of the mandible.
  ii. In the case of decreased facial height.
  iii. Patients who have well-aligned or protrusive, but not retroclined mandibular incisors.

## BIBLIOGRAPHY

1. Baalack IB, Poulsen A. Occipital anchorage for distal movement of the maxillary first molars. Acta Odontol Scand. 1966;24(3):307-25.
2. da Silva Filho OG, Magro AC, Capelozza Filho L. Early treatment of the class II malocclusion with rapid maxillary expansion and maxillary protraction. Am J Orthod Dentofacial Orthop. 1998;113(2):196-203.
3. Dewel BF. Class treatment in the mixed dentition with the Edgewise appliance and extraoral traction. Rep Congr Eur Orthod Soc. 1968;44:307-19.
4. Firouz M, Zernik J, Nanda R. Dental and orthopedic effects of high-pull headgear in treatment of class II, division 1 malocclusion. Am J Orthod Dentofacial Orthop. 1992;102(3):197-205.
5. Graber TM. Extra-oral force—facts and fallacies. Am J Orthod. 1955;41:490-505.
6. Greenspan RA. Reference charts for controlled extraoral force application to maxillary molars. Am J Orthod. 1970;58(5):486-91.
7. Gregorak W. Eruption path of permanent maxillary molars in class 2, division 1 malocclusion using headgear. Am J Orthod. 1962;48(5):367-81.
8. Henry RG. Cervical anchorage and the upper first permanent molar. Aust Dent J. 1961;6:260-8.
9. Kuhn RJ. Control of anterior vertical dimension and proper selection of extraoral anchorage. Angle Orthod 1968;38(4):340-9.
10. Marcotte MR. Biomechanics in Orthodontics. Philadelphia: BC Decker Inc, 1990.
11. Nanda R. Biomechanical and clinical considerations of a modified protraction headgear. Am J Orthod. 1980;78(2):125-39.
12. Proffit WR. Contemporary Orthodontics, St Louis: CV Mosby, 1986.
13. Poulton DR. Changes in class II malocclusions with and without occipital headgear therapy. Angle Orthod. 1959;29:232-50.
14. Poulton DR. The influence of extraoral traction. Am J Orthod. 1967;53(1):8-18.
15. Poulton DR. A three year survey of class II malocclusions with and without headgear therapy. Angle Orthod. 1964;34:181-93.
16. Rosenstein SW. A new concept in the early orthopedic treatment of cleft lip and palate. Am J Orthod. 1969;55(6):765-75.
17. Seward S. Extraoral anchorage. Aust Dent J. 1964;9:419-25.

## EXAM-ORIENTED QUESTIONS

### Long Essay or Long Questions
1. What are orthodontic appliances? Write down basis of orthodontic appliance therapy, principles of orthopedic appliance and discuss in detail about headgear.
2. What are the reverse pull headgear or face mask. Write down indication, mode of action, principles, components, types and effects of face mask therapy.
3. Compare and contrast delaire and petit face mask therapy.

### Short Notes
1. Orthodontic force vs Orthopedic force
2. Chin cup appliance
3. What is chin cup appliance? Discuss the types, fabrication, indication and effects of chin cup appliance.

## CHAPTER OVERVIEW

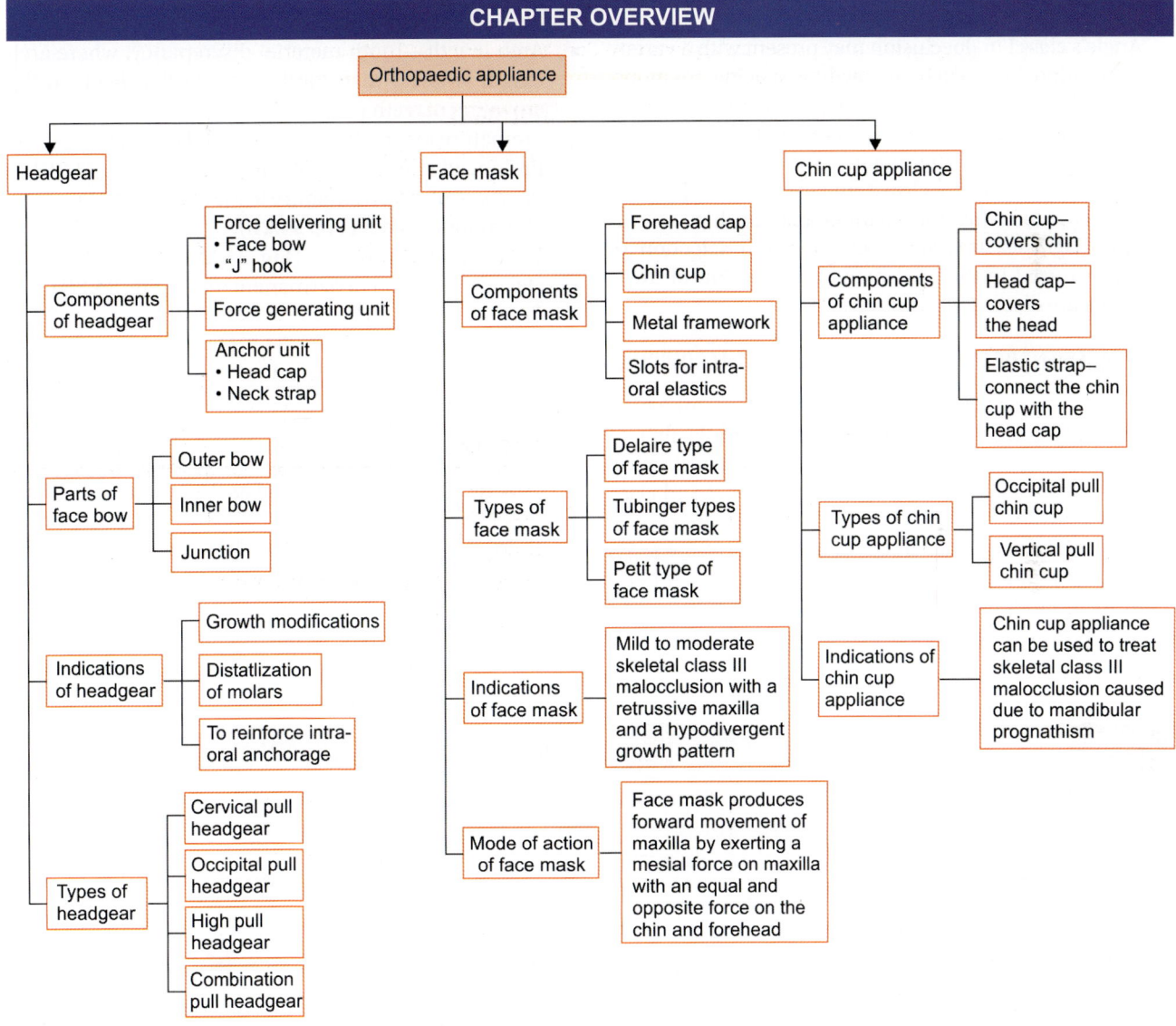

# CHAPTER 34
# Management of Class I Malocclusion

*Phulari BS, Shah A*

Class I malocclusion is the most common type of malocclusion observed in most population groups. Angle's class I malocclusion is a condition in which malalignment of teeth is present with a class I molar relationship (mesiobuccal cusp of permanent maxillary first molar occludes in the mesiobuccal developmental groove of mandibular first permanent molar).

Angle's class I malocclusion may present with a variety of tooth malpositions such as crowding, spacing, rotations, bimaxillary protrusion, bimaxillary retrusion, crossbite and open bite. Management of class I malocclusion is aimed at correcting the malocclusion present, while maintaining the existing class I molar relationship which is considered to be the normal molar relationship.

The diagnosis, treatment planning and selection of appliances used in the treatment and retention of these problems are discussed in this chapter.

## MANAGEMENT OF CLASS I MALOCCLUSION WITH CROWDING

Crowding is by far the most common complaint for which patients seeks orthodontic treatment, especially that of the anterior region which compromises facial aesthetics. crowding may be associated with class I, class II and class III malocclusion. Management of crowding in class I malocclusion is described in this chapter.

Arch length—Tooth material discrepancy where, tooth material is more than the arch length can lead to crowding. Crowding may be seen in anterior or posterior regions of one or both the dental arches. It may be mild or severe, unilateral or bilateral, localized or generalized **(Figs 34.1A to D)**.

### Etiological Factors

Crowding may be caused due to a number of causes. Multiple factors act together in many cases.

- Arch length—Tooth material discrepancy, where arch length is lesser than tooth material that leads to the crowding of teeth **(Fig. 34.2A)**.
- Premature loss of deciduous teeth **(Fig. 34.2B)**.
- Prolonged retention of deciduous teeth **(Fig. 34.2C)**.
- Presence of supernumerary teeth **(Fig. 34.2D)**.
- Macrodontic teeth **(Fig. 34.2E)**.
- Altered path of eruption **(Fig. 34.2F)**.
- Delayed eruption of permanent teeth **(Fig. 34.2G)**.
- Trauma
- Gemination of teeth **(Fig. 34.2H)**.

### Clinical Features

- Crowding may be present unilaterally **(Figs 34.3A)** or bilaterally **(Fig. 34.1D)** in the dental arches.
- Crowding may be localized **(Fig. 34.3B)** or generalized **(Fig. 34.2A)**.
- There is often difficulty in maintenance of good oral hygiene due to inaccessibility of certain tooth surfaces in crowded areas to toothbrush.
- Food impaction may occur.

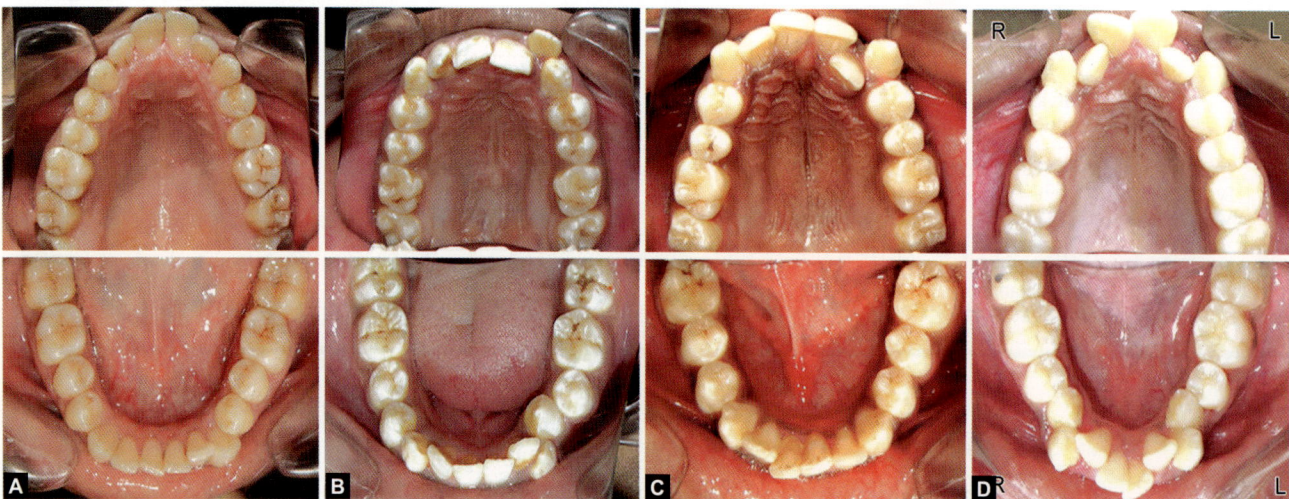

**Figs 34.1A to D:** Different cases of Class I malocclusion with varying degrees of crowding. (A) Mild localized crowding; (B and C) Moderate and localized crowding; (D) Severe and generalized crowding

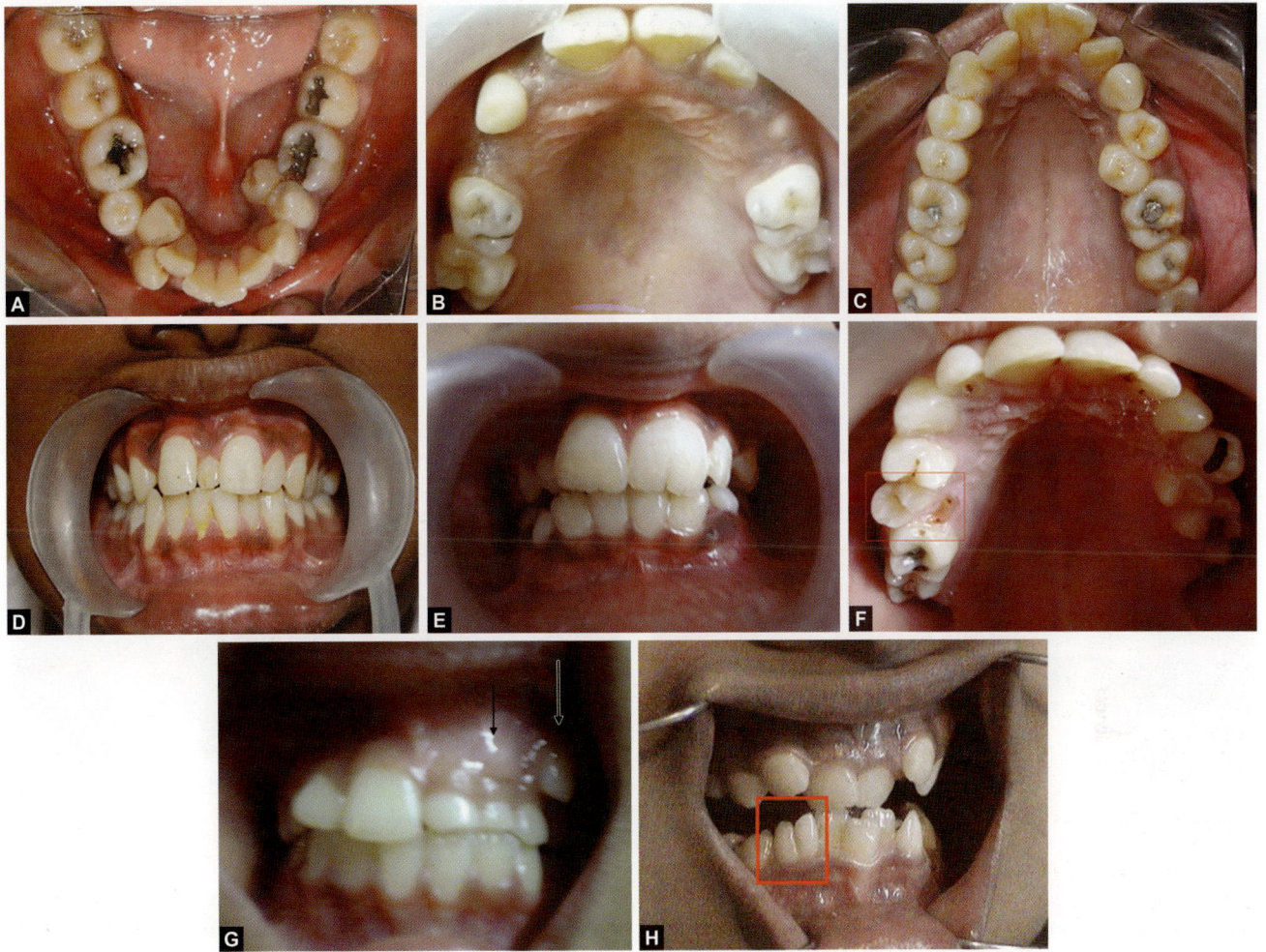

**Figs 34.2A to H:** Etiological factors of dental crowding: **(A)** Severe crowding in the maxillary and mandibular arches due to arch length—tooth material discrepancy. **(B)** Premature loss of deciduous teeth. **(C)** Crowding in the maxillary arch caused due to prolonged retention of right and left deciduous canines (53, 63) and second deciduous molar (55). **(D)** Intraoral frontal and occlusal view photographs showing crowding in the maxillary arch caused due to presence of supernumerary tooth (mesiodens), **(E)** Intraoral frontal view showing crowding in the arch due to macrodontic right and left permanent central incisors. **(F)** Altered path of eruption of right permanent second premolar due to retained root stumps of deciduous right second molar. **(G)** Delayed eruption permanent left anterior teeth due to over retained deciduous left central incisor, lateral incisor and canine. Note labially erupting permanent left canine and labial bulge of the erupting permanent left lateral incisor. **(H)** Gemination of left permanent lateral incisor

- Halitosis may be present.
- Gingivitis and periodontitis may occur.

## Diagnosis

- Clinical examination reveals the extent and location of crowding **(Fig. 34.4)**.
- Model analysis is needed for determining the arch length and tooth material discrepancy.
- Radiographic examination helps in evaluating any trauma, bony pathology and unerupted teeth.

## Treatment

### Relief of Crowding by Gaining Space

Space is required for the relief of crowding in the arch. The required amount of space may be gained by proximal stripping, arch expansion (e.g. Quad helix appliance) **(Fig. 34.5)**, distalization of molars and proclination of anteriors or extraction of teeth.

I. Treatment using removable orthodontic appliance: The following removable orthodontic appliances are used to relieve crowding in the arches:
   a. Removable orthodontic appliances with Jack screw.
   b. Removable orthodontic appliances with canine retractor.
   c. Removable orthodontic appliances with "Z" spring.
   a. Removable orthodontic appliances with Jack screw: Removable orthodontic appliance incorporates a Jack screw in the midpalatal raphe region. On activation of screw, there will be opening up of mid-palatal suture and spacing in the midline between centrals, later this space can be utilized to relieve crowding in the dental arches **(Fig. 34.6)**.

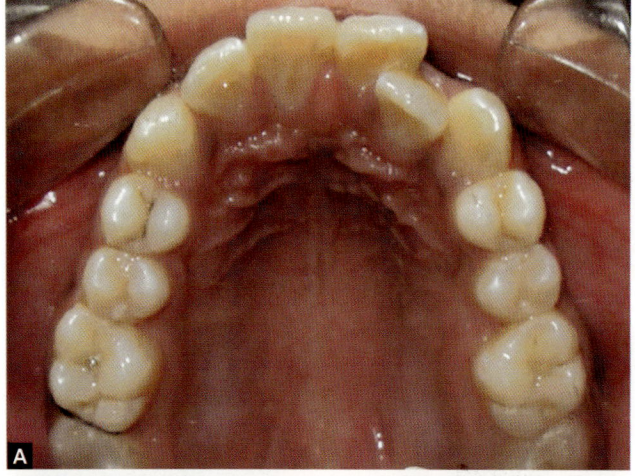
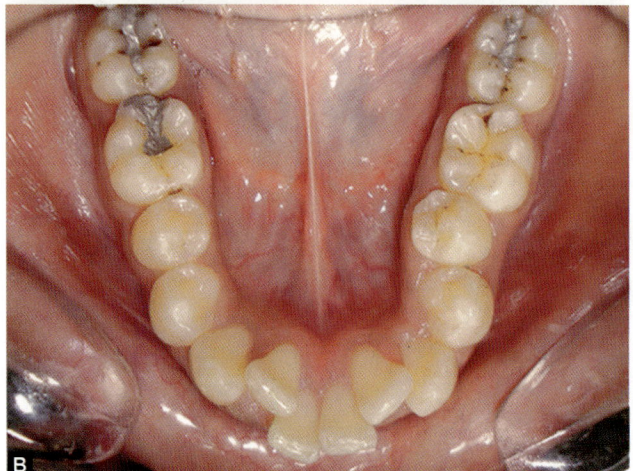
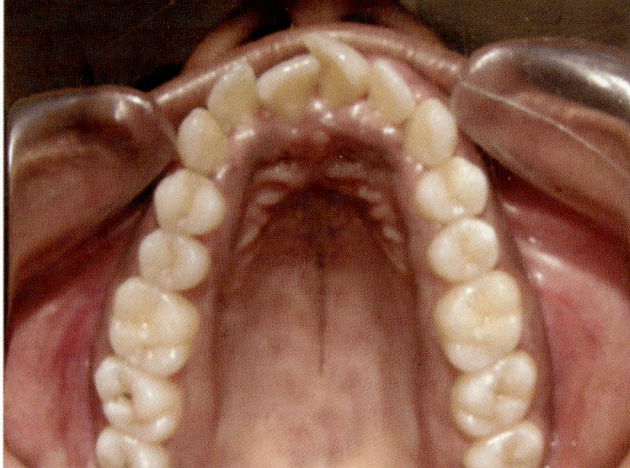
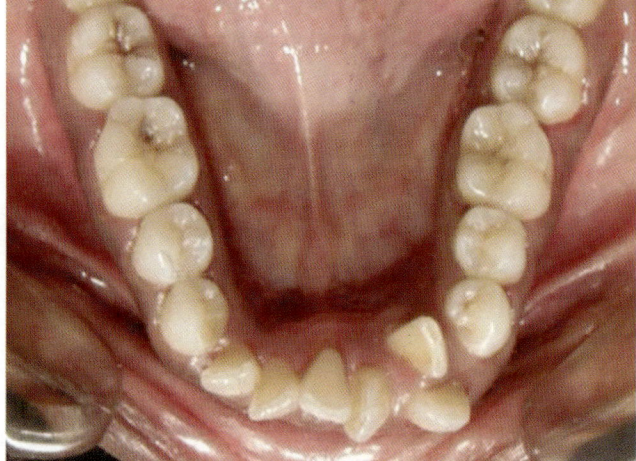

**Figs 34.3A to B:** Clinical features of crowding: **(A)** Unilateral crowding involving crowding only on the right quadrant in the anterior region. **(B)** Generalized crowding in the mandibular arch and Gingivitis

**Fig. 34.4:** Maxillary and mandibular anterior crowding

    b. Removable orthodontic appliances with canine retractor: Removable orthodontic appliance with canine retractors can be used in selected cases. Activation of canine retractor brings about distal movement of canine leaving behind space distal to lateral incisor and mesial to canine, this space later can be used to relieve crowding in the dental arches **(Fig. 34.7)**.

    c. Removable orthodontic appliances with "Z" spring: Crowding in the anterior segments caused due to palatally erupted lateral incisor can be managed with removable orthodontic appliance with "Z" springs. "Z" spring fabricated on lateral incisor, on activation brings about labial movement of lateral incisor to the final alignment on the dental arches **(Fig. 34.8)**.

 II. Treatment using fixed orthodontic appliance: Fixed orthodontic appliance with NiTi arch wire or open coil spring can be used to relieve crowding in the arch **(Figs 34.9A to C)**. Therapeutic extraction of certain teeth may be needed to gain the required space.

## MANAGEMENT OF CLASS I MALOCCLUSION WITH SPACING

Arch length—Tooth material discrepancy where, tooth material is less than arch length can lead to spacing. Spacing may be seen in one or both dental arches. Spacing may be localized or generalized, unilateral or bilateral in the dental arches. Spacing present between the two permanent maxillary centrals in the midline is referred as midline diastema. Management of midline diastema is discussed separately in Chapter 37.

Spacing may be caused by oral habits such as thumb sucking/digit sucking and tongue thrusting. Other causes of spacing include large tongue, relative microdontia and macrognathia. Correction of spacing involves identification and removal of etiological factors followed by consolidation of space using removable or fixed orthodontic appliance or by conservative approach.

### Etiological Factors

1. Arch length—Tooth material discrepancy, where arch length is more than the tooth material can lead to spacing **(Fig. 34.10A)**.

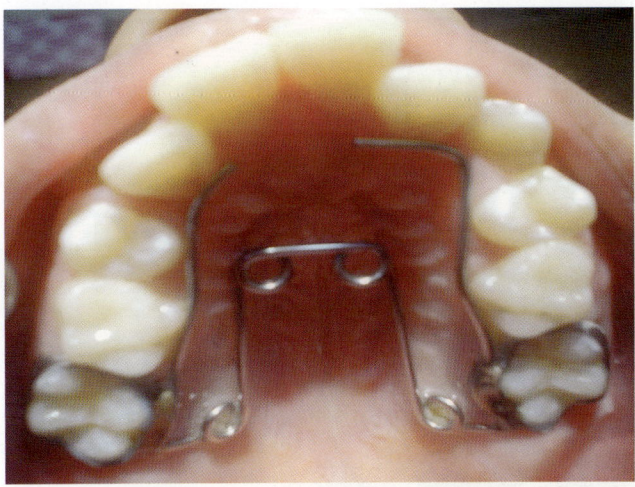

Fig. 34.5: By gaining space by using Quad helix expansion appliance

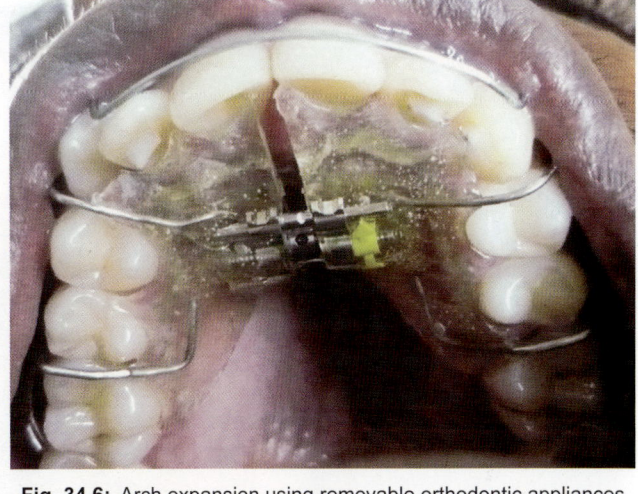

Fig. 34.6: Arch expansion using removable orthodontic appliances with Jack screw

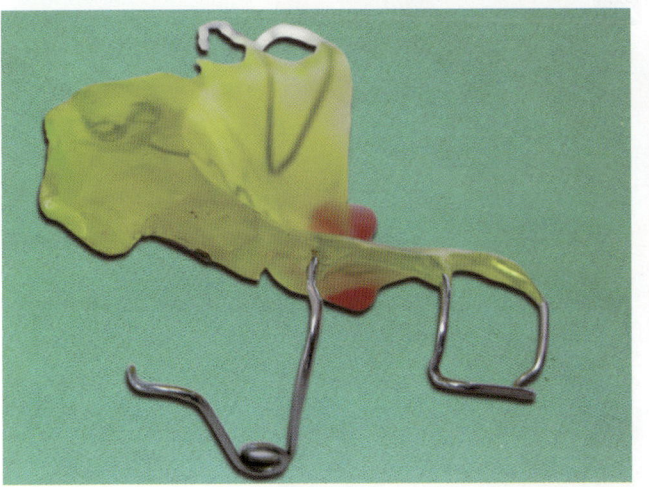

Fig. 34.7: Removable orthodontic appliances with canine retractor

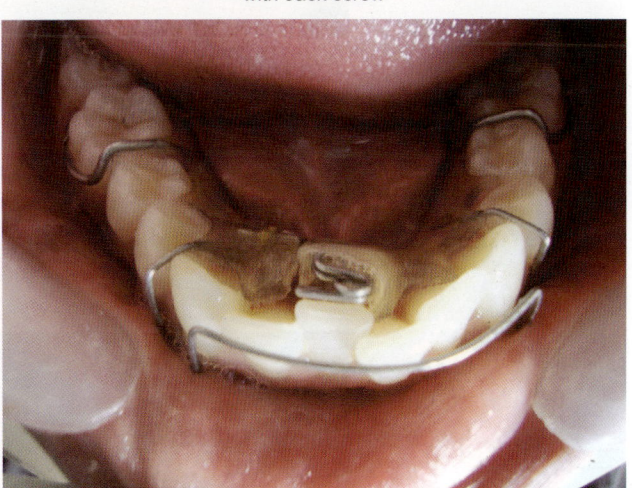

Fig. 34.8: Removable orthodontic appliances with "Z" spring.

2. Oral habits:
   - Thumb sucking (**Fig. 34.10B**).
   - Tongue thrusting.
3. Abnormal tooth form:
   - Peg-shaped maxillary permanent lateral incisors (**Fig. 34.10C**).
4. Abnormally large tongue exerting pressure on teeth may cause spacing:
   - Macroglossia
5. Abnormal tooth size:
   - Microdontia (**Fig. 34.10D**).
6. Anomalies in number of teeth:
   - Oligodontia
   - Partial anodontia (**Fig. 34.10G**).
7. Bony pathologies like cystic lesions, odontomes.
8. Congenitally missing teeth (**Figs 34.10E**).
9. Premature loss of permanent teeth.
10. Soft tissue abnormalities:
    - Abnormal labial frenum attachment (**Fig. 34.10G**).
11. Prolonged retention of deciduous teeth.

## Clinical Features of Class I Malocclusion with Spacing

- Spacing may be present in one or both the dental arches (**Figs 34.11A i and ii**).
- Spacing may be localized or generalized (**Fig. 34.11B**).
- Spacing may be unilateral or bilateral (**Fig. 34.11C**).
- Spacing between two permanent maxillary central incisors in the midline is often referred to as midline diastema (**Fig. 34.11D**).

## Diagnosis of Class I Malocclusion with Spacing

For diagnosis of this condition, a thorough examination should be supplemented with routine orthodontic diagnostic aids such as orthodontic study models to evaluate arch length—tooth material discrepancy and radiographic examination (**Fig. 34.12**) to rule out bony pathologies and unerupted teeth in the jaws.

## Treatment of Class I Malocclusion with Spacing

I. Removal of the etiologic causes (**Box 34.1**):

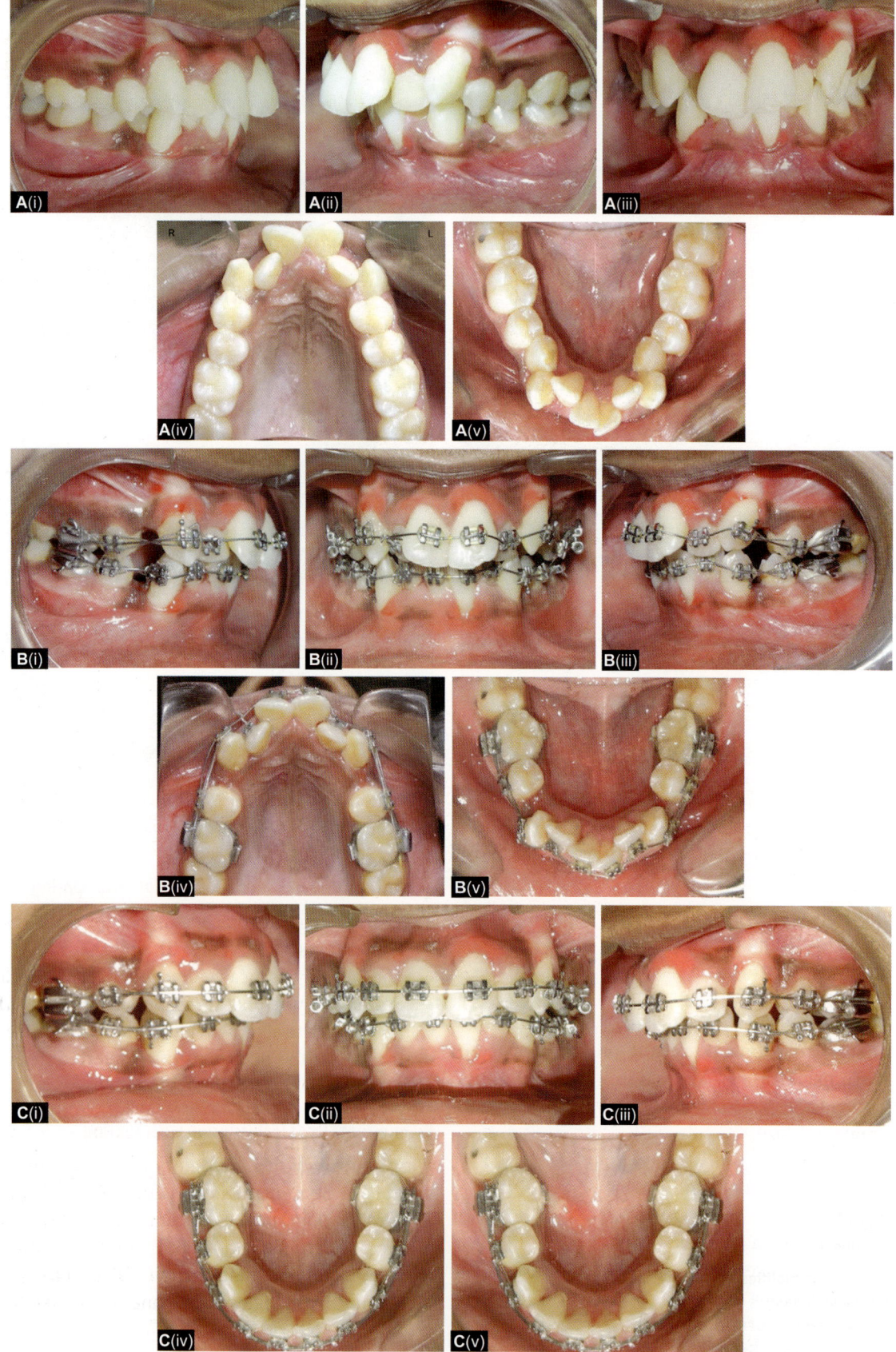

**Figs 34.9A to C:** A patient with class I malocclusion with severe crowding treated with fixed mechanotherapy using NiTi arch wire: (A) Pretreatment intraoral photographs. (B) Initial phase of fixed orthodontic treatment after extraction of all 4 first premolars. (C) Near completion of treatment

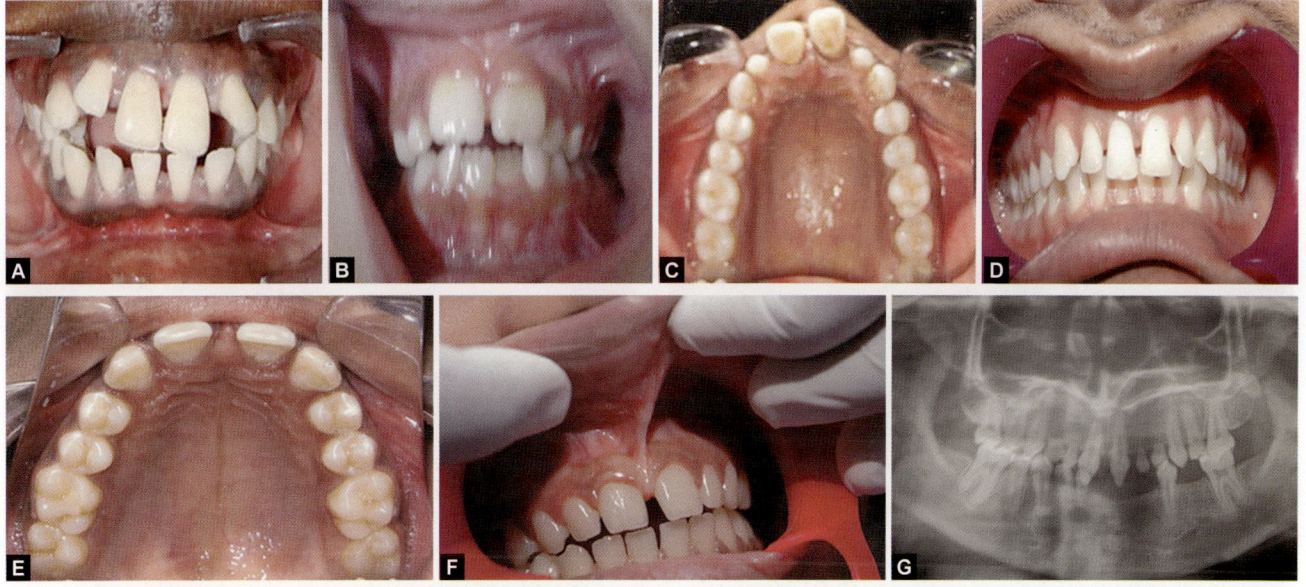

**Figs 34.10A to G:** Causes of spacing in the arches: (A) Spacing in the arches due to arch length –tooth material discrepancy. (B) Spacing in the maxillary anterior region due to thumb sucking habit. (C) Spacing in the maxillary anterior segment due to bilateral peg shaped lateral incisors. (D) Spacing in the maxillary and mandibular anterior segments due to microdontic teeth. (E) Bilateral congenitally missing lateral incisors causing spacing: Intraoral occlusal view. (F) Midline diastema caused by high labial frenum attachment. (G) Partial anodontia causing spacing in the arches.

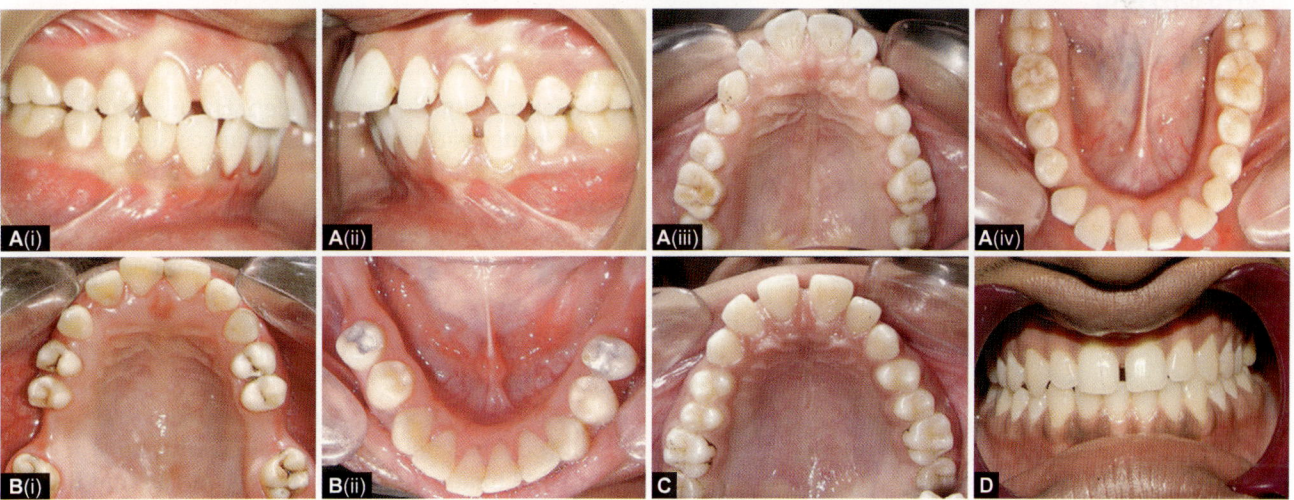

**Figs 34.11A to D:** Clinical features of Class I malocclusion with spacing: (A) Spacing in both the arches. (C) Spacing in the maxillary anterior region. (B) Bilateral spacing in the arches. (D) Midline diastema

**Box 1.1: Etiologic factors**

| | |
|---|---|
| **1. Oral habits**<br>• Thumb sucking<br>• Digit sucking<br>• Tongue thrusting | **Treatment**<br>Habit breaking appliance with crib **(Fig. 34.13)** or rake. |
| **2. Bony pathologies**<br>• Cystic lesions, odontomes | Surgical removal of the cystic lesion |
| **3. Soft tissue abnormalities**<br>• Abnormal labial frenum attachment Prolonged retention of deciduous teeth. | Frenectomy<br>Extraction of retained deciduous teeth and facilitating the eruption of unerupted permanent teeth. |

II. Treatment of Class I malocclusion with spacing by using removable orthodontic appliances

Simple removable orthodontic appliance with labial bow or finger springs may be used to close the spacing in the arch.

III. Treatment of Class I malocclusion with spacing by using fixed orthodontic appliances

Fixed orthodontic appliance **(Figs 34.14A to C)** can be used to close the spaces by employing any of the following active components:
- E-chain (short or long)
- Closed coil spring
- Elastics
- Elastic thread

IV. Treatment of Class I malocclusion with spacing by conservative approach.

In cases of minor spacing in the arch, conservative approach can also be employed using appropriately

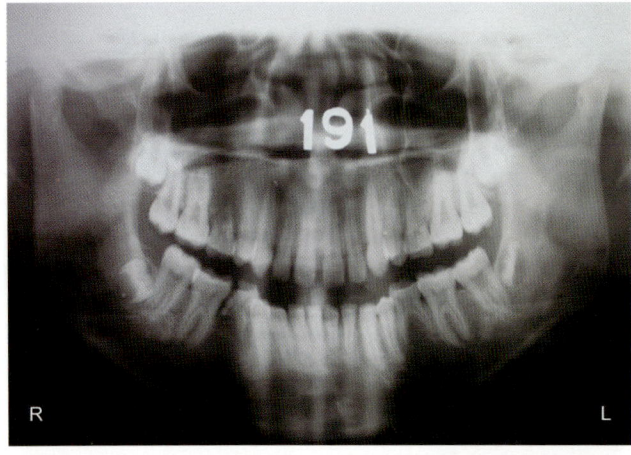

Fig. 34.12: OPG used to evaluate underlying pathology associated with the spacing in the arches

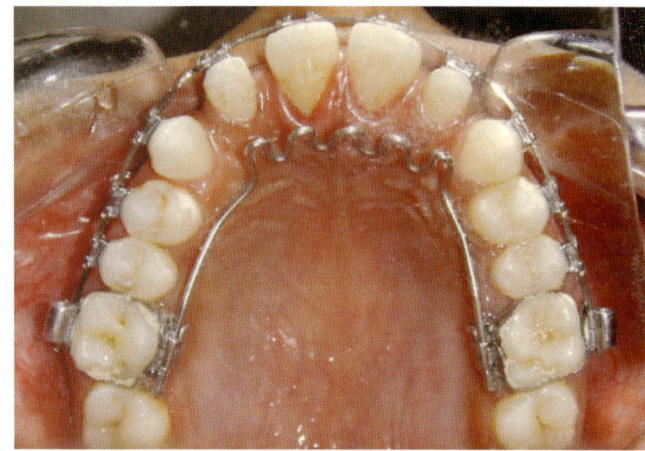

Fig. 34.13: Removable crib in conjunction with fixed mechanotherapy used to intercept the tongue thrusting habit while simultaneously correcting the existing malocclusion

shade-matched composite resin restorations **(Figs 34.15A and B)**.

## MANAGEMENT OF CLASS I MALOCCLUSION WITH ROTATION

Movement of teeth around their long axis is termed as rotation. Rotation may involve a single tooth, multiple teeth and one or both the arches. It may be mild or severe. Rotated anterior teeth occupy less space, whereas rotated posterior teeth occupy more space in the arch. Thus, some amount of space is gained followed by de-rotation of posterior teeth; while correction of rotated anterior teeth requires space creation.

Correction of rotated teeth can be done by using removable orthodontic appliances or fixed mechanotherapy. There is high risk of relapse associated with de-rotated teeth due to stretching of the supra-alveolar and trans-septal gingival . Thus precision (circumferential supra-crestal fiberotomy) followed by long-term retention is often required to achieve stability of the treatment.

### Types of Rotations

Rotations are essentially of two types and are as follows:
1. Mesiolingual or distobuccal rotation **(Fig. 34.16A)**
2. Distolingual or mesiobuccal rotation **(Fig. 34.16B)**

### Clinical Features of Class I Malocclusion with Rotation

- Rotation may involve anterior **(Fig. 34.16A)** or posterior teeth **(Fig. 34.16C)**; single tooth/multiple teeth, one or both the arches. It may be mild or severe **(Fig. 34.16D)**.
- Unesthetic facial appearance when anterior are involved.
- Food impaction.
- Prone for dental caries.
- Difficulty in maintaining good oral hygiene.

### Diagnosis of Class I Malocclusion with Rotation

Diagnosis of rotation of teeth can be easily done by proper clinical examination. However, orthodontic study models may be needed to evaluate the extent of rotation and they also aid in treatment planning.

### Treatment of Class I Malocclusion with Rotation

Although mild rotation with single or few teeth involvement can be treated with removable appliances, severe rotations are best treated with fixed mechanotherapy. De-rotation of rotated teeth requires application of a force couple **(Fig. 34.17)**. Rotations are often easier to treat than to retain. Retention should be carefully planned to prevent future relapse.

#### Treatment of Class I Malocclusion with Rotation Using Removable Orthodontic Appliance

Removable orthodontic appliance incorporating "Z" spring (double cantilever spring) along with labial bow can be used to treat mild rotations **(Figs 34.18A and B)**. Only upper helix of the Z spring is activated for achieving de-rotation of tooth or teeth.

#### Treatment of Class I Malocclusion with Rotation Using Fixed Orthodontic Appliance

- When there is severe rotation of a single or multiple teeth, fixed orthodontic appliance is the treatment of choice **(Figs 34.19A to D)**. Space required for derotation of anterior teeth can be obtained by arch expansion, proximal stripping, etc. depending on the case.
- NiTi arch wire and derotation springs are often used for derotation of teeth.

### Retention Following Correction of Rotation

A noticeably high risk of relapse is seen among these cases due to the resiliency of gingival fibers. The supracrestal gingival fibers take relatively longer time to reorganize

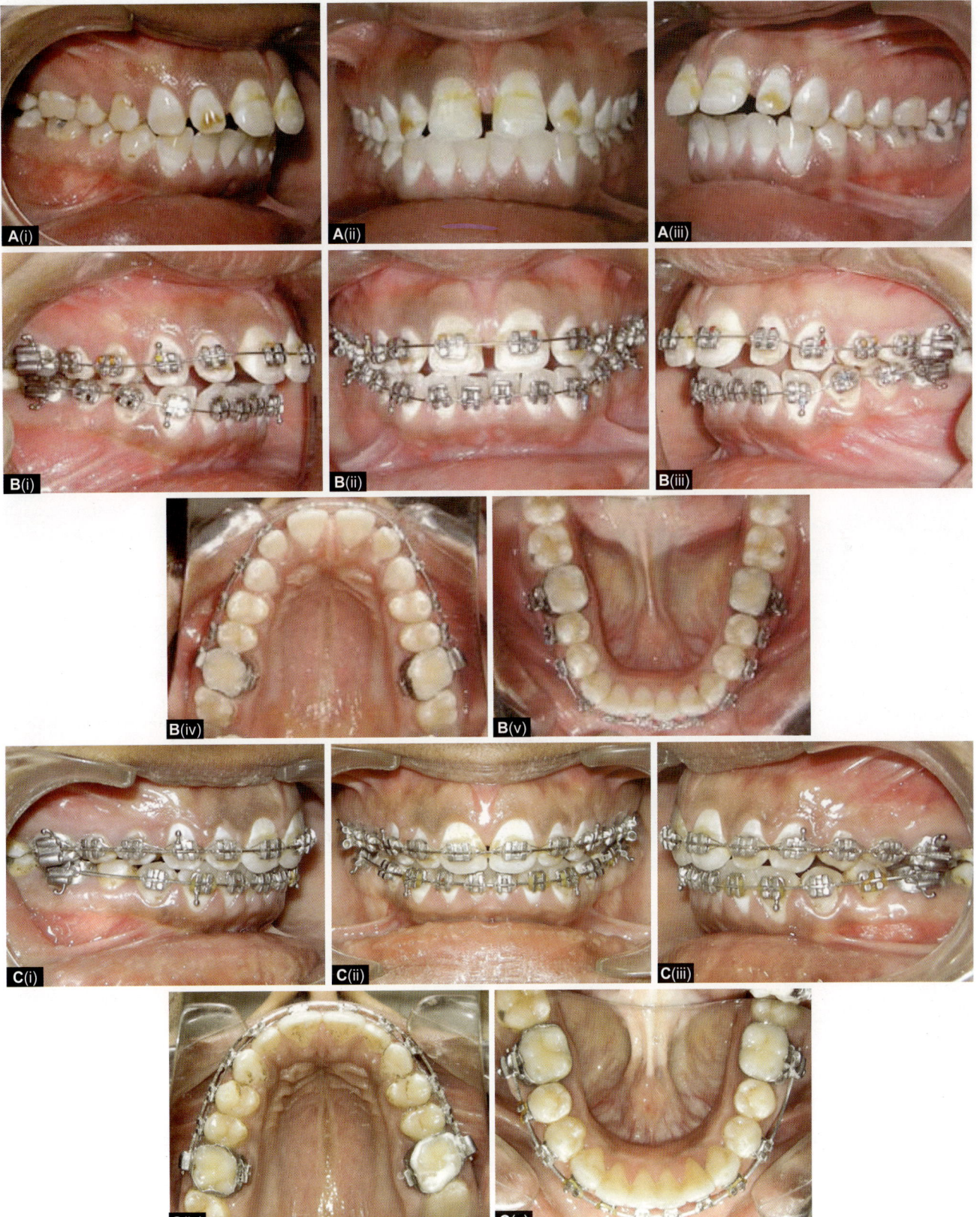

**Figs 34.14A to C:** Treatment of Class I malocclusion with spacing by using fixed orthodontic appliance: **(A)** Pre-treatment intraoral photographs. **(B)** During treatment. **(C)** Intra-oral photographs after treatment

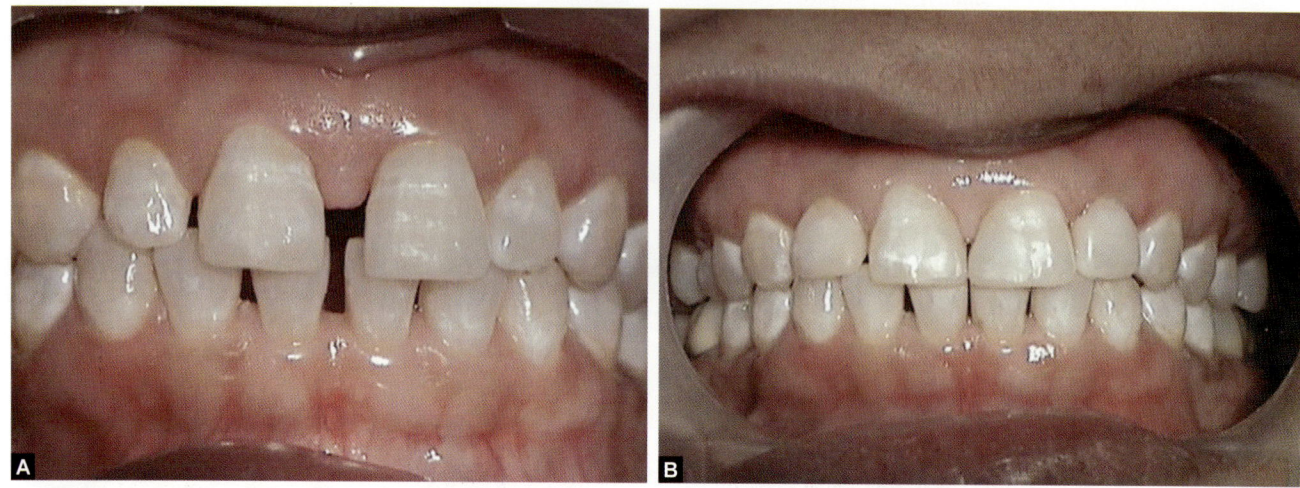

**Figs 34.15A and B:** Minor spacing in the arch can be treated by conservative approach using appropriately shade-matched composite resin restoration: (A) Before treatment. (B) After treatment

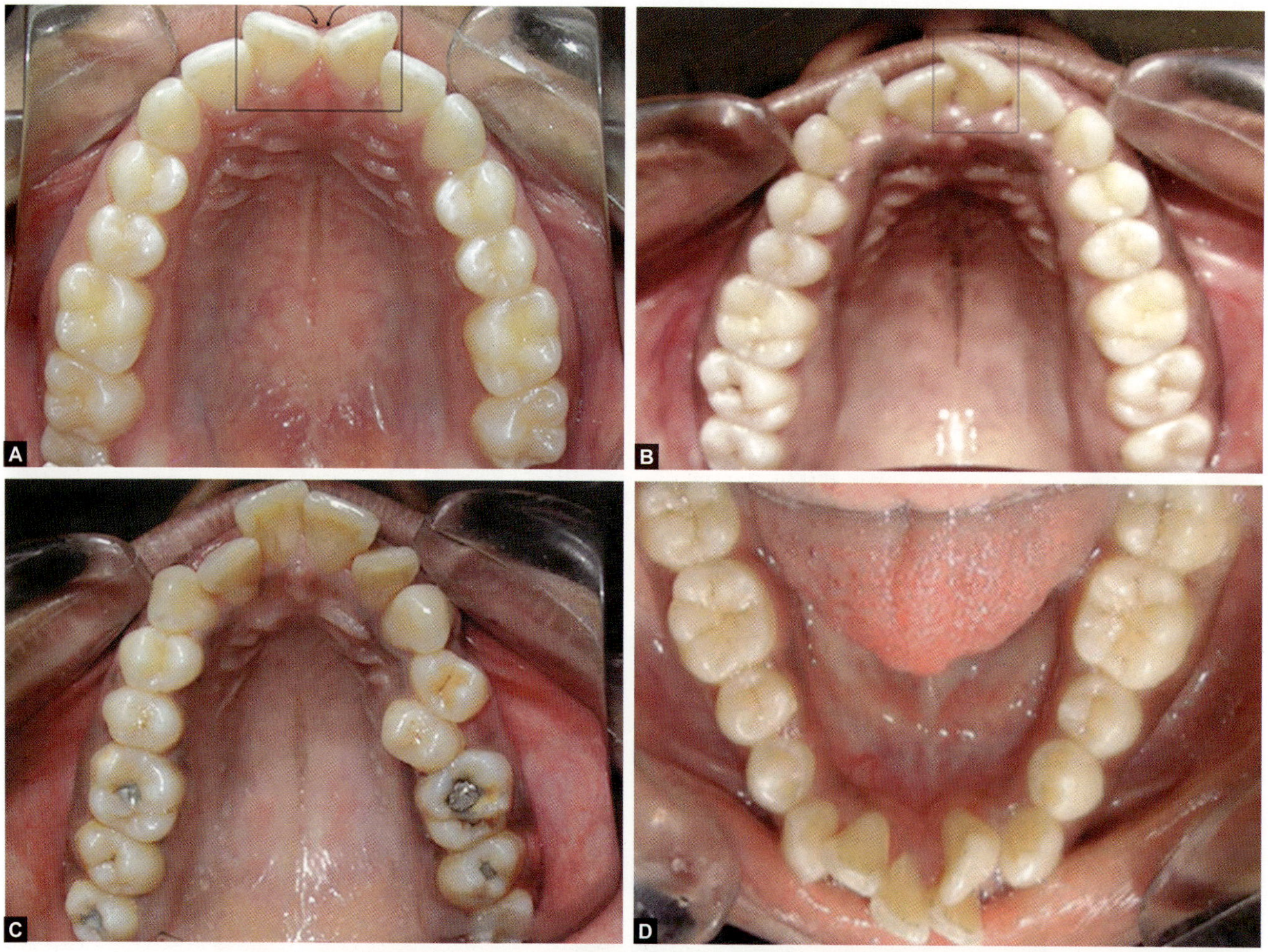

**Figs 34.16A to D:** Types of rotations: (A) Mesiolingual or distolabial rotation of maxillary right and left central incisors. (B) Distolingual or mesiolabial rotation of a maxillary central incisor. (C) Rotations involving anterior and posterior teeth. (D) Severe rotation of the mandibular anterior teeth

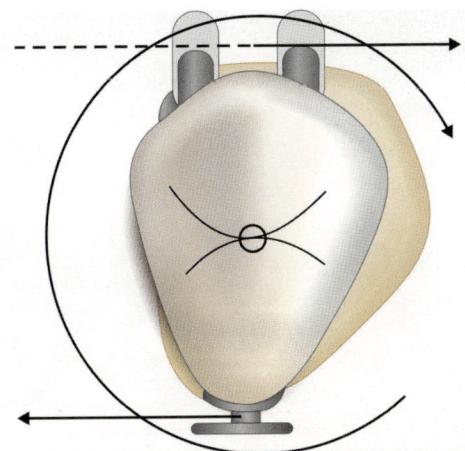

**Fig. 34.17:** Derotation of rotated teeth requires application of a force couple A

after derotation of the tooth **(Fig. 34.20A)**. Hence, the importance of proper retention following treatment of such cases cannot be overemphasized.

- Long-term retention is required.
- Circumferential supracrestal fiberotomy or pericision **(Fig. 34.20B)** is a useful adjunctive surgical procedure where the gingival fibers are incised to prevent relapse. The following methods are recommended for retention following derotation of teeth:
- Recommended retention following derotation of single tooth: In case of correction of single tooth rotation, band and spur is the retainer of choice **(Fig. 34.21A)**.
- Recommended retention following derotation of multiple teeth: In cases of correction of multiple rotations, banded canine-to-canine or bonded canine-to-canine lingual retainer can be used **(Fig. 34.21B)**.

## MANAGEMENT OF BIMAXILLARY PROTRUSION

Bimaxillary dentoalveolar protrusion is a malocclusion characterized by dentoalveolar flaring of both the maxillary and the mandibular anterior teeth, with resultant protrusion of the lips and convexity of the face. Bimaxillary protrusion is quite commonly seen in Asian population. For these patients, in Orthodontic field, it is accepted that extraction of the four first premolars is the most viable and effective means of reducing their facial convexity. In addition, maximum anchorage is believed to be the most critical part of the treatment plan. It is well-known that, closure of the extraction sites can occur by retraction of the anterior segments, protraction of the posterior segments or a combination of the two. When it is indicated to prevent mesial movement of the posterior segments in the anteroposterior dimension, this is termed as maximum anchorage.

## CLINICAL FEATURES OF BIMAXILLARY PROTRUSION

### Extra-oral Features

A patient with bimaxillary protrusion **(Fig. 34.22)** may exhibit the following features:

- Decreased nasolabial angle due to proclined maxillary anterior **(Fig. 34.22A)**.
- Shallow mentolabial sulcus due to proclined mandibular anterior **(Fig. 34.22B)**.
- Lips may be potentially incompetent **(Fig. 34.22C)**.
- Convex facial profile **(Fig. 34.22D)**.

### Intra-oral Features

Intra-oral examination may reveal the following features **(Fig. 34.23):**

- Maxillary and mandibular anterior proclination.
- Class I molar relationship.
- Class I canine relationship.
- Class I incisor relationship.
- Bimaxillary protrusion may be seen.

### Cephalometric Findings

- Decreased interincisal angle.
- Increased incisor mandibular plane angle.

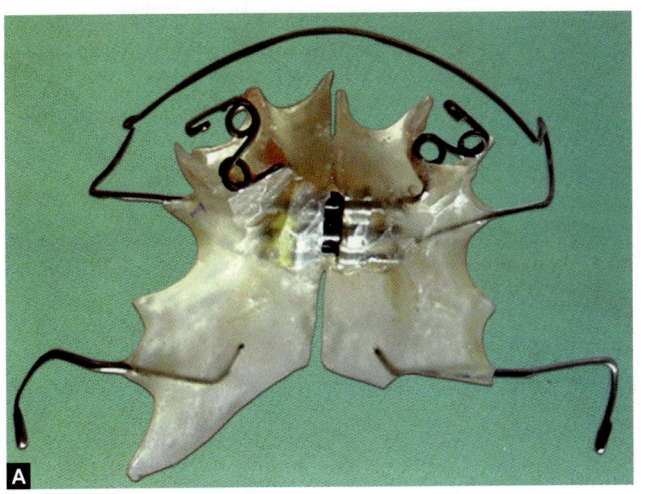
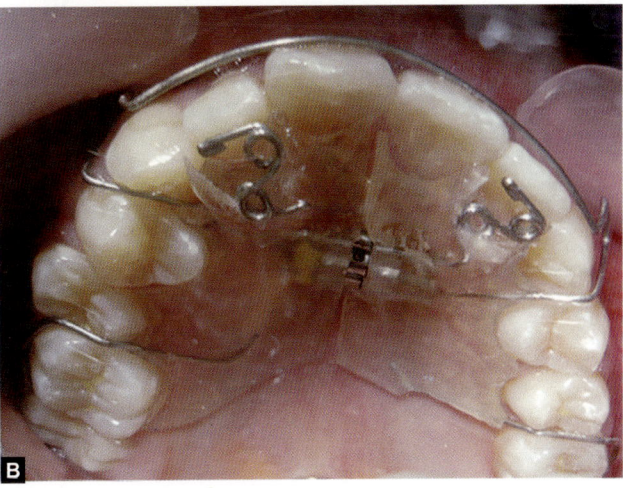

**Figs 34.18A and B:** Removable orthodontic appliance incorporating "Z" spring (double cantilever spring) along with labial bow can be used to treat mild rotations

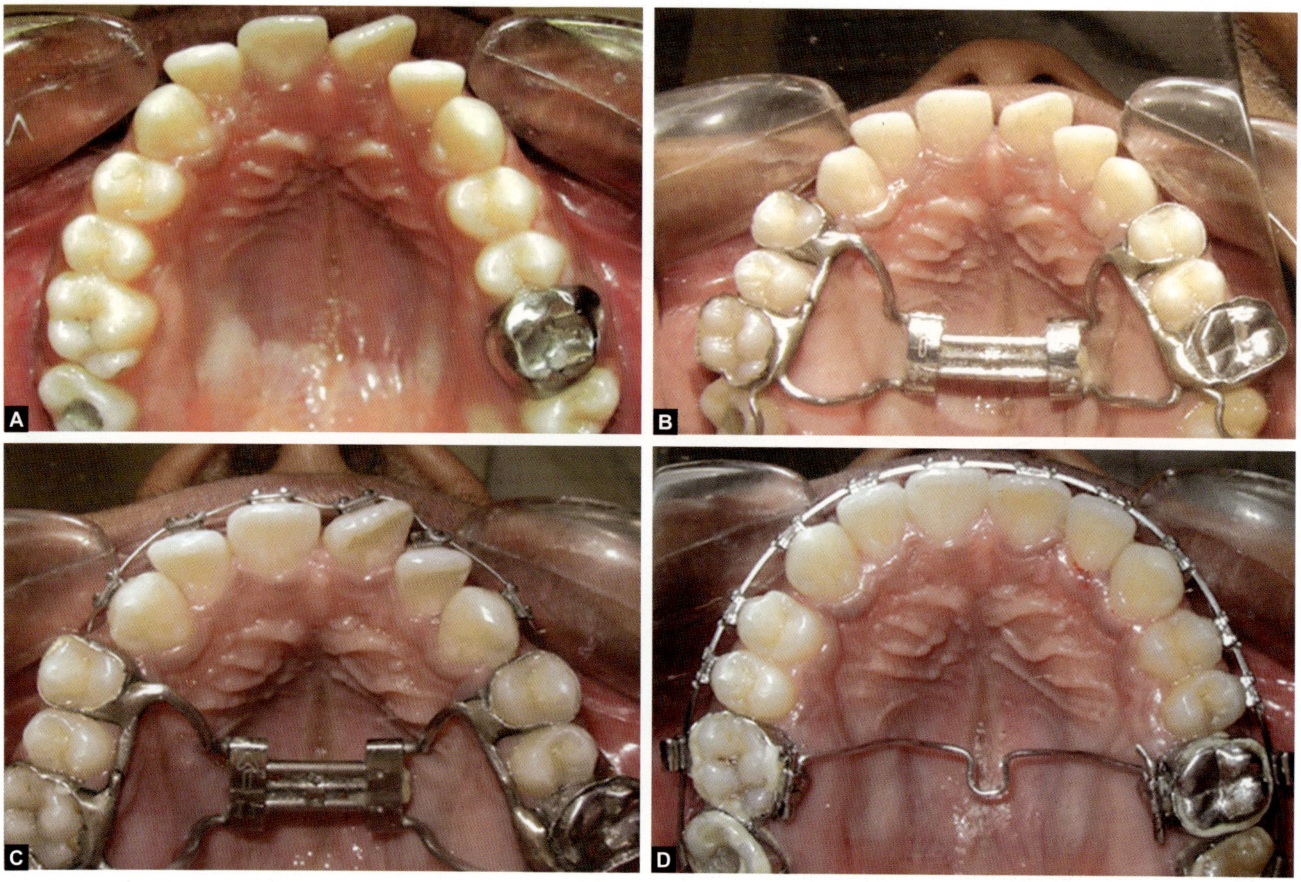

**Figs 34.19A to D:** Fixed orthodontic appliances with RME can be used to treat multiple rotations: (A) Pretreatment intraoral occlusal photograph showing multiple rotations. (B and C) Hyrax used to create space for derotation of teeth. (D) Nearing the completion of treatment

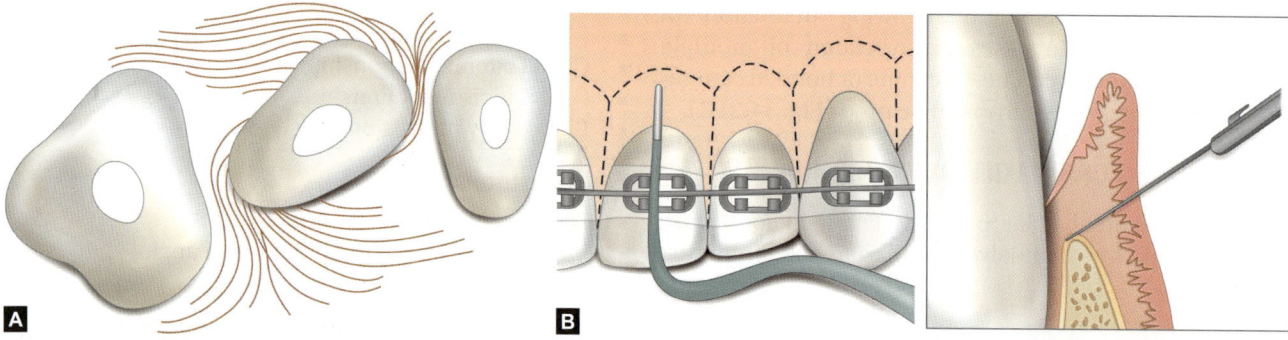

**Figs 34.20A and B:** (A) Supracrestal gingival fibers take longer time to reorganize after orthodontic derotation of the tooth. (B) Circumferential supracrestal fibrotomy or pericision is a useful adjunctive surgical procedure in which the gingival fibers are incised to prevent relapse

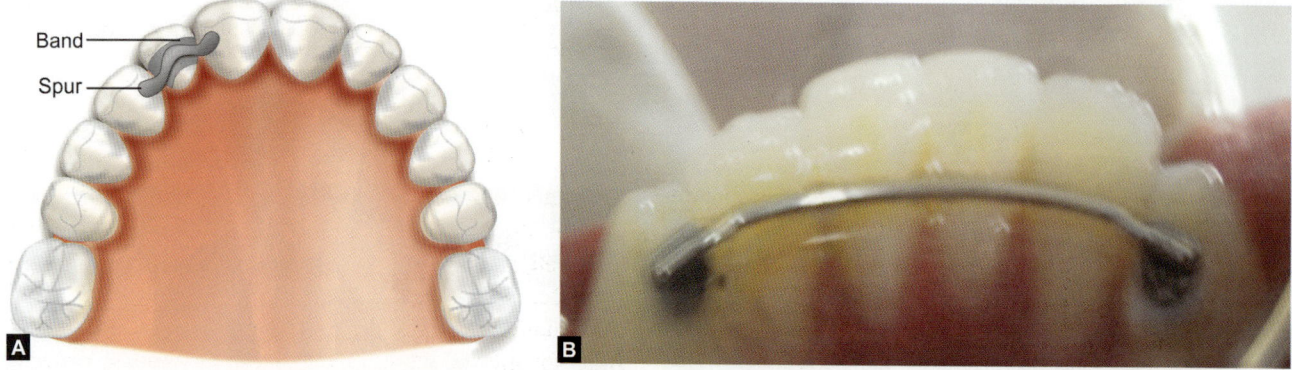

**Figs 34.21A and B:** Retention following derotation of teeth: (A) Band and spur is the retainer of choice in cases of correction of single tooth rotation. (B) Bonded canine to canine lingual retainer

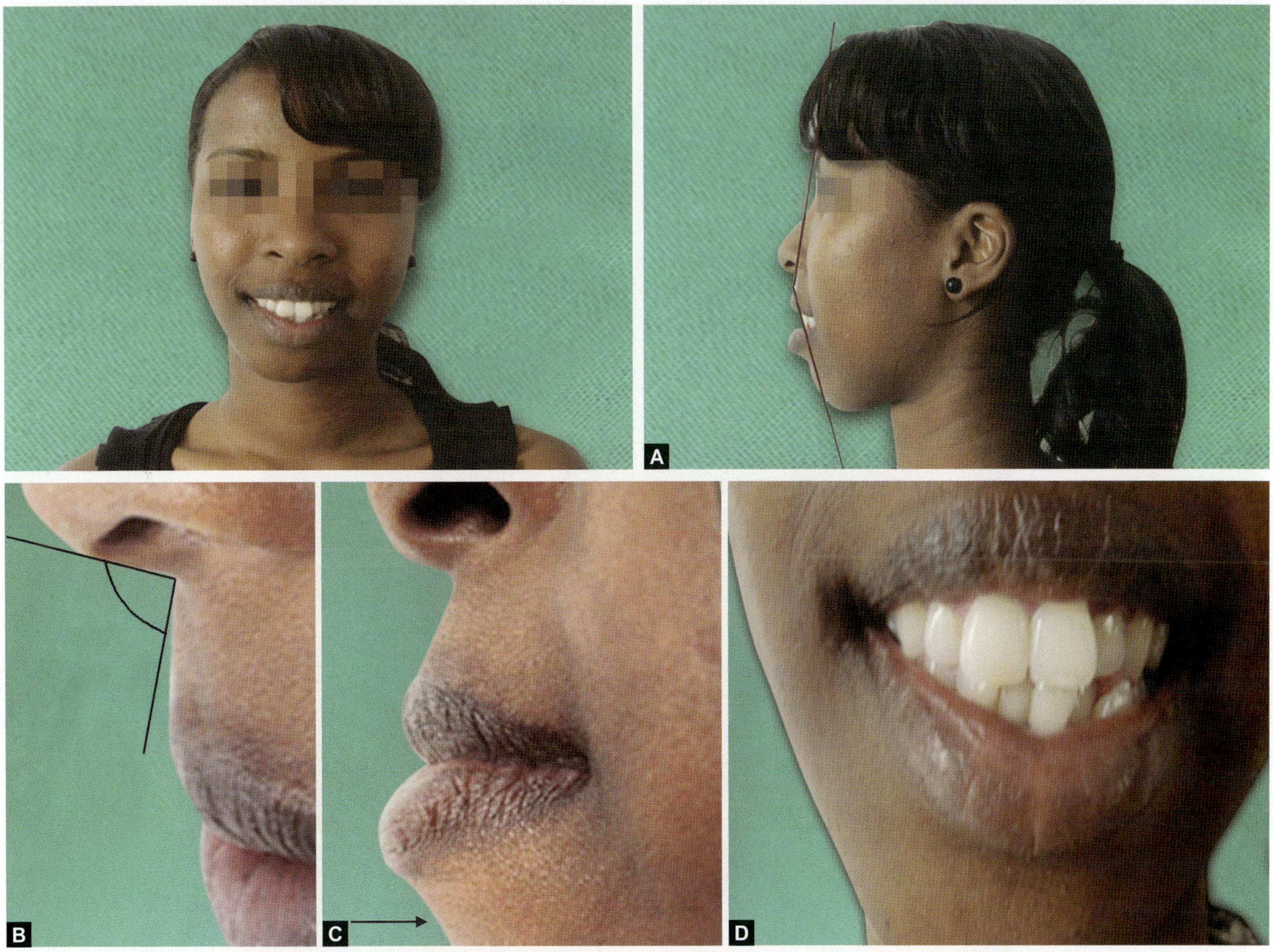

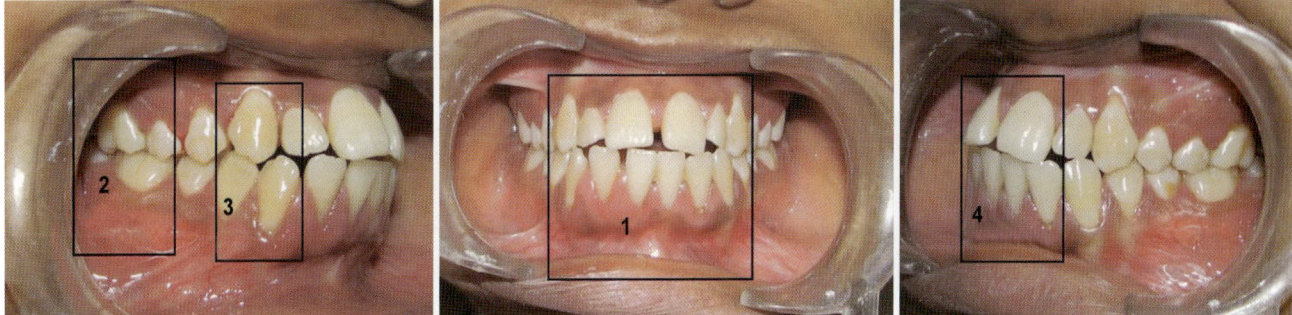

**Figs 34.22A to D:** Extra-oral features of bimaxillary protrusion: (A) Convex facial profile (B) Decreased nasolabial angle due to proclined maxillary anteriors. (B) Shallow mentolabial sulcus due to proclined mandibular anteriors. (C) Lips incompetent.

**Fig. 34.23:** Intra-oral features of another case of bimaxillary protrusion: (1) Maxillary and mandibular anterior proclination. (2) Class I molar relationship. (3) Class I canine relationship. (4) Class I incisor relationship

- Increased SNA and SNB angle, if there is prognathism of the jaws.
- Increased S-N-Pr and S-N-Id angle in cases associated with bimaxillary prognathism.

## TREATMENT OF BIMAXILLARY PROTRUSION

### Treatment of Bimaxillary Protrusion Using Either Removable Orthodontic Appliances or Fixed Orthodontic Appliances

Bimaxillary protrusion can be well managed by either removable orthodontic appliances or fixed orthodontic appliances depending upon the inclination of canines. Removable orthodontic appliance is the choice of appliance in cases where there are distally inclined canines. On the other hand, cases with mesially inclined canines are well managed with fixed orthodontic appliances **(Figs 34.24A to F)**.

Usually first premolars are extracted to gain enough space for anterior retraction. The maxillary and mandibular anterior are retracted while maintaining the existing Class I molar and canine relationships.

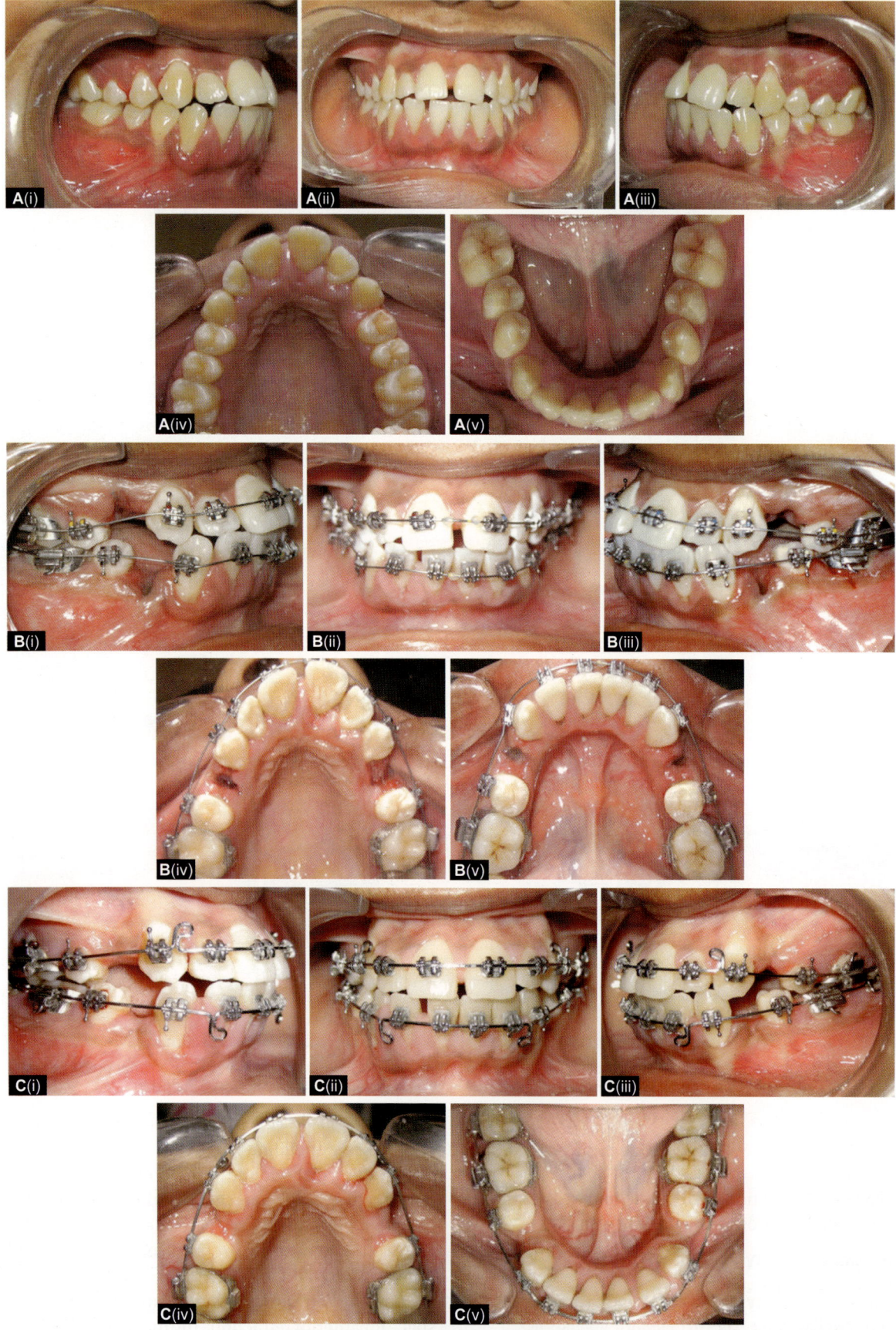

**Figs 34.24A to C:** Treatment of bimaxillary protrusion with fixed mechanotherapy. All first premolars are extracted to gain enough space for anterior retraction. The maxillary and mandibular anterior are retracted while maintaining the existing Class I molar and canine relationships

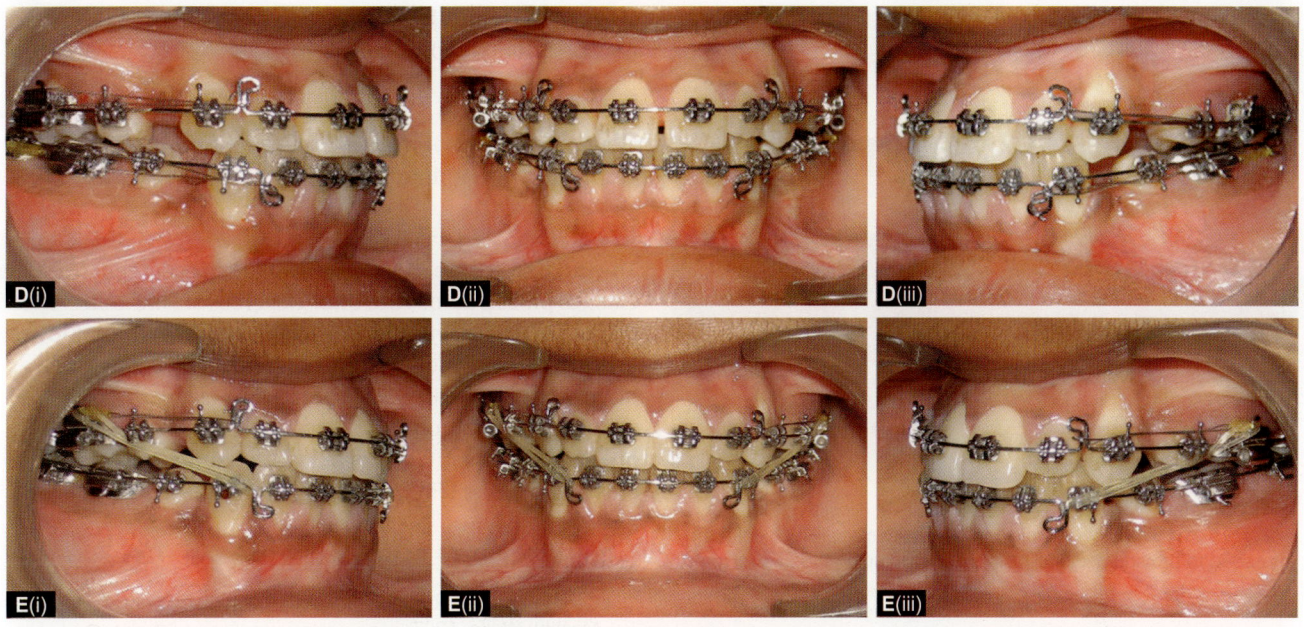

**Figs 34.24D to E:** Treatment of bimaxillary protrusion with fixed mechanotherapy. All first premolars are extracted to gain enough space for anterior retraction. The maxillary and mandibular anterior are retracted while maintaining the existing Class I molar and canine relationships

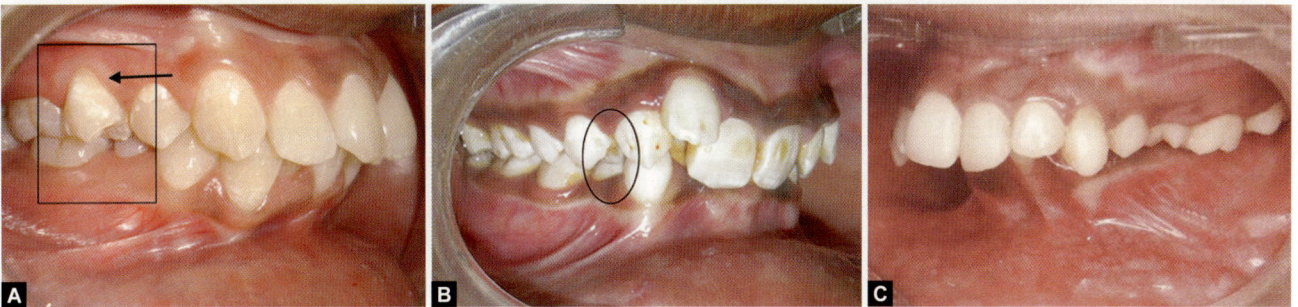

**Figs 34.25A to C:** Scissors bite: (A) Scissors bite in relation to right permanent second premolar. (B) Scissors bite in relation to right permanent first premolar. (C) Segmental scissors bite on left side.

## MANAGEMENT OF BIMAXILLARY RETRUSION

Bimaxillary retrusion is a condition characterized by retrusion of both upper and lower anterior teeth resulting in a concave facial profile.

### Clinical Features of Bimaxillary Retrusion

#### Extraoral Features
A patient with bimaxillary retrusion may have the following features:
- Increased nasolabial angle due to retruded maxillary anteriors.
- Deep mentolabial sulcus due to retruded lower anteriors.
- Mild concave facial profile.

#### Intra-oral Features
The following findings may intraorally be observed:
- Maxillary and mandibular anterior retroclination.
- Class I molar relationship.
- Class I canine relationship.
- Retrognathic bimaxillary arches may be seen.

#### Cephalometric Findings
- Increased interincisal angle.
- Decreased incisor mandibular plane angle.
- Decreased SNA and SNB angles in cases with retrognathic bimaxillary arches associated with bimaxillary retrusion.
- Decreased S-N-Pr and S-N-Id angles in cases associated with retrognathic bimaxillary arches.

### Treatment of Bimaxillary Retrusion

#### Treatment of Bimaxillary Retrusion Using Removable Orthodontic Appliances
- *Removable orthodontic appliance with expansion screw*: Removable orthodontic appliances with incorporated expansion screw can be used. Activation of expansion screw following Timms schedule of activation (wherein the screw is turned up to 90° twice in a week in growing patient) brings about forward placement/labial placement of anteriors thereby correcting of bimaxillary retrusion.
- *Removable orthodontic appliances with modified double cantilever spring*: Removable orthodontic

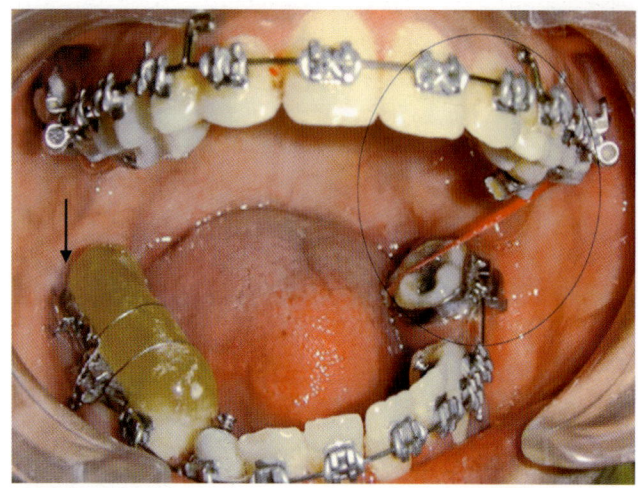

**Fig. 34.26:** The treatment of scissors bite is done by placement of cross elastics placed across the bite (encircled). Bite blocks are needed to provide occlusal clearance for jumping the bite (arrow)

appliance with modified double cantilever spring fabricated from canine to canine can also be used. Activation of modified double cantilever spring by opening the helices brings about labial movement of anteriors, thereby correcting of bimaxillary retrusion.

## MANAGEMENT OF SCISSOR BITE

Scissor bite is the buccal crossbite where, the upper posterior teeth are placed completely buccal to their lower counterparts. It may involve a single tooth (Figs 34.25A and B) or group of teeth (Fig. 34.25C) and may be unilateral or bilateral.

### Diagnosis

Diagnosis of scissors bite is done by thorough clinical and study model examination.

### Treatment

The treatment of scissors bite is done by placement of cross elastics placed across the bite. The cross elastic is stretched from buccal aspect of upper tooth to the lingual of lower tooth involved in scissor bite. Lingual attachments such as lingual button are used to engage the elastic on the lingual aspect of lower tooth involved in scissor bite. Bite blocks are needed to provide occlusal clearance for jumping/clearing the bite (Fig. 34.26).

## BIBLIOGRAPHY

1. Cameron AC, Widmer RP. Handbook of pediatric dentistry London, Mosbby-Wolfe, 1997.
2. Graber M, Vanarsdall L. Orthodontic Current Principles and Techniques. Mosby Year Book Inc., 1994.
3. Graber TM, Vanarsdall RL. Orthoontic: Current principles and techniques, 3rd edn., St Louis, Mosby, 2000.
4. Graber TM. Orthodontics: Principles and Practice. WB Saunders, 1988.
5. Popovich F ,Thompson GW. Craniofacial templates for orthodontic case analysis. Am J Orthod 1977;71:406-20.
6. Profitt WR. Contemporary Orthodontics. St. Louis: CV Mosby, 1986.
7. Rocke RA. Management of a severe Class I Division I Malocclusion. Begg J Orthod Theory and Treat 1963; 2:37-47.

---

### EXAM-ORIENTED QUESTIONS

**Long Essay or Long Questions**

1. Management of class I and malocclusion with crowding in detail in dental arches.
2. Management of class I and malocclusion with spacing in detail in dental arches.
3. Management of class I and malocclusion with rotation in detail in dental arches.
4. Management of bimaxillary protrusion.

**Short Notes**

1. Management of bimaxillary protrusion
2. Management of scissor's bite.

# CHAPTER 34: Management of Class I Malocclusion

## CHAPTER OVERVIEW

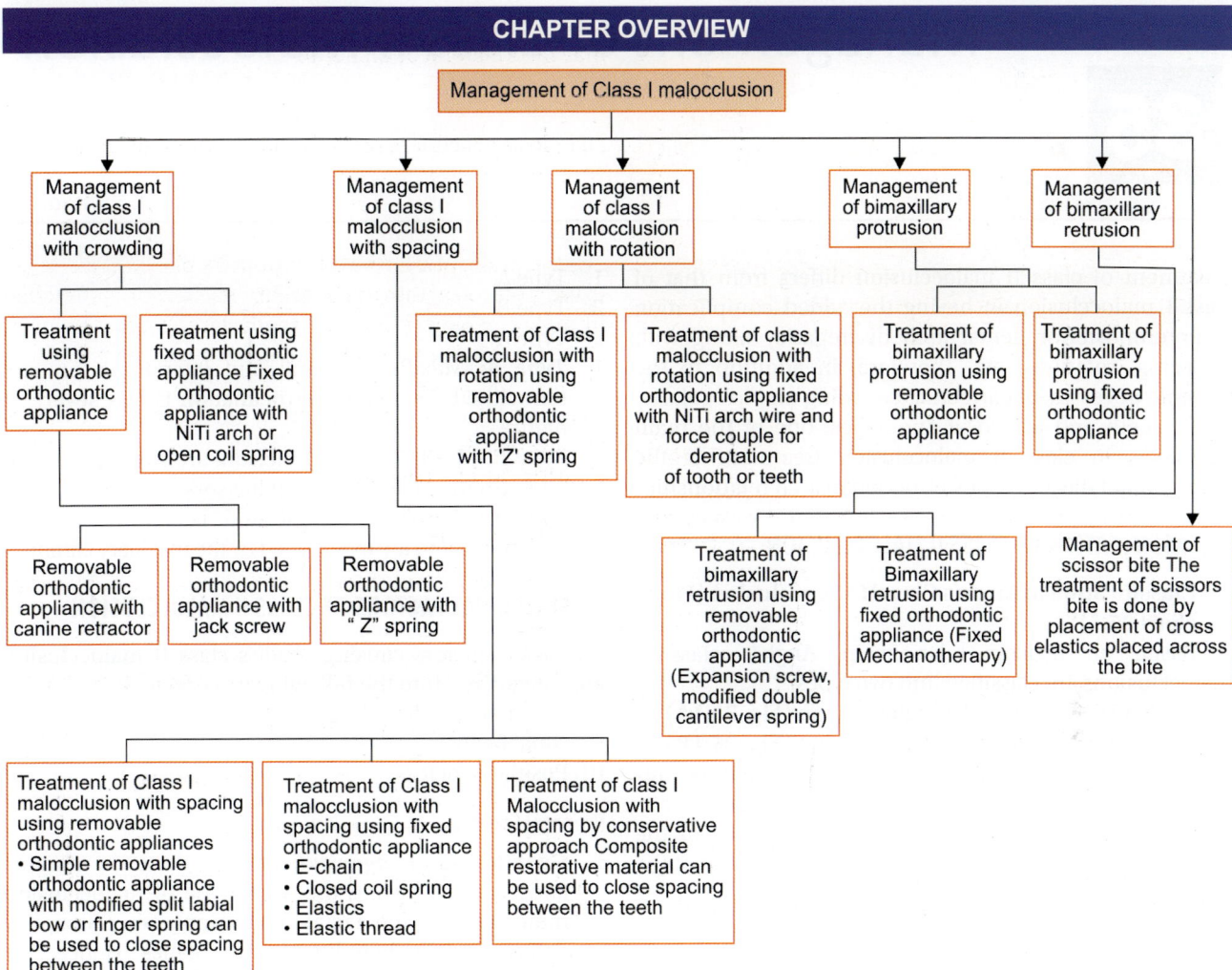

# CHAPTER 35: Management of Class II Malocclusion

*Phulari BS*

Treatment of class II malocclusion differs from that of class I malocclusion in having the added complication of anteroposterior dental arch discrepancy along with crowding, rotations, etc. Therefore, in addition to the possible necessity of correcting crowding and irregularity of the teeth and any local anomalies, one of the main objectives in class II malocclusion treatment is the correction of the anteroposterior dental arch relationship.

## CLASSIFICATION OF CLASS II MALOCCLUSION

I. **Classification of Angle's Class II Malocclusion (Flowchart 35.1)**

Based on incisors relationship, Angle's class II malocclusions are classified into two types:
- Angle's class II division 1 malocclusion **(Fig. 35.1A)**
- Angle's class II division 2 malocclusion **(Fig. 35.1B)**

II. **Classification Based on Abnormal Skeletal Relationship**

Based on the abnormal skeletal relationship of the maxilla and mandible, class II malocclusion can be of the following two types:
- Skeletal class II division 1 malocclusion
- Skeletal class II division 2 malocclusion

Skeletal class II malocclusion may be caused due to any one of the following features:
- Maxillary prognathism **(Fig. 35.1C)**
- Mandibular retrognathism **(Fig. 35.1D)**
- Maxillary prognathism and mandibular retrognathism **(Fig. 35.1E)**.

III. **Classification Based on Severity of Incisor Relationship**

Von-der-Linden classified Angle's class II division 2 malocclusion into the following three types based on severity of incisor relationship **(Flowchart 35.2)**:

1. Type A
2. Type B
3. Type C

1. **Type A:** Maxillary central and lateral incisors are retroclined. Degree of retroclination is less severe in nature.
2. **Type B:** Maxillary lateral incisors are overlapping the retroclined maxillary central incisors.
3. **Type C:** Maxillary central and lateral incisors are retroclined and are overlapped by the maxillary canines.

## ETIOLOGICAL FACTORS OF CLASS II MALOCCLUSION

Etiological factors causing Angle's class II malocclusion are categorized into the following three factors:
I. Prenatal factors
II. Natal factors
III. Postnatal factors.

### Prenatal Factors

1. **Genetic and congenital:** Studies done on parents and children having the same type of malocclusion indicates that the facial dimensions are principally determined by heredity through genes. Hence, the dimensions of the basal bones which can contribute to skeletal class II malocclusion can be inherited.
2. **Teratogenesis:** Administration of certain drugs during pregnancy has a potential of yielding abnormal development of arches leading to class II malocclusion. Such drugs are referred to as teratogens.
3. **Irradiation:** Irradiation therapy during fetal life can also be a causative factor for class II malocclusion.
4. **Intrauterine fetal posture:** Abnormal posture of the fetus such as hands across the face is found to affect mandibular growth.

### Natal Factors

Improper forceps application during delivery can lead to condylar damage/fracture causing internal hemorrhage into the joint area. TMJ can get ankylosed or fibrosed later, leading to underdevelopment of the mandible.

### Postnatal Factors

Certain conditions that can influence the normal development of the craniofacial skeleton are:
- Traumatic injuries during play
- Long-term irradiation therapy
- Oral habits such as thumb sucking
- Congenitally missing teeth
- Anomalies in the shape of teeth.

**Flowchart 35.1:** Angle's class II malocclusion

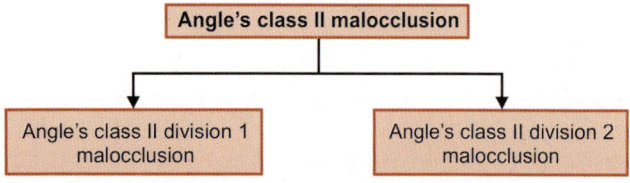

**Flowchart 35.2:** Von-der-Linden's classification

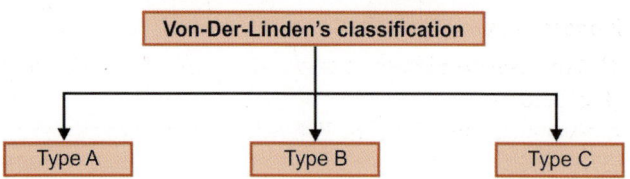

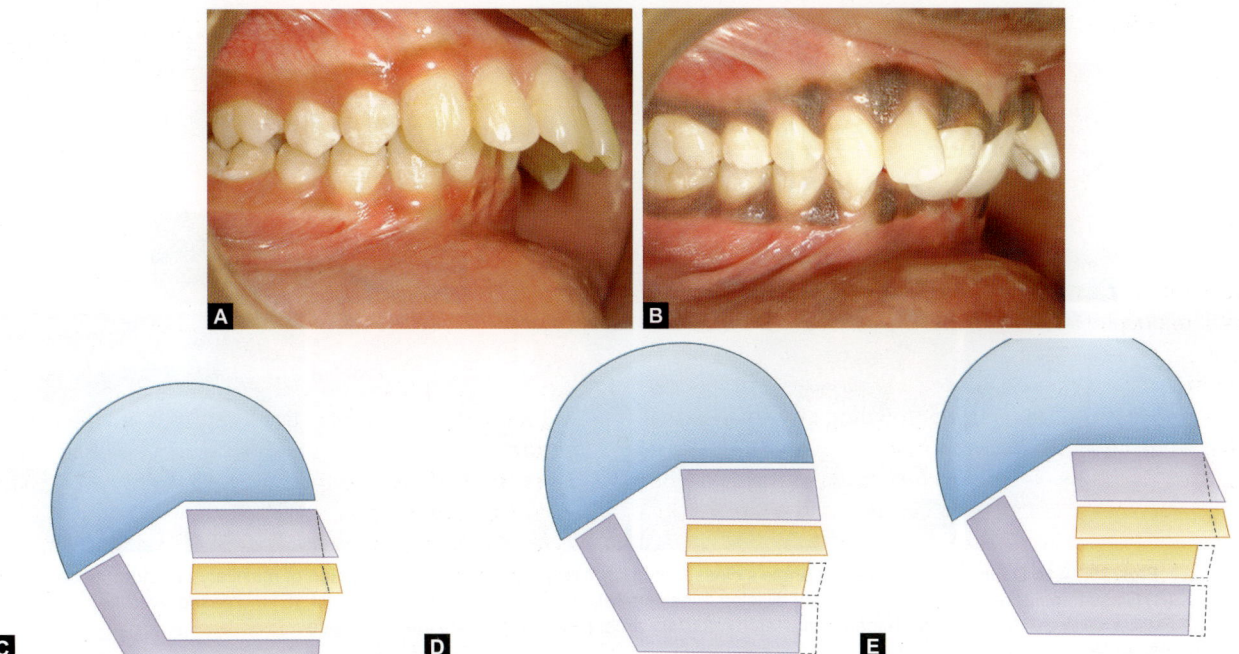

**Figs 35.1A to E:** Angle's class II malocclusion: (A) Angle's class II division 1 malocclusion; (B) Angle's class II division 2 malocclusion; (C) Skeletal class II malocclusion due to maxillary prognathism; (D) Skeletal class II malocclusion due to mandibular retrognathism; (E) Skeletal class II malocclusion due to maxillary prognathism and mandibular retrognathism

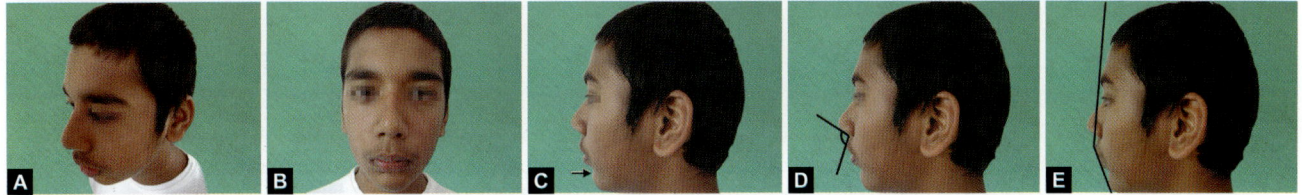

**Figs 35.2A to E:** Extraoral features of Angle's class II division 1 malocclusion: (A) Shape of the head: Mesocephalic or dolichocephalic; (B) Facial form: mesoprosopic or euryprosopic; (C) Deep mentolabial sulcus; (D) Decreased nasolabial angle; (E) Convex facial profile

## CLINICAL FEATURES

### Clinical Features of Class II Division 1 Malocclusion

#### Extraoral Features

***Shape of the head:*** Mesocephalic or Dolichocephalic **(Fig. 35.2A)**.
***Facial form:*** Mesoprosopic or Euryprosopic **(Fig. 35.2B)**.
***Facial divergence:*** Posterior facial divergence.
***Lips:*** Incompetent lips.
***Mentolabial sulcus:*** Deep **(Fig. 35.2C)**.
***Nasolabial angle:*** Decreased **(Fig. 35.2D)**.
***Mentalis:*** Hyperactive.
***Lower facial height:*** Decreased.
***Profile:*** Convex facial profile **(Fig. 35.2E)**.

#### Intraoral Features

***Maxillary anteriors:*** Proclination of maxillary anterior **(Fig. 35.3A)**.
***Molar relationship:*** Class II molar relationship **(Fig. 35.3B)**.
***Incisor relationship:*** Class II division 1 incisor relationship **(Fig. 35.3C)**.

***Overjet:*** Increased **(Fig. 35.3D)**.
***Overbite:*** Increased **(Fig. 35.3E)**.
***Shape of the maxillary arch:*** V-shaped arch **(Fig. 35.3F)**.
***Curve of Spee:*** Exaggerated **(Fig. 35.3G)**.
***Anterior open bite:*** May or may not be present. Depends on the persistence of deleterious oral habits.
***Posterior crossbite and scissor bite:*** Presence depends on persistence of habit.

### Clinical Features of Class II Division 2 Malocclusion

#### Extraoral Features

***Shape of the head:*** Brachycephalic.
***Facial form:*** Euryprosopic **(Figs 35.4Ai and ii)**.
***Facial profile:*** Straight to mildly convex **(Fig. 35.4B)**.
***Mentolabial sulcus:*** Deep **(Fig. 35.4C)**.
***Mentalis:*** Hyperactive.

#### Intraoral Features

***Molar relationship:*** Class II molar relationship **(Fig. 35.5A)**.
***Incisor relationship:*** Class II division 2 incisor relationship **(Fig. 35.5B)**.

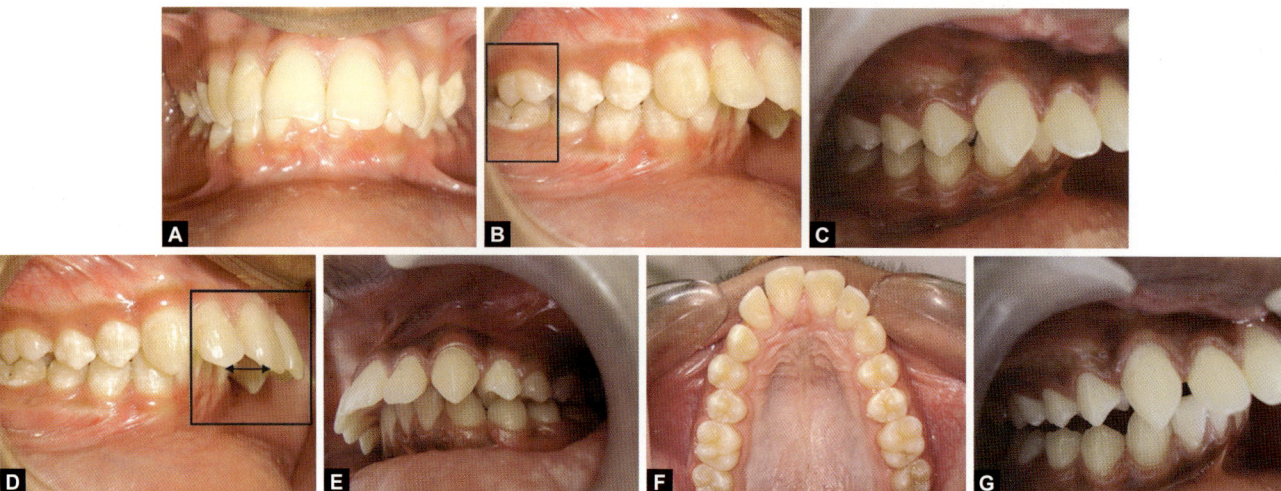

**Figs 35.3A to G:** Intraoral features of Angle's class II division 1 malocclusion: (A) Proclination of maxillary anteriors; (B) Class II molar relationship; (C) Class II division 1 incisors relationship; (D) Increased overjet; (E) Increased overbite; (F) V-shaped dental arch maxillary arch; (G) Exaggerated curve of Spee

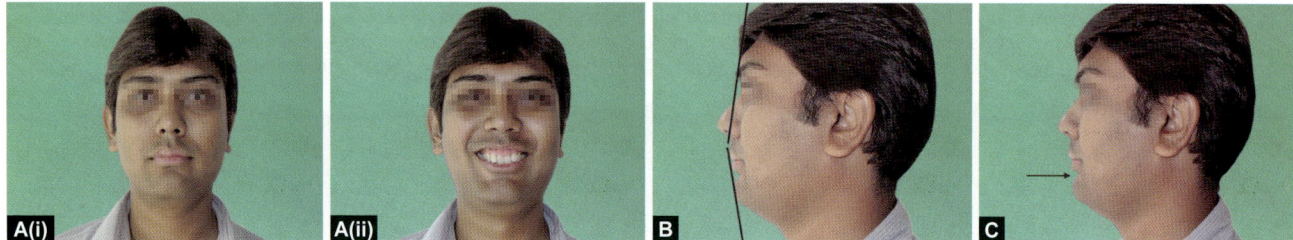

**Figs 35.4A to C:** Extraoral features of class II division 2 malocclusion. (A i and ii) Facial form: Euryprosopic; (B) Facial profile: Straight to mildly convex; (C) Deep mentolabial sulcus

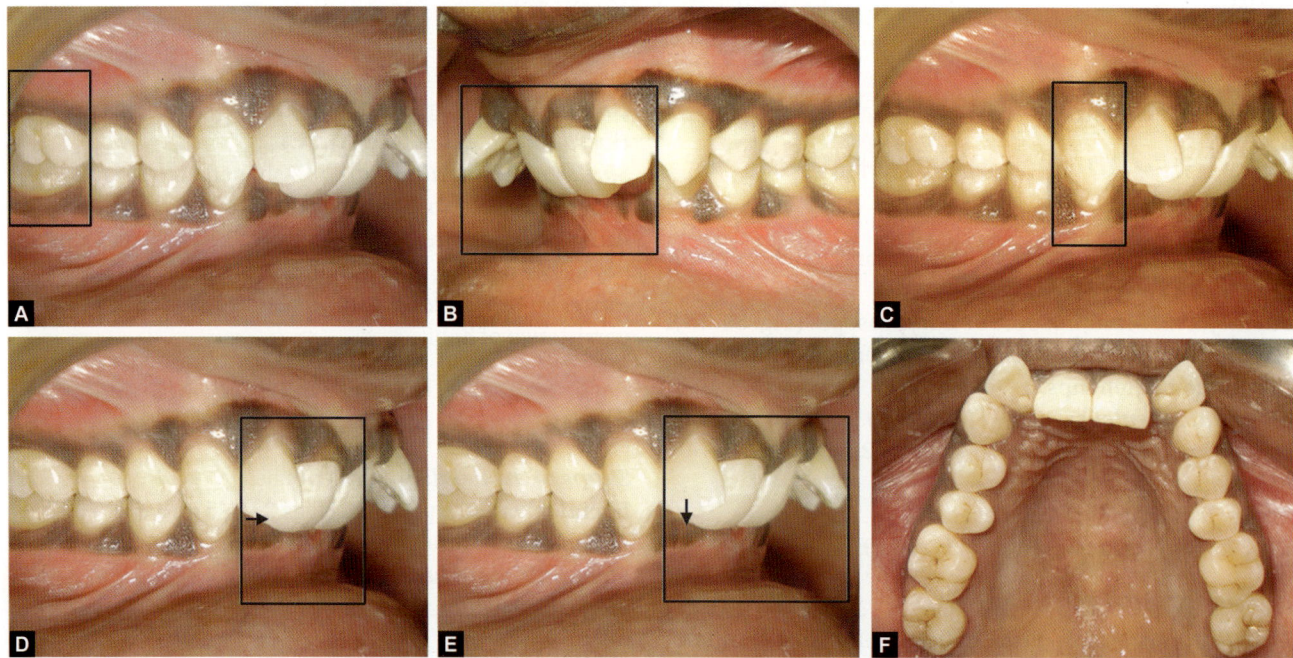

**Figs 35.5A to F:** Intra-oral features of class II division 2 malocclusion: (A) Class II molar relationship; (B) Class II division 2 incisors relationship; (C) Class II canine relationship; (D) Decreased overjet; (E) Increased overbite; (F) U-shaped maxillary arch

*Canine relationship:* Class II canine relationship **(Fig. 35.5C)**.
*Overjet:* Decreased **(Fig. 35.5D)**.
*Overbite:* Increased **(Fig. 35.5E)**.
*Maxillary arch:* "U" shaped arch **(Fig. 35.5F)**.
*Dental calculus:* More prone on labial surface of mandibular anteriors.

## TREATMENT OF CLASS II DIVISION 1 MALOCCLUSION

### Treatment Objectives

The objective of treatment in patients with Angle's class II division 1 malocclusion includes:
- Relief of crowding and local irregularities
- Reduction of incisal overbite
- Reduction of incisal overjet
- Correction of class II relationship of the buccal teeth.

### Strategies of Class II Division 1 Malocclusion Treatment

There are two strategies used in the treatment of class II division 1 malocclusion:
I. Two-phase treatment (early and late)
II. One phase treatment (late)
I. Two-phase treatments (early and late)
  Two treatment strategies of Angle's class II division 1 malocclusion treatment involve early and late treatment;
- Early treatment at the age of 8–10 years.
- Late treatment at the age of 11–14 years.
II. One phase treatment (Late)
  Here, treatment of Angle's class II division 1 malocclusion is carried out during the age of 11–14 years and treatment will be finished in one phase.

### Treatment of Angle's Class II Division 1 Malocclusion with No Extraction in Mixed Dentition

In some children with severe proclination of the maxillary anteriors, early reduction of the incisal overjet has been advocated, since proclined incisors are thought to be vulnerable to accidental trauma. Treatment with functional appliances such as activator is often carried out in the mixed dentition, before premolars and permanent canines erupt, which greatly reduces the overjet and improves the skeletal pattern **(Figs 35.6A to F)**.

### Treatment of Angle's Class II Division 1 Malocclusion with Extraction of Teeth in Permanent Dentition

Treatment of Angle's class II division 1 malocclusion with extraction of teeth is carried out after the eruption of permanent premolars and molars in permanent dentition **(Figs 35.7A to D)**.

### Relief of Crowding

Extraction in Angle's class II division 1 malocclusion treatment:
Extraction of teeth helps in the following:
I. To relieve crowding in both arches, i.e. maxillary and mandibular arches.
II. To provide space in the maxillary arch for the retraction of the anterior segment.
III. To provide space in the lower arch for intermaxillary traction.

### Reduction of Overbite

If the incisal overbite is excessive, it is not possible to reduce the overjet completely, without reducing the overbite. Reduction of overbite is, therefore, a frequent part of Angle's class II division 1 malocclusion treatment and usually carried out as one of the first stages.
There are three ways of reducing overbite:
1. Removable orthodontic appliance or fixed orthodontic appliance with anterior bite plane **(Figs 35.8A and B)**. Anterior bite plane with removable orthodontic appliances causes reduction of overbite by allowing vertical development of the posterior dentoalveolar segment.
2. Fixed orthodontic appliance with downward force by using a mandibular fixed appliance to apply direct downward force to the mandibular incisors. Mandibular fixed orthodontic appliance reduces overbite by causing intrusion of anterior segment with extrusion of the posterior segment.
3. Fixed orthodontic appliance with upward force by using a fixed appliance to apply direct upward force to the maxillary incisors. Maxillary fixed orthodontic appliance reduces overbite by causing intrusion of the anterior segment with extrusion of the posterior dento-alveolar segment.

### Reduction of Overjet

Overjet reduction is usually brought about by retraction of the maxillary anterior segment **(Fig. 35.9)**. Occasionally, overjet reduction may be achieved by moving the mandibular incisor forward or by moving the whole maxillary arch backward.

### Method of Retraction of Maxillary Anteriors

The method of retraction of maxillary anterior depends essentially on the degree of Angle's class II skeletal discrepancy.

### In Mild Skeletal Class II Division 1 Malocclusion

A simple tipping movement of the incisor should be sufficient to produce a satisfactory incisor relationship **(Fig. 35.10)**. This can be brought about by removable orthodontic appliance using intramaxillary traction.

### In Severe Skeletal Class II Division 1 Malocclusion

In severe skeletal class II division 1 malocclusion it is necessary to produce bodily movement of the incisors to reduce the overjet without producing excessive retroclination **(Figs 35.11A to C)**. Fixed orthodontic appliance using intermaxillary traction may be used to reduce the increased overjet.

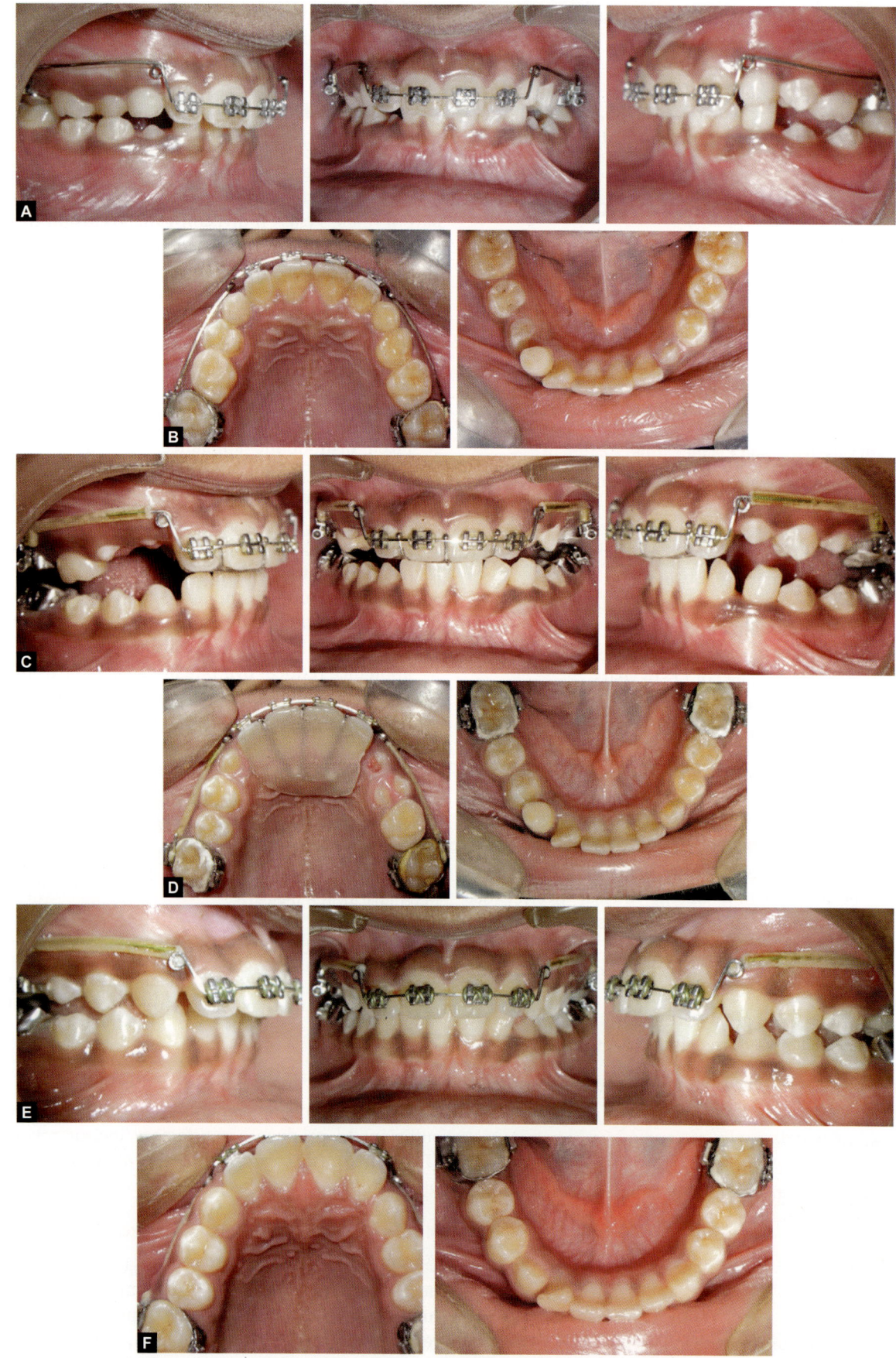

**Figs 35.6A to F:** Treatment of Angle's class II division 1 malocclusion with no extraction in mixed dentition

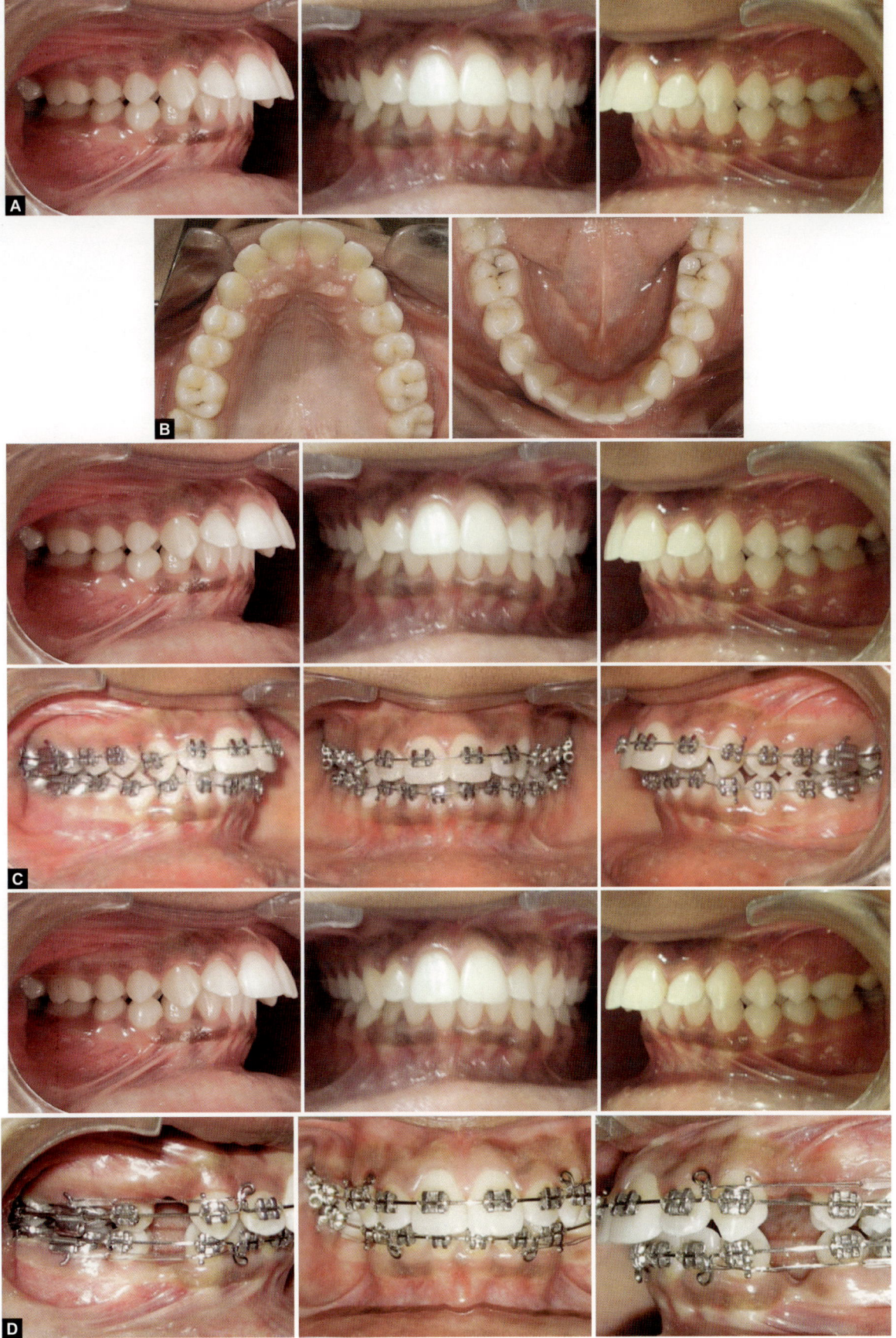

**Figs 35.7A to D:** Treatment of Angle's class II division 1 malocclusion with extraction of teeth in permanent dentition

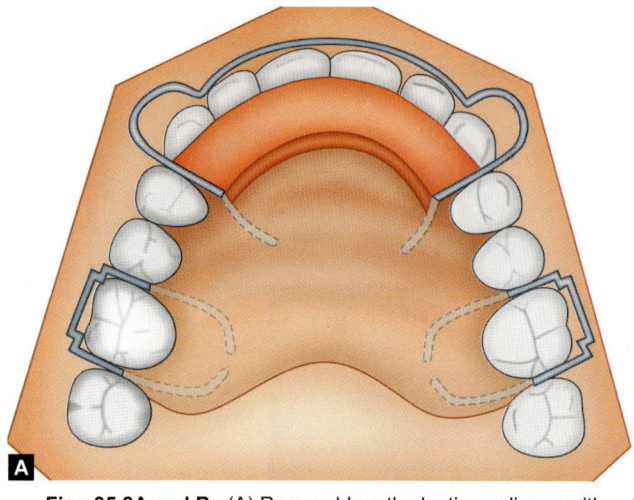 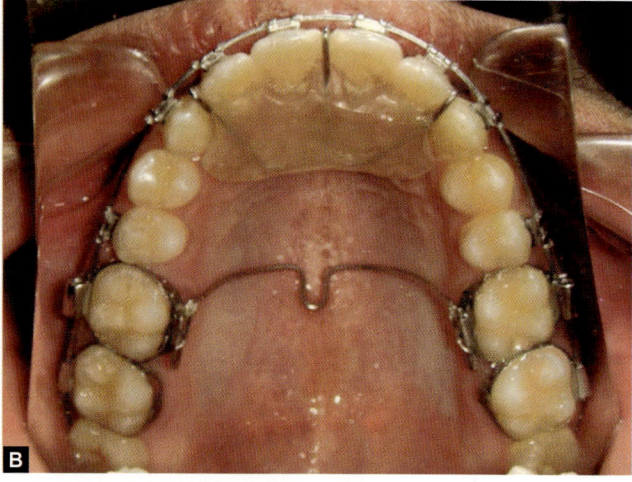

**Figs 35.8A and B:** (A) Removable orthodontic appliance with anterior bite plane; (B) Fixed orthodontic appliance with anterior bite plane

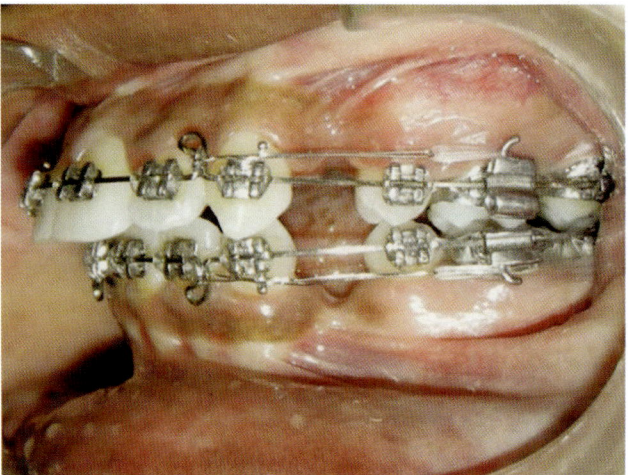 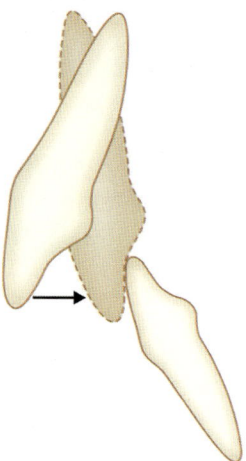

**Fig. 35.9:** Reduction of overjet by retraction of anterior segment

**Fig. 35.10:** A simple tipping movement of the incisor should be sufficient to produce a satisfactory incisor relationship

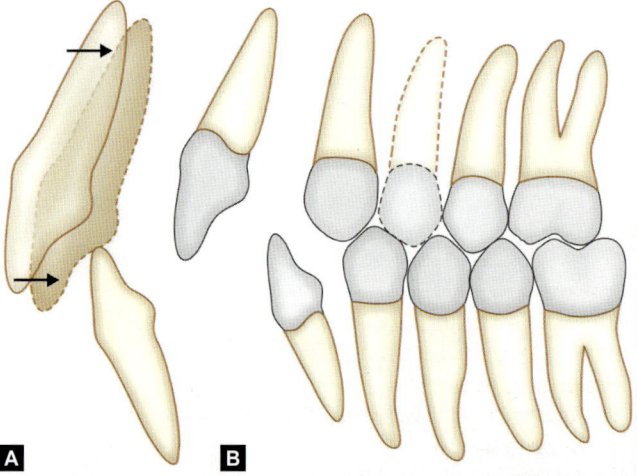 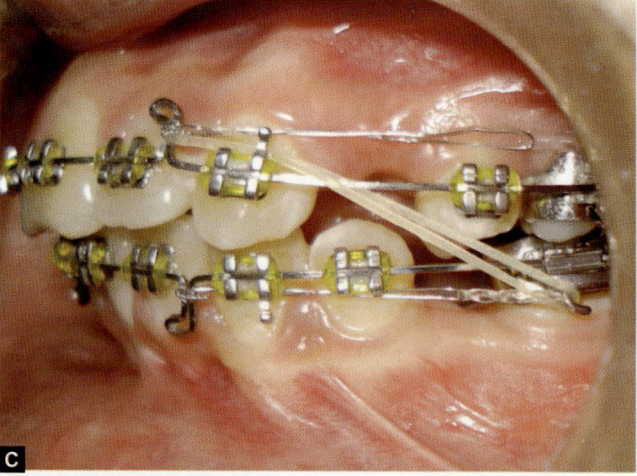

**Figs 35.11A to C:** In severe skeletal class II division 1 malocclusion, it is necessary to produce bodily movement of the incisors to reduce the overjet without producing excessive retroclination

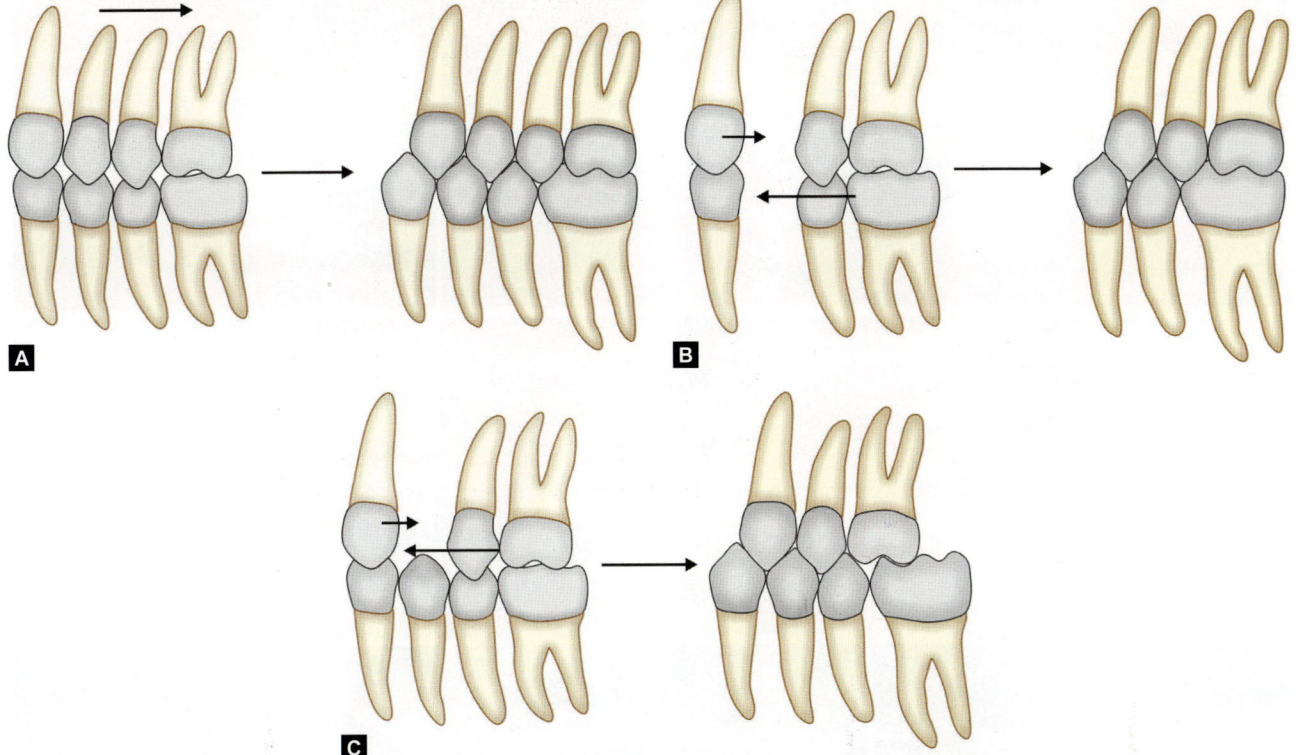

**Figs 35.12A to C:** (A) Distal movement of upper posterior teeth—this will produce class I relationship; (B) Mesial movement of lower posteriors will also produce class I relationship. It is frequently carried out following removal of a premolar from each side of the upper and lower arches; (C) Mesial movement of upper posterior teeth produces class II relationship with cuspal inter-digitalization and is appropriate to the less severe class II division 1 malocclusion where the lower arch is satisfactory

## Correction of Buccal Segment Relationship (Molar Relationship)

Three basic ways for correction of buccal segment relationship:
I. Distal movement of the upper posterior teeth.
II. Mesial movement of lower posterior teeth.
III. Mesial movement of upper posterior teeth

I. *Distal movement of the upper posterior teeth*
   This will produce class I relationship, but can only be done if the jaw is large enough to accommodate the teeth in a more distal position. It is occasionally achieved following extraction of the upper second molar **(Fig. 35.12A)**.

II. *Mesial movement of lower posterior teeth*
   This will also produce class I relationship. It is frequently carried out following removal of a premolar from each side of the upper and lower arches. Intramaxillary traction is applied to move the upper anterior segment back and the lower posterior segment forward **(Figs 35.12)**.

III. *Mesial movement of upper posterior teeth*
   In some cases where it is difficult to acheive class I molar relationship, a compromised line of treatment is to retain the class II molar relationship with correction of anterior relationship.
   This produces class II relationship with cuspal interdigitation and is appropriate in less severe cases of class II division 1 malocclusion, where the lower arch is satisfactory. An upper premolar is extracted on each side of the jaw. The upper anterior segment is moved back and the upper posterior segment is forwarded to the space of extraction using intramaxillary traction **(Fig. 35.12C)**.

## Management of Angle's Class II Division 2 Malocclusion

The main differences between treatment of Angle's class II division 1 malocclusion and Angle's class II division 2 malocclusion lies in the correction of the incisor relationship **(Figs 35.13A to G)**.

### Treatment Objectives

I. Relief of crowding and local irregularities
II. Relief of anterior gingival trauma and correction of incisal inclinations
III. Correction of buccal segment relationship.

### Correction of Incisor Relationship

In a mild class II division 2 malocclusion with no gingival trauma, treatment may be confined to correction of crowding and local irregularities.
When gingival trauma exists, treatment includes:
- Reduction of incisal overbite with anterior bite plane or fixed orthodontic appliances.
- Alteration of incisal inclinations to achieve contact between upper and lower incisors.

Severe class II division 2 skeletal discrepancies may prevent the attainment of incisal contact and if there is gingival trauma, a permanent retainer may be necessary after reduction of the overbite.

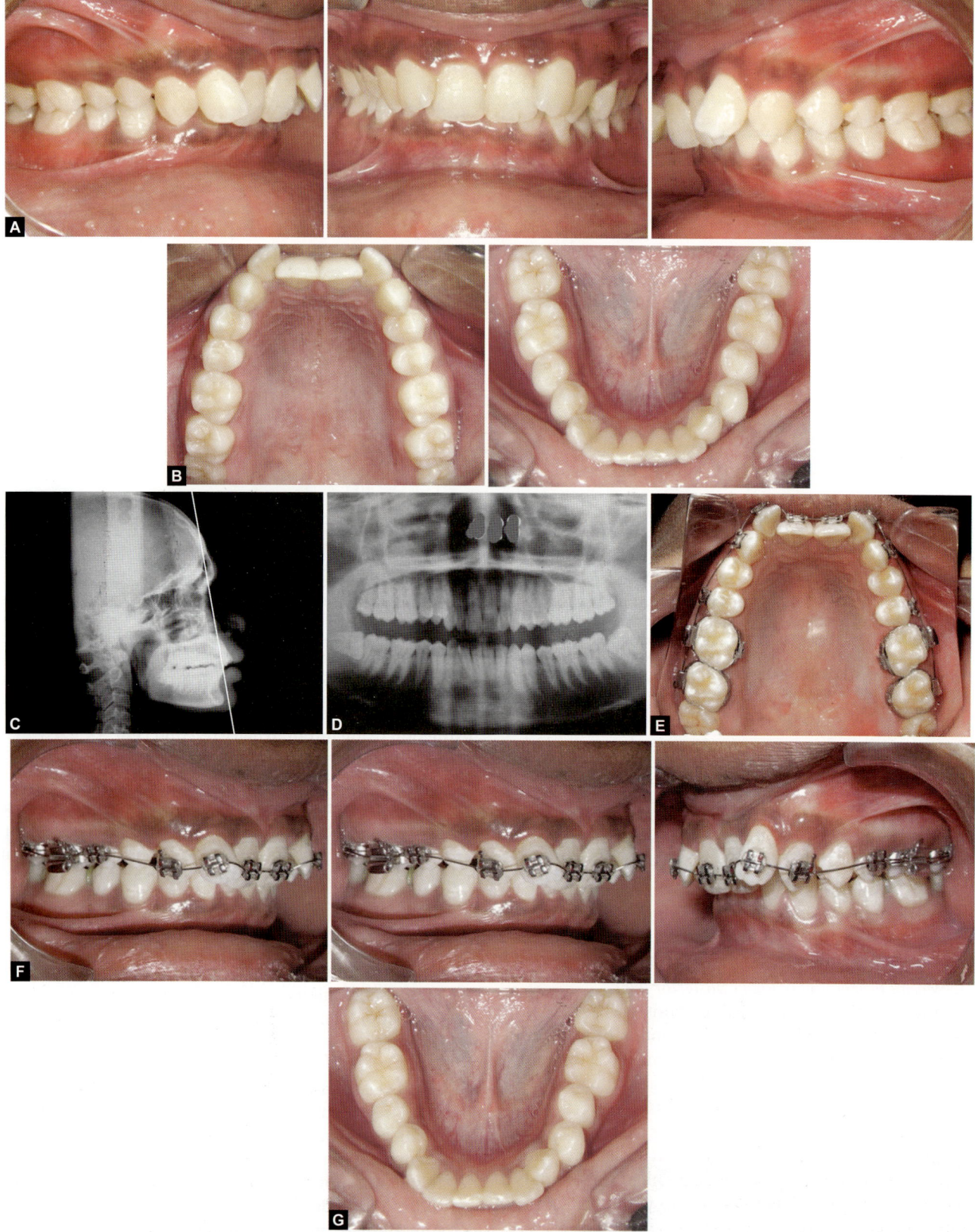

Fig. 35.13A to G: Management of class II division 2 malocclusion using fixed orthodontic appliances

**Flowchart 35.3:** Management of class II malocclusion

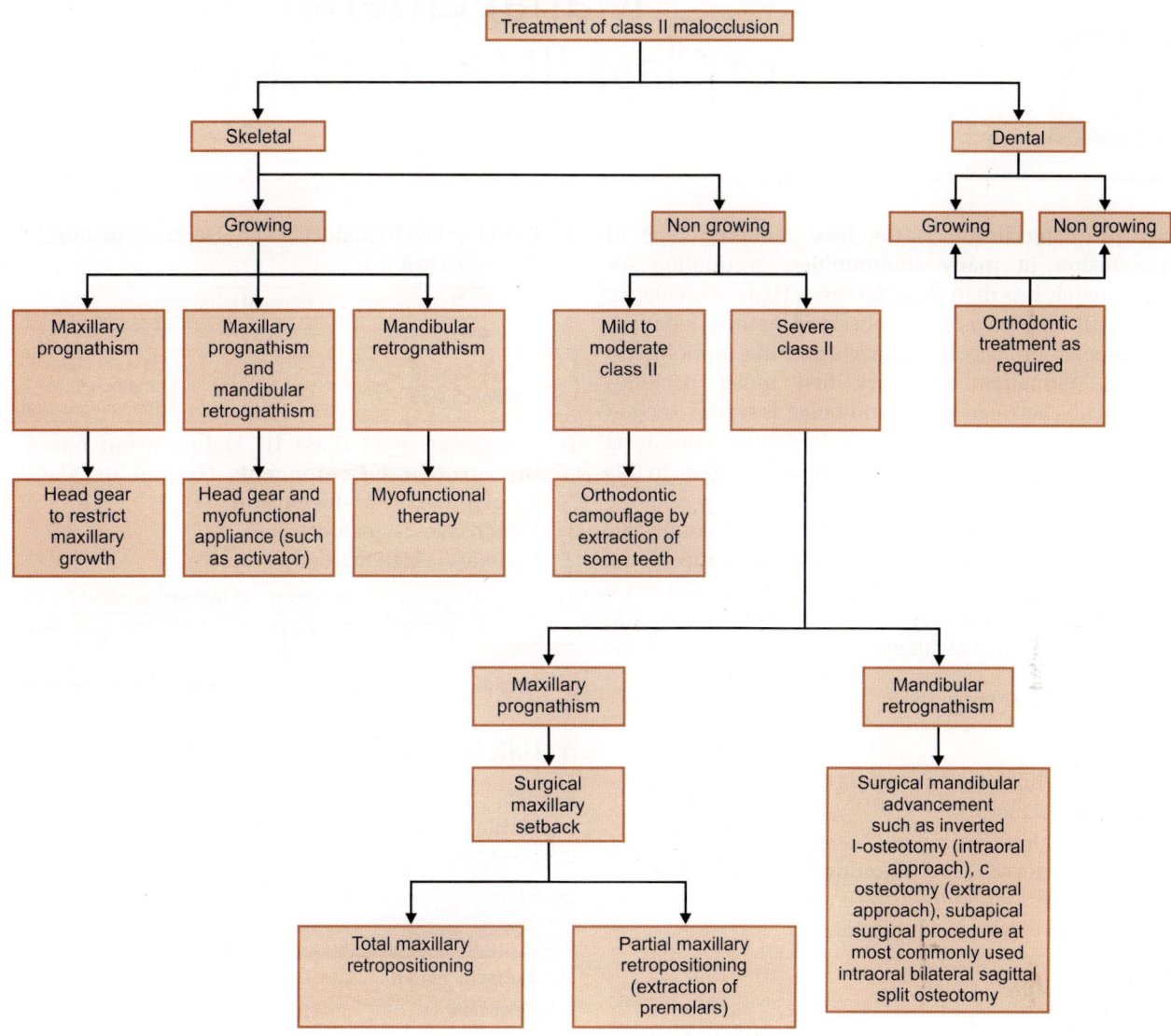

Management of class II malocclusion is summarized in **Flowchart 35.3**.

## BIBLIOGRAPHY

1. Delivanis HP, Kuftinec MM. Variation in morphology of maxillary central incisors found in class II, division 2 malocclusions. Am J Orthod. 1980;78(4):438-43.
2. Hitchkock HP. The cephalometric distinction of class II, division 2 malocclusion: Am J Orthod. 1976;69:447-54.
3. McNumara JA, Howe RP, Dischinger TG. A comparison of the Herbst and Franel appliances in the treatment of class II malocclusion. Am J Orthod Dentofacial Orthop. 1990;98:134-44.
4. Profitt. Contemporary Orthodontics, St Louis: CV Mosby, 1986.
5. Ruf S, Panherz H. Class II division 2 malocclusion: genetics or environment? A case report of monozygotic twins, Angle Orthod. 1999;69:321-4.
6. Seely DM. An American Board of Orthodontics case report: treatment of a crowded Class II malocclusion in an adult. Am J Orthod. 1993;298-303.
7. Ward DM. Angle class II, division 1 malocclusion. Am J Orthod. 1994;428-33.

## EXAM-ORIENTED QUESTIONS

### Long Essay or Long Questions

1. Discuss the different treatment modalities of class II div 1 malocclusion.
2. Discuss the different treatment modalities of class II div 2 malocclusion.
3. Management of class II malocclusion.

### Short Notes

1. Discuss about the retention followed by active mechanotherapy of class II malocclusion.

# CHAPTER 36
# Management of Class III Malocclusion

*Phulari BS*

Class III malocclusion is the least common type of malocclusion in many communities, accounting for approximately less than 5% of all cases. Highest incidence of class III malocclusion is observed among Japanese and Koreans. In class III malocclusion the mesiobuccal cusp of permanent maxillary first molar occludes interdentally between the mandibular first and second permanent molars, instead of occluding with mesiobuccal developmental groove of the permanent first molar. In this type of malocclusion, the mandibular incisors overlap the maxillary incisors instead of the other way around. This reverses the normal anteroposterior relationship of the incisors and sometimes called as "reverse overjet". In class III malocclusion, maxillary and mandibular canines do not exhibit any contact with each other.

## ETIOLOGICAL FACTORS

- Heredity
- Unilateral/bilateral hyperplasia of mandibular condyle
- Occlusal prematurities
- Enlarged adenoids
- Habitual forward positioning of the mandible predisposes to pseudo-class III malocclusion
- Premature loss of deciduous molars.

## CLASSIFICATION

**I. Class III Malocclusion can be Classified into the following Two Types Based on True or Habitual:**
1. True class III malocclusion
2. Pseudo-class III malocclusion (Habitual/postural class III malocclusion)

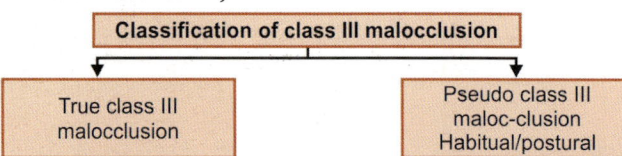

**II. Classification of Class III Malocclusion based on the Structural Components (Dental or Skeletal) Involved in the Malocclusion**
1. Dental class III malocclusion
2. Skeletal class III malocclusion

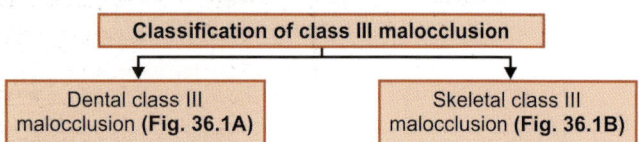

## CLINICAL FEATURES

Clinical features of Dental Class III malocclusion See **Tables 36.1** and **36.2**.

**Table 36.1:** Extraoral features of dental class III malocclusion

| Extraoral features | Findings | Figures |
|---|---|---|
| Lower facial height | Increased | Fig. 36.2A |
| Facial profile | Straight/concave | Fig. 36.2B |
| Facial divergence | Anterior facial | Fig. 36.2C |
| Lips | Divergence incompetent/potentially incompetent | |

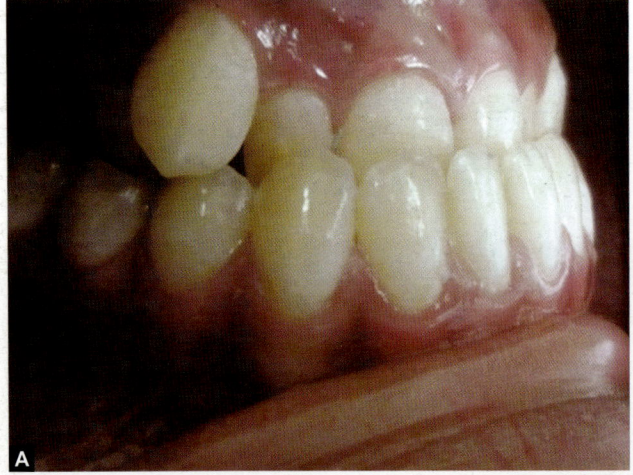
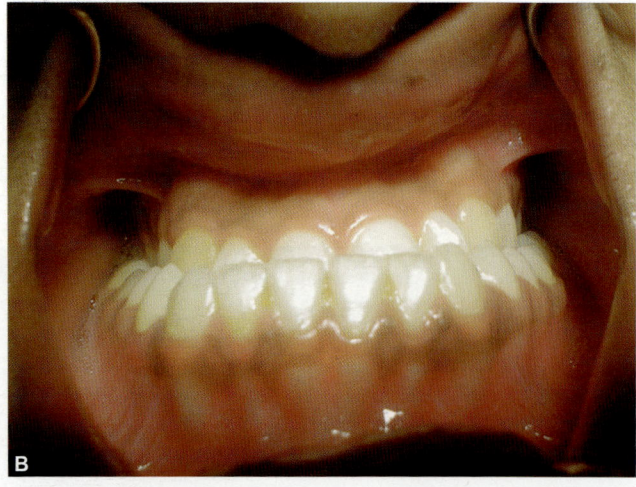

**Figs 36.1A and B:** Class III malocclusion: (A) Dental class III malocclusion; (B) Skeletal class III malocclusion

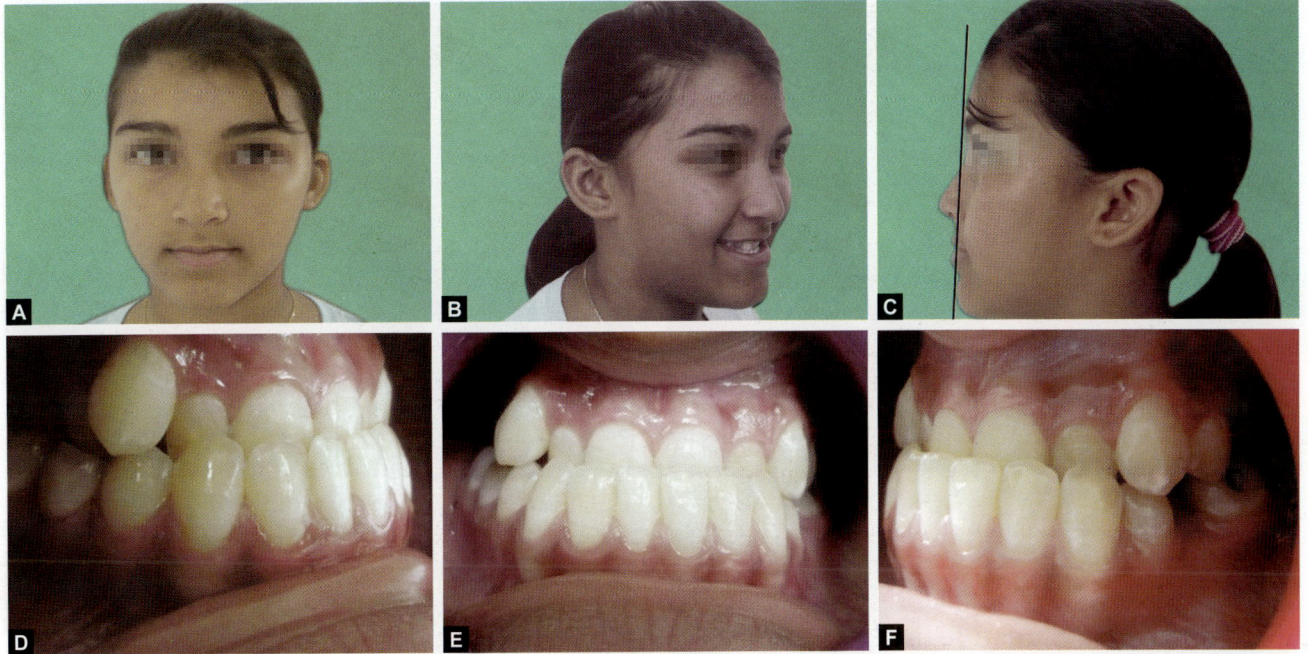

**Figs 36.2A to F:** Extraoral features of dental class III malocclusion: (A) Increased lower facial height; (B) Straight profile; (C) Anterior facial divergence; (D to F) Intraoral photographs

### Clinical Features of Skeletal Class III Malocclusion
See Tables 36.3 and 36.4.

### DIAGNOSIS OF ANGLE'S CLASS III MALOCCLUSION

Diagnosis of class III malocclusion should be aimed at evaluating whether the condition is dental or skeletal and true or pseudo-class III malocclusion. The diagnosis should be based on clinical examination and radiographic evaluation of skeletal growth pattern using lateral cephalogram.

**Table 36.2:** Intraoral features of dental class III malocclusion

| Intraoral features | Findings | Figures |
| --- | --- | --- |
| Incisor relationship relation with reverse overjet | Class III incisor | Fig. 36.3A |
| Canine relationship | Class III | Fig. 36.3B |
| Molar relationship | Class III | Fig. 36.3C |
| Transverse relationship of the arches | Posterior crossbite | Fig. 36.3D |

**Table 36.3:** Extra-oral features of skeletal class III malocclusion

| Extraoral features | Findings | Figures |
| --- | --- | --- |
| Facial profile | Concave | Fig. 36.4A |
| Facial form | Leptoprosopic | Fig. 36.4B |
| Facial divergence | Anterior facial divergence | Fig. 36.4C |
| Mandible | Prognathic | Fig. 36.4D |
| Lips | Competent lips | Fig. 36.4E |
| Mentolabial sulcus | Shallow | |
| Chin | Prominent | Fig. 36.4F |
| Lower facial height | Increased | Fig. 36.4D |

### TREATMENT OF CLASS III MALOCCLUSION

#### Treatment Objectives and Limitations

The main treatment objectives in Angle's class III malocclusion may include:
- Reduction of crowding
- Correction of the reverse overjet
- Correction of incisor overbite
- Correction of molar relationship.

#### Reduction of Crowding
Reduction of crowding may be done by using removable or fixed appliance or with or without extraction of teeth.

#### Correction of Reverse Overjet
Reverse overjet can be corrected by moving the maxillary incisors anteriorly and mandibular incisors posteriorly.

**Table 36.4:** Intraoral features of skeletal class III malocclusion (Figs 36.5 and 36.6)

| Intraoral features | Findings | Figures |
| --- | --- | --- |
| Incisor relationship | Class III | Fig. 36.5A |
| Canine relationship | Class III | Fig. 36.5B |
| Molar relationship | Class III | Fig. 36.5C |
| Transverse relationship of the arches | Posterior crossbite | Fig. 36.5C |
| Mandible | Prognathic | Fig. 36.6A |
| Maxilla | Retrognathic | Fig. 36.6B |
| Combined maxilla and mandible | Prognathic mandible and retrognathic maxilla | Fig. 36.6C |

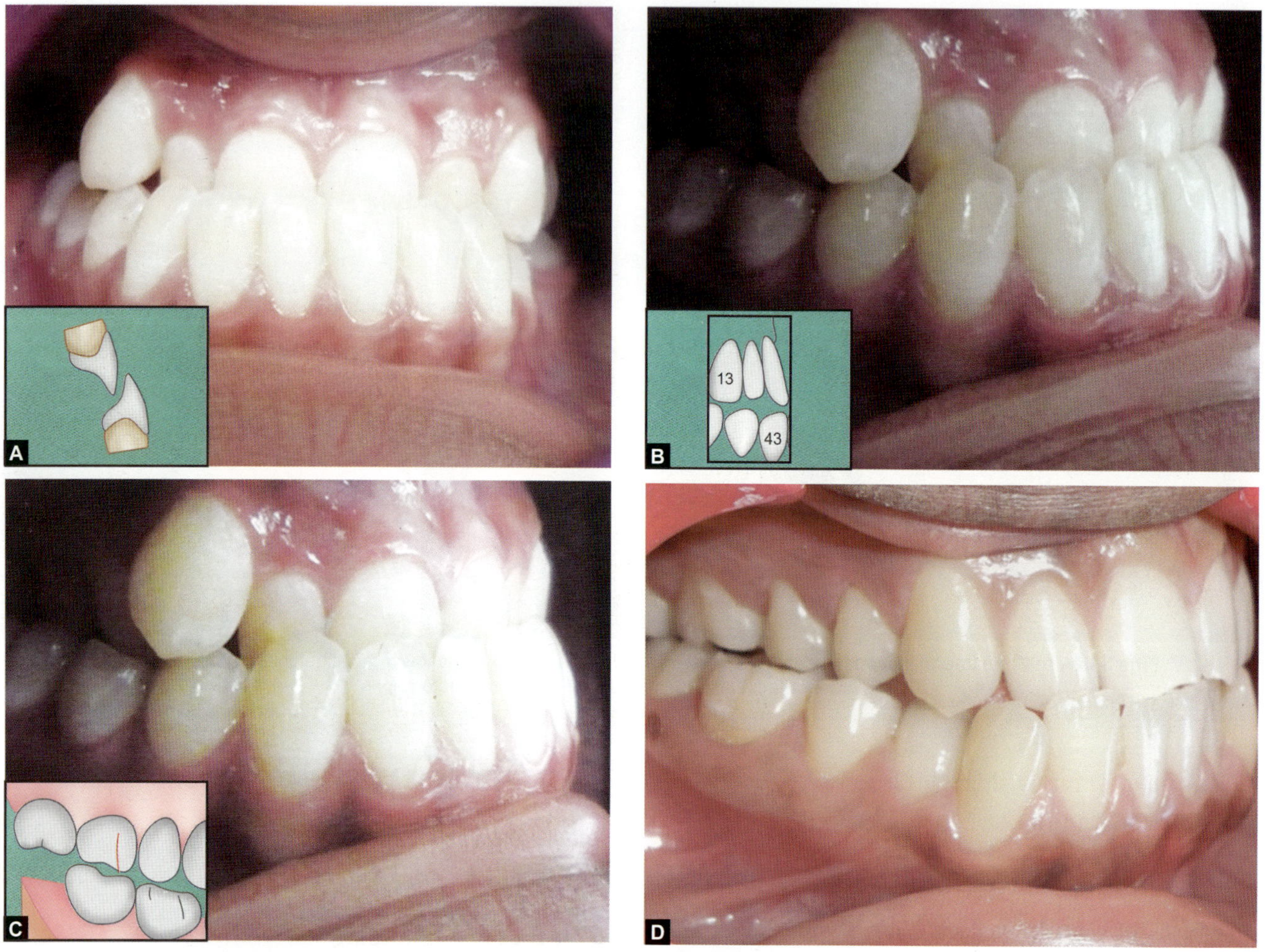

**Figs 36.3A to D:** Intraoral features of dental class III malocclusion: (A) Incisor relationship; (B) Canine relationship; (C) Molar relationship; (D) Posterior crossbite

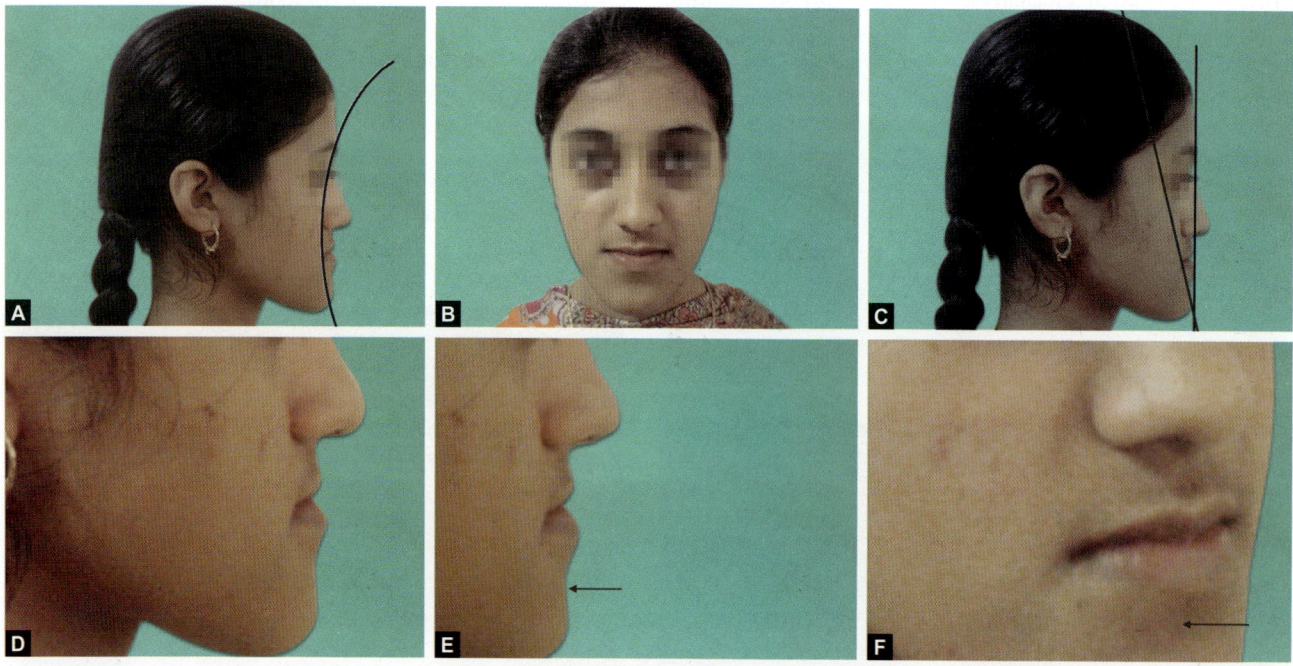

**Figs 36.4A to F:** Extraoral features of skeletal class III malocclusion: (A) Concave facial profile; (B) Leptoprosopic facial form; (C) Anterior facial divergence; (D) Prognathic mandible and increased lower facial height; (E) Shallow mentolabial sulcus; (F) Prominent chin

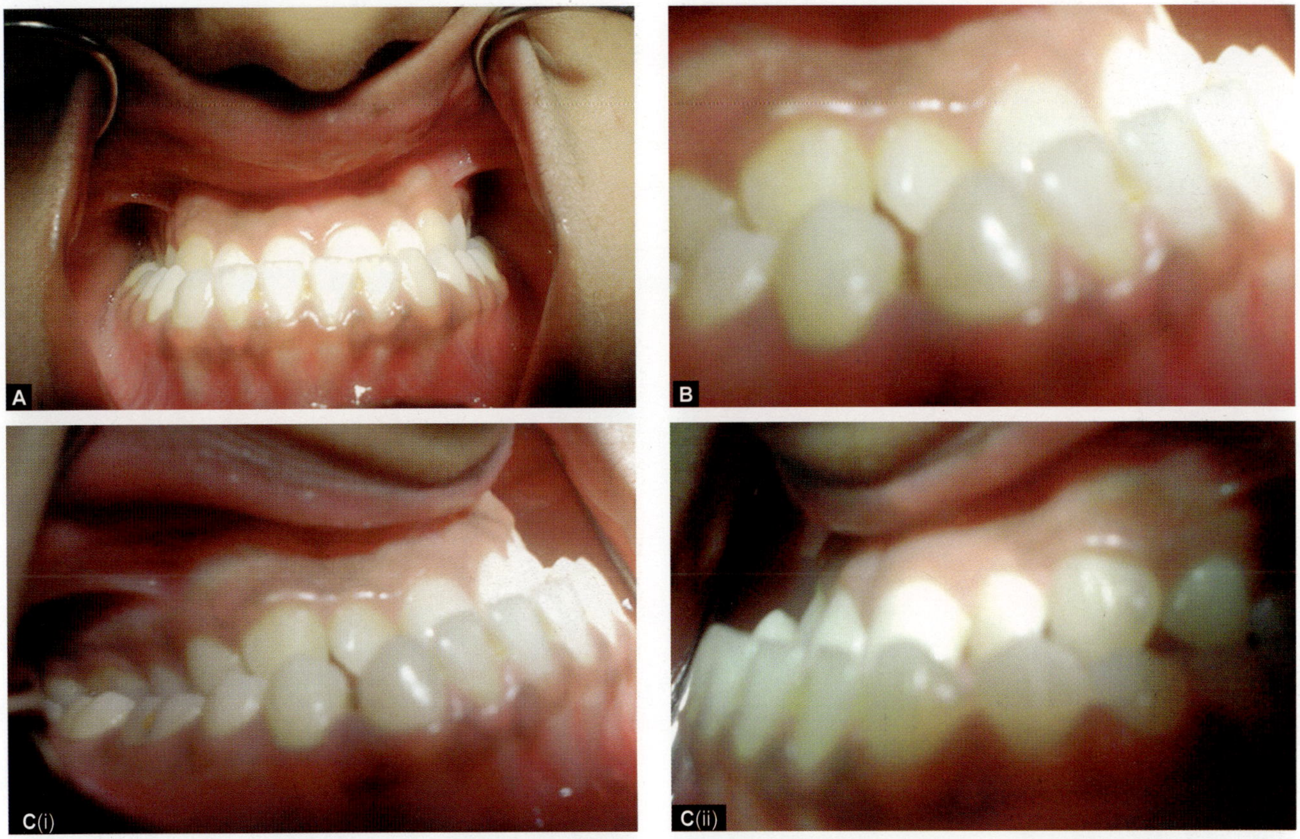

**Figs 36.5A to C:** Intraoral features of skeletal class III malocclusion: (A) Anterior crossbite and class III incisor relationship; (B) Class III canine relationship; (C i and ii) Class III molar relationship

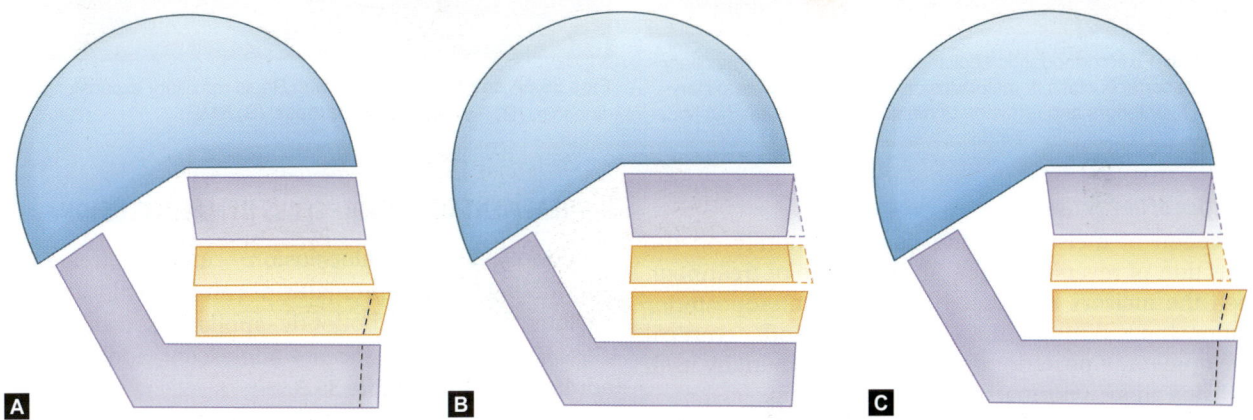

**Figs 36.6A to C:** (A) Prognathic mandible; (B) Retrognathic maxilla; (C) Prognathic mandible and retrognathic maxilla

| Table 36.5: Appliances used to treat class III malocclusion | | | | | |
|---|---|---|---|---|---|
| **Stage** | **Surgery** | **Removable orthodontic appliances** | **Myofunctional orthodontic appliances** | **Fixed orthodontic appliances** | **Orthopedic orthodontic appliances** |
| Pre-adolescent | — | 3D screw expansion appliance | a. Frankel III appliance **(Fig. 36.7)**<br>b. Reverse activator | Fixed orthodontic appliance | a. Chin cup<br>b. Anterior face mask with RME **(Figs 36.8A and B)** |
| Adolescent | — | 3D screw expansion appliance | a. Frankel III appliance<br>b. Reverse activator<br>c. Class III bionator | Fixed orthodontic appliance with class III intermaxillary elastics **(Fig. 36.9)**<br>Dental camouflage using fixed mechanotherapy | a. Chin cup<br>b. Anterior face mask<br>c. High pull headgear |
| Adult | Orthognathic surgery | — | — | Fixed orthodontic appliance for dental correction | — |

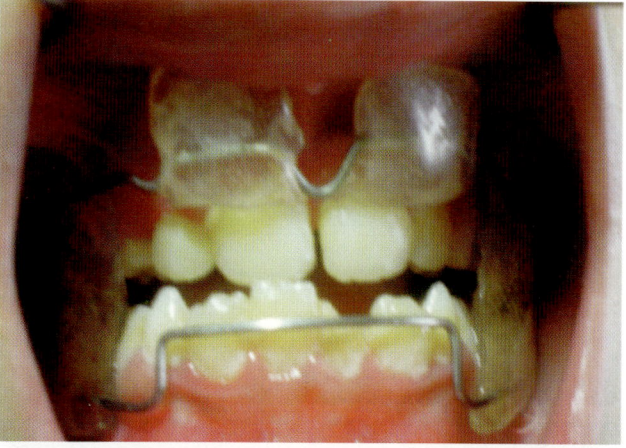

**Fig. 36.7:** Frankel III appliance photo change

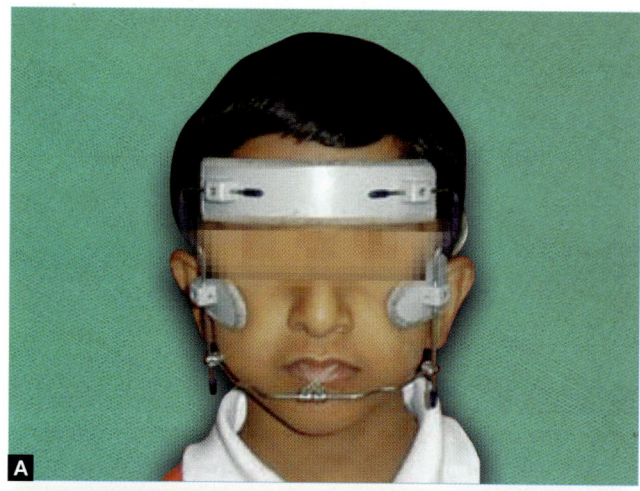

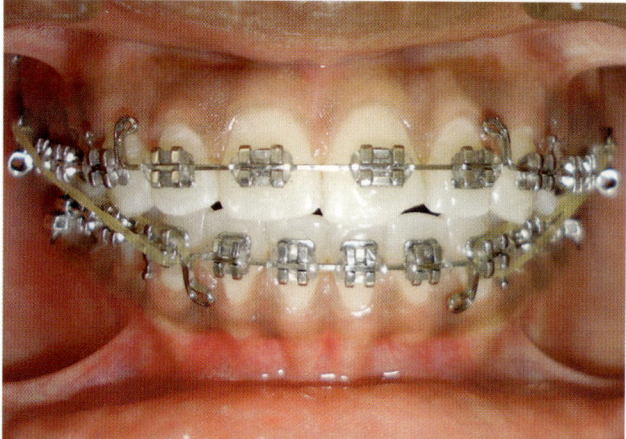

**Fig. 36.9:** Fixed orthodontic appliance with class III intermaxillary elastics corrects class III malocclusion by protrusion of maxillary anteriors and retrusion of mandibular anteriors

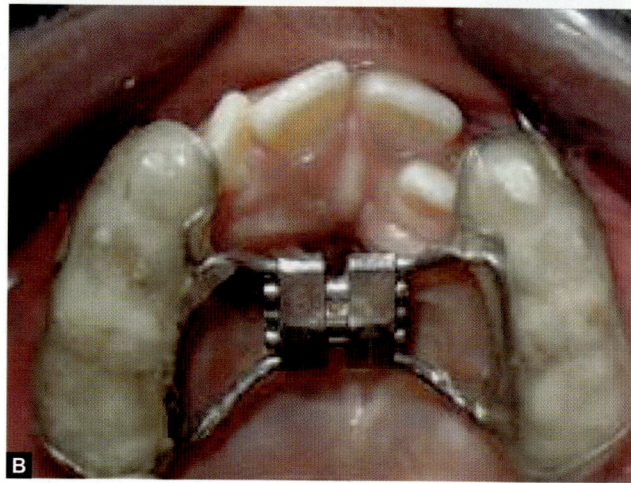

**Figs 36.8A and B:** Face mask with Rapid maxillary expansion (RME): (A) Face mask; (B) RME

### Correction of Incisor Overbite

Correction of incisor overbite depends entirely on the correction of reverse overjet. In the course of treatment, when the incisors are placed in correct anteroposterior relationship during the growth period, vertical development of posterior dentoalveolar segment by itself will bring about a normal overbite relationship.

*Correction of anterior open bite:* Correction of anterior open bite is much more difficult and is limited by the size and function of the tongue and the vertical dimension of the face. A minor degree of anterior open bite may be corrected by producing vertical movement of upper and lower incisors but with any major discrepancy, orthodontic treatment may not be sufficient to overcome the limiting factors.

### Correction of Molar Relationship or Posterior Segment Relationship

Maxillary teeth are moved forward with backward movement of mandibular teeth will bring about correction of molar relationship.

## TREATMENT OF PSEUDO-CLASS III MALOCCLUSION

Pseudo-class III malocclusion can be treated by eliminating occlusal prematurities and other local factors. Various types of orthodontic appliances used to treat class III malocclusions in pre-adolescent, adolescent and adults are given in **Table 36.5**.

## TREATMENT OF ANTERIOR CROSSBITE

Anterior crossbite in class III malocclusion can be treated by using lower anterior inclined planes or removable orthodontic appliance incorporating expansion screw designed for anterior expansion.

## TREATMENT OF POSTERIOR CROSSBITE

Posterior crossbite in class III malocclusion can be treated by rapid maxillary expansion.

## TREATMENT OF SKELETAL CLASS III MALOCCLUSION

Severe class III malocclusions after the cessation of growth are treated by surgical and corrective orthodontic procedures.
- Treatment of skeletal class III malocclusion ( maxillary retrognathism with mandibular prognathism):
- Skeletal class III malocclusion due to maxillary retrognathism and mandibular prognathism can be treated by maxillary advancement procedures such as Le Fort I osteotomy.
- Treatment of skeletal class III malocclusion (severe mandibular prognathism):
  Skeletal class III malocclusion due to severe mandibular prognathism can be treated by surgical procedures such as mandibular setback procedure.

## BIBLIOGRAPHY

1. Fränkel R. Maxillary retrusion in class III and treatment with the function corrector III. Trans Euro Orthod Soc. 1970;249-59.
2. Graber TM. Orthodontics: Principles and Practice. WB Saunders, 1998.
3. Graber TM, Vanarsdall RL. Orthodontics, Current Principles and Techniques. Mosby Year Book, Inc, 1994.
4. McNamara JA. An orthopedic approach to the treatment of class III malocclusion in young patients. J Clin Orthod. 1987;22:598-608.
5. Tollaro, Baccetti, Franchi. Early functional treatment of class III malocclusion. Am J Orthod. 1995;525-32.

### EXAM-ORIENTED QUESTIONS

*Long Questions*

1. Discuss different treatment modalities for class III malocclusion.
2. Appliance used to treat class III malocclusion.
3. Angle's class III malocclusion and write down etiological factors of class III malocclusion.

# Management of Midline Diastema

*Modley D, Phulari BS*

CHAPTER 37

Midline diastema is a common esthetic problem in mixed and early permanent dentitions. The diastema can occur either as a transient malocclusion during developmental years (ugly duckling stage), hereditary/racial feature or may occur due to pathological (abnormal labial frenum attachment) or iatrogenic factors (rapid maxillary expansion). Apart from orthodontic tooth movement, midline diastema can also be treated by conservative approach or prosthesis in suitable cases. Midline diastema is often easy to treat, but difficult to retain.

## DEFINITION

Spacing between two permanent maxillary central incisors in the midline is referred to as "midline diastema" **(Fig. 37.1)**.

## ETIOLOGICAL FACTORS

- Racial predisposition
- Hereditary factors
- Transient malocclusion
- Arch length: Tooth material discrepancy
  - Microdontia (peg laterals)
  - Congenitally missing teeth, especially maxillary laterals
  - Mesiodens.
- Abnormal frenum attachment
- Habits
  - Thumb-sucking habit
  - Tongue-thrusting habit
  - Mouth-breathing habit
- Midline pathologies
  - Cystic lesions
  - Midline tumors
  - Odontomas
- Iatrogenic.

### Hereditary

Midline diastema is often seen to be transferred from parents to offsprings although it is not a rule **(Figs 37.2A and B)**.

### Racial Predisposition

Highest incidence of midline diastema is seen in Negroid race groups **(Fig. 37.3)**.

### Transient Malocclusion

Midline diastema, seen in the ugly duckling stage **(Fig. 37.4)**, is transient, self-correcting one, as the eruption of canines will automatically correct the midline diastema.

### Arch Length–Tooth Material Discrepancy

An excess of arch length compared to tooth material due to conditions such as missing lateral incisors, macrognathia, microdontia **(Fig. 37.5)** can result in midline diastema.

### Abnormal Frenum Attachment

Abnormal labial frenum attachment is one of the most common causes of midline diastema. Presence of a thick fibrous labial frenum prevents approximation of maxillary

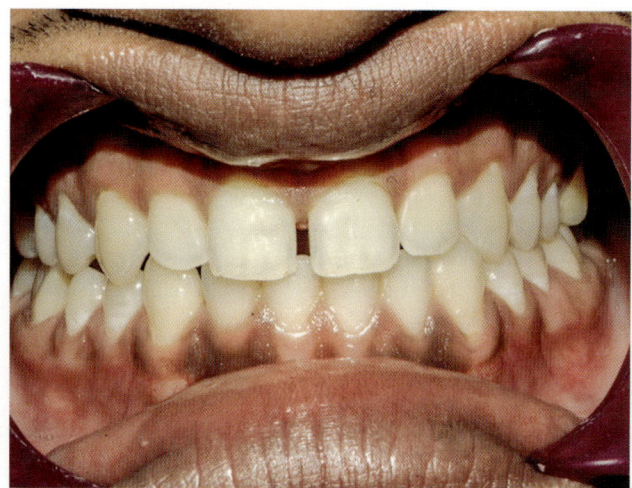

**Fig. 37.1:** Midline diastema is spacing between two permanent maxillary central incisors in the midline

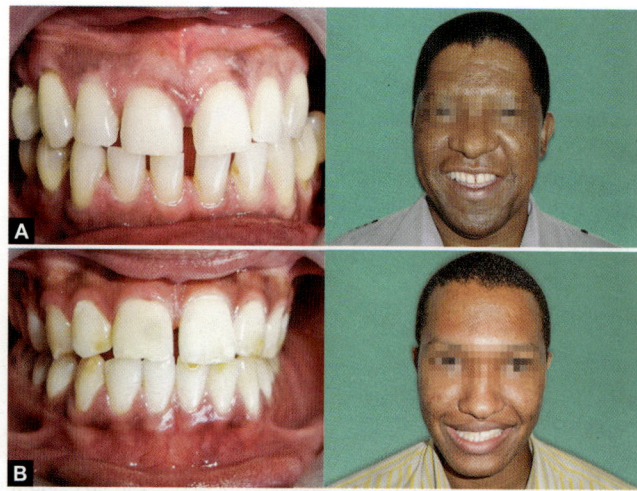

**Figs 37.2A and B:** Midline diastema of hereditary origin. (A) Midline diastema in father. (B) Midline diastema seen in his son

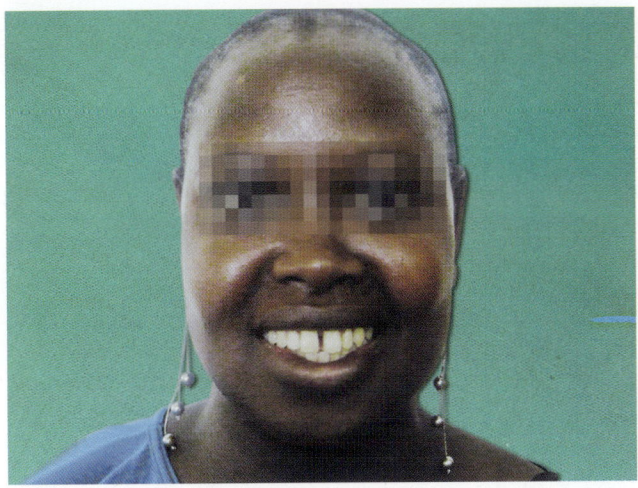

Fig. 37.3: Midline diastema is fairly common in Negroid race group

central incisors and thus can lead to spacing between these two teeth **(Fig. 37.6)**.

### Abnormal Oral Habits

Abnormal pressure habits, such as thumb-sucking habit **(Fig. 37.7)**, tongue-thrusting habit and mouth-breathing habit, may predispose to the occurrence of midline diastema.

### Midline Pathologies

Soft tissue and hard tissue pathologies of maxillary jaw in the midline such as cystic lesions, tumors and odontomes, may lead to midline diastema. Impacted or erupted mesiodens can also cause midline diastema **(Fig. 37.8A)**.

### Iatrogenic

Rapid maxillary expansion, when employed as a method of gaining space, may lead to midline diastema **(Fig. 37.8B)**. The removable/fixed expansion appliances cause a fan-shaped splitting of the mid-palatine suture causing separation of central incisors.

Therapeutic extraction of mesiodens can also lead to midline diastema.

## CLINICAL FEATURES

Clinical features of midline diastema are as follows:
(a) There is spacing between maxillary central incisors.
(b) Localized papillary gingivitis in relation to permanent central incisors may occur.
(c) Esthetics is affected as midline diastema becomes evident during conversation and smiling.
(d) There is hampered phonation and saliva may escape during speech.

## DIAGNOSIS

Diagnosis of midline diastema should be followed with a thorough assessment of its etiology using proper history, clinical examination (Blanch test) and radiographic evaluation **(Table 37.1)**.

### Blanch Test

*Steps*
1. Upper lip is pulled upward and forward
2. Observe for blanching of the tissue in the incisive papilla region on palatal side of the permanent maxillary central incisors **(Fig. 37.9)**.

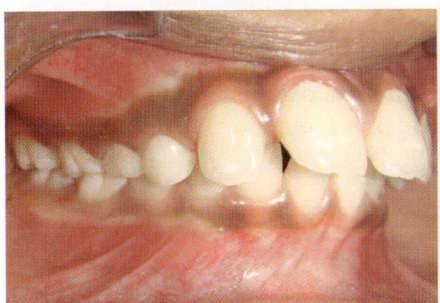 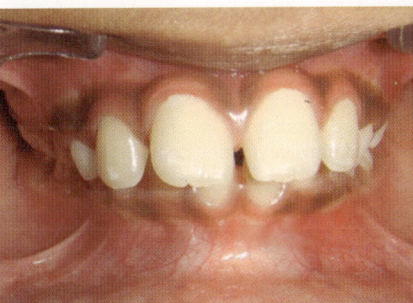 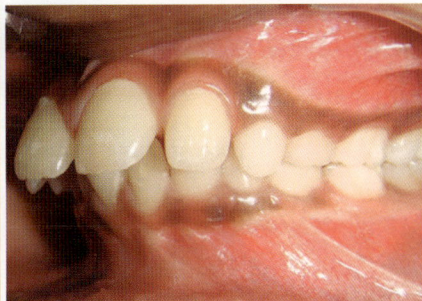

Fig. 37.4: Ugly duckling stage. Transient midline diastema as a result of erupting canines

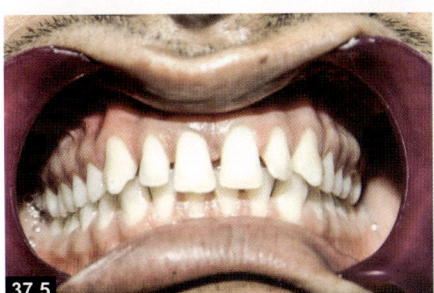 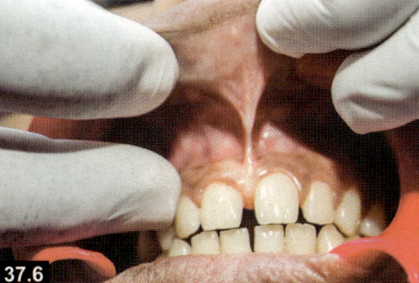 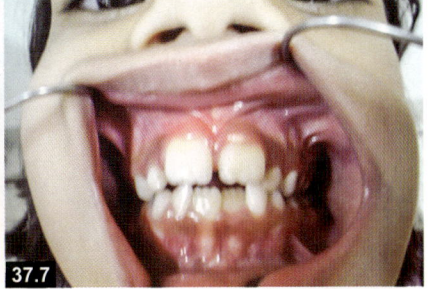

**Fig. 37.5:** Microdontic teeth causing midline diastema along with spacing between other anterior teeth; **Fig. 37.6:** Midline diastema due to thick fibrous abnormal maxillary labial frenum, which prevents approximation of the central incisors;
**Fig. 37.7:** Thumb-sucking habit causing midline diastema

| Table 37.1: Diagnosis of midline diastema | | |
|---|---|---|
| **History and clinical examination** | **Radiographic examination** | **Blanch test (For diagnosing abnormal labial frenum attachment)** |
| Familial History<br>Trauma<br>Evaluation of etiological factors such as:<br>• Supernumerary<br>• Peg lateral<br>• Missing tooth<br>• Abnormal labial frenum attachment | • Radiographic evaluation of midline pathologies such as cysts, tumors and odontomas.<br>• Radiographic evaluation of high labial frenum attachment shows notch-like radiolucent area in the interdental region between two permanent maxillary central incisors in the midline (Fig. 37.9). | Steps:<br>• Upper lip is pulled upward and forward.<br>• Observe for blanching of the tissue in the incisive papilla region on palatal side of the permanent maxillary central incisors (Fig. 37.10).<br>**Blanch present–Blanch test positive**<br>Presence of thick and fleshy frenum<br>**Blanch absent–Blanch test negative**<br>Absence of thick and fleshy frenum |

### Blanching Present–Blanch Test Positive
Presence of thick and fleshy frenum

### Blanching Abscent–Blanch Test Negative
Absence of thick and fleshy frenum

### Radiographic Examination
Radiographic evaluation of midline pathologies such as cysts, tumors and odontomas.

Radiographic evaluation of high labial frenum attachment shows notch-like radiolucent area in the interdentally region between two permanent maxillary central incisors (**Fig. 37.10**).

## TREATMENT

**Treatment of Midline Diastema by Removable Orthodontic Appliances (Flowchart 37.1 and Table 37.2)**

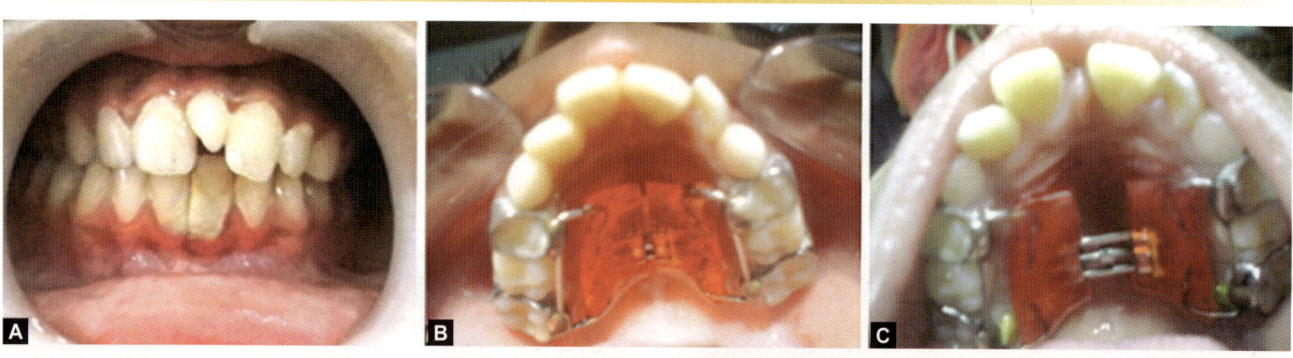

**Figs 37.8A and B:** (A) Erupted mesiodens causing midline diastema. (B) Midline diastema seen in a patient undergoing rapid maxillary expansion, (Bi) Before expansion, (B ii) After expansion

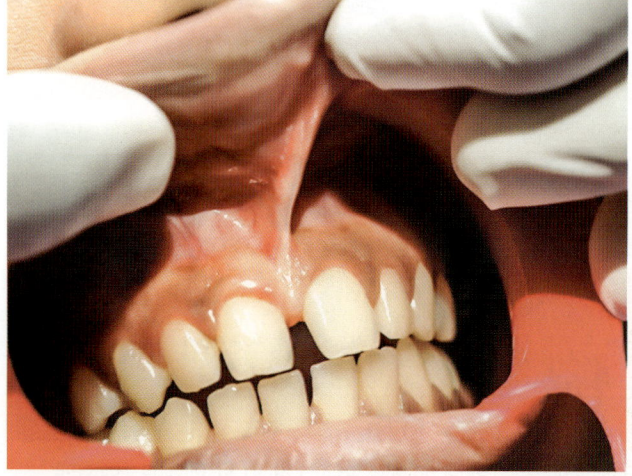

**Fig. 37.9:** Blanch test

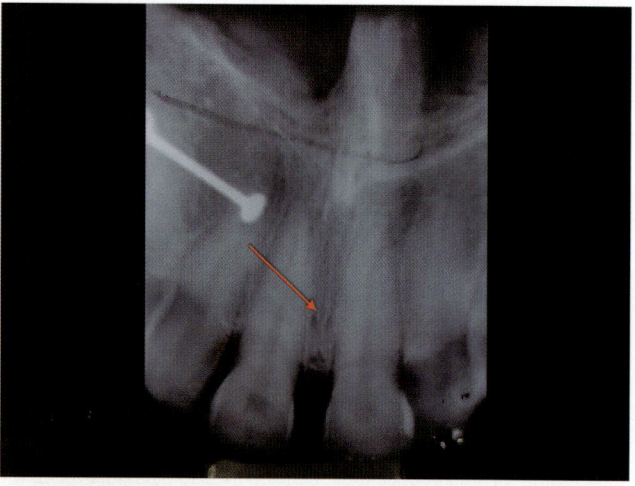

**Fig. 37.10:** Intraoral periapical radiograph showing notch-like radiolucent area in the midline

**Table 37.2:** Removal of etiological factors causing midline diastema using various orthodontic appliances

| Removal of etiological factors causing midline diastema | Treatment of midline diastema using orthodontic appliances |
|---|---|
| A. Habits | |
|    1. Thumb-sucking habit | Habit-breaking appliances<br>• Habit-breaking appliances with crib<br>• Habit-breaking appliances with rake<br>• Removable or fixed habit-breaking appliances |
|    2. Tongue-thrusting habit | • Removable or fixed tongue rake<br>• Double oral screen |
|    3. Mouth-breathing | Oral screen |
| B. Abnormal labial frenum attachment | Frenectomy followed by removable or fixed orthodontic treatment |
| C. Supernumerary tooth | Extraction of supernumerary tooth followed by removable or fixed orthodontic treatment to close the diastema |
| D. Congenital missing tooth | • Implant-orthodontic mechanotherapy may be required for space redistribution before the placement of the implant<br>• Crown/bridge |

**Flowchart 37.1:** Treatment of midline diastema

- Removable orthodontic appliance with finger springs on both maxillary central incisors can be used to close midline diastema **(Fig. 37.11)**.
- Activation of finger spring is done by opening its helix and bending the active arm by 2–3 mm towards the tooth to be moved. Activated finger spring moves the central incisors towards midline thereby closing midline diastema.

***Disadvantage:*** A disadvantage of this method, however, is that there may be a space created between central and lateral permanent incisors.

### Removable Orthodontic Appliance with Modified Split Labial Bow

Removable orthodontic appliance with modified split labial bow can also be used to close midline diastema **(Fig. 37.12)**. Compression of U loops of modified split labial bow brings about mesial movement of both the central incisors, thereby closes the midline diastema similar to finger springs. However, this appliance may also create space distal to central incisors.

## Treatment of Midline Diastema by Fixed Orthodontic Appliances

### Fixed Orthodontic Appliance with Closed Coil Spring

Fixed orthodontic appliance with closed coil spring placed between the brackets of left and right permanent central incisors bring about closure of midline diastema **(Fig. 37.13)**.

### Fixed Orthodontic Appliance with E-chain

Fixed orthodontic appliance with E-chain placed on the brackets of all teeth (right first molar to left first molar) can effectively close the midline diastema **(Fig. 37.14)**.

### Fixed Orthodontic Appliance with Elastic Thread

An elastic thread wrapped around the brackets of left and right maxillary permanent central incisors in the fashion of figures of eight can affect the closure of midline diastema **(Fig. 37.15)**.

### Fixed Orthodontic Appliance with M Spring

M spring consists of three helices. Its free arms are engaged in the slots of brackets of the permanent central incisors and when activated by closing its three helices, a force is exerted, which results in closure of midline diastema **(Fig. 37.16)**.

## Treatment of Midline Diastema by Conservative Approach

A conservative approach can be opted for those patients who are unwilling for orthodontic treatment, when midline diastema is minimal up to 2 mm **(Figs 37.17A and B)**. Discoloration of the composite restoration over a period of time is a frequent problem associated with such a procedure.

## Treatment of Midline Diastema by Fixed Prosthesis

Selected cases of mild-to-moderate midline diastema can also be treated using fixed prosthesis like full ceramic

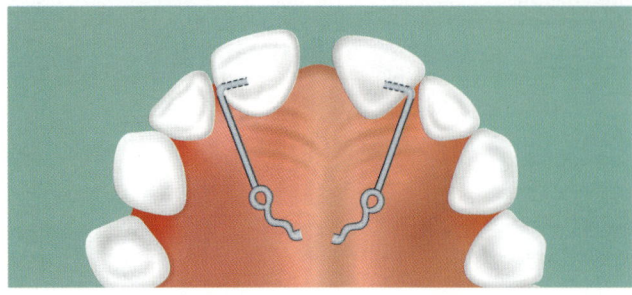

**Fig. 37.11:** Removable orthodontic appliance with finger springs on both maxillary central incisors can be used to treat midline diastema

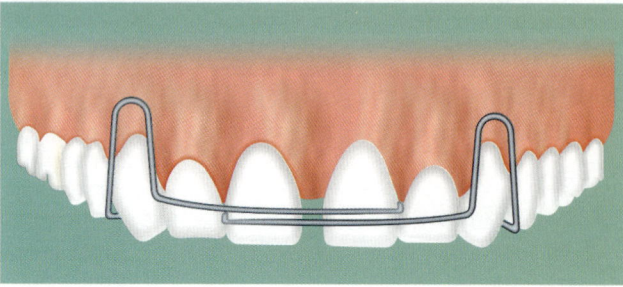

**Fig. 37.12:** Removable orthodontic appliance with modified split labial bow can also be used to close midline diastema

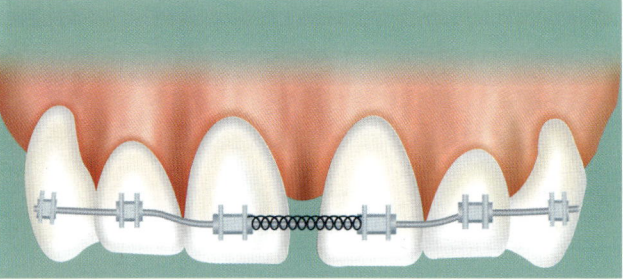

**Fig. 37.13:** Fixed orthodontic appliance with closed coil spring placed between the brackets of left and right permanent central incisors can be used to bring about closure of midline diastema

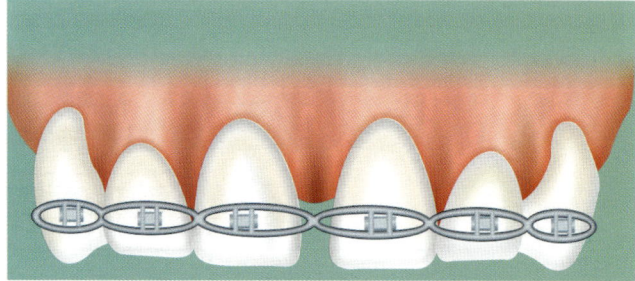

**Fig. 37.14:** Fixed orthodontic appliance with E-chain placed on brackets can be used to treat midline diastema

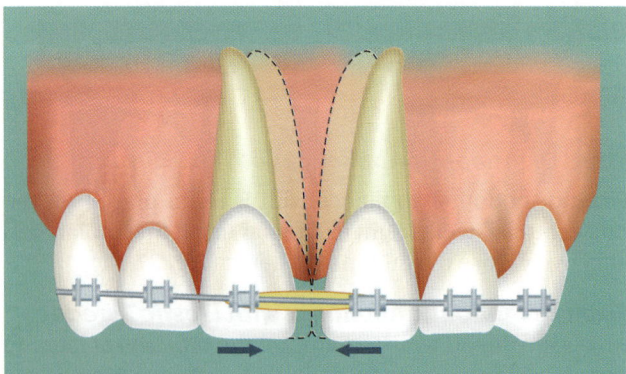

**Fig. 37.15:** An elastic thread wrapped around the brackets of central incisors to achieve closure of midline diastema

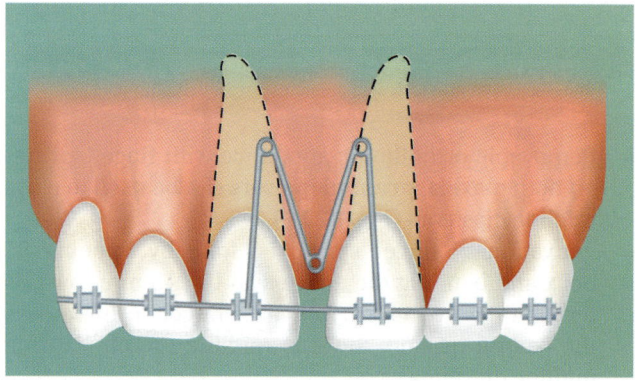

**Fig. 37.16:** Activating the free arms of the M spring engaged in the brackets slots to achieve closure of midline diastema

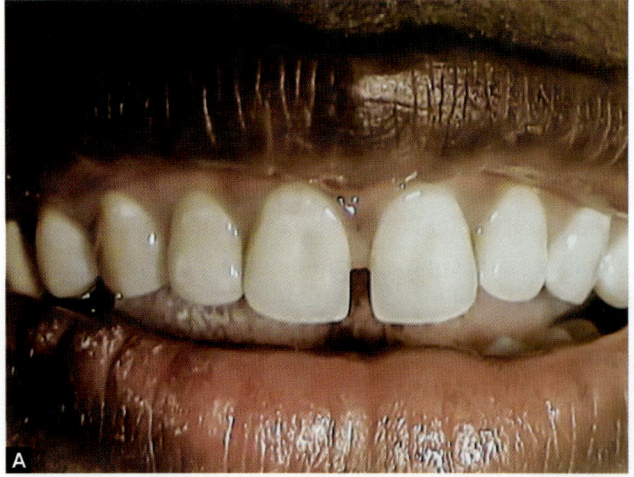
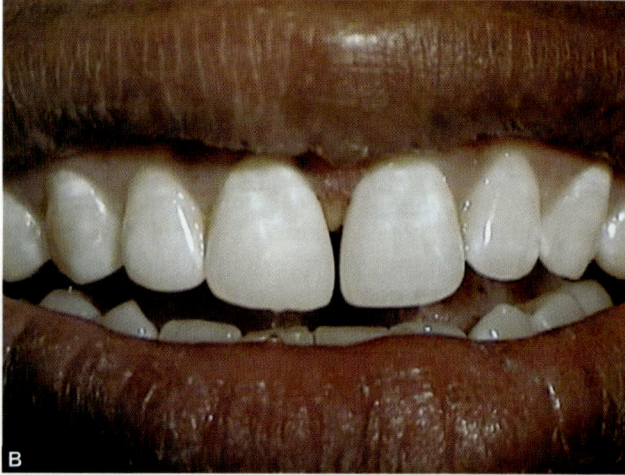

**Figs 37.17A and B:** Treatment of midline diastema by conservative approach using composite build-up: (A) Before composite restoration. (B) After composite restoration (*Courtesy:* Dr Anil Shah, Innovate Dental Clinic, Surat, India)

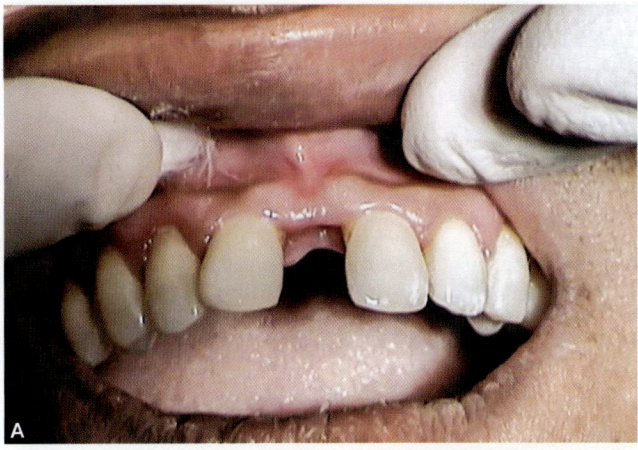
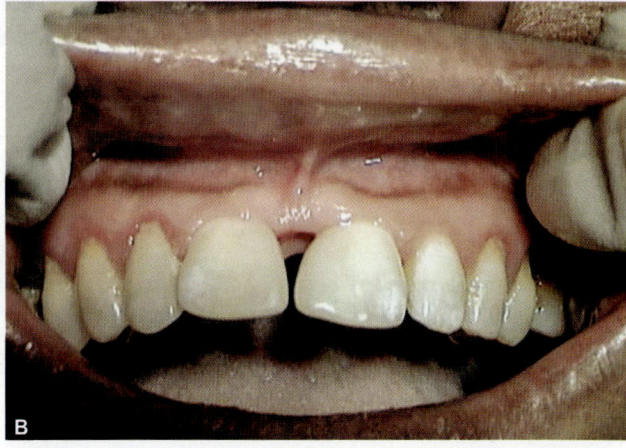

**Figs 37.18A and B:** Treatment of midline diastema by fixed prosthesis, like full ceramic crowns. (A) Before treatment. (B) After treatment
(*Courtesy:* Dr Anil Shah, Innovate Dental Clinic, Surat, India)

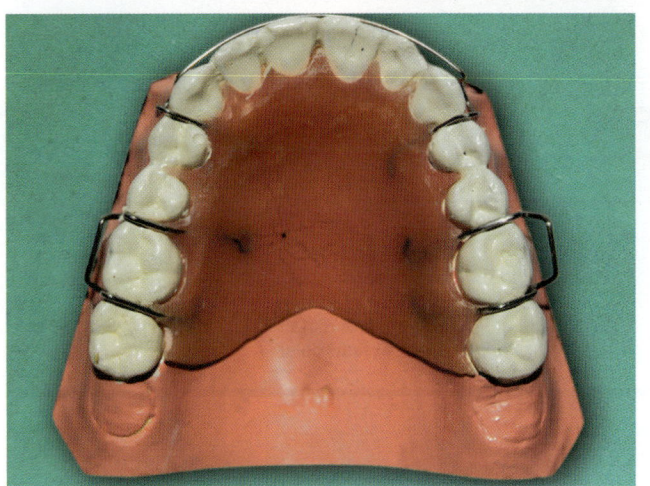

**Fig. 37.19:** Hawley's retainer (passive labial bow from canine to canine and Adam's clasps on first molars)

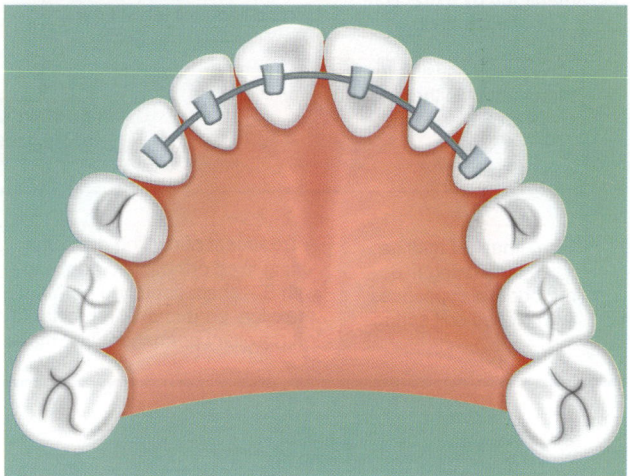

**Fig. 37.20:** Fixed bonded retainer from canine to canine

crowns on permanent maxillary central incisors, provided their periodontal support is favorable **(Figs 37.18A and B)**.

## RETENTION FOLLOWED BY THE TREATMENT

Although midline diastema is relatively easy to treat, it is difficult to retain the correction over a long period. Thus, a long-term retention program is usually followed by correction of midline diastema.

When conservative approach is used to correct midline diastema, composite build up of central incisors can be joined lingually in the midline to prevent opening of the diastema.

A removable simple Hawley's retainer **(Fig. 37.19)** or fixed bonded retainer from canine to canine **(Fig. 37.20)** on palatal side can be used as a retainer followed by the treatment of midline diastema to prevent opening of the diastema.

## BIBLIOGRAPHY

1. Graber TM. Orthodontics: Principles and Practice. WB Saunders, 1988.
2. Graber TM, Vanarsdall RL. Orthodontics, Current Principles and Techniques. Mosby Year Book Inc, 1994.
3. Profitt WR. Contemporary Orthodontics. St louis: CV Mosby, 1986.

### EXAM-ORIENTED QUESTIONS

*Long Notes or Long Questions*

1. Define midline diastema. Discuss in detail about etiology, clininical features, diagnosis and management of midline diastema.
2. Management of midline diastema.

*Short Notes*

1. Removal of etiological factors causing midline diastema using various orthodontic appliances.
2. Blanch test.
3. Retention followed by the treatment of midline diastema.

# CHAPTER OVERVIEW

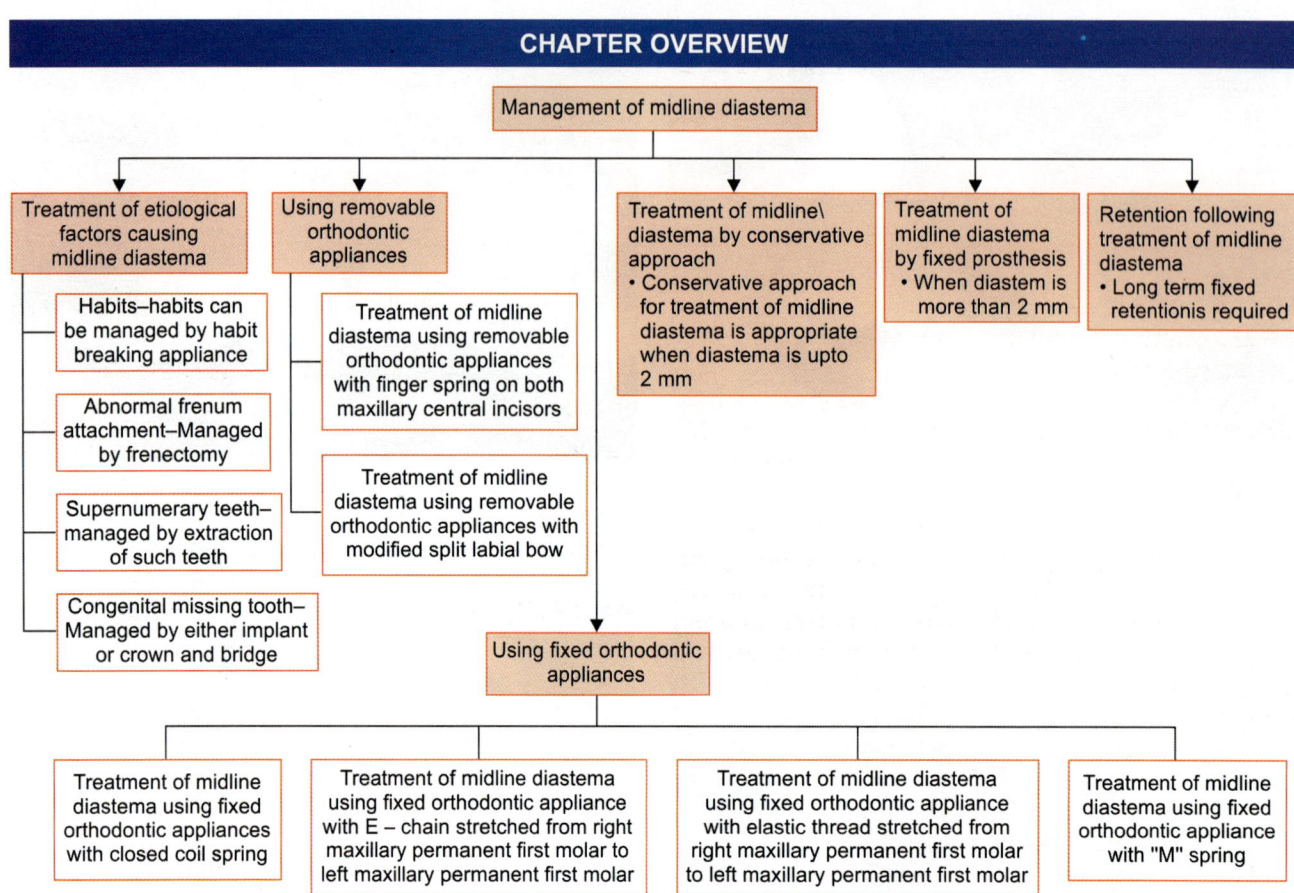

# CHAPTER 38

# Management of Open Bite

*Phulari BS*

Lack of vertical overlap between maxillary and mandibular teeth in centric occlusion is referred to as open bite. Open bite may be dental or skeletal in origin. It can occur in anterior or posterior segment of the dental arches and are called as anterior open bite and posterior open bite respectively. Posterior open bite may be unilateral or bilateral.

Anterior open bite is often caused by oral habits, such as thumb sucking/digit sucking, tongue thrusting and mouth breathing; while posterior open bite is usually caused by ankylosed/submerged posterior teeth or lateral tongue thrusting habit. Unfavourable growth patterns of the jaws may contribute to the development of skeletal open bite.

Anterior open bite is unesthetic and may pose difficulties during speech and swallowing. Posterior open bite may affect mastication depending on the severity.

Any abnormal oral habits causing open bite should be identified and eliminated and then followed with correction of open bite using fixed mechanotherapy. Correction of open bite involves extrusion of the maxillary and mandibular anterior and intrusion of maxillary and mandibular posterior teeth. In cases of skeletal open bite caused by unfavourable jaw-growth pattern, growth modification using functional appliances or surgical intervention may be required.

## CLASSIFICATION OF OPEN BITE MALOCCLUSIONS

- Based on dental or skeletal components
  - Dental
  - Skeletal
- Based on location
  - Anterior
  - Posterior
- Working classification of open bite (**Flowchart 38.1**)

## ANTERIOR OPEN BITE

The vertical overlap of permanent maxillary anteriors over the mandibular anterior in normal occlusion is referred to as "overbite," which is ideally about 2 mm. When there is no overlap of upper anterior over the lower anterior, such a condition is known as "Anterior open bite (**Fig. 38.1**)."

Anterior open bite may be of dental (**Fig. 38.2**) or skeletal (**Fig. 38.3**) origin and can be caused by a number of etiological factors.

### Etiological Factors of Anterior Open Bite

- Habits
  - *Thumb/Digit sucking habit*: Abnormal pressure habits like thumb/digit sucking cause forward placement of pre-maxilla, narrowing of the maxillary arch and proclination of maxillary anterior thereby disturbing the normal vertical relationship of anterior teeth.

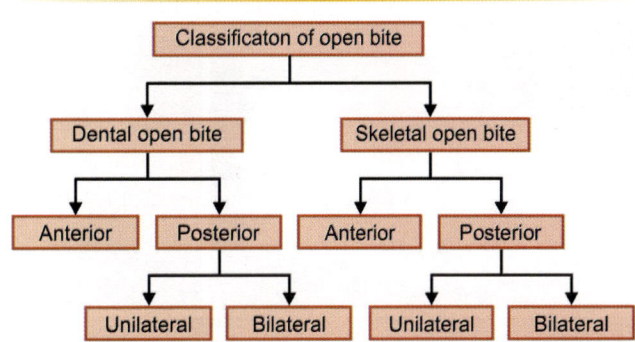

**Flowchart 38.1:** Classification of open bite

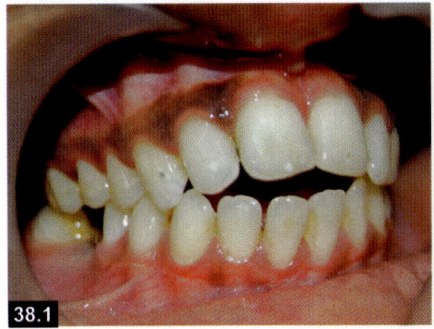
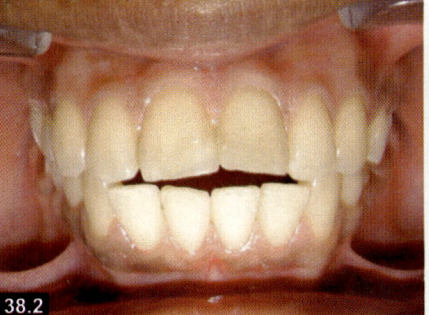
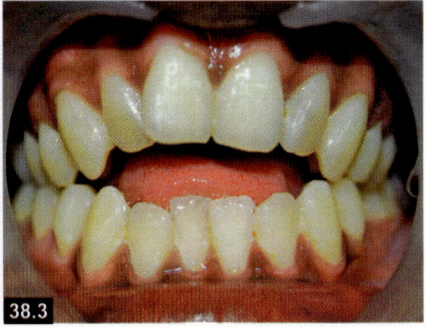

**Fig. 38.1:** Anterior open bite is the lack of vertical overlap between upper and lower anterior;
**Fig. 38.2:** Dental anterior open bite; **Fig. 38.3:** Skeletal anterior open bite

- *Anterior tongue thrusting habit*: Habitual tongue thrusting causes proclination and flaring of upper anterior, leading to anterior open bite.
- *Mouth breathing*: Mouth breathing habit due to any nasopharyngeal obstruction may also cause prognathic premaxilla, proclined upper anterior and thus anterior open bite.

■ Abnormally increased tongue size
  • Inherited
  • Acquired

Macroglossia caused due to hereditary or acquired factors may also lead to anterior open bite by exerting pressure on the lingual surfaces of upper anterior.

■ Abnormal growth pattern **(Figs 38.4A to D)**
Any abnormalities in the growth pattern of maxilla, mandible or both may lead to anterior open bite:

- Abnormal skeletal growth pattern of the maxilla: Counter-clockwise rotation of the maxilla.
- Abnormal skeletal growth pattern of the mandible: Clockwise rotation of the mandible.
- Abnormal skeletal growth pattern of both maxilla and mandible: Counter-clockwise rotation of the maxilla and clockwise rotation of the mandible.
- Vertical maxillary excess.

## Clinical Features of Dental Anterior Open Bite

Patients with dental anterior open bite may reveal the following features **(Fig. 38.5)**:

■ Open bite confined to anterior segment only.
■ Maxillary anterior proclination.
■ Proclination of mandibular anterior.
■ Spacing may be present in maxillary and/or mandibular

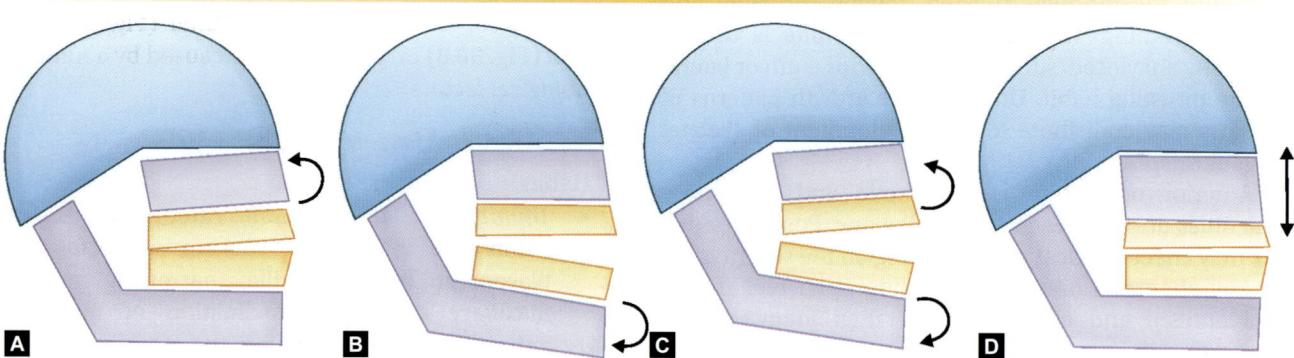

**Figs 38.4A to D:** Abnormal growth pattern causing open bite: (A) Skeletal anterior open bite due to counter-clockwise rotation of the maxilla. (B) Skeletal anterior open bite due to clockwise rotation of the mandible. (C) Skeletal anterior open bite due to counter–clockwise rotation of the maxilla and clockwise rotation of the mandible. (D) Skeletal open bite due to vertical maxillary excess

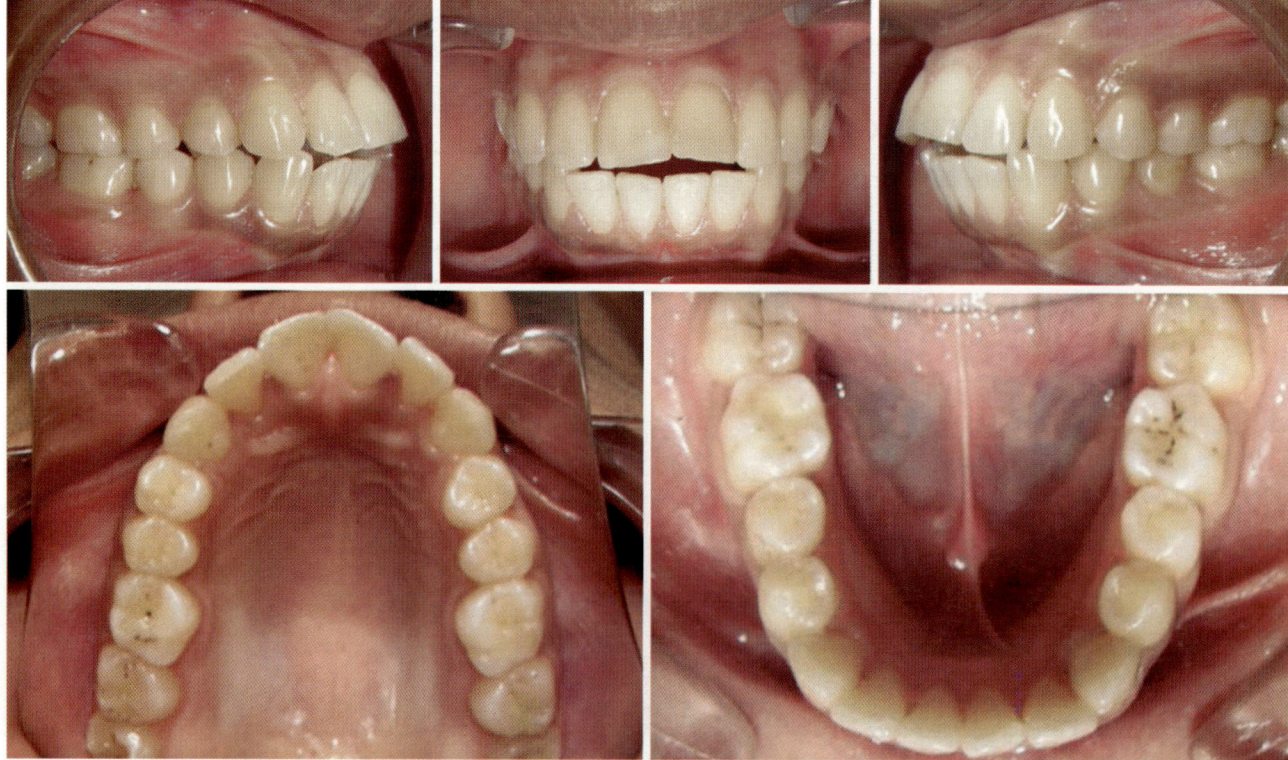

**Fig. 38.5:** Clinical features of dental anterior open bite

anterior segments.
- Narrow maxillary arch.
- Fish-mouth appearance may be present.

## Clinical Features of Skeletal Anterior Open Bite

### I. Extraoral Features of Skeletal Open Bite
- Lips
  - Incompetent lips
  - May show hyper tonicity
  - May be averted **(Fig. 38.6A)**
- Increased anterior facial height and decreased posterior facial height.
- Increased lower anterior facial height **(Fig. 38.6A)** and decreased upper anterior facial height **(Fig. 38.6B)**.
- A steep mandibular plane angle.
- Decreased nasolabial angle **(Fig. 38.6C)**.
- Shallow mentolabial sulcus **(Fig. 38.6D)**.
- Cephalometric examination may show
  - Clockwise rotation of mandible and/or anticlockwise rotation of maxilla, or
  - Vertical maxillary excess.
  - Steep anterior cranial base.

### II. Intraoral features of skeletal open bite
They are as listed below **(Figs 38.6E to G)**:
- Narrow maxillary arch
- Anterior or posterior open bite
- Excessive gingival display
- Decreased freeway space

## Diagnosis of Anterior Open Bites

Diagnosis of anterior open bite should include thorough clinical examination and radiographic evaluation to decide whether the condition is dental or skeletal in origin. Lateral cephalogram aids in assessing the skeletal growth pattern. An increased Frankfort mandibular plane angle (high angle case) indicates a vertical type of growth pattern **(Fig. 38.7)**. The diagnosis should also include detection of the etiological factors in a given case to make a suitable treatment plan.
- Intraoral photographs (right lateral, frontal and left lateral views) showing:
  - Open bite confined to anterior segment only.
  - Proclination of maxillary and mandibular anteriors
- Intraoral occlusal photographs showing:
  - Mild maxillary and mandibular anterior crowding
  - Constricted maxillary arch
A. Everted lower lip
B. Decreased upper anterior facial height
C. Decreased nasolabial angle
D. Shallow mentolabial sulcus
E. Anterior open bite
   i. Increased lower anterior facial height
F. Right lateral intra-oral view showing open bite
G. Left lateral intra-oral view showing open bite

## Treatment of Dental Anterior Open Bite

### Removal of the Cause (Table 38.1)

### Treatment of Anterior Open Bite using Fixed Orthodontic Appliance
Open bites are more difficult to treat and are more unpredictable in their prognosis than deep bites. Open bites are ideally treated by intrusion of posterior teeth, thereby permitting counter clockwise rotation of the mandible. Extrusion of anterior teeth represents a dental compensation and is achieved with box elastics or extrusion arch wire.

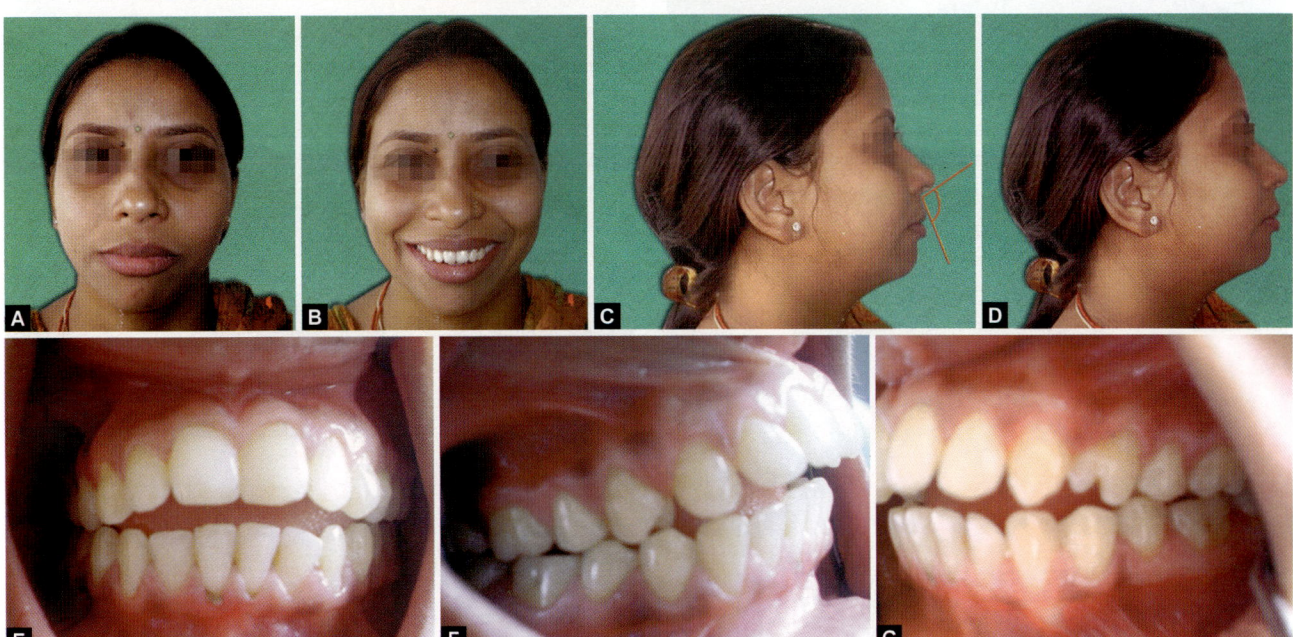

**Figs 38.6A to G:** Clinical features of skeletal anterior open bite

| Table 38.1: Treatment of dental anterior open bite | |
|---|---|
| **Etiological Factors** | **Treatment** |
| Habit | Habit breaking appliances **(Figs 38.8)** |
| a. Thumb/Digit sucking habit | |
| b. Anterior tongue thrusting habit **(Fig. 38.9)**. | |
| c. Mouth breathing. | |

| Table 38.2: Treatment of posterior open bite | |
|---|---|
| **Etiological factors** | **Treatment** |
| Lateral tongue thrusting habit | Lateral tongue spikes |

Mild to moderate dental anterior open bite can be successfully treated using fixed orthodontic appliance with box elastics. The elastic is stretched in the form of a box encircling all the four canine teeth **(Fig. 38.10)**. This causes extrusion of the anterior, thereby closing the anterior open bite. However, this method is not advisable in skeletal anterior open bite.

### Myofunctional Orthodontic Appliances

Skeletal anterior open bite can be successfully treated during growth period using Franckel IV or modified activator. Posterior bite blocks incorporated in these appliances cause intrusion of maxillary and mandibular posterior teeth thereby improving the anterior open bite.

### Orthopedic Appliance

A chin cup with vertical pull head cap can be used for treating skeletal anterior open bite, caused due to clockwise rotation of the mandible during mixed dentition period.

### Surgical Correction

Skeletal open bite in adults can be treated surgically after correction of the habit by Le Fort I ostectomy of the maxilla.

## POSTERIOR OPEN BITE

Posterior open bite is characterized by the lack of contact between the posteriors when the teeth are in centric occlusion **(Fig. 38.11)**. Posterior open bite can be unilateral or bilateral.

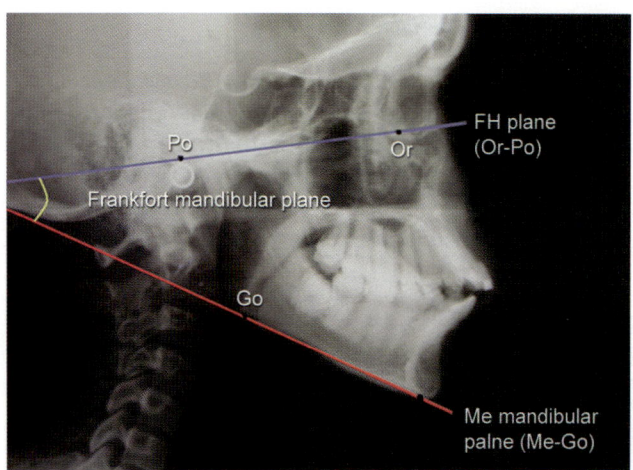

Fig. 38.7: Lateral cephalogram showing increased Frankfort mandibular plane angle indicating vertical growth pattern

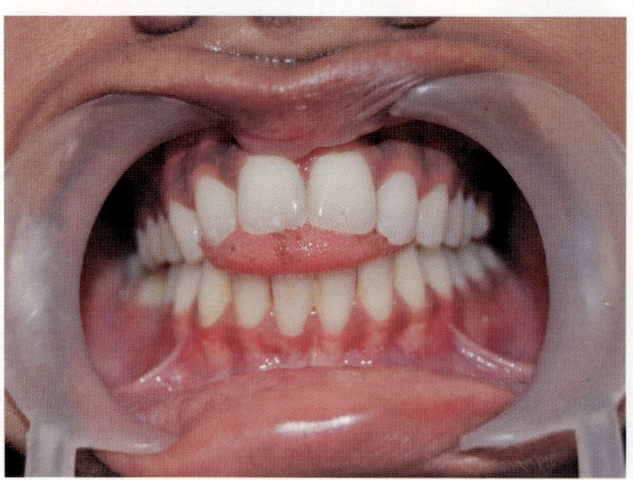

Fig. 38.9: Anterior tongue thrusting habit

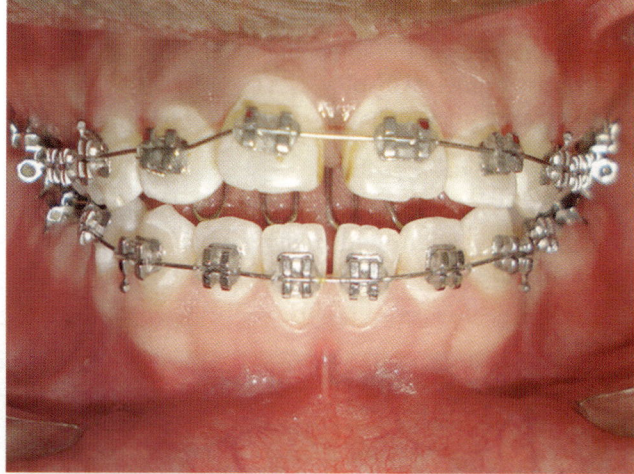

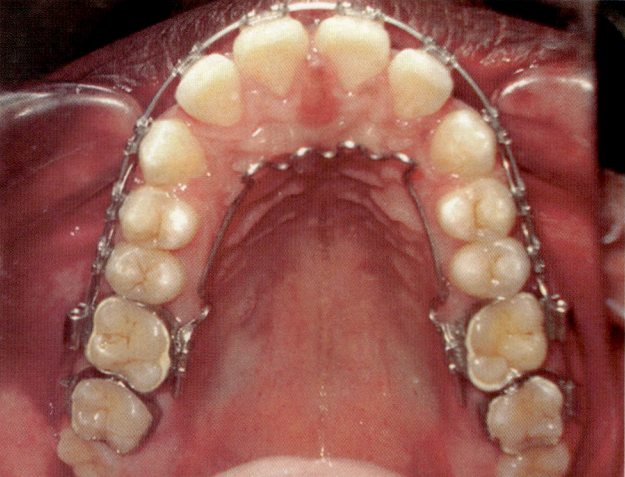

Fig. 38.8: Habit-breaking appliance with fixed orthodontic appliance (Fixed tongue crib) is used to eliminate tongue thrusting habit

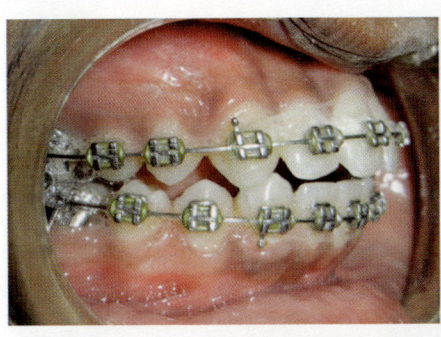 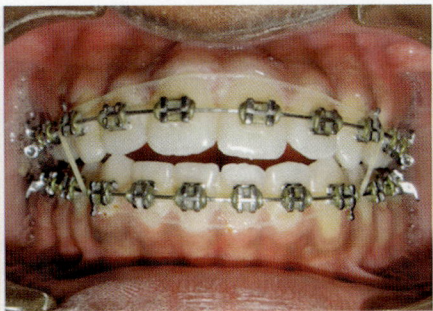 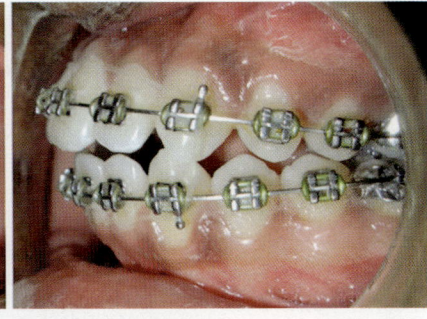

**Fig. 38.10:** Anterior open bite treated using box elastic with fixed orthodontic appliance

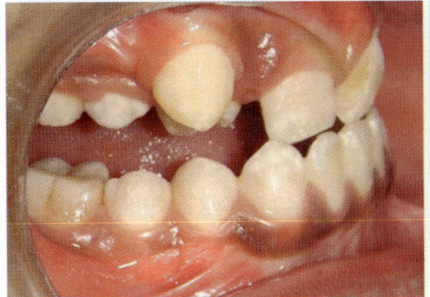 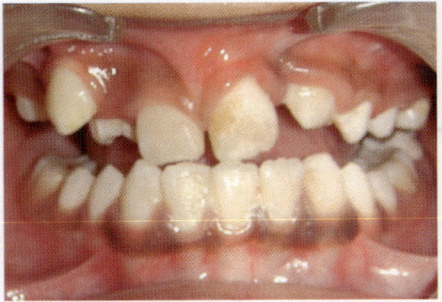 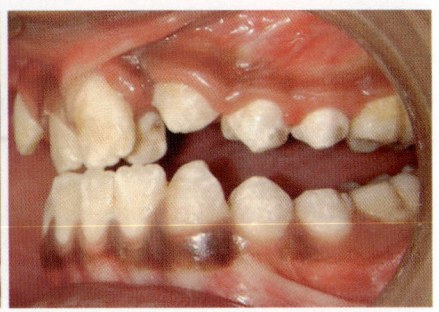

**Fig. 38.11:** Bilateral posterior open bite

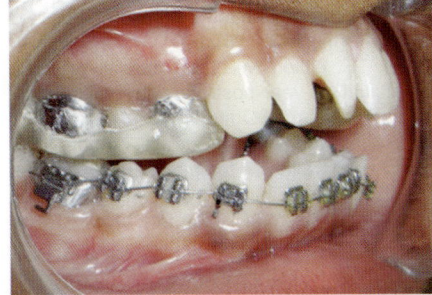 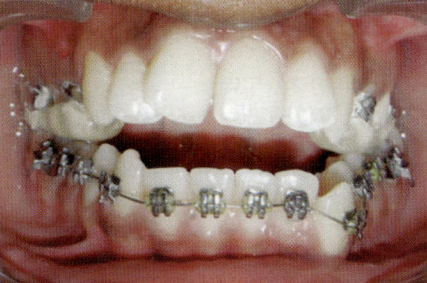 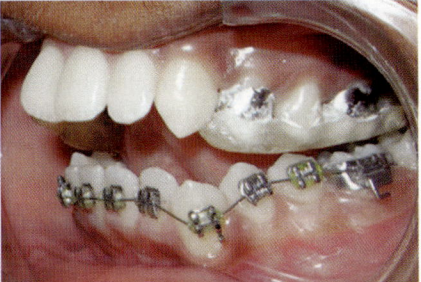

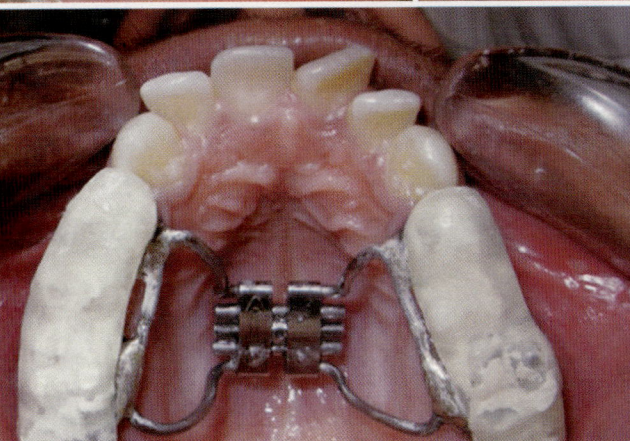 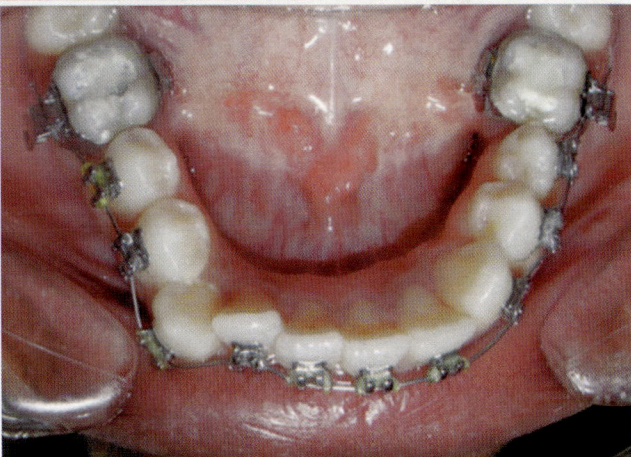

**Fig. 38.12:** Treatment of posterior open bite using fixed orthodontic appliance

1. *Unilateral posterior open bite*: Occurrence of posterior open bite on one side of the arch is referred as unilateral posterior open bite.
2. *Bilateral posterior open bite*: Occurrence of posterior open bite on both sides of dental arches is termed as bilateral posterior open bite **(Fig. 38.11)**.

### Etiological Factors Causing Posterior Open Bite

1. Lateral tongue thrusting habit.
2. Ankylosed/submerged posterior teeth fail to reach the occlusal plane and thus may cause posterior open bite.

**Table 38.3:** Management of open bite

| Condition/cause | Management |
|---|---|
| **Anterior Open Bite** | |
| Anterior open bite caused due to abnormal oral habits | Habit breaking appliance followed by removable or fixed Orthodontic treatment |
| Skeletal open bite in mixed dentition | FR-IV (Frankel appliance) chin-cup appliance with high-pull headgear |
| Mild dental/skeletal open bite in permanent dentition Skeletal open bite in permanent dentition | Fixed orthodontic treatment with box elastics Surgical correction |
| **Posterior open bite** | |
| Lateral/posterior open bite caused due to lateral tongue thrust habit | Habit breaking appliance followed by removable or fixed orthodontic treatment |
| **Skeletal open bites** | |
| Growing patients | <ul><li>Bionator</li><li>Frankel appliance</li></ul> |
| Non-growing patients | <ul><li>Orthognathic surgery</li></ul> |

### Treatment of Posterior Open Bite

#### Removal of the Cause

In most cases eventual closure of posterior open bite occurs followed with cessation of the tongue thrusting habit **Table 38.2**.

#### Treatment of Posterior Open Bite using Fixed Orthodontic Appliance

Posterior open bite caused due to ankylosed/submerged teeth that can be corrected by forced extrusion of the antagonistic teeth using fixed orthodontic appliance **(Fig. 38.12)**, or by restoring the normal occlusal level using crowns on submerged teeth.

The management of open bite is given in **Table 38.3**.

#### Treatment of Skeletal Open Bite

Skeletal open bite in growing patients can be treated using functional appliance such as bionator or Frankel appliance. A skeletal open bite in non-growing patients is best treated by orthognathic surgery.

## BIBLIOGRAPHY

1. Fränkel R, Fränkel C. A functional approach to treatment of skeletal open bite. Am J Orthod 1983;84(1):54-68.
2. Kim YH. Anterior open bite and its treatment means of multiloop edgewise archwire. Angle Orthod 1987; 57:290-321.
3. Lopez-Gavito G, Wallen TR, Little RM, et al. Anterior open-bite malocclusion: a longitudinal 10-year postretention evaluation of orthodontically treated patients. Am J Orthod 1985; 175-86.
4. Reitzik M, Barer PG, Wainwright WM. Surgical treatment of skeletal anterior open bite deformities with rigid internal fixation in mandible. Am J Orthod 1990; 52-57.
5. Worms F, Meskin L, Isaacson R, et al. Open bite. Am J Orthod 1971; 59:589-95.

### EXAM-ORIENTED QUESTIONS

#### Long Note
1. Describe in detail about the management of open bite.

#### Short Notes
1. Management of posterior open bite
2. Treatment of anterior open bite
3. Treatment of posterior open bite
4. Treatment of skeletal open bite
5. Classifications of open bite.

## CHAPTER OVERVIEW

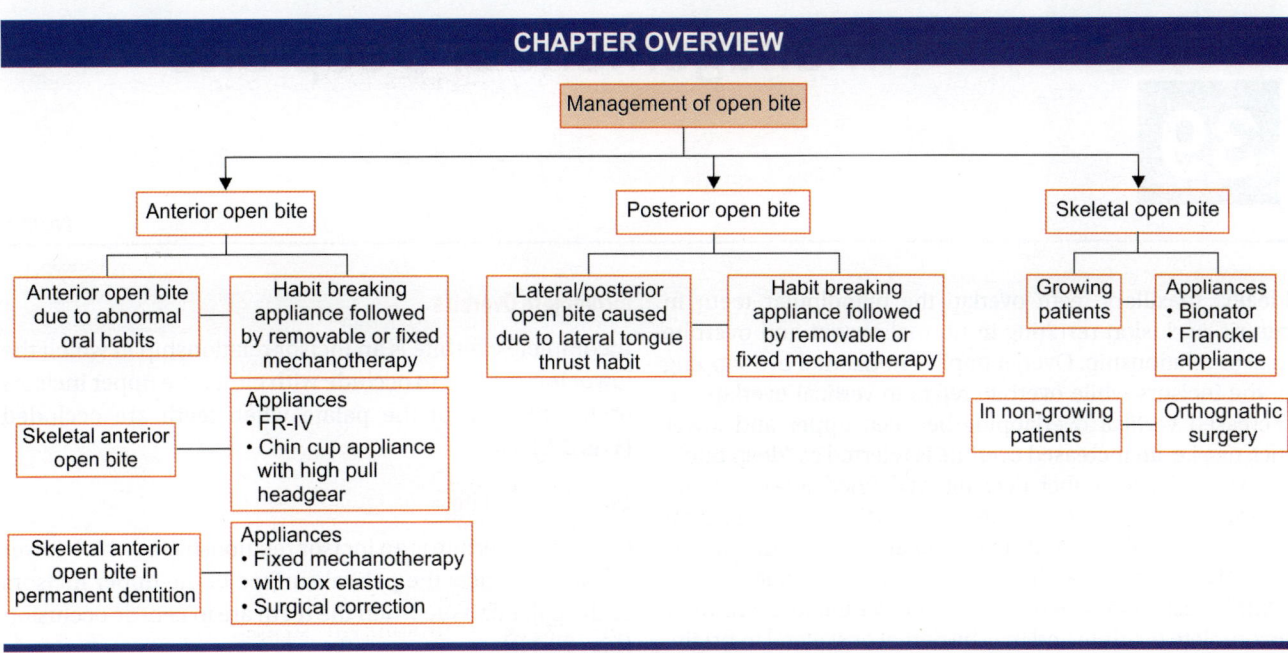

# Management of Deep Bite

*Naik P*

Ideally, maxillary teeth overlap the mandibular teeth in centric occlusion resulting in normal overjet and overbite incisor relationship. Overjet implies horizontal overlapping of the incisors while overbite refers to vertical overlap. An increased vertical overlapping between upper and lower incisors, i.e. an increased overbite is referred as "deep bite".

According to Graber, deep bite is defined as 'a condition of excessive overbite, where the vertical measurement between maxillary and mandibular incisal margins is excessive when mandible is brought into habitual or centric occlusion'. Deep bite may be complete overbite or incomplete overbite and may be dental or skeletal in origin.

Correction of deep bite involves intrusion of maxillary and mandibular anteriors and extrusion of maxillary and mandibular posterior teeth. Deep bite cases can be treated by removable orthodontic appliances such as anterior bite plane, myofunctional appliances such as activator or bionator and fixed orthodontic appliances.

## CLASSIFICATION

I. Deep bite can be classified into the following two types:
   1. Incomplete overbite
   2. Complete overbite.

### Incomplete Overbite

Incomplete overbite is an incisor relationship in which the lower incisors fail to occlude with either the upper incisors or the mucosa of the palate when teeth are occluded (Fig. 39.1A).

### Complete Overbite

Complete overbite is an incisor relationship in which lower incisors contacts the palatal surface of the upper incisors or the palatal tissue when the teeth are in centric occlusion (Fig. 39.1B).

II. Deep bite can further be classified into the following two types:
   1. Dental deep bite
   2. Skeletal deep bite.

### Dental Deep Bite

Dental deep bite is confined to the dentition where there is extrusion of anterior and intrusion of molars. Dental deep bite is often seen in Angle's class II division 2 malocclusion (Figs 39.2A to C).

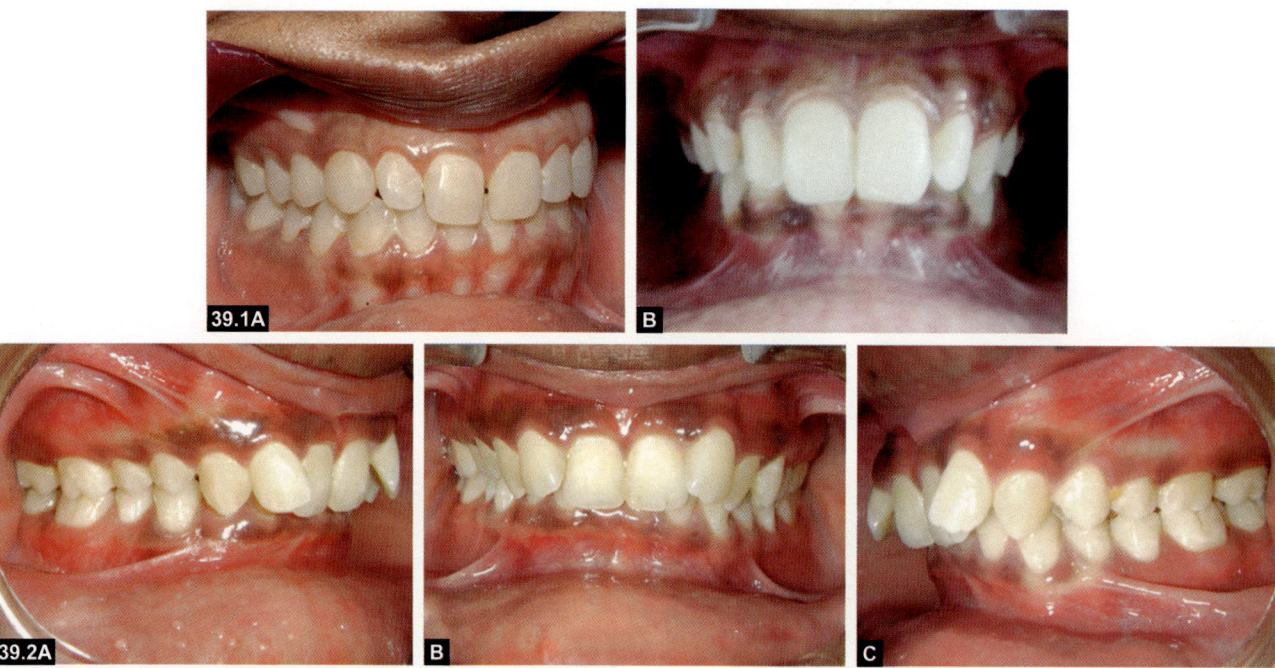

**Figs 39.1A and B:** Types of deep bite: (A) Incomplete overbite; (B) Complete overbite;
**Figs 39.2A to C:** Dental deep bite is commonly seen in Angle's class II division 2 malocclusion

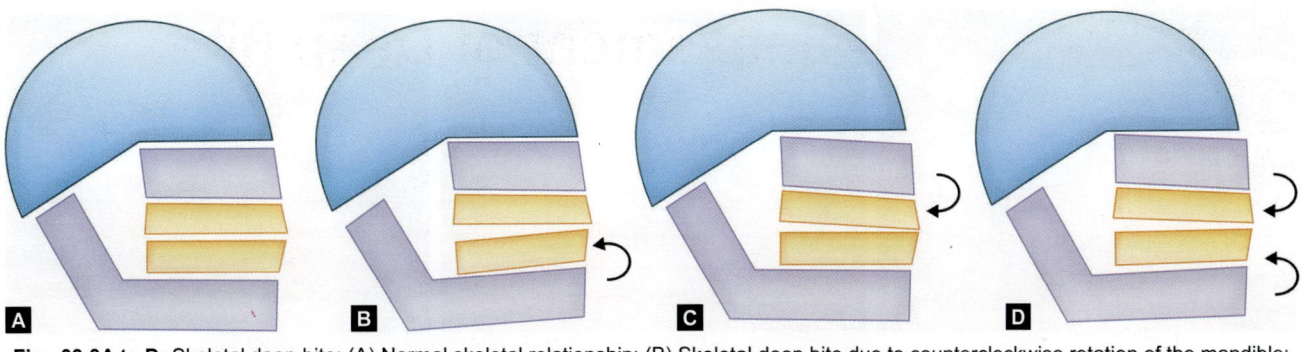

**Figs 39.3A to D:** Skeletal deep bite: (A) Normal skeletal relationship; (B) Skeletal deep bite due to counterclockwise rotation of the mandible; (C) Skeletal deep bite due to clockwise rotation of the maxilla; (D) Skeletal deep bite due to combination of (B) and (C)

### Skeletal Deep Bite

Skeletal deep bites are usually of genetic origin **(Fig. 39.3A)** caused by upward and forward rotations, i.e. counterclockwise rotation of the mandible **(Fig. 39.3B)**. It can also be caused by clockwise rotation of maxilla or a combination of both **(Figs 39.3C and D)**. Skeletal deep bites are seen in Angle's skeletal class II division 2 malocclusion.

## CLINICAL FEATURES

Clinical features of dental deep bites are listed below:

### Extraoral Features

Decreased lower facial height **(Fig. 39.4)**.

### Intraoral Features (Fig. 39.5)

- Increased overbite **(Fig. 39.5A)**.
- Decreased overjet **(Fig. 39.5B)**.
- Extruded maxillary anteriors **(Fig. 39.5C)**.
- Intruded maxillary posteriors.
- Increased susceptibility to food impaction and resultant gingivitis in lower anterior region.

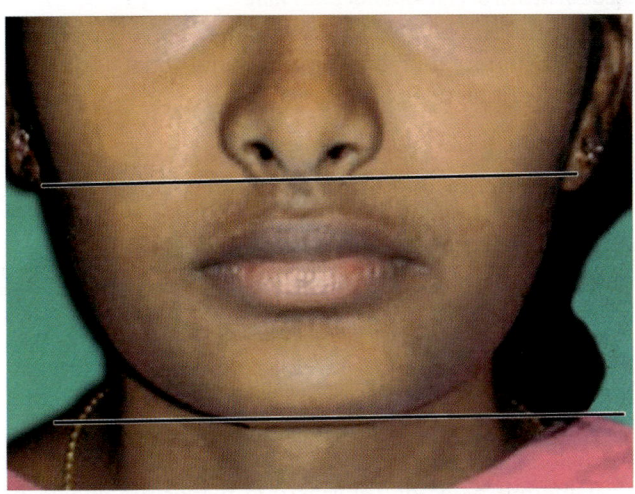

**Fig. 39.4:** Decreased lower facial height

### Cephalometric Findings

Increased interincisal angle **(Fig. 39.6)**.
Clinical features of skeletal deep bite are listed below:

### Extraoral Feature

Decreased lower facial height.

### Intraoral Features

- Increased overbite.
- Decreased overjet.
- Increased risk of gingivitis in the mandibular anterior region.

### Cephalometric Findings

- Increased ramus height.
- Decreased FMA angle.
- Upward and forward rotations of the mandible **(Fig. 39.3B)**.

## DIAGNOSIS

Extraoral and intraoral examinations of the patient should thoroughly be done and history of oral habits should also be noted. Following diagnostic aids are used in the diagnosis of deep bite:
- Clinical examinations.
- *Orthodontic study models:* To evaluate the extent of severity of deep bite.
- *Lateral cephalograms:* To evaluate ramus height, interincisal angle and Frankfort mandibular plane angle.

## TREATMENT

Management of deep bites can be brought about by maxillary anterior intrusion, maxillary posterior extrusion, mandibular anterior intrusion, mandibular posterior extrusion or combination of these. Depending upon the specific problems and treatment objectives for an individual patient, any or all of these above tooth movements may be used for deep bite management. Light forces are used for incisors intrusion (recommended

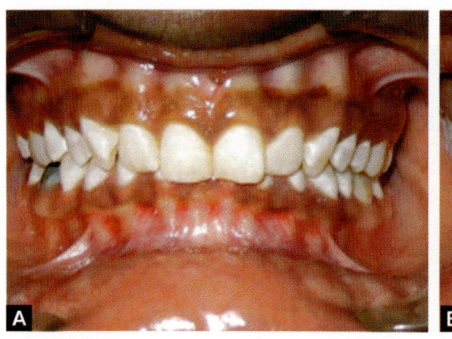
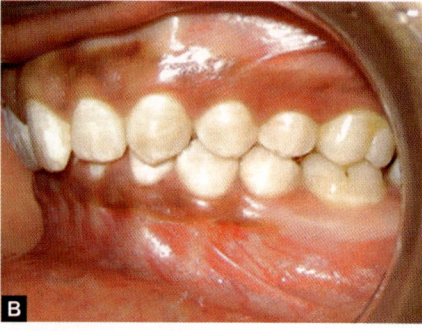
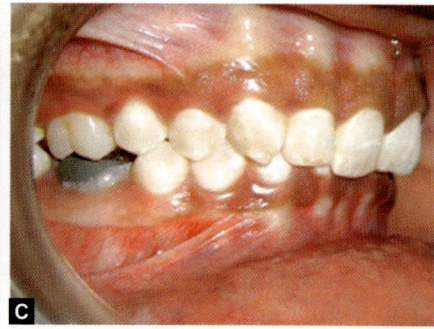

**Figs 39.5A to C:** Intraoral features of deep bite: (A) Increased overbite; (B) Decreased overjet and extrusion of maxillary anteriors; (C) Occlusal view of the dental arches

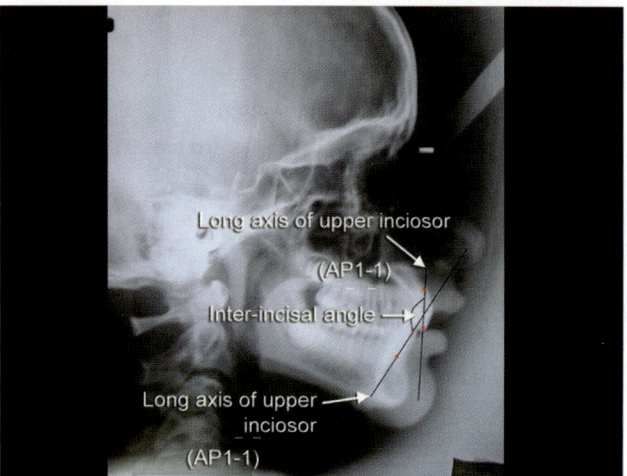

**Fig. 39.6:** Increased interincisal angle

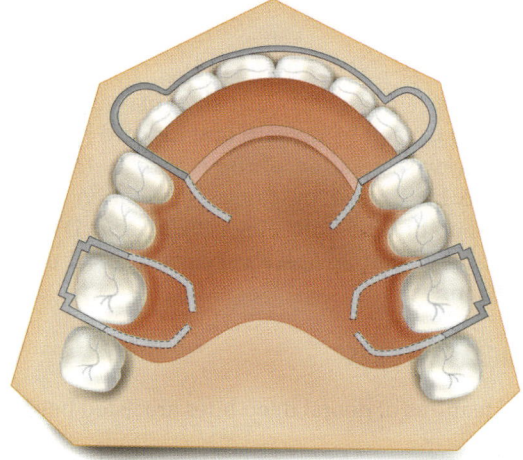

**Fig. 39.7:** Hawley's retainer with anterior bite plane corrects deep bite

forces for lower incisors intrusion are in the range of 12.5 g/tooth and for maxillary incisors about 15–20 g/tooth) whereas heavier forces for extrusion of posteriors.

Deep bite can be treated by using removable, myofunctional appliances or fixed orthodontic appliances.

## REMOVABLE ORTHODONTIC APPLIANCES TO CORRECT DEEP BITE

### Anterior Bite Plane

Anterior bite plane can effectively be used to treat deep bite. It is often used in conjunction with fixed mechanotherapy to treat deep bite along with other malrelations of teeth. Anterior bite plane is a modified version of Hawley's removable orthodontic appliance with the following features **(Fig. 39.7) (Table 39.1)**:
- Adam's clasps on molars—aid in retention of the bite plane.
- Labial bow—prevents maxillary anterior proclination.
- Bite plane should be—1.5–2.0 mm.

### Flat Anterior Bite Plane

The flat anterior bite plane is used with maxillary removable orthodontic appliance and is made by building up of acrylic base material behind the maxillary incisors so that the mandibular incisors touch the bite plane before the buccal teeth come into occlusion **(Figs 39.8A and B)**.

The main purpose of flat anterior bite plane is to reduce the incisal overbite (deep bite). It is mainly used to reduce incisal overbite in Angle's class II division 2 malocclusion and Angle's class I malocclusion with deep bite.

#### Mode of Action of Flat Anterior Bite Plane

The flat anterior bite plane induces extrusion of upper and lower posteriors thereby it brings about reduction of the incisal overbite (deep bite).

### Inclined Anterior Bite Plane

Inclined anterior bite plane on the maxillary removable orthodontic appliance is also used for the correction of deep bite cases. It is mainly used in the correction of deep bite in Angle's class II division 1 malocclusion **(Fig. 39.9)**.

#### Mode of Action of Inclined Anterior Bite Plane

The inclined anterior bite plane induces a forward mandibular posture and reciprocal backward force on the maxillary appliance from the masticatory forces and extrusion of lower posteriors.

Different types of anterior bite planes are shown in **Flowchart 39.1**.

Table 39.1: Different types of anterior bite planes, their effects and use in malocclusion

| Type of anterior bite plane | Effect of anterior bite planes | Mechanotherapy | Use in condition |
|---|---|---|---|
| Hawley's retainer with anterior bite plane | Extrusion of posteriors and intrusion of anteriors | Often used in conjunction with fixed mechanotherapy<br>And also used in removable appliance therapy | Angle's class I malocclusion with deep bite |
| Flat anterior bite plane | Extrusion of upper and lower posteriors | Used in removable appliance therapy | Angle's class II division 2 malocclusion |
| Inclined anterior bite plane | Forward mandibular posture<br>Backward maxillary posture<br>Extrusion of lower posteriors | Used in removable appliance therapy | Angle's class II division 1 malocclusion |

## MYOFUNCTIONAL ORTHODONTIC APPLIANCE TO CORRECT DEEP BITE

Thin layer activation (TLA) following myofunctional orthodontic appliances, such as activator can be used for correction of deep bite. In both the appliances interocclusal acrylic is trimmed to facilitate extrusion of posteriors followed by intrusion of anteriors (**Figs 39.10A and B**). Bionator or Frankel appliance (FR Ia) can also be used for the management of deep bite cases.

## FIXED ORTHODONTIC TREATMENT APPLIANCE TO CORRECT DEEP BITE

Fixed orthodontic appliances can be used to treat deep bites. The intrusion arches and utility arches when used bring about correction of deep bites by intrusion of incisors and are indicated in patients with excessive maxillary incisor visibility at rest or when smiling (gummy smiles) (**Figs 39.11A to E**).

## FIXED ORTHODONTIC APPLIANCE WITH UTILITY ARCHES

Utility arches are arch wires used with fixed orthodontic appliance for the correction of deep bite cases. They are bent in such a way that they bypass the premolars and are engaged on the incisors. These arch wires can be used to perform a number of tooth movements including incisors protrusion or retraction, intrusions of incisors (**Figs 39.12A to E**). They are activated by giving a V bend in the buccal segment of the wire mesial to molar to generate an intrusive force on the incisors (**Fig. 39.13**).

## ARCH WIRES WITH REVERSE CURVE OF SPEE

The use of arch wires with reverse curve of Spee is another common approach to the management of deep bite. These arch wires provide both an intrusive force on the anterior teeth and an eruptive force on the posterior teeth (**Fig. 39.14**).

## USE OF ANCHORAGE BENDS

Anchorage bends are given in the arch wire mesial to the molar tubes so that the anterior part of the wire lies

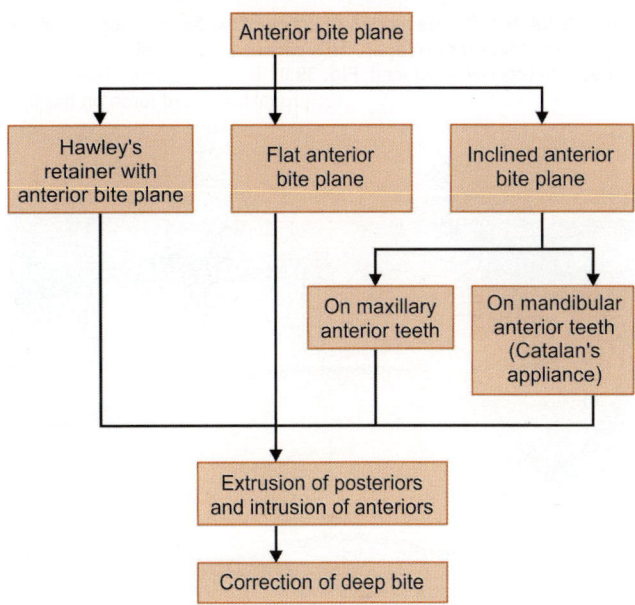

Flowchart 39.1: Anterior bite planes

gingival to the bracket slot (**Fig. 39.15**). Thus, when these wires are pulled occlusally and engaged into the brackets, a gingivally directed intrusive force is exerted on the incisors which reduce the deep bite.

## RETENTION FOLLOWED BY DEEP BITE CORRECTION

If the deep bites are corrected by intrusion of maxillary anteriors then a bite plate on maxillary retainers is desirable. The patient is instructed to wear such retainer continuously for the period of minimum 4-6 months. In deep bite cases, overcorrection is usually desirable, and equilibration and adjustment to functional occlusion are necessary.

Principles of management of deep bite are summarized in **Flowchart 39.2**.

## BIBLIOGRAPHY

1. Bell, Jacobs, Legan. Treatment of Class II deep bite by orthodontic and surgical means. Am J Orthod. 1984;19:1-20.
2. Engel. Treatment of deep bite cases. Am J Orthod. 1980;1-13.

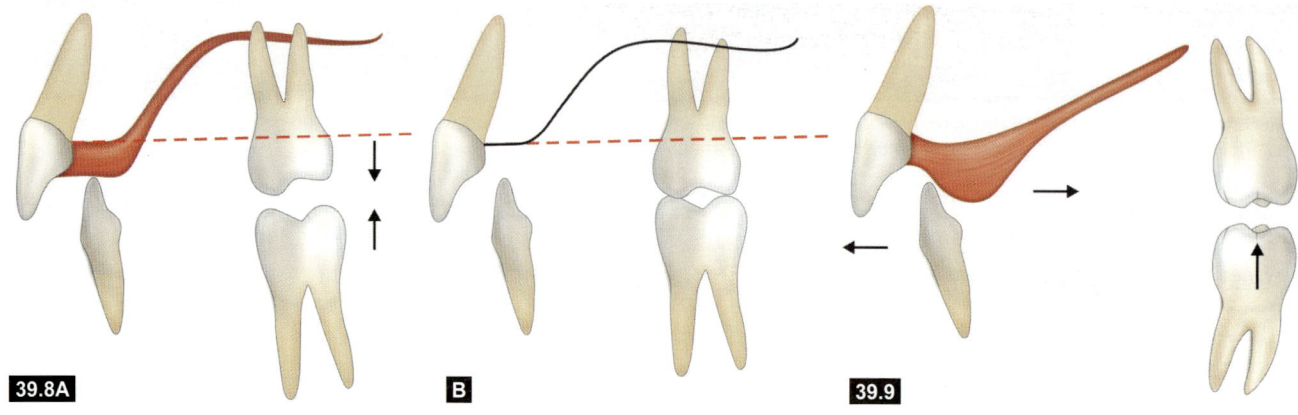

**Figs 39.8A and B:** The modeS of action of the flat anterior bite plane: (A) with the appliance fitted, the lower incisors touch the bite plane and posterior teeth remain apart. This causes intrusion of anteriors and extrusion of posteriors; (B) when the bite plane is removed, the incisal overbite has been reduced; **Fig. 39.9:** Inclined anterior bite plane. The incline of the bite plane induces a forward mandibular posture and reciprocal backward force on the upper appliance from the masticatory forces

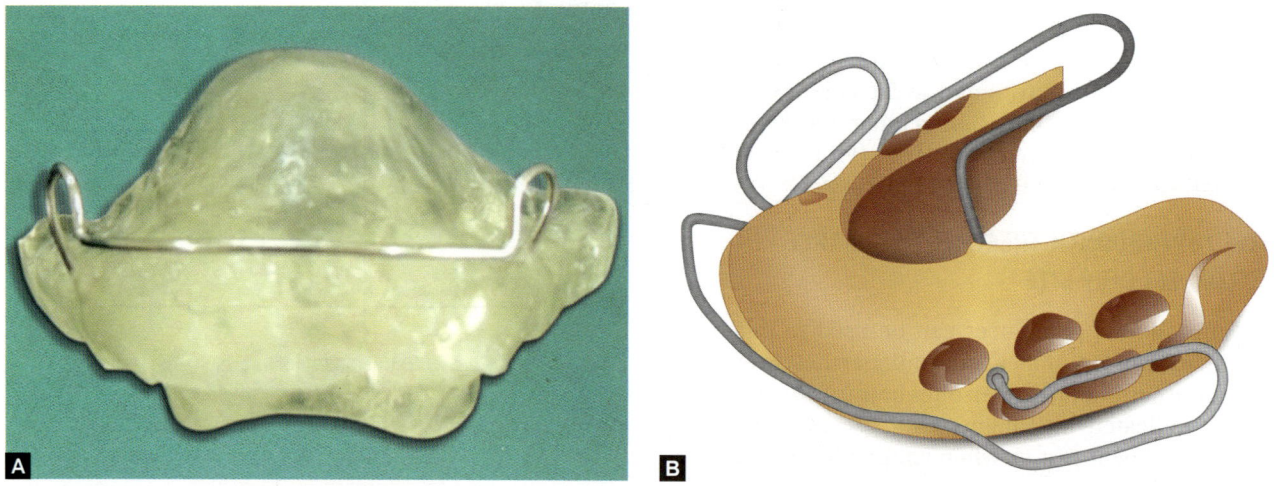

**Figs 39.10A and B:** Myofunctional orthodontic appliances used for correction of deep bite: (A) Activator; (B) Bionator. In both the appliances, the interocclusal acrylic is trimmed to facilitate extrusion of posteriors followed by intrusion of anteriors for the correction of deep bite

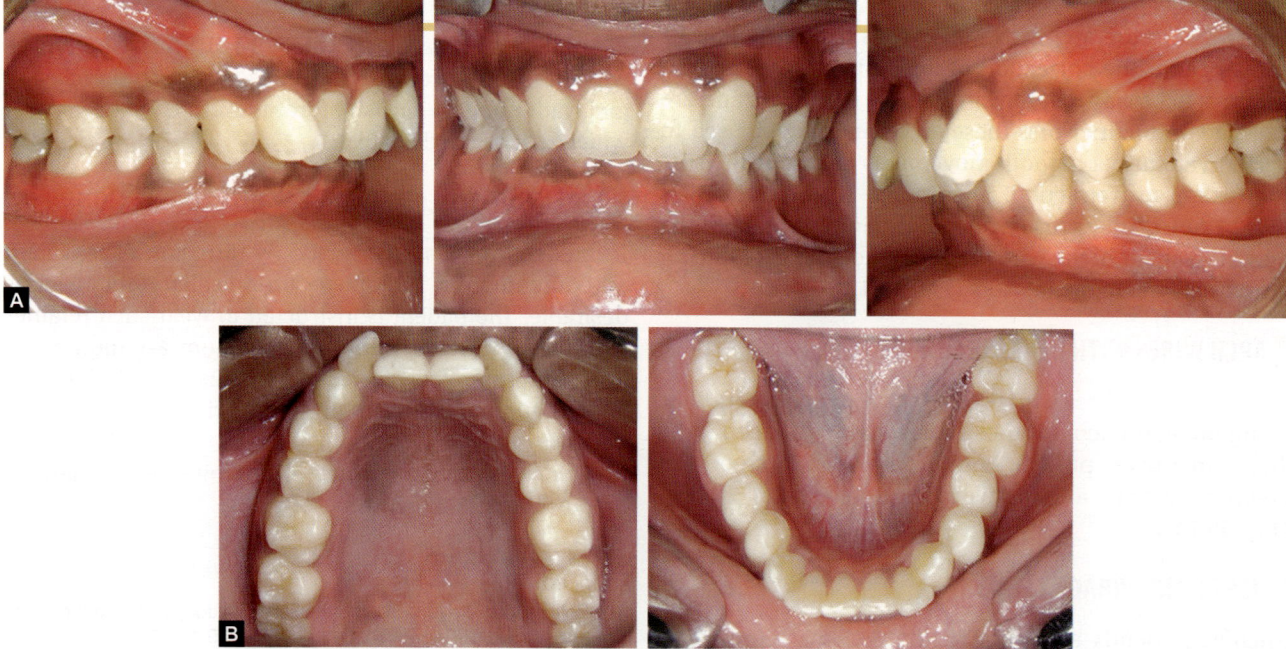

**Figs 39.11A and B**

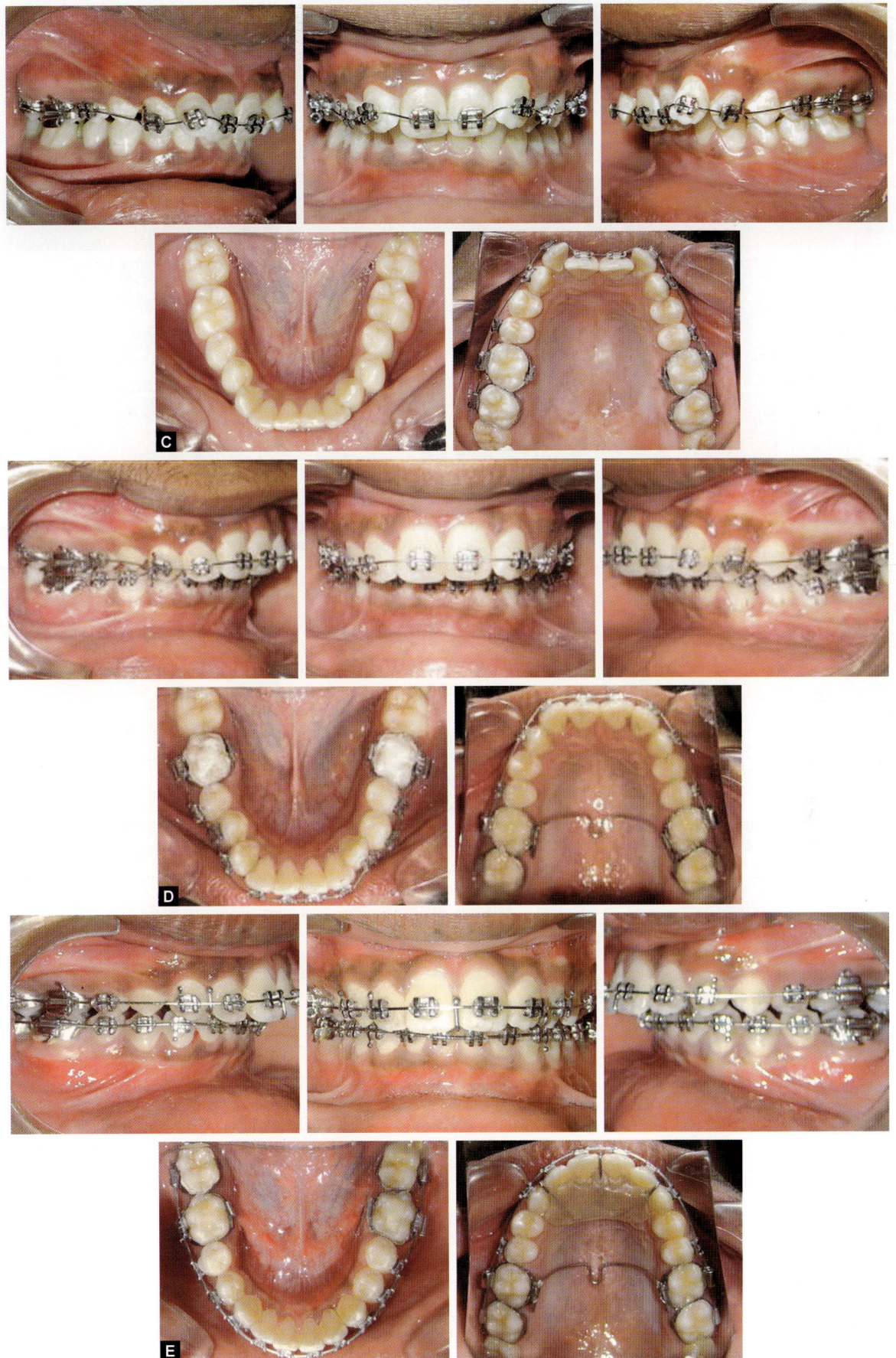

Fig. 39.11C to E

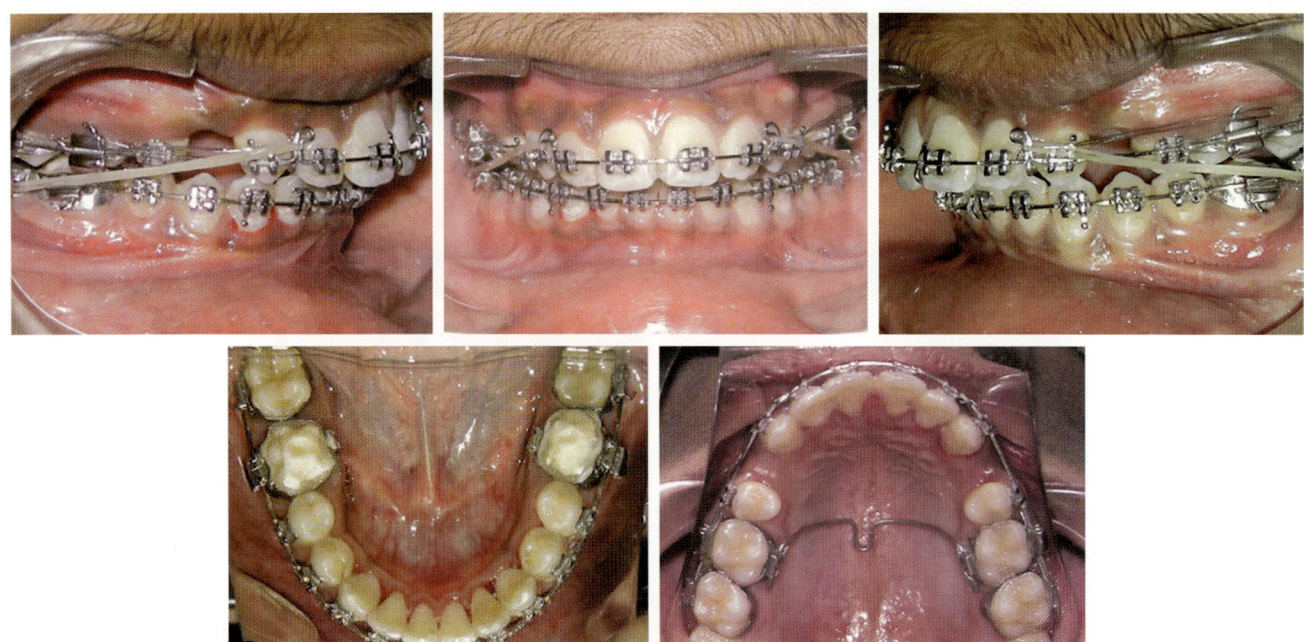

**Figs 39.11A to F:** Fixed orthodontic appliances can be used to correct deep bite (A and B) pre-treatment; (C and D) during the treatment; (E and F) nearing the completion of correction of deep bite

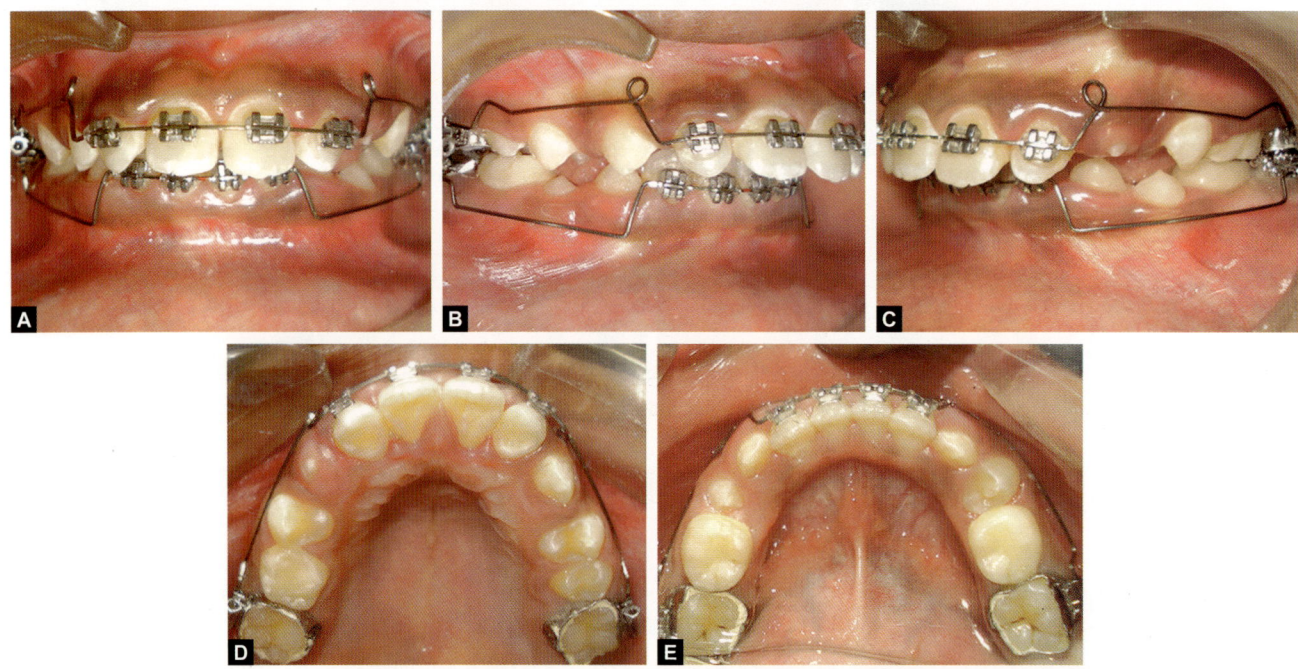

**Figs 39.12A to E:** Fixed orthodontic appliances with utility arches bring about correction of deep bite by intrusion of upper and lower anteriors and extrusion of upper and lower posteriors

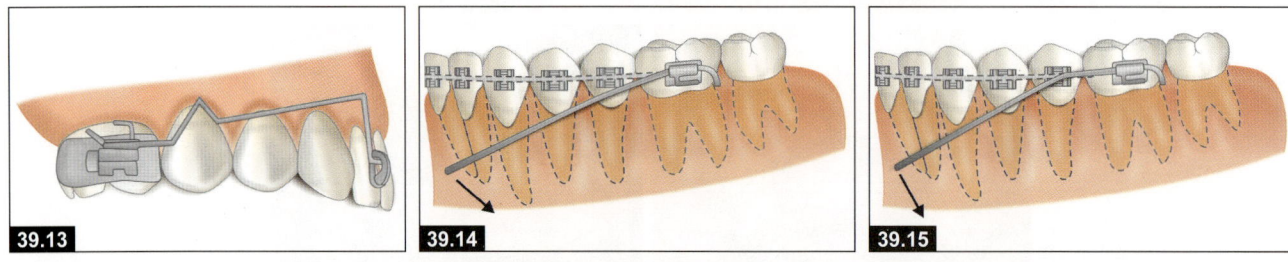

**Fig. 39.13:** Utility arches are activated by giving a V bend in the buccal segment of the wire mesial to molar to generate an intrusive force on the incisors; **Fig. 39.14:** Arch wires with reverse curve of Spee produce intrusive force on the anterior teeth and an eruptive force on the posterior teeth; **Fig. 39.15:** Anchorage bends for intrusion of anterior teeth

3. Graber M, Vanarsdall L. Orthodontic Current Principles and Techniques. Mosby Year Book Inc. 1994.
4. Graber TM. Orthodontics: Principles and Practice. WB Saunders, 1988.
5. Hinkle. Surgical treatment of class II, Division 2 malocclusion. Am J Orthod. 1989;185-91.
6. Ligthelm-Baker, Wattel, Uljee, Prahl-Andresen. Vertical growth. Am J Orthod. 1992;509-13.
7. McDowell and Baker. Skeletodental Appliances in Deep bite Correction. Am J Orthod. 1991;370-5.
8. Ortial. Vertical dimension and therapeutic choices. Am J Orthod. 1995;432-41.
9. Parker, Nanda and Currier. Treatment of deepbite malocclusion changes. Am J Orthod. 1995;382-93.
10. Pfeiffer and Groberty. Combined orthopedic—orthodontic treatment. Am J Orthod. 1982;185-201.
11. Profitt WR. Contemporary Orthodontics. St Louis: CV Mosby, 1986.
12. Robert E Moyers. Hand Book of Orthodontics. Year Medical Publishers, Inc; 1988.
13. Salzman JA. Practice of Orthodontics. JB Lippincott Company, 1966.

## EXAM-ORIENTED QUESTIONS

### Long Note
1. Management of deep bite.

### Short Notes
1. Reverse curve arch wire
2. Use of anchorage bends in management of deep bite.

## CHAPTER OVERVIEW

```
Management of deep bite
├── Removable orthodontic appliances
│   └── Anterior bite plane
│       └── Extrusion of posteriors and some extent of intrusion of anteriors
├── Myofunctional appliances
│   ├── Activator
│   │   └── Trimming of acrylic to allow extrusion of posteriors
│   └── Frankle 1A
│       └── Extrusion of posteriors and intrusion of anteriors
└── Fixed orthodontic appliances
    ├── Intrusion arches
    │   ├── Intrusion arch wires
    │   └── Utility arches
    │       └── Intrusion of incisors
    └── Bite planes
        └── Extrusion of posteriors

→ Correction of deep bites
```

# CHAPTER 40

# Management of Crossbite

*Phulari BS, Naik P*

According to Graber crossbite is defined as a condition where one or more teeth may be abnormally malposed buccally or lingually or labially with reference to the opposing tooth or teeth.

## Classification of Crossbite

I. **According to their location in the arch**
   A. Anterior crossbite
      1. Single tooth crossbite
      2. Segmental crossbite
   B. Posterior crossbite
      1. Single tooth crossbite
      2. Segmental crossbite.

II. **Classification of posterior crossbite on the basis of its presence on one or both sides of arch.**

   According to presence of posterior crossbite on one side or both sides of the arch, posterior crossbite can be classified into following two types:
   1. Unilateral posterior crossbite
   2. Bilateral posterior crossbite.

III. **According to the extent of crossbite**
   1. Simple posterior crossbite
   2. Buccal nonocclusion (scissor bite)
   3. Lingual nonocclusion.

IV. **Classification of crossbite based on structure involved.**

   Crossbite can be classified into following three types based on structure involved:
   1. Dental crossbite
   2. Skeletal crossbite
   3. Functional crossbite.

## ANTERIOR CROSSBITE

Anterior crossbite is a condition, where mandibular anteriors overlap the maxillary anteriors (**Figs 40.1A to C**). The condition is often due to lingual position of maxillary anterior teeth in relation to the mandibular anterior teeth.

### Classification of Anterior Crossbite

Anterior crossbite may be further classified into the following two types, based on number of teeth involved in the crossbite:

1. ***Single tooth crossbite:*** Single tooth anterior crossbite is a condition, where there is overlapping of one of the mandibular anterior teeth over one of the maxillary anterior teeth (**Fig. 40.2**).
2. ***Segmental anterior crossbite:*** Segmental anterior crossbite is a condition where there is overlapping of a group of mandibular anterior teeth over a group of maxillary teeth (**Fig. 40.3**).

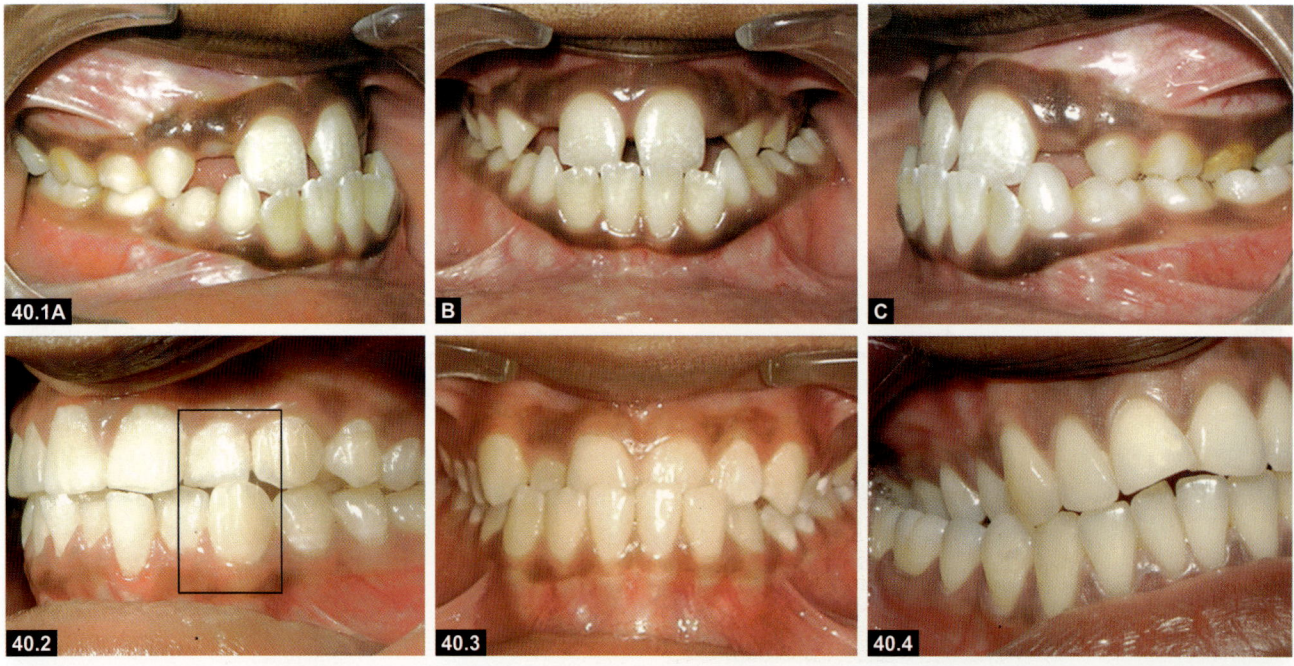

**Fig. 40.1A to C:** Anterior crossbite is a condition where mandibular anteriors overlap the maxillary anteriors; **Fig. 40.2:** Single tooth anterior crossbite related to left permanent lower canine; **Fig. 40.3:** Segmental anterior crossbite; **Fig. 40.4:** Posterior crossbite

# POSTERIOR CROSSBITE

Posterior crossbite refers to a condition where there is an abnormal transverse relationship between upper and lower posterior teeth **(Fig. 40.4)**.

## Classification of Posterior Crossbite

A. Based on the number of teeth involved posterior crossbite can be further classified into following two types:
   1. ***Single tooth posterior crossbite:*** Single tooth posterior crossbite is a condition where there is an overlapping of one of the mandibular posteriors over one of the maxillary posterior teeth **(Fig. 40.5A)**.
   2. ***Segmental posterior crossbite:*** Segmental posterior crossbite is a condition where there is overlapping of group of mandibular posterior teeth over group of maxillary posterior teeth **(Fig. 40.5B)**.
B. According to the presence of posterior crossbite on single or both sides of the dental arch, crossbites are classified into two types:
   1. ***Unilateral crossbite:*** It is a condition where there is posterior crossbite on one side of the dental arch **(Fig. 40.6A)**. Unilateral crossbite involves deviation in the path of mandibular closure, usually warrants orthodontic treatment.
   2. ***Bilateral posterior crossbite:*** It is a condition where posterior crossbite is present on both sides of the dental arch **(Fig. 40.6B)**.
C. Posterior crossbites are classified into the following three types, based on the extent of crossbite:
   1. ***Simple posterior crossbite:*** Simple posterior crossbite is referred to as a condition where buccal cusps of one or more maxillary posterior teeth occlude lingual to buccal cusps of the mandibular teeth **(Fig. 40.7)**.
   2. ***Buccal nonocclusion (Scissor bite):*** Here the palatal cusps of maxillary teeth in occlusion are placed buccal to the mandibular posterior teeth, referred to as buccal nonocclusion **(Fig. 40.8)**.
   3. ***Lingual nonocclusion:*** Here the maxillary posterior tooth or teeth are placed completely palatal to the lingual aspect of the mandibular posterior teeth, i.e. the buccal cusp of the maxillary tooth is palatal/lingual to the lingual cusp of the mandibular posterior teeth **(Fig. 40.9)**.

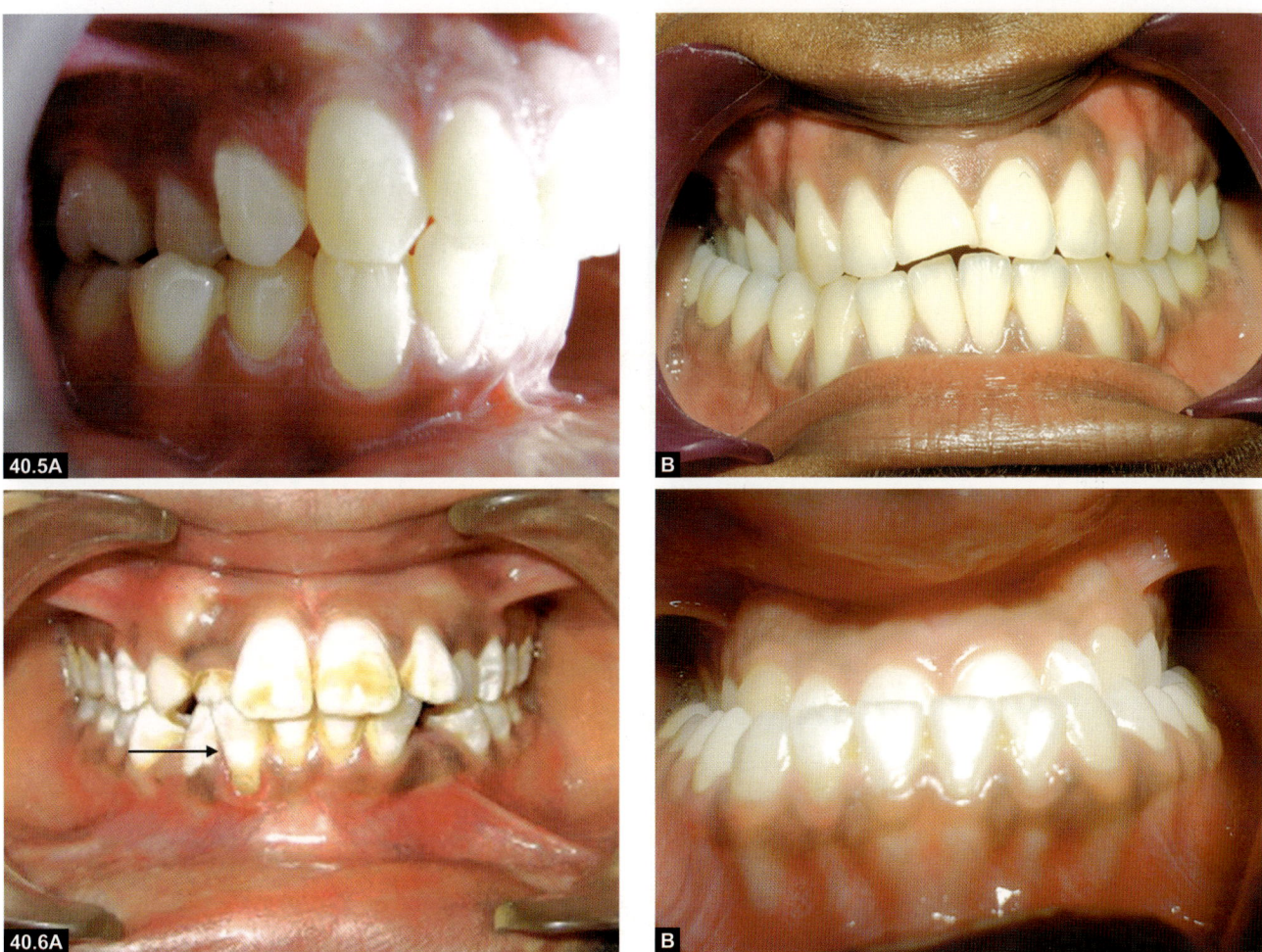

**Figs 40.5A and B:** Types of posterior crossbite: (A) Single tooth posterior crossbite; (B) Segmental posterior crossbite;
**Figs 40.6A and B:** (A) Unilateral posterior crossbite; (B) Bilateral posterior crossbite

D. Crossbites are classified into the following three types:
1. **Dental crossbite:** When crossbite is confined to the dentition is referred to as dental crossbite **(Fig. 40.10)**.
2. **Skeletal crossbite:** Crossbite involving the skeletal structures such as maxillary and mandibular arches are referred to as skeletal crossbite. Maxillary retrognathism, mandibular prognathism or a combination of both can result in skeletal crossbite, e.g. skeletal class III malocclusion **(Fig. 40.11)**.
3. **Functional crossbite:** Functional crossbites are usually caused due to the presence of occlusal interference or premature loss of deciduous molars, e.g. pseudo class III malocclusion. In such situation, patient tends to habitually move the mandible forward, so as to achieve maximum intercuspation. This may lead to pseudo class III malocclusion **(Fig. 40.12)**.

## ETIOLOGY OF CROSSBITE

### Etiology of Dental Crossbite
I. **Anomalies of number of teeth**
   1. Supernumerary teeth
   2. Missing teeth.
II. **Anomalies of tooth shape**
III. **Anomalies of tooth size**
   1. Microdontia
   2. Macrodontia **(Fig. 40.13)**.

### Etiology of Skeletal Crossbite
I. Habits—Thumb sucking, mouth breathing, etc.
II. Trauma at birth (ankylosis of the TMJ by forceps injury during delivery).

## TREATMENT (TABLE 40.1)

### Correction of Anterior Crossbite
I. **Correction of anterior crossbite in the preadolescent age group:**
The following appliances are used to correct the anterior crossbite in the preadolescent age groups:
1. Tongue blade
2. Catlan's appliance or lower anterior inclined plane
3. Removable orthodontic appliances such as:
   a. Removable orthodontic appliances with double cantilever spring or "Z" spring

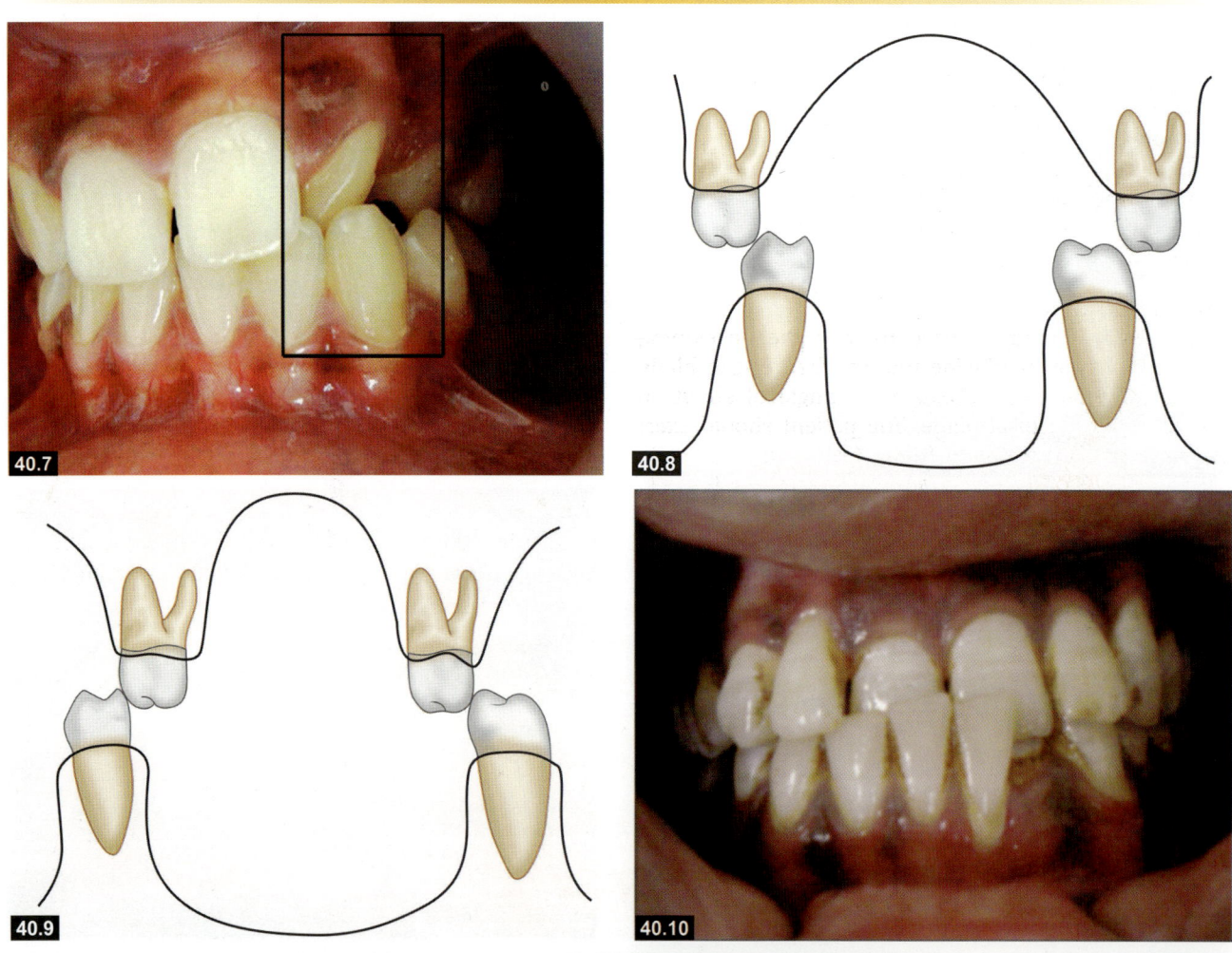

**Fig. 40.7:** Simple posterior crossbite; **Fig. 40.8:** Buccal nonocclusion;
**Fig. 40.9:** Lingual nonocclusion; **Fig. 40.10:** Dental crossbite

| Table 40.1: Management of crossbites | |
|---|---|
| **Type of crossbite** | **Management** |
| Developing anterior crossbite | • Tongue blade therapy<br>• Lower inclined plane therapy |
| Anterior crossbite | • Z spring with posterior bite planes<br>• Telescopic expansion screw<br>• Segmental expansion screw with posterior bite plane<br>• Multilooped arch wire with fixed appliances |
| Single tooth posterior crossbite | • Cross elastics<br>• Sectional fixed appliances<br>• Removable orthodontic appliance with expansion screw |
| Unilateral posterior crossbite | • Removable orthodontic appliance with unilateral expansion screw<br>• Fixed orthodontic appliance |
| Bilateral posterior crossbite | • Coffin spring<br>• Quad helix<br>• Hyrax<br>• Symmetrical expansion screw |

b. Removable orthodontic appliances with expansion screw
4. Orthopedic appliances:
   a. Face mask along with RME
   b. Chin cup appliance
5. Myofunctional appliance such as Frankel III appliance.

**II. Correction of anterior crossbite in adolescents and adults**
1. *Removable orthodontic appliances:* Removable orthodontic appliances with expansion screw (mini expansion screw or medium expansion screw).
2. Fixed orthodontic appliances.

### Tongue Blade Therapy
Tongue blade therapy is used to treat the developing anterior crossbite by placing the wooden tongue blade behind the tooth in crossbite at an angle of about 60 degrees to the occlusal plane. The patient should exert force by biting on it using the lower teeth as a fulcrum for a period of 5–10 minutes. Usually the tooth will erupt into normal position over a period of time **(Figs 40.14A and B)**.

Catalan's Appliance or Lower Anterior Inclined Plane **(Figs 40.15A and B)**.

Catalan's appliance is also called as "lower anterior inclined plane", which explains the design of this appliance. Catalan's appliance consists of an inclined plane cemented to the lower incisor.

### Fabrication
Acrylic resin or cast metal is used to fabricate Catalan's appliance. The lower anterior inclined plane is designed in such a way that, it is at 45 degree angle to the maxillary occlusal plane. Catlan's appliance can be fabricated on a single lower anterior tooth for the correction of single tooth crossbite or for the whole anterior segment.

### Indication
a. Sufficient space in the arch for the alignment of the maxillary teeth in crossbite.
b. Crossbite due to palatally displaced maxillary incisor.

### Disadvantages
a. Patient may have hampered speech during treatment.
b. Catalan's appliance cannot be constructed if mandibular anterior teeth are crowded.
c. Periodontal problem of the mandibular teeth associated with prolonged use of appliance may cause periodontal ligament problems.
d. Occurrence of anterior open bite is reported in patients with prolonged usage of this appliance due to supra-eruption of posterior teeth.
e. It is contraindicated in patients with periodontally compromised mandibular anterior teeth.

Patient has to follow the dietary restrictions during treatment.

### Removable Orthodontic Appliances
a. Removable orthodontic appliances with "z" spring:
   Anterior crossbite involving one or two maxillary teeth can be treated by using a double cantilever spring or "z" spring **(Fig. 40.16)**.
• In case of single tooth anterior crossbite, "Z" spring on tooth involved in corssbite can be used for correction of such a condition.
• In case of anterior crossbites involving two teeth in crossbite, "Z" spring on two teeth is used to correct the anterior crossbite by involving group of teeth by labial movement.

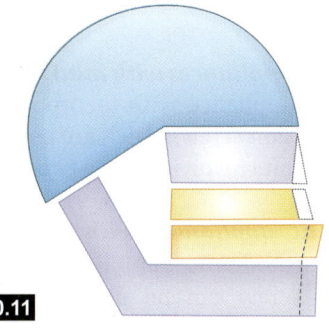
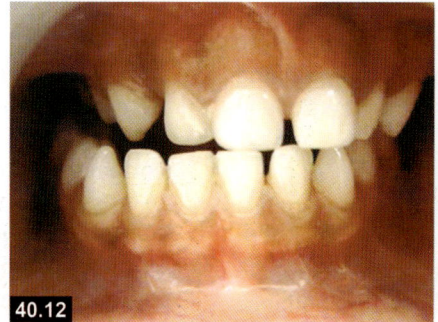
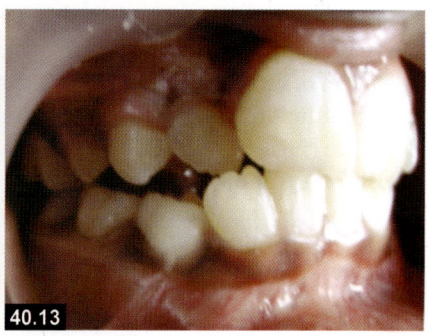

**Fig. 40.11:** Skeletal crossbite; **Fig. 40.12:** Functional crossbite; **Fig. 40.13:** Macrodontic maxillary central incisors causing mesopalatal rotation of right lateral incisor resulting in single tooth anterior crossbite

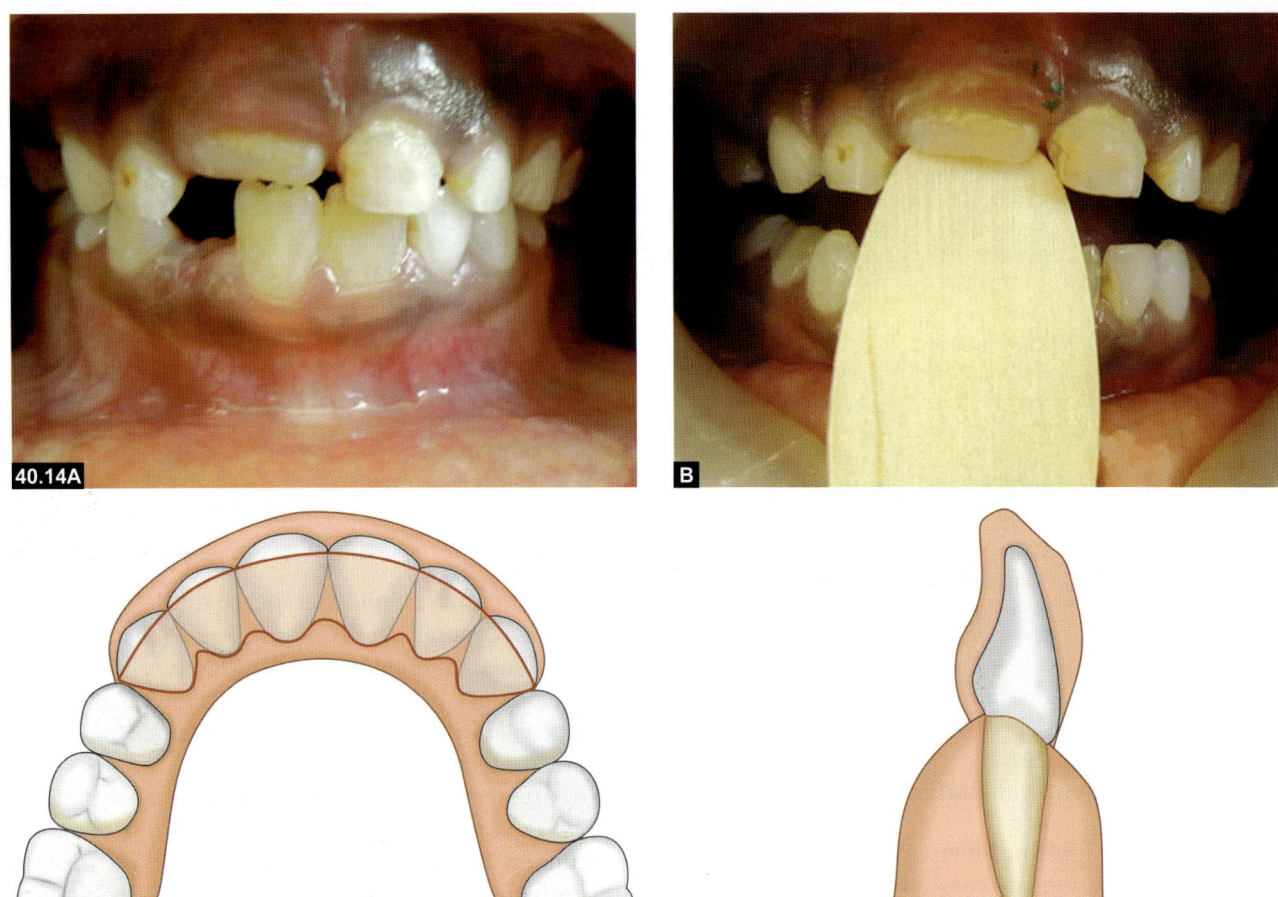

**Figs 40.14A and B:** (A) Patient indicated for tongue blade therapy; (B) Tongue blade can be used to correct developing anterior crossbite; **Figs 40.15A and B:** Catalan's appliance (Lower anterior inclined plane) can be used to single and segmental anterior correct crossbite: (A) Catalan's appliance; (B) Side view of the Catalan's appliance

b. Removable orthodontic appliances with expansion screw:

Removable orthodontic appliance incorporates expansion screw of various types, which can be used to correct either single tooth crossbite or segmental tooth crossbite **(Fig. 40.17)**.

### Orthopedic Appliances

a. Face mask along with RME:

Face mask (reverse headgear) is used in the treatment of skeletal anterior crossbite during growth period, before cessation of growth. Face mask helps in protraction of the retrognathic premaxilla, thereby normalizing the skeletal crossbite **(Figs 40.18A and B)**.

b. Chin-cup appliance:

Chin-cup appliance is one of the orthopedic, orthodontic appliance and is used to redirect the growth of the mandible to prevent or correct the anterior crossbite due to excessive mandibular growth. Chin cup appliance tends to rotate the mandible posteriorly and inferiorly **(Fig. 40.19)**.

### Myofunctional Appliances or Functional Appliances

Frankel III appliance may be used to correct a developing class III skeletal jaw in relation with anterior crossbite **(Fig. 40.20)**.

### Correction of anterior crossbite in adolescent and adults

Removable orthodontic appliance incorporated expansion screw of either mini or medium, which may also be used to correct anterior crossbite; involving single tooth or group of teeth in adults.

### Removable Orthodontic Appliances

a. ***Removable orthodontic appliances with mini screw:*** Removable orthodontic appliance with incorporated mini screw type of expansion screw, which are used to correct the anterior crossbite involving up to two teeth in crossbite.

b. ***Removable orthodontic appliances with medium screw:*** Removable orthodontic appliance with incorporated medium screw can be used to treat anterior crossbite involving up to 4–6 teeth in crossbite **(Fig. 40.21)**.

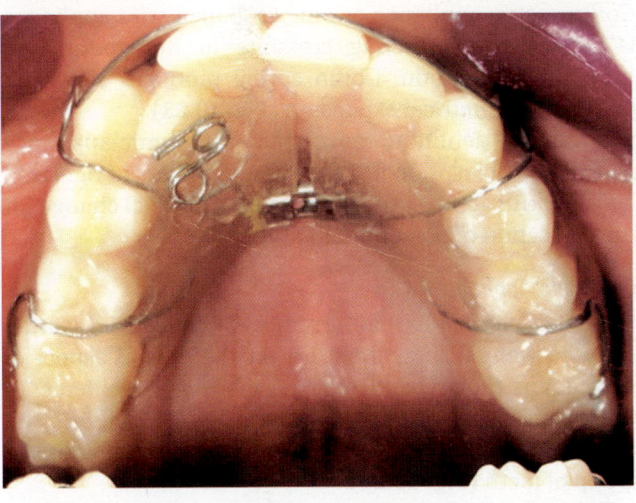

**Fig. 40.16:** Anterior crossbite involving one or two maxillary teeth can be treated by using a double cantilever spring or "z" spring

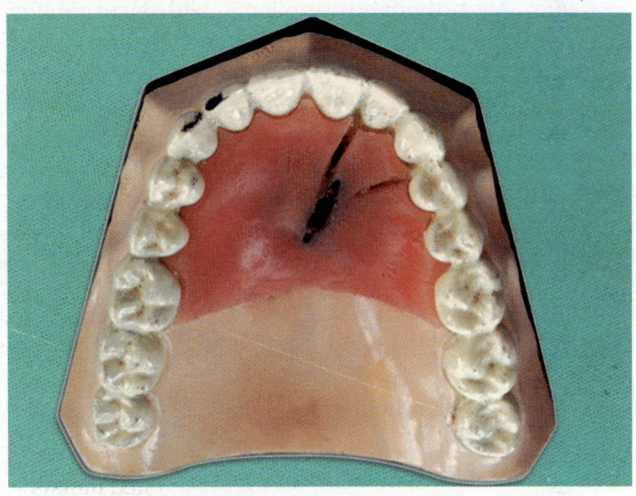

**Fig. 40.17:** Removable orthodontic appliance incorporated expansion screw of various types can be used to correct either single tooth crossbite or segmental tooth crossbite

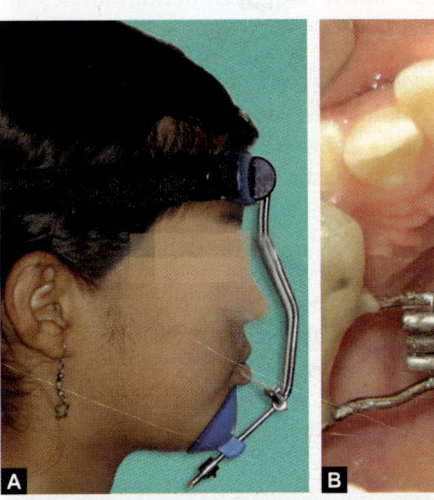
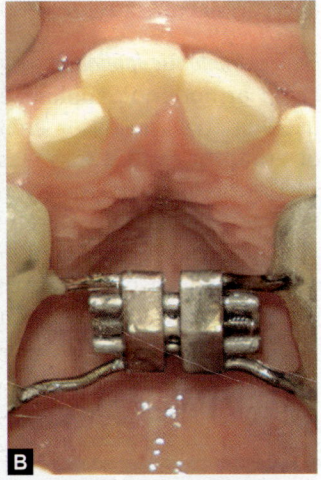

**Figs 40.18A and B:** Face mask along with RME: (A) Face mask side view; (B) Acrylic bonded rapid maxillary expansion appliance

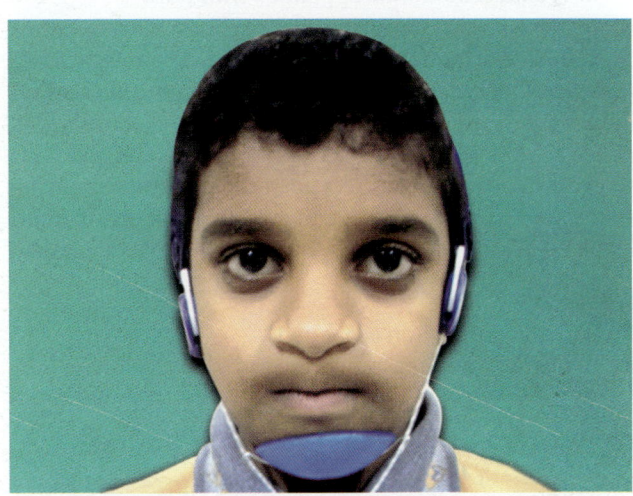

**Fig. 40.19:** Chin-cup appliance

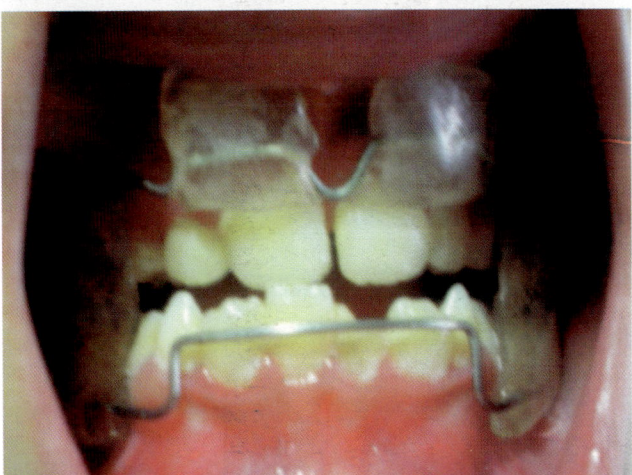

**Fig. 40.20:** Frankel III appliance may be used to correct a developing class III skeletal jaw relation with anterior crossbite

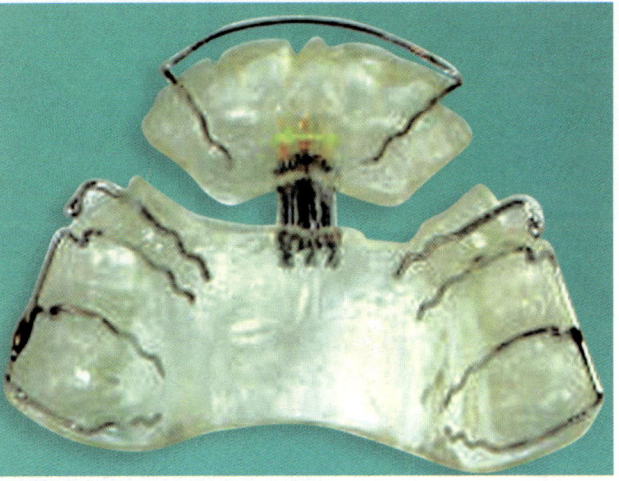

**Fig. 40.21:** Removable orthodontic appliance with incorporated medium screw can be used to treat anterior crossbite involving up to 4–6 teeth in crossbite

c. **Removable orthodontic appliances with 3D screw:** Removable orthodontic appliance with incorporated three dimensional expansion screws in the midline can be used in the treatment of anterior crossbite associated with pseudo class III malocclusion.

### Fixed Orthodontic Appliances

Fixed orthodontic appliance can be used to correct anterior crossbite involving single tooth or group of teeth **(Figs 40.22A to F)**.

### Correction of Posterior Crossbites

1. By removable orthodontic appliance, which are as follows
   a. Removable orthodontic appliances with expansion screw
   b. Removable orthodontic appliances with coffin spring
   c. Quad helix appliance.
2. By fixed orthodontic appliance
   a. Fixed orthodontic appliance with RME
   b. Fixed orthodontic appliance with NiTi expanders
   c. Fixed orthodontic appliance with cross elastics.

***Removable orthodontic appliance with expansion screw:*** Removable orthodontic appliance with incorporated various types of screws such as mini, medium and 3D screws can be used to correct posterior crossbite involving single tooth or group of teeth by labialization of tooth involved in crossbite.

### Drawbacks

- Patient cooperation is needed.
- Activation requires frequent visits.

### Removable orthodontic appliances with coffin spring

Coffin spring appliance or omega shaped wire appliance is capable of correcting crossbite in the young and developing dentition. Coffin spring produces slow and bilateral symmetrical expansion **(Fig. 40.23)**.

In mixed dentition, removable orthodontic appliance with Adam's clasps on first permanent molars of right and left side with coffin spring brings about skeletal change for the correction of posterior crossbite.

### Quad Helix Appliance

Quad helix appliance may be removable when it is inserted into the welded lingual sheath on the palatal aspect of permanent molar band or fixed when it is soldered to the palatal aspect of the molar band, which can be used to correct the posterior crossbite involving single tooth or group of teeth **(Fig. 40.24)**.

Activation of Quad helix appliance is done by using a prong plier, which produces skeletal changes in the preadolescents and slowly expands dental arches in adolescents and adults.

### Fixed orthodontic appliances with cross elastics

Fixed orthodontic appliances with cross elastics can be used to treat posterior crossbite involving single tooth or group of teeth. Cross elastic is stretched from palatal surface of maxillary posterior teeth to the buccal surface of the mandibular teeth. Here, cross elastics is stretched from lingual button or lingual attachment, welded or soldered on the palatal aspect of maxillary tooth in crossbite to the bracket tube on buccal surface of the mandibular tooth. These appliances are used to correct single tooth crossbite

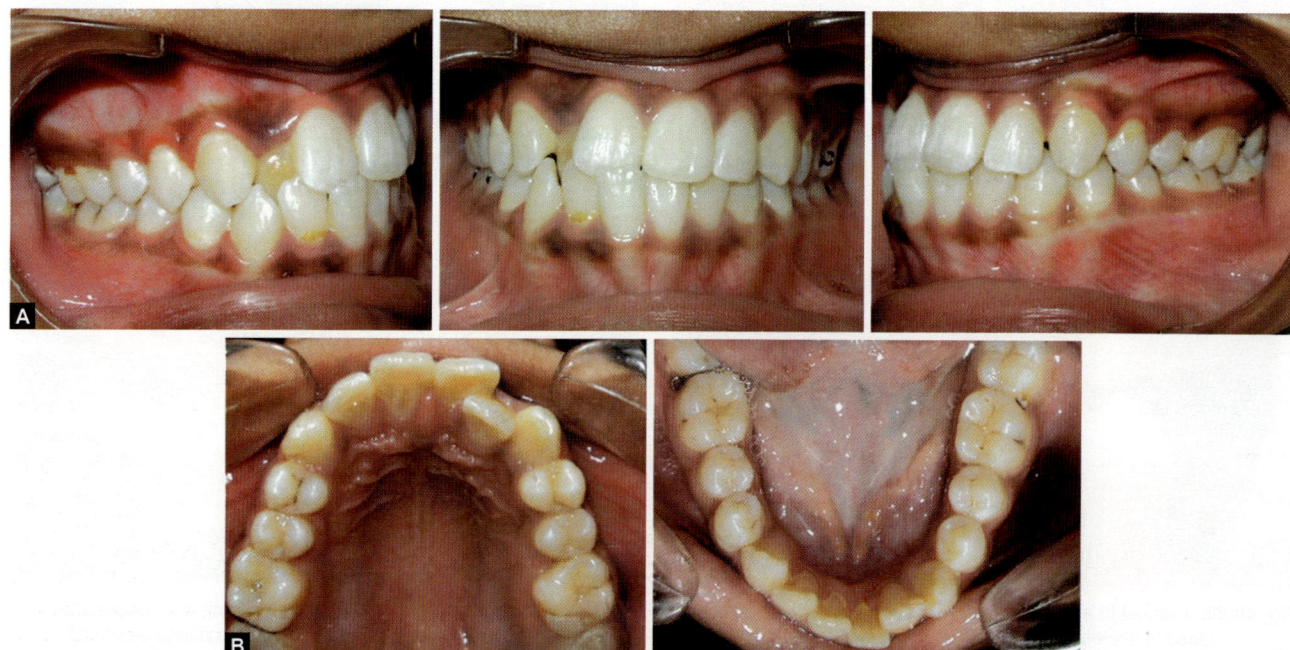

**Fig. 40.22A:** Pretreatment intraoral photographs (Right lateral, frontal and left lateral) of single tooth cross bite;
**Fig. 40.22B:** Intraoral occlusal photograph

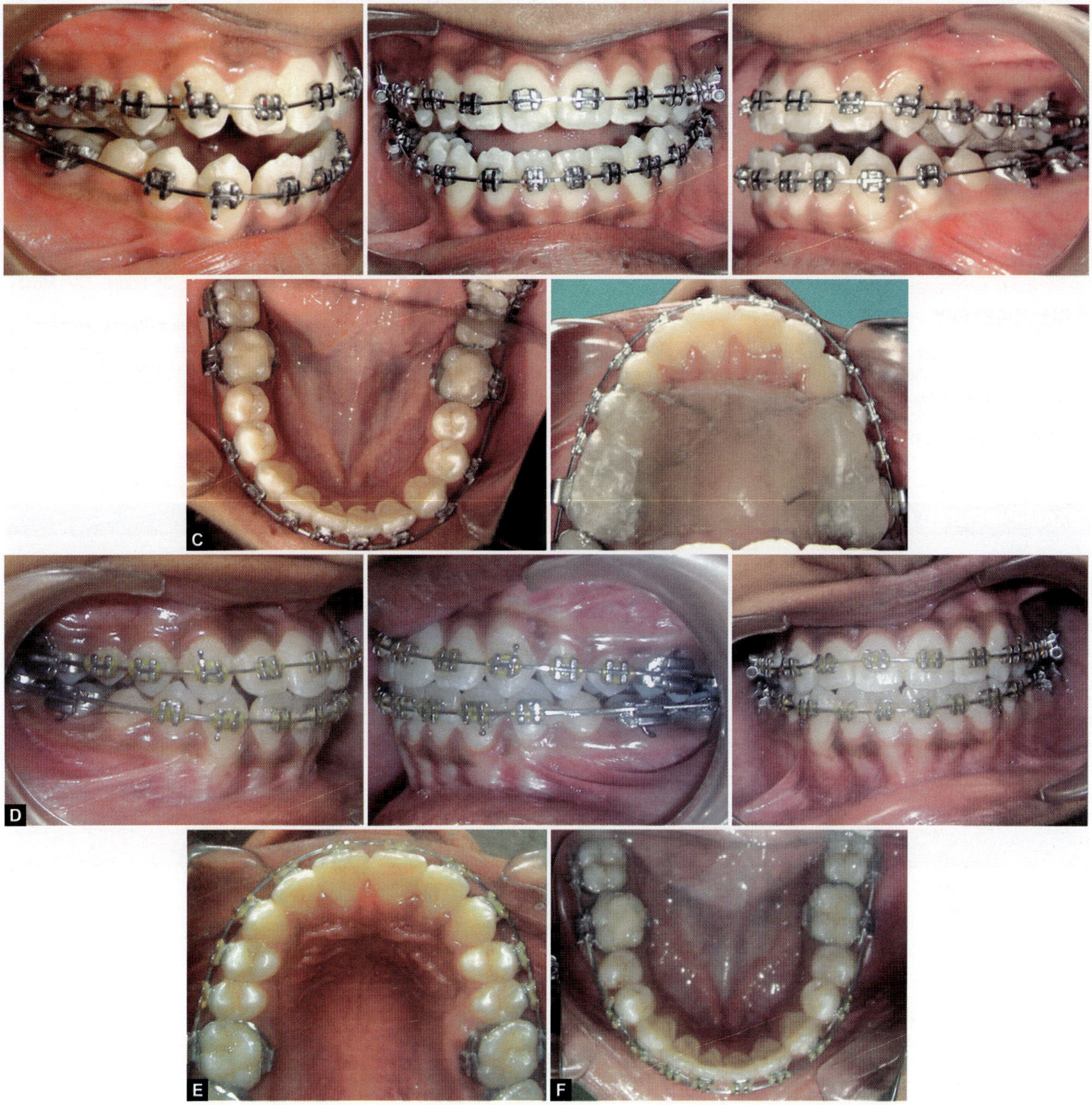

**Figs 40.22C and D:** Fixed orthodontic appliance with posterior maxillary bite plane, during treatment; **Fig. 40.22E and F:** After correction of crossbite
**Figs 40.22A to F:** Fixed orthodontic appliances can be used to correct anterior crossbite involving single tooth

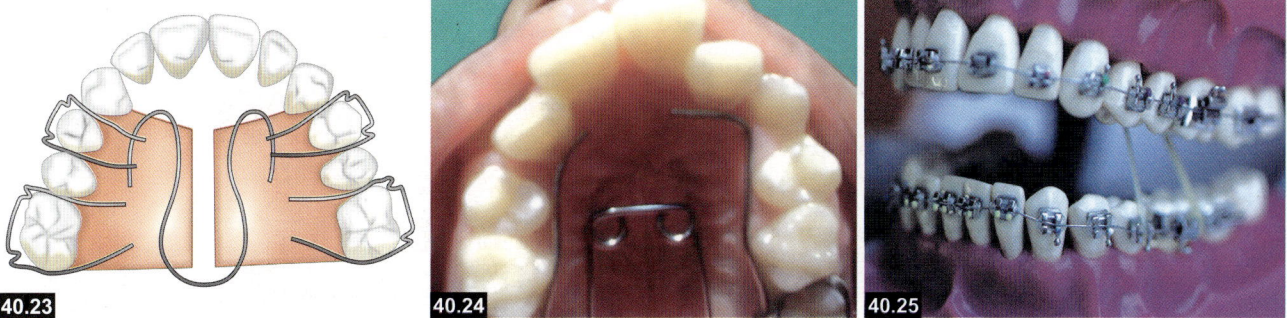

**Fig. 40.23:** Removable orthodontic appliances with coffin spring. Coffin spring corrects crossbite by producing slow and bilateral symmetrical expansion; **Fig. 40.24:** Fixed quad helix appliance; **Fig. 40.25:** Fixed orthodontic appliances with cross elastics for the correction of segmental posterior teeth crossbite. Cross elastic is stretched from palatal surface of maxillary posterior teeth to the buccal surface of the mandibular teeth

by buccal movement of maxillary tooth and the lingual movement of the mandibular tooth.

### Segmental Teeth Posterior Crossbite

Here fixed orthodontic appliance with cross elastics is stretched from lingual attachment, which involves the maxillary posterior teeth and welded buccal tube on the molar band. The bracket on involved teeth in the crossbite is used to correct the segmental tooth posterior crossbite by buccal movement of maxillary posterior teeth and lingual movement of mandibular teeth **(Fig. 40.25)**.

## BIBLIOGRAPHY

1. Bell RA. A review of maxillary expansion in relation to rate of expansion and patient's age. Am J Orthod. 1982;81(1):32-7.
2. Bell RA, Lecompte EJ. The effect of maxillary expansion using a quad-helix appliance during the deciduous and mixed dentitions. Am J Orthod. 1981;79(2):152-61.
3. Graber M, Vanarsdall L. Orthodontic Current Principles and Techniques. Mosby Year Book Inc., 1994.
4. Graber TM. Orthodontics: Principles and Practice. WB Saunders, 1988.
5. Haas AJ. Palatal expansion: Just the beginning of dentofacial orthopedics. Am J Orthod. 1970;57(3):219-55.
6. Hass AJ. Rapid expansion of the maxillary dental arch and the nasal cavity by opening the mid palatal suture. Angle Orthod. 1961;31:73-90.
7. Hass AJ. Rapid expansion: just the beginning of dentofacial orthopedics. Am J Orthod. 1970;219-55.
8. Raymond P Howe. Palatal expansion using a bonded appliance. Am J Orthod 1982;464-8.
9. Profitt WR. Contemporary Orthodontics. St Louis: CV Mosbj, 1986.
10. Robert E Moyers. Hand Book of Orthodontics. Year Book Medical Publishers, Inc, 1988.
11. Urbaniak, Brantley, Pruhs, Zussman, and Post. In vitro force delivery of quad-helix appliance. Am J Orthod 1988; 311-6.

---

### EXAM-ORIENTED QUESTIONS

**Long Note**

1. Management of crossbite.

**Short Notes**

1. Catalan's appliance
2. Management of Functional crossbite
3. Tongue blade therapy
4. FR III in management of cross bite
5. Enumerate and write in brief removable orthodontic appliances used in the treatment of crossbite.

---

## CHAPTER OVERVIEW

- **Management of cross bite**
  - **Anterior cross bite**
    - Developing anterior cross bite
      - Tongue blade therapy
      - Lower inclined plane therapy
    - Anterior cross bite
      - Z spring with posterior bite planes
      - Telescopic expansion screw
      - Segmental expansion with poster bite plane
      - Multilooped arch wire with fixed appliances
  - **Posterior cross bite**
    - Single tooth posterior cross bite
      - Cross elastics
      - Sectional fixed appliances
      - Removable orthodontic appliance with expansion screw
    - Unilateral posterior cross bite
      - Removable appliance with unilateral screw
      - Fixed orthodontic appliances
    - Bilateral posterior cross bite
      - Coffin spring
      - Quad helix
      - Hyrax
      - Symmetrical expansion screw

# CHAPTER 41
# Management of Cleft Lip and Palate

*Naik P, Phulari BS*

The word 'cleft' literally means a crack, split or a gap. Orofacial clefts are congenital deformities, which manifest at birth. Cleft lip and cleft palate are the most common congenital malformations of the head and neck region. The term cleft lip and cleft palate are commonly used to represent the following two types of malformation which are embryologically distinct:
1. Cleft lip with or without associated cleft palate (CL ± CP) **(Fig. 41.1A** and **B)**.
2. Isolated cleft palate (CP) **(Fig. 41.2)**.

The term harelip is often used to denote cleft lip. Cleft lip and cleft palate exhibit wide range of presentation with varying degrees of severity; from a small notch in the lip vermillion to a complete bilateral cleft lip and cleft palate. Cleft may occur in isolation or as a part of syndrome.

Management of these patients is quite challenging since cleft lip and cleft palate are usually associated with impaired facial appearance, speech, hearing, mastication, deglutition, dental occlusion and treatment should address these problems. Thus, management of cleft lip and cleft palate requires a multidisciplinary approach with a long-term treatment plan and individualized rehabilitation program designed to address the treatment of the patients. Malocclusion is usually present and an orthodontic therapy with or without corrective jaw surgery is frequently indicated.

The defects generally have profound psychosocial implications on the afflicted children and their parents. It is reassuring that with a team approach, the defects are fairly correctable and need not adversely affect the child's future.

## DEMOGRAPHIC DATA

### Race

The reported incidence of cleft lip and palate varies from 1 in 500 to 1 in 2500 live births depending on geographic origin, racial and ethnic backgrounds. The incidence of cleft lip and palate is reported to be highest in Asians (Mongoloids—1 in 500), intermediate in Caucasians and least in Negroid populations (1 in 2000 to 2500).
- Jones C (2000) estimated the occurrence of oral clefts in UK to be 1 in 700 births.
- Fough-Anderson (1956) cited 1 in 665 as incidence of cleft lip and palate in Denmark.
- Overall incidence of cleft lip and palate in human appears to be 1 in 700 live births.

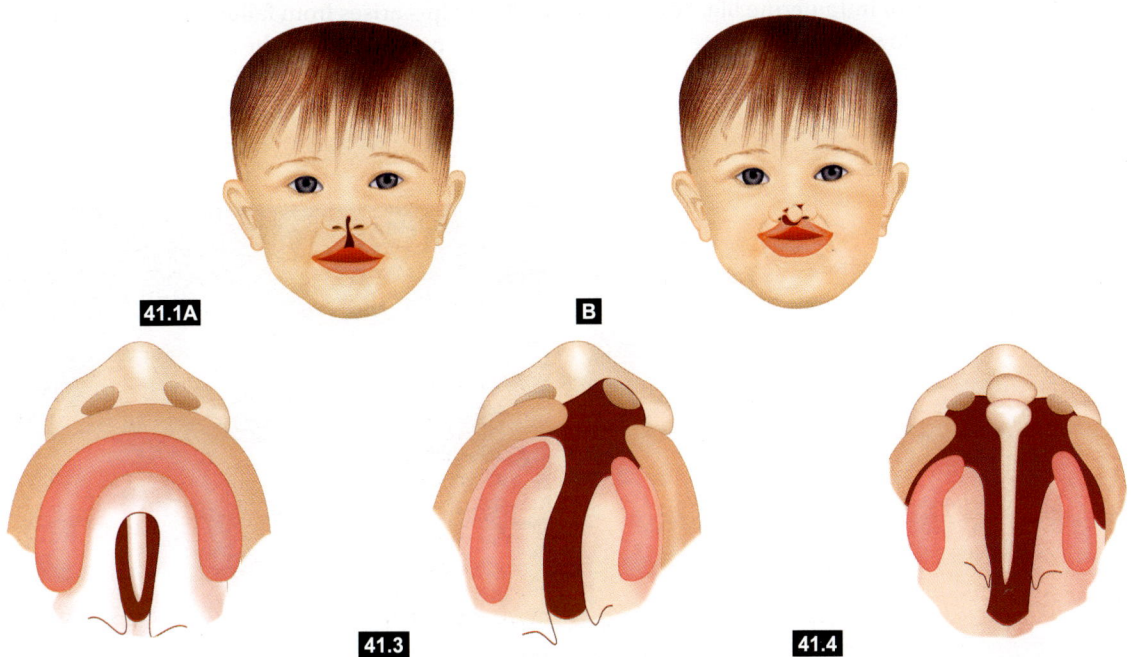

**Figs 41.1A and B:** Cleft lip and cleft palate; (A) Unilateral cleft lip; (B) Bilateral cleft lip;
**Fig. 41.2:** Isolated cleft palate; **Fig. 41.3:** Unilateral cleft lip with cleft palates; **Fig. 41.4:** Bilateral cleft lip with cleft palate

### Sex

Males are more commonly affected by orofacial clefts than females by a ratio of 3:2.

Cleft lip with or without cleft palate is more common in males than in females (2:1), whereas isolated cleft palate is observed to be more common in females.

### Type and Side

- Cleft lip with or without cleft palate is more common than isolated cleft palate.
- Unilateral clefts are more common as compared to that of bilateral clefts **(Figs 41.3 and 41.4)**.
- Unilateral clefts account for 75% of all clefts seen, while bilateral clefts account for the remaining 25%.
- In cases of unilateral clefts, left side **(Figs 41.5 and 41.6)** is more commonly affected than the right side. The reason why left side is more frequently involved is still unknown.

### Syndromic and Nonsyndromic

As stated earlier, orofacial clefts can occur alone (nonsyndromic) or as part of syndrome with congenital deformities of other parts of the body (syndromic). Over 300 syndromes are known to be associated with orofacial clefts. However, clefting syndromes are rare and make up only 5% of all clefts.

## EMBRYOLOGICAL ASPECTS

An understanding of the embryological development of these structures is essential so as to appreciate the etiology of these clefts.

The embryonic development of palate takes place between 6th and 9th weeks of intrauterine life. The entire palate develops from the following two structures:
- Primary palate (premaxilla)
- Secondary palate.

### Primary Palate

- The primary palate is the triangular shaped part of the palate anterior to the incisive foramen. It is developed from frontonasal process by fusion of two medial nasal processes; primary palate forms the premaxilla which carries the incisor teeth.

### Secondary Palate

- The secondary palate gives rise to the hard and soft palates posterior to the incisive foramen. It develops from the fusion of the following three parts:
- Two palatine shelves, which extend from left and right maxillary process toward the midline.
- Nasal septum which grows downward from the frontonasal process along the midline.

After the descent of the tongue, the elongated palatine shelves become horizontally oriented and are in close proximity to each other by 8th week. They fuse with each other in the midline and is represented by the median palatine raphe. The palatine shelves also fuse with primary palate and the nasal septum.

Incisive foramen is present at the junction of primary and secondary palates. Fusion between palatine shelves and nasal septum proceeds from incisive foramen in a posterior direction ending at uvula; whereas, fusion between the primary palate and the anterior borders of the palatine shelves progress in an anterior direction toward the lip.

### Cleft Lip and Palate Formation

Cleft lip and palate occur when mesenchymal connective tissues from various embryological structures fail to merge with each other.
- Cleft lip—arises from failure of fusion between medial nasal processes and the maxillary process. It can be unilateral or bilateral; and can be extended into the alveolar process (CL ± CP).

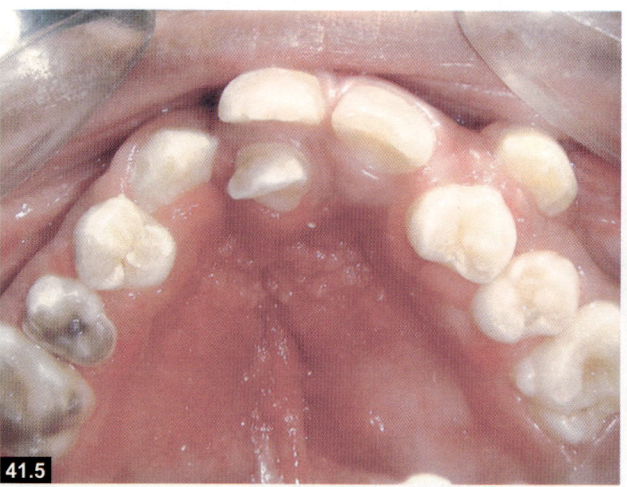
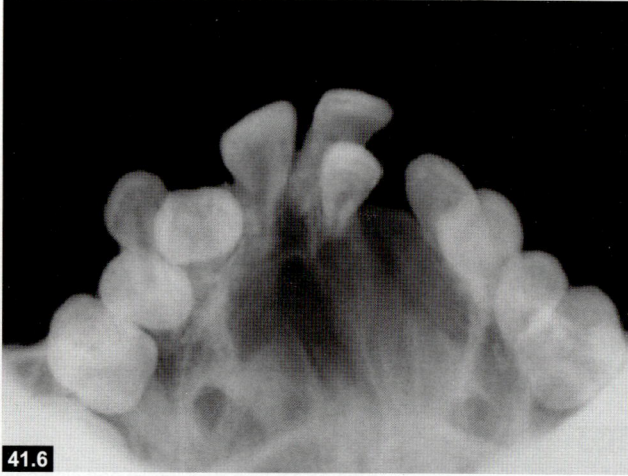

**Fig. 41.5:** Intraoral occlusal view showing unilateral cleft palates on left side; **Fig. 41.6:** Occlusal radiograph of the same patient

- Cleft palate—arises from failure of palatine shelves to fuse with each other, or with the nasal septum or with the primary palate.

## CLASSIFICATION

There are many classifications of clefts. Few commonly used ones are given below:

### Embryologic Classification

Patients with cleft lip and palate can be divided into two groups which are embryologically distinct.
1. Cleft lip with or without cleft palate (CL ± CP)
   Include:
   - Patients with cleft lip and cleft palate (CL ± CP)
   - Patients with cleft lip without cleft palate (CL)
2. Isolated cleft palate (CP)
   Include: Patient with cleft palate alone.

### Classification by the International Confederation for Plastic and Reconstructive Surgery (1968)

This classification has the following three main groups:
**Group 1:** Cleft of anterior primary palate:
a. Lip:
   - Right side
   - Left side
   - Both
b. Alveolus:
   - Right side
   - Left side
   - Both

**Group 2:** Clefts of anterior and posterior palate:
a. Lip:
   - Right side
   - Left side
   - Both
b. Alveolus:
   - Right side
   - Left side
   - Both
c. Hard palate:
   - Right side
   - Left side
   - Both

**Group 3:** Clefts of posterior secondary palate:
a. Hard palate:
   - Right
   - Left
b. Soft palate: Median

### Veau's Classification

This classification is morphological and described as four types of clefts:
**Group I:** Clefts of the soft palate only.
**Group II:** Clefts of the hard and soft palates extending up to the incisive foramen (**Fig. 41.2**).
**Group III:** Complete unilateral clefts involving the soft palate, hard palate, alveolar ridge and the lip on one side.
**Group IV:** Complete bilateral clefts of the soft and hard palates, alveolar ridge and the lip.

### Kernahan's Stripped 'Y' Classification

Kernahan proposed a symbolic classification of cleft lip and palate deformity using a stripped 'Y' having numbered blocks. The incisive foramen is symbolically represented by a small circle with the dividing points between the primary and the secondary palates (**Fig. 41.7**).

Each right and left limb is divided into three portions representing respectively the lip, alveolus and area between alveolus and incisive foramen. The stem of the Y is similarly divided into three portions representing hard palate and soft palate. Each block represents a specific area of the oral cavity:

| Block 1 and 4 | - lip |
| Block 2 and 5 | - alveolus |
| Block 3 and 6 | - hard palate anterior to the incisive foramen |
| Block 7 and 8 | - hard palate posterior to the incisive foramen |
| Block 9 | - soft palate |

Each individual can diagrammatically be represented by stippling appropriate areas of clefting. In submucous cleft of palate, the appropriate section is cross hatched.

## ETIOLOGY OF CLEFT LIP AND PALATE

Despite numerous clinical and experimental investigations, the etiology of cleft lip and palate in humans is still largely unknown. In most cleft cases, no single factor can be identified as the cause. Heredity with superimposed environmental factors is considered to be the most probable cause of cleft formation.

It is important here to distinguish between two forms of clefts—Nonsyndromic clefts with no other related health problem and syndromic clefts associated with other birth disorders or syndromes.

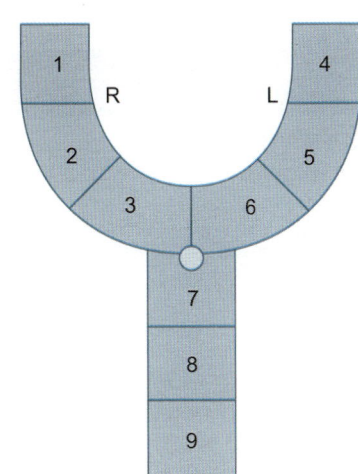

**Fig. 41.7:** Kernahan's stripped 'Y' classification

### Syndromic Cleft Cases

In syndromic cases, cleft occurs by monogenic mode of transmission, i.e. by a single mutant gene producing a large effect. Over 300 syndromes have been reported in the literatures which have associated clefts along with other defects. Most of these syndromes are rare. Some of the relatively common syndromes associated with cleft lip and palate are listed in **Box 41.1**.

Velocardiofacial syndrome (velum = palate, cardia = heart, facies = face) is the most common syndrome to exhibit clefts. The features include the following:
- Cleft palate
- Cardiac defects
- Characteristic facial appearance
- Learning problems and speech
- Feeding problems

### Non-syndromic Clefts

Recent investigations show that both heredity and environmental factors act together in causation of non-syndromic clefts. Such a mode of transmission of a defect/trait caused by interaction of multiple genes and multiple environmental factors is known as multifactorial inheritance.

### Heredity (Genetic Predisposition)

In contrast to syndromic clefts caused by single mutant gene, clefts in non-syndromic patients are caused by multiple genes (polygenic), each producing small effects which together create this condition.

Every individual carries some genetic liability for clefting, but there is no cleft formation until the threshold level for expression is reached. When the total genetic liability of an individual reaches a certain level, the threshold for expression is reached and cleft occurs.

Genetic basis of cleft lip and palate is significant but not predictable. Studies reveal that less than 40% of cleft lip with or without cleft palate is genetic in origin; less than 20% of isolated cleft palates (CP) are genetically determined.

---

**Box 41.1:** Common syndromes associated with cleft lip and palate

*Craniofacial Syndromes*
- Velocardiofacial syndrome
- Apert's syndrome
- Crouzon's syndrome
- Carpenter's syndrome
- Down syndrome
- Encephalocele
- Goldenhar syndrome
- Hypertelorism
- Pfeiffer syndrome
- Pierre Robin syndrome
- Saethre-Chotzen syndrome
- Treacher Collins syndrome
- van der Woude's syndrome

---

### Environmental Factors

Earlier, heredity was thought be single most important causative factor. However, recent studies have shown that, environmental factors play a significant contributory role at the critical time of embryogenic development when lip and palatal shelves are fusing.

A number of environmental factors have been suggested as causative factors including:
- A defective vascular supply to the area involved during critical time of embryonic development.
- A mechanical disturbance in which size of the tongue may prevent union of parts.
- Excessive concentration of circulating substances such as alcohol, certain drugs (antibiotics, steroids, insulin) and toxins.
- Viral infections.
- Exposure to radiation.
- Hypoxia.
- Vitamin deficiencies.
- Stress.

### Risk of Producing a Child with Cleft Deformity

- Every parent has approximately 1 in 700 risk of having a child with a cleft.
- Parents having a child with a cleft have increased risk of having the 2nd child affected—2–5%.
- If more than one person in immediate family has a cleft—risk rises to 10–12%.
- A parent having a cleft—has 2–5% chance of having a child with a cleft.
- If a syndrome is involved, the risk for recurrence within a family can be as high as 50%.
- Maternal age—increased risk of clefting is observed when age of conceiving is late.

## CLINICAL FEATURES

Oral clefts commonly affect the upper lip, alveolar ridge and hard and soft palates.
- The clefting anterior to the incisive foramen is defined as the cleft of primary palate.
- The clefting posterior to the incisive foramen is defined as a cleft of secondary palate.
- A patient may have clefting of primary palate, secondary palate or both.
- The clefts can be complete, i.e. extending the entire distance from the lip to the soft palate or incomplete.
- CL ± CP can be unilateral or bilateral; isolated cleft palate occurs in midline.
- Severity of CL ± CP may range from a small notch on the edge of the vermilion border to a wide cleft extending into the nasal cavity.
- Isolated cleft palate may also present with varying degrees of severity. Mildest form is the bifid uvula. A more severe form is a cleft of the soft palate. A complete cleft palate constitutes a cleft of the hard palate, soft palate and cleft uvula.

# CLEFT LIP AND PALATE ASSOCIATED PROBLEMS

Most patients with cleft lip and cleft palate (CL ± CP) and isolated cleft palate (CP) present with a myriad associated problems:
- Dental problems
- Occlusal problems (malocclusion and impaired facial esthetics)
- Feeding problems
- Nasal deformity
- Ear problems
- Speech difficulties
- Psychological problems.

## Dental Problems

Cleft involving alveolus often affects the development of primary and permanent teeth and the jaw. The cleft usually extends between the lateral incisor and the canine area. Teeth may be congenitally absent in the area of cleft or even supernumerary teeth may also be present. Teeth present near the region of cleft may morphologically be deformed or hypomineralized. Crowding or severe displacement of the teeth near the region is a common finding. The patient with cleft lip and palate may show the following features **(Figs 41.8A and B)**:
- Lateral incisor on the cleft side may be absent
- Presence of supernumerary teeth
- Fusion of teeth
- Enamel hypoplasia
- Multiple missing teeth
- Ectopically erupting teeth
- Anterior and/or posterior crossbite
- Periodontal complications
- Crowding may be seen
- Spacing may be present.

## Occlusal Problems

- Clefts involving alveolus and palate invariably show malocclusion. Patients with clefts, especially of the palate, show discrepancies in size, shape and position of their jaws **(Fig. 41.9)**.
- Most patients exhibit class III malocclusion with hypoplastic maxilla and relative prognathism of the mandible.
- Along with missing teeth or supernumerary teeth, retardation of maxillary growth significantly contributes to the development of malocclusion. Scar contracture following early closure of cleft palate significantly retards the growth and development of maxilla in all three planes of space. Narrow high arch palate with constricted and retruded maxilla is a common finding.
- Crowding in the arches
- Space presents between left permanent central incisor and left permanent lateral incisor
- Ectopic eruption of right second permanent premolar

## Feeding Problems

Structural defects of cleft lip and palate prevent negative oral pressure required for effective sucking. Feeding is a major problem in these patients as food and liquids regurgitate through the nose. Thus, breast or bottle feeding by sucking is difficult. However, babies can swallow normally, if they are fed directly toward the hypopharynx. The problem can

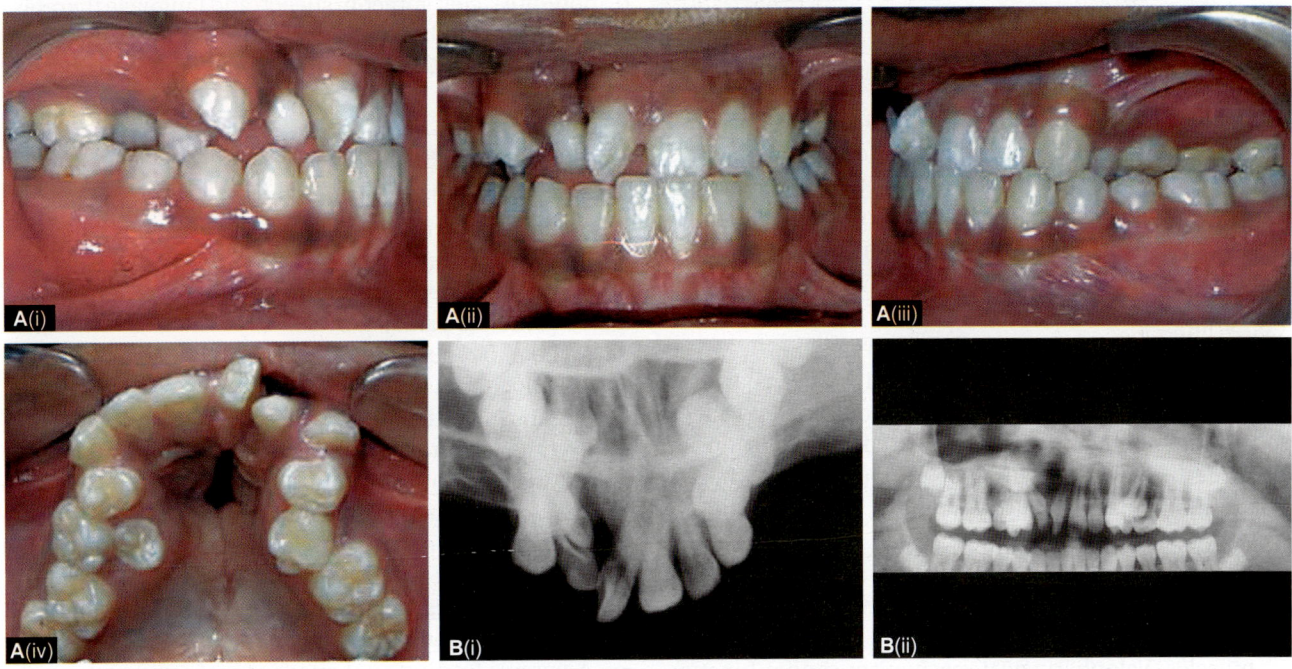

**Figs 41.8A and B:** (A) A patient with unilateral cleft palate on the left side associated with following dental problems: (B) OPG and occlusal radiographs of the same patient

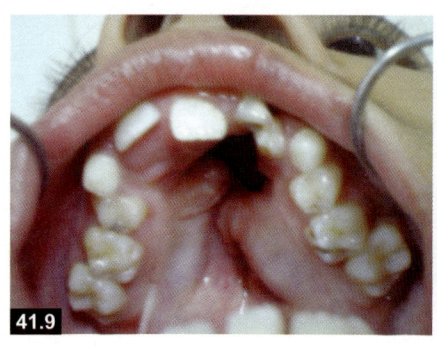 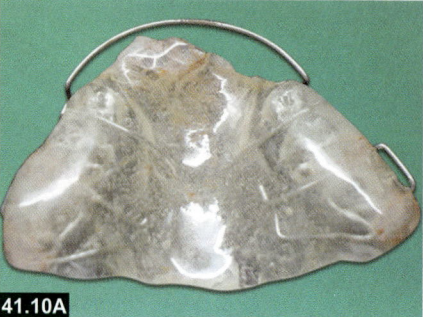 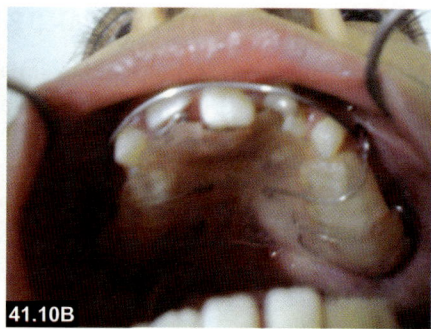

**Fig. 41.9:** Intraoral occlusal view showing unilateral cleft palate on the right side, crowding in the arch and high arch palate; **Figs 41.10A and B:** Obturator without wings used to cover the hard palate defect and a soft acrylic extension is used to cover the soft palate defects: (A) Obturator. (B) Obturator on patient

be overcome through the use of specially designed nipples that are elongated and have bigger opening which extend directly into the hypopharynx. Child may inhale a lot of air during swallowing and need frequent burping.

### Nasal Deformity

Patients with cleft lips often exhibit deformities of nasal architecture, especially when the cleft extends into the floor of the nose. Plastic surgery of nose is usually done at later stage and treatment after correction of all clefts and associated problems.

### Ear Problems

Clefts involving soft palate predispose to middle ear infections. This is because the levator and tensor veli palatine, the muscles of soft palate are left unattached in case of soft palate clefts. These muscles have their origins near the auditory tube and under normal circumstances allow opening of the auditory tube into the nasopharynx facilitating equilibrium and the pressure.

In palatine clefts this function is disrupted, the middle ear becomes a closed space without a drainage mechanism. When tube opening mechanism is impaired, there is greater susceptibility of middle ear infections. Accumulation of serious fluids and then bacteria can lead to serious otitis media. Chronic otitis media causes hearing impairment that is common in patients with cleft palate.

### Speech Difficulties

During normal speech, the tongue, lips, lower jaw and soft palate work together in a highly coordinated fashion to produce the sounds. The soft palate is raised during the speech, preventing air escape from the nose. The soft palate functions as a valve to control the distribution of escaping air between oropharynx and nasopharynx. This is called valopharyngeal mechanism (valo = soft palate).

During speech and deglutition, soft palate is elevated toward the posterior pharyngeal wall by contraction of its muscles. Valopharyngeal mechanism cannot function when a soft palate is involved by the cleft. The soft palate cannot elevate to make contact with the pharyngeal wall, and this results in escape of air into the nasal cavity producing hypernasal speech.

Hearing impairment may further aggravate the speech problem. Retardation of consonant sounds (e.g. p, b, t, d, k, g) is the most common problem. Speech problem should be addressed at the earliest, and several years of speech therapy may be needed to achieve intelligible speech.

### Psychosocial Problems

Impaired facial esthetics, hearing and speech problems often produce psychosocial problems in these patients. Support of the family, professional help and social worker are all necessary to the normal well-being of these patients.

## MANAGEMENT OF CLEFT LIP AND CLEFT PALATE

Management of cleft lip and cleft palate requires a team-based approach; main team members include orthodontist, cleft surgeon, speech and language therapist, ENT specialist. Other disciplines involved at various stages include health visitor, oral surgeon, restorative dentist and psychologist.

### Stages in the Management of Cleft Lip and Cleft Palate

*Stage 1:* Predental treatment/pre-surgical orthopedics: Predental treatment of cleft lip and palate helps:
- To facilitate feeding.
- To establish normal tongue posture.
- To stimulate palatal growth.
- To help to reduce the chances of ear infections.
- To guide tooth eruption.
- To reposition the premaxilla.
- To establish proper sutural growth pattern early when sutures are most responsive.

Presurgical orthopedic appliances:
- The aim of presurgical orthopedics to align the displaced cleft segments
- Lip repair is carried out at about 3 months and cleft palate is carried out at 9–18 months.
- A passive feeding appliance incorporated with acrylic or wire wings.

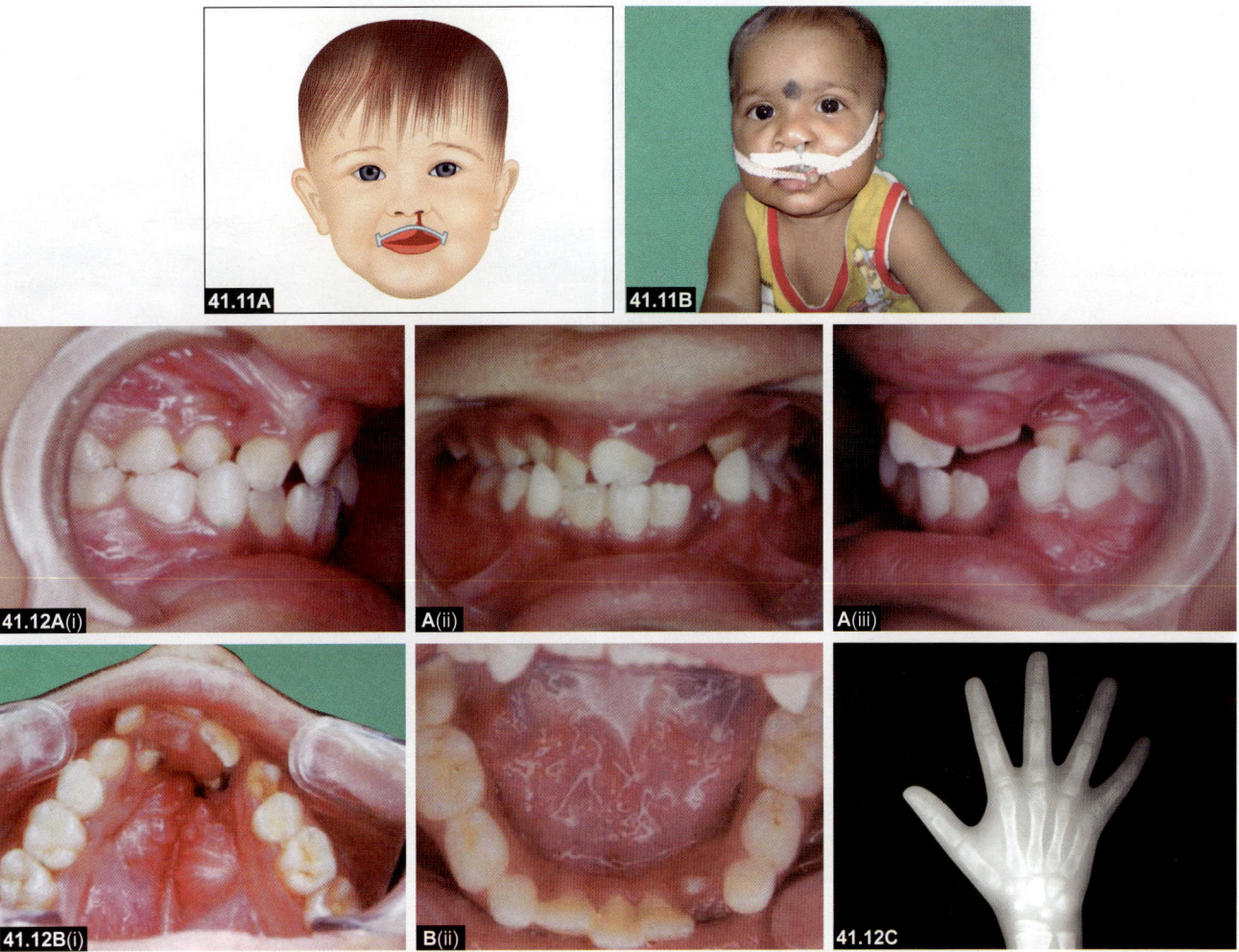

**Figs 41.11A and B:** Extraoral strapping [*Courtesy:* Dr Nikunj Patel MDS (Ortho)]; **Figs 41.12A to C:** (A) Intraoral pre-treatment photographs. i—Right lateral view, ii—Frontal view, iii—Left lateral view (B) Intraoral occlusal view of maxilla and mandibular arches (C) Hand-wrist radiograph

- Duyzing plate is used for patients with cleft lip hard and soft palates. Hard palate is blocked and a soft acrylic extension is used to cover the soft palate defects **(Figs 41.10A and B)**.
- **Extraoral strapping:** The main objective of the extraoral strapping is to reposition the premaxillary portion of jaw by means of pressure from extraoral strapping when an appliance is worn in the month **(Figs 41.11A and B)**.

***Stage 2:*** Treatment of cleft lip and cleft palate during deciduous dentition: Orthodontic treatment should not be undertaken because of its limited advantage at this stage.

***Stage 3:*** Treatment of cleft lip and cleft palate during mixed dentition:

*Treatment of cleft lip and cleft palate during early mixed dentition:* Permanent incisors may erupt into linguo-occlusion. This should be corrected if feasible but may be delayed until the next phase of development.

*Treatment of cleft lip and cleft palate during mid-mixed dentition:* If an alveolar cleft is evident, secondary alveolar bone graft is routinely performed at age 9–10 years. Cancellous bone from the iliac crest is placed in the alveolar cleft and it will:

- Facilitate eruption of the permanent canine.
- Allow alignment of teeth adjacent to the cleft.
- Promote orthodontic treatment rather than prosthodontic repair.
- Help to stabilize maxillary segments.
- Assist closure of fistulae.
- Improves vestibular anatomy.

***Stage 4:*** Treatment of cleft lip and cleft palate during permanent dentition:

- If the cleft lip and cleft palate are not associated with skeletal discrepancy, then conventional fixed mechanotherapy is carried out **(Figs 41.12A to H)**. A significant proportion of cleft cases will have a severe skeletal class III pattern, the full correction of which requires combined orthodontic treatment and orthognathic surgeries.
- Class III incisor relationship has to be corrected by fixed appliance to decompensate and coordinate the dental arches prior to orthognathic surgeries (Le Fort I osteotomy. Genioplasty may also be indicated).

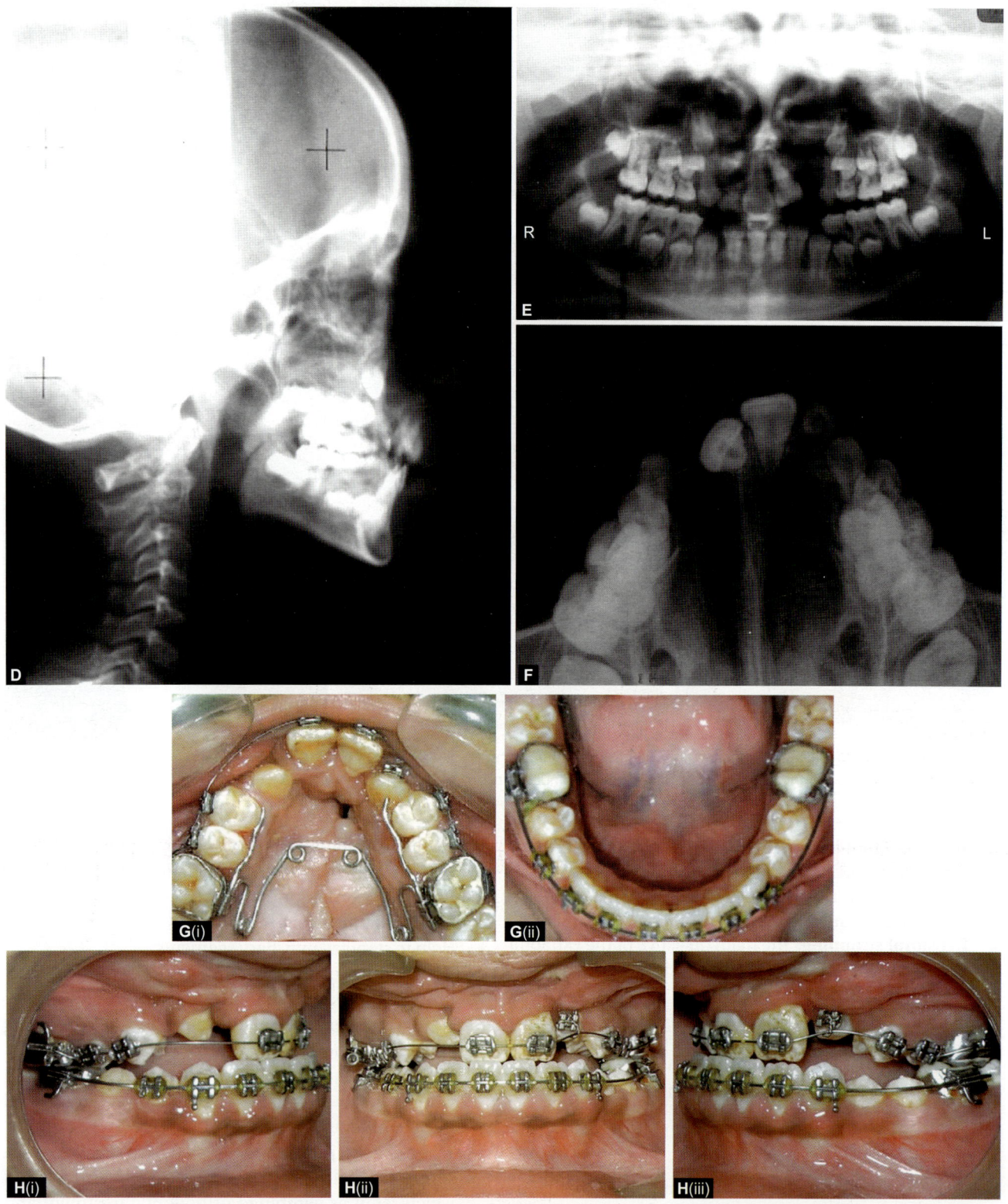

**Figs 41.12D to H:** (D) Lateral cephalogram; (E) OPG; (F) Occlusal radiograph; (G) Druing treatment with fixed straight wire appliance; (H) During treatment with fixed straight wire appliances (Management of a patient with cleft palate using fixed orthodontic appliances)

## BIBLIOGRAPHY

1. Andin-Sobocki, Eleasson, and Paulin. Bone grafting in patients with cleft lip and cleft palate. Am J Orthod. 1995;144-52.
2. Balkhi, Fadanelli, Subtelny. Treatment of bilateral cleft lip and palate. Am J Orthod. 1991;297-305.
3. Bergland O, Semb G, Abyholm FE. Elimination of the residual alveolar cleft by secondary bone grafting and subsequent orthodontic treatment. Cleft Palate J. 1986;23(3):175-205.
4. Bishara, Wilson, Perez, et al. Dentofacial findings in child with unrepaired median cleft of lip. Am J Orthod. 1985;157-62.
5. Boyne PJ, Sands NR. Combined orthodontic-surgical management of residual palato-alveolar cleft defects. Am J Orthod. 1976;70(1):20-37.
6. Cohen MM, Bankier A. Syndrome delineation involving orofacial clefting. Cleft Palate Craniofac J. 1991;28(1):119-20.
7. FitzPatrick DR, Raine PA, Boorman JG. Facial clefts in the west of Scotland in the period 1980-1984: Epidemiology and genetic diagnoses. J Med Genet. 1994;31(2):126-9.
8. James DR, Brook K. Maxillary hypoplasia in patients with cleft lip and palate deformity—The alternative surgical approach. Eur J Orthod. 1985;7(4):231-47.
9. Markus T, Booth PW. Managing cleft lip and palate. BMJ. 1995;311(7008):765-6.
10. Mars M, Asher-McDade C, Brattström V, et al. A six-center international study of treatment outcome in patients with clefts of the lip and palate: Part 3. Dental arch relationships. Cleft Palate Craniofac J. 1992;29(5):405-8.
11. Mars M, Plint DA, Houston WJ, et al. The Goslon Yardstick: A new system of assessing dental arch relationships in children with unilateral clefts of the lip and palate. Cleft Palate J. 1987;24(4):314-22.
12. Moyers RE. Handbook of Orthodontics. Year Book Medical Publishers, Inc, 1988.
13. Pigott RW. Organisation of cleft lip and palate services—results of a questionnaire. Br J Plast Surg. 1992;45(5):385-7.
14. Profitt WR. Contemporary Orthodontics. St Louis: CV Mosby, 1986.
15. Rosenstein. A new concept in the early orthopedic treatment of cleft lip and palate. Am J Orthod. 1969;219-29.
16. Sell D, Harding A, Grunwell P. A screening assessment of cleft palate speech (Great Ormond Street Speech Assessment). Eur J Disord Commun. 1994;29(1):1-15.
17. Shprintzen RJ, Golding-Kushner KJ. Evaluation of velopharyngeal insufficiency. Otolaryngol Clin North Am. 1989;22(3):519-36.
18. Ten cate AR. Oral Histology: Development Structure and Function. St Louis: CV Mosby; 1980.
19. Williams A, Shaw WC, Devlin HB. Provision of services for cleft lip and palate in England and Wales. BMJ. 1994;309(6968):1552.
20. Winters JC, Hurwitz DJ. Presurgical orthopedics in the surgical management of unilateral cleft lip and palate. Plast Reconstr Surg. 1995;95(4):755-64.
21. Witzel MA, Salyer KE, Ross RB. Delayed hard palate closure: The philosophy revisited. Cleft Palate J. 1984;21(4):263-9.

## EXAM-ORIENTED QUESTIONS

### Long Question
1. Classify cleft Lip and palate; describe the role of orthodontist in the treatment of the same.

### Short Questions
1. Classify cleft lip and palate
2. Obturators
3. Extraoral strapping
4. Kernahan's stripped 'Y' classification of cleft lip and palate.

## CHAPTER OVERVIEW

Management of cleft lip and palate

- **Stage 1–pre-surgical phase**
  - Lip repair–3 months
  - Cleft palate closure–9-18 months
  - Extra-oral strapping

- **Stage 2–management Of cleft lip and palate In deciduous dentition**
  - No any kind of orthodontic treatment is given during this stage because of limited Advantages

- **Stage 3–management of cleft lip and cleft palate in mixed dentition**
  - Early mixed dentition
    - Correction of permanent incisors
  - Mid mixed dentition period
    - Secondary alveolar bone graft is performed at age 9-10 years

- **Stage 4- management of cleft lip and cleft palate In permanent dentition**
  - Le-fort I osteotomy genioplasty

# CHAPTER 42

# Surgical Orthodontics

*Tsahannerr F, Zakaullah S, Phulari BS*

Oral and maxillofacial surgical procedures are sometimes necessary to optimize the results of orthodontic treatment. Surgical orthodontics encompasses all those surgical procedures that are carried out as an adjunct to, or in conjunction with orthodontic treatment. These procedures may range from minor surgeries, such as tooth extraction to major procedures such as orthognathic surgeries of maxilla and/or mandible.

In cases of crowding due to arch length tooth material discrepancy, it may be necessary to extract some teeth to obtain proper alignment of teeth. Unerupted teeth may require surgical exposure to facilitate bracket placement and their subsequent alignment. Adult patients with narrow maxilla may need surgically assisted rapid maxillary expansion to correct malocclusion in transverse plane.

Patients with significant skeletal discrepancies and dentofacial deformities cannot be treated satisfactorily by orthodontic management alone. In such cases surgical correction by means of orthognathic surgeries of maxilla and mandible may be indicated to obtain optimal occlusal and esthetics results. Adult patients with significant skeletal malocclusion in whom growth modification procedures cannot be carried out may also benefit from orthognathic surgery.

Children with congenital malformations, such as cleft lip and palate, often require surgical procedures along with orthodontic treatment for their rehabilitation.

In recent times new surgical approaches have been adapted in orthodontic management such as implant placement to gain anchorage and distraction osteogenesis for advancement of maxilla or mandible.

## SURGICAL ORTHODONTIC PROCEDURES

### Minor Procedures

A. Soft tissue procedures
   - Frenectomy
   - Circumferential supracrestal fibrotomy (pericision)
B. Dentoalveolar procedures
   - Tooth extraction for orthodontic treatment purposes
   - Surgical exposure of impacted teeth
   - Transplantation of teeth
   - Corticotomy.

### Major Procedures

- Orthognathic surgeries
- Surgically assisted rapid maxilla expansion
- Cosmetic surgeries
- Distraction osteogenesis
- Surgical procedures in the management of cleft lip and palate.

## MINOR SURGICAL PROCEDURES

### Soft Tissue Procedures

*Frenectomy*

Frenectomy is the surgical excision of frenum with its fibrous attachment. Frenectomy of maxillary labial and lingual frena may sometimes be indicated as explained below.

**Maxillary labial frenectomy**: A midline diastema between the maxillary central incisors can be associated with an abnormal maxillary labial frenum. Abnormal labial frenum is thick, fibrous tissue having its insertion into the palatal soft tissues lingual to the incisors (incisive papilla region) that may prevent approximation of the two maxillary central incisors, thereby causing diastema between these two teeth **(Fig. 42.1A)**.

Frenectomy **(Fig. 42.1B)** in such cases greatly increases the long-term stability of the orthodontic closure of midline diastema. However, other causes of midline diastema must be carefully ruled out before undertaking frenectomy procedure. Most clinicians advocate orthodontic closure of the diastema before frenectomy so that the scar tissue does not impede closure of the diastema.

Following points should be checked during frenectomy:
- The frenum should be completely excised up to the bone, rather than merely be "clipped".
- Any fibrous tissue attached palatally into the intermaxillary suture area should also be removed.

***Lingual frenectomy:*** An abnormal lingual frenum attachment consists of mucosa, dense fibrous tissue and sometimes superior fibers of the genioglossus muscle. Such abnormal attachment binds the top of the tongue to the posterior surface of the mandibular alveolar ridge and may restrict free movement of the tongue and thus may affect patient's phonetics. Such a condition is often referred to as "ankyloglossia" or "tongue tie" **(Fig. 42.2)**.

Frenectomy is indicated in such cases as the patient may also develop abnormal tongue behavior/tongue thrusting and can thus impede occlusal stability after orthodontic treatment.

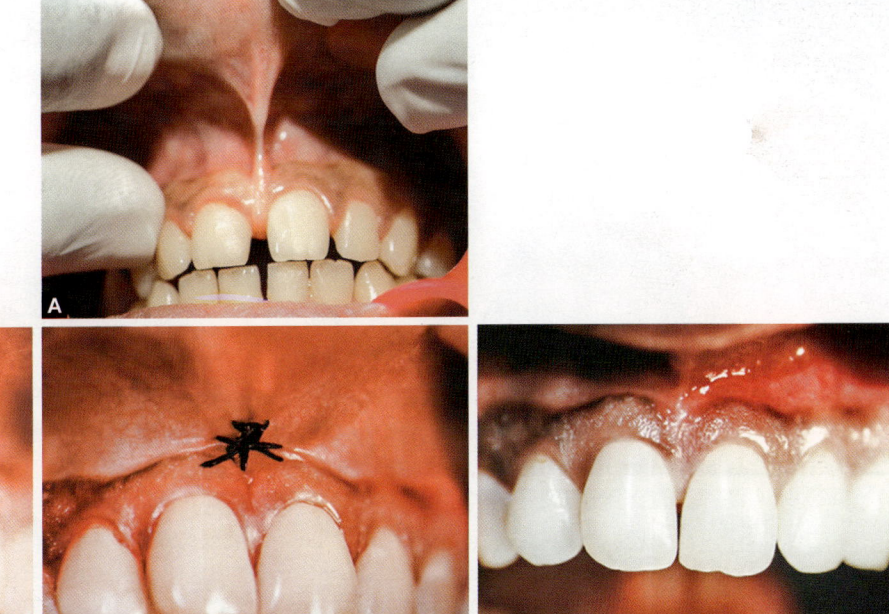

**Fig. 42.1A and B:** **(A)** Thick fibrous labial frenum attachment causing midline diastema; **(B)** Frenectomy

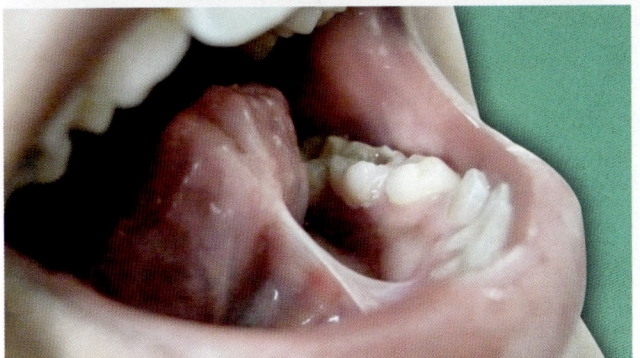

**Fig. 42.2:** Ankyloglossia (tongue tie)

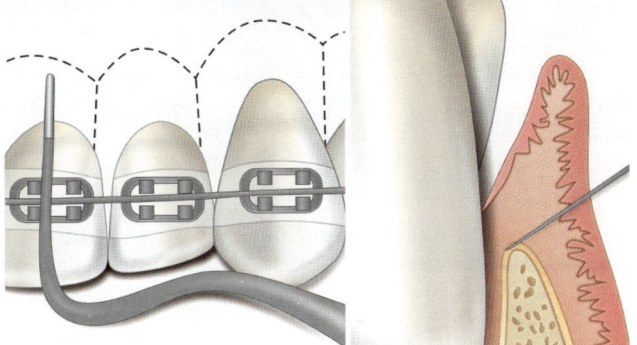

**Fig. 42.3:** Circumferential supracrestal fibrotomy (pericision)

### *Circumferential Supracrestal Fibrotomy (Pericision)*

Orthodontic correction of rotated teeth is associated with a high tendency of relapse due to the slow process of reorganization of the gingival and transseptal fibers. Surgical sectioning of these fibers, 'circumferential supracrestal fibrotomy' (pericision), when done following derotation, appears to be effective in reducing the relapse tendencies of the derotated teeth **(Fig. 42.3).**

### Dentoalveolar Procedures

### *Extraction of Teeth for Orthodontic Treatment Purposes*

Extraction of teeth may be indicated during orthodontic treatment in the following conditions:
- Therapeutic extraction of permanent teeth.
- Surgical removal of ankylosed primary teeth.
- Removal of retained primary teeth which may prevent or deflect the eruption path of succedaneous teeth.
- Removal of supernumerary teeth and odontomes which may impede the progress of orthodontic tooth movement.
- Serial extraction procedure.
- Extraction of impacted third molars.

**Therapeutic extraction of permanent teeth**: Some sound permanent teeth may have to be sacrificed to gain enough space for proper alignment of other teeth in cases of crowding. The choice of teeth to be sacrificed depends on the amount of arch length tooth material discrepancy which is determined by model analysis.

It is a common practice to remove first premolars or sometimes second premolars for therapeutic reasons.

**Surgical removal of ankylosed primary teeth**: Ankylosed primary teeth may prevent eruption of their successors. They may need surgical extraction as the roots are directly fused with the underlying bone.

**Removal of retained primary teeth**: Prolonged retention of the primary teeth may delay the eruption or may even deflect the eruption pathway of their successors. Maxillary permanent canines are often observed to erupt labially or lingually due to retained primary canines **(Figs 42.4).** Such retained primary teeth have to be extracted during orthodontic therapy.

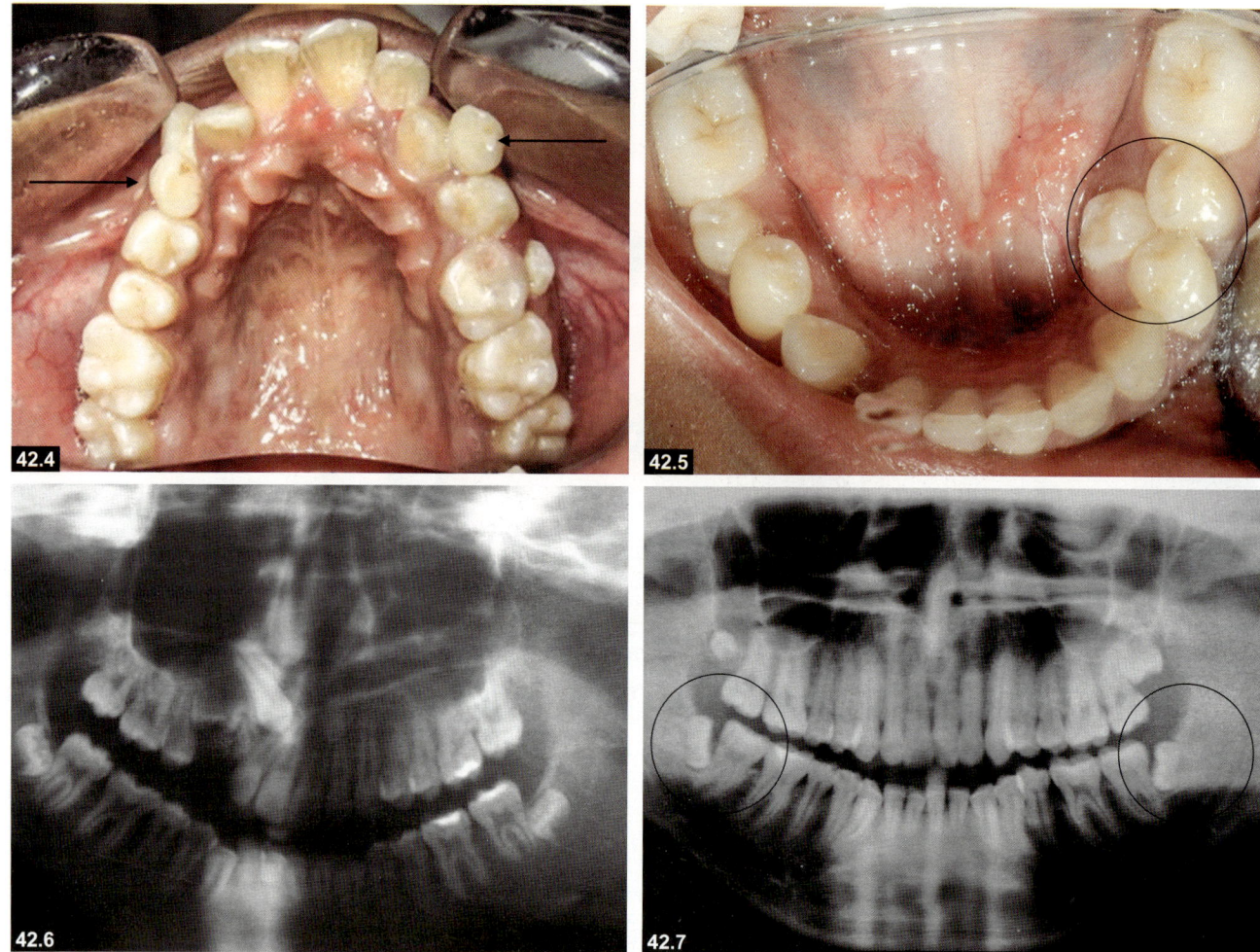

**Fig. 42.4:** Retained primary canines deflecting the permanent successors indicated for extraction; **Fig. 42.5:** Supernumerary premolars causing crowding in the arch; **Fig. 42.6:** Compound odontome preventing eruption of maxillary canine and first premolar; **Fig. 42.7:** Impacted third molars

**Removal of supernumerary teeth and odontomes:** Presence of supernumerary teeth and odontomes may be causing certain malocclusions and may impede the progress of orthodontic tooth movement and thus have to be removed. Mesiodens when erupted may deflect the erupting central incisors while impacted mesiodens may cause midline diastema. Supernumerary premolars can cause crowding in the arch **(Fig. 42.5).**

**Compound odontomes** often occur in the anterior region and may prevent eruption of canines and other adjacent teeth **(Fig. 42.6).** Impacted canines need to bring to occlusion after removal of odontomes.

**Serial extraction:** Serial extraction is an interceptive procedure which involves removal of certain deciduous teeth followed by specific permanent teeth in an orderly sequence so as to guide the rest of the permanent teeth into a favorable position. It is usually done in mixed dentition and may not require orthodontic treatment in future or the treatment period may get shortened.

***Extraction of third molars:*** Third molars are the most commonly impacted teeth, as few individuals have adequate arch length for proper eruption and long-term maintenance of all third molars **(Fig. 42.7).** They often get completely or partially impacted and thus less likely to become fully functional.

Some orthodontists advocate prophylactic removal of third molar germs at an early stage of development. They believe that crowding of lower anterior is caused by ineffectual attempts of impacted mandibular third molars to erupt. Whether impacted third molars contribute to the relapse of anterior mandibular crowding has been a matter of controversy in orthodontics. Some orthodontist's advice removal of third molars at the end of orthodontic treatment when retainers are being placed.

### Exposure of Impacted Teeth

The most common teeth to be impacted other than the third molars are the maxillary canines followed by premolars and maxillary second molars. Other teeth may also be impacted although less common and need surgical exposure during orthodontic treatment for their proper alignment.

**Radiographic location**: Precise radiographic location of the impacted tooth is necessary to plan the surgical approach. For example, maxillary canine may be impacted labially/lingually and needs to be located precisely before undertaking the procedure. The tooth is usually located by referring two radiographs taken at different angles (SLOB rule) or by using more than one radiographic technique (one IOPA view and one occlusal view).

**Surgical exposure of the tooth**: The crown of the impacted tooth is exposed by excision of the overlying soft tissue and careful removal the bone covering the crown.

Once the tooth is exposed a bondable bracket with an attached chain or ligature is placed on the exposed surface of the tooth. Orthodontic forces can then be applied to the tooth with the help of these attachments and the tooth is brought into the line of occlusion **(Figs 42.8 to 42.10)**.

### Transplantation of Teeth

Teeth can be transplanted from one position to another in the dental arch. This may particularly be useful in patients with several missing teeth. Transplantation of misplaced/impacted teeth into a desirable position in the arch may be a good alternative for an adult patient who cannot undergo conventional orthodontic movement of an impacted tooth.

The technique involves careful wide exposure of the impacted tooth and its subsequent movement into its position within the dental arch. The transposed tooth is stabilized with a segmental orthodontic appliance. The tooth may be treated endodontically at a later stage, if needed.

### Corticotomy

Corticotomy is sometimes undertaken in patients having dental proclination with spacing. Such a procedure can hasten the orthodontic tooth movement, and duration of the appliance therapy can be shortened.

The technique involves the sectioning of the dentoalveolar region into multiple small units. Labial and palatal flaps are raised and vertical cuts of predetermined width are made on either side of each tooth parallel and away from the roots **(Fig. 42.11)**. The apical ends of these cuts are joined by a horizontal cut made only through the compact bone having the cancellous bony support of the teeth. Flaps are replaced and sutured.

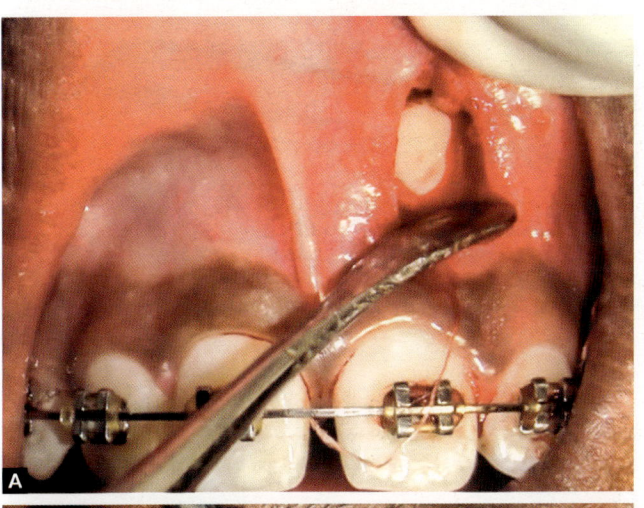
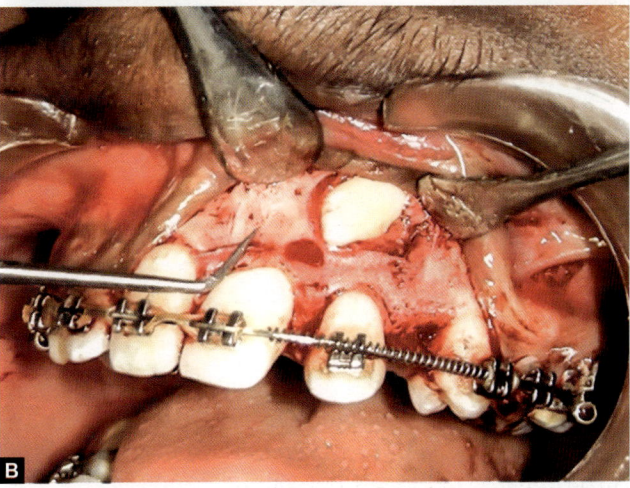

**Figs 42.8A and B:** Surgical exposure of impacted maxillary canine. Bondable bracket is attached on the exposed surface of the impacted tooth and is pulled toward occlusion using a ligature wire;

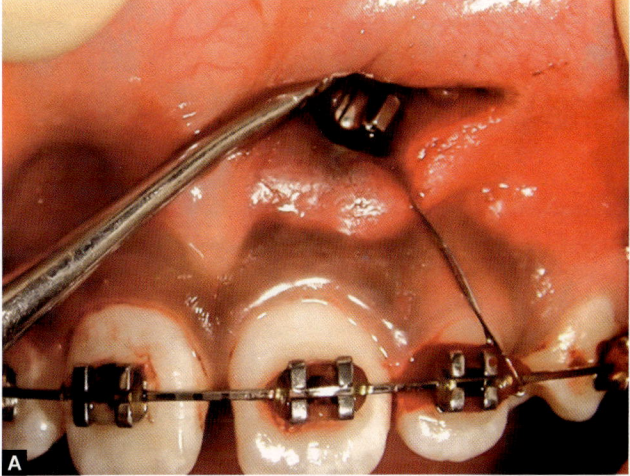
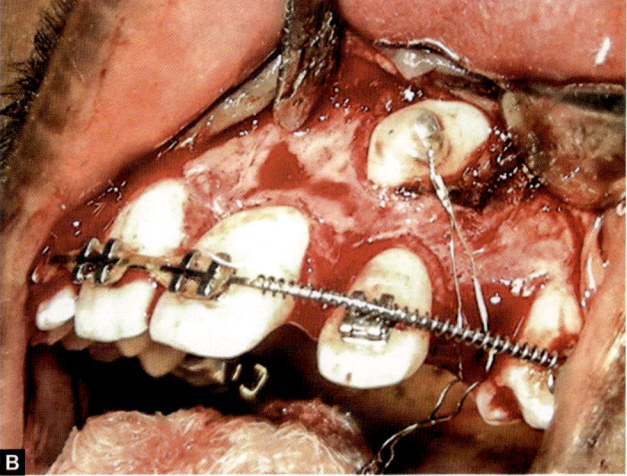

**Figs 42.9A and B:** Another case of impacted maxillary canine surgically exposed. A bondable lingual button is attached to the exposed surface of the tooth and occlusal force is applied using a ligature wire

Fixed orthodontic appliance can be fitted after 2–3 days and the tooth movement rapidly occurs. Retention period of 6 months is usually required to stabilize the result.

## MAJOR PROCEDURES

### Orthognathic Surgeries

Dentofacial deformities may occur due to hereditary, congenital, developmental or acquired causes. Dental camouflage with orthodontic tooth movement may be sufficient to improve facial esthetics in cases of mild skeletal discrepancy. However, patients with severe dentofacial deformities require orthodontic alignment as well as surgical movement of one or both jaws to achieve acceptable occlusion and facial esthetics.

Patients with facial discrepancies are best managed by a team approach including oral and maxillofacial surgeon, orthodontist, periodontist and restorative dentist. This integrated approach should be used throughout the evaluation, presurgical and post-surgical phases of patient care to obtain the best possible results for these patients.

### Timing and Rationale of Orthognathic Surgery

Orthodontic treatment alone may be sufficient when the skeletal discrepancy is minimal and orthodontic compensation does not adversely affect dental or facial esthetics or the post-treatment stability.

However, surgery combined with orthodontic treatment is necessary in some cases with severe skeletal discrepancy and facial deformities where orthodontic movement alone cannot achieve adequate facial and dental esthetics.

In a growing child with a developing dentofacial deformity, growth modification with functional appliances may be the preferred line of treatment. Surgery is usually undertaken in patients who do not respond to growth modification. As a rule of thumb, orthognathic surgery should be delayed until growth is complete in patients who have problems of excess growth, although surgery can be considered earlier for patients with growth deficiencies.

### Steps in Orthognathic Surgery

Orthognathic surgery requires thorough patient evaluation and methodical treatment planning. The following are the sequential steps involved in orthognathic surgery:

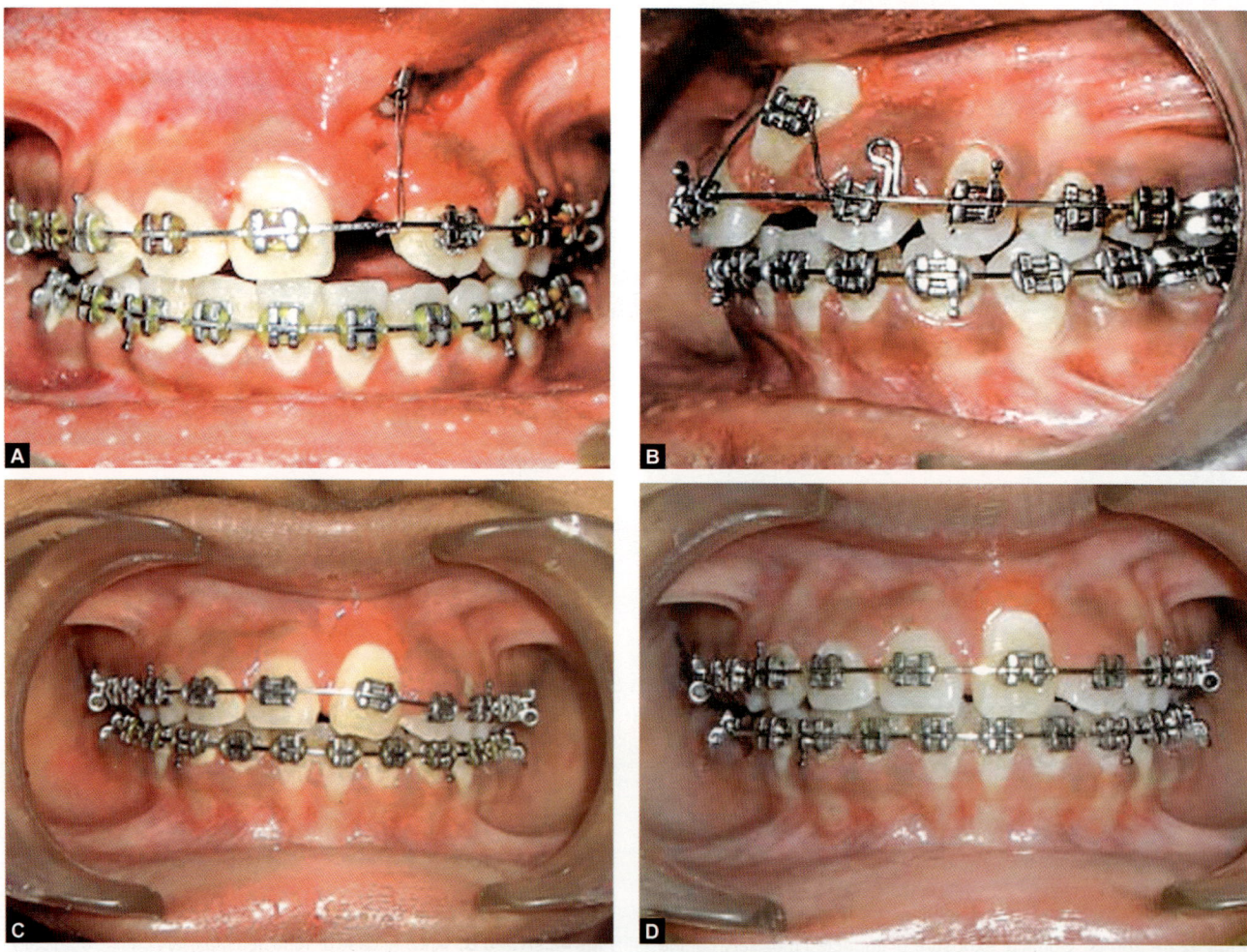

**Figs 42.10A to D:** Surgical exposure of impacted maxillary central incisor. After surgical exposure the tooth is brought to occlusion using attachments

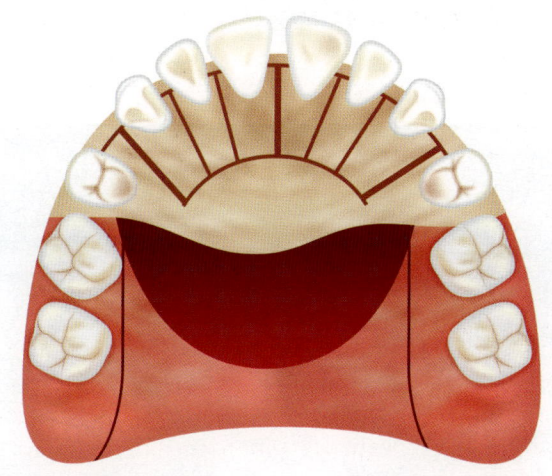

**Fig. 42.11:** Corticotomy undertaken in patients having dental proclination with spacing can hasten the orthodontic tooth movement and duration of the appliance therapy can be shortened

- Patient evaluation
- Presurgical orthodontics
- Final planning of surgery with mock surgery and visual treatment objective (VTO)
- Surgery and stabilization
- Post-surgical orthodontics
    i. Evaluation of the patient: The treatment planning for orthognathic surgery begins with a thorough patient evaluation. Evaluation is aimed at assessing the nature and severity of the dentofacial deformity.
a. Medical and psychological evaluation: The interview is conducted to know the patients' perception of the problems and to set goals of the treatment keeping in mind the patients' expectation from the surgery. Patients' health status and any medical or psychological problems that may affect the treatment are noted.
b. Evaluation of facial esthetics: Orthodontists and oral maxillofacial surgeon should conduct a thorough examination of facial structures with consideration of full face and profile esthetics. Overall facial balance is assessed, noting the presence of any asymmetries. Full face view and profile photographs of the pretreatment condition of the patient are taken for evaluation of facial morphology. Computerized images where appropriable may be used.
c. Cephalometric evaluation: The lateral cephalometric radiograph is evaluated using various analyses to assess the nature and severity of skeletal abnormality **(Fig. 42.12A)**.
Anteroposterior cephalograms are useful to assess presence of asymmetry **(Fig. 42.12B)**.
d. OPG and other radiographs: Panoramic evaluation is used as a screening for TMJ anomalies, gross abnormalities of dentition and presence or absence of impacted teeth **(Fig. 42.12C)**. TMJ projection may also be needed in certain patients **(Fig. 42.12D)**.
e. Dental examination: A complete dental examination should include assessment of dental arch form, symmetry, tooth alignment and occlusal abnormalities in all three planes of space. Patients' hygiene and periodontal ligament health status should be evaluated. Teeth are also evaluated for carious lesions and faulty restorations, and are treated before surgery. Muscles of mastication and temporomandibular joint (TMJ) function should also be evaluated. Evaluation for dental compensation is extremely important. Teeth may have tipped to compensate for the abnormal jaw positions and these need to be corrected in the presurgical orthodontic phase.
    f. Diagnosis: A thorough diagnosis should be made after careful evaluation of the patient. The diagnosis should include presence or absence of skeletal abnormalities, dental and occlusal abnormalities and other findings such as presence or absence of impacted 3rd molars.

Skeletal diagnosis should include the jaw or jaws involved, the direction of the problem and whether the problem is an excess or a deficiency. The skeletal discrepancy may be due to problem in one or both the jaws. For example, a typical diagnosis might be maxillary sagittal deficiency or mandibular sagittal excess. The diagnosis should also include presence or absence of dental compensation which has to be corrected during presurgical orthodontic phase.

  ii. Presurgical orthodontics: Undesirable angulations of the anterior teeth occur as a compensatory response to a developing dentofacial deformity. Patients with maxillary deficiency, mandibular excess, or both often have flared upper incisors and retroclined lower incisors **(Figs 42.13A to C)**. Similarly, patients with mandibular deficiency may show flaring of lower incisors.

Such dental compensation in response to skeletal deformity should be corrected orthodontically before surgery so that both skeletal and dental components are in an ideal position after surgical treatment. The decompensation is aimed at improving the angulations of teeth over underlying basal bone after which skeletal problems are corrected.

Decompensation is done by orthodontically repositioning the teeth properly over the underlying skeletal bone without consideration of the bite relationship to the opposing arch. This presurgical orthodontic movement accentuates the patient's deformity, but is necessary for achievement of normal occlusal relationships when skeletal bones are properly positioned at surgery.

The amount of presurgical orthodontics can vary ranging from only appliance placement in few patients to approximately 12-month active appliance therapy in those with severe crowding and incisor malposition.

  iii. **Final treatment planning before surgery**: After presurgical orthodontics, the actual surgical approach is planned using mock surgery and VTO. Presurgical photographs, radiographs and presurgical models are taken. A centric relation bite registration is recorded and computerized images are obtained when available.

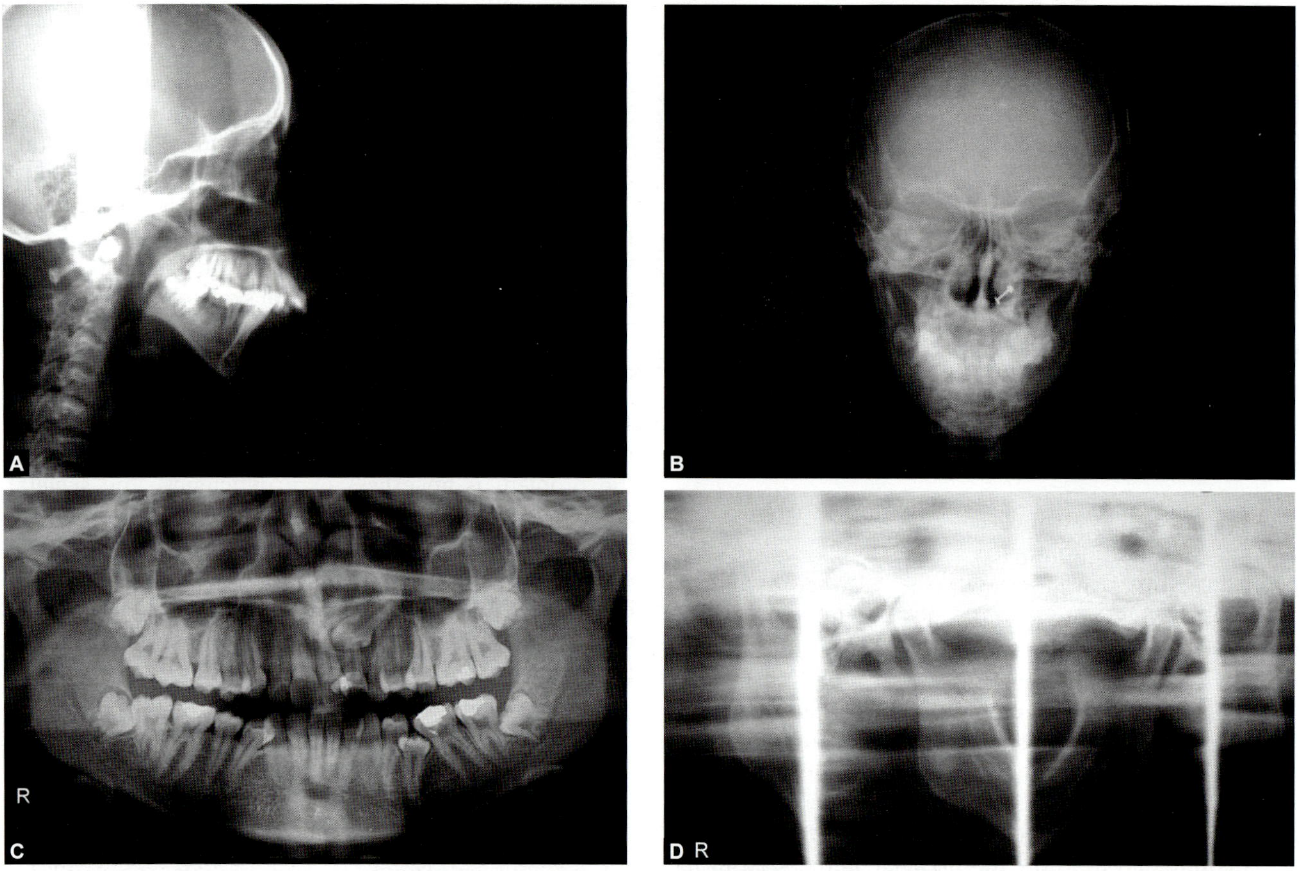

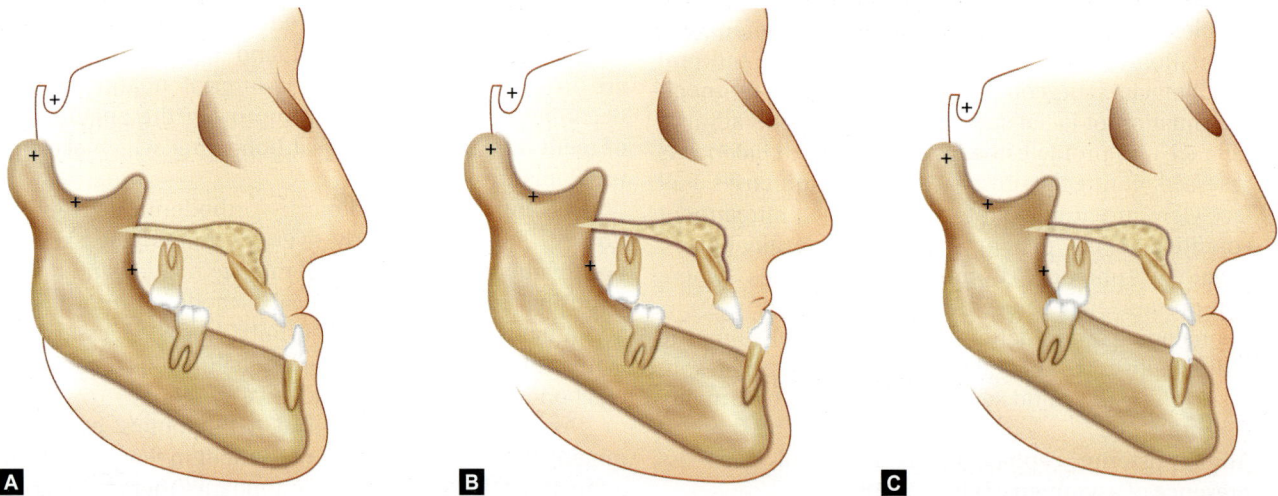

**Figs 42.12A to D:** Radiographic evaluation: (A) Lateral cephalogram showing skeletal discrepancy. Cephalometric analysis is done to determine the nature and extent of skeletal discrepancy. (B) Anteroposterior cephalogram useful in assessment of facial asymmetry. (C) OPG is examined to screen for gross abnormalities of dentition and presence of impacted teeth. (D) TMJ projection

**Figs 42.13A to C:** Presurgical orthodontics: (A) Dental compensation seen in a class III patient, with maxillary deficiency and mandibular excess, includes—flaring of upper incisors and retroclined lower incisors. (B) Dental compensation is corrected in presurgical orthodontic phase by retroclination of upper incisors and slight proclination of lower incisors. This accentuates the facial discrepancy. (C) Ideal facial profile is achieved after surgical correction with proper positioning of mandible and advancement of maxilla

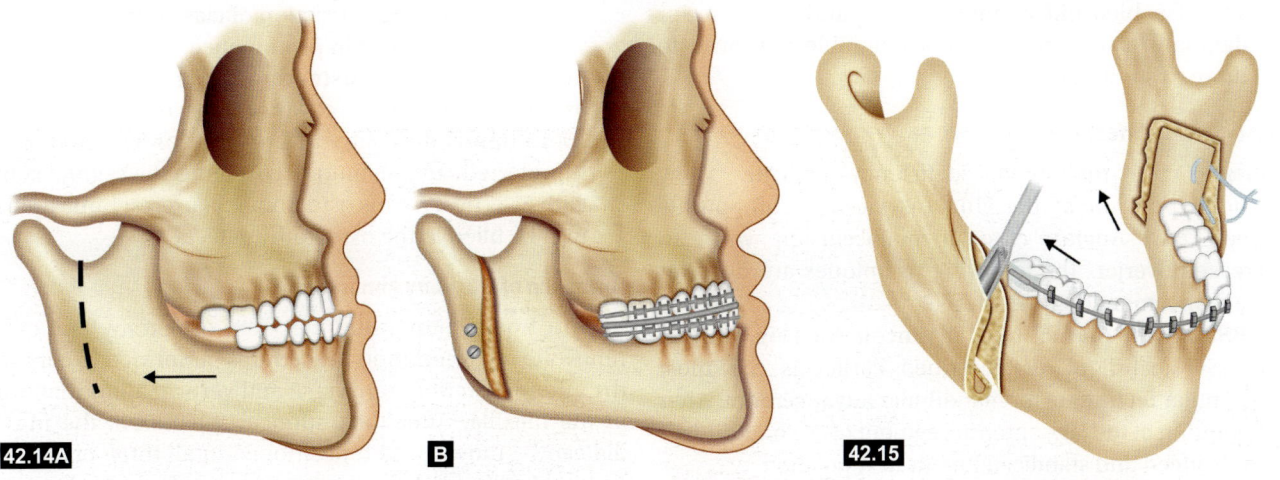

**Figs 42.14A and B:** Vertical ramus osteotomy. Class III malocclusion resulting from mandible excess is treated by vertical ramus osteotomy with posterior positioning of mandible; **Fig. 42.15:** Bilateral sagittal split osteotomy (BSSO) technique. It involves sagittal splitting of ramus and posterior body of mandible; anterior mandibular segment is then repositioned anteriorly or posteriorly as desired

---

a. **Mock surgery (model surgery):** Mock surgery is done on a duplicate set of presurgical dental casts to determine the exact surgical movements necessary to achieve the desired postoperative occlusion.
b. **VTO:** Visualized treatment objective is designed to provide organized and simplified information to help in diagnosis, treatment planning and the extraction/non-extraction decisions. It should be used as an adjunct to, but not a substitute for, conventional cephalometric analysis.
   iv. **Surgical treatment phase:** Severe skeletal malocclusion and dentofacial abnormalities are treated by isolated osteotomies involving surgical repositioning of one of the jaws, or by combination procedures involving surgeries of both the jaws when abnormalities are present in both maxilla and mandible.

Several major jaw procedures are commonly used to correct skeletal abnormalities including bilateral sagittal split osteotomy (BSSO), transoral vertical ramus osteotomy and Le Fort osteotomy among others. Usually the repositioned bones are held in their new positions using plates, screws and wires. In some cases, adjunctive procedures, such as genioplasty, molar augmentation and reconstructive rhinoplasty, may be needed to optimize the esthetics results.

Possible options of surgical procedures in cases of excess/deficiency of jaws are discussed below.

### Correction of Mandibular Abnormalities

#### Mandibular Excess
Mandibular excess was one of the first dentofacial deformities treated by a combination of orthodontics and surgery.

Excess growth can occur in anteroposterior (sagittal) or vertical dimension. Mandibular excess frequently results in Angle's class III malocclusion with reverse overjet.

The following are some of the commonly used surgical techniques to treat patients with mandibular excess.

1. **Vertical ramus osteotomy (Fig. 42.14):** Transoral vertical ramus osteotomy was popularized by Caldwell and Letterman in the early 1950s, where lateral aspect of ramus was exposed through a submandibular incision. Intraoral incision is used in recent times. The technique can be utilized for mandibular setback.
   In this technique, the ramus is sectioned in a vertical fashion and the entire body and anterior ramus section of the mandible are moved posteriorly. The proximal segment containing condyle is overlapped on the posteriorly positioned anterior portion of the ramus; the jaw is then stabilized during healing phase.
2. **Bilateral sagittal split osteotomy (BSSO) with mandibular setback (Fig. 42.15):** BSSO technique has become one of the most popular methods for treatment of both mandibular deficiency and mandibular excess. This technique can be used to either advance or retrude the mandible. Class III patients with mandibular excess are treated by BSSO with mandibular setback.
   BSSO was first described by Trauner and Obswegerer and later modified by Dalpont, Hunsuck and Epker. The technique involves the splitting of the ramus and posterior body of the mandible in a sagittal fashion, which allows either advancement or setback of the mandible. This type of splitting produces large area of bony overlap that provides flexibility necessary to move the mandible in several directions. The significant bony overlap also allows for adequate bone healing and improved postoperative stability.
3. **Mandibular subapical osteotomy (Figs 42.16A and B):** When the reverse overjet relationship is isolated to the anterior dentoalveolar area of the mandible, a subapical osteotomy technique can be used for correction of mandibular dental prognathism. In this technique, bone is removed in the area of an extraction

site of a bicuspid or molar tooth, and the anterior dentoalveolar segment of the mandible is moved to more posterior position.

### Mandibular Deficiency

Patients with mandibular deficiency typically show retruded position of the chin (as viewed from profile aspect) and Angle's class II malocclusion with an increased overjet. The following techniques are used for the advancement of the mandible:

1. **BSSO with mandibular advancement (Fig. 42.17):** BSSO technique as described earlier is the most popular technique for mandibular advancement. After splitting of the jaw, anterior segment of the mandible is advanced and stabilized into its new position.
2. **Mandibular total subapical osteotomy (Fig. 42.18):** Total subapical osteotomy may be an option for mandibular advancement when chin prominence is adequate in a patient with class II malocclusion. Dentoalveolar segment of mandible is moved anteriorly allowing correction of class II malocclusion without increasing chin prominence.
3. **Vertical 'L' or 'C' osteotomy (Fig. 42.19):** When extreme mandibular advancement of greater than 10–15 mm is necessary a vertical 'L' or 'C' osteotomy is preferred. The technique combines the sagittal split with a vertical ramus osteotomy. Iliac crest bone grafts may be filled in the osteotomy defect.

### Correction of Maxillary Abnormalities

Le Fort I osteotomy (total maxillary osteotomy) are currently the most common procedures performed to correct the anteroposterior, transverse and vertical abnormalities of the maxilla. After total surgical separation, the maxilla can be moved and repositioned in all three planes of space. Maxilla can be moved in upward, downward or forward direction after Le Fort I osteotomy **(Fig. 42.20)**.

### Maxillary Excess

Maxillary excess can occur in transverse, anteroposterior and vertical dimensions.

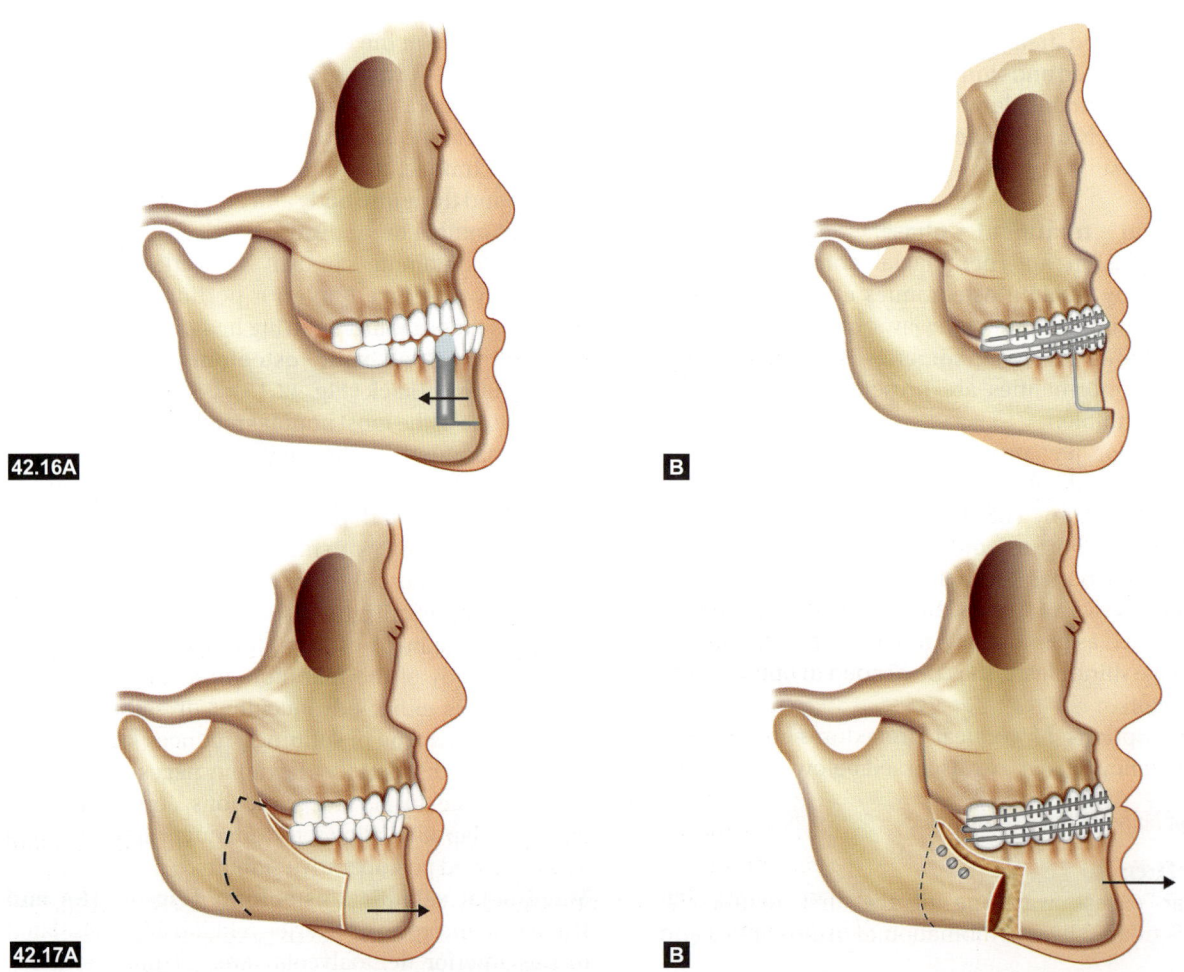

**Figs 42.16A and B:** Anterior mandibular subapical osteotomy: **(A)** Removal of premolar teeth and bone in the area of extraction sites.; **(B)** After separation, anterior dentoalveolar segment is repositioned posteriorly extraction sites are closed, and anterior reverse overjet relationship is corrected; **Figs 42.17A and B:** Bilateral sagittal split osteotomy (BSSO) with mandible advancement to correct class II malocclusion mandible deficiency

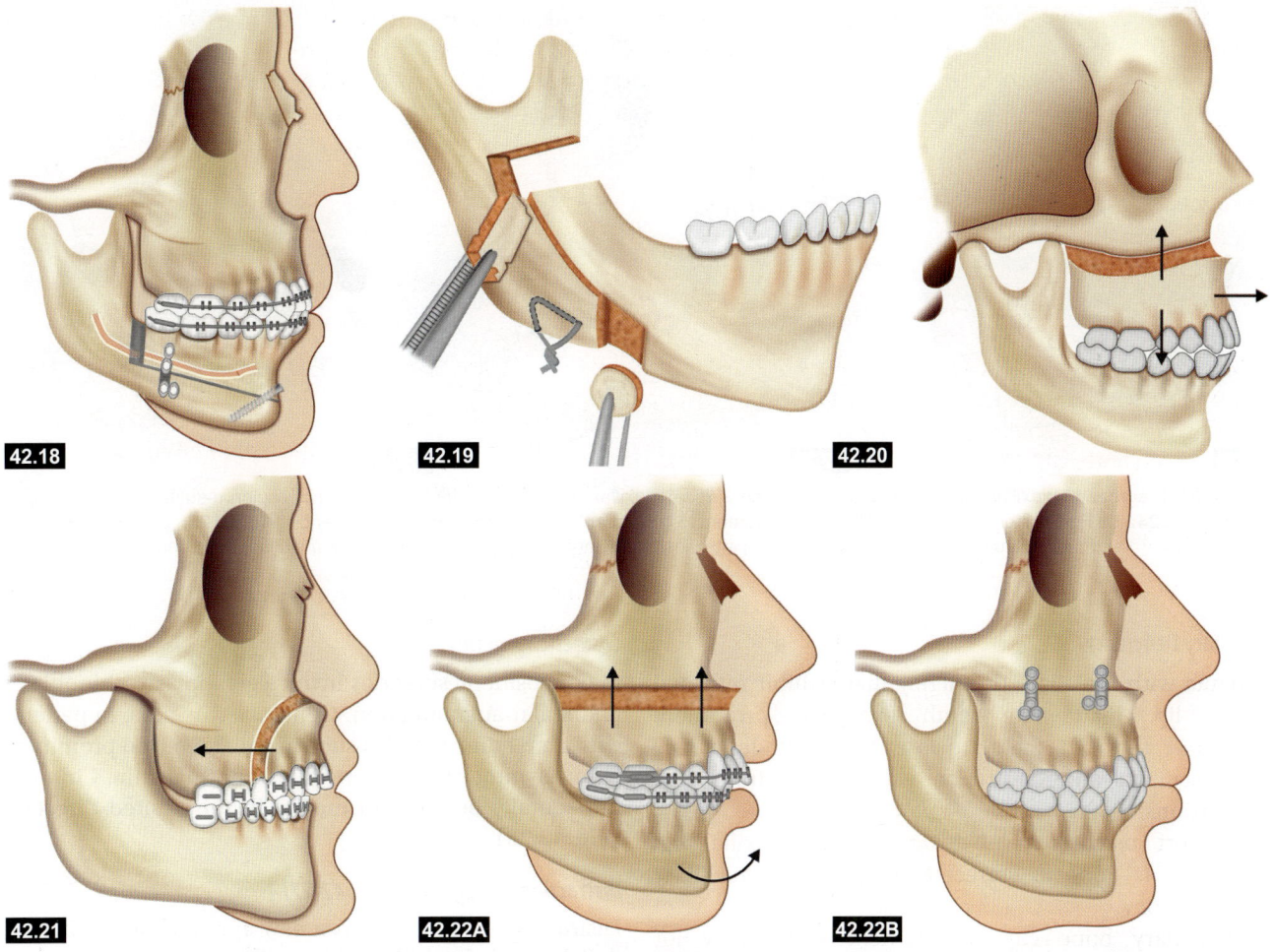

**Fig. 42.18:** Mandibular total subapical osteotomy: The dentoalveolar segment is moved anteriorly to correct class II malocclusion without increasing the chin prominence; **Fig. 42.19:** Vertical "L" or "C" osteotomy can be used when large mandibular advancement is needed. Iliac crest bone grafts are used to fill the gaps created; **Fig. 42.20:** Le Fort I osteotomy (total maxillary osteotomy) is the most common procedure to correct maxillary abnormalities. After total separation maxilla can be moved and repositioned in all three planes of space; **Fig. 42.21:** Anterior maxillary subapical setback to correct skeletal class II malocclusion caused by sagittal maxillary excess. Premolar teeth and bone removed in the area and maxillary anterior segment is positioned posteriorly utilizing the extraction space; **Figs 42.22A and B:** Le Fort I osteotomy with maxillary impaction indicated in case of vertical maxillary excess in anterior as well as posterior segments

### Maxillary Excess in Anteroposterior Dimension

1. **Anterior maxillary subapical setback (Fig. 42.21):** This technique is used when skeletal class II malocclusion is caused by a maxillary excess limited to the anteroposterior dimension with no vertical increase of the maxilla. Patient typically exhibits midface protrusion. Maxillary excess in the anterior region can effectively be treated with surgical retraction of the maxillary anterior segment by utilizing the maxillary first premolar extraction space.
2. **Le Fort I osteotomy (Fig. 42.20) with maxillary setback:** Le Fort I osteotomy (total maxillary osteotomy) is the most common procedure to correct maxillary abnormalities. After total separation maxilla can be moved and repositioned in all three planes of space.

### Vertical Maxillary Excess

Vertical maxillary excess may result in excessive lower facial height, incompetent lips, excessive vertical display of incisors and gingival or skeletal anterior open bite. In skeletal anterior open bite, posterior portion of maxilla show excessive downward growth. Thus, when molar teeth are in occlusion of this anatomic abnormality, the anterior teeth are left without contact.

1. **Le Fort I osteotomy with maxillary impaction (Figs 42.22A and B):** It is done when the excess is present in anterior as well as posterior segments. Bone is removed at osteotomy site to permit superior repositioning of the maxilla.
2. **Segmental maxillary osteotomy (Fig 42.23):** A maxillary excess which is mostly in posterior region causing anterior open bite can be treated by bilateral posterior segmental maxillary osteotomies. Maxillary first premolar is removed and maxilla is sectioned into posterior and anterior dentoalveolar segments. Excess bone is cut at the osteotomy sites and segments are moved superiorly and posteriorly to allow even contact between all the teeth.

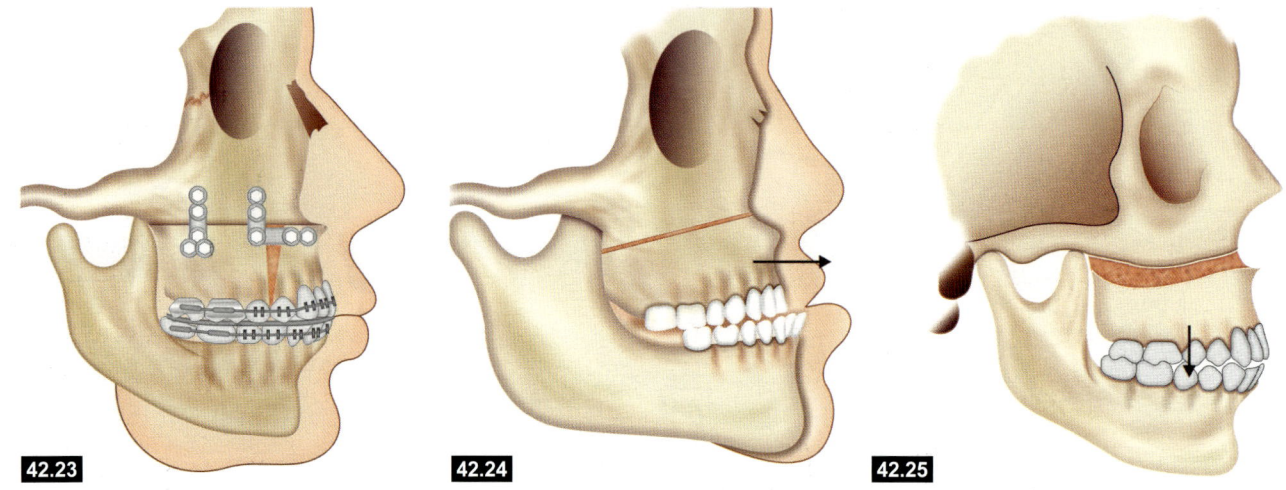

**Fig. 42.23:** Segmental maxillary osteotomy indicated when vertical maxillary excess is restricted to posterior region resulting in anterior open bite; **Fig. 42.24:** Le Fort I osteotomy with maxillary advancement to correct anteroposterior maxillary deficiency; **Fig. 42.25:** Le Fort I osteotomy and downward repositioning of maxilla with interpositional bone grafting to correct vertical maxillary deficiency

### Maxillary Deficiency

Patients with maxillary deficiency may exhibit retruded upper lip, inadequate tooth exposure, prominent chin and class III malocclusion. Maxillary deficiency can occur in anteroposterior, vertical and transverse dimensions.

1. Le Fort I osteotomy with advancement of maxilla **(Fig. 42.24)** is done to correct anteroposterior maxillary deficiency.
2. Maxillary bone can be segmented to allow for transverse expansion when maxilla is constricted.
3. In case of vertical maxillary deficiency, elongation of lower 3rd of face can be achieved by inferior positioning of maxilla with bone grafts using a Le Fort I osteotomy **(Fig. 42.25)**.

***Post-surgical orthodontics:*** After a period of healing, final alignment and positioning of teeth and closure of any extraction space is accomplished by orthodontic tooth movement. The final setting of occlusion occurs rapidly within 6–10 months. Retention after surgical orthodontics is similar to routine orthodontic management.

### Surgical Assisted Rapid Palatal Expansion

A transverse deficiency of the maxilla in adult patients can be treated with surgically assisted rapid maxillary expansion. This procedure involves the techniques of orthodontic palatal widening with a modification of the Le Fort I osteotomy.

A cut is made along the lateral surface of the maxilla, which is similar to the Le Fort I cut in this area. Then a vertical cut is made in the anteronasal spine above the apices of central incisors to open/split the midpalatal suture. Activation of the maxillary expansion appliance is now begun. When the maxilla reaches its desired width, the expansion appliance is stabilized for 3 months in a retention phase.

### Cosmetic Surgeries

Major cosmetic surgeries involve genioplasty, rhinoplasty and malar augmentation. Genioplasty is done in patients with chin abnormalities such as too flat or too prominent chin; asymmetrical or vertically abnormal chin. Chin can horizontally be cut and moved in the desired direction **(Fig. 42.26)**.

### Distraction Osteogenesis (Fig. 42.27)

Distraction osteogenesis is a new approach to correct the deficiencies of maxilla and mandible.

Conventional osteotomy techniques have several limitations:
- Associated soft tissues cannot adapt to the changes when large skeletal movements are done and stretching occurs after surgical repositioning of bony segment
- The failure of tissue adaptation can result in surgical relapse
- Excessive loading of TMJ structure
- Increased risk of neurosensory loss due to stretching of nerve
- Bone grafts may be needed to fill gaps from secondary surgical sites, e.g. iliac crest.

Distraction osteogenesis is developed to overcome these limitations of conventional osteotomy techniques.

### Technique

- Distraction osteogenesis involves cutting osteotomy to separate the segments of bone and the application of a traction appliance that will facilitate the gradual and incremental separation of bone segments.
- The gradual tension placed on the bony segments produces continuous bone formation.
- Along with new bone formation, the surrounding tissues also adapt to this gradual tension, producing adaptive changes in the surrounding muscles and tendons, nerves, cartilages, blood vessels and skin.

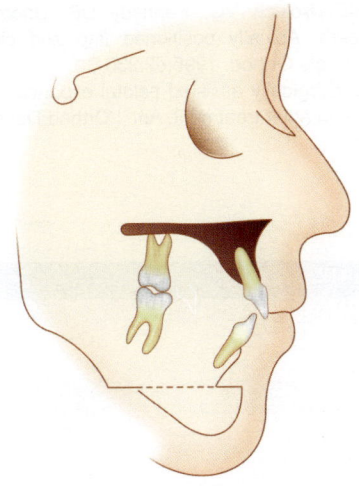
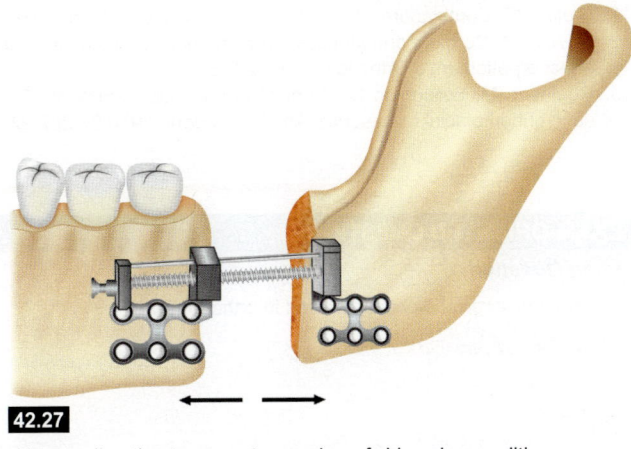

**Fig. 42.26:** Genioplasty—chin can be cut horizontally and moved in any direction to correct a number of chins abnormalities;
**Fig. 42.27:** Distraction osteogenesis involves surgical separation of the segments of bone and application of a traction appliance that will facilitate the gradual and incremental separation of bone segments

- Distraction osteogenesis can be applied to both maxilla and mandible.

### Advantages
- Can produce larger skeletal movements without stretching of tissues.
- Eliminates the need for bone grafts and the associated secondary surgical sites.
- Better long-term stability.
- Less chances of trauma to TMJ structures.
- Decreased risk of neurosensory loss.

### Disadvantages
- Procedure is very technique sensitive.
- Needs two surgical procedures: placement and removal.
- Increased cost.
- Longer treatment period.
- Can be used for treating only skeletal discrepancies with deficiencies cannot be used for treating excesses of the jaws.

### Combined Surgical Procedure

In certain cases, surgery may be needed in both maxilla and mandible. A female patient with maxillary deficiency and mandibular advancement treated by combined surgical approach is shown in **Figures 42.28A and B**.

### Surgical Procedures in the Management of Cleft Lip and Palate

Rehabilitation of the patients with cleft lip and palate requires long-term treatment by multidisciplinary team. Depending on the type and severity of the deformity, multiple surgical procedures are often required at different age of the patient. Management of cleft lip and palate is discussed separately in Chapter 40.

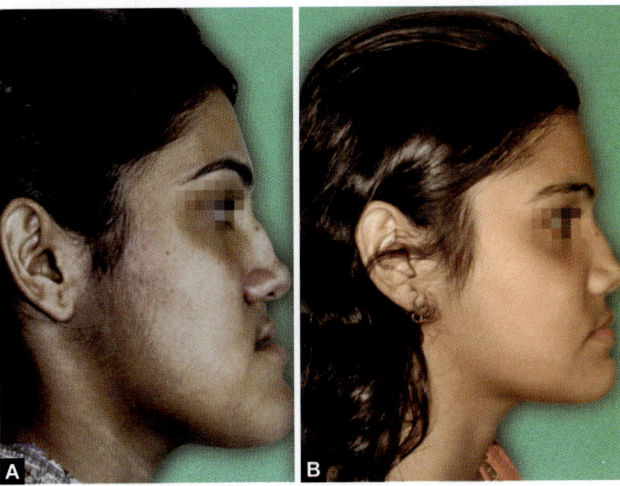

**Figs 42.28A and B:** A female patient with maxillary deficiency and mandibular prognathism is treated with maxillary advancement (Le Fort-I), mandibular set bak and genioplasty. **(A)** Pre-treatment, **(B)** Post-treatment (*Courtesy*: Dr Nikunj Patel MDS [Ortho])

## BIBLIOGRAPHY

1. Bell WH, Alessanda PA, Condit CL. Surgical orthodontic correction of class 2 malocclusion. J Oral Surg. 1968;26:265-72.
2. Boese LR. Fibrectomy and reproximation without lower retention, nine years in retrospect: Art 1. Angle Ortho. 1980;50:88-97.
3. Charest A, Maranda G. New method for surgical correction of maxillary protrusion. J Canada Dent Ass. 1968;34:630-5.
4. Edwards JG. A surgical procedure to eliminate rotational relapse. Am J Orthodont. 1970;57:35-46.
5. Graber TM. Orthodontics: Principles and Practice. WB Saunders, 1988.
6. Graber TM, Vanarsdall RL. Orthodontic Current Principles and Techniques. Mosby Year Book Inc, 1994.
7. Graber TM. Team effort--Oral ssurgery and orthodontics. J Oral Surg. 1967;25:210-24.
8. Herren P. The surgical pre-orthodontic treatment of impacted tooth using the 'looping' technique. Europ Orthodont Soc Trans. 1964:245-7.
9. MacIntosh RB. The surgical approach to class 2, division 1 Malocclusion. JADSA. 1971;28:796-804.

10. Nordenram A. Vertical subcondylar osteotomy in the treatment of mandibular protrusion. Norseke Tanlaeg Tid. 1968;78:394-407.
11. Profitt WR. Contemporary Orthodontics, St Louis: CV Mosby 1986.
12. Revell JH. Surgical orthodontics. New method to stimulate and direct eruption. Int J Orthodont. 1964;2:5-20.
13. Robinson M, Stoughton D. Surgical orthodontic treatment of a case of hemefacial microsomia. Am J Orthodont. 1970;57:287-92.
14. Vermette ME, Kokich VG, Kennedy DB. Uncovering labially impacted teeth. Apically positioned flap and closed eruption techniques. Angle Orthod. 1995;62:230-3.
15. Wintner ML. Surgically assisted palatal expansion: An important consideration in adult treatment. Am J Orthod Dentofacio Orthop. 1991;85-90.

## EXAM-ORIENTED QUESTIONS

### Long Question
1. Common surgical procedures used in orthodontics.

### Short Questions
1. Corticotomy
2. BSSO
3. Osteotomy Le Fort 2
4. Distraction osteogenesis.

# CHAPTER 43

# Retention and Relapse

*Phulari BS*

Retention is the phase of orthodontic treatment, which maintains the teeth in their orthodontically corrected positions following the cessation of active orthodontic tooth movement. Orthodontic retainer resists the tendency of teeth to return to their original position under the influence of periodontal, occlusal and soft tissue forces and continuing dentofacial growth.

## WHY IS RETENTION NECESSARY?

Retention is necessary for the following reasons:
1. The gingival and periodontal tissues are affected by orthodontic tooth movement and require time for reorganization when the appliances are removed.
2. The teeth may be in an inherently unstable position after the treatment so that soft tissue pressures constantly produce a relapse tendency.
3. Changes produced by growth may alter the orthodontic treatment result.

## SCHOOLS OF RETENTION

Over the years, various philosophies have been put forward to explain post-treatment stability.

These are referred to as schools of retention.

### The Occlusion School

According to Kingsley, proper occlusion is a key factor in determining the stability of the newly moved teeth. The importance of this factor in safeguarding the stability in the new position has been agreed upon by several other authors and research workers.

### The Apical Base School

- The apical base school has been formulated around the writings of several authors, including Alex, Lundstrom, Mc Cauley and Nance.
- Alex Lundstrom suggested that the apical base is an important factor in the correction of malocclusion and maintenance of the stability of the treated cases.
- Mc Cauley added that the intercanine and intermolar widths should be maintained during orthodontic treatment to minimize retention problems.
- Nance noted that the arch length cannot be permanently increased to a major extent.

### The Mandibular Incisor School

Grieves and Tweed have suggested that post-treatment stability was increased when the mandibular incisors were placed upright or slightly retroclined over the basal bone.

### The Musculature School

The dentition is encapsulated from outside and inside by muscles. According to Rojers, functional muscle balance is necessary in order to ensure post-treatment stability.

## CAUSES OF RELAPSE

Numerous are the causes attributed to relapse. No single factor can be said the sole cause of relapse. In most cases relapse occurs due to a combination of causes **(Flowchart 43.1)**.

### Periodontal Ligament Traction

Whenever teeth are moved orthodontically, the periodontal principal fibers and the gingival fibers that encircle the teeth are stretched. These stretched fibers can contract and should be a potent cause of relapse. The principal fibers of the periodontal ligament rearrange themselves quite rapidly to the new position. Studies have shown that principal fibers reorganize in about four week's time. The supra-alveolar gingival fibers on the other hand take as much as 40 weeks to rearrange around the new position and thus predispose to relapse. After comprehensive orthodontic treatment, teeth require 4–5 months of full-time retention so as to allow the reorganization of periodontal ligament fibers. After this period, retention should be continued on a reduced basis for a further 7–8 months so as to allow the more sluggish gingival fibers to readapt to the new tooth positions.

### Relapse due to Growth-related Changes

Patients with skeletal problems associated with class II, class III, open bite or deep bite malocclusion may exhibit response due to continuation of the abnormal growth pattern after orthodontic therapy. Studies have shown that the original growth pattern resurfaces or dominates,

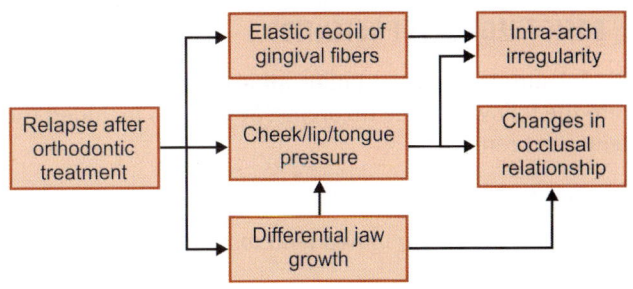

**Flowchart 43.1:** Causes of relapse arter orthodontic treatment

if the orthodontic treatment is completed prior to the completion of growth. Hence, prolonged retention is indicated until active growth is completed.

### Bone Adaptation

Teeth that have been moved recently are surrounded by lightly calcified osteoid bone. Thus, the teeth are not adequately stabilized and have a tendency to move to their original position. The bony trabeculae are normally arranged perpendicular to the long axis of the teeth. However, during orthodontic treatment, they get aligned parallel to the direction of force. During the retention phase, they revert back to their normal arrangement.

### Muscular Forces

Teeth are encapsulated in all directions by a blanket of muscles. Muscle imbalance at the end of the orthodontic therapy can result in the reappearance of malocclusion. The orthodontist should aim at harmonizing the muscles at the conclusion of the orthodontic treatment so as to increase the stability of the treatment results achieved.

### Failure to Eliminate the Original Cause

The cause of the malocclusion should be determined at the time of diagnosis and adequate treatment steps should be planned to eliminate the same or reduce its severity. Failure to remove the etiology can result in relapse.

## ROLE OF THIRD MOLARS

The third molars erupt very late in the development of dentition. They erupt in most cases between the age 18 and 21 years. By this time most patients would have completed their orthodontic treatment. The pressure exerted by the erupting third molars is believed to cause late anterior crowding, predisposing to relapse.

## ROLE OF OCCLUSION

Good intercuspation of the upper and the lower teeth is an important factor in maintaining the stability of treated cases. The centric relation and the centric occlusion should coincide or the slide from centric should not be more than 1.5–2 mm in order to have greater stability of the treatment results. Presence of certain occlusal mannerisms, such as clenching, grinding, nail biting, lip biting, etc. is important causes of relapse.

## BASIC THEOREMS OF RETENTION

Riedel summarized the philosophies regarding retention into the following nine theorems. Moyer has included the tenth theorem.

### Theorem 1

*"Teeth that have been moved tend to return to their former position."*

It is proved beyond doubt that orthodontically moved teeth have a tendency to return to their original position. Factors, such as muscular forces, bone morphology and periodontal ligament and gingival fibers contribute to this tendency.

### Theorem 2

*"Elimination of the causes of malocclusion will prevent relapse."*

All the possible causes of existing malocclusion should be identified at the time of diagnosis and all efforts should be made to eliminate them wherever possible. It is especially true for abnormal muscle forces aggravating the existing malocclusion, e.g. Thumb sucking, tongue thrusting and other abnormal pressure habits.

### Theorem 3

*"Malocclusion should be over corrected as a safety factor."*

Although there is little evidence about its effectiveness, overcorrection appears to be helpful in the management of certain conditions, such as rotations, class II and class III malocclusions.

It is a common practice to over correct class II malocclusion into an edge-to-edge incisor relationship and to overcorrect rotations by slightly rotating the tooth in an opposite direction.

In this way, over correction allows some amount of relapse without deleteriously affecting function and esthetics.

### Theorem 4

*"Proper occlusion is a potent factor in holding teeth in their corrected positions."*

Orthodontic treatment should aim at achieving harmonious centric, as well as functional occlusions of mandible. Proper intercuspation of teeth may aid in retention as one tooth in the arch is related to two teeth of the opposing arch.

### Theorem 5

*"Bone and adjacent tissues must be allowed to reorganize around newly positioned teeth."*

During orthodontic tooth movement, there occurs bone remodeling, as well as reorganization of periodontal ligament fibers.

Considerable time is needed for the maturation of the newly deposited osteoid bone and reorganization of the fibers of the periodontal ligament. Retention appliances are aimed at providing sufficient time for this reorganization.

### Theorem 6

*"If the lower incisors are placed upright over basal bone, they are more likely to remain in good alignment."*

It has been observed that post-treatment stability increases when the mandibular incisors are placed upright over the basal bone (perpendicular to the mandibular plane) or slightly inclined in a lingual direction.

## Theorem 7

*"Corrections carried out during periods of growth are less likely to relapse."*

Orthodontic treatment should be initiated at the earliest possible age so that the changes occurring during active growth periods can be positively influenced by the treatment.

By initiating the treatment early during periods of growth, orthodontist can retard or change the direction of growth of maxilla/mandible when indicated (by using headgear/functional appliances). Hence, institution of early treatment allows growth modulations, interception of developing malocclusion and correction of skeletal malrelationships.

Treatment carried out during active growth periods is more stable because the tissue systems are adapted well.

## Theorem 8

*"The farther the teeth have been moved, the less likelihood of relapse."*

Although, it is logical to think that the teeth moved farther away are less likely to return to their original position, such a measure may not always be justified and may even cause root resorption. It is more desirable to guide the proper eruption of teeth and intercept developing skeletal discrepancies rather than carrying out extensive tooth movement at a later stage.

## Theorem 9

*"Arch form, particularly in the mandibular arch, cannot be altered permanently by appliance therapy."*

Studies have shown that the alteration of mandibular arch form carry an increased risk of relapse.

It is advisable to maintain the existing molar width and canine width and build the arches around them.

## Theorem 10

*"Many treated malocclusions require permanent retaining devices."*

Some type of malocclusions require very long period of retention.

## THE RETAINERS USED IN ORTHODONTICS

A number of removable and fixed retainer designs are available, which suite different needs.

The retainer appropriate for a clinical situation and the level of patient cooperation must be used. Although conductive to good oral hygiene, successes of removable retainers depend entirely on patient compliance. Fixed retainers make a good choice in patients with questionable compliance. Types of retainers are given in **Box 43.1**.

## REMOVABLE RETAINERS

### Hawley's Retainer

Hawley's retainer, designed by Hawley in 1920, is one of the most routinely used removable retainers. It has a simple design and accepts a number of modifications to suite various clinical needs. Although generally used as a passive retainer, it can bring about minor tooth movement when desired by activating the labial bow.

#### Design of Hawley's Retainer

Hawley's retainer consists of a retentive clasp on molar teeth and a characteristic labial bow with adjustment U loop, spanning from canine to canine (**Fig. 43.1**).

#### Wire Components
- **Clasp:** Adam's clasp
- **Bow:** Short passive labial bow.

#### Acrylic Components
- Acrylic base material.

**Box 43.1:** Classification of retainers

**Removable Retainers**
1. Hawley's retainer
   Modifications of Hawley's retainer:
   i. Hawley's retainer with C clasp on molar teeth.
   ii. Hawley's retainer with long labial bow.
   iii. Hawley's retainer with contoured labial bow.
   iv. Hawley's retainer with light elastic across the incisor teeth.
   v. Hawley's retainer with labial bow soldered to bridge of Adams clasp.
   vi. Hawley's retainer with bite plane.
   vii. Hawley's retainer with lingual extension clasps on molar.
   viii. Hawley's retainer with occlusal rest.
2. Begg's retainer
3. Clip-on retainer/spring aligner
4. Wrap around retainer
5. Kesling's tooth positioner
6. Invisible retainer

**Fixed Retainers**
1. Band and spur fixed retainer
2. Banded canine-to-canine fixed retainer
3. Bonded canine-to-canine fixed retainer

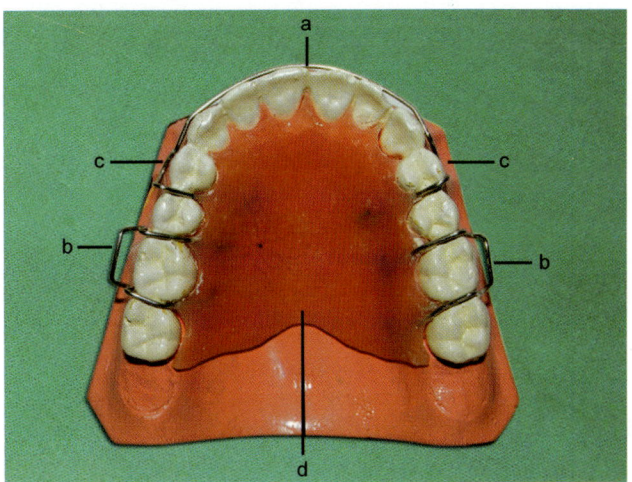

**Fig. 43.1:** Parts of Hawley's retainer: (a) Passive labial bow, (b) Adam's clasp, (c) U loop of the passive labial bow, (d) Acrylic base material

### Advantages

1. Easy to fabricate because of its simple design.
2. Offers good patient compliance due to its reduced bulk.
3. A Hawley's retainer can be used for the maxillary or mandibular arches.
4. Its acrylic component provides a potential bite plane to control overbite.

### Disadvantages

1. It is susceptible to fracture or loss.
2. Hawley's retainer constructed on mandibular arch is sometimes fragile and may be difficult to insert because of undercut in premolar and molar region.

#### Modifications of the Hawley's Retainer

Over the years a number of modifications have been devised to suit various conditions, some of these modifications are listed below.
   i. Hawley's retainer with C clasp on molar teeth.
   ii. Hawley's retainer with long labial bow.
   iii. Hawley's retainer with contoured labial bow.
   iv. Hawley's retainer with light elastic across the incisor teeth.
   v. Hawley's retainer with labial bow soldered to bridge of Adam's clasp.
   vi. Hawley's retainer with bite plane.
   vii. Hawley's retainer with lingual extension clasps on molar.
   viii. Hawley's retainer with occlusal rest.

i. ***Hawley's retainer with C clasp on molar:*** Hawley's retainer with C clasp on molars is a modification of Hawley's retainer in which circumferential clasps are used instead of Adam's clasps (**Fig. 43.2**). This type of retainer is indicated when there is tight occlusal contact and occlusal arms of clasps might cause occlusal interference. However, retention of this appliance may be less than that of conventional Hawley's retainer with Adam's clasp.

#### Indications

- This type of modification of Hawley's retainer is indicated when there is tight occlusal contact.

ii. ***Hawley's retainer with long labial bow:*** This modification incorporates a long labial bow from premolar to premolar rather than from canine to canine (**Fig. 43.3**). This helps to keep the extraction space closed in premolar extraction case.

#### Indication

- It is indicated when space exists distal to canine.
- Compression of U loop of the long labial bow can bring about closure of the space.

iii. ***Hawley's retainer with contoured labial bow:*** In this modification, the labial bow is contoured or fitted in the cervical margins of the anterior teeth (**Fig. 43.4**). It is sometimes used when retention is needed in the anterior segment and it gives better control over the anterior teeth. However, fabrication of contoured labial bow may pose some difficulties.

iv. ***Hawley's retainer with light elastics:*** Instead of the labial bow, light elastic is stretched across the anterior teeth in this modification (**Fig. 43.5**). It can be used for closure of minor spaces in the anterior segment. Although it is more esthetic, the position of elastic on anterior teeth cannot be controlled properly.

v. ***Hawley's retainer with labial bow soldered to the bridge of Adam's clasp:*** In this modification, terminal ends of labial bow are soldered to the bridge of Adam's clasp instead of terminating as retentive arms in the acrylic base material (**Fig. 43.6**). This design allows closure of space in the anterior segment, as well as any residual space in premolar extraction site. This design also avoids the risk of space opening up between canine and premolar due to the crossover wires.

vi. ***Hawley's retainer with bite plane:*** Here, a bite plane is incorporated lingual to the maxillary incisors while the rest of the features are similar to the standard design Hawley's retainer (**Fig. 43.7**). It is indicated in deep bite cases where the added feature of anterior bite plane aids in the establishment and maintenance of normal overbite by encouraging supraeruption of the posterior teeth.

vii. ***Hawley's retainer with lingual extension clasp on molars:*** This modification of Hawley's retainer has lingual extension clasp on molars instead of 'C' clasp or Adam's clasp (**Fig. 43.8**). Retentive capacity of the lingual extension clasp is comparatively less when compared to that of the Adam's clasp in the standard Hawley's retainer.

This type of modification of Hawley's retainer is indicated when there is tight occlusal contact.

viii. ***Hawley's retainer with occlusal rest:*** This modification of Hawley's retainer has occlusal rest on molars instead of 'C' clasp or Adam's clasp (**Figs 43.9**). This type of retainer is indicated when there is tight occlusal contact and occlusal arms of clasps might cause occlusal interference.

## Begg's Retainer

It was designed by PR Begg.

### Design of the Appliance

Begg's retainer consists of a labial bow wire that extends till the last erupted molar and curves around it to get embedded in acrylic base material that spans the palate (**Fig. 43.10**).

### Wire component

- Extended labial bow.

### Acrylic component

- Acrylic base material.

### Advantages

1. There is no crossover wire between any teeth, thus, eliminates the risk of space opening up.

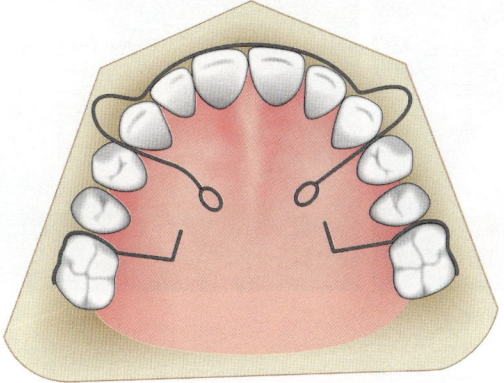

**Fig. 43.2:** Hawley's retainer with C clasp on molar

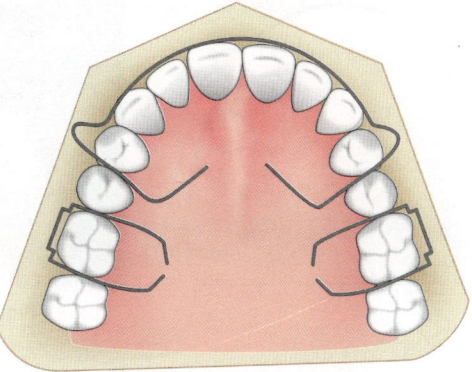

**Fig. 43.3:** Hawley's retainer with long labial bow

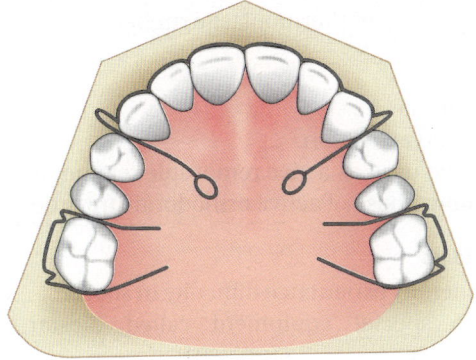

**Fig. 43.4:** Hawley's retainer with contoured labial bow

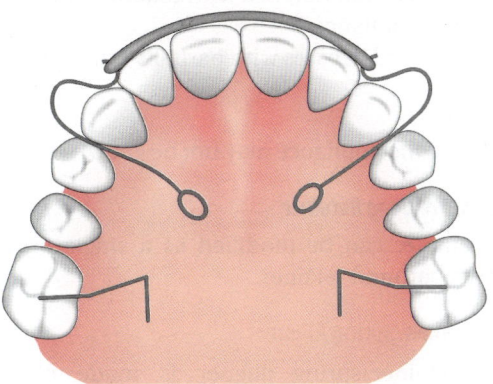

**Fig. 43.5:** Hawley's retainer with light elastics

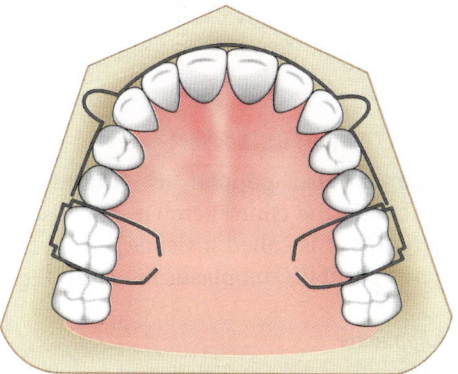

**Fig. 43.6:** Hawley's retainer with labial bow soldered to the bridge of Adam's clasp

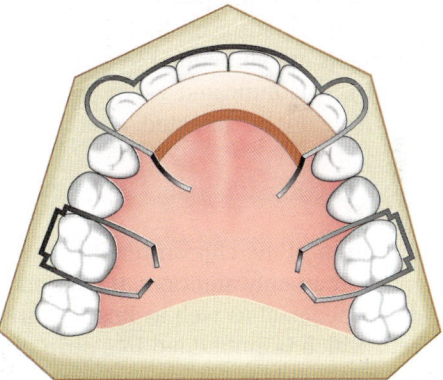

**Fig. 43.7:** Hawley's retainer with anterior bite plane

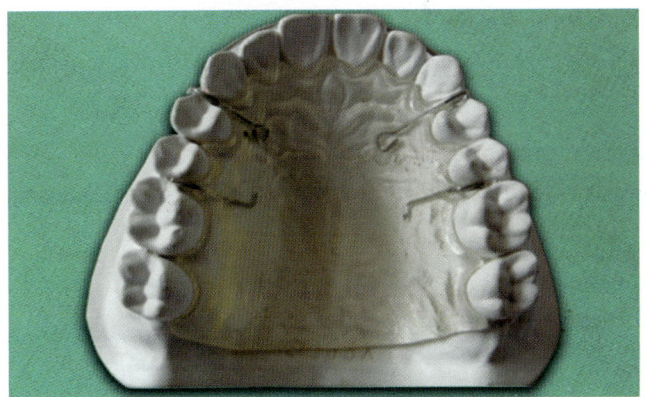

**Fig. 43.8:** Hawley's retainer with lingual extension clasp on molars

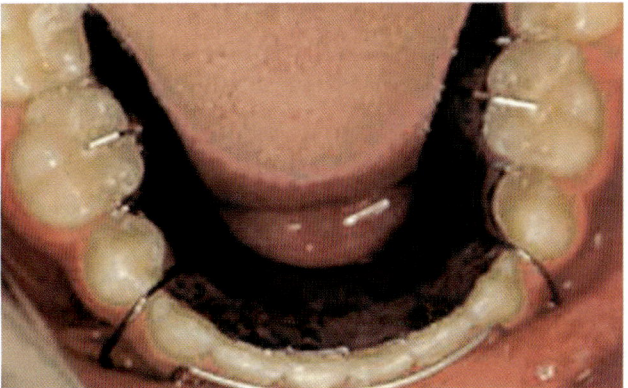

**Fig. 43.9:** Hawley's retainer with occlusal rest

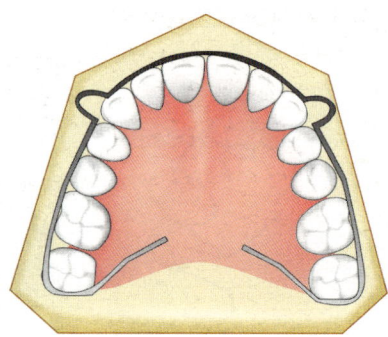 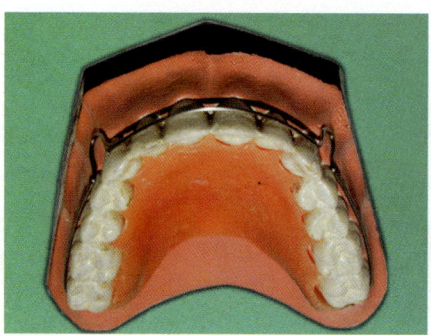 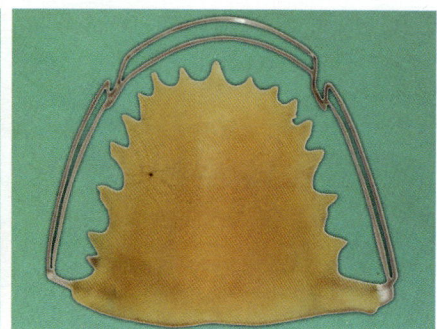

**Fig. 43.10:** Begg's retainer

2. Less occlusal interference with retainer and increased patient compliance.
3. It can be used in cases with partially erupted molars.

### Disadvantages
Retention of the appliance may not be good.

### Modification of Begg Retainer
Begg's retainer can be modified as a single arrowhead partial wraparound retainer.

### Clip-on Retainer/Spring Aligner
Clip-on retainer/spring aligner is made of a wire framework that runs labially over the incisors and then passes between the canine and premolar and is recurved to lie over the lingual surface. Both the labial and lingual wire segments are embedded in a strip of acrylic **(Figs 43.11A to C)**. It is indicated when position of the lower anteriors have to be retained after orthodontic correction.

### Wrap Around Retainer
This is a modification of the clip-on retainer that covers all the teeth rather than only anteriors. It consists of wire that passes along the labial as well as lingual surfaces of all erupted teeth which is embedded in a strip of acrylic **(Figs 43.12A and B)**.

### Kesling's Tooth Positioner
Kesling's tooth positioner was developed by HD Kesling in 1945. It covers the clinical crowns of maxillary and mandibular teeth sparing interocclusal space and a small portion of gingiva.

### Design of the Appliance
Kesling tooth positioner covers the clinical crowns of maxillary and mandibular teeth but spares the inter-occlusal space and a small portion of gingiva **(Fig. 43.13)**.

### Wire component
- There is no wire component in this type of removable retainer.

### Acrylic component
- It is made up of thermoplastic rubber-like material.

### Advantages
1. It is durable.
2. Needs no activation.
3. It can be used as active removable retainer in the final finishing phase of active orthodontic treatment.

### Disadvantages
1. Patient may experience difficulty in speech.
2. Needs special equipment called biostar for its fabrication.

### Indication
1. Can be used as an active removable retainer when minor adjustment for the settling of occlusion is required.

### Invisible Retainer (Osamu's Invisible Retainer)
Invisible retainer, also popular as Osamu's invisible retainer fully covers the clinical crowns and also a part of the gingival tissue. It is called invisible as it is fabricated from thin transparent thermoplastic material **(Fig. 43.14)**.

### Design of the Appliance
Invisible retainer fully covers the clinical crown and also a part of the gingival tissue.

### Wire component
- There is no wire component in this type of removable retainer.

### Acrylic component
- It is made up of ultra thin transparent thermoplastic sheets

### Advantages
1. They are esthetic and often go unnoticed.
2. Well accepted by patients.

### Disadvantages
It requires equipment called biostar for its fabrication.

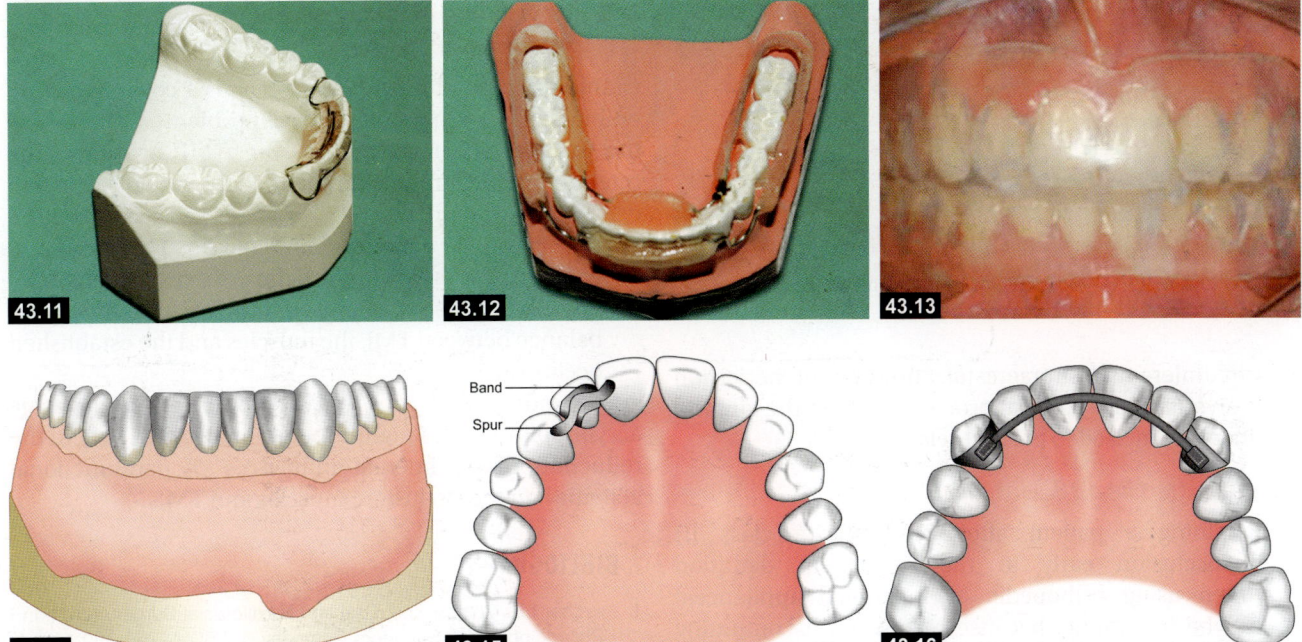

**Fig. 43.11:** Clip on retainer; **Figs 43.12:** Wrap around retainer: **Fig. 43.13:** Kesling tooth positioner; **Fig. 43.14:** Invisible retainer (Osamu's invisible retainer): **Fig. 43.15:** Band and spur retainer; **Fig. 43.16:** Banded canine-to-canine retainer

## FIXED RETAINERS

### Band and Spur Retainer

The tooth that has been rotated is banded using anterior band material and spurs are soldered onto bands so as to overlap the adjacent teeth **(Fig. 43.15)**. In derotation cases one spur is placed labially and the other lingually to prevent relapse.

#### Indications

It's a choice of retainer in case of Angle's class I malocclusion with single tooth rotation treated.

#### Advantages

1. It is very conventional in design.
2. Design permits good oral hygiene maintenance.

#### Disadvantages

It is unesthetic because metallic band and spur is visible.

### Banded Canine-to-canine Retainer

Banded canine-to-canine retainer is frequently used in mandibular anterior region.

#### Design

The left and right canines are banded and a thick wire is contoured over the lingual aspect and soldered to the canine bands **(Fig. 43.16)**.

#### Disadvantages

1. It is unesthetic because bands are visible.
2. Predisposes to poor oral hygiene because of the framework.

### Bonded Canine-to-canine

Bonded canine-to-canine retainer is a fixed type of retainer in which the retainer is bonded on the palatal/lingual surfaces of maxillary and mandibular anterior teeth **(Fig. 43.17)**. The bar of the retainer is made from a round 0.032 inch stainless steel wire or plain blue Elgiloy wire or 0.030 inch gold-coated wire. The wire is adapted palatally for upper anteriors and lingually for lower anteriors to follow the curvature of anterior teeth. Each terminal end is curved over the canines where it is bonded with a chemical cure or light cure composite resin because such adhesives provides the strongest bonds and show comparatively little abrasion over extended periods.

*Indications:* The purpose of lingual bonded retainer is as follows:

- To prevent incisor recrowding
- To hold the achieved lower incisor position in space
- To keep the rotation center in the incisor area where a mandibular anterior growth rotation tendency is present.

## RETENTION FOLLOWING CERTAIN TYPES OF ORTHODONTIC TREATMENT

### Retention following Correction of Rotation

A noticeably high risk of relapse is seen after rotation type of tooth movement, due to the resiliency of gingival fibers. Hence, the importance of proper retention following treatment of such cases cannot be overemphasized.

- Long-term retention is required.

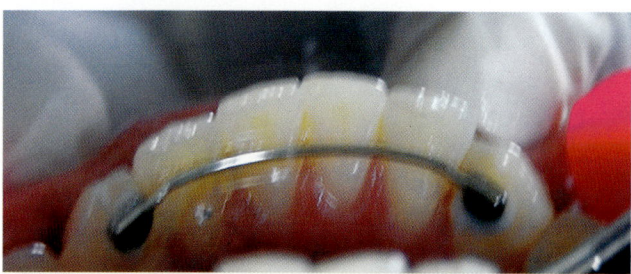

**Fig. 43.17:** Bonded canine-to-canine retainer

- Circumferential supracrestal fibrotomy or pericision is an adjunctive surgical procedure where the gingival fibers are incised to prevent relapse.

### Retention after Class III Malocclusion

- Retaining a patient after correcting a class III malocclusion early in the permanent dentition (often using orthopedic or functional appliances) can be frustrating, because relapse from continuing mandibular growth is very likely to occur and such growth is extremely difficult to control. Thus, night time wear of the appliance until cessation of growth is advised to prevent relapse.
- Applying a restraining force to the mandible, as from a chin cup, is not nearly as effective in controlling growth in a class III patient as applying a restraining force to the maxilla as in class II problems.
- In mild class III problems, a functional appliance, or a positioner may be enough to maintain the occlusal relationship during post-treatment growth.

### Retention followed by Treatment of Midline Diastema

A removable simple Hawley's retainer or fixed bonded retainer from canine to canine on palatal side is used as a retainer followed by the treatment of midline diastema to prevent opening up of the diastema.

### Retention after Deep Bite Correction

- Retention after deep bite is accomplished most readily by using a removable retainer.
- Bite depth can be maintained by wearing the retainer only at the night, after stability in other regards has been achieved.

### Retention in Cleft Palate Cases

Retention in cleft palate cases should be of longer duration than the duration normally used for noncleft patients and sometime it may be necessary to maintain for a lifetime.

### Retentions followed by the Orthodontic Treatment of Craniomandibular Disorders

Craniomandibular disorders (CMDs) is a collective term, embracing a number of clinical problems that involve the masticatory musculature, the TMJ or both. The retention procedures, recommended for patients who had orthodontic treatment and also presented earlier with a craniomandibular disorder should have a dual purpose:
- First purpose is to minimize the orthodontic relapse.
- Second purpose is to preserve the existing functional balance between TMJ, the muscles and the established occlusion.

Retention appliances that incorporate a full coverage acrylic splint for the night-time use may contribute to the reduction of detrimental influences of parafunctional activities on the occlusion, muscles and TMJs.

## BIBLIOGRAPHY

1. Archer LE. Composites, Oral and Maxillofacial Surgery (5th edn.) Philadelphia: WB Saunders Company, 1975; pp. 250-390.
2. Atherton JD, Wynne THM. Long-term assessment of the facial pattern in children who had received orthodontic treatment. D Pract 1964;14:317-22.
3. Becker A. Early treatment for impacted maxillary incisors. Am J Orthod Dentofacial Orthop. 2002;121(6):586-7.
4. Bishara SE. Impacted maxillary canines: A review. Am J Orthod Dentofacial Orthop. 1992;101:159-71.
5. Edwards JG. The prevention of relapse in extraction cases. Am J Orthod. 1971;60:128-41.
6. Graber Thomas M, Vanarsdall Robert L. Orthodontic Current Principles and Techniques. Mosby Year Book Inc, 1994.
7. Graber TM. Orthodontics: Principles and Practice. WB Saunders, 1988.
8. Jacobs RM. Treatment objectives and case retention: cybernetic and "myometric" considerations. Am J Orthod. 1970;58:552-64.
9. Khouw FE. Band space closure and retention. J Pract Orthod. 1969;3:424-5.
10. Levitt H. High labial retainer. J Clin Orthod. 1972;6:35-9.
11. Lin YT. Treatment of an impacted dilacerated maxillary central incisor. Am J Orthod Dentofacial Orthop. 1999;115:406-9.
12. Muchnic HV. Retention and continuing treatment. Am J Orthod. 1970;57:23-35.
13. Profitt WR. Contemporary Orthodontics. St Louis: CV Mosby, 1986.
14. Riedel RA. A review of the retention problem. Angle Orthod 1960; 30:179-99.
15. Rosenstein SW, Jacobson BN. Retention: An equal partner. Am J Orthod. 1971;59:323-32.
16. Steadman SR. A philosophy and practice of orthodontic retention. Angle Orthod. 1967;37:175-85.
17. Wasserstein A, Tzur B, Brezniak N. Incomplete canine transposition and maxillary central incisor impaction—a case report. Am J Orthod Dentofacial Orthop. 1997;111:635-9.
18. Weiss H, Gurman M. The tooth aligner. J Clin Orthod. 1971;5:655-7.

## EXAM-ORIENTED QUESTIONS

### Long Questions
1. Define relapse and describe various orthodontic appliances used to prevent it.
2. Retainers used in orthodontics

### Short Questions
1. Relapse
2. Hawley's retainer
3. School of retention
4. Retention followed by treatment of craniomandibular disorders.

## CHAPTER OVERVIEW

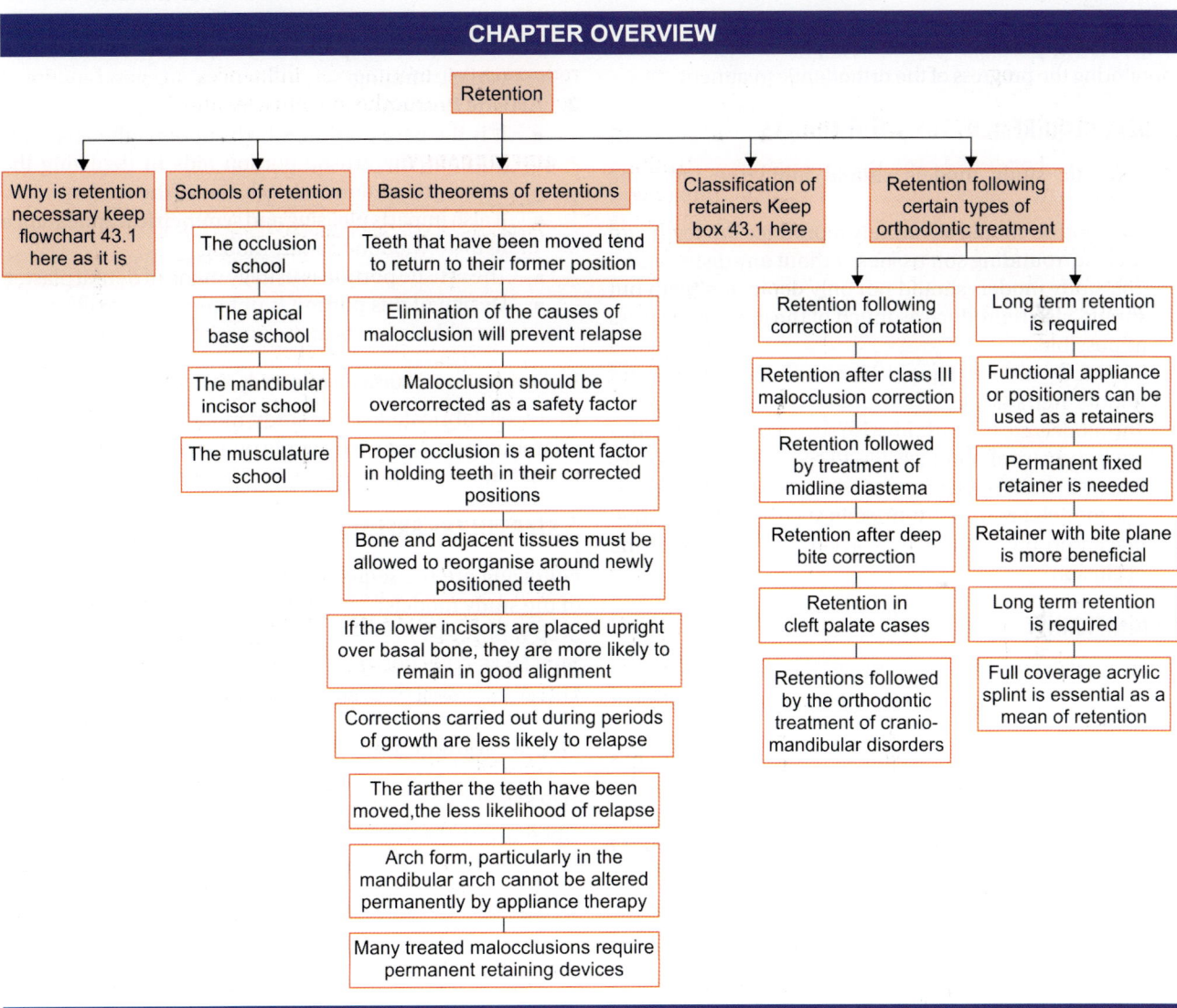

# CHAPTER 44

# Orthodontic Study Model

*Phulari BS, Tsipova V*

The study models are the accurate plaster reproductions of the teeth, alveolar process and their surrounding soft tissues. They are essential diagnostic records, which allow examination of teeth and the occlusion from all the directions. They aid in diagnosis, treatment planning and fabrication of selected appliances, as well as in patient education and monitoring the progress of the orthodontic treatment.

## IDEAL REQUIREMENTS OF STUDY MODELS

Orthodontic study models should fulfill the following criteria:
1. The models should accurately reproduce the teeth and their surrounding soft tissues without any distortion.
2. The study models should not only depict the teeth but should also reproduce as much of the alveolar process as possible.
3. The study models should have a clean, smooth and nodule-free surface.
4. The models are to be trimmed in such a manner that they are symmetrical and pleasing to the eyes. This enables instant identification of asymmetries in the arch form.
5. The models are to be trimmed in such a way that, when placed on their backs, they accurately reproduce the occlusion.

## SIGNIFICANCE

- Orthodontic study models are important and essential tools needed for orthodontic diagnosis and treatment planning.
- They are the three dimensional replica of the patient's dentition and simulate accurately the occlusion present in the patient's oral cavity.
- They provide a means of accurate assessment of occlusion as the occlusion can be viewed from all the directions, including lingual aspect.
- They act as visual guide for the clinician in planning the appropriate line of treatment.
- They serve as important visual aids for education and motivation of the patients.
- They act as permanent record of the pre-treatment state of dentition and occlusion, and thus serve as a reference to compare the post-treatment changes and are also important for medicolegal purposes.

## PARTS

Orthodontic study model consist of two parts (**Fig. 44.1**):
1. Anatomic portion.
2. Artistic portion.

1. **Anatomic Portion**
   - Anatomic portion of a orthodontic study model is that part of the study model which is the actual replica of the dental arch and surrounding tissues.
   - This part is usually made of dental stone.
   - The anatomic portion should not be disturbed while trimming.
2. **Artistic Portion**
   - It is the base portion, which supports the anatomic portion. The artistic portion aids in depicting the actual orientation and occlusion of the study models.
   - It also imparts pleasing and symmetrical appearance to the orthodontic study model.
   - The artistic portion is usually made of dental plaster.
   - Design of this portion is different for maxillary and mandibular casts in the anterior segment.

### Ratio of Portions of Orthodontic Study Model

In a well-fabricated set of study models, the ratio of the anatomic portion to artistic portion is 3:1, i.e. three parts of anatomic portion and one part of artistic portion.

## STEPS IN THE PREPARATION

Following are the sequential steps involved in fabrication of the study models:
**Step I:** Impression making
**Step II:** Disinfection of the impression
**Step III:** Casting the impression
**Step IV:** Basing and trimming of the cast
**Step V:** Finishing and polishing

### Step I: Impression Making

Obtaining a good impression of the hard and soft tissues of the dentoalveolar region is an important factor in the proper fabrication of orthodontic study models.
- The maxillary impression should cover the hard palate but should not extend on the soft palate.
- Mandibular impression should extend to the limits of the buccal and lingual sulcii.

### Armamentarium Required for Impression Making
- Impression trays (**Fig. 44.2A**)
- Irreversible hydrocolloids (alginate) impression material (**Fig. 44.2B**)

### Selection of Impression Tray
- Dentist should select the impression tray of appropriate size and extension that covers the entire hard palate and buccal sulcus in case of maxillary arch and both

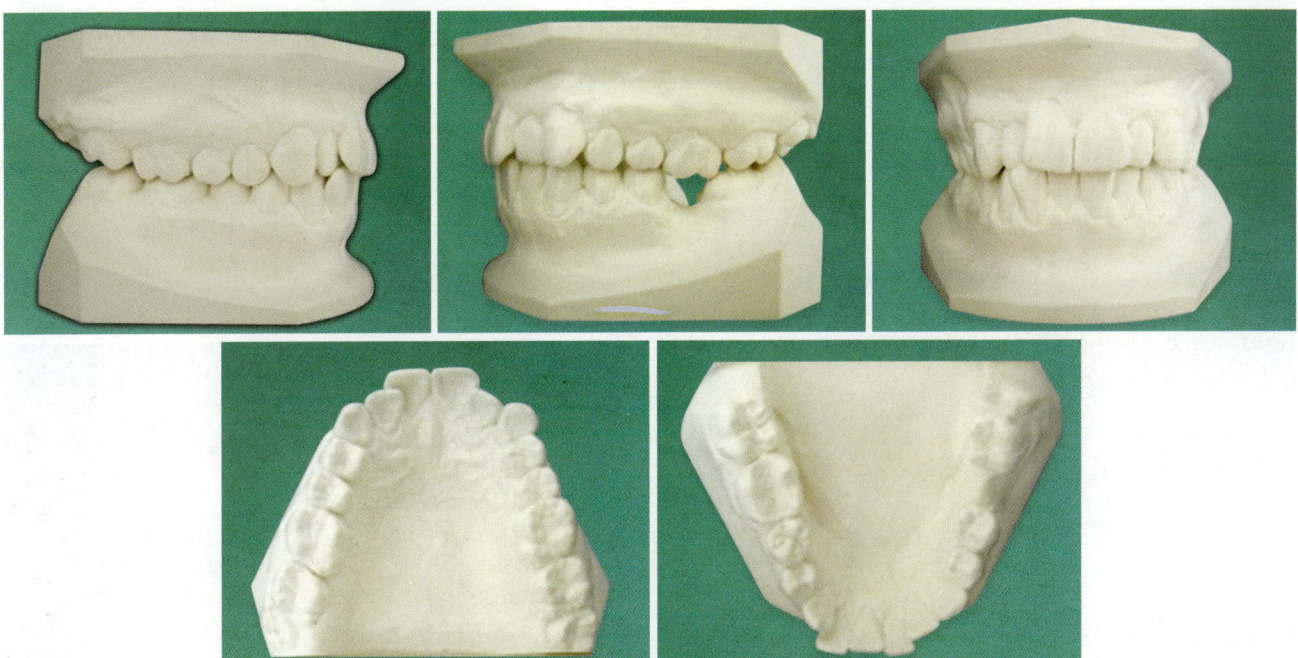

**Fig. 44.1:** Orthodontic study models

the buccal and lingual sulcii in case of mandibular arch.
- It is advisable to use high flange orthodontic trays that extend deep into the sulcii so as to reproduce as much of the supporting structures as possible.
- Selected impression trays should also include the posterior most erupted teeth.
- A clearance of 3 mm should exist between teeth and the tray to accommodate the impression material.

*Preparation of the Patient*
- Patient should be asked to rinse the mouth to eliminate food particles, etc.
- The patient is asked to sit upright on the dental chair to cover the problems of entering impression material in the pharynx and to avoid gagging reflex (**Fig. 44.3A**).
- Maxillary and mandibular impressions are made using alginate impression material (**Fig. 44.3B**).

## Step II: Disinfection of the Impression
- Impression is rinsed thoroughly in running water to free the impression from plaque and local secretions (**Fig. 44.4A**).
- Then the impression is soaked in a disinfectant solution such as biocide (**Fig. 44.4B**).
- After disinfection, the impression is once again rinsed in water to clear them of any residual disinfectant.

## Step III: Casting the Impression
The impression is then poured with finely mixed dental stone to obtain the cast (**Fig. 44.5**). Use of a vibrator while pouring eliminates incorporation of air bubbles in the cast.

## Step IV: Basing and Trimming of the Cast to Obtain the Artistic Portion

After the impression tray is poured to get the anatomic portion of the study model, the base is built up using thickly mixed dental plaster. The cast with the impression tray attached is set aside for 30-60 minutes to allow the setting of dental stone and plaster.

The base is then trimmed in a systematic manner to obtain the artistic portion of the study model (**Figs 44.6A to J**). Trimming of the cast is done using an electric plaster trimming machine with a carborandum wheel.

The following are the steps involved in trimming of the study models:

*Step 1:* Base of the mandibular cast trimmed in such a way that it should be parallel to the occlusal plane. To achieve this, the mandibular cast is placed inverted over T-shaped piece of rubber and marking is done circumferentially using a pencil marker mounted over a vertical stand (**Fig. 44.6A**). Base of the cast is then trimmed up to the marking to obtain parallelism with its occlusal plane.

*Step 2:* Back of the mandibular cast is trimmed so that it is perpendicular to the base and a line drawn between two central incisors. While trimming the back of the cast, 5 mm of plaster base should be left distal to the most posterior teeth (**Fig. 44.6B**).

*Step 3:* Occlude the upper and lower models together and trim the maxillary back surface, so that the maxillary back is in flush with the mandibular back (**Fig. 44.6C**).

*Step 4:* The upper and lower models are occluded together and are placed on their backs on the model trimmer. The base of maxillary cast should be trimmed

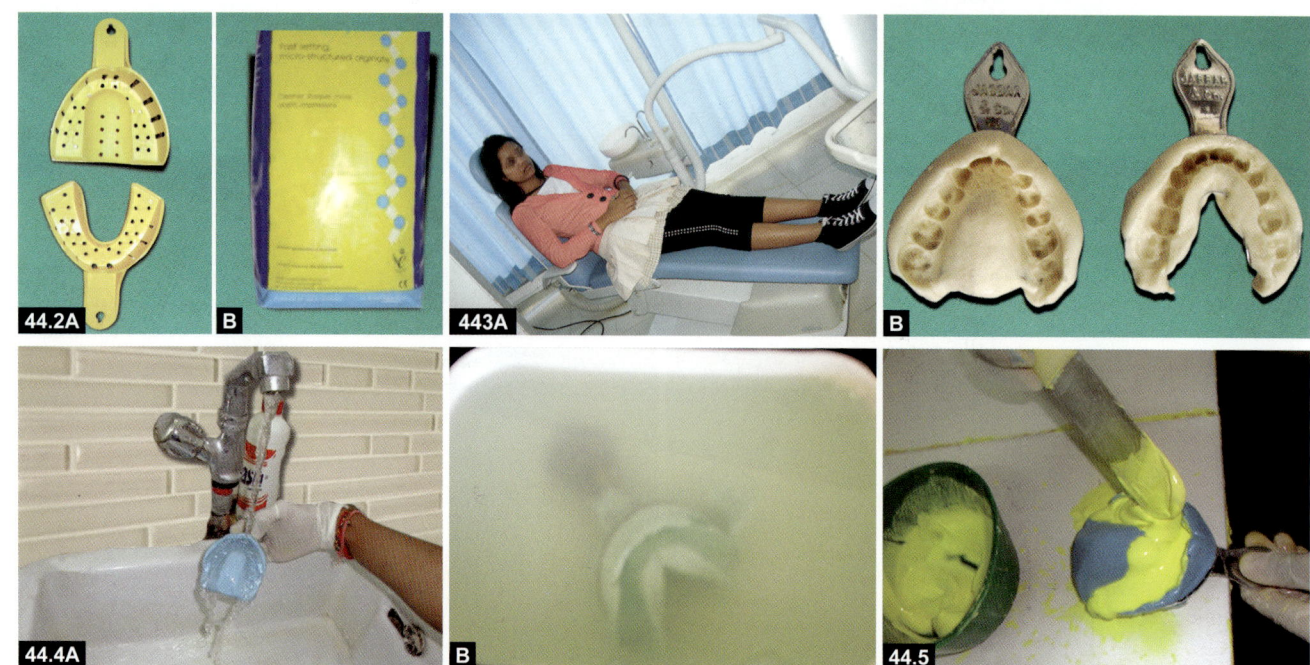

**Figs 44.2A and B:** Armamentarium required for impression making: (A) Impression trays; (B) Alginate impression trays; **Figs 44.3A and B:** (A) The patient is asked to sit in upright position on a dental chair; (B) Maxillary and madibular impression made with alginate impression material; **Figs 44.4A and B:** (A) Impression is rinsed thoroughly in running water to free the impression from plaque and local secretions; (B) Impressions kept in biocide solution for disinfection; **Fig. 44.5:** The impression is then poured with finely mixed dental stone to obtain the cast

in such a way that it is parallel to the base of mandibular cast **(Fig. 44.6D)**. After this step, the bases of maxillary and mandibular casts should be parallel to each other and to the occlusal plane, and the backs of both the casts should be perpendicular to their bases.

*Step 5:* The buccal cuts are made on the mandibular cast 5–6 mm away from the buccal surface of the posterior teeth. The buccal cuts are to be made 60° to the back of the model **(Fig. 44.6E)**.

*Step 6:* The anterior segment of the lower arch is trimmed into a curve that follows the curvature of the lower anterior teeth. The anterior curve should be (5–6 mm) away from the labial surface of the anterior teeth **(Fig. 44.6F)**.

*Step 7:* The posterior cuts of the mandibular model are made at approximately 115° to the back of the model. The linear measurement of the posterior cuts should be 13–15 mm **(Fig. 44.6G)**.

*Step 8:* The buccal cuts are made on the maxillary cast 5 mm away from the buccal surface of the most posterior teeth. The buccal cuts should be 65° to the back of the maxillary cast **(Fig. 44.6H)**.

*Step 9:* The anterior cuts are made on the maxillary cast. The cuts on either side should be of equal length and should lay 5–6 mm ahead of the labial surface of the anterior teeth. The anterior cuts on either side should meet at the midline of the cast and should extend till the midline of the canine. The anterior cuts are made 30° to the back of the cast **(Fig. 44.6I)**.

*Step 10:* The posterior cuts of the maxillary cuts are made in such a way that they are in flush with the posterior cuts of the mandibular cast. This is done by occluding the model and trimming the maxillary cuts till they are in line with the mandibular posterior cuts **(Fig. 44.6J)**.

Commercially available rubber base formers **(Figs 44.7 A and B)** can also be used to obtain the artistic base portion of the study models. These base formers have standard size and incorporate the cut design specific for maxillary and mandibular models.

After the anatomic portion is poured, the impression tray is placed inverted over the base former filled with thickly mixed dental plaster. Excess plaster is removed and cast is allowed to set.

### Trimming of Gnathostatic Models

Gnathostatic models are the orthodontic study models in which the base of the maxillary cast is trimmed to correspond to the Frankfort horizontal plane. By trimming in this fashion; the study models give an approximate idea about the inclination of the occlusal plane to the patient's face. Although valuable, such information can be easily and more accurately gained by lateral cephalogram.

### Step V: Finishing and Polishing

The artistic portion of the study models is polished using the grained sand paper to obtain a smooth finish. The casts are soaked in soap solution for about an hour. They are then rinsed in fresh water and buffed after they are dried to obtain a smooth and shiny finish. While finishing and

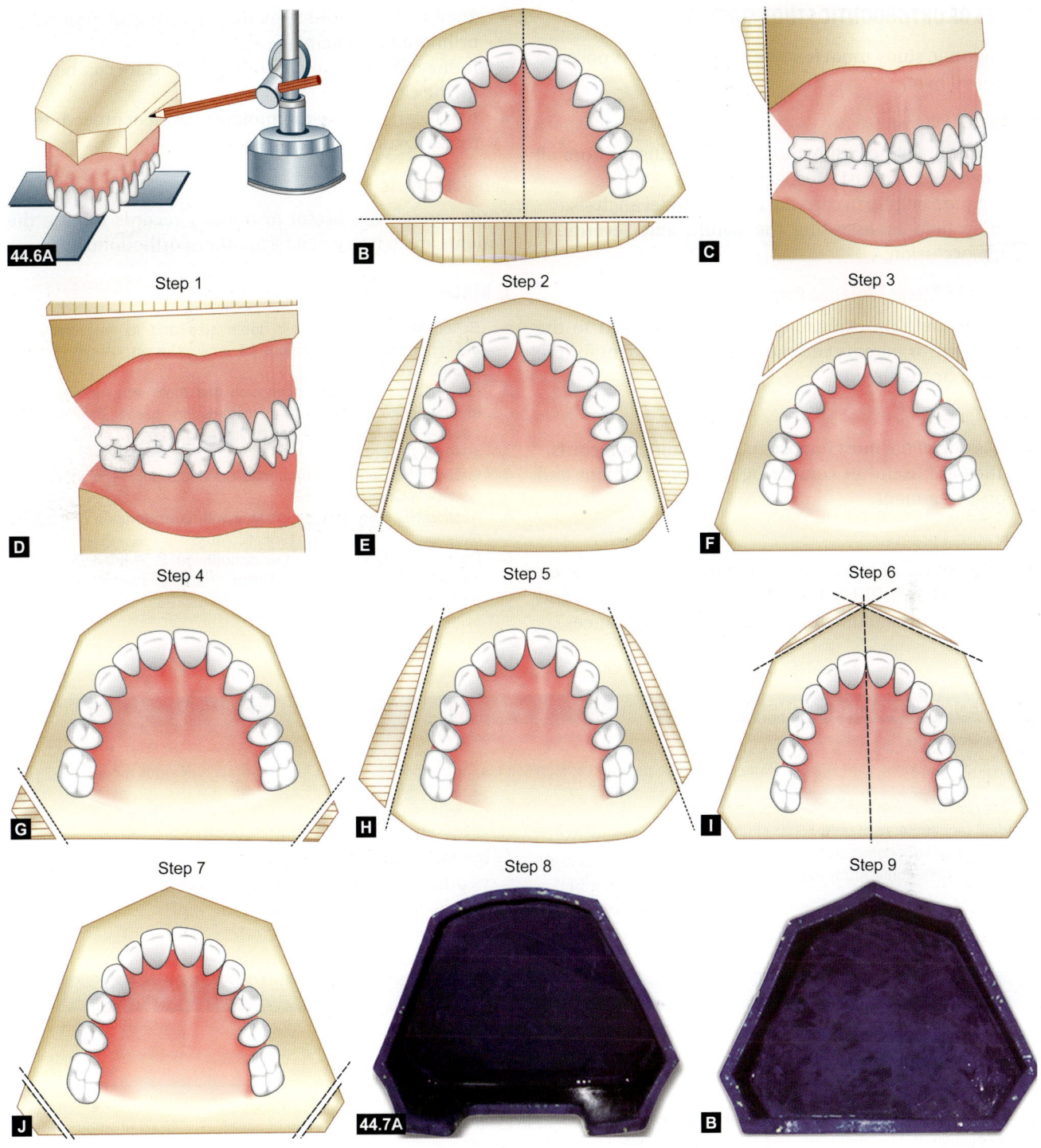

**Figs 44.6A to J:** (A to J) Steps involved in trimming of study models; **Fig. 44.7 A and B:** Base formers

polishing the models, care should be taken not to disturb the acute angles of the artistic portion.

## STORAGE OF THE STUDY MODELS

- The finished orthodontic study models are labelled with patient's name, reference number and date on the back of both upper and lower casts.

- The models should be stored on a flat surface placing the upper and lower models together on their back. It is advisable to always pick and return the upper and lower models together so as to avoid damage to the anatomic portion.

- The study models are usually stored in special racks designed for this purpose.

## USES OF ORTHODONTIC STUDY MODELS

Orthodontic study models serve a number of purposes as described here:

### Diagnostic Purpose
- With the help of study models, the occlusion from all aspects can be easily inspected.
- They are helpful in carrying out the model analysis.
- They help in assessing the nature and severity of malocclusion.

### Patient and Parent Education Purpose
They are useful in explaining the treatment plan to the patient and/or parents and motivating the patient for the orthodontic treatment.

### Record Purpose
- It is one of the most important pre-treatment records.
- They are useful in comparing the pre-treatment and post-treatment.

### Laboratory Purpose
- Fabrication of removable orthodontic appliances on the models. (All kind of labial bows and springs and expansion, myofunctional and retentive appliances).
- They are also useful in the repairing of removable orthodontic appliances.
- Indirect banding and bonding procedure can be done on the cast.
- It makes it possible to simulate treatment procedure on the cast, such as mock surgery.

### Referral Purpose
Study models are useful to transfer records in case the patients are to be treated by anothern orthodontist.

## BIBLIOGRAPHY

1. Bolton WA. Disharmony in tooth size and its relationship to the analysis and treatment of malocclusion. Angle Orthod. 1958;28:113-30.
2. Carey CW. Linear arch dimension and tooth size; an evaluation of the bone and dental structures in cases involving the possible reduction of dental units in treatment. Am J Orthod. 1949;35:762-75.
3. Graber TM. Current Orthodontic Concepts and Techniques. WB Saunders Company, 1969.
4. Kesling HD. The diagnostic setup with consideration of the third dimension. Am J Orthod. 1956;42:740-8.
5. Pont A. Der Zahn Index in Der orthodontia. Z. Zahnaerztl; 1909.
6. Tanaka, Johnston. The prediction of size of unerupted canines and premolars. Jam Dent Asso. 1974;88:798.

---

### EXAM-ORIENTED QUESTIONS

*Long Question*

1. Define orthodontic study model. Write the ideal requirements, significance, parts and the steps in the preparation of study models.

*Short Notes*

1. Ideal requirements of orthodontic study models.
2. Storage of orthodontic study models.
3. Uses of orthodontic study models.

---

### CHAPTER OVERVIEW

Orthodontic study models
- Accurate plaster reproduction of teeth, alveolar process and their surrounding soft tissues
- Parts
  a. Anatomic portion
  b. Artistic portion
- Ratio of portions of study model (anatomic portion to artistic portion is 3:1)
- Steps in the preparation of study models
  A. Impression making
  B. Disinfection of the impression
  C. Casting the impression
  D. Basing and trimming of the cast
  E. Finishing and polishing
- Storage of study models Special racks designed for this purpose
- Uses of study models
  a. Diagnostic purpose
  b. Record purpose
  c. Laboratory purpose
  d. Education purpose
  e. Referral purpose

# Welding and Soldering

*Phulari BS*

## WELDING

Welding is defined as the process of fusing two or more metal parts through the application of heat, pressure or both without a filler metal to produce a localized union across an interface between the parts.

Welding involves the joining of two or more metal pieces directly under pressure without the introduction of an intermediary or filler material.

### Types of Welding

Following are three types of welding:
1. Cold welding
2. Hot welding
3. Spot welding.

### Cold Welding

Cold welding is a process of plastically deforming a metal (usually at room temperature) accompanied by strain hardening.

For example, Gold foil filling.

### Hot Welding

Hot welding uses the heat of sufficient intensity to melt the metals being joined.

### Spot Welding

Spot welding involves both heat and pressure, these two are the basic principles involved in the process of spot welding.

For example, joining of orthodontic components.

**Principles of spot welding:** Following are the two principles involved in the process of spot welding:
 i. Heat
 ii. Pressure

- Electric current (A/C) is made to pass through a step-down transformer to obtain a low voltage of high amperage current that is conducted through two copper electrodes on either side of the metals being joined.
- Resistance offered by stainless steel to the current of high amperage generates very high temperature at the electrodes.
- Thus, the area of metal under the electrodes becomes plastic.
- The copper electrodes simultaneously apply pressure on the metals and, therefore, squeeze the metals into each other.

**Copper electrodes:** The copper electrodes (**Figs 44.1A and B**) in a welding unit serve the following purposes:

- Transmit current to the metals to be joined so as to cause a rapid increase in temperature.
- The electrodes help in conducting the heat produced away from the area so as to preserve the properties of stainless steel around the weld spot.
- The two electrodes also help in holding together the two metals to be joined.
- The electrodes are designed to apply pressure on the metals being joined. As soon as the temperature increases, the pressure exerted by the electrodes helps in squeezing the metal into each other.

**Duration of current:** It includes-

- It is very important that this passage of current at the weld spot be of very short duration, i.e. not more than 1/10th of a second.
- In case, the current is passed for a longer duration of time, it results in weld decay due to the precipitation of carbides from the metal.

### Procedure of Spot Welding

i. **Selection of proper electrodes:** Select the proper *electrodes for the thickness or shape* of the material to be welded.
   a. *For welding thin materials:* A broad electrode should be used for thin materials.
   b. *For welding thick materials:* A narrow electrode should be used for thick materials.
ii. **Cleansing the electrodes:** The electrodes of the welder are cleaned so as to remove any carbide precipitates.
iii. **Surface of electrodes:** Surface of electrodes must be smooth, flat and perpendicular to its long axis.
iv. **The metals being joined:** The metals being joined are placed between the electrodes (**Fig. 45.2**).
v. **Switch is turned on:** The electrode pressure can be maintained for a few seconds to help to obtain a good joint.

### Factors Influencing Welding of Stainless Steel

Welding of stainless steel depends on the proper use of each of the following variables:
a. The current flowing through the circuit.
b. The time during which the current is allowed to flow.
c. The mechanical pressure applied at the welding heads.

### Application of Welding in Orthodontics

1. Joining of metal strips during banding.
2. Fixing attachments, such as brackets and molar tubes to the bands (**Figs 45.3A and B**).

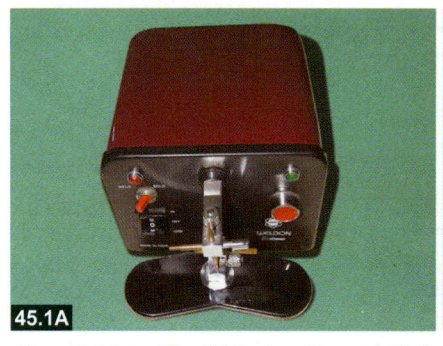 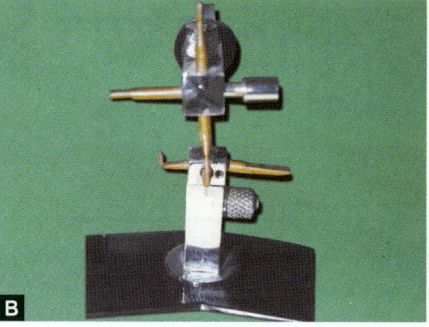 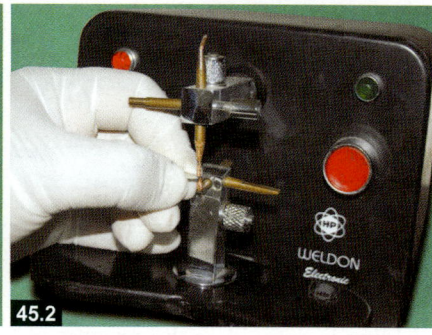

**Figs 45.1A and B:** (A) Spot welder and (B) Copper electrodes of different diameters in the spot welder; **Fig. 45.2:** Both the ends of the band material are assembled and placed between the two electrodes for welding

## SOLDERING

Soldering is defined as a process of joining metals by the use of a filler metal, which has a substantially lower fusion temperature than that of the metals being joined. If the fusion temperature of the filler metal used exceeds 440°C and then the procedure is called as brazing.

### Dental Solders (Fig. 45.4)

Dental solders are alloys that are used as intermediary or a filler metal to join two or more metallic parts.

### Ideal Requirements

1. The solder should exhibit excellent tarnish and corrosion resistance in the oral environment.
2. The fusion temperature of the dental solder should be lower than that of the parts being joined.
   Ideally fusion temperature of the dental solder should be 50–100°C less than its parts being joined.

### Definitions

#### Soldering
Soldering is defined as the process of joining metals by the use of a filler metal, which has a substantially lower fusion temperature than that of the metals being joined.

#### Brazing
If the fusion temperature of the filler metal used exceeds 440°C, then the procedure is termed as brazing.

*Types of soldering:*
There are two types of soldering:
a. Investment soldering
b. Free-hand soldering

**a. Investment Soldering**
It is carried out whenever its area of contact between the metallic parts being joined is large and whenever precision is needed in joining the metal.

### Procedure

- Procedure involves the embedding of metallic parts in an investment, leaving a gap of about 0.013 between its metals.
- Flux dissolves any surface impurities, prevents oxidation of its metals and also significantly reduces the melting point of its dental solder.

### Antiflux

Antiflux is a material that is used to confine the flow of the molten solder over the metal surfaces being joined.

### Commonly Used Antifluxes

- Lead pencil
- Graphite lines
- Iron rogu

### Flux

Flux is a Latin word meaning flow.
Composition:
Borax glass: 55%
Boric acid: 35%
Silica: 10%

### Fluoride Fluxes

- Boric acid and potassium fluoride (1:1) produces excellent soldered joints.

### Functions

1. The flux aids in removal of the oxide coating so as to increase the flow of the molten solder.
2. It should be free flowing and should adequately wet the metal parts; it unites so that good adhesion is achieved.
3. The strength of the solder should be similar to that of the metals being joined.
4. The color of the dental solder should match with that of the parts to be soldered.

### Composition

Dental solder is composed of–
- Gold
- Silver
- Copper – Yellow appearance to its solder
- Zinc
- Tin
- Nickel – White color to its solder

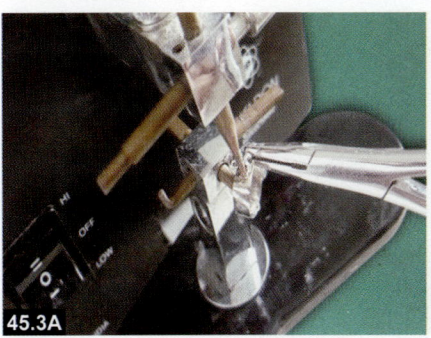 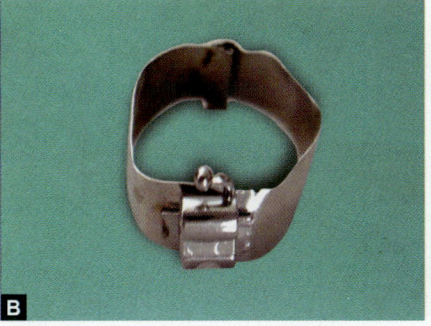 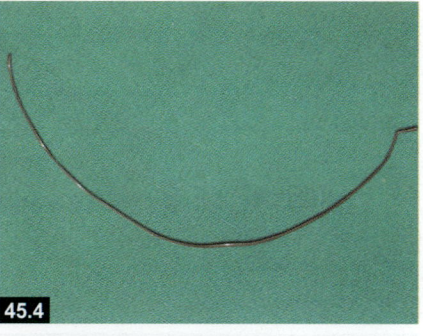

**Figs 45.3A and B:** Welding applications in orthodontics: (A) Welding of double buccal tube to molar band; (B) Figure showing double buccal tube welded to molar band; **Fig. 45.4:** Dental solder

**b. Free Hand Soldering**

The process involves soldering two metallic parts together after adequate stabilization, without the use of investment to precisely hold its parts together.

**Steps in soldering:** Following are the steps involved in the process of soldering:

1. Cleansing the surfaces to be joined
2. Assembling the parts to be joined
3. Selection of the appropriate solder and flux
4. Selection of a proper joint
5. Application of flux
6. Heat and introduction of solder
7. Quenching.

### Steps in Soldering

1. **Cleansing the Surfaces to be Joined:** Prior to the soldering, the parts to be joined should be adequately cleaned to remove dirt and other surface contaminants. Any surface impurities like dust may weaken the solder joint **(Fig. 45.5A)**.
2. **Assembling the Parts to be Joined:** Dental plaster or stone is used to stabilize the parts to be joined while maintaining 0.5 mm gap between the parts to be soldered **(Fig. 45.5B)**.
3. **Selection of the Appropriate Solder and Flux:** The appropriate dental solder and flux should be selected based on the metallic parts to be soldered. The selected solder should have a fusion temperature less than that of the metallic parts to be soldered.
4. **Selection of Proper Joint:** A proper joint required to have a good soldering joint for example, when two wires are being joined together it would be beneficial to wrap one of the wires around the other rather than having a point contact **(Fig. 45.5C)**.
5. **Application of Flux:** The flux is applied on the assembled units forming the joint and also over an extended portion of the metals to be joined. Antiflux is used to confine the flow of the flux **(Fig. 45.5D)**.
6. **Healing and Introduction of Solder:** The parts of the assembled units to be joined in healed using a soldering torch **(Figs 45.5E)**. The dental solder is introducing once the flux begins to fuse. The solder melts due to heat and filler. The joint is encasing it. The flame is maintained until the filler metal has flowed completely into the joint **(Fig. 45.5F)**.
7. **Quenching:** The soldered assembly is immediately quenched in water so as to limit the spread of heat **(Fig. 45.5G)**.

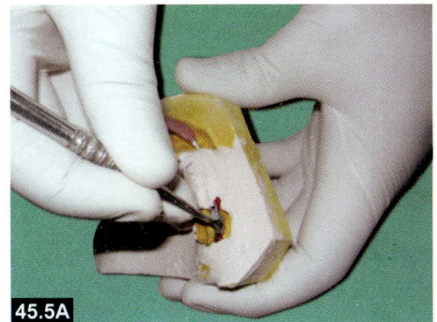 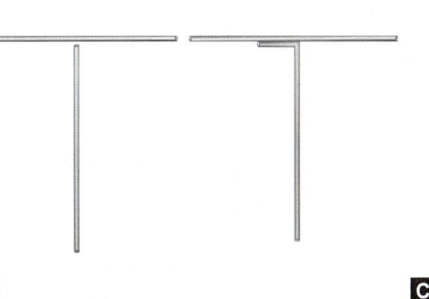

**Figs 45.5A to C:** Steps in soldering procedure; (A) Cleansing the surfaces to be joined: Prior to the soldering, the parts to be joined should be adequately cleaned to remove dirt and other surface contaminants; (B) Assembling the parts to be joined: Dental plaster or stone is used to stabilize the parts to be joined while maintaining 0.5 mm gap between the parts to be soldered; (C) Selection of proper joint: A proper joint required to have a good soldering joint

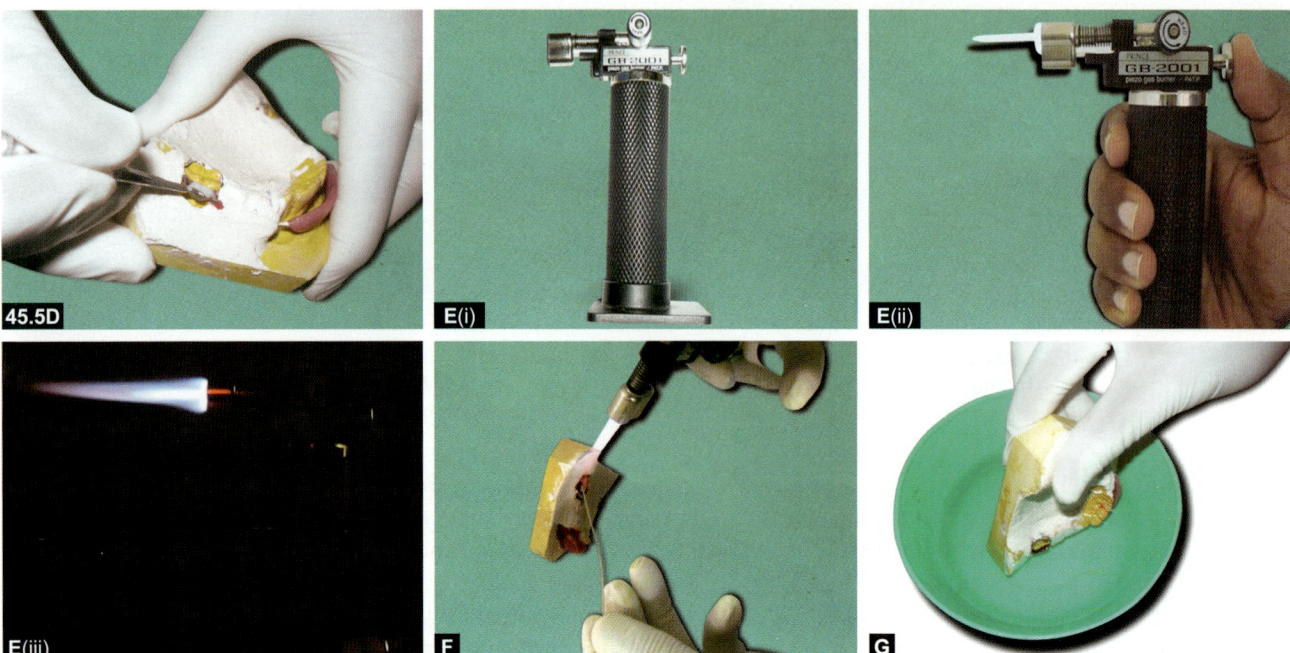

**Figs 45.5D to G:** Steps in soldering procedure; (D) Application of flux: The flux is applied on the assembled units forming the joint and also over an extended portion of the metals to be joined; (E) Soldering torch; (F) The flame of the soldering torch is maintained until the filler metal has flowed completely into the joint; (G) Quenching: The soldered assembly is immediately quenched in water so as to limit the spread of heat;

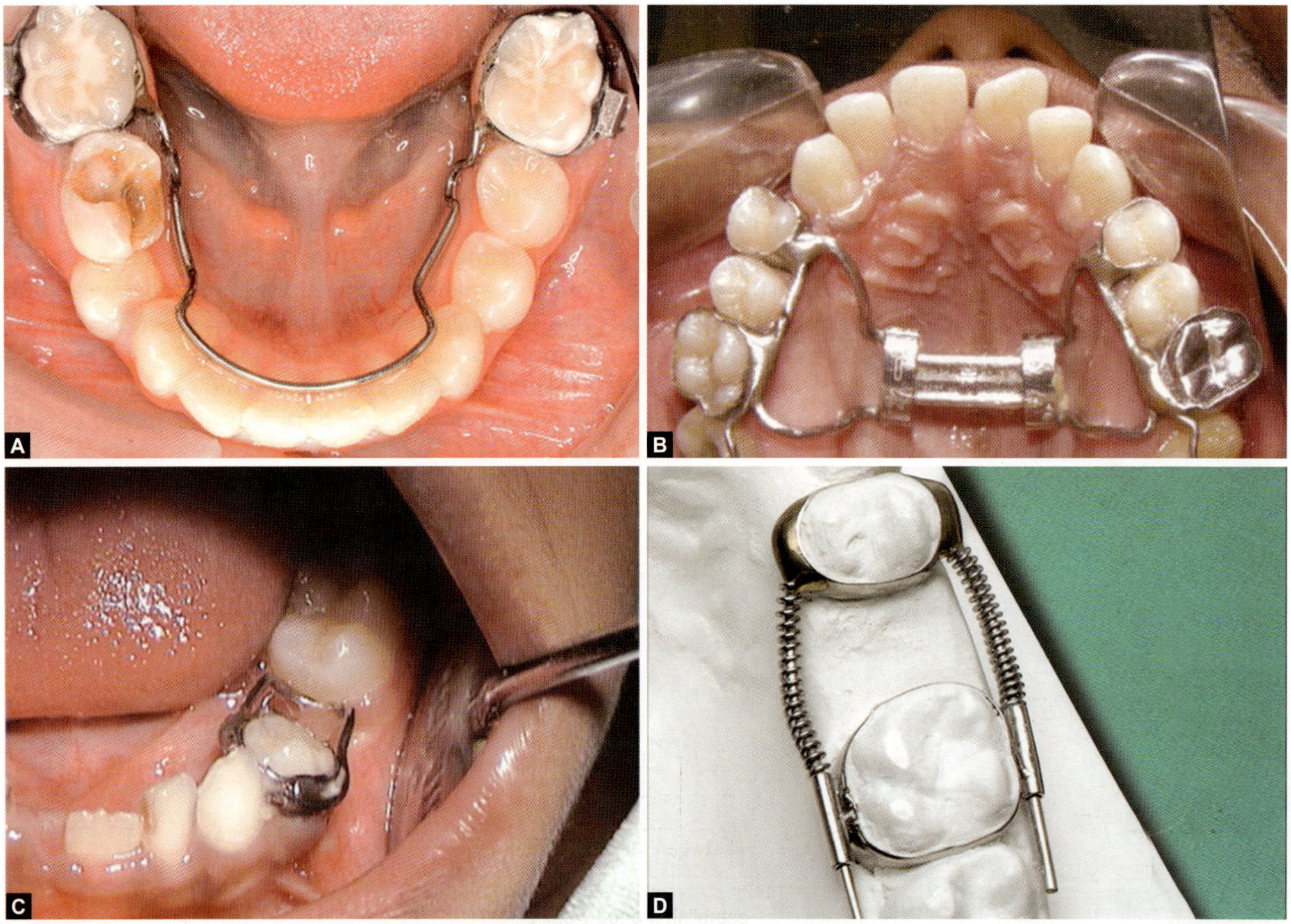

**Figs 45.6A to D:** Clinical application of soldering in orthodontics: (A) Lingual arch: Note that the lingual arch is soldered to the mesolingual line angle of the mandibular molar band; (B) Hyrax rapid maxillary expander; (C) Band and loop space maintainer in which a loop is soldered to the molar band on its buccal and lingual surfaces; (D) Gerber's space regainer.

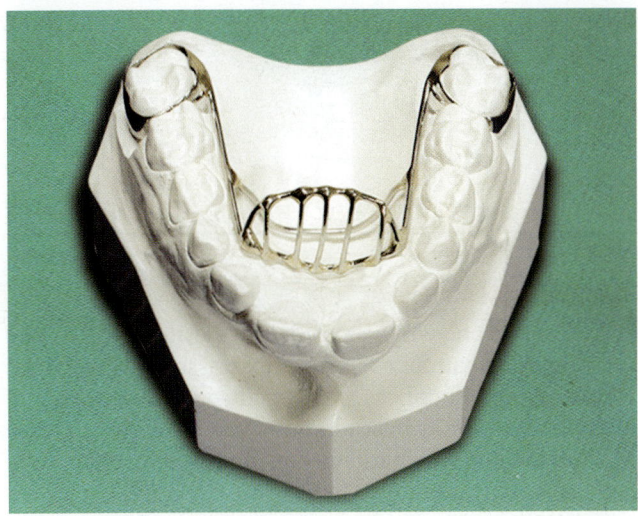

**Fig. 46.6E:** Fixed crib in which the crib is soldered to the palatal surface of the molar bands

### Clinical Application of Soldering in Orthodontics

Soldering is used to fasten the attachments to the molar band, such as:
- Quad helix
- Lingual arch (**Fig. 45.6A**)
- Hyrax maxillary expander (**Fig. 45.6B**)
- A loop in case of band and loop space maintainer (**Fig. 45.6C**)
- Gerber's space regainer (**Fig. 45.6D**)
- Transpalatal arches
- A fixed crib (**Fig. 45.6E**)
- W arch appliance.

## BIBLIOGRAPHY

1. Craig. Dental Materials. Mosby, 1998.
2. Profitt WR. Contemporary Orthodontics. St Louis: CV Mosby, 1986;228-44.
3. White TC, Gardiner JH, Leighton BC. Orthodontics for dental students. MacMillan, 1985.

---

### EXAM-ORIENTED QUESTIONS

#### Long Questions
1. Define welding. Write the types, procedure and applications of welding in orthodontics.
2. Define soldering. Write the types of solders, procedure and applications of soldering in orthodontics.
3. Soldering, welding & brazing.

#### Short Notes
1. Weld decay
2. Clinical applications of soldering in orthodontics
3. Clinical applications of welding in orthodontics
4. Dental solders
5. Brazing
6. Flux and Antiflux.

---

## CHAPTER OVERVIEW

Welding procedure
- Types of welding
  - Cold welding e.g gold foil filling
  - Hot welding
  - Spot welding e.g joining orthodontic components
- Principles of welding
  - Heat
  - Pressure
  - Welding
- Welding procedure
  - First step-selection of proper electrodes
  - Second step–cleansing the electrodes
  - Third step-surface of electrodes must be smooth and flat
  - Fourth step–metals being joined are assembled and placed between the electrodes
  - Fifth step-switch is turned on to establish a good weld joint
- Applications of welding
  - Joining of metal strips during banding
  - Fixing attachments such as weldable brackets, cleat, button to the band

# Adult Orthodontics

*Phulari BS*

Traditionally, orthodontic treatment has been rendered to children and adolescents. However, the ratio of adults seeking orthodontic treatment has been on the rise in the last few years. Progressively better understanding of bone cell reactions to orthodontic forces has lead to the success of adult orthodontics. Today, healthy teeth can be moved at almost any age. The American Association of Orthodontists estimates that nearly one in five orthodontic patients is an adult.

Major reasons for this emerging trend include an increased social awareness of the availability of orthodontic treatment for adults, an increased appreciation of how orthodontist can facilitate other dental treatments, such as prosthetic and restorative procedures to maintain the dentition; and improvements in the design of orthodontic appliances.

Adults are those who are past their growing years. Generally, individuals above 18 years of age are considered as adults. Young adults are essentially treated as other adolescent patients. However, middle aged and older adults with medical factors and compromised dentition (e.g. periodontal disease, tooth loss) often require an integrated multidisciplinary approach to obtain the best possible results.

This chapter describes the essential aspects of adult orthodontics.

## REASONS OF INCREASED NUMBER OF ADULT PATIENTS

The number of adult patients is overwhelming in certain parts of the world that some orthodontists have restricted their practices only to them. Various factors have contributed to an increased percentage of adult patients in today's orthodontic practice.

### Increased Public Awareness

Increased awareness about the significance of dental health and about the availability of orthodontic treatment for adults is one of the main reasons for the increased adult orthodontic patients. Media in the form of newspapers, health magazines and advertisement has contributed to the heightened awareness among public.

### Esthetics Conscious Society

In today's society, a person's dentition is an important component of facial attractiveness, which can markedly affect his or her self esteem and self image. Several studies have shown that the primary motivation for adults who seek orthodontic care by their own wish is to improve their dental and facial appearance.

### Increased Social Acceptance

Primary reason why most adult hesitate to obtain orthodontic treatment is the embarrassment associated with wearing appliances. Increased social acceptance of orthodontic therapy in adults associated with the increase in adult orthodontic patients has diminished some of the fears of embarrassment.

### Advances in Appliance Design and Technique

Recent advances in orthodontic appliance design have increased patient acceptance. Direct bonding technique has significantly decreased the bulk of the appliances. Today's metal appliances are much smaller and thus are esthetically less objectionable.

In addition, ceramic brackets and tooth color wires have made orthodontic appliances less noticeable. Lingual placement of brackets (lingual orthodontics) and invisalign (invisible orthodontics) techniques have only increased the scope of adult orthodontics.

### Increased Affluence

As adults become economically independent they can afford the expenses of orthodontic treatment.

### Advances in the Field of Surgical Orthodontics

Advancement in surgical orthodontics has widened the possibilities of correcting severe skeletal discrepancies in adults who are past growing age. Treatment of severe skeletal malocclusions in nongrowing adult is now possible with orthogenetic surgeries.

### General Dentist Awareness

Now, general dentists are more aware of the scope of orthodontics in adult patient and appreciate how orthodontics can facilitate other dental procedures to maintain the dentition. General dentist often refer the adult patient for orthodontic consultation.

## DIFFERENCES BETWEEN ADOLESCENT AND ADULT PATIENTS

A number of differences can be appreciated between adult and adolescent patients in terms of growth changes, medical and dental status, motivation, hygiene maintenance, etc. **(Table 46.1)**. These differences have to be kept in mind for achieving optimal result in adult patients.

In contrast to children and adolescents, who exhibit significant craniofacial growth, adults has minimal or no growth potential left and thus, they cannot be treated

| Table 46.1: Differences between child/adolescent patient and adult patient | | |
|---|---|---|
| **Factors** | **Child/adolescent patient** | **Adult patient** |
| 1. Growth potential | <ul><li>Significant growth is still occurring</li><li>Possible to treat skeletal discrepancies with growth modification</li></ul> | <ul><li>No/limited growth potential. Only tooth movement possible</li><li>Growth modification not possible</li><li>Skeletal discrepancies need surgical approach</li></ul> |
| 2. General health | <ul><li>Seldom a concern, chronic medical problems are less likely to be present</li></ul> | <ul><li>Major concern (e.g. diabetes, osteoporosis, renal failure, etc.)</li></ul> |
| 3. Dental status | <ul><li>Sound dentition</li></ul> | <ul><li>Compromised dentition with edentulous spaces, caries, failing old restorations, abrasion, attrition</li></ul> |
| 4. Periodontal health | <ul><li>Good periodontal health</li></ul> | <ul><li>Increased prevalence of periodontitis</li></ul> |
| 5. Motivation and cooperation | <ul><li>Ranges from poor to excellent</li><li>Hygiene maintenance may be a major problem when cooperation is lacking</li></ul> | <ul><li>Highly motivated and cooperative, good oral hygiene maintenance</li></ul> |
| 6. Appliance design and esthetics | <ul><li>Rarely a concern</li></ul> | <ul><li>Of major concern</li><li>Ceramic brackets, lingual bracket placement preferred</li></ul> |
| 7. Appliance tolerance | <ul><li>Usually tolerate most appliances readily</li></ul> | <ul><li>May take more time to adjust. Appliances should be well designed to prevent trauma and soft tissue irritation</li></ul> |
| 8. Speech | <ul><li>Learn to adjust quickly</li></ul> | <ul><li>Adjustment takes time and effort</li></ul> |
| 9. Anchorage planning | <ul><li>Less challenging.</li><li>Extra oral anchorage feasible</li></ul> | <ul><li>More challenging</li><li>May require mini-implants in case of multiple tooth loss</li></ul> |
| 10. Retention | <ul><li>Short- 6 months retention sufficient in most cases</li></ul> | <ul><li>Long term/ permanent retention may be required</li></ul> |
| 11. Appreciation of treatment outcome | <ul><li>Ranges from hardly concerned to highly appreciative</li></ul> | <ul><li>Usually highly appreciative</li></ul> |

with growth modification procedures. Consequently, orthognathic surgery may be required in adults with skeletal discrepancies, such as severe class II or class III malocclusions.

Cooperation is often a problem with children and adolescents, especially when they are not motivated and are compelled to take treatment by their parents. Adults usually make wonderful patients as they are highly motivated, cooperative, keep up appointments and are appreciative of the treatment outcome. Children and adolescents generally have intact dentition with few restorations and a healthy periodontium **(Fig. 46.1)**. Adults may have old failing restorations, tooth loss with migration of adjacent teeth into edentulous spaces, abraded teeth, periodontal bone defects, and a variety of other restorative and periodontal problems that would compromise the orthodontic result **(Fig. 46.2)**.

## BIOMECHANICAL CONSIDERATIONS IN ADULT PATIENTS

Adults may have problems other than malposed teeth and jaws that make their orthodontic treatment more challenging. The following are some of the important factors to be considered while treating adult patients.

### Systemic Health

Chronic medical problems are more likely to be present in older adults. Certain conditions, such as renal and

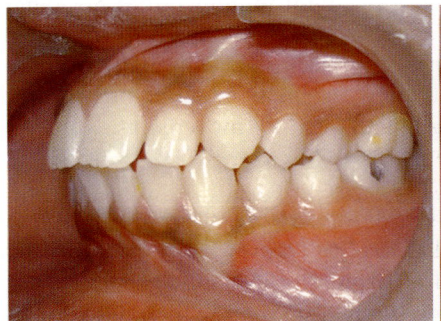 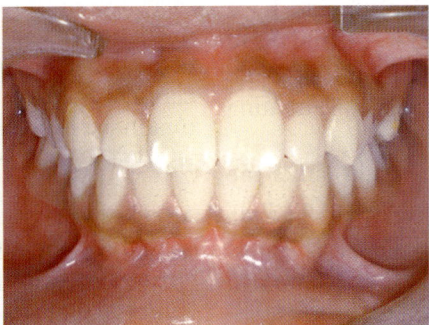 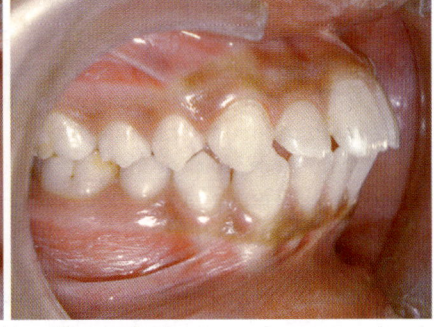

**Fig. 46.1:** Healthy periodontium in a female adolescent patient with bimaxillary protrusion

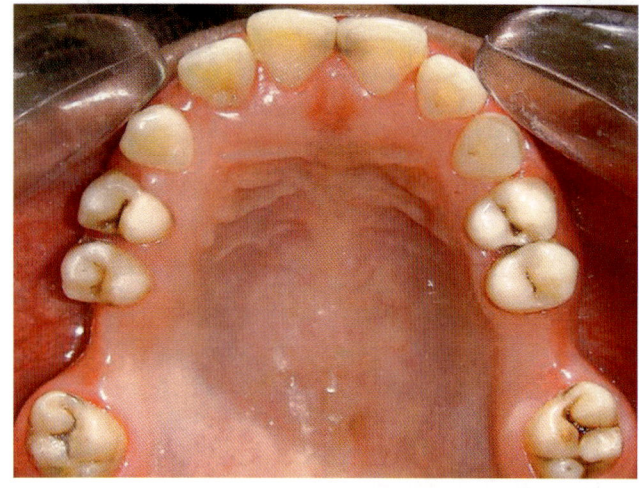 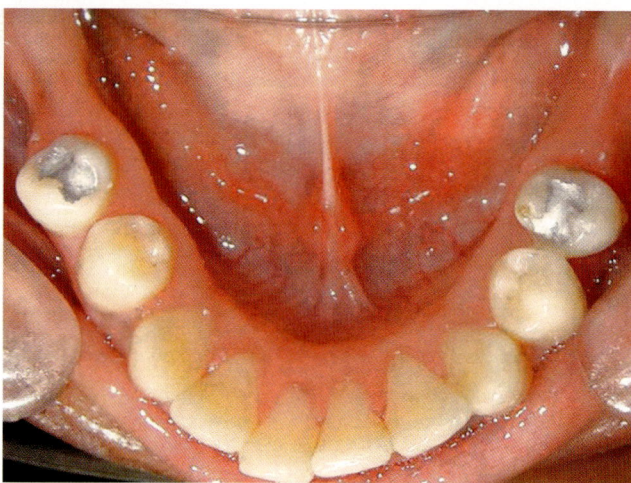

**Fig. 46.2:** Adults may have old restorations, tooth loss with migration of adjacent teeth into edentulous spaces, abraded teeth and periodontal bone defects that would compromise the orthodontic outcome

liver diseases, osteoporosis, which affect vitamin D and calcium metabolism may complicate orthodontic tooth movement. Patients with uncontrolled diabetes often exhibit periodontal disease, resulting in a severe bone loss. Orthodontic treatment in such patients may result in significant complications. Orthodontic treatment can be performed if diabetes is well controlled and periodontium is healthy. With advances in medical care, most conditions do not preclude orthodontics treatment as long as they are under control and the patient is receiving regular medical care.

**Age Related Changes**

Ageing is associated with myriad biochemical changes that could affect the feasibility and duration of orthodontic therapy. Reduced cell population and often reduced vascularity of alveolar bone mean slower initial tooth movement but otherwise movement is as efficient as in adolescents. Retention is often lengthy as there is slower tissue remodelling and it must be permanent, if there is reduced periodontal ligament support.

**Periodontal Disease**

Adults have increased prevalence of periodontal disease. Periodontal disease should be under control before orthodontic therapy is begun and patient should have regular periodontal follow up. Decrease in the height of alveolar bone decreases the periodontal support of teeth. Thus, lighter orthodontic forces are required while treating adults with reduced periodontium.

Furthermore, loss of alveolar bone height shifts the center of resistance of the tooth more apically. This may necessitate alteration in the bracket placement so as to direct the forces as near to the center of resistance as possible. Otherwise more tipping movement of teeth occurs, which may not be desirable.

Alveolar bone loss in adults often causes disproportionate crown/root ratio of teeth. Orthodontist may have to reduce the clinical crown length of these teeth to improve the crown/root ratio before the placement of brackets.

### Lack of Growth Potential

Lack of growth in adult means that skeletal discrepancies other than mild ones are often best dealt with orthognathic surgeries rather than by dental camouflage.

### Drugs

Orthodontic tooth movement may be impeded by certain drugs used primarily by adults, such as inhibitors of bone resorption used to treat osteoporosis (e.g. alendronate, calcitonin, bisphosphates) and potent prostaglandin inhibitors used for arthritis (e.g. indomethacin).

### Anchorage Planning

Anchorage planning is more demanding in adult due to previous tooth loss and/or reduced bony support. Extra oral anchorage is not realistic instead; palatal and lingual arches have to be used. In case of multiple missing teeth and mini- implants may have to be used to obtain good anchorage and better control over tooth movements **(Fig. 46.3)**.

### Mechanics of Tooth Movement

Mechanics of tooth movement in adults does not differ much from that of adolescent, but may have to be modified to their specific goals. Root resorption **(Fig. 46.4)** is a more commonly encountered problem in adult orthodontic treatment, especially with intrusive movements.

### Lack of Functional Adaptability

Adults have less adaptive ability to disruption in occlusion, so stable functional occlusion post-treatment must be ensured. Occlusal disruption and abnormal occlusal contacts may lead to temporomandibular joint (TMJ) problems.

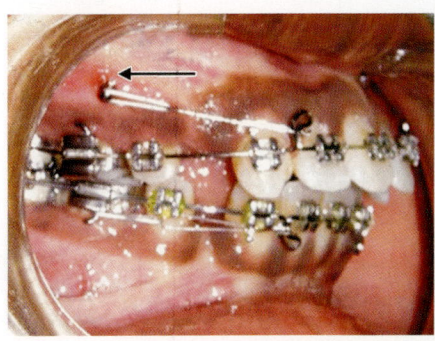 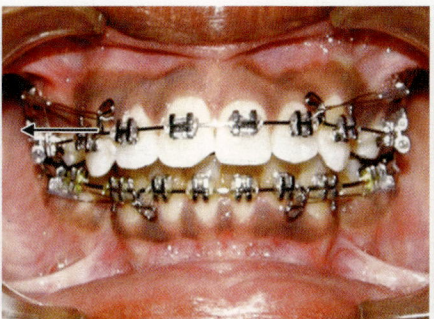 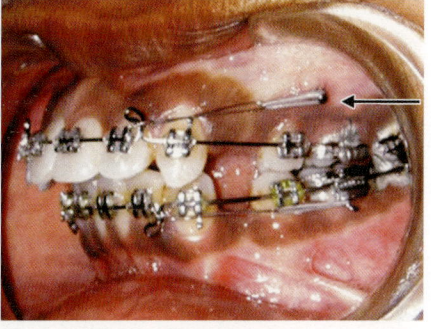

**Figs 46.3:** Mini-implants may have to be used to obtain good anchorage and better control over tooth movements

## DIAGNOSIS AND TREATMENT PLANNING IN ADULT ORTHODONTICS

### Systematic Evaluation

Compared to the management of children and adolescent, adult orthodontic treatment is more challenging as there is a higher probability of medical and dental compromise. Adult patients seek orthodontic treatment not only to improve occlusion but also for esthetic reasons, psychosocial factors and improvement of periodontal health, general health and speech. Thus, it is important to follow a disciplined evaluation process to prevent overlooking significant problems.

The evaluation process should begin with an overall consideration of patient's health by considering medical factors, psychological factors and lifestyle and then progress through an orderly evaluation of the face, TMJ, oral cavity, periodontal status, restorative status and other factors before reaching the target malocclusion. Along with routine diagnostics aids, additional diagnostic procedures, such as TMJ projection radiographs, muscle examination and stress evaluation may have to be done.

### Setting Realistic Treatment Goals

In adolescent patients with complete dentitions, orthodontic treatment objectives tend to be idealistic. Idealistic treatment objectives may not be appropriate and even not possible in adult patients with compromised dentition. Not all existing occlusal irregularities in adult patient need to be corrected to an adolescent ideal. Thus while treating adult patients, it is important to set realistic goals by considering occlusal, periodontal, restorative, esthetic and economic factors.

### Appliance Selection

Appliance selection is an important aspect of treatment planning for adult patients. Esthetically pleasant and less noticeable appliances are important for adults as they often have active professional and social lives. Lingual orthodontic technique **(Fig. 46.5A)** is an excellent choice. Ceramic brackets **(Fig. 46.5B)** and tooth colored wires are preferred to metal appliances **(Fig. 46.5C)**.

### Multidisciplinary Approach

Usually orthodontist makes most of the decisions about treatment plan for a child or adolescent patient. However, adult patients with compromised general and dental health require a multidisciplinary approach for optimal results. A team of orthodontist, oral and maxillofacial surgeon, periodontist, endodontist and prosthodontist must interact to make prudent treatment decisions for the patient.

## TYPES OF ORTHODONTIC TREATMENT IN ADULTS

Adult orthodontic treatment **(Table 45.2)** has been classified by Profitt as:
1. Adjunctive orthodontic treatment
2. Comprehensive orthodontic treatment
3. Surgical orthodontic treatment.

## ADJUNCTIVE ORTHODONTIC TREATMENT

Adjunctive orthodontic treatment is the movement of teeth to facilitate other dental procedures necessary to control disease and restore function. For instance, tilted, drifted and rotated abutment teeth may have to be orthodontically corrected before prosthetic replacement of the missing teeth. Since the goals of an adjunctive therapy are usually limited, orthodontic appliances are typically required in only a portion of the dental arch, i.e. segmental treatment.

**Fig. 46.4:** Mild root resorption following orthodontic treatment

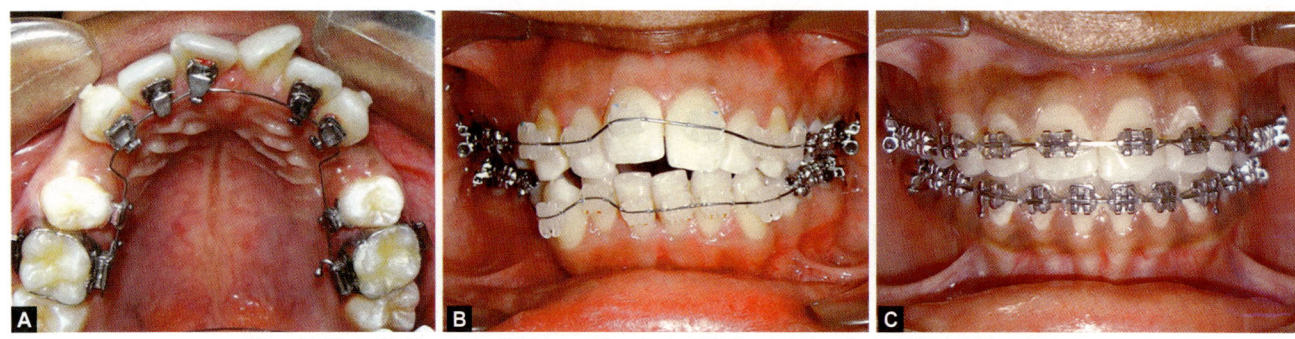

**Figs 46.5A to C:** Brackets: (A) Lingual brackets, (B) Ceramic brackets, (C) Metal brackets

Adjunctive orthodontic treatment requires less time as compared to comprehensive orthodontic treatment. With efficient use of orthodontic appliances, most of the adjunctive orthodontic treatments can be completed within six months duration.

### Indications of Adjunctive Orthodontic Treatment

Adjunctive orthodontic treatment includes the following procedures done as an adjunct to cosmetic, prosthetic restorative and periodontal procedures.

#### Restorative Indications

- Closure of midline diastema by composite build up **(Figs 46.6A and B)**: Most adult patient seeks orthodontic treatment for esthetic reasons. Anterior diastemas may compromise one's facial esthetic greatly. Space closure or space redistribution by orthodontic tooth movement can simplify restorative procedures and greatly improve the esthetics. Orthodontic space redistribution improves access and permits placement of well adapted and contoured restorations. For example, when composite resin build up to recontour incisors are planned.
- Anterior alignment: Mild anterior crowding or proclination can be successfully treated with adjunctive orthodontic treatment using segmental fixed mechanotherapy **(Fig. 46.7)**. Overlapping incisors, rotated anterior teeth, when corrected orthodontically will restore esthetics and function.

- Correction of unesthetic gingival level discrepancies: A common problem in adult patient is wear or abrasion of central incisors causing uneven gingival levels, which is unesthetic. Gingival level discrepancy can also be caused by unilateral gingival recession. In such a situation, facial esthetic can be improved by orthodontic extrusion of longer tooth to bring the gingival margin to same level and then reducing the incisal edge of the extruded tooth or by intrusion of shorter tooth and then restoring its incisal position to increase the crown height.
- Elimination of interproximal "Black Spaces": Presence of open gingival embrasures between central incisors creates "black space," which is unesthetic. Poor embrasure form may be due to divergent root of incisors or abnormal crown shape with incisal edges much wider than cervical portion. "Black spaces" can be eliminated by orthodontically correcting the divergent roots or by recontouring the mesial surfaces of central incisors and then orthodontically closing the space.

#### Prosthodontic Indications

- Uprighting of tilted teeth and regaining the extraction space: Loss of posterior teeth (usually first permanent molars) is a frequent problem in adults. When a tooth is lost the adjacent teeth usually tip, drift or rotate. This makes prosthetic replacement of missing teeth difficult due to insufficient space for pontic placement. Orthodontic correction of tipped, drifted and rotated teeth will result in increased space for prosthetic replacement of teeth by fixed/removable partial dentures **(Fig. 46.8)**.
- Paralleling of abutment teeth: One of the common prosthodontic indications of orthodontic treatment is to achieve parallelism of the abutment teeth when bridgework is planned. Occlusal forces are better distributed when abutment teeth are upright and parallel with each other.
- Space opening for insertion of single tooth implant: Another common situation requiring adjunctive orthodontic treatment involves congenitally missing one or two maxillary lateral incisors and patient may need implants to replace missing tooth or teeth. Often

**Table 46.2:** Types of adult orthodontic treatment

| Factors | Adjunctive treatment | Comprehensive treatment |
|---|---|---|
| Goal | To facilitate disease control and restoration of function | To achieve ideal occlusion |
| Extent of application | Less than full arch | One or both the arches |
| Timeframe Type of problem | 6 month or less<br>• Extrusion<br>• Molar uprighting<br>• Space redistribution<br>• Incisor alignment | 8 to 36 months<br>• Open bite<br>• Deep bite<br>• Skeletal excess or deficiency<br>• Class II or class III malocclusion |

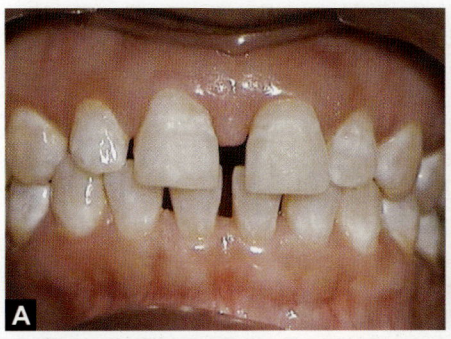
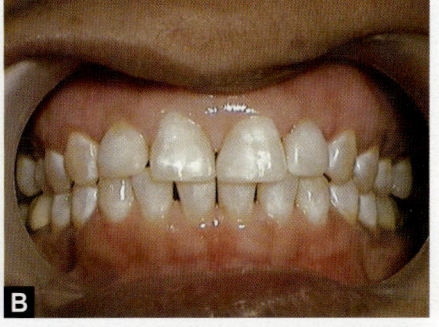

**Figs 46.6A and B:** Management of midline diastema in adults by composite build up (Courtesy: Dr Anil Shah, Innovate Dental Clinic, Surat, India)

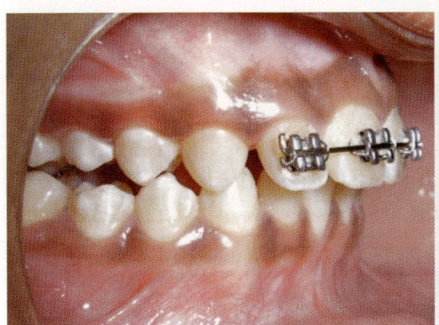
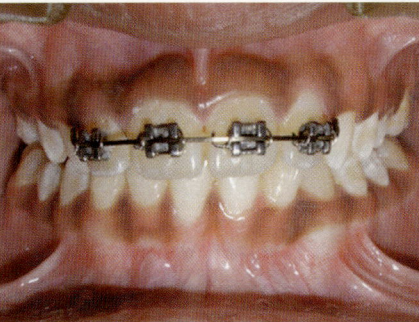
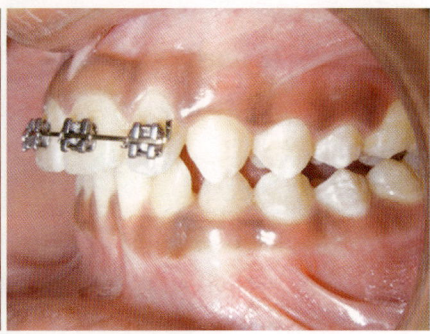

**Fig. 46.7:** Segmental fixed mechanotherapy used to treat mild anterior proclination

canines drift next to central, leaving insufficient space for implants. Space can be gained by orthodontic tooth movement to facilitate implant placement. Orthodontic space regaining may also be indicated for restorative build up of peg-shaped or malformed lateral incisors.

- Intrusion of supraerupted teeth: When a tooth is lost, the antagonistic tooth tends to supraerupt. Supraerupted teeth may have to be intruded to facilitate prosthetic rehabilitation of the patient.

### *Periodontal Indications*

Tilted teeth can be uprighted orthodontically to eradicate pseudoperiodontal pockets, which may progress to periodontitis and bone loss due to the accumulation of subgingival plaque. Orthodontic uprighting will restore the periodontal ligament health.

- Slow orthodontic extraction: When a compromised tooth is indicated for extraction and implant is planned for its replacement, slow extrusion of the tooth by orthodontic force application facilitates alveolar bone generation. Thus, when eventually the mutilated tooth is extracted, there is sound bone ready to receive implant rather than an empty extraction socket.

### *Endodontic Indications*

- Forced eruption of endodontically treated fractured teeth: When clinical crown length is less due to fracture or carious destruction, crown placement after endodontic treatment becomes difficult. Forced eruption in such cases increases the clinical crown height and gives proper retention for the crown.

## COMPREHENSIVE ORTHODONTIC TREATMENT

The objectives of comprehensive orthodontic treatment are to achieve the best balance between dental and facial esthetics, ideal occlusal relationships and long-term dentoalveolar stability. Consequently, complete fixed appliances are used to reposition all or nearly all of the teeth in one or both arches.

Comprehensive orthodontic treatment is usually carried out in young adults **(Figs 46.9A to C)** and is similar to orthodontic treatment performed in adolescent patients. It involves full-fledged orthodontic treatment with or without extraction of teeth. It typically takes longer than 6 months to complete and may extend up to 18 months.

### Indications

Comprehensive orthodontic treatment is indicated for malocclusions that lead to:
- Unacceptable esthetics
- Reduced masticatory function
- Increased predisposition to trauma (for example, protruded incisors are more prone for traumatic injury)
- Increased predisposition to caries and periodontal ligament diseases

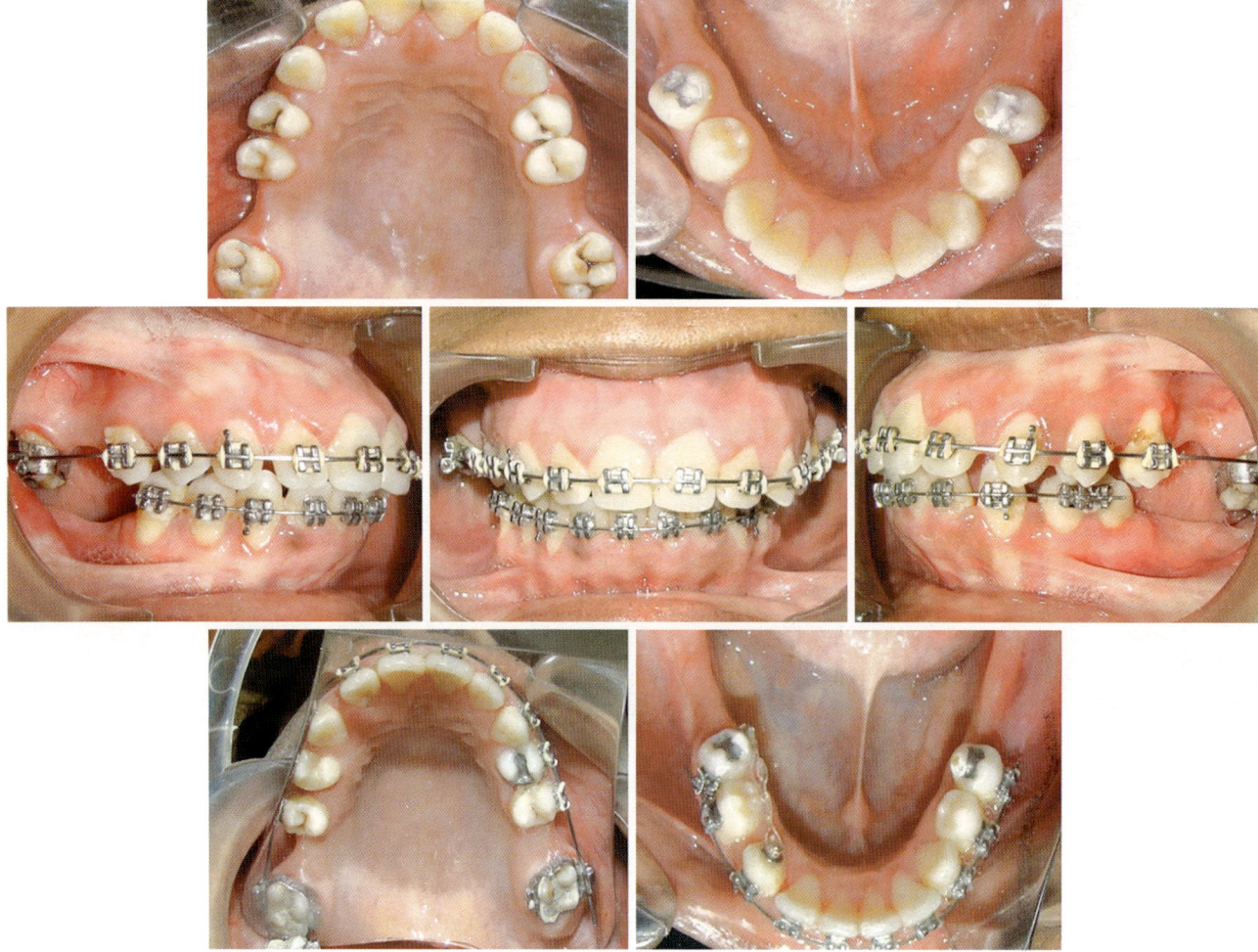

**Fig. 46.8:** An adult with multiple tooth loss, spacing in the arches and drifting of teeth into the space will make difficult for prosthetic replacement. Hence, orthodontic correction for spacing and drifted teeth will result in increased space for prosthetic replacement of teeth by fixed/removable partial dentures

- Deep, impinging overbite predisposes to periodontal ligament breakdown
- Class II malocclusion, crossbite or open bite may predispose to temporomandibular dysfunction.

Comprehensive orthodontic treatment in adult is essentially similar to orthodontic treatment in adolescent except that the previously mentioned biochemical considerations have to be borne in mind. Comprehensive treatment of adults may or may not require surgical orthodontic correction.

### SURGICAL ORTHODONTIC TREATMENT FOR ADULTS

As growth modification has little value in case of adults, more severe skeletal discrepancies need orthognathic surgeries to obtain optimal results. Surgical orthodontic approach involves the following phases of treatment:
- Pre-surgical phase: Involving orthodontic decompensation of teeth
- Surgical phase: Involving planned surgical fracturing of maxilla and/or mandible followed by their repositioning and stabilization using bone plates or wires
- Post-surgical phase: Involving achievement of final occlusal balance, stability and esthetics.

Surgical orthodontic procedures are dealt in detail in a separate chapter 41.

### RETENTION FOLLOWING ORTHODONTIC TREATMENT IN ADULTS

Appropriate retention after completion of active orthodontic mechanotherapy is an important consideration in adult orthodontics. In adults who require prosthetic replacement of missing tooth after orthodontic correction, the retainer should also include a temporary replacement for the missing tooth until permanent prosthesis or implant is placed. As adults often have prior bone loss and periodontally compromised teeth,

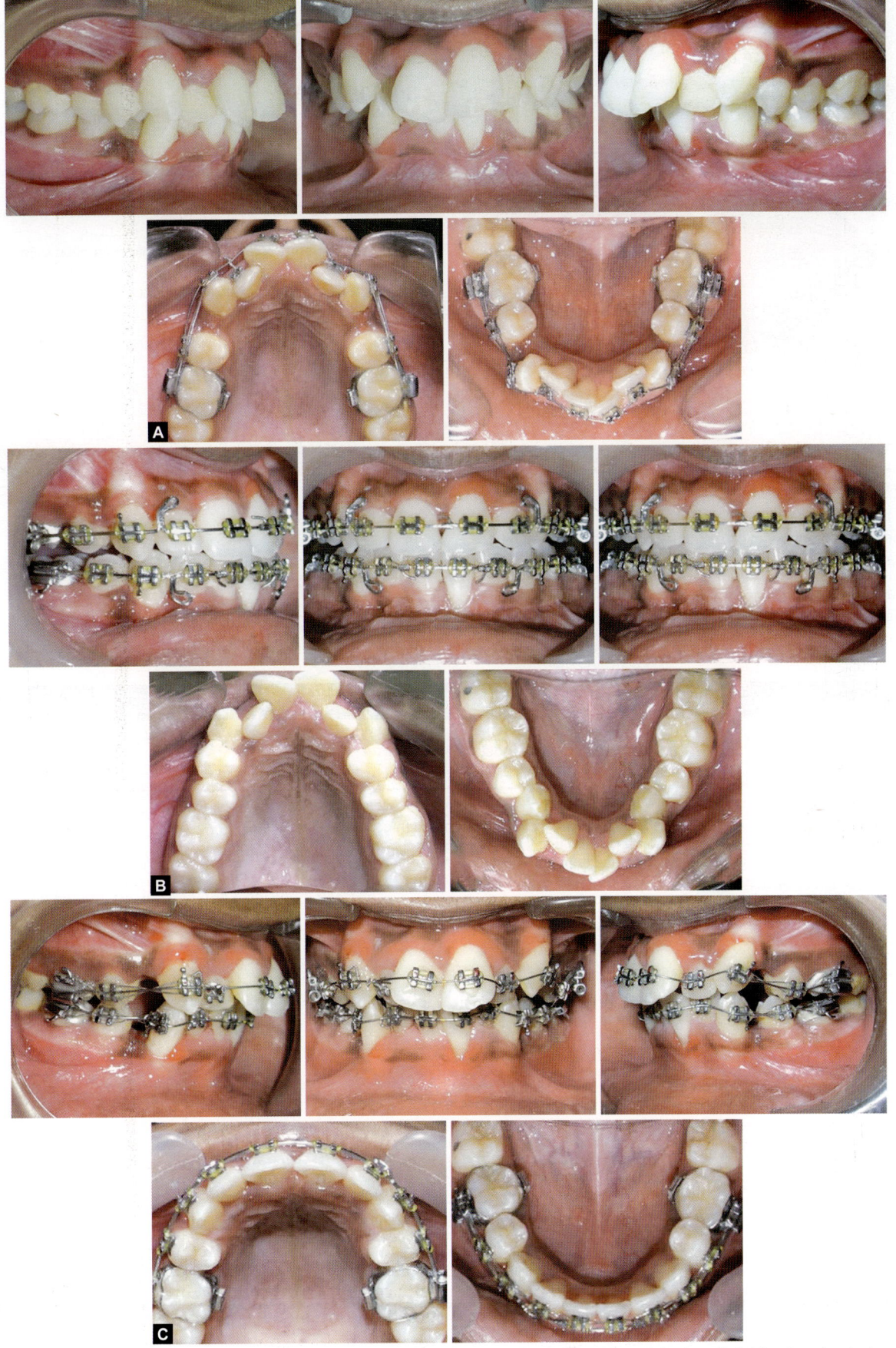

**Figs 46.9A to C:** Comprehensive orthodontic treatment carried out in a young adult with Angle's class II division 2 malocclusion. (A) Pretreatment intraoral photographs. (B) During treatment with fixed orthodontic appliance. (C) Nearing completion of treatment

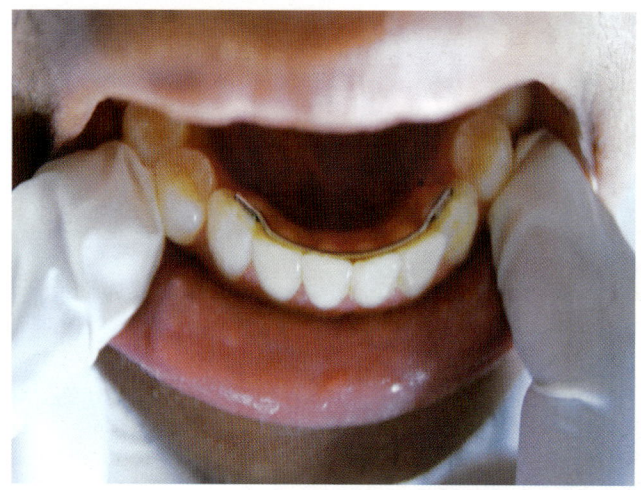

**Fig. 46.10:** Fixed lingual bonded retainer from canine to canine

the retention should also aim at stabilizing the teeth and reducing mobility. Permanent lingual bond type of retainer is often beneficial **(Fig. 46.10)**.

## BIBLIOGRAPHY

1. Graber TM, Vanarsdall RL. Orthodontic Current Principles and Techniques. Mosby Year Book Inc., 1994.
2. Graber TM. Craniofacial morphology in cleft palate and cleft lip deformities. Surg Gynecol Obstet. 1949;88:359-69.
3. Graber TM. Orthodontics: Principles and Practice. WB Saunders, 1988.
4. Nattrass C, Sandy JR. Adult orthodontics—a review. Br J Orthod. 1995;22:331-7.
5. Profitt WR. Contemporary Orthodontics. St Louis: CV Mosby, 1986;228-45.

## EXAM-ORIENTED QUESTIONS

### Long Questions
1. Adult Orthodontics
2. Types of adult orthodontic treatment.

### Short Notes
1. Adjunctive v/s Comprehensive treatment
2. Retention in adult orthodontic treatment.

## CHAPTER OVERVIEW

Adult orthodontics

- Reasons of increased number of adult patients
  - Increased public awareness
  - Esthetic conscious society
  - Increased social acceptance
  - Advance in appliance design and technique
  - Increased affluence
  - Advance in field of surgical orthodontics
  - General dentist awareness
- Difference between adolescent and adult patient Keep table 46.1
- Biomechanical considerations in adult patients
  - Systemic health: Renal and liver disease, osteoporosis affects vitamin D deficiency and calcium metabolism and may complicate orthodontic tooth movement
  - Age related changes: Affects feasibility and duration of orthodontic therapy
  - Periodontal disease: Causes disproportion of crown/root ratio of teeth
  - Drugs: Yalendronate, calcitonin, bisphophate and indomethacin may impede orthodontic tooth movement
  - Anchorage planning: TPA and lingual arches are used
  - Mechanics of tooth movement: Intrusive force causes more root resorption
  - Lack of functional adaptability: Occlusal disruption and abnormal occlusal contacts may lead to TMJ problems
- Types of orthodontic treatment
  - Table 46.2
- Retention in adult orthodontics
  - Permanent lingual bonded retainer is often more beneficial in adult orthodontics

# CHAPTER 47

# Implants in Orthodontics

*Vernon MD*

With the advent of osseointegrated oral implants in the latter half of the 20th century, a permanent and independent alternative to conventional fixed prosthodontics was born. The orthodontic premise of conserving the natural dentition was bolstered by the ability to treat hypodontia and space closure with endosseous implants.

Though it remains important to seek the ideal outcome with orthodontics alone, in particular circumstances combinative therapy of implant placement and orthodontics may give a better result. A good grasp of implant therapy is required to allow comprehensive orthodontic treatment planning.

A second significant development is the use of implants for orthodontic anchorage. The ankylosed nature of endosseous implants creates an immovable platform from which true (or total) anchorage may be achieved.

Mini-implants have evolved from past implant principles to provide the orthodontist with a simple placement implant with which to achieve this anchorage.

## IMPLANT THERAPY

Endosseous implants form an intimate abutment with bone by osseointegration, a term first described by the orthopedic surgeon Professor Brenamark. Though a number of materials have demonstrated osseointegration ability, commercially pure titanium is considered the most effective. Modern-day implants consist of a threaded cylinder with a rough titanium oxide surface. A coronal lumen allows the insertion of either a screw-retained crown or an abutment onto which a crown is cemented (**Fig. 47.1**).

High success rates and long-term predictability may be achieved with ideal selection criteria. Few absolute medical contraindications exist to prohibit implant placement. Both short- and long-term success may be compromised by aggressive periodontal disease, poor oral hygiene and smoking. Naturally, a pragmatic and holistic approach should be adopted on a case by case basis, considering all the relevant factors.

Placement requires sufficient bone volume to encapsulate the implant. A number of bone augmentation techniques exist to overcome an insufficiency of bone. Such procedures include guided bone regeneration, ridge expansion, ridge splitting, intraoral and extraoral bone grafts and sinus floor elevation.

Careful assessment of the bone volume is critical to provide predictable surgery. Inspection of the recipient alveolar site along with palpation will start to build a picture of the ridge morphology.

Ridge mapping using callipers to pierce the mucosa and measure the bone width may be used in accessible regions but is generally unreliable. True preoperative 1:1 mapping may only be achieved by computed topography. The advent of low dose high accuracy Cone Beam CT (CBCT) scanning has led to a greater prescription of such mapping techniques. MRI scanning is also used with growing popularity.

Though implants can be loaded immediately with a restoration, more commonly a period of 3–6 months is required to allow for osseointegration. This is a two stage-approach and once osseointegrated, the implant may be restored.

## INFRAOCCLUSION

As implants remain dimensionally static, care must be given when considering implant placement with the adolescent. Continued remodeling of the alveolus will result in an apparent vertical withdrawal of the implant, a process called infraocclusion. For this reason, implant placement should be withheld until the mainstay of dentoalveolar growth has occurred. This growth cessation varies between individuals but a perhaps crude rule is 18 years. Infraocclusion may occur at any age given the

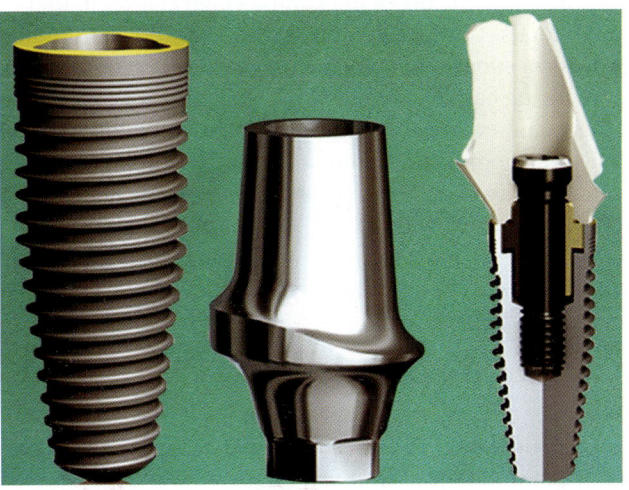

**Fig. 47.1:** Replace Select Nobel Biocare™—Implant, abutment and Abutment/Implant

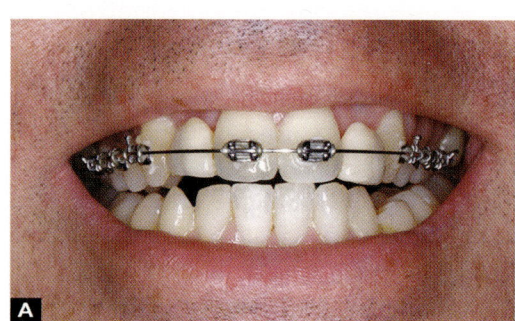 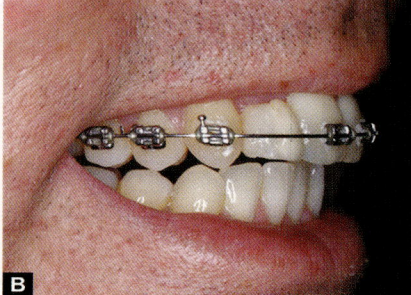 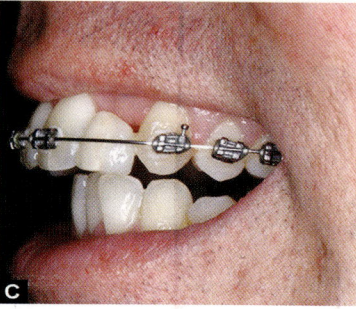

**Figs 47.2A to C: (A)** 12, 22 space expansion 7 mm (front view); **(B)** Lateral view (left side); **(C)** Lateral view (right side)

continued remodeling of the alveolus throughout life and care should be taken to accommodate this when deciding on the gingival level of the implant-retained crown.

The presence of tooth buds and the relatively poor bone density in patients under 15 years is a further contraindication. Generally, 17–18 years of age is considered safe, however, growth assessment must be made on an individual basis. For these reasons, single implant placement in conjunction with orthodontics is generally restricted to adults.

With sensible planning and with careful case selection, implant success is considered to be high. Many studies report success rates between 95% and 100% in the long term. Mandibular implants appear to carry a marginally higher success rate than in the maxilla.

### Congenitally Missing Maxillary Lateral Incisors

A common indication for the use of endosseous implants in combination with orthodontics is congenitally missing lateral incisors. It is the view of the author, however, that in the majority of cases, space closure with careful and convincing camouflage of the maxillary anterior segment is preferable. A purely orthodontic approach will avoid infraocclusion of the implant-retained crowns over time.

Once space closure is achieved between the canines and the central incisors, slight extrusion of the canines is required to bring down the canine gingival level to that of the laterals. Conversely, intrusion of the first premolars will allow subsequent gingival recontouring to establish a convincing canine gingival level. Reduction of the canine length and composite addition can create a good lateral incisor camouflage. Often a slight lengthening of the central incisors is also required to establish an esthetic crown length to width ratio. Composite addition to the maxillary first premolars should be performed in order to create "canine" guidance and, therefore, a favorable occlusal scheme.

### Tooth Movement and Composite Camouflage

Maxillary incisors fail to develop in 2% of the population. Though uncommon, the resultant malocclusion is the most noticeable. The decision must be made whether to orthodontically close the space and camouflage the canines or to place endosseous implants. Patient's expectations, esthetics and the occlusal scheme will influence the decision. Due to infraocclusion concerns, combinative orthodontic/implant therapy should generally be limited to adult orthodontics preferably with a nongingival smile line.

Natural space closure will generally prohibit implant placement. Orthodontic expansion is required to achieve sufficient width for both implant placement and the provision of a well-proportioned crown. Care must be taken to ensure the adjacent roots do not converge and restrict the mesiodistal corridor along the length of the implant **(Figs 47.2A to C)**.

6 mm mesiodistal width is required for the placement of a narrow implant along with 5 mm thickness of the alveolar ridge and 6 mm interdental space.

Once space has been achieved, a temporary rochette bridge may be used for interim esthetics and space maintenance. A bisacryl pontic will allow the addition of composite resin as the space increases. Use of an orthodontic bracket cement will allow the removal and replacement of the bridge for implant placement. An alternative and perhaps more simple solution is attached to a free pontic to the orthodontic wire with a bracket.

### Rochette Temporary Bridges

Following orthodontic expansion, the alveolar ridge thickness will become thin. Assessment of the bone volume, including ridge thickness must be made both before and after orthodontic treatment.

Ridge expansion **(Figs 47.3 to 47.6)** may be performed, if the cortical plates are not fused and sufficient alveolar

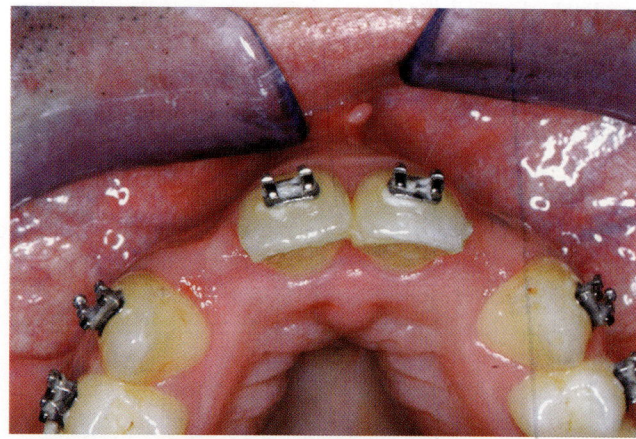

**Fig. 47.3:** Preoperative state, note labial plate concavity

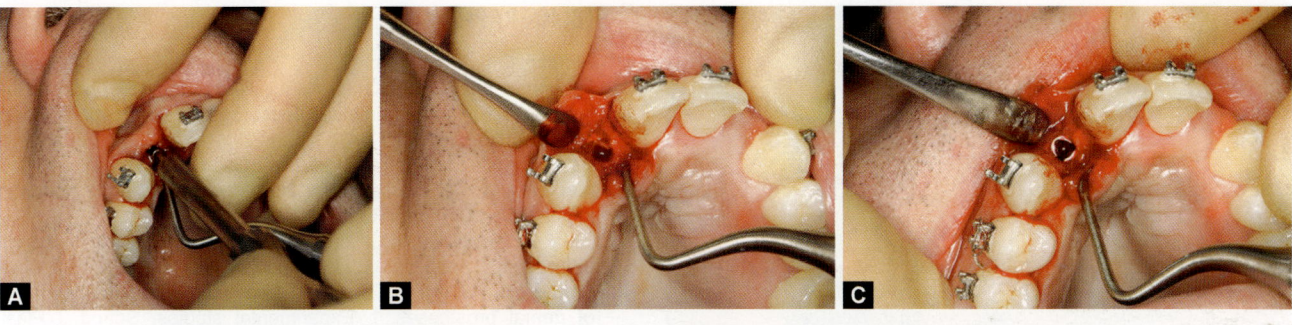

**Figs 47.4A to C:** (A) Osteotomey technique for ridge expansion; (B) Tissue retraction; (C) Implant in situ

height present. If the cortical plates have fused, then an intraoral autogenous bone graft is recommended.

Given the immaturity of the new bone from the osteogenic space expansion a two-stage approach is required with a 4–6 month period of unloaded healing. Orthodontic retention throughout this stage is recommended to prevent the closure of the prosthetic space.

## MINI-IMPLANTS (FIGS 47.7A TO C)

The value of true anchorage achievable from endosseous implants is of great value in the realms of orthodontics. Conventional modern-day implants though used for such anchorage give a number of drawbacks when purely as an anchoring fixture. The need for multistage invasive surgery breeds concerns for patients and may impact on treatment uptake. Such surgical procedures are not routine in the orthodontic office and as such less likely to be widely adopted. Implant placement is greatly restricted as sufficient space is required for placement. The majority of orthodontic management is concerned with fully dentate mouths absent of suitable sites for implant placement and restoration. This is further compounded by the common need for bilateral anchorage.

In order to overcome these pitfalls a new "mini-implant" has been developed providing true anchorage yet allow for discrete placement with minimal surgery and subsequent morbidity.

The mini-implants have the following advantages:
1. Narrow to allow placement between roots
2. Self-tapping for minimally invasive placement
3. Single-stage procedure
4. Reduced osseointegration to allow easy removal at the end of the treatment.

### Placement

Mini-implant placement is simple, one stage and of minimum discomfort for the patient. Once treatment planned, the placement site is anesthetized with local anesthetic. A pilot 2 mm twist drill is used to depth and the self-tapping mini-implant placed leaving the fixture head supramucosal. The mini-implant may then be gently loaded with full reciprocal anchorage.

Given the reduced surface area of anchorage mini-implants compared to conventional endosseous implants, removal may be achieved simply with the handheld driver. Often topical anesthetic alone is sufficient for comfort.

### Sites

Mini-implants provide true anchorage allowing movement of individual, segment or bilateral movement of the dentition. Site placement is restricted mainly by teeth but also key structures, such as the inferior dental nerve. Location is naturally critical to the direction of intended force.

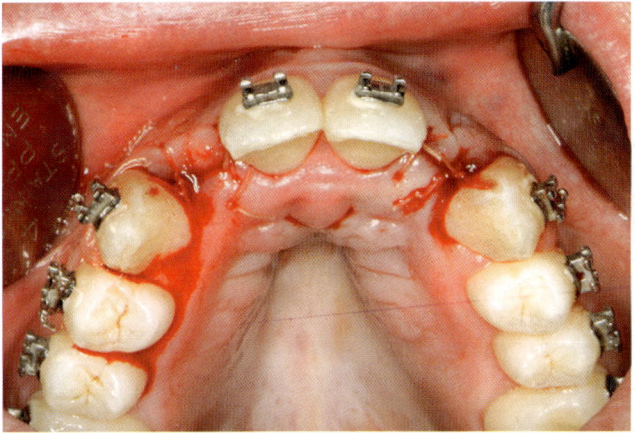

**Fig. 47.5:** Postoperative view—note improvement in labial plate contour

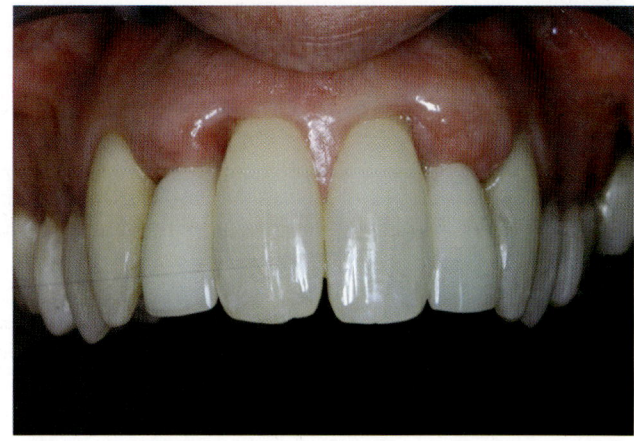

**Fig. 47.6:** Two weeks post second-stage with provisional crowns in situ. Note labial soft tissue augmentation

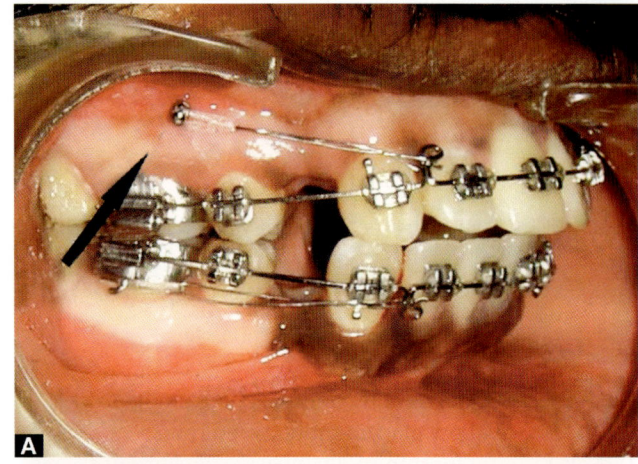
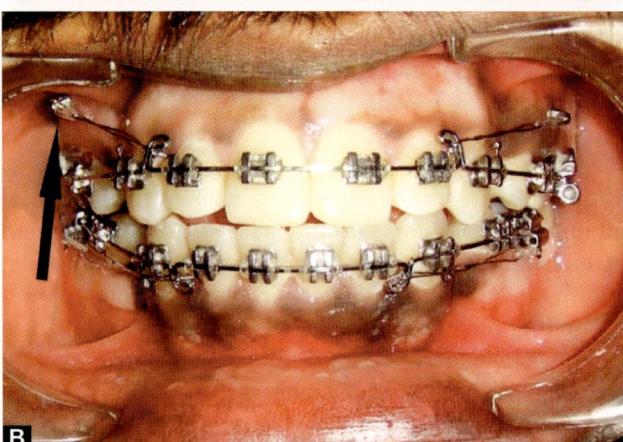
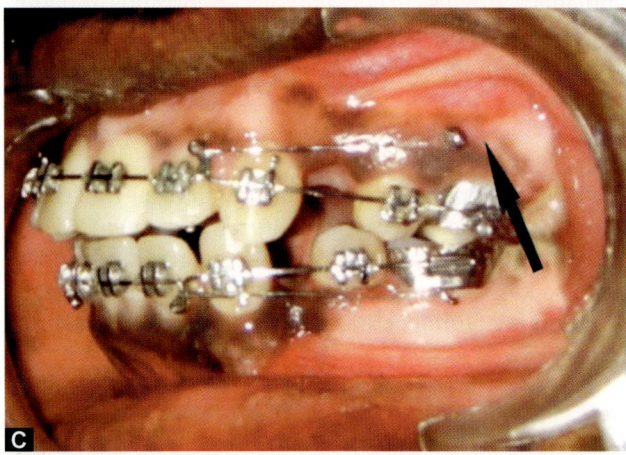

**Figs 47.7A to C:** Mini-implant

## BIBLIOGRAPHY

1. Albrektsson T, Branemark P-I, Hansson HA, et al. Osseo-integrated titanium implants. Requirements for ensuring a long-lasting, direct bone-to-implant anchorage in man. Acta Orthop Scan 1981;52:155-70.
2. Bernhart T, Vollgruber A, Dortbudak O, et al. Alternative to the median region of the palate for the placement of an orthodontic implant. Clin Oral Impl Res 2000;11:595-601.
3. Block MS, Hoffman DR. A new device for absolute anchorage for orthodontics. Am J Orthod Dento Fac Orthop 1995;107:251-8.
4. Branemark P-I, Adell R, Breine U, et al. Intra-osseous anchorage of dental prostheses. I. Experimental studies. Scand J Plast Reconstr Surg 1969;3:81-100.
5. Gainsforth BL, Higley LB. A study of orthodontic anchorage possibilities in basal bone. Am J Orthod Oral Surg 1945;31:406-17.
6. Lekholm U, Zarb GA. Patient selection and preparation. In: Brånemark PI, Zarb GA, Albrektsson T (Eds). Tissue-integrated prostheses: Osseointegration in clinical dentistry. Chicago: Quintessence;1985;199-209.
7. Lindh T, Gunne J, Tillberg A, et al. A meta-analysis of implants in partial edentulism. Clin Oral Implants Res 1999;10:139-48.
8. Linkow LI. The endosseous blade implant and its use in orthodontics. Int J Orthod 1969;18:149-54.
9. Melsen B, Verna C. A rational approach to orthodontic anchorage. Prog Orthod 1999;1:10-22.
10. Oesterle LJ. Implant considerations in the growing child. In: KW Higuchi (Ed). Orthodontic applications of oseointegrated implants. Illinois: Quintessence; 2000;156-7.
11. Rasmussen RA. The Branemark System of Oral Reconstruction: A Color Atlas. Tokyo: Ishiyaku EuroAmerica Inc., 1992.
12. Roberts WE, Marshall KJ, Mozsary PG. Rigid endosseous implant utilized as anchorage to protract molars and close an atrophic extraction site. Angle Orthod 1989;60:135-51.
13. Sherman JA. Bone reaction to orthodontic forces on vitreous carbon dental implants. Am J Orthod 1978;74:79-87.
14. Siegel D, Soletsz U. Numerical investigations of the influence of implant shape on the stress distribution in jaw bone. Int J Oral Maxillofac Impl 1989;4:333-9.
15. Thilander B, Odman J, Lekholm U. Orthodontic aspects of the use of oral implants in adolescents: a 10-year follow-up study. Eur J Orthod 2001;23:715-31.
16. Triaca A, Antonin M, Wintermantel E. Ein neues Titan-Flaschrauben-implantat zur orthodontischen Verankerung am anterion Gaumen. Int Orthod Kieferorthop 1992;24:251-7.
17. Turley PK, Kean C, Schur J, et al. Orthodontic force application to titanium endosseous implants. Angle Orthod 1988;58:151-62.
18. Turley PK, Shapiro PA, Moffett BC. The loading of bioglass-coated aluminium oxide implants to produce sutural expansion of the maxillary complex in the pigtail monkey. Macaca Nemestrina. Arch Oral Biol 1980;25:459-69.
19. Wehrbein H, Merz BR. Aspects of the use of endosseous palatal implants in orthodontic therapy. J Esth Dent 1998;10:315-24.
20. Worthington P, Lang BB, Lavelle WE. Osseo-integration in dentistry: an introduction. Illinois: Quintessence, 1994.

## EXAM-ORIENTED QUESTIONS

### Long Note
1. Implants in orthodontics.

### Short Note
1. Mini-implants used in orthodontics.

## CHAPTER OVERVIEW

**Mini-implants**

**Advantages of miniplants**
- Narrow to allow placement between roots
- Self tapping for minimally invasive placement
- Single stage procedure
- Reduced osseointegration to allow easy removal at the end of the treatment

**Placement**
- Simple
- One stage
- Minimal discomfort for the patient
- Spray local anesthesia
- Pilot 2 mm twist drill is used
- Mini-implant loaded gently with full reciprocal anchorage

**Site**
- Location is naturally critical to the direction of intended force

CHAPTER 47 Implants in Orthodontics

# CHAPTER 48

# Invisalign Techniques

*Phulari BS*

For a long time now, orthodontists and patients have wanted to correct the teeth inconspicuously and without the use of fixed dental brackets. New technology has turned this dream into reality; the new type of treatment is called invisalign **(Fig. 48.1)**.

## INVISIBLE

Invisalign (Invisible/Align) technique was introduced in 1999. Invisalign incorporates a series of invisible (clear) plastic aligners that fit comfortably over teeth and are designed to move teeth gradually into the desired position. Invisalign aligners are manufactured at the align technologies dental laboratory using Computer-aided Design/Computer-aided Manufacturing (CAD/CAM) processes.

According to researchers and align technologies, invisalign can be used to correct the following types of mild malocclusions:
1. Malocclusion with mild crowding
2. Malocclusion with mild spacing
3. In cases of mild relapse-after traditional braces have been removed, when some relapsing tooth movement has occurred.

## TECHNIQUE

The technique for using the invisalign system is as follows:
- The clinician sends a rubber base impression of maxillary and mandibular arches to align technology laboratories along with patient facial photographs, radiographs and a detailed treatment plan.
- The impression is inspected by the laboratory to ensure that patient's dentition has been fully captured. Then the impression is scanned using computer tomography to create a highly accurate and detailed three-dimensional study model.
- Based on the clinician's treatment plan, technician generates a virtual correction of the malocclusion that is then reviewed by the clinician. This process is called clincheck.
- The clinician reviews the planned corrections and if necessary, sends any revisions to align technology. The final step of clincheck must be approved by the treating clinician.
- After final approval, the treatment sequence is divided into a series of algorithmic stages. Each stage has a maximum tooth movement potential of 0.25 mm per appliance.
- Models of each stage of treatment are made by process called stereolithography.
- Individual appliances (aligners) are made from the computer-generated models of each stage.
- A typical invisalign treatment requires 20 to 30 aligners for the maxillary and mandibular arches.
- In most of the cases, treatment with invisalign is done in less than a year; however, treatment time depends on the specific alignment problem.

## PROCEDURE OF TREATMENT WITH INVISALIGN

### First Evaluation
- Orthodontist evaluates and creates a program of treatment.
- Records and impressions of arches are done.

### Invisalign Aligners are Made and Delivered
- A CT scan (computed tomography or CAT scan), is made from the dental impressions that produces an extremely accurate, 3D digital model of patient's teeth.
- CAD (Computer-aided Design) software is then used to simulate the movement of the teeth desired during treatment.
- The treatment plan is reviewed, modified and approved before the aligners are created.
- Invisalign then uses advanced stereolithography (SLA) technology to build precise moulds of teeth at each stage of treatment.
- Individualized, custom-created clear aligners are made from these models and sent to orthodontist.

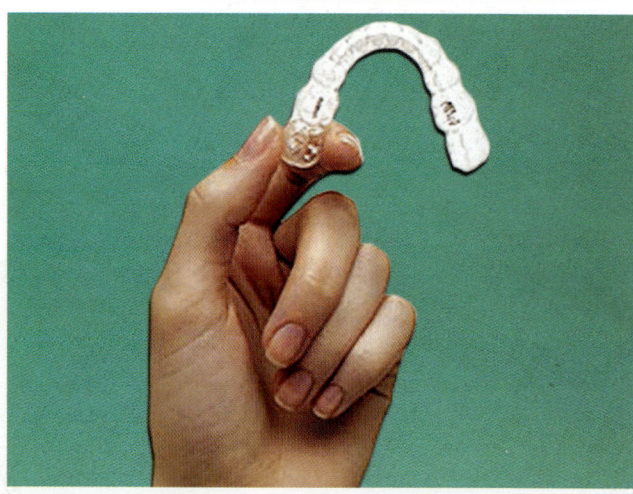

**Fig. 48.1:** Invisalign (Invisible/Align)

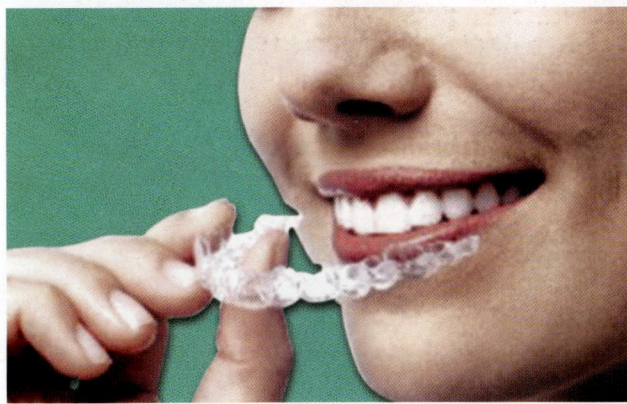
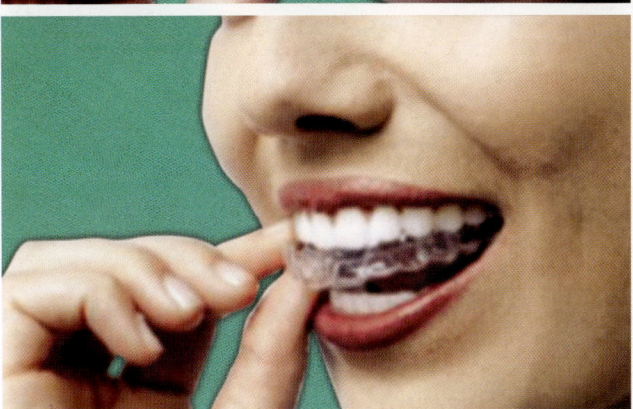
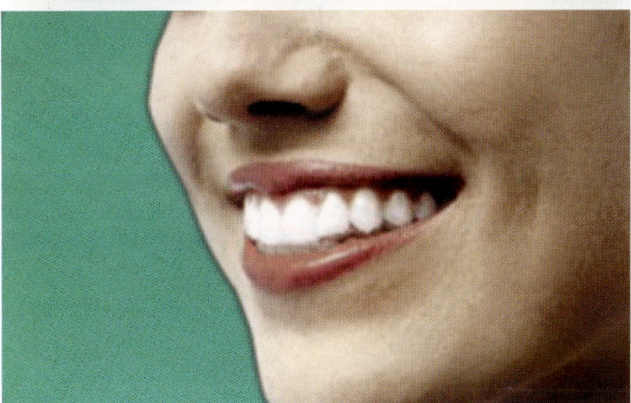

**Fig. 48.2:** Wearing of Invisalign

### Wearing of Invisalign (Fig. 48.2)

- Visits are made to orthodontist for adjustments and to check progress on a monthly basis.
- At regular intervals, a new set of custom-moulded clear aligners are given to the patient to continue the straightening process.

The total number of clear aligners is specific to each patient and is determined by orthodontist for the course of treatment.

### BENEFITS

1. Invisible thus no unwarranted attention drawn to patient's mouth.
2. Removable thus easy-to-eat, brush and floss.
3. No brackets to accumulate food debris and plaque.
4. Healthier gums from properly aligned teeth that help gums to "fit" properly around each tooth.
5. Easier cleaning helps in maintaining a good oral hygiene program that reduces chances of plaque buildup, tooth decay and periodontal disease.

### LIMITATIONS OF INVISALIGN TREATMENT

1. Severe malocclusions cannot be satisfactorily treated by Invisalign alone.
2. Class II div 1 malocclusion cannot be treated by Invisalign.
3. Invisalign is not useful in treating skeletal malocclusions.
4. It is expensive and facility may not be available at all places.

### CARE OF TEETH WITH INVISALIGN

1. Teeth and the aligners would need to be kept cleaned everyday, if the teeth and gums are to be healthy during and after orthodontic treatment.
2. Patints need to follow the instructions on how often to brush, how often to floss and use of other cleaning aids to help maintain good dental health.

Like brackets and arch wires, invisalign aligners move teeth through the appropriate placement of controlled force on the teeth. The principal difference is that invisalign not only controls forces, but also controls the timing of the force application. At each stage, only certain teeth are allowed to move and these movements are determined by the orthodontic treatment plan for that particular stage. This results in an efficient force-delivery system.

### BIBLIOGRAPHY

1. Boyd RL, Miller RJ, Vlaskalic V. The Invisalign System in Adult Orthodontics: Mild Crowding and Space Closure Cases. J Clin Orthod 2000;34:203-12.
2. Boyd RL, Vlaskalic V. Three-dimensional diagnosis and orthodontic treatment of complex malocclusions with the invisalign appliance. Semin Orthod 2001;7:274-93.
3. Ellis CP. Invisalign and changing relationships. Am J Orthod 2004;126:20A21A.
4. Miller RJ, Derakhshan M. The Invisalign System: Case report of a patient with deep bite, upper incisor flaring, and severe curve of Spee. Semin Orthod 2002;8:43-50.
5. Miller RJ, Duong T, Derakhshan M. Lower incisor extraction treatment with the Invisalign System. J Clin Orthod 2002;36:95-102.
6. Vlaskalic V, Boyd RL. Orthodontic treatment of a mildly crowded malocclusion using the Invisalign System. Austral Orthod J. 2001;17:41-6.
7. Wheeler TT. Invisalign material studies. Am J Orthod 2004;125:19A.

## EXAM-ORIENTED QUESTIONS

### Long Question
1. Invisalign technique.

### Short Notes
1. Benefits of Invisalign
2. Limitations of invisalign technique
3. Care of teeth with invisalign.

## CHAPTER OVERVIEW

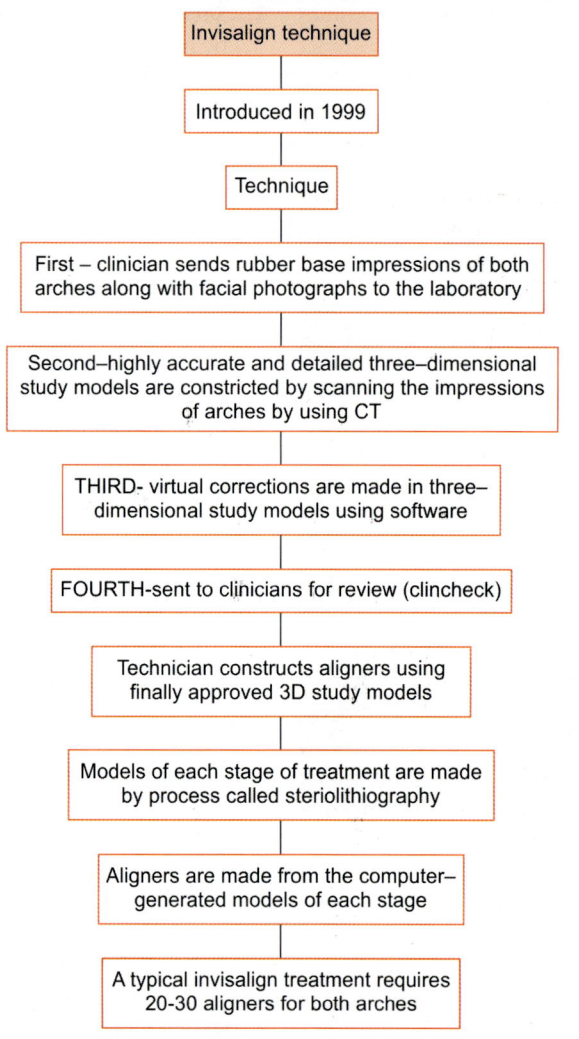

# CHAPTER 49

# Lasers in Orthodontics

*Shah A, Thukral N, Vakade M*

Dental lasers have been used in dentistry since 1960s. The basic idea is to treat dental pathologies involving hard and soft tissues with minimal vibration and pain. Today various dental lasers are available of different wavelengths, which can be used safely on both hard and soft tissues with maximum efficacy giving much comfort and benefits to the patient. Modern research has perfected this technology that has become almost indispensable in day-to-day dentistry, in accordance with the philosophy of minimally invasive therapy.

Lasers have significant applications in various fields of dentistry and their scope in orthodontics is discussed in this chapter. Soft-tissue lasers have numerous applications in orthodontic practice which are listed in **Box 49.1**.

**Box 49.1: Applications of lasers in orthodontics**
- Gingivectomy
- Frenectomy
- Operculectomy
- Papilla flattening
- Uncovering temporary anchorage devices
- Ablation of apthous ulcerations
- Exposure of impacted teeth
- Crown lengthening
- Debonding of brackets
- Removal of redundant gingival tissue during orthodontic treatment
- Reduction of pain following the application of separators
- Controlling the growth of facial structures
- caries control during orthodontic treatment
- Tooth whitening as an adjunctive procedure

Today laser surgery has helped many orthodontists to enhance the design of a patient's smile and improve treatment efficacy. Use of different wavelengths of laser energy is a noticeable aid in the surgical management of soft tissues before or during orthodontic treatment. The benefits of laser treatment include reduced bleeding during surgery with consequent reduction in operating time and rapid postoperative hemostasis, thus eliminating the need for sutures. The lack of need for anesthetics and sutures, as well as improved healing and postoperative comfort, make this technique particularly useful for very young patients. Advantages of lasers are listed in **Box 49.2**.

**Box 49.1: Benefits of Lasers treatment**
- Reduced bleeding during surgery with consequent reduction in operating time
- Rapid postoperative hemostasis, thus eliminating the need for sutures
- Painless
- Faster healing
- Less / no scaring
- Minimum postoperative pain

Before incorporating lasers into clinical practice, the clinician must fully understand the basic science, safety protocol, and risks associated with them. Before proceeding further, it is important to understand the fundamentals of laser physics.

## LASER PHYSICS

Today various dental lasers are available of different wavelengths which encompass the entire oral cavity. Lasers can be used safely for both—hard and soft tissues. Laser, as we all know, is an acronym for light amplification by stimulated emission of radiation (**Fig. 49.1**). Light is a form of electromagnetic energy and its basic unit of energy is called a photon. Normal light bulb produces light which is a spectrum of violet, indigo, blue, green, yellow, orange, and red. In other words, it is polychromatic and divergent.

The three main characteristics of light are:
1. Amplitude (**Fig. 49.2**) is the total height of the wave oscillation from the top of the peak to the bottom on the vertical axis. This is an indication of the amount of intensity in the wave: the larger the amplitude, the greater the amount of energy generated.
2. Wavelength (**Fig. 49.2**) is the distance between any two corresponding points on the wave on the horizontal axis. This is one single aspect which is important in determining how the laser light is delivered to the surgical site and how it reacts with tissue.
3. Frequency is oscillation per second and is inversely proportional to the wavelength: shorter the wavelength, higher is the frequency, and vice versa.

## STIMULATED EMISSION

- The term stimulated emission has its basic in the quantum theory of physics, introduced in 1900 and further conceptualized as relating to atomic architecture by Niels Bohr.
- Photon, the smallest unit of energy, is released after an atom has absorbed energy and releases it.
- Albert Einstein used this theory and substantiated that if already charged atom is energized, it releases two photons. This emission or radiated identical photons travel as coherent wave. These photons energize more atoms which release identical photons resulting into amplified light energy called stimulated emission (**Fig. 49.3**).

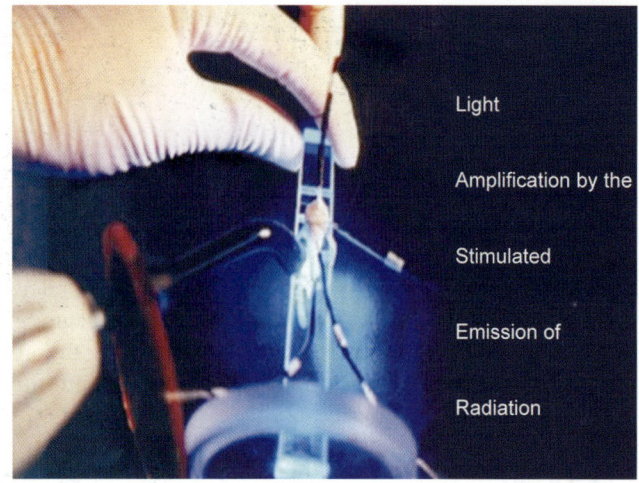

Fig. 49.1: Laser: Light amplification by stimulated emission of radiation

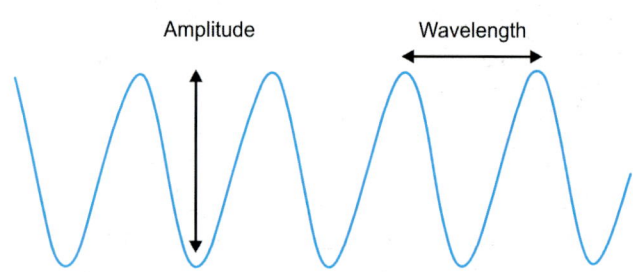

Fig. 49.2: Showing amplitude, wavelength and frequency

**Note:**

- Amplitude is the total height of the wave oscillation from the top of the peak to the bottom on the vertical axis
- Wavelength is the distance between any two corresponding points on the wave on the horizontal axis
- Frequency is oscillation per second

In laser, the light beam is created by stimulation of actively charged photons. These photons generate more and more number of photons creating a beam. This controlled stimulated emission has certain characteristics:

1. **Monochromatic (Fig. 49.4)**—The beam of light thus created, has a single color ranging from infrared to invisible spectrum.
2. **Collimation (Fig. 49.5)**—This means that the laser beam travels within specific spatial boundaries. This particular characteristic ensures that there is a constant size and shape of the beam emitted from the laser cavity. X-ray is one such example.
3. **Coherency (Fig. 49.6)**, which means that the light waves are all in the same phase and have identical wavelength.

## COMPONENTS OF LASER UNIT

1. Laser medium or active medium—They are classified as **(Figs 48.7A to C):**
   Gas—$CO_2$, Argon, Krypton
   Solid—Nd:YAG, Er:YAG, Ruby
   Liquid—It is an organic dye, i.e. Rhodium
   Semiconductor crystals—Diode.

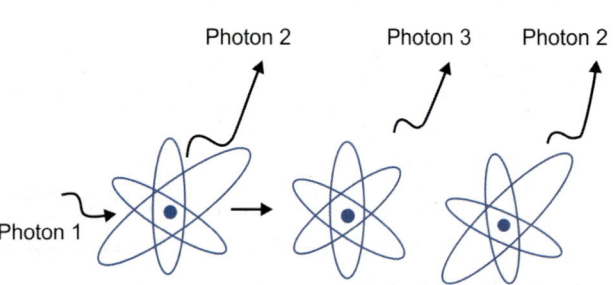

Fig. 49.3: Stimulated emissions

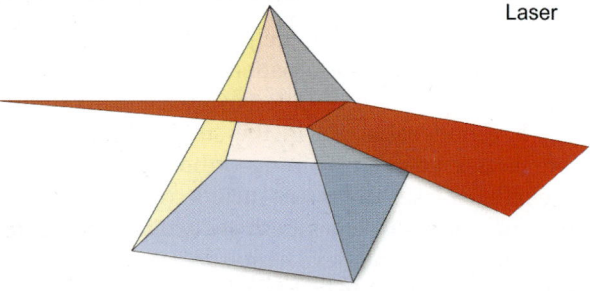

Fig. 49.4: Monochromatism—the beam of light generated with one color

Fig. 49.5: Collimation—a beam having specific spatial boundaries with constant beam size and shape emitted from laser unit

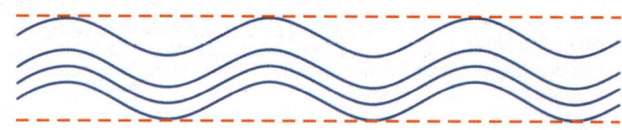

Fig. 49.6: Coherency—which means that the light waves are all in the same phase and have identical wavelength

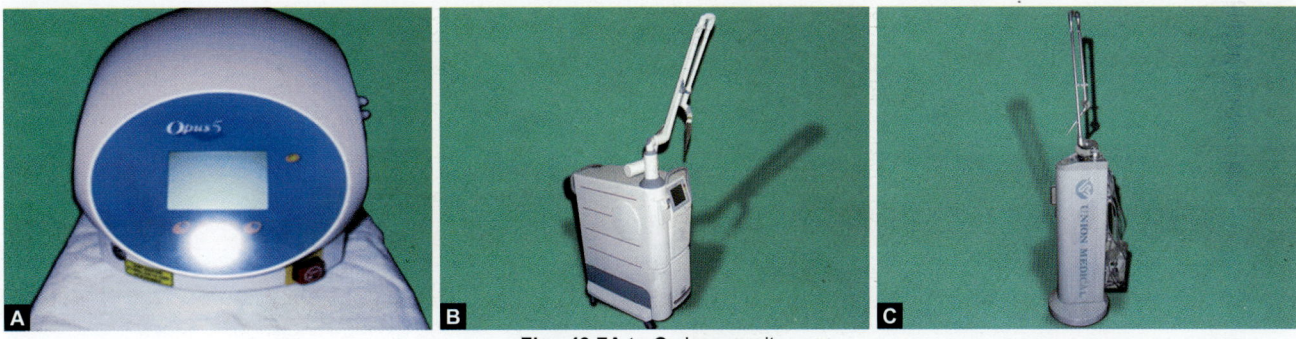

**Figs 49.7A to C:** Laser units

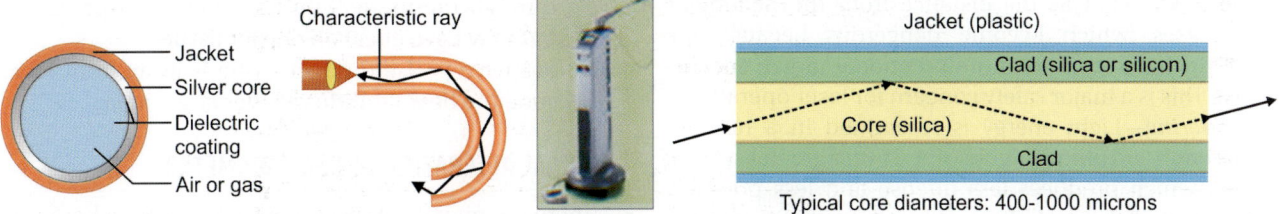

**Fig. 49.8:** Laser beam delivery system

2. Laser resonator—Active medium is contained within an optical enclosure.
3. Power source—Active medium needs to be changed to release photons, external source of energy may be either electrical, chemical or flash lamp.

## LASER BEAM DELIVERY SYSTEMS

The beam of laser light should be delivered to the target tissue in a manner that is ergonomic and precise (**Fig. 49.8**). Two types of delivery systems are:
1. Fibro-optic: Quarts silica fibers with a handpiece—diode, Nd:YAG, newer Er:YAG.
2. Hollow tube waveguide: It is hollow tube lined with series of well-aligned mirrors which reflect the laser beam from the unit to the handpiece—$CO_2$, Er:YAG.
3. The development of these delivery systems in inaccessible areas of oral cavity makes more and more applications possible.

## USE OF LASER BEAM

1. *Contact mode*—Distal end of fibro-optic is placed in direct contact of the target tissue. Here tactile feedback is perceived.
2. *Non-contact mode*—Handpiece is held away from the tissue and the operator has to adjust the focus of the beam by varying distance between the headpiece and the target to have the desired effect.

## MODE OF LASER BEAM

1. *Pulsed mode*—It emits the energy from laser beam in series of pulses with burst of peak energy at each pulse with a resting time in between. This allows the tissue to cool in between each energy delivery and minimize heat conduction with optimum benefits.
2. *Continuous mode*—Laser wave emits energy in continuous mode at average power till they are cut off using external source like foot switch of pre-settings in the laser unit. This type of energy is useful in ablative procedure or coagulation.

## LASER TISSUE INTERACTION

When laser light emerges from a laser, it usually does in the form of pencil thin beam of laser energy traveling at the speed of light. This beam travels in a straight line until it hits something that reflects or refracts it or until it hits something that stops it and absorbs its energy. The laser beam diverges gradually as it travels away from the laser, which means that the beam's diameter increases with the distance between the headpiece and target tissue.

Laser light has either of four different interactions with the target tissue, depending on the optical properties of that tissue (**Fig. 49.9**):
1. *Absorption*—Laser light is converted into effective thermal energy. The amount of energy that is absorbed by the tissue depends on the tissue characteristics, such as pigmentation and water content, and on the laser wavelength and emission mode. In general, the shorter wavelengths are readily absorbed in pigmented tissue and blood elements. Longer wavelengths are more interactive with water and hydroxyapatite.
2. *Transmission*—Light energy passes freely through the tissue, without interaction of any kind and has little or no effect. It is an inverse of absorption.

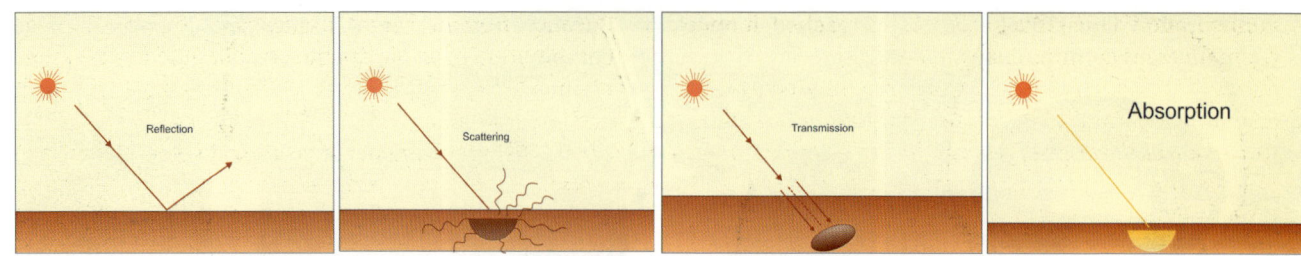

**Fig. 49.9:** Action of lasers on the tissue

3. *Reflection*—Light energy reflects off tissue surface with little or no absorption and consequently has no effect on tissue. The laser beam generally becomes more divergent as the distance from the headpiece increases, which become dangerous because the energy is directed to an unintentional target, such as eye. This is a major safety concern for laser operation.

4. *Scattering*—Light energy is re-emitted in a random direction and ultimately absorbed over a greater surface area which produces less intense and less precisely distributed thermal effect. When laser light emerges from a laser it usually does in the form of pencil thin beam of laser energy traveling at the speed of light. This beam travels in a straight line until it hits something that reflects or refracts it or until it hits something that stops it and absorbs its energy. The laser beam diverges gradually as it travels away from laser, which means that the beam's diameter increases with the distance between he headpiece and target tissue.

- Absorption—when the target tissue absorbs the beam, desired result and energy acts at the focal spot depending upon the tissue
- Reflection—the beam is reflected from the tissue with no result
- Transmission—the light energy is transmitted through the tissue with no effect on target tissue but may have effect on deeper tissues
- Scattering—if the target tissue is away from focal spot, the beam is diffused over larger area.

## OPTICAL ALTERATION OF BEAM DIAMETER

- There are many instances in laser dentistry where one needs a different beam diameter from that generated by laser, one typically uses an optical lens to deliberately introduce positive or negative divergence.
- Passing a well-collimated laser beam through a negative or diverging lens can drastically increase the divergence of the beam.
- On the other hand, a positive or converging lens causes beam diameter to decrease with distance, until it reaches a desired distance from the lens. This is known as focal length, where the beam is reduced to its minimum diameter depending upon optical

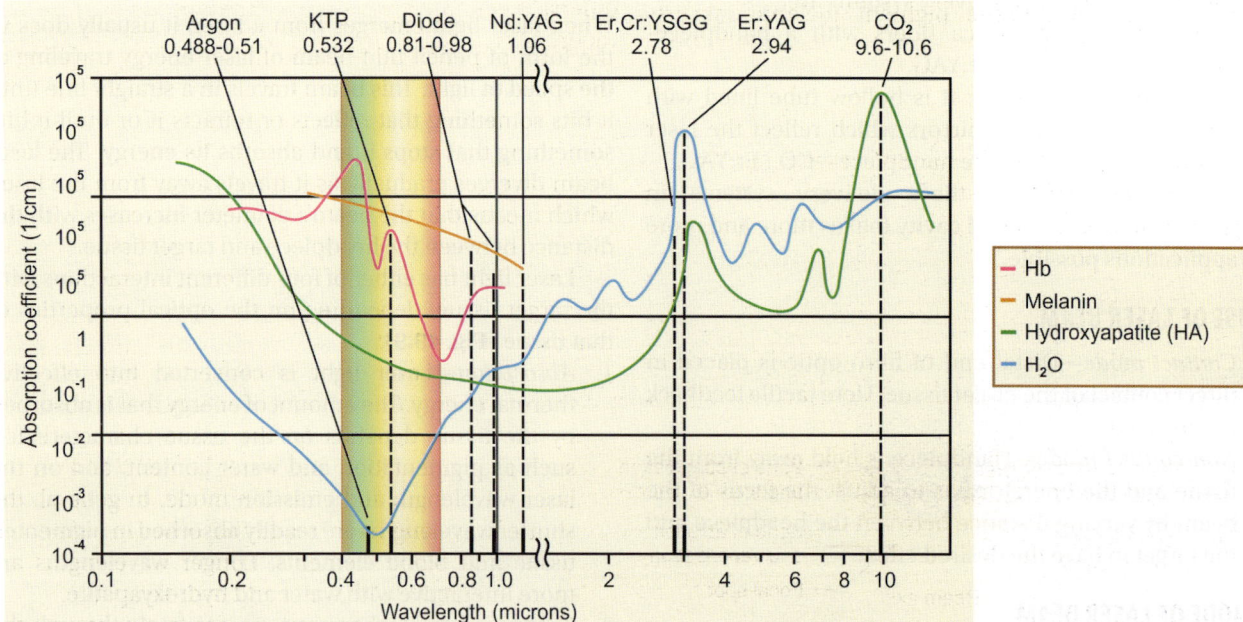

**Fig. 49.10:** Absorption curves of various tissue components

configuration. Once this focal point is reached, it once again diverges continuously outward.
- *Spot size*—This is the measure of surface area on which laser is concentrated. Spot size, partially determines the localization of laser energy to the intended areas of treatment without affecting adjacent tissue and, therefore, effect precision.
- Spot size is also directly related to efficiency and speed of tissue interaction with radiant laser energy.
- Smaller laser spot diameters are ideal for procedures that require high precision to remove very small tissue structures without damaging nearby structures, manly applied in incision and excision.
- Lasers with bigger spot size may save time as less repositioning is required, mainly in ablation and hemostatic procedure.

## WAVELENGTH SPECIFIC INTERACTION WITH TISSUES

- Molecules involving in biological systems are extremely complex and can maintain vital activity only under certain well-defined conditions. Depending on the laser wavelength used, different tissue interactions will occur. Thermal changes which occur when light energy is absorbed by tissue vary according to the degree of temperature rise which is produced **(Fig. 49.10)**.
- Water which is present in all biological tissues, best absorbs Er wavelengths followed by $CO_2$ wavelength. Conversely, water allows the transmission of shorter wavelength lasers like Ar, Diode and Nd:YAG.
- Apatite crystals which form the structure of the teeth and bone, readily absorb $CO_2$ wavelength and to a lesser degree, those in Er group of lasers. Apatite, however, does not absorb the shorter wavelength of Ar, diode and Nd:YAG. Hemoglobin and other blood components and tissue pigment melanin, absorb shorter wavelength.
- Because human dental tissues are composed of a combination of water, apatite crystal, blood and tissue pigment, the clinician must choose the best laser for each treatment.

Lasers using wavelength in the visible portion of spectrum, lead to two forms of interaction:
1. Energy of laser absorbed is converted into heat since temperature is critical parameter of the normal operation of living cell. Even a small increase in temperature can lead to thermal changes or irreversible damage.
2. The laser can provide energy that results in photo-chemical reaction such as photosynthesis or photodynamic therapy.

The type of damage caused by photocoagulation is thermal and is associated with denaturalization of proteins and deactivation of enzymes. This type of interaction is involved in all photocoagulation application with Ar, krypton and dye lasers in ophthalmology. Visible wavelength laser depends upon the presence of some chromophore like melanin, hemoglobin or dye to promote absorption of energy. Without the substance present, visible light energy is either reflected or transmitted with little or no tissue effect. For laser in UV part of spectrum, abiotic changes would be expected. UV radiation generally causes non-thermal reaction in biological tissue resulting in photoablation. If tissue is exposed to higher energy densities of UV radiation in a very short time interval, surface will be removed layer by layer with each pulse.

For laser in mid and far infrared part of spectrum, interactions with tissue are thermal in effect because they are highly absorbed by water. Tissue temperature can reach the boiling point of water. This results in vaporization and rapidly expanding water vapor will cause ablation on the borders of the interaction. The photocoagulation effect differs, depending on the particular wavelength used. The vaporization tends to stabilize tissue temperature until all the

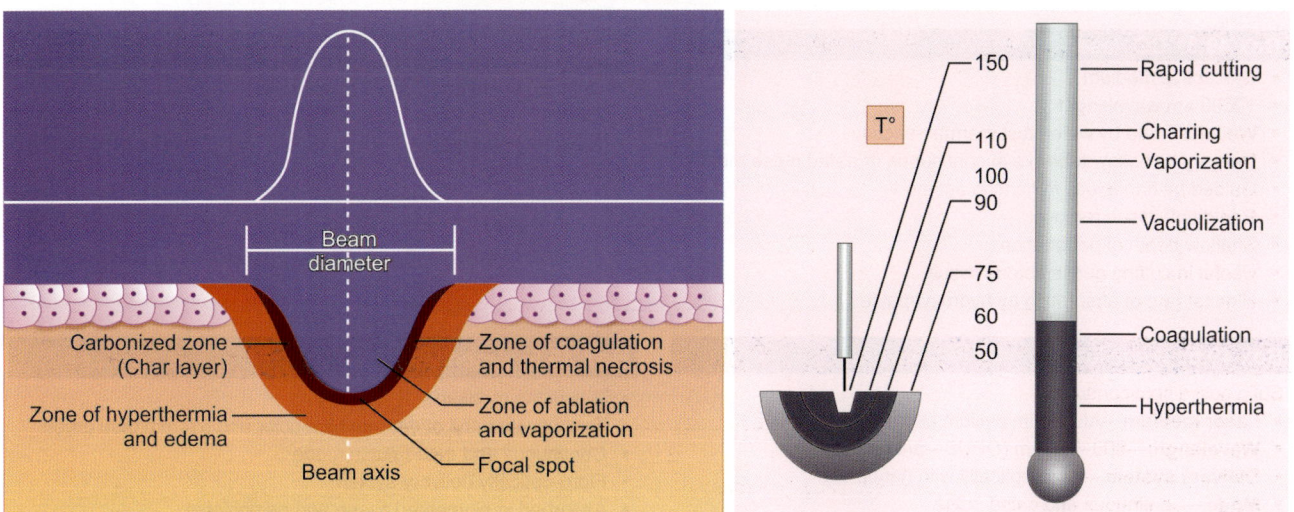

**Fig. 49.11:** Laser energy and tissue temperature: When intracellular temperature reaches 60°, e.g. proteins begin to degenerate
• At 100°, the vaporization of water within the tissue occurs; • At 200°, tissue is dehydrated burned and carbonization occurs

| Table 49.1: Types of lasers | | |
|---|---|---|
| State | Soft tissue lasers | Hard tissue lasers |
| Gas state | • CO$_2$<br>• He-Ne<br>• Argon<br>• Krypton | |
| Solid state | • Nd:YAG<br>• Ruby<br>• KTP<br>• Diode<br>• Ho: YAG | • Er:YAG Er<br>• Cr: YSGG |
| Liquid state | • Rhodium | |

water is boiled off at which point the temperature, if increased further, then carbonization can occur (**Fig. 49.11**).

- At 100°, the vaporization of water within the tissue occurs.
- At 200°, tissue is dehydrated, burned and carbonization occurs.

## TYPES OF LASERS

Lasers are mainly of two types—hard and soft tissue lasers and are listed in the **Table 49.1**.

## CO$_2$

The CO$_2$ is a non-contact mode laser. The beam does not contact the tissue during the cutting phase; thus there is no tactile feedback during the surgical incision. CO$_2$ laser is well-absorbed by water, and has fast thermal reaction. It operates with the wavelength of 10600 nm. It has an advantage of rapid soft tissue removal and shallow depth of penetration. It is useful in cutting dense fibrous tissue (**Box 49.3**). New technology enables us to give precise cut in super pulse mode making it extremely less traumatic and efficient in soft tissue surgeries.

*Disadvantages:* Less hemostasis compared to Nd:YAG/Diode.

## ERBIUM LASER

The Erbium laser has a wavelength of 2790 to 2940 nm, which makes ideal for absorption by both hydroxyapatite and water. It is used for caries removal, tooth preparation, soft tissue surgeries and bone ablation (**Box 49.4**). New technology is slowly making the Erbium family into all tissue lasers where it can effectively perform soft issue surgeries.

*Disadvantages:* Less hemostasis compared to Nd:YAG/Diode.

## DIODE LASER

Diode laser is a solid active semiconductor. It has a wavelength of 812 to 980 nm. The laser energy is absorbed by pigmentation in the soft tissues and this makes the diode laser an excellent hemostatic agent. Diode laser is used in contact mode and it also provides tactile feedback during the surgical procedure.

The diode laser can deliver energy in continuous or pulsed mode. In continuous mode, the tissue tends to absorb more energy, resulting in greater heat. The pulsed mode permits intermittent cooling between pulses of energy.

The diode laser can often be used without anesthesia to perform very precise anterior soft tissue esthetic surgery or surgery in other areas of the mouth without bleeding or discomfort (**Box 49.5**). It is an excellent all purpose laser in dentistry. It can be used in bleaching, endodontics, soft tissue surgeries and periodontics. Good hemostasis can be achieved but it has to be judiciously used as it may cause damage to adjacent tissues due to rapid absorption.

## ARGON LASER

Argon laser has two wavelengths of 488 nm blue color and 514 nm blue green. It delivers the energy in either

---

**Box 49.3:** CO$_2$ laser

- Gas active medium
- 10600 nm wavelength
- Well-absorbed by water, fast thermal reaction
- Delivery by hollow tube like in continuous or gated pulse mode
- Guided by handpiece in noncontact mode
- Rapid soft tissue remover
- Shallow depth of penetration
- Useful in cutting dense fibrous tissue
- Highest rate of absorption by hydroxyapatite.

**Box 49.5:** Diode laser

Solid active semiconductor
- **Laser medium**—Aluminum gallium and arsenide
- **Wavelength**—800–980 nm (OPUS—5/810 nm)
- **Delivery system**—Fibro-optically with handpiece
- **Mode**—Continuous and gated pulse
- **Absorption**—By pigmented tissues, water
- Portable and compact

**Box 49.4:** Er: YAG laser

- Yittrium aluminium Garnet doped with Erbium
- 2790 nm wavelength
- Free running pulse
- High affinity for hydroxyapatite
- Can be used for carious lesion
- Ablation of soft tissue

**Box 49.6:** Argon laser

- Gas is the medium
- Two wavelengths of 488 nm blue color and 514 nm blue green
- Continuous and gated pulse mode
- Fibro-optically delivery system
- Absorbed in pigmented tissue and hemoglobin
- Useful as good hemostatic activity and in acute inflammatory soft tissue lesions
- Caries detection—orange-red color

continuous or gated pulse mode. It is well-absorbed in pigmented tissue and hemoglobin. It is useful as good hemostatic activity and in acute inflammatory soft tissue lesions and it is also useful in vascular lesion **(Box 49.6)**.

## ND: YAG LASER

Nd:YAG has an wavelength of 1064 nm and it can be easily absorbed by pigmented tissues. It delivers the energy in free running pulse mode. It is useful in periodontal surgery, sulcular debridement, cutting and coagulation, root canal sterilization **(Box 49.7)**.

## APPLICATIONS OF LASERS IN ORTHODONTICS

Lasers have wide range of applications in dentistry. In this chapter only few important applications in orthodontics are discussed.

### Exposure of Impacted Tooth by Laser

Canine is the most commonly impacted tooth in the anterior segment of the dental arches due to arch length—tooth material discrepancy, this may delay the progress of orthodontic treatment. Exposure of impacted tooth by laser facilitates accessibility and decreases the risk of bond failure **(Figs 49.12A and B)**.

### Frenectomy by Laser

As permanent maxillary central incisors erupt in the oral cavity, the labial frenum shifts apically; in some instances frenum may persist even after complete eruption of permanent maxillary central incisors termed as high labial frenum attachment. Abnormal frenum attachment prevents approximation of maxillary central incisors resulting in midline diastema. Frenectomy by laser **(Fig. 49.13A)** prevents recurrence and facilitates diastema closure. Patient acceptance with laser application is very high even in condition like tongue tie, as it facilitates healing, reduces the discomfort and no sutures are required **(Fig. 49.13B)**.

### Reduction of Pain in Orthodontic Patient by Application of Laser

Procedures like separators placement and banding procedures are considered to be painful in the whole course of orthodontic treatment. Studies proved that the application of laser in patient with separators reduces the level of pain threshold.

### Application of Laser in Bonding Orthodontic Bracket

Nowadays laser is used in curing of orthodontic bracket in bonding procedure. Curing of orthodontic bracket by laser

---

**Box 49.7:** Nd: YAG laser

- Solid active media: Crystal of Yittrium Aluminium Garnet doped with Neodymium
- First laser to be designed for extensive dental treatment
- Large published scientific data and research
- 1064 nm wavelength
- 10000 more absorbed by water than argon, easily absorbed by pigmented tissues
- Free running pulse mode
- Fibro-optic delivery system
- Periodontal surgery, sulcular debridement
- Cutting and coagulating

**Box 49.8:** Advantages of lasers

- No pain
- No bleeding
- Better visualization
- Less/no scarring
- Facilitates healing
- The laser cut is more precise than that of a scalpel
- Minimum postoperative pain
- Laser application reduces the risk of postoperative infections
- The laser sterilizes as it cuts
- Laser application reduces the risk of blood-borne transmission of diseases
- Less damage occurs to adjacent tissue following the use of lasers.

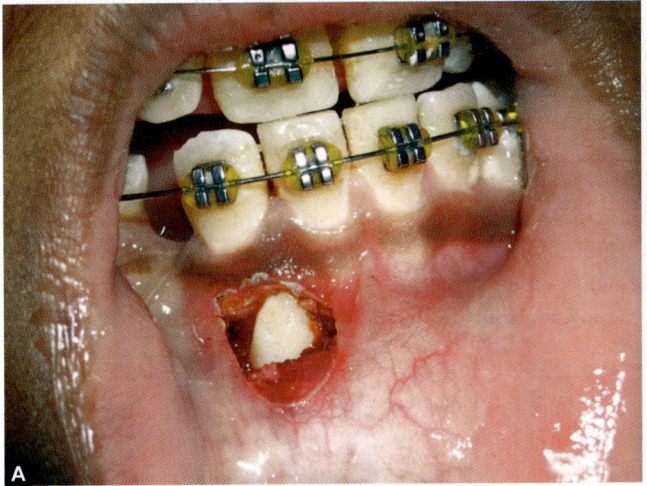
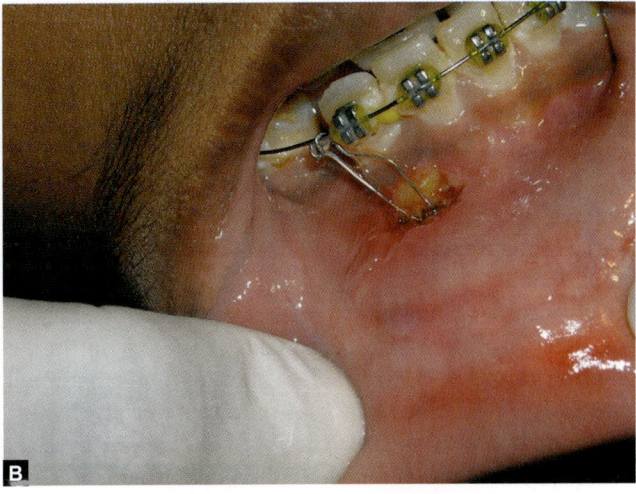

**Figs 49.12A and B:** Exposure of impacted tooth by laser: (A) Exposure of impacted canine with laser; (B) Exposed canine is bonded and ligated to the arch wire

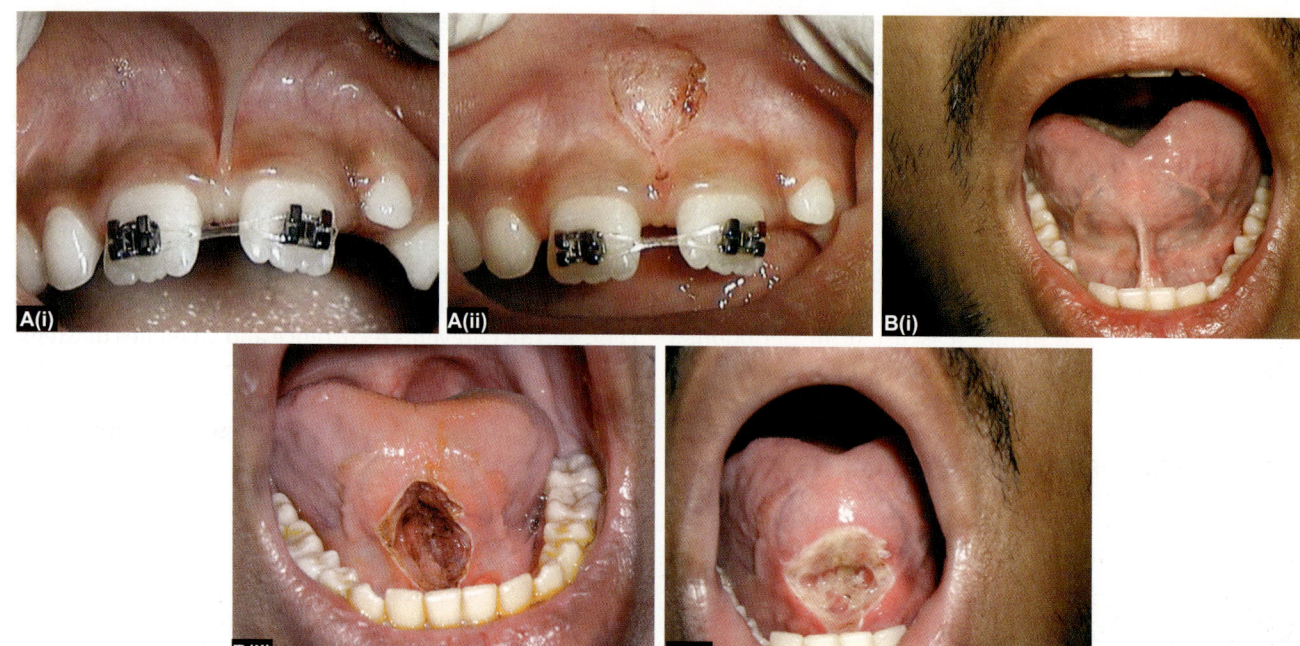

**Figs 49.13A and B:** (A) Frenectomy by laser (i) Abnormal frenum attachment prevents approximation of maxillary central incisors resulting in midline diastema; (ii) Frenectomy by laser followed by active fixed mechanotherapy; (B) Tongue tie excision by laser (i) Tongue tie; (ii) Excised tongue tie with laser; (iii) Nearly completion of healing

takes approximately (3–5) seconds. It reduces the chair time and increases the efficiency of bonding especially in uncooperative and very apprehensive patients.

### Laser Ablation of Surface Enamel for Orthodontic Bracket Placement

Laser ablation has been proposed as an alternative method to acid etching. Common problems during orthodontic treatment after acid etching the enamel, are demineralization and susceptibility to caries around brackets. Er: YAG laser ablation might overcome this drawback while offering other benefits like reduction in clinical time, good moisture control during bonding and bond strength similar to that of acid etching.

### Gaining Access for Bracket Placement on Partially Erupted Teeth

In certain cases, the orthodontic treatment is often prolonged due to incomplete or delayed eruption of the tooth, because the labial surface is covered by the gingival, which hinders the bracket placement. In such cases either we have to wait until tooth erupts completely till the occlusal plane or refer the patient to periodontist for removal of tissue to gain access for bracket placement. Either choice could add significant time to the overall treatment.

Exposure of teeth by laser facilitates accessibility and decreases the risk of bond failure. The patient in the **Figures 49.14A** to **F**, the progress of orthodontic treatment was delayed by thick mucosal barrier covering the left permanent central incisor. The tooth is exposed by laser and then bracket is bonded, thereby bringing it into alignment.

### Removal of Redundant Gingival Tissue by Laser during Orthodontic Treatment

Poor oral hygiene in orthodontic patient results in swollen gingival tissue, which delays the orthodontic treatment. Laser can be used in the removal of redundant tissue, which fastens the progress of orthodontic treatment.

### Management of Aphthous Ulcer by Laser during Orthodontic Treatment

One of the most uncomfortable experiences for orthodontic patients is the formation of aphthous ulcer. Application of laser for aphthous ulcer (**Figs 49.15A and B**) helps in reducing the pain and also promotes healing. Healing usually takes place in a day. Laser irradiates the surface nerve ending and eliminates the painful stimuli.

### Removal of Operculae on Second Molar by Laser

In some cases, second permanent molar is also bonded to provide additional anchorage and to avoid excessive repair visits. If second permanent molar is the last tooth in the arch, it is often associated with operculum. Presence of operculum hinders the band placement. Removal of operculum by soft tissue laser facilitates the exposure of tooth, later providing accessibility for band placement (**Figs 49.16A** and **B**).

### Use of Laser in Controlling the Growth of Facial Structure

Orthodontics is one of the important domains with interests in human growth and development with the advent of "high-energy lasers" (that are not deleterious), it may prove that research could lead to the use of lasers in the practice

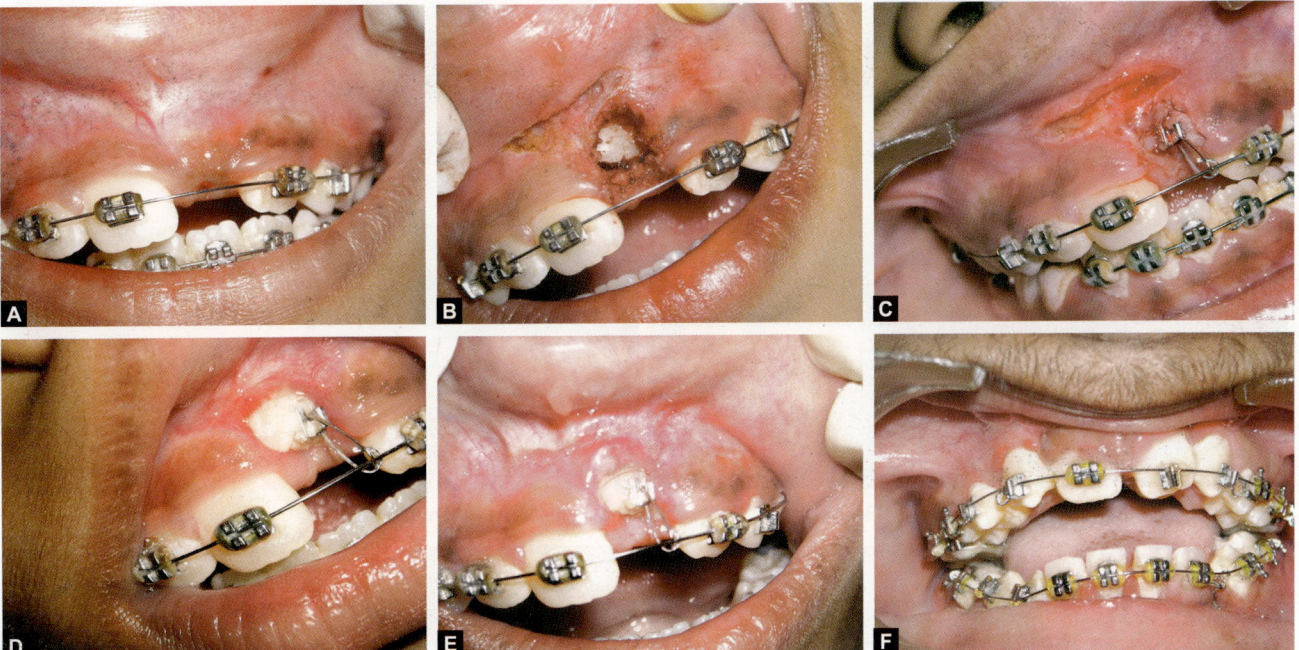

**Figs 49.14A to F:** Gaining access for bracket placement on partially erupted teeth (A) Mucosal barrier covering the permanent central incisor and preventing it from erupting; (B) Exposure of permanent central incisor by laser; (C) Begg bracket bonded on the exposed permanent central incisor and ligated to the arch wire; (D and E) Nearing the alignment of permanent central incisor; (F) Almost the permanent central incisor has brought into alignment

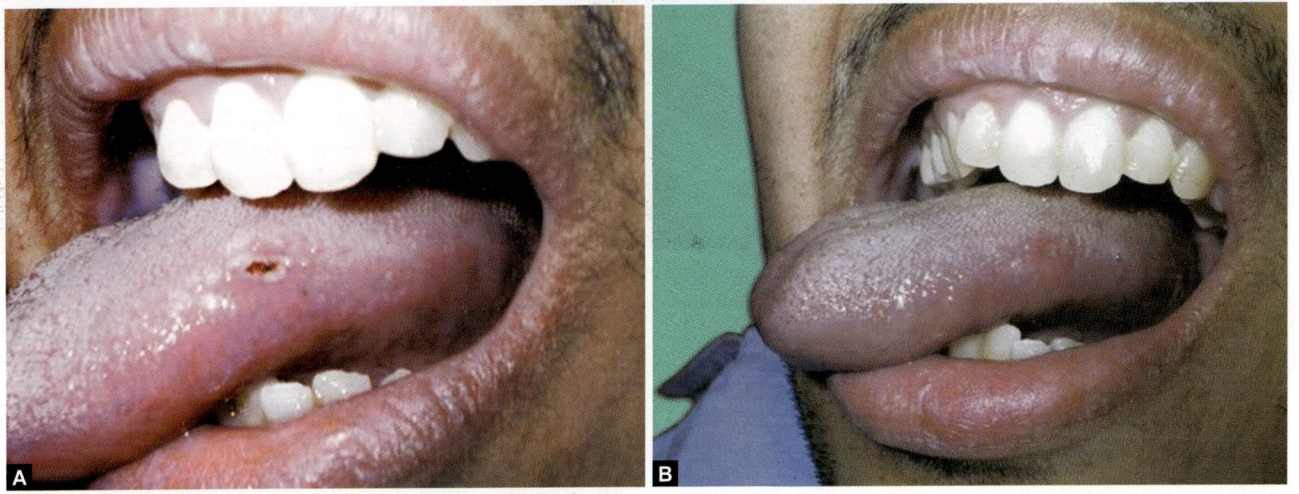

**Figs 49.15A and B:** Management of aphthous ulcer by laser (A) Aphthous ulcer on the lateral borer of the tongue; (B) Healing of the aphthous ulcer followed by laser therapy

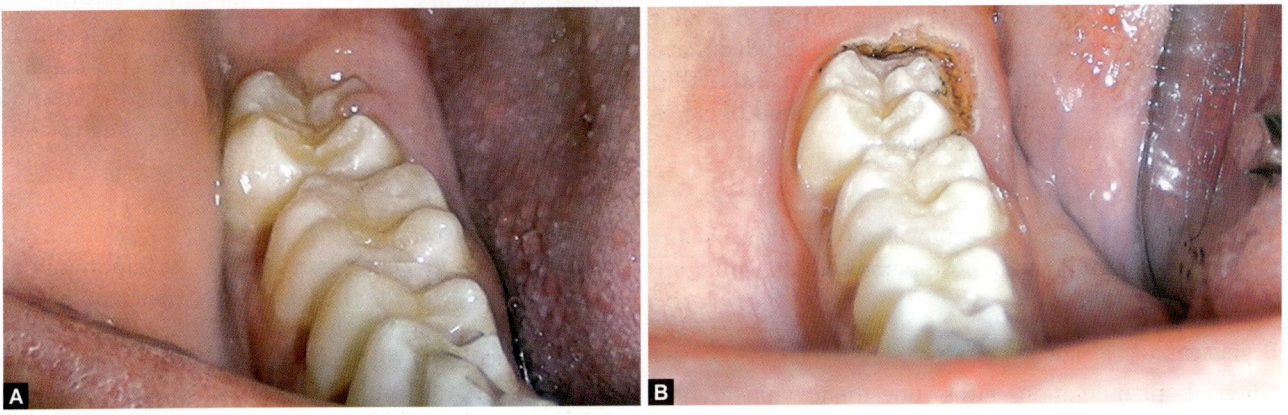

**Figs 49.16A and B:** Removal of operculae on second molar by laser (A) Showing operculum in relation to second molar; (B) Operculum has been removed with the laser

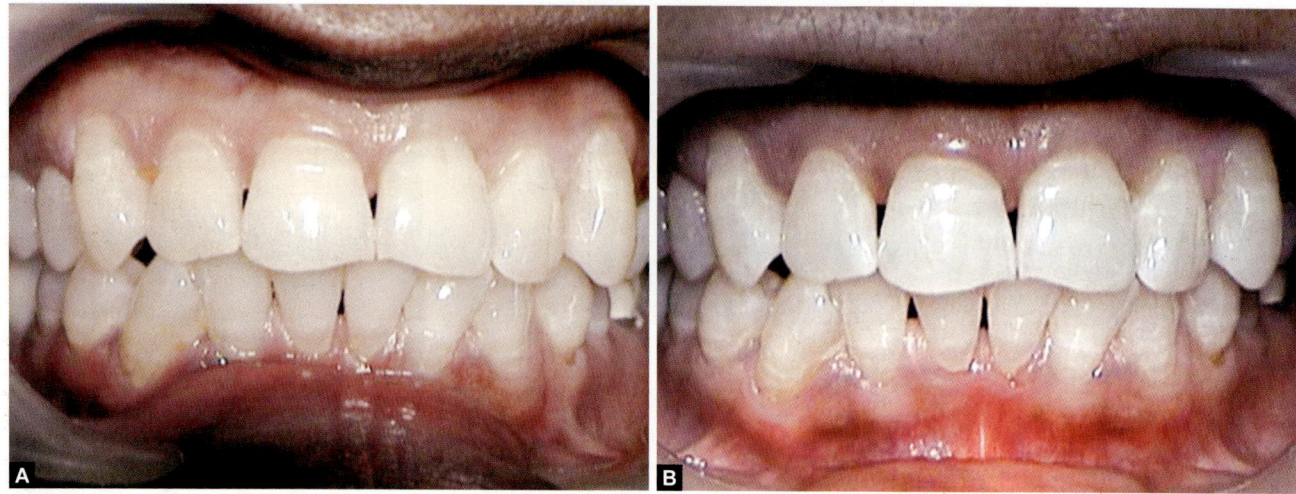

**Figs 49.17A and B:** Tooth whitening by laser (A) Before (B) After

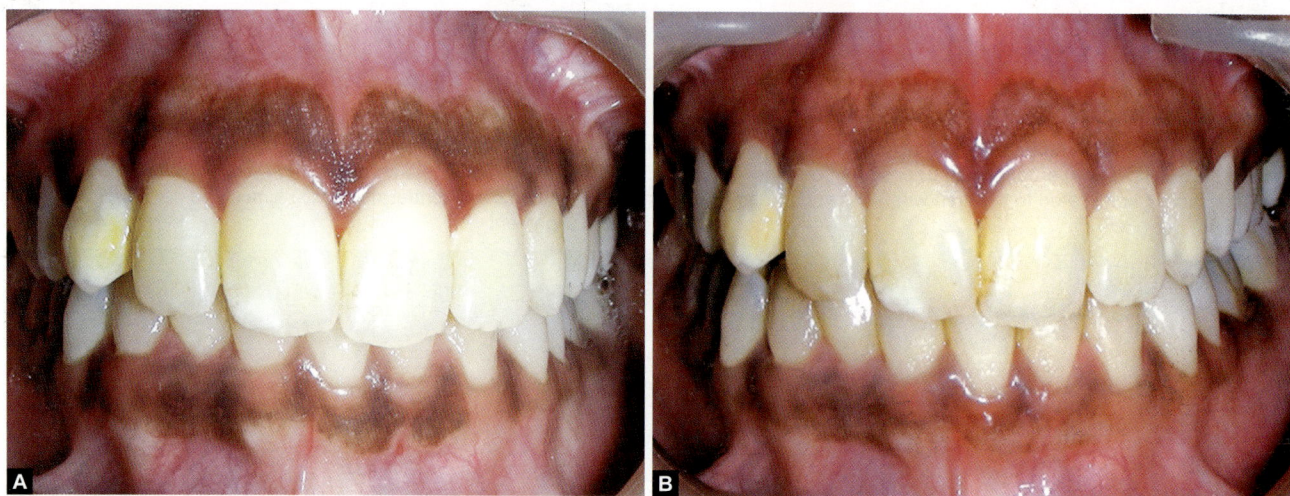

**Figs 49.18A and B:** Depigmentation of gingiva by laser (A) Before (B) After

of orthodontics. "High-energy lasers" might be applied to manipulation of human facial growth leading to new methods to cope with problems either overgrowth or undergrowth.

### Caries Control during Orthodontic Treatment

Development/occurrence of dental caries is not an uncommon complication in orthodontic patient especially around brackets and in interproximal area after proximal stripping of teeth to gain space. Studies have demonstrated that Nd: YAG laser irradiation with (APF) fluoride application acts as an effective method of caries control during orthodontic treatment.

### Tooth Whitening by Laser

Laser can be used for removal of intrinsic stains **(Figs 49.17A and B)** and or postoperative tooth whitening to brighten the smile.

### Depigmentation of Gingiva by Laser

Gingival pigmentation gives unesthetic appearance, especially during smiling and seen more commonly in black race groups. Lasers can be used to remove gingival pigmentation and helps in restoring the lost esthetics **(Figs 49.18A and B)**.

### Crown Lengthening Procedure by Laser

An excellent application of crown lengthening is when a canine is substituted for a congenitally missing lateral incisor. When first premolar is the canine position, its crown height looks too short. Some clinicians recommend intrusion of the premolar and placement of a laminate veneer to restore length. Another option, however, is to lengthen the premolar crown by laser gingivectomy **(Figs 48.19A and B)**.

### Debonding of Brackets by Laser

Debonding of brackets is one of the most important procedures carried out after the active fixed mechanotherapy. Debonding of ceramic bracket is difficult and often results in fracture of brackets. Studies proved that application of lasers in debonding of brackets not only helps in debonding of metal brackets but also makes easy of ceramic bracket debonding and prevents fracture of enamel.

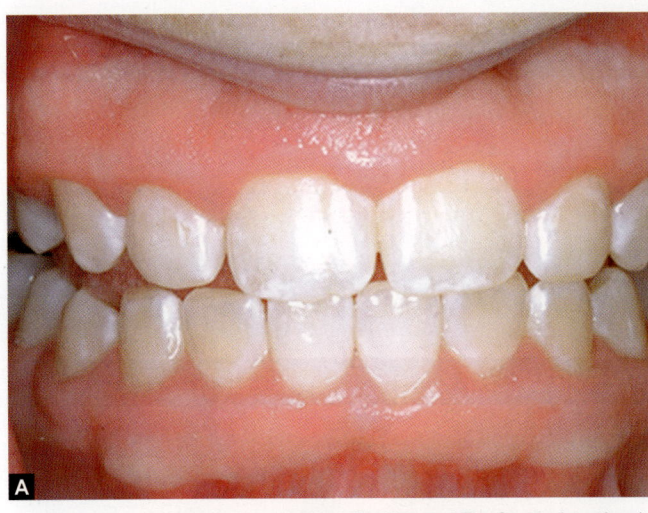
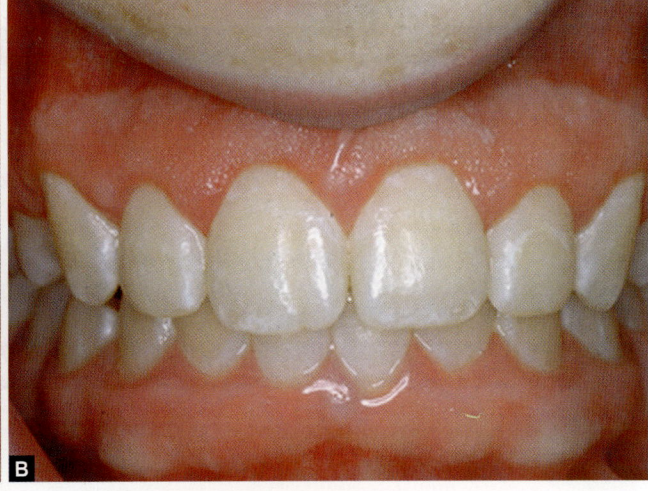

**Figs 49.19A and B:** Crown lengthening procedure by laser (A) Before (B) After

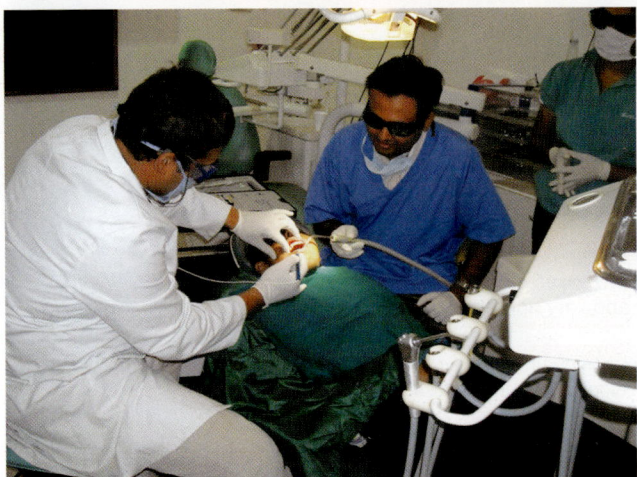

**Fig. 49.20:** Always put on the protective eye glasses prior to the application of lasers. It is recommended to use only laser specific protective eye glasses

## LASER SAFETY

Lasers are excellent tools, but they also bear a very high risk for severe injury and damage. Laser radiation mainly endangers eyes, the retina, cornea and the lens are concerned. Damage of the retina usually is permanent. Thus just a slight carelessness can impair your vision.

The second affected organ is skin although it is much less sensitive than eyes and damages occur only at high energies. Hence, the high risks require suitable protective measures; their strict observation is the responsibility of the clinician and the management.

## PRECAUTIONARY MEASURES

Following are the important precautionary measures prior to the handling and clinical applications of lasers:

1. Always put on the protective eye glasses prior to the application of lasers. It is recommended to use only laser specific protective eye glasses **(Fig. 49.20)**.
2. Make sure the door of the operatory room should always be closed.
3. Use of nonreflective instrument is recommended to avoid indirect hazard.
4. Cover the endotracheal tube with wet gauge piece or use special stainless steel tube to avoid combustion of anesthetic gases by laser beam.
5. Use of high vacuum suction or smoke evacuator for evacuations of toxic gases.

## BIBLIOGRAPHY

1. Hall RR, Hill DW, Beach AD. A carbon dioxide surgical laser. Ann R Coll Surg Engl. 19771;48;181-8.
2. Hicks MJ, Flaitz CM, Westernman GH, Blakenau RJ, Powell GL, Berg JH. Enamel caries initiation and progression following low energy. Argon Laser J Clin Dent. 1995;20(1):9-13.
3. Jost-Brinkman PG, Stien H, et al. Histological investigation of the human pulp after thermodebonding of metal and ceramic brackets. Am J Orthod. 1992;102:410.
4. Li ZZ, Code JE, Van De Merwe WP. Er: YAG laser ablation of enamel and dentin of human teeth. Determination of ablation rates at various influences and pulse repetition rates. Laser Surg Med. 1992;12:625-30.
5. Midda M. The use of laser in periodontology. Curr opin Dent. 1992;2;104-8.
6. Oliver RG. The effect of different methods of bracket removal on the amount of residual asdhesive. Am J Orthod Dentofacial Orthop. 1988;93:196-200.
7. Pick RM, Pecaro BC, Silberman CJ. The laser gingivectomy. The use of the CO2 laser for removal of phytoin hyperplasia.
8. Rossman JA, Cobb CM. Laser in periodontal therapy. Periodontology. 2000;1995:150-64.
9. Rufenacht CR. Fundamentals of esthetics.Chicago; quintessence; 1990.
10. Sarver DM, Yanosky M. Principles of cosmetic dentistry in orthodontics; part 3. Laser treatment for tooth eruption and soft tissue problems. Am J Orthod Dentofacial Orthop. 2005; in press.
11. Von Fraunhofer JA, Allen DJ, Orbell GM. Laser etching of enamel for direct bonding. Angle Orthod. 1993;63:73-6.
12. Walsh LJ, Abood D, Brockhurst PJ. Bonding of resin composites to carbon dioxide laser—modified human enamel. Dent Mater. 1994;10:162-6.

## EXAM-ORIENTED QUESTIONS

### Long Questions
1. Lasers in orthodontics
2. Applications of Lasers in orthodontics.

### Short Notes
1. Advantages of Lasers in orthodontics
2. Precautionary measures during lasers application in Orthodontics.

## CHAPTER OVERVIEW

**Applications of lasers in orthodontics**

- **Exposure of impacted tooth** → Accessibility and decreases the risk of bond failure
- **Frenectomy by laser** →
  - Faster healing
  - Reduces discomfort
  - No suture
  - No pain
- **Reduction of pain in orthodontic patient by applications of laser** → Applications of laser in patient with separator reduces the level of pain threshold
- **Applications of laser in bonding brackets** →
  - Laser bonding takes only 3-5 seconds
  - Reduces chain time
  - Increases efficiency of bonding in uncooperative and very apprehensive patients
- **Laser ablation of surface enamel for orthodontic bracket placement** →
  - Less chair time
  - Good moisture control
  - Bond strength
- **Removal of redundant gingival tissue by laser during orthodontic treatment** → Lasers can be used in the removal of redundant tissue which fasten the progress of orthodontic treatment
- **Management of apthous ulcers by laser during orthodontic treatment** → Helps in reducing pain and promotes healing
- **Removal of perculae on second molar by laser** → Facilitates exposure of teeth and accessibility for band placement
- **Use of laser in controlling the growth of facial structure** → Controls overgrowth or under growth by application of lasers
- **Caries control during orthodontic treatment** → Nd: YAG laser irradiation with APF fluoride application acts as an effective method of caries control during orthodontic treatment
- **Tooth whitening by lasers** → Lasers can be used for removal of intervene stain and post-operative tooth whitening to brightens the smile
- **Depigmentation of gingiva by laser** → Lasers can be used to remove gingival pigmentation and helps in restoring the lost esthetics

# CHAPTER 50: MCQs in Orthodontics

*Phulari BS*

## 1. INTRODUCTION AND HISTORY

### INTRODUCTION AND HISTORY OF ORTHDONTICS

1. Orthodontics is the branch of dentistry concerned with
   A. Prevention and correction of malocclusion
   B. Prevention, interception and correction of malocclusion and other dentofacial abnormalities
   C. Interception and correction of malocclusion
   D. Prevention and interception of malocclusion

2. 'Odontos' is the Greek word for
   A. Odontology          B. Tooth anomalies
   C. Tooth/teeth         D. Orthodontics

3. In which year has the British society for the study of orthodontics put forward the definition of orthodontics?
   A. 1922      B. 1923
   C. 1932      D. 1924

4. The term orthodontics is derived from
   A. Greek     B. Latin
   C. French    D. Spanish

5. The aims of orthodontics have been summarised by
   A. Le Felon           B. Jackson
   C. Emerson C Angell   D. Edward H angle

6. Orthodontic treatment brings about changes in
   A. Dentition only
   B. Facial and jaw musculature only
   C. Dentofacial structure only
   D. All of the above

7. What are the aims/objectives of orthodontic treatment?
   A. Functional efficiency   B. Structural balance
   C. Esthetic harmony        D. All of the above

8. What is the most common reason for seeking orthodontic care?
   A. Inability to chew properly
   B. Aesthetic harmony
   C. Pain in the temporomandibular joint
   D. Predisposition to periodontal diseases and dental caries

9. Who is the father of modern orthodontics?
   A. Edward Hartley Angle
   B. Emerson C Angel
   C. John Farrar
   D. Pierre Fauchard

10. Who advocated the use of finger pressure to align irregular teeth?
    A. Edward Hartley Angle
    B. Calvin Case
    C. Aulius Cornelius Celsius
    D. PR Begg

11. Edward H Angle brought forward
    A. Jackson's triad
    B. Classification of malocclusion
    C. Rapid maxillary expansion
    D. Inter-maxillary elastics

12. Who is the founder of modern dentistry?
    A. Edward H angle
    B. Norman Kingsley
    C. Aulius Cornelius Celsius
    D. Pierre Fauchard

13. Emerson C Angel is credited for the development of which appliance?
    A. Bandelette
    B. Inter-maxillary elastics
    C. Straight wire appliance
    D. Band and loop

14. Angle's classification of malocclusion was modified by whom?
    A. Laurence Andrews
    B. Lischer
    C. Dewey
    D. Both (B) and (C)

15. Bandelette is an orthodontic appliance used
    A. To band molars
    B. To expand the dental arch
    C. To align molars
    D. As a space maintainer

16. Pierre Fauchard was
    A. A French dentist     B. An American dentist
    C. A Greek dentist      D. A German dentist

17. Baker's anchorage was introduced in
    A. 1983      B. 1893
    C. 1896      D. 1898

18. Who first advocated the opening of mid palatal suture to expand the dental arch?
    A. Emerson C Angel     B. Pierre Fauchard
    C. Edward H Angle      D. Raymond Begg

19. Who is considered to be the pioneer of cleft palate management?
    A. Emerson C Angel     B. Pierre Fauchard
    C. Norman Kingsley     D. Raymond Begg

20. Who promoted orthodontics as a speciality rather than part of dentistry?
    A. Le Felon
    B. Aulius Cornelius Celsius
    C. Pierre Fauchard
    D. Edward H Angle
21. Which classification of malocclusion is most commonly used?
    A. Simon's classification of malocclusion
    B. Angle's classification of malocclusion
    C. Ackermann-Profitt classification of malocclusion
    D. Bennet's classification of malocclusion
22. Who was the first to band the teeth for active tooth movements?
    A. Pierre Fauchard      B. Henry A. Baker
    C. William E. Magill    D. Emerson C. Angel
23. Raymond Begg was a
    A. Australian    B. British
    C. American      D. German
24. Who started the first school for specialisation in orthodontics?
    A. Calvin case      B. Norman Kingsley
    C. John Farrar      D. E.H. Angle
25. Who of the following orthodontists advocated extraction of some teeth to achieve a stable post-treatment occlusion?
    A. Edward H. Angle    B. Martin Dewey
    C. Calvin Case        D. Lawrence Andrews
26. Who first introduced acid etch technique in 1955?
    A. Magill    B. Buonocore
    C. Cruz      D. Baker
27. Acid etch technique was introduced by Buonocore in the year
    A. 1956    B. 1955
    C. 1954    D. 1953
28. Who of the following was a critic of Angle's philosophy of arch expansion?
    A. Martin Dewey    B. Raymond Begg
    C. Calvin Case     D. Lawrence Andrews
29. Cephalometric radiography was introduced in the year
    A. 1931    B. 1831
    C. 1921    D. 1941
30. In which year Le felon coined the term orthodontics?
    A. 1839    B. 1939
    C. 1739    D. 1838
31. Currently the faculty of orthodontics is called as
    A. Orthodontia
    B. Orthodontics
    C. Orthodontics and dentofacial orthopaedics
    D. Specialisation in orthodontics
32. Who introduced the E-Arch technique?
    A. Edward Hartley Angle
    B. P Raymond Begg
    C. Calvin Case
    D. Cruz

33. Who introduced the monobloc appliance?
    A. Pierre Robin    B. Viggo Andresen
    C. Hapul           D. Edward H Angle
34. In which year Pierre Robin introduced monobloc?
    A. 1902    B. 1903
    C. 1901    D. 1904
35. Monobloc is used for
    A. Protrude the mandible forward
    B. Retrude the mandible backward
    C. Rotate the mandible forward
    D. Rotate the mandible backward
36. Monobloc is used in patients with
    A. Glossoptosis
    B. Class III malocclusion
    C. Skeletal class III
    D. Skeletal class II
37. The term orthodontics is derived from;
    A. Orthos and Odontos
    B. Orthod and Dontos
    C. Orthodontia
    D. Orthodons and dontics
38. Who developed the appliance called activator?
    A. Viggo Andresen    B. Pierre Robin
    C. Hapul             D. E H Angle
39. In which year Viggo Andresen developed the activator?
    A. 1911    B. 1910
    C. 1909    D. 1908
40. Who introduced the functional regulator?
    A. Walter Coffin    B. Rolf Frankel
    C. Newell           D. Andresen
41. In which year Rolf Frankel developed function regulator?
    A. 1969    B. 1968
    C. 1967    D. 1966
42. Who was the first to introduce the use of extra-oral force to correct protruding teeth?
    A. Norman Kingsley    B. Pierre Fauchard
    C. Angle              D. Celsus
43. Where did Angle started his school of orthodontics for the first time in the world?
    A. New York      B. New Jersey
    C. St. Louis     D. London
44. Who is the pioneer of medical sciences?
    A. Aristotle
    B. Hipppocrates
    C. Leonardo Da Vinci
    D. Aulius Cornelius Celsus
45. Who first coined the word orthodontics?
    A. Aulius Cornelius Celsus
    B. Le Felon
    C. Edward H. Angle
    D. Emerson C Angel
46. Who was against extraction of teeth for achievement of stable results?
    A. Martin Dewey    B. Edward H. Angle
    C. Calvin Case     D. Lawrence Andrews

47. Which scientist introduced cephalometric radiography
    A. Richard A. Riedel
    B. Alexander Jacobson
    C. Herbert I Margolis
    D. Holly Broadbont and Hofarath
48. The department of orthodontia is referred to as orthodontics up to
    A. 1930        B. 1940
    C. 1950        D. 1960
49. Who was the first surgeon to devise an obturator for the treatment of cleft palate?
    A. Paul Aegina      B. Ambrose Pare
    C. John Hunter      D. Norman Kingsley
50. Who introduced the expansion screw?
    A. William Lintott    B. JS Tunnel
    C. Emerson C Angel   D. William and Magill
51. Who introduced the chin strap as occipital anchorage for the treatment of mandibular protrusion?
    A. JS Gunnell         B. Emerson C Angel
    C. William and Magill D. Norman Kingsley
52. In which year JS Gunnell introduced chin strap as an occipital anchorage for the treatment mandibular protrusion?
    A. 1940        B. 1840
    C. 1640        D. 1540
53. Who published 2 volumes entitled 'Irregularities of the teeth and their correction' in 1888 and 1889
    A. Norman Kingsley
    B. John Nutting Farrar
    C. John Hunter
    D. John Kennedy
54. Who introduced the philosophy of tooth movement by using a rubber tooth positioning device in which the teeth were moved into a more ideal cuspal relationship after major correction has been accomplished?
    A. H.D.Kesling
    B. Charles A Hawley
    C. Henry A Baker
    D. William and Magill
55. Who introduced ANB angle?
    A. Richard A. Riedel   B. Alexander Jacobson
    C. William B Downs     D. Herbert I Margolis
56. Wit's analysis was given by:
    A. Richard A Riedel    B. Alexander Jacobson
    C. William B Downs     D. Herbert I Margolis
57. Who developed the pin and tube appliance?
    A. Raymond Begg        B. Emerson C. Angel
    C. Edward H. Angle
    D. Henry Baker
58. Who suggested the first mechanical treatment for correcting irregularities?
    A. Aulius Cornelius Celsus
    B. Gaius Pliuius Secundus
    C. Hippocrates
    D. Paul of Aegina
59. Plaster of Paris for impressions of the cast was first exported by?
    A. Phillip Pfall
    B. Matthacus Gottfried Purmana
    C. EH Angle
    D. Norman kingsley
60. Who was the first to mention supernumerary teeth?
    A. Paul of Aegina
    B. Piette Dionis
    C. Gains plinius Secundus
    D. Norman kingsley
61. In 1825, who recognised habit as a factor in malocclusion?
    A. Gaius Plinius Sewndus
    B. E.H. Angle
    C. Bennet
    D. Joseph Sigmond
62. The term orthodontics is derived from:
    A. Orthos meaning correction and odontos meaning a tooth or teeth
    B. Orthos meaning tooth or teeth and odontos meaning correction
    C. Orthos meaning straightening and odontos meaning tooth tissue structures
    D. Orthos meaning aesthetic and odontos meaning oral tissues
63. Branches of orthodontics are
    A. Preventive orthodontics
    B. Interceptive orthodontics
    C. Corrective orthodontics
    D. All of the above
64. Preventive orthodontics refers to
    A. Prevention of oral diseases
    B. Action taken to preserve the integrity of what appears to be normal occlusion at a specific time
    C. Space maintainers
    D. Parent and child education
65. According to Noyes, orthodontics is defined as:
    A. The study of the relation of teeth to the development of the face, and the correction of arrested and perverted development
    B. The study of the relation of the teeth to the development of the face
    C. The correction of arrested and perverted development
    D. None of the above
66. Who was the first to advocate the use of removable orthodontic appliance?
    A. Der Schiefetand Der Zahox
    B. Kneisel
    C. Robin
    D. Andrew
67. In which year has Noyes defined the term orthodontics?
    A. 1910        B. 1911
    C. 1912        D. 1913

68. In which year Salzmann defined the term orthodontics
    A. 1943
    B. 1944
    C. 1945
    D. 1946
69. The abbreviation ABO means?
    A. American Board of Orthodontics
    B. American Board of Orthodontists
    C. American Board of Orthodontia
    D. American Board of Orthodontic society
70. Edward H Angle was basically an
    A. Orthodontist
    B. Prosthodontist
    C. Orthognatic surgeon
    D. Cosmetic dentist
71. Angle's contribution to orthodontics
    A. E-arch technique
    B. Pin-tube technique
    C. Edgewise technique
    D. All of the above
72. What is Andrew's fourth key to normal occlusion in adult dentition?
    A. Molar relationship
    B. Crown inclination
    C. Absence of space
    D. None of the above
73. What are the radiographs used for orthodontic diagnosis and treatment planning?
    A. OPG
    B. Lateral cephalogram
    C. Sialography
    D. Both of (a) and (b)
74. Malocclusion refers to
    A. Abnormal deviation to normal occlusion
    B. Abnormal deviation in face
    C. Abnormal deviation of only skeletal structures
    D. All of the above
75. Which type of malocclusion contributes to the highest prevalence?
    A. Class I malocclusion
    B. Class II malocclusion
    C. Class III malocclusion
    D. All of the above
76. Midline diastema refers to:
    A. Spacing between two maxillary central incisors in the midline in permanent dentition
    B. Spacing between two central mandibular incisors in the midline in permanent dentition
    C. Spacing between two central maxillary incisors in the midline in deciduous dentition
    D. Spacing between two central mandibular incisors in the midline in deciduous dentition
77. Who was the first to use the term orthopedics in connection with the correction of malocclusions?
    A. Bunon
    B. Angle
    C. Le Felon
    D. John Hunter
78. In which journal and year did Edward H Angle publish the landmark article introducing his classification of malocclusion?
    A. 1886
    B. 1884
    C. 1885
    D. 1889
79. Who was a proponent of the nonextraction school of thought?
    A. Calvin Case
    B. John Farrar
    C. Edward H. Angle
    D. John Hunter
80. Is driftodontics a branch of orthodontics?
    A. Yes
    B. No
    C. A branch of adult orthodontics
    D. None of the above
81. Unfavourable sequelae of malocclusion are
    A. Poor facial appearance
    B. Abnormalities of function
    C. Risk of periodontal diseases
    D. All of the above
82. Benefits of orthodontic treatment are
    A. To improve confidence
    B. Well aligned teeth that are easier to maintain clean and healthy
    C. Ideally positioned teeth which lessen the chance of gingivitis and advanced gum disease
    D. All of the above
83. Angle's classification of malocclusion was published in Dental Cosmos in
    A. 1899
    B. 1888
    C. 1887
    D. 1886
84. PR Begg was a disciple of
    A. E H Angle
    B. Calvin Case
    C. John Farrar
    D. John Hunter
85. Who said the following famous line? "I have finished my work. It is as perfect as I can make it."
    A. Calvin Case
    B. John Hunter
    C. John Farrar
    D. Edward H Angle
86. In which year and what was the first orthodontic society and who has developed it?
    A. In 1935-American Association of Orthodontists- E.H.Angle
    B. In 1935-The society of Orthodontists- E.H.Angle
    C. In 1935-American orthodontists- E.H.Angle
    D. Combination of A,B and C
87. First successful closure of soft palate defect was reported by
    A. Le Monnier, a French dentist
    B. Le Felon, a French dentist
    C. Norman Kingsley, an American orthodontist
    D. Neither of all
88. First successful closure of hard palate defect was reported by
    A. Le Monnier, a French dentist
    B. Le Felon, a French dentist
    C. Norman Kingsley, an American orthodontist
    D. Dieffenbach, a German dentist
89. Orthodontic appliances are
    A. Removable orthodontic appliance
    B. Fixed orthodontic appliance
    C. Brackets, Labial Bow and Adam's clasp
    D. Both (a) and (b)

90. Dimensional light wire appliance was introduced by
    A. Edward H. Angle
    B. Emerson C Angel
    C. Raymond Begg
    D. Norman kingsley
91. At what age can orthodontic treatment begin?
    A. 6 years
    B. 7 years
    C. 8 years
    D. At any age
92. Who was the chief proponent of removable orthodontic appliances?
    A. Victor Hugo Jackson
    B. George Crozat
    C. Robbin
    D. Adams
93. How many keys of occlusion has Andrews put forward?
    A. 6
    B. 3
    C. 5
    D. 8
94. Andrews's first key to normal occlusion deals with
    A. Incisal relationship
    B. Canine relationship
    C. Molar relationship
    D. Third molar relationship
95. Andrews's first key to normal occlusion in adult dentition is characterised by
    A. Crown angulation
    B. Crown inclination
    C. Incisal guidance
    D. None of the above
96. According to Andrews's six keys of occlusion, crown angulations should be present?
    A. True
    B. False
    C. Gingival part of the long axis of crown must be distal to occlusal part of the line
    D. Gingival part of the long axis should be in line with occlusal part of the line.
97. According to Andrews's fifth key of occlusion, presence of spacing between teeth is physiological to normal occlusion, in adult dentition?
    A. The spaces are called primate spaces.
    B. There should be tight contacts between adjacent teeth.
    C. Spacing between teeth should be present to allow eruption of third molars.
    D. None of the above.
98. Curve of Spee should not exceed 1.5 mm according to
    A. Andrews's first key
    B. Andrews's second key
    C. Andrews's third key
    D. None of the above
99. According to Andrews's key 3 to normal occlusion is
    A. Mandibular incisor show a pronounced negative crown inclination.
    B. Mandibular incisor show a mild negative crown inclination.
    C. Mandibular incisor show a pronounced positive crown inclination.
    D. Mandibular incisor show a mild positive crown inclination.
100. Who was the first to develop functional orthodontic appliance?
    A. Walter Coffin
    B. Rolf Frankel
    C. Newell
    D. Andresen.

Ans: 1. B  2. B  3. A  4. A  5. B  6. D  7. D  8. B  9. A  10. C  11. B  12. D  13. A  14. D  15. B
16. A  17. B  18. A  19. C  20. D  21. B  22. C  23. A  24. D  25. C  26. B  27. B  28. C  29. A  30. A
31. C  32. A  33. A  34. A  35. A  36. D  37. A  38. A  39. B  40. B  41. D  42. A  43. C  44. B  45. B
46. B  47. D  48. A  49. B  50. A  51. A  52. B  53. B  54. A  55. A  56. B  57. C  58. B  59. A  60. A
61. A  62. A  63. D  64. B  65. A  66. A  67. B  68. A  69. A  70. B  71. D  72. D  73. D  74. A  75. A
76. A  77. A  78. D  79. C  80. D  81. D  82. D  83. A  84. A  85. D  86. B  87. A  88. D  89. D  90. C
91. A  92. A  93. A  94. C  95. D  96. C  97. B  98. D  99. B  100. D

## 2. GROWTH AND DEVELOPMENT

### GENERAL PRINCIPLES OF GROWTH AND DEVELOPMENT

1. Mixed dentition growth spurts in Boys
    A. 6-8 years
    B. 8-11 years
    C. 14-17 years
    D. 19-21 years
2. Mixed dentition growth spurts in Girls
    A. 6-8 years
    B. 8-11 years
    C. 14-17 years
    D. 7-9 years
3. Prepubertal growth spurts in Boys
    A. 6-8 years
    B. 8-11 years
    C. 12-14 years
    D. 19-21 years
4. Prepubertal growth spurts in Girls
    A. 6-8 years
    B. 10-12 years
    C. 14-17 years
    D. 19-21 years
5. Growth is
    A. The self multiplication of living substance
    B. Increase in size, change in proportion and progressive complexity
    C. Both A and B
    D. None of the above
6. Followings are the theories of growth, except
    A. Functional matrix theory
    B. Cartilaginous theory
    C. Sutural theory
    D. Bolton's theory
7. The genetic theory was antagonized by
    A. Moss and other investigators
    B. Sicher
    C. James scott
    D. Enlow

8. Who was the main proponent of sutural dominance theory?
   A. Moss and other investigators.
   B. Sicher
   C. James scott
   D. Enlow
9. Points raised against Sutural dominance theory were
   A. Growth does not continue after transplantation of an area of suture to another location. This shows a lack of innate growth potential of sutures.
   B. Growth at suture cannot be halted by mechanical forces.
   C. Both A and B
   D. None of the above
10. Which of the followings evidence supports the cartilaginous theory?
    A. Many bones grow by cartilaginous growth, where a precursor cartilage is replaced by bone.
    B. A part of epiphyseal plate continues to grow on transplantation to a different location indicating intrinsic growth potential of the cartilage.
    C. Experimental studies on rabbit showed retarded mid-face development when nasal septal cartilage was removed.
    D. All of the above
11. The components of Functional matrix are
    A. Capsular matrix     B. Periosteal matrix
    C. Both A and B        D. None of the above
12. Example of capsular matrices are;
    A. Neurocranial capsule (skin and dura mater) which is controlled by the growing brain thrusting the bony calvarial plates outward.
    B. Orofacial capsules (comprising of skin and oral mucosa) within which the facial bone arise, grow and are maintained.
    C. Both A and B
    D. None of the above
13. Examples of the periosteal matrices include
    A. Muscles,
    B. Tendon,
    C. Nerves, blood vessels and glands
    D. All of the above
14. The data derived from accurate quantitative measurements are the most appropriate scientifically. Measurements can be made
    A. Direct data
    B. Indirect data
    C. Derived data
    D. All of the above
15. Von Limborgh's theory
    A. It is a multifactorial theory
    B. It explains the process of growth and development in a view that combines all three existing theories
    C. Both A and B
    D. None of the above
16. Enlow expanding 'V' principle
    A. Many facial bones or parts or bones have a "V" shaped pattern of growth
    B. The growth movements and enlargement of these bones occur towards the wide ends of the "V" as a result of differential deposition and selective absorption
    C. Both A and B
    D. None of the above

Ans: 1. B  2. D  3. C  4. B  5. C  6. D  7. A  8. B  9. C  10. D  11. C  12. C  13. D  14. D  15. C  16. C

## PRENATAL GROWTH AND DEVELOPMENT OF HEAD, FACE AND ORAL CAVITY

1. What are the three successive prenatal phases in human development?
   A. Period of ovum, embryo, morula
   B. Period of embryo, ovum, foetus
   C. Period of ovum, embryo, foetus
   D. Foetus, embryo, ovum
2. Period of ovum in prenatal development of human spans from
   A. Ovulations to 14th day
   B. Fertilization to 3 weeks
   C. Fertilization to 14 days
   D. Implantation to 2 weeks
3. Period of embryo in prenatal development of human spans from
   A. 4 to 8 weeks
   B. 5 to 9 weeks
   C. 6 to 10 weeks
   D. 3 to 8 weeks
4. Period of foetus in prenatal development of human spans from
   A. 80 days to birth     B. 56 days to birth
   C. 50 days to birth     D. 55 days to birth
5. Which of the following statements are not true regarding the period of ovum in human prenatal developmental stage?
   A. Implantation of ovum to the uterine wall
   B. Rapid proliferation of cells occurs with no little differentiation
   C. Rapid differentiation of cells with proliferation
   D. Fertilization to implantation of ovum
6. Which of the following statements is not true regarding period of embryo during prenatal human development stage?
   A. All proliferation and differentiation occur during the stage
   B. Organogenesis occurs
   C. Differentiation of all major organ and systems
   D. There is no proliferation and differentiation during this period

7. Which of the following statements is not true regarding period of foetus during prenatal human development stage?
   A. The embryo is called foetus
   B. Growth and maturation
   C. There is rapid differentiation
   D. Overall increase in size of foetus
8. Which of the following statements is not true in early embryonic events?
   A. Fertilization is a process by which male and female gametes fuses
   B. Fertilization occurs in the ampulla of uterine tube
   C. Fertilization is a period of blastocyst formation
   D. Fertilized egg undergoes rapid division to form a ball of cells called morula
9. Which are the cell populations seen in blastocyst
   A. Trophoblast and myloblast
   B. Myloblast and embryoblast
   C. Trophoblast or embryoblast
   D. Inner cell mass and erythroblast
10. During which period of human prenatal development does the congenital defects occur
    A. Period of ovum
    B. Period of embryo
    C. Period of morula
    D. Period of fetus
11. What are the causes for congenital defects during the period of embryo
    A. Virus infection    B. Bacterial
    C. Drugs              D. Both A and C
12. Which of the following cells are responsible for embryo proper
    A. Inner cell mass/embryoblast
    B. Myloblast
    C. Trophoblast
    D. Blastocyte
13. Which of the following statements is true during implantation?
    A. Embryoblast is associated with implantation of embryo and formation of placenta
    B. Blastocyte is associated with implantation
    C. Trophoblast cells are associated with implantation of embryo and formation of placenta
    D. Myloblast cells are associated with formation of placenta and embryo
14. Bilaminar disc is formed during which period of embryonic events
    A. 1st week
    B. 3rd week
    C. 2nd week
    D. 4th week
15. Bilaminar disc is comprised of following
    A. Epiblast and hypoblast
    B. Myloblast and epiblast
    C. Embryoblast and hypoblast
    D. Trophoblast and myloblast
16. During which period does the trilaminar disk is formed
    A. 2nd week
    B. 3rd week
    C. 6th week
    D. 8th week
17. Gastrulation refers to the following
    A. Trilaminar embryo is converted into bilaminar embryo
    B. Bilaminar embryo is converted into trilaminar embryo
    C. Myeloblast embryo is converted into bilaminar embryo
    D. Embryoblast embryo is converted into trilaminar embryo
18. During gastrulation, all the three germ layers are formed by following cell layer
    A. Trophoblast cell layer
    B. Myeloblast cell layer
    C. Epiblast cell layer
    D. Embryoblast cell layer
19. Which of the following structures are derived from ectoderm
    A. Nervous system with neural crest tissue
    B. Enamel
    C. Dentin
    D. Both A and B
20. Primitive oral cavity is bounded by the following processes
    A. Ventral frontal prominence
    B. Cranially by frontal prominence and ventrally by developing cardiac bulge
    C. Lateral prominence and frontally by developing cardiac bulge
    D. Laterally developing cardiac bulge
21. Foregut is separated from stomatodeum by which of the following
    A. Pharyngeal membrane
    B. Buccopharyngeal membrane
    C. Linguopharyngeal membrane
    D. Mesiopharyngeal membrane
22. During which period does the pharyngeal branchial arches are formed
    A. 2 weeks        B. 3 weeks
    C. 4 weeks        D. 5 weeks
23. How many pharyngeal arches are seen during embryonic development of humans
    A. 12             B. 6
    C. 8              D. 5
24. The fourth pharyngeal arch is formed by fusion of following archs during embryo development of human
    A. 1 and 2        B. 4 and 6
    C. 5 and 6        D. 2 and 3
25. Which of the pharyngeal arches completely regresses during the embryonic development in human?
    A. vi             B. iv
    C. v              D. iii

26. First arch is also called
    A. Hyoid arch
    B. Mandibular arch
    C. Maxillary arch
    D. Pharyngeal arch
27. Second arch is also called
    A. Hyoid arch
    B. Mandibular arch
    C. Maxillary arch
    D. Pharyngeal arch
28. Third and fourth arch is also called as
    A. Hyoid arch
    B. Mandibular arch
    C. Maxillary arch
    D. None of the above
29. Which of the pharyngeal arch completely regresses without contribution to development of any structures during development in humans?
    A. iv
    B. v
    C. vi
    D. iii
30. Which specific nerve passes through the first arch or mandibular arch?
    A. Vagus nerve
    B. Glossopharyngeal
    C. Trigeminal nerve
    D. Facial nerve
31. Which specific nerve passes through the second arch or hyoid arch?
    A. Optic nerve
    B. Vagus nerve
    C. Facial nerve
    D. Trigeminal nerve
32. Mandibular arch gives rise to the following structures except
    A. Maxillary process
    B. Mandibular process
    C. Frontonasal process
    D. None of the above
33. Hyoid arch gives rises to the following structures except
    A. Muscles of facial expression
    **B. Muscles of mastication**
    C. Sytohyoid ligament
    D. Stylopharyngeus muscle
34. Which specific nerve passes through the 3rd arch
    A. Occulomotor nerve
    B. Glossopharyngeal nerve
    C. Facial nerve
    D. Trigeminal nerve
35. The following structures are derived from 3rd arch expect
    A. Larygenal cartilage
    B. Circothyroid cartilage
    C. Intrinsic muscles of pharynx
    D. Muscles of facial expression
36. Which specific nerve passes through the 4th and 6th arch
    A. Hypoglossal nerve
    B. Trigeminal nerve
    C. Vagus nerve
    D. Glossopharyngeal nerve
37. Development of face usually occurs at
    A. 4-6 weeks
    B. 2-6 weeks
    C. 4-8 weeks
    D. 2-4 weeks
38. During the development of face stomatodeum is surrounded by the following
    A. Laterally by the lateral nasal process, medially by the medial nasal process, ventrally by the frontonasal process
    B. Crainally by the frontonasal process, caudally by the cardiac bulge and laterally by the first branchial arch
    C. Caudally by the frontonasal process, laterally by the cardiac bulge and cranially by the medial nasal process
    D. Caudally by the lateral nasal process, cranially by the medial nasal process and laterally by the frontonasal process
39. Lower lip is formed by the following processes
    A. Merging of two mandibular processes
    B. Merging of maxillary process
    C. Merging of lateral nasal process
    D. Merging of medial nasal process
40. The maxillary process gives rises to the following structures except
    A. Lateral portion of upper lip
    B. Secondary palate
    C. Most of the maxilla
    D. Premaxilla
41. Which of the following structures is derived from frontonasal process
    A. Forehead
    B. Dorsum bridge of nose
    C. Both A and B
    D. None of the above
42. The following structures are derived from medial nasal process except
    A. Midline of the nose
    B. Nasal septum
    C. Middle portion of upper lip
    D. Lower lip
43. Which of the following facial structures is derived from mandibular process?
    A. Entire mandible
    B. Lower lip
    C. Both A and B
    D. None of the above
44. Development of palate occurs in
    A. 8-9 weeks
    B. 6-9 weeks
    C. 6-10 weeks
    D. 7-9 weeks
45. Primary palate is derived from
    A. Maxillary process
    B. Frontonasal process
    C. Mandibular process
    D. Lateral nasal process
46. Secondary palate is derived from
    A. Two palatine shelves from right and left maxillary process and nasal septum
    B. Two palatine shelves from medial nasal process
    C. Two medial nasal process and lateral nasal process
    D. None of the above

47. Which of the following is true
    A. Palatine shelves oriented horizontally and later assumes vertically downwards.
    B. Palatine shelves oriented ventrally and later assumes horizontally downwards with the tongue interposed between them
    C. Palatine shelves first direct vertically downwards with the tongue interposed and later assumes horizontally
    D. Palatine shelves first direct medially downwards with tongue interposed and later assumes ventrally
48. Development of tongue occurs during
    A. 3rd week
    B. 4th week
    C. 2nd week
    D. 5th week
49. Tongue is derived from
    A. Copula, two lingual swelling and hypobranchial eminence
    B. Tuberculum impar, one lingual swelling and hypobranchial eminence
    C. Tuberculum impar, two lingual swellings and hypobranchial eminence
    D. Copula and hypobranchial eminence
50. Tongue mainly develops from the following pharyngeal arches
    A. 1, 2, 3
    B. 2, 3, 4
    C. 1, 3, 4
    D. 2, 4, 5
51. Epiglottis is derived from
    A. 1 arch
    B. 3 arch
    C. 4 arch
    D. 2 arch
52. During the development of tongue the first pharyngeal arch give rise to
    A. Tuberculum impar
    B. Hypobranchial eminence
    C. Two lingual swelling
    D. A and C
53. Which pharyngeal arch does not contribute to the development of tongue?
    A. 1 arch
    B. 2 arch
    C. 3 arch
    D. 4 arch
54. Anterior two third of tongue is derived from
    A. 2 arch
    B. 1 arch
    C. 3 arch
    D. 4 arch
55. Posterior one third of the tongue is derived from
    A. 1 arch
    B. 3 arch
    C. 2 arch
    D. 6 arch
56. Muscles of the tongue are derived from
    A. 4 arch
    B. 3 arch
    C. Occipital myotomes
    D. 1 arch
57. Anterior two third of tongue or body is formed
    A. Tuberculum impar and hypobranchial eminence
    B. Copula and two lingual swelling
    C. Two lingual swellings and tuberculum impar
    D. Hypobranchial eminences and copula
58. Posterior one third of the tongue or base is formed by
    A. Two lingual swelling
    B. Hypobranchial eminence
    C. Copula
    D. Tuberculum impar
59. Hypobranchial eminence is derived from
    A. 1 arch
    B. 3 arch
    C. 2 arch
    D. 4 arch
60. Sensory nerves supply to the body of the tongue
    A. Optic nerve
    B. Trigeminal nerve
    C. Facial nerve
    D. Glossopharyngeal nerve
61. Sensory nerve supply to the base of the tongue
    A. Facial nerve
    B. Trigeminal nerve
    C. Glossopharyngeal nerve
    D. Optic nerve
62. Motor nerve supply to the muscles of the tongue
    A. Glossopharyngeal nerve
    B. Hypoglossal nerve
    C. Trigeminal nerve
    D. Facial nerve
63. Cranium is divided into
    A. Neurocranium
    B. Viscerocranium
    C. Both A and B
    D. None of the above
64. Neuro cranium includes
    A. Cranial vault
    B. Cranial base
    C. Both A and B
    D. None of the above
65. Viscerocranium includes
    A. Cranial base
    B. Maxilla
    C. Mandible
    D. Both B and C
66. Following develop mainly from intramembranous ossification expect
    A. Cranial vault
    B. Cranial base
    C. Maxilla
    D. Mandible
67. Following develop mainly from endochondral ossification
    A. Maxilla
    B. Cranial vault
    C. Cranial base
    D. Mandible
68. Following are secondary cartilages in the development of mandible expect
    A. Condylar cartilage
    B. Coronoid cartilage
    C. Meckles cartilage
    D. Symphysial cartilage
69. Primary cartilage of the 1st arch is
    A. Coronoid cartilage
    B. Meckels cartilage
    C. Reichert cartilage
    D. Condylar cartilage
70. Primary cartilage of the second pharyngeal arch is
    A. Condylar cartilage
    B. Reichert cartilage
    C. Symphysial cartilage
    D. Meckels cartilage
71. The inital site of ossification of mandible occurs at
    A. Division of mandible nerve into lingual and inferior alveolar nerve
    B. At the division inferior alveolar nerve into incisive and mental nerve
    C. Division of glossopharyngeal nerve
    D. Division of facial nerve

72. Meckels cartilage forms the following structures except
    A. Incus and malleus
    B. Spine of the sphenoid
    C. Stylomandibular ligament
    D. Sphenomandibular ligament
73. Secondary cartilages of develop mandible at
    A. 10-16 weeks
    B. 10-14 weeks
    C. 10-12 weeks
    D. 12-16 weeks
74. Following areas of mandible are derived from endochondrial ossification expect
    A. Condylar process, coronoid process, alveolar process
    B. Frontal process, condylar process, mental process
    C. Condylar process, coronoid process, mental process
    D. Symphysial process, condylar process, mental process
75. Development of coroniod process of mandible occurs at
    A. 10-12 weeks    B. 12-16 weeks
    C. 10-14 weeks    D. 14-16 weeks
76. During development of maxilla the centre of ossification occurs
    A. Posterior superior alveolar nerve and inferior alveolar nerve
    B. Anterosuperior alveolar nerve and lingual nerve
    C. Angle between anterosuperior and infraorbital nerve
    D. Superoinferior and superior orbital nerve
77. Secondary cartilage during the development of maxilla
    A. Condylar cartilage    B. Malar cartilage
    C. Zygomatic cartilage   D. Both B and C
78. Development of maxillary sinus occurs at
    A. 2nd month    B. 3rd month
    C. 4th month    D. 5th month
79. All the tissue of tooth and its supporting structures are derived from ectomesechymal cells expect
    A. Pulp         B. Enamel
    C. Dentin       D. Cementum
80. Ectomesenchyme essential for craniofacial development is derived from
    A. Endoderm germ layer
    B. Neural crest cells from ectoderm germ layer
    C. Both A and B
    D. None of the above
81. Each pharyngeal arch has
    A. Specific nerve that supplies muscles and mucosa derived from that arch
    B. A specific cartilage that forms the skeleton of that of secondary cartilage
    C. Muscular components termed as branchiomere and arteries termed aortic arch
    D. All of the above

Ans: 1. C  2. C  3. D  4. B  5. C  6. D  7. C  8. C  9. C  10. B  11. D  12. A  13. C  14. C  15. A  16. B
17. B  18. C  19. D  20. B  21. B  22. C  23. B  24. B  25. C  26. B  27. A  28. D  29. B  30. C  31. C  32. A
33. C  34. B  35. D  36. B  37. C  38. B  39. A  40. D  41. C  42. D  43. C  44. B  45. B  46. A  47. C  48. B
49. C  50. C  51. C  52. D  53. B  54. B  55. B  56. C  57. C  58. B  59. B  60. B  61. C  62. B  63. C  64. C
65. D  66. B  67. C  68. C  69. B  70. B  71. B  72. C  73. B  74. C  75. C  76. C  77. D  78. B  79. B  80. B
81. D

## POSTNATAL GROWTH AND DEVELOPMENT OF HEAD, FACE AND ORAL CAVITY

1. Infant skull at birth consists of how many bony elements?
   A. 42      B. 22
   C. 35      D. 45
2. Total number of bones in adult skull is
   A. 22
   B. 45
   C. 35      D. 45
3. Around 90% of growth of cranial vault occurs by
   A. 7 years    B. 6 years
   C. 5 years    D. 4 years
4. Growth of cranial vault follows
   A. Genital growth curve
   B. Neural growth curve
   C. Somatic growth curve
   D. All of the above
5. Cranial base is formed by the following bones except
   A. Occipital    B. Ethmoid
   C. Zygomatic
   D. Sphenoid
6. Post natal growth of cranial base mainly occurs at
   A. Intra ethmoidal synchondrosis
   B. Inter-sphenoid synchondrosis
   C. Spheno-occipital synchondrosis
   D. Sphenoid synchondrosis
7. Spheno-occipital synchondrosis fuses at what age?
   A. At birth       B. 13-15 years
   C. 5 years
   D. Before birth
8. Which of the following synchondrosis fuses before birth?
   A. Spheno-ethmoid synchondrosis
   B. Intra ethmoid and Inter-sphenoid synchondrosis
   C. Spheno-occipital synchondrosis
   D. Intra-occipital synchondrosis

9. Intra occipital synchondrosis fuses at
   A. 4 years
   B. 6 years
   C. 5 years
   D. 7 years
10. Sphenoid synchondrosis fuses at
    A. 5 years
    B. 7 years
    C. 6 years
    D. 8 years
11. Growth of nasomaxillary complex occurs by which of the following mechanisms?
    A. Translation/Displacement
    B. Growth at sutures
    C. Surface remodeling
    D. All of the above
12. Translation/displacement of bone refers to
    A. Growth occurs at surface of bones
    B. Change in special position of bone
    C. Surface remodeling of bone
    D. Resorption of bone
13. Primary translation refers to
    A. Actual enlargement of bone will change its position in space
    B. Displacement of bone is brought about by its own enlargement
    C. Both A and B
    D. None of above
14. Secondary translation refers to
    A. Growth of a bone causing its displacement
    B. Growth of one bone results in change in the spatial position of an adjacent bone
    C. Both A and B
    D. None of above
15. Postnatal growth of nasomaxillary complex occurs by
    A. Growth of sutures.
    B. Primary translation.
    C. Secondary translation.
    D. All the above.
16. Nasomaxillary complex is surrounded by the following sutures except
    A. Fronto-maxillary suture
    B. Zygomatico-temporal and zygomatico-maxillary suture
    C. Squamo-tympanic suture
    D. Pterygopalatine suture
17. V-shaped palatal growth occurs by
    A. Resorption of zygomatic and deposition at nasal floor
    B. Resorption of nasal floor and bone deposition on oral side of palatal vault
    C. Deposition at maxillary tuberosity
    D. Resorption of maxillary tuberosity
18. Postnatal growth of following bones follow the expanding "V" principle except
    A. Palate
    B. Zygoma
    C. Mandible
    D. Coronoid process
19. Growth of mandible follows
    A. Downwards and backwards
    B. Downwards and forwards
    C. Upwards and downwards
    D. Backwards and upwards
20. Which of the following statement about postnatal growth of ramus is true?
    A. Bone deposition at anterior border and resorption at posterior border occurs
    B. Bone resorption at the anterior border and resorption at posterior border occurs
    C. Bone deposition at anterior and posterior boders
    D. Both B and C.
21. Postnatal growth of coronoid process occurs on an expanding "V" by
    A. Periosteal deposition an lingual surface and resorption of buccal surface
    B. Deposition of posterior border
    C. Basal part of ramus shows deposition on buccal side and with contralateral resorption from lingual surface
    D.
22. Postnatal growth of face (maxilla and mandible) follows
    A. General growth curve
    B. Neural growth curve
    C. Lymphoid curve
    D. Genital growth curve

Ans: 1. **D**  2. **A**  3. **C**  4. **B**  5. **C**  6. **C**  7. **B**  8. **B**  9. **C**  10. **D**  11. **D**  12. **B**  13. **C**  14. **B**  15. **D**  16. **C**  17. **B**  18. **B**  19. **B**  20. **B**  21. **A**  22. **A**

## DEVELOPMENT OF DENTITION AND OCCLUSION

1. The embryonic oral cavity is lined by:
   A. Stratified Squamous Epithelium
   B. Squamous Cell Epithelium
   C. Dental Lamina
   D. Mesenchymal Cells
2. Development of teeth can be divided into:
   A. Cap Stage, Bud Stage, Bell Stage
   B. Bell Stage, Cap Stage, Bud Stage
   C. Bud Stage, Cap Stage, Bell Stage
   D. None of the above
3. Ectomesenchymal condensation surrounding tooth bud and dental papilla is:
   A. Dental Lamina
   B. Dental Sac
   C. Enamel Organ
   D. Oral Ectoderm
4. The central area of enamel organ between the outer and inner enamel epithelium in cap stage:
   A. Dental Papilla
   B. Dental Sac
   C. Stellate Reticulum
   D. Stratum Intermedium

5. **Flat squamous cells seen between inner enamel epithelium and stellate reticulum is:**
   A. Outer Enamel Epithelium
   B. Dental Lamina
   C. Stratum Intermedium
   D. None of the above

6. **Hetwig's Epithelial root sheath is formed by:**
   A. Outer and Inner enamel epithelium
   B. Stratum Intermedium
   C. Stellate Reticulum
   D. Outer Enamel Epithelium

7. **Alveolar processes at the time of birth is known as:**
   A. Gingival Pads      B. Gum Pads
   C. Oral Cavity        D. Gums

8. **Teeth present at time of birth are known as:**
   A. Neonatal Teeth
   B. Prenatal Teeth
   C. Postnatal Teeth
   D. Natal Teeth

9. **Teeth which erupt during first month of age are known as:**
   A. Natal Teeth        B. Neonatal Teeth
   C. Prenatal Teeth     D. All of the above

10. **Initiation of primary tooth occurs during:**
    A. First six weeks of intrauterine life
    B. Third month of
    C. Second Trimester
    D. First week of

11. **Eruption sequence of deciduous dentition is:**
    A. A-B-C-D-E         B. D-A-B-C-E
    C. E-A-B-D-C         D. A-B-D-C-E

12. **Spacing between deciduous dentition is:**
    A. Physiological Spacing
    B. Developmental Spaces
    C. Both A and B
    D. None of the above

13. **Physiological space seen mesial to maxillary canine and distal to mandibular canines is:**
    A. Primate Space     B. Simian Space
    C. Anthropoid Space  D. All of the above

14. **Mesiodistal relation between the distal surfaces of upper and lower second deciduous molars is:**
    A. Flush Terminal Plane
    B. Mesial Step
    C. Distal Step       D. Terminal Plane

15. **Flush terminal plane is:**
    A. Normal feature of deciduous dentition
    B. Plane where distal surfaces of upper and lower second deciduous molars are in same plane
    C. Maxillary deciduous molar is ahead of mandibular
    D. Both A and B

16. **First transition period in mixed dentition is:**
    A. Characterized by emergence of first permanent molars
    B. Eruption of permanent canines
    C. None of the above
    D. All of the above

17. **Shift in molars from a flush terminal plane to a Class I relation occurs by:**
    A. Early Shift       B. Late Shift
    C. Mesial Shift      D. Early and Late Shift

18. **Early mesial shift utilizes:**
    A. Primate Space     B. Leeway Space
    C. Both of the above D. None of the above

19. **Leeway Space is utilized by:**
    A. Early Shift       B. Late Mesial Shift
    C. Mesial Shift      D. Distal Shift

20. **Vertical plane in mixed dentition also denotes:**
    A. Terminal Plane
    B. Mesial step terminal plane
    C. Distal step terminal plane
    D. Flush terminal plane

21. **Mesial step terminal plane usually gives way to:**
    A. Angle's Class I malocclusion
    B. Angle's Class II occlusion
    C. Angle's Class I occlusion
    D. Angle's Class II division II malocclusion

22. **Distal step terminal plane usually gives way to:**
    A. Angle's Class I malocclusion
    B. Angle's Class III malocclusion
    C. Angle's Class II malocclusion
    D. None of the above

23. **Incisal liability is:**
    A. Difference in space between maxillary and mandibular incisors
    B. Difference in space between primary and permanent incisors
    C. Both A and B
    D. None of the above

24. **Incisal liability is corrected by:**
    A. Utilization of interdental spaces
    B. Increase in inter-canine width
    C. Change in incisor inclination
    D. All of the above

25. **Incisor liability is:**
    A. 7 mm in maxillary arch and 5 mm in mandibular arch
    B. 5 mm in mandibular arch and 7 mm in maxillary arch
    C. 5-7 mm in maxillary arch
    D. 5-7 mm in mandibular arch

26. **Ugly Duckling Stage was termed by:**
    A. Broadbent
    B. Nance
    C. Lawrence F Andrews
    D. Calvin Case

27. **Leeway Space was determined by:**
    A. Nance             B. Edward Angle
    C. Calvin Case       D. Martin Dewey

28. **Ugly Duckling Stage**
    A. Needs Fixed Orthodontic Therapy at a later stage
    B. Self Correcting
    C. Transient
    D. Both B and C

29. Which of the below is true?
    A. Leeway Space is greater in maxillary arch
    B. Leeway Space is 3.4 mm in maxillary arch
    C. Leeway Space is greater in mandibular arch than maxillary arch
    D. Leeway Space in mandinular arch is 1.7 mm
30. Leeway Space in maxillary arch is:
    A. 0.9 mm
    B. 1.8 mm
    C. 1.7 mm
    D. 3.4 mm
31. Leeway Space in mandibular arch is:
    A. 0.9 mm
    B. 1.7 mm
    C. 1.8 mm
    D. 3.4 mm
32. Frequently seen eruption sequence in permanent dentition in maxillary arch is:
    A. 6-1-2-4-3-5-7
    B. 6-1-2-3-4-5-7
    C. Both (A) and (B)
    D. None of the above
33. Eruption sequence in mandibular arch is:
    A. 6-1-2-3-4-5-7
    B. 6-1-2-4-3-5-7
    C. 6-1-4-2-3-5-7
    D. Both (A) and (B)
34. Ugly Duckling Stage is corrected by:
    A. Eruption of permanent Lateral Incisors
    B. Eruption of permanent maxillary canines
    C. Eruption of permanent mandibular canines
    D. Eruption of second molar
35. First tooth to erupt in primary dentition is:
    A. First Premolars
    B. Mandibular central incisors
    C. Canine
    D. First Molars
36. Calcification of first permanent molars begin
    A. Before birth
    B. At Birth
    C. 1 year after birth
    D. 2 years after birth

Ans: 1. A  2. C  3. B  4. C  5. C  6. A  7. B  8. D  9. B  10. A  11. D  12. C  13. D  14. D  15. D  16. A
17. D  18. A  19. B  20. D  21. C  22. C  23. B  24. D  25. A  26. A  27. A  28. D  29. C  30. B  31. D  32. C
33. D  34. B  35. B  36. A

## 3. CLASSIFICATION OF ETIOLOGY

### OCCLUSION—BASIC CONCEPTS

1. **Ideal occlusion can be defined as**
    A. Occlusion that deviates in one or more ways
    B. Arrangement of teeth which will provide highest efficiency during the excursive movement of the mandible
    C. Preconceived theoretical concept of occlusal structural and functional relationships that include idealized principles and characteristics than an occlusion should be
    D. Occlusal relationship in which all posterior teeth on a side contact evenly as the jaw is moved towards that side.
2. **Unilateral balanced occlusion can be termed as**
    A. Occlusion that deviates in one or more ways
    B. Arrangement of teeth which will provide highest efficiency during the excursive movement of the mandible
    C. Preconceived theoretical concept of occlusal structural and functional relationships that include idealized principles and characteristics than an occlusion should be
    D. Occlusal relationship in which all posterior teeth on a side contact evenly as the jaw is moved towards that side.
3. **Balanced occlusion can be termed as**
    A. Occlusion in which balanced and equal contacts are maintained throughout the entire arch during all excursions of mandible.
    B. Arrangement of teeth which will provide highest efficiency during the excursive movement of the mandible
    C. Preconceived theoretical concept of occlusal structural and functional relationships that include idealized principles and characteristics than an occlusion should be
    D. Occlusal relationship in which all posterior teeth on a side contact evenly as the jaw is moved towards that side.
4. **Centric occlusion can be termed as**
    A. Abnormal occlusal stress which is capable of producing or has produced an injury to the periodontium
    B. Maximum intercuspation or contact attained between maxillary and mandibular posterior teeth
    C. Most posterior position of the mandible relative to the maxilla at a given vertical dimension
    D. Deflection of mandible forward and to the left in any contact of opposing teeth
5. **Centric relation can be termed as**
    A. Abnormal occlusal stress which is capable of producing or has produced an injury to the periodontium
    B. Maxillary intercuspation or contact attined between maxillary and mandibular posterior teeth
    C. Most posterior position of the mandible relative to the maxilla at a given vertical dimension
    D. Deflection of mandible forward and to the left in any contact of opposing teeth

6. **Lingual cusps of the maxillary posterior teeth and the buccal cusps of the mandibular posterior teeth are referred to as**
   A. Supporting cusps
   B. Non-supporting cusps
   C. Both of the above
   D. None of the above

7. **Supporting cusps are also called as**
   A. Centric holding cusps
   B. Stamp cusps
   C. Combination of A and B
   D. None of the above

8. **Centric occlusal contacts are classified into**
   A. Anterior centric occlusal contact
   B. Posterior centric occlusal contact
   C. Both A and B
   D. None of the above

9. **Cusp-fossa occlusion is termed as**
   A. Supporting cusp of a tooth occludes in a single fossa of a single opposing tooth
   B. Supporting cusp of a tooth occludes with two opposing teeth
   C. Downward movement of both the condyles along with the slopes of the articular eminence
   D. None of the above

10. **Curve of Spee is termed as**
    A. Cusp tips of the posterior teeth follows a gradual curve from left side to right side
    B. Cusp tips of the posterior teeth follows a concave curve anteroposteriorly
    C. Highest point of a curve or greatest convexity or bulge
    D. None of the above

11. **Curve of Wilson is termed as**
    A. Cusp tips of the posterior teeth follows a gradual curve from left side to right side
    B. Cusp tips of the posterior teeth follows a concave curve anteroposteriorly
    C. Highest point of a curve or greatest convexity or bulge
    D. None of the above

12. **Ideal tooth relationships were described an classified as class I relation by**
    A. Anderson
    B. Goldberg
    C. Edward H Angle
    D. Both (a) and (c)

13. **Ideal tooth relationships were described an classified by EH Angle in**
    A. 1800 s
    B. 1850s
    C. 1900s
    D. 1960s

14. **Maxillary anterior teeth overlaps the mandibular teeth by**
    A. Horizontal overlap
    B. Vertical overlap
    C. Both of the above
    D. None of the above

15. **Horizontal overlap refers to**
    A. Incisal edges of the maxillary anterior teeth extend below the incisal edges of the mandibular teeth
    B. Incisal edges of the mandibular anterior teeth extend below the incisal edges of the maxillary teeth
    C. Incisal edges of maxillary anterior teeth are labial to the incisal edges of the mandibular teeth
    D. Incisal edges of maxillary anterior teeth are buccal to the incisal edges of the mandibular teeth

16. **Angle for crown inclination is**
    A. 45 degree
    B. 180 degree
    C. 90 degree
    D. 270 degree

17. **Lawrence F Andrew described how many keys of normal occlusion**
    A. 3
    B. 4
    C. 5
    D. 6

18. **Excessive curve of Spee**
    A. Restricts amount of space available for upper teeth
    B. Creates excessive space in the upper jaw
    C. Both (a) and (b)
    D. None of the above

19. **Reverse curve of Spee**
    A. Restricts amount of space available for upper teeth
    B. Creates excessive space in the upper jaw
    C. Both (a) and (b)
    D. None of the above

20. **According to Lawrence F Andrew curve of Spee should be**
    A. Be deeper than 1.5 mm
    B. Not be deeper than 1.5 mm
    C. Be deeper than 1.0 mm
    D. Not be deeper than 1.0 mm

21. **Lawrence F Andrew's key 4 of normal occlusion is**
    A. Presence of tight contacts
    B. Flat occlusal plane
    C. Absence of rotations
    D. Crown inclination

22. **Several concepts of an ideal or optional occlusion of natural dentition have been suggested by**
    A. Friel, Ramfjord, and Angle
    B. Goldberg, Andrew and Friel
    C. Goldberg, Andrew and Angle
    D. None of the above

23. **Which of the following combinations include Lawrence F Andrew's keys of normal occlusion?**
    A. Presence of rotations, premolar relationship, straight occlusal plane
    B. Absence of rotations, molar relationships, flat occlusal plane
    C. Absence of tight contacts, molar relationships, absence of rotations
    D. None of the above

24. **Human dentition presents two types of cusps as follows**
    A. Supporting and non-supporting
    B. Guiding and shear
    C. Centric holding and stamps
    D. None of the above

25. **Normal occlusion is a**
    A. Class II relationship

B. Class I relationship
C. Class II division 2 relationsip
D. Both A and C

26. **Anterior centric occlusal contacts consist of**
    A. Mesial and buccal range of contacts of maxillary and mandibular anterior
    B. Lingual and mesial range of contacts of maxillary and mandibular anterior
    C. Labial and lingual range of contacts of maxillary and mandibular anteriors
    D. Both B and C

27. **In which year Andrew put forward the six keys to normal occlusion**
    A. 1960      B. 1970
    C. 1999      D. 2000

28. **Acquired occlusion is also called as**
    A. Habitual occlusion
    B. Normal occlusion
    C. Canine guided occlusion
    D. All of the above

29. **Centric contacts have been classified into**
    A. Anterior centric contacts of maxillary and mandibular posteriors
    B. Posterior centric contacts of maxillary and mandibular posteriors
    C. Both A and B      D. None of the above

30. **Posterior centric contacts consist of**
    A. Facial range of contacts of maxillary and mandibular posteriors
    B. Lingual range of contacts of maxillary and mandibular posteriors
    C. Both A and B
    D. None of the above

31. **Facial range of posterior centric contact involves**
    A. Mandibular facial cusps tips contacting the central fossae and mesial marginal ridge of the opposing teeth
    B. Maxillary facial cusp tips contacting the central fossae and mesial marginal ridge of the opposing teeth
    C. Both A and B
    D. None of the above

32. **Lingual range posterior centric contact involves**
    A. The maxillary lingual cusp tips contacting the central fossae and distal marginal ridge of the opposing mandibular teeth
    B. The mandibular lingual cusp tip contacting the central fossae and distal marginal ridge of the opposing maxillary teeth
    C. Both A and B      D. None of the above

33. **According to Hellman, there are how many anterior centric occlusal contacts?**
    A. 14      B. 24
    C. 12      D. 52

34. **There are how many posterior centric occlusal contacts?**
    A. 42      B. 126
    C. 100     D. 52

35. **Tri-poded contact is**
    A. Contact occurs on three inclines
    B. Contact occurs on two inclines
    C. Contact occurs on two-four inclines
    D. Contact occurs on 7 inclines

36. **Bi-poded contact is**
    A. Contact occurs on three inclines
    B. Contact occurs on two inclines
    C. Contact occurs on two-four inclines
    D. Contact occurs on 7 inclines

37. **Functional occlusion is also called as**
    A. Working side occlusion
    B. Side occlusion
    C. Non working side occlusion
    D. No occlusion

38. **Functional occlusion can be**
    A. Lateral functional occlusion
    B. Protrusive functional occlusion
    C. Non functional occlusion
    D. Both A and B

39. **Lateral functional occlusion can be of**
    A. Canine guided occlusion
    B. Grouped lateral occlusion
    C. Both A and B
    D. None of the above

40. **Centric holding cusps are also called as**
    A. Stamp cusp      B. Non stamp cusp
    C. Stepped cusp    D. Steppled cusp

41. **Non supporting cusps are also called as**
    A. Shearing cusps  B. Guiding cusps
    C. Both A and B
    D. None of the above

42. **Centric holding cusps are**
    A. Facial cusps of mandibular posterior teeth
    B. Palatal cusps of maxillary posterior teeth
    C. Both A and B
    D. None of the above

43. **Centric holding cusp occludes into**
    A. The central fossae of opposing teeth
    B. Marginal ridge of opposing teeth
    C. Both A and B
    D. None of the above

44. **Non supporting cusps are**
    A. Mandibular lingual cusps and maxillary buccal cusps
    B. Maxillary and mandibular buccal cusps
    C. Maxillary lingual and mandibular buccal cusp
    D. Mandibular lingual and maxillary buccal cusp

45. **Human dentition exhibits**
    A. Four types of tooth arrangement
    B. Two types of tooth arrangement
    C. Six types of tooth arrangement
    D. Eight types of tooth arrangement

46. **Tooth to tooth arrangement is an synonym for**
    A. Cusp-fossa occlusion
    B. Cusp-embrassure occlusion
    C. Both A and B
    D. None of the above

**47. Which of the following statement is true**
   A. Rotated posterior teeth occupy more space in the dental arch wile rotated incisors occupy less space in the arch
   B. Rotated anterior teeth occupy more space in the dental arch wile rotated posteriors occupy less space in the arch
   C. Both A and B
   D. None of the above

Ans: 1. C  2. D  3. A  4. B  5. C  6. A  7. C  8. C  9. A  10. B  11. A  12. C  13. C  14. C  15. C  16. C  17. B  18. A  19. B  20. B  21. C  22. A  23. B  24. A  25. B  26. C  27. B  28. A  29. C  30. C  31. A  32. A  33. C  34. B  35. A  36. B  37. A  38. D  39. C  40. A  41. C  42. C  43. C  44. A  45. B  46. A  47. A

## CLASSIFICATION OF MALOCCLUSIONS

1. **Malocclusion can be broadly classified into**
   A. Intra-arch malocclusion
   B. Inter-arch malocclusion
   C. Skeletal malocclusion
   D. All of the above

2. **Intra-arch malocclusion is the malocclusion that occurs**
   A. Within the same arch in maxillary or mandibular arch
   B. Involving both the arches
   C. Involving underlying skeletal structures
   D. All of the above

3. **Inter-arch malocclusion is the malocclusion involving**
   A. Within the same arch in maxillary or mandibular arch
   B. Involving both the arches
   C. Involving underlying skeletal structures
   D. All of the above

4. **Skeletal malocclusion is the malocclusion involving**
   A. Within the same arch in maxillary or mandibular arch
   B. Involving both the arches
   C. Involving underlying skeletal structures
   D. All of the above

5. **Intra-arch malocclusion can be in the form of**
   A. Abnormal inclination
   B. Displacement
   C. Rotations
   D. All of the above

6. **Abnormal inclination refers to**
   A. Abnormal tilting of the crown with the root being in normal position
   B. Abnormal tilting of the root with the crown being in normal position
   C. Abnormal titling of crown as well as root
   D. All of the above

7. **Buccal inclination of a tooth refers to**
   A. Buccal or labial tilting of the tooth crown
   B. Lingual tilting of the tooth crown
   C. Mesial titling of the tooth crown
   D. Distal tilting of the tooth crown

8. **Lingual inclination of a tooth refers to**
   A. Buccal or labial tilting of the tooth crown
   B. Lingual tilting of the tooth crown
   C. Mesial titling of the tooth crown
   D. Distal tilting of the tooth crown

9. **Mesial inclination of a tooth refers to**
   A. Buccal or labial tilting of the tooth crown
   B. Lingual tilting of the tooth crown
   C. Mesial titling of the tooth crown
   D. Distal tilting of the tooth crown

10. **Distal inclination of a tooth refers to**
    A. Buccal or labial tilting of the tooth crown
    B. Lingual tilting of the tooth crown
    C. Mesial titling of the tooth crown
    D. Distal tilting of the tooth crown

11. **A tooth can be displaced in how many directions**
    A. 5 directions
    B. 2 directions
    C. 3 directions
    D. 4 directions

12. **Buccal displacement of a tooth refers to**
    A. Bodily movement of the tooth in labial/buccal direction
    B. Bodily movement of the tooth in lingual/palatal direction
    C. Bodily movement of the tooth mesial direction towards the midline
    D. Bodily movement of the tooth in distal direction away from the midline

13. **Lingual displacement of a tooth refers to**
    A. Bodily movement of the tooth in labial/buccal direction
    B. Bodily movement of the tooth in lingual/palatal direction
    C. Bodily movement of the tooth mesial direction towards the midline
    D. Bodily movement of the tooth in distal direction away from the midline

14. **Mesial placement of a tooth refers to**
    A. Bodily movement of the tooth in labial/buccal direction
    B. Bodily movement of the tooth in lingual/palatal direction
    C. Bodily movement of the tooth mesial direction towards the midline
    D. Bodily movement of the tooth in distal direction away from the midline

15. **Distal displacement of a tooth refers to**
    A. Bodily movement of the tooth in labial/buccal direction
    B. Bodily movement of the tooth in lingual/palatal direction

C. Bodily movement of the tooth mesial direction towards the midline
D. Bodily movement of the tooth in distal direction away from the midline

16. **Rotation of a tooth in orthodontics refers to**
    A. Movement of a tooth around its long axis
    B. Movement of a tooth in labio-lingual direction
    C. Movement of a tooth in mesio-distal direction
    D. All of the above

17. **Inter- arch malocclusion can occur in**
    A. Sagittal plane
    B. Vertical plane
    C. Transverse plane
    D. All of the above

18. **Pre-normal occlusion in orthodontics refers to**
    A. Lower arch is placed more anterior when the teeth meet in centric occlusion
    B. Lower arch is placed more posterior when the teeth meet in centric occlusion
    C. Both A and B
    D. None of the above

19. **Malocclusion in vertical plane includes**
    A. Open bite      B. Deep bite
    C. Cross bite     D. Both A and B

20. **Malocclusion in sagittal plane includes**
    A. Angle's class I malocclusion
    B. Angle's class II malocclusion
    C. Angle's class III malocclusion
    D. All of the above

21. **Malocclusion in transverse plane includes**
    A. Scissor bite    B. Open bite
    C. Cross bite      D. Both A and B

22. **According to British standard classification, in class 1 incisor relationship**
    A. Lower incisal edges occlude with/or lie immediately below the cingulum plateau of the upper incisor
    B. The lower incisal edge lies posterior to the cingulum plateau of the upper incisors
    C. The lower incisal edge lies anterior to the cingulum plateau of the upper incisors
    D. All of the above

23. **According to British standard incisor classification class 2 incisor relationship is**
    A. Lower incisal relationship is with/or lies immediately below the cingulum plateau of the upper incisor
    B. The lower incisal edges lie posterior to the cingulum plateau of the upper incisors
    C. The lower incisal edge lies anterior to the cingulum plateau of the upper incisors
    D. All of the above

24. **In British standard incisor classification, class 3 incisor relationship is**
    A. Lower incisal relationship is with/or lies immediately below the cingulum plateau of the upper incisor
    B. The lower incisal edge lies posterior to the cingulum plateau of the upper incisors
    C. The lower incisal edges lie anterior to the cingulum plateau of the upper incisors
    D. All of the above

25. **In British standard incisor classification class II division 1 incisal relationship is**
    A. The upper central incisor are retroclined
    B. The upper central incisors are proclined
    C. The upper central incisors are rotated
    D. The upper central incisors are transpositioned

26. **In British standard incisor classification class II division 2 incisal relationship is**
    A. The upper central incisor are retroclined
    B. The upper central incisors are proclined
    C. The upper central incisors are rotated
    D. The upper central incisors are transpositioned

27. **Class I canine relationship means**
    A. Mesial cuspal inclination of upper canine overlaps the distal cuspal inclination of lower canine
    B. Distal cuspal inclination of upper canine overlaps the mesial cuspal inclination of lower canine
    C. No relationship exist between upper and lower canine
    D. All of the above

28. **Class II canine relationship means**
    A. Mesial cuspal inclination of upper canine overlaps the distal cuspal inclination of lower canine
    B. Distal cuspal inclination of upper canine overlaps the mesial cuspal inclination of lower canine
    C. No relationship exist between upper and lower canine
    D. All of the above

29. **Class III canine relationship means**
    A. Mesial cuspal inclination of upper canine overlaps the distal cuspal inclination of lower canine
    B. Distal cuspal inclination of upper canine overlaps the mesial cuspal inclination of lower canine
    C. **No relationship exist between upper and lower canine**
    D. All of the above

30. **Class I molar relationship is**
    A. **Mesiobuccal cusp of permanent maxillary 1st molar occludes with mesiobuccal developmental groove of permanent mandibluar 1st molar**
    B. Distobuccal cusp of permanent maxillary 1st molar occludes with mesiobuccal developmental groove of permanent mandibular molar
    C. Mesiobuccal cusp of maxillary molar occludes interdentally between 1st and 2nd mandibular molar
    D. All of the above

31. **Class II molar relationship is**
    A. Mesiobuccal cusp of permanent maxillary 1st molar is in mesiobuccal developmental groove of permanent mandibluar 1st molar
    B. **Distobuccal cusp of permanent maxillary 1st molar occludes with mesiobuccal developmental groove of permanent mandibular molar**

C. Mesiobuccal cusp of maxillary molar occludes interdentally between 1st and 2nd mandibular molar
D. All of the above

32. Class III molar relationship is
    A. Mesiobuccal cusp of permanent maxillary 1st molar is in mesiobuccal developmental groove of permanent mandibluar 1st molar
    B. Distobuccal cusp of permanent maxillary 1st molar occludes with mesiobuccal developmental groove of permanent mandibular molar
    C. **Mesiobuccal cusp of maxillary molar occludes interdentally between 1st and 2nd mandibular molars**
    D. All of the above

33. In which year did Angle introduce his classification of malocclusion
    A. **1898**            B. 1989
    C. 1789            D. 1689

34. Angle's classification of malocclusion was published in the journal
    A. Angle orthodontist
    B. **Dental cosmos**
    C. American journal of orthodontics
    D. None of the above

35. Angle categorized malocclusion into
    A. 2 classes       B. 3 divisions
    C. **3 classes**       D. 3 subdivisons

36. In Angle's classification, malocclusions are divided into the following classes, except
    A. Angle's class I malocclusion
    B. Angle's class II malocclusion
    C. Angle's class III malocclusion
    D. **Angle's class VII malocclusion**

37. Angle's class II malocclusion is further divided into
    A. Class II division 1 malocclusion
    B. Class II division 2 malocclusion
    C. Class II division 3 malocclusion
    D. **Both A and B**

38. In Angle's classification, class II malocclusion is further divided into class II division 1 and division 2 based on
    A. Molar relationship
    B. Canine relationship
    C. **Incisor relationship**
    D. All of the above

39. Subdivision of Angle's class II malocclusion include
    A. Class II subdivision division 1 malocclusion
    B. Class II subdivision division 2 malocclusion
    C. Class II subdivision division 3 malocclusion
    D. **Both A and B**

40. Class III malocclusion can be
    A. True            B. Pseudo
    C. Unilateral      D. Both A and B

41. Following are extra-oral features of class I malocclusion except
    A. Mesocephalic
    B. Mesoprospic
    C. Orthognatic facial profile
    D. Convex facial profile

42. Following are the intra-oral features of class I malocclusion except
    A. Class I molar relationship
    B. Class I canine relationship
    C. Class I incisor relationship
    D. Q shaped dental arch

43. Which is the most commonly used classification of malocclusion
    A. Angle's         B. Dewey's
    C. Ballard's       D. Bennett's

44. Following are the extra-oral features of class II division 1 malocclusion except
    A. Concave facial profile
    B. Decreased nasolabial angle
    C. Incompetent lips
    D. Shallow mentolabial sulcus

45. Intra-oral features of class II division 1 malocclusion include the following except
    A. Convex facial profile
    B. V shaped maxillary arch
    C. Increased over jet
    D. Increased over bite

46. Intra-oral features of class II division 2 malocclusion include
    A. Decreased over jet
    B. Increased over bite
    C. U shaped maxillary arch and Maxillary anterior crowding
    D. All of the above

47. Following are the extra-oral features of Angle's class III malocclusion except
    A. Concave facial profile
    B. Decreased nasolabial angle
    C. Shallow mentolabial sulcus
    D. Anterior facial divergence

48. Who modified Angle's classification
    A. Dewey           B. Lischer
    C. Both A and B    D. None of the above

49. Dewey's modified Angle's class I malocclusion into
    A. 5 types         B. 4 types
    C. 5 divisions     D. 2 divisions

50. Dewey's modification for Angle's class III malocclusion includes how many types
    A. 5 types         B. 4 types
    C. 3 types         D. 2 divisions

51. Dewey did not propose any modification to Angle's
    A. Class I malocclusion
    B. Class II malocclusion
    C. Class III malocclusion
    D. None of the above

52. Dewey's class I type 1 malocclusion is
    A. Crowding in the anterior segment
    B. Proclination of anterior teeth
    C. Anterior cross bite
    D. Posterior cross bite

53. Dewey's class I type 2 malocclusion is
    A. Crowding in the anterior segment
    B. Proclination of anterior teeth
    C. Anterior cross bite
    D. Posterior cross bite
54. Dewey's class I type 3 malocclusion is
    A. Crowding in the anterior segment
    B. Proclination of anterior teeth
    C. Anterior cross bite
    D. Posterior cross bite
55. Dewey's class I type 4 malocclusion is
    A. Crowding in the anterior segment
    B. Proclination of anterior teeth
    C. Anterior cross bite
    D. Posterior cross bite
56. Dewey's class I type 5 malocclusion is
    A. Anterior cross bite
    B. Posterior cross bite
    C. Mesial displacing of molars
    D. Proclination of anteriors
57. Dewey's class III type 1 malocclusion is
    A. Normal incisor overlapping
    B. Edge to edge incisor relationship
    C. Incisor are in cross bite
    D. All of the above
58. Dewey's class III type 2 malocclusion is
    A. Normal incisor overlapping
    B. Edge to edge incisor relationship
    C. Incisor are in cross bite
    D. All of the above
59. Dewey's class III type 3 malocclusion is
    A. Normal incisor overlapping
    B. Edge to edge incisor relationship
    C. Incisor are in cross bite
    D. All of the above
60. Following are the Lischer's modifications of Angle's classification except
    A. Neutro-occlusion
    B. Disto occlusion
    C. Mesio occlusion
    D. Cross bite
61. Who classified malocclusion in all 3 planes of space
    A. Angle
    B. Andrew
    C. Simon
    D. Ackerman and Proffit
62. Simon's classification of malocclusion is based on
    A. Sagittal plane
    B. Transverse plane
    C. Vertical plane
    D. All of the above
63. According to Simon's classification of malocclusion the term 'attraction' means
    A. If a dental arch or part of it is closer than normal to the FH plane
    B. If a dental arch or part of it is further away from the FH plane
    C. Both A and B
    D. None of the above
64. According to Simon's classification of malocclusion the term 'abstraction' denotes
    A. If a dental arch or part of it is closer than normal to the FH plane
    B. If a dental arch or part of it is further away from the FH plane
    C. Both A and B
    D. None of the above
65. According to Simon's classification of malocclusion the term 'protraction' means
    A. If dental arches or part of it is further from orbital plane
    B. If the dental arches or part of it is closer to vertical plane
    C. Both A and B
    D. None of the above
66. According to Simon's classification of malocclusion the 'retraction' denotes
    A. If dental arches or part of it is further from orbital plane
    B. If the dental arches or part of it is closer to orbital plane
    C. Both A and B
    D. None of the above
67. According to Simon's classification of malocclusion the term 'contraction' means
    A. If the dental arches or part of it is closer to the mid sagittal plane
    B. If dental arches or part of it is further away from the mid sagittal plane
    C. Both A and B
    D. None of the above
68. According to Simon's classification of malocclusion the term distraction means
    A. If the dental arches or part of it is closer to the mid sagittal plane
    B. If dental arches or part of it is further away from the mid sagittal plane
    C. Both A and B
    D. None of the above
69. Sir Norman Bennett classification of malocclusion is based on
    A. Etiology
    B. Chemical features
    C. Management
    D. All of the above
70. Bennett's class I malocclusion is
    A. Abnormal position of one or more teeth due to local causes
    B. Abnormal position of a part or whole of either arch due to developmental defects of bone
    C. Abnormal relationship between upper and lower arches
    D. All of the above
71. Bennett's class II malocclusion is
    A. Abnormal position of one or more teeth due to local causes

B. Abnormal position of a part or whole of either arch due to developmental defects of bone
C. Abnormal relationship between upper and lower arches
D. All of the above

72. Bennett's class III malocclusion is
    A. Abnormal position of one or more teeth due to local causes
    B. Abnormal position of a part or whole of either arch due to developmental defects of bone
    C. Abnormal relationship between upper and lower arches
    D. All of the above

73. Following are the characteristics of Ackerman and Profit system of classification except
    A. Alignment
    B. Profile
    C. Type
    D. Overjet

74. Ackerman and Proffit classification of malocclusion is based on
    A. Trigonometry
    B. Venn diagrams
    C. Three planes
    D. All of the above

75. Group 1 in Ackerman and Proffit's classification includes
    A. Intra arch alignment
    B. Symmetry
    C. Alignment
    D. All of the above

76. Group 2 in Ackerman and Profit classification includes
    A. Profile
    B. Divergent
    C. Both A and B
    D. None of the above

77. Ackerman and Profit classified malocclusion into
    A. 4 groups
    B. 9 groups
    C. 5 classes
    D. 3 classes

78. Which group of Ackerman and Profit system of classification represents malocclusion in three planes of space that is transverse, sagittal and vertical plane
    A. Group 1, 2, 7
    B. Group 3, 4, 5
    C. Group 6, 7, 8
    D. None of the above

Ans: 1. D  2. A  3. B  4. C  5. D  6. A  7. A  8. B  9. C  10. D  11. D  12. A  13. B  14. C  15. D  16. A  17. D  18. A  19. D  20. D  21. D  22. A  23. B  24. C  25. B  26. A  27. A  28. B  29. C  30. A  31. B  32. C  33. A  34. B  35. C  36. D  37. D  38. C  39. D  40. D  41. D  42. D  43. A  44. A  45. A  46. D  47. B  48. C  49. A  50. C  51. B  52. A  53. B  54. C  55. D  56. C  57. A  58. B  59. C  60. D  61. C  62. D  63. A  64. B  65. A  66. B  67. A  68. B  69. A  70. A  71. B  72. C  72. D  73. D  74. C  75. C  76. B  77. B  78. B

## GENERAL ETIOLOGICAL FACTORS OF MALOCCLUSION

**General Etiology:**

1. General etiological factors of malocclusion include
   A. Hereditary
   B. Congenital
   C. Abnormal pressure habits
   D. All of the above

2. The hereditary factors causing malocclusion can be those influencing the following
   A. Dentition
   B. Skeletal base
   C. Neuromuscular
   D. All of the above

3. Which of the following characteristic of dentition is influenced by heredity
   A. Shape and size of the tooth
   B. Number of teeth
   C. Arch dimension
   D. All of the above

4. Cleft lip and palate may have profound influence on the craniofacial development, can cause
   A. Malocclusion and dental caries
   B. Malocclusion of skeletal origin
   C. Both A and B
   D. None of the above

5. Cleft lip and palate shows a number of dental abnormalities such as
   A. Supernumerary tooth
   B. Crowding of teeth in the area of cleft
   C. Crossbite due to narrow maxillary arch
   D. All of the above

6. Congenital syphilis can present with
   A. Hutchinson's incisors
   B. Mulberry molars
   C. Maxillary deficiency in relation to mandible
   D. All of the above

7. Features of cleidocranial dysostosis include
   A. Maxillary retrusion and possible mandibular protrusion
   B. Retained deciduous teeth
   C. Rotational eruption of permanent teeth
   D. All of the above

8. Hypothyrodism can cause
   A. Retardation in the rate of calcium deposition in bone and teeth
   B. Irregularities in tooth arrangement and crowding of teeth may occur
   C. Prolonged retention of deciduous and delayed eruption of permanent teeth
   D. All of the above

9. Hyperthyrodism
   A. This condition is associated with the increased metabolic rate and increased rate of maturation
   B. May exhibit premature eruption of deciduous and permanent teeth
   C. Combination of A and B
   D. None of the above

10. **Hypoparathyrodism**
    A. Is often associated with with delayed eruption of teeth
    B. Altered morphology
    C. Hypoplasia of teeth
    D. All of the above
11. **Hyperparathyrodism**
    A. Can cause an increase in blood calcium level by resorption of bone
    B. Osteoporosis in such parts contraindicates the dentin tooth movement
    C. Can cause disturbance in tooth eruption and shedding pattern and this may predispose to malocclusion
    D. All of the above
12. **Dietary problems cause malocclusion by**
    A. Primarily by upsetting the dental developmental time-table of resulting in premature loss of teeth
    B. Nutritional deficiency during pregnancy has been associated with certain malformation after in the child including cretinism and cleft lip and palate
    C. Combination of A and B
    D. None of the above
13. **Abnormal pressure habits include**
    A. Thumb sucking
    B. Tongue thrusting
    C. Lip biting
    D. All of the above
14. **Accident and trauma to the teeth can cause**
    A. Non vital deciduous teeth that do not resorb
    B. Deflection of permanent tooth germ
    C. Abnormal eruption of path of permanent successors
    D. All of the above
15. **Overjet is the**
    A. Horizontal overlapping of upper incisors over the lower incisors
    B. Vertical overlapping of upper incisors over the lower incisors
    C. Horizontal overlapping of lower incisors over the upper incisors
    D. Vertical overlapping of lower incisors over the upper incisors
16. **Overbite is the**
    A. Horizontal overlapping of upper incisors over the lower incisors
    B. Vertical overlapping of upper incisors over the lower incisors
    C. Horizontal overlapping of lower incisors over the upper incisors
    D. Vertical overlapping of lower incisors over the upper incisors
17. **Micrognathism**
    A. Means small jaw
    B. Can affect either of the jaws
    C. Often associated with congenital heart disease and Robin syndrome
    D. All of the above
18. **Oligodontia is also called as**
    A. Hypodontia
    B. Anodontia
    C. Combination of A and B
    D. None of the above
19. **Features of gonadal dysfunction**
    A. Delayed sexual development
    B. Dental age is normal
    C. Premature sexual development
    D. All of the above
20. **Vitamin C deficiency can cause**
    A. Disturbed collagen fiber formation
    B. Red, edematous tender bleeding gums
    C. Loosening of teeth
    D. All of the above
21. **Vitamin B Complex deficiency can cause**
    A. Disturbed digestion    B. Retarded growth
    C. Pernicious anemia    D. All of the above
22. **Post-natal trauma can**
    A. Occur at any age
    B. May affect any region of the orofacial complex
    C. Both A and B
    D. Displacement
23. **Trauma to the teeth often results in**
    A. Dilaceration    B. Deformation
    C. Displacement    D. All of the above
24. **Prenatal trauma**
    A. Is often associated with hypoplasia of the mandible
    B. Associated with facial asymmetries
    C. Both A and B
    D. None of the above

**Ans:** 1. **D**  2. **D**  3. **D**  4. **B**  5. **D**  6. **D**  7. **D**  8. **D**  9. **C**  10. **D**  11. **D**  12. **C**  13. **D**  14. **D**  15. **A**  16. **B**  17. **D**  18. **A**  19. **D**  20. **D**  21. **D**  22. **C**  23. **D**  24. **C**

## LOCAL ETIOLOGICAL FACTORS OF MALOCCLUSION

1. **Supernumerary teeth refers to**
    A. Extra teeth in relation to the normal compliment of teeth
    B. Extra teeth in relation to the abnormal compliment of teeth
    C. Combination of A and B
    D. None of the above
2. **Supernumerary teeth cause**
    A. Spacing in the arches
    B. Crowding in the arches
    C. May or may not cause crowding
    D. Both B and C
3. **Supernumerary teeth present in the midline between two maxillary central incisors is called as**
    A. Para incisor    B. Mesiodens
    C. Both A and B    D. None of the above

4. Which is the most common type of supernumerary teeth seen?
   A. Para-premolar   B. Mesiodens
   C. Both A and B    D. None of the above
5. Most common site of supernumerary teeth is
   A. In the midline between two maxillary central incisors
   B. In the midline between two mandibular central incisors
   C. In the midline between two deciduous maxillary central incisors
   D. In the midline between two deciduous mandibular central incisors
6. Mesiodens can be
   A. Erupted         B. Impacted
   C. Both A and B    D. None of the above
7. Erupted or impacted mesiodens can cause malocclusion by
   A. Preventing eruption of maxillary central incisor
   B. Delaying the eruption of maxillary central incisors
   C. Displacing one or both maxillary central incisors
   D. All of the above
8. Extra tooth adjacent to molar is called as a
   A. Para molar
   B. Distomolar
   C. Combination of A and B
   D. None of the above
9. Extra tooth present distal to the last molar is called as
   A. Distomolar      B. Mesomolar
   C. Labiomolar      D. Linguomolar
10. Extra tooth present in the premolar region is called as
    A. Parapremolar   B. Distopremolar
    C. Mesopremolar   D. Labiopremolar
11. The occurrence of supernumerary teeth may be
    A. Single or multiple   B. Unilateral or bilateral
    C. Erupted or impacted  D. All of the above
12. Erupted supernumerary teeth can cause
    A. Arch length—Tooth material discrepancy
    B. May delay the eruption of adjacent teeth
    C. May prevent or deviate the path of eruption of adjacent teeth
    D. All of the above
13. Unerupted supernumerary teeth show a tendency for
    A. Cyst formation     B. Midline diastema
    C. Both A and B       D. None of the above
14. Occurrence of congenitally missing teeth may be
    A. Single or multiple    B. Unilateral or bilateral
    C. In maxilla or mandible D. All of the above
15. Microdontia can cause
    A. Spacing in the arch
    B. Localized or generalized spacing depending upon the teeth involved in microdontia
    C. Crowding in the arch
    D. Both A and B
16. Macrodontia can cause
    A. Crowding in the arch and it depends upon number of teeth involved
    B. Spacing in the arches
    C. Both A and B
    D. None of the above
17. Talon's cusp is a
    A. Anomalous structure projecting from cingulum of maxillary permanent incisors
    B. Anomalous structures projecting from the lingual fossa of maxillary permanent incisor
    C. Anomalous structure projecting from the incisal edge of maxillary permanent incisor
    D. Anomalous structure projecting from the labial surface of maxillary permanent incisor
18. Peg-shaped lateral incisors can cause
    A. Spacing in the arch
    B. Migration of adjacent teeth
    C. Abnormal incisors relationships
    D. All of the above
19. Talon's cusp can cause
    A. Disturbance in establishment of normal overbite and overjet
    B. Forces from the antagonistic tooth in occlusion
    C. Labial tipping of affected tooth
    D. All of the above
20. Premature loss of deciduous second molar can cause crowding in the posterior segment by
    A. Mesial migration of the permanent first molar
    B. Loss of arch length
    C. Lack of space for permanent second premolar to erupt
    D. All of the above
21. Prolonged retention of deciduous teeth can occur due to
    A. Absence of underlying permanent tooth
    B. Non-vital deciduous tooth which fails to resorb
    C. Ankylosed deciduous tooth that do not resorb
    D. All of the above
22. Delayed eruption of permanent teeth can be due to
    A. Presence of supernumerary teeth, e.g. mesiodens can delay eruption of maxillary centrals
    B. Retained deciduous root fragments in the jaw may delay or displace the erupting successor tooth
    C. Presence of thick mucosal barrier overlying the erupting permanent teeth
    D. All of the above
23. Delayed eruption of permanent teeth can be due to
    A. Premature loss of deciduous root
    B. Ankylosed deciduous tooth that do not resorbs
    C. Endocranial disturbances like hypothyroidism
    D. All of the above
24. Causes of midline diastema
    A. Abnormal frenum attachment
    B. Mesiodens
    C. Congenitally missing or microdontic teeth
    D. All of the above

25. Proximal caries or complete loss of a tooth due to dental caries may cause:
    A. Premature loss of the affected tooth
    B. Loss of arch length due to drifting of teeth
    C. Over eruption of antagonistic teeth
    D. All of the above

26. A permanent tooth may assume an abnormal path of eruption due to
    A. Presence of supernumerary tooth
    B. Retained deciduous root fragments
    C. Retained deciduous predecessor tooth
    D. All of the above

27. Abnormal eruptive teeth can cause
    A. Crowding in the arch
    B. Cross bite
    C. Impaction
    D. All of the above

28. According to Graber, local factors causing malocclusion include
    A. Anomalies of number
    B. Anomalies of tooth size
    C. Anomalies of tooth shape
    D. All of the above

29. According to Graber, local factors causing malocclusion include:
    A. Premature loss of deciduous teeth
    B. Prolonged retention of deciduous teeth
    C. Delayed eruption of permanent tooth
    D. All of the above

30. According to Graber, local factors causing malocclusion can be:
    A. Dental Caries
    B. Improper dental restoration
    C. Ankylosis
    D. All of the above

31. Over contoured occlusal restoration can cause
    A. Functional shift of the mandible during jaw closure
    B. Functional shift of the mandible during jaw opening
    C. Combination of A and B
    D. None of the above

32. Under contoured occlusal restoration can lead to
    A. Supra-eruption of the opposing dentition
    B. Infra-eruption of the opposing dentition
    C. Supra-eruption of the tooth with under-contoured occlusal restoration
    D. Infra-eruption of the tooth with under contoured occlusal restoration

33. In blanch test
    A. The upper lip is pulled superiorly and anteriorly
    B. The upper lip is pulled superiorly and posteriorly
    C. The upper lip is pulled inferiorly and anteriorly
    D. The upper lip is pulled inferiorly and posteriorly

34. Is blanch test the only test to confirm midline diastema?
    A. Yes
    B. No
    C. There are other like IOPA
    D. A and C

35. Dens in dente is a
    A. Developmental variation which radiographically may ressembles a tooth within a tooth
    B. It rarely has any clinical significance from an orthodontic point of view
    C. Both A and B
    D. None of the above

36. True fusion is seen when the tooth arises through the
    A. Union of two abnormally separated tooth germs
    B. Union of two normally separated tooth germs
    C. A and B
    D. None of the above

37. True fusion can cause
    A. Spacing
    B. Complicate its movement by orthodontic means
    C. Both A and B
    D. None of the above

38. Gemination of teeth arises from
    A. Division of two germs by invagination
    B. Division of a single tooth germ by invagination
    C. A and B
    D. None of the above

39. Concrescence refers to
    A. Fusion of teeth which occurs before root formation has been completed
    B. Fusion of teeth which occurs after root formation has been completed
    C. Just fusion of two teeth completely throughout the length of the tooth
    D. All of the above

40. Peg-shaped lateral incisor can be
    A. Associated with congenital syphilis
    B. Can cause spacing in the arch
    C. Commonly associated with maxillary lateral incisor
    D. All of the above

41. Congenitally missing teeth in decreasing frequency
    A. Third molar > Upper lateral > Mandibular 2nd premolar
    B. Lateral incisor > Maxillary canine > Macillary 1st molar
    C. Mandibular premolar > Third molars > Canines
    D. All of the above

42. Supplemental tooth is
    A. Supernumerary tooth
    B. One that bears a close resemblance to a particular group of teeth
    C. Erupt close to the regional sight of teeth commonly seen in premolar and lateral regions
    D. All of the above

43. The most common tooth affected with microdontia except third molars is
    A. Maxillary lateral incisors
    B. Maxillary canines
    C. Both A and B
    D. Mandibular lateral incisors

### 44. Dilacerated tooth
A. Is an anomaly of the tooth
B. Is a sharp bend or curve in the root or crown
C. Can complicate orthodontic treatment
D. All of the above

### 45. Midline diastema may be caused by
A. Abnormal high labial frenum attachement
B. Presence of mesiodens
C. Congenital absence of lateral incisors
D. All of the above

### 46. Midline diastema during ugly duckling stage in
A. Transient malocclusion
B. Malocclusion that cannot be treated
C. Can be treated with myofunctional orthodontic appliance
D. None of the above

### 47. Local etiological factors causing malocclusion include
A. Delayed eruption of permanent teeth
B. Trauma or accident
C. Endocrence imbalance
D. Both A and B

### 48. Completely erupted mesiodens
A. Has to be extracted and followed by ortho treatment for midline diastema
B. Extract the mesiodens
C. Both A and B
D. None of the above

Ans: 1. A   2. D   3. B   4. B   5. A   6. C   7. D   8. A   9. A   10. A   11. D   12. D   13. C   14. D   15. D   16. A   17. A   18. A   19. D   20. D   21. D   22. D   23. D   24. D   25. D   26. D   27. D   28. D   29. D   30. D   31. A   32. A   33. A   34. C   35. C   36. B   37. C   38. B   39. B   40. D   41. A   42. D   43. A   44. D   45. D   46. A   47. D   48. A

## GENETICS IN ORTHODONTICS

1. **Who is called founder of human genetics?**
   A. Adam Joseph   B. Gregor Mendel
   C. Charles Darwin   D. Pythagoras

2. **Who is the father of modern genetics?**
   A. Gregor Mendel   B. Adam Joseph
   C. Charles Darwin   D. Harvey

3. **Gregor Mandel was a**
   A. Scientist   B. Scholar
   C. Monk   D. Dentist

4. **Law of segregation was put forward by**
   A. Adam Joseph   B. Watson and Crick
   C. Salton and Boven   D. Gregor Mendel

5. **Who proposed the structure of DNA molecule?**
   A. Watson and Crick   B. Gregor Mandel
   C. Sulton and Boven   D. Finch and Klung

6. **Chromosome theory of inheritance was proposed by**
   A. Watson and Crick   B. Finch and Klung
   C. Sulton and Boveri   D. Adam Joseph

7. **Solenoid model of chromosome structure was proposed by**
   A. Watson and Crick
   B. Finch and Klung
   C. Sulton and Boven   D. Gregor Mendel

8. **Number of chromosomes present in every cell of an organism**
   A. Constant
   B. Changes from one species to another
   C. Both (A) and (B)
   D. None of the above

9. **Chromosomes are made up of**
   A. Long chains of DNA only
   B. Long chains of RNA only
   C. Both (A) and (B)
   D. None of the above

10. **Process by which information is transmitted from DNA to messenger RNA at initial stage of replication is called as**
    A. Translation   B. Transcription
    C. Transmission   D. All of the above

11. **Process by which genetic information is actually converted into protein synthesis is termed as**
    A. Transcription   B. Translation
    C. Transmission   D. None of the above

12. **Pattern of genetic transmission is**
    A. Repetitive   B. Discontinuous
    C. Variable   D. All of the above

13. **Protein synthesis for the process of replication is controlled by**
    A. Cell   B. Chromosome
    C. Gene   D. DNA

14. **Gene mutation can be of**
    A. Visible mutation   B. Detrimental mutation
    C. Lethal mutation   D. All of the above

15. **Different types of mutagens are**
    A. Ionizing radiation
    B. Certain drugs, chemicals and food additives
    C. Certain viruses
    D. All of the above

16. **Who demonstrated the presence of 23 pairs of chromosomes in man?**
    A. Ford and Hamerton
    B. Watson and Crick
    C. Gregor Mendel
    D. Sulton and Boweri

17. **Which of the below is numerical disorder of chromosome?**
    A. Klinefelters syndrome
    B. Turner's syndrome
    C. Trisomy and Monosomy
    D. All of the above

18. Structural disorder of chromosome are
    A. Translocation
    B. Deletions
    C. Ring chromosomes
    D. All of the above
19. Who reported that malocclusion may be skeletal and dental can be transmitted from one generation to another?
    A. Frederick G Kussel
    B. Gregor Mendel
    C. Adam Joseph
    D. Darwin
20. Dentofacial disturbances of genetic origin can be
    A. Cleft lip and cleft palate
    B. Down's syndrome
    C. Gardner's syndrome
    D. All of the above
21. Two individuals developed from a single fertilized ovum are
    A. Monozygotic twins   B. Dizygotic twins
    C. Both A and B        D. None of the above
22. Two individuals developed from two separate ova, ovulated and fertilized at the same time is termed as
    A. Monozygotic Twins   B. Dizygotic Twins
    C. Both A and B        D. None of the above
23. A trait can be
    A. Monogenic           B. Polygenic
    C. Multifactorial      D. All of the above
24. Monogenic traits can be
    A. Autosomal           B. Autosomal recessive
    C. X-linked            D. All of the above
25. Penetrance denotes
    A. The degree to while a gene is expressed
    B. The proportion of individuals that show an expected phenotype
    C. Both A and B
    D. None of the above
26. Expressivity refers to
    A. The degree to which a gene is expressed in the same/different individuals
    B. Trait expressed in all subjects
    C. Both A and B
    D. None of the above
27. Which type of malocclusion is often considered as a genetic trait
    A. Class I malocclusion
    B. Class II division 1 malocclusion
    C. Class II division 2 malocclusion
    D. Both A and B
28. Hapsburg jaw refers to
    A. Class I malocclusion
    B. Class III malocclusion with prognathic mandible
    C. Class II malocclusion
    D. Both B and C
29. According to Butter's field theory the stable key tooth in molariform field in
    A. 1st premolar        B. 1st molar
    C. 3rd molar           D. 2nd molar
30. In molar-premolar field maximum variability is seen for
    A. 1st molars          B. 2nd premolars
    C. 2nd molars          D. 3rd molars

Ans: 1. A  2. A  3. C  4. D  5. A  6. C  7. B  8. C  9. A  10. B  11. B  12. D  13. C  14. D  15. D  16. A  17. D  18. D  19. A  20. D  21. A  22. B  23. D  24. D  25. B  26. A  27. C  28. B  29. B  30. D

# EPIDEMIOLOGY OF MALOCCLUSION

1. HLD index stands for
    A. Handicapping labio-lingual deviation index
    B. Handy linguo-labial deviation index
    C. Hygiene labio-lingual deviation index
    D. None of above
2. HLD index was developed by
    A. Master and Frankel   B. Vankirk and Pennel
    C. Poulton and Aaronson D. Harry L Draker
3. HLD index is applicable to
    A. Only permanent dentition
    B. Only deciduous dentition
    C. Permanent dentition as well as deciduous dentition
    D. None of the above
4. Which index was the first index designed to meet the administrative needs of program planners?
    A. DAI                 B. IOIN
    C. HLD                 D. TPI
5. The main intention of the HLD index is to measure the
    A. Presence or absence and the degree of the handicap caused by the components of the index
    B. To assess the severity of malocclusion
    C. Both (A) and (B)    D. None of the above
6. The HLD index is based on
    A. Five components     B. Seven components
    C. Nine components     D. Six components
7. Followings are the conditions of HLD, except
    A. Condition 1- cleft palate
    B. Condition 2- traumatic deviation
    C. Condition 3- open bite
    D. Condition 4- overbite
8. Codes used in HLD are
    A. O- condition absent  B. X- condition present
    C. A- clinical apparent D. All of the above
9. Codes used in HDL are following except
    A. M- mixed dentition   B. D- clinical disapproval
    C. A- clinical absent   D. X- condition present

10. **TPI stands for**
    A. Treatment priority index
    B. Tendency priority index
    C. Treatment prior index
    D. Treatment priority improvement
11. **TPI was developed by**
    A. Grainger RM
    B. Master and Frankel
    C. Harry L Draker
    D. Poulton and Aaronson
12. **In which year Grainger RM developed TPI**
    A. 1940       B. 1967
    C. 1980       D. 1950
13. **The range of low score in TPI is**
    A. 0-2.5      B. 2.5-4.5
    C. 4.5-5.5    D. None
14. **The range of middle score in TPI is**
    A. 0-2.5      B. 2.5-4.5
    C. 4.5-5.5    D. None
15. **High score of TPI is**
    A. 0-2.5      B. 2.5-4.5
    C. 4.5-5.5    D. None
16. **The manifestations of malocclusion measured in TPI are**
    A. Bi-molar relationship
    B. Maxillary over jet
    C. Open bite
    D. All of the above
17. **The manifestations of malocclusion measured in TPI are followings except**
    A. Over bite
    B. Tooth displacement
    C. Congenitally missing teeth
    D. Oral habits
18. **Malalignment Index was developed by**
    A. Master and Frankel    B. Vankirk and Pennel
    C. Henry Draker          D. Poulton and Aaronson
19. **Occlusal features Index was developed by**
    A. Master and Frankel    B. Vankirk and Pennel
    C. Draker                D. Poulton and Aaronson
20. **Occlusal index was developed by**
    A. Vankirk and Frankel   B. Draker
    C. Poulton and Aaronson  D. Summers
21. **Measurement of Occlusal feature Index includes**
    A. Lower anterior crowding
    B. Cuspal inter-digitation
    C. Vertical over bite
    D. All of the above
22. **Measurement of HLD index by Draker includes**
    A. Cleft palate          B. Traumatic deviation
    C. Over jet              D. All of the above
23. **Handicapping malocclusion assessment record by**
    A. Salzmann              B. Draker
    C. Summer
    D. Pennel
24. **Least prevalence malocclusion in India is**
    A. Angel's class I malocclusion
    B. Angel's class II malocclusion
    C. Angel's class III malocclusion
    D. None of the above
25. **The commonest malocclusion seen is**
    A. Angel's class I malocclusion
    B. Angel's class II malocclusion
    C. Angel's class III malocclusion
    D. None of the above
26. **Jamison H D and McMillan R S have proposed a list of requirements for an ideal orthodontic index that can be used in the epidemiological studies of orthodontic problems are as follows**
    A. The index should be simple
    B. Must be usable either on patients and on study models
    C. The index must be designed as to differentiate between handicapping and non-handicapping malocclusion
    D. All of the above

**Ans:** 1. A  2. D  3. A  4. C  5. A  6. B  7. C  8. D  9. C  10. A  11. A  12. B  13. A  14. B  15. C  16. D  17. D  18. B  19. D  20. D  21. D  22. D  23. A  24. C  25. A  26. D

## 4. DIAGNOSIS AND DIAGNOSTIC AIDS

### ORTHODONTIC DIAGNOSIS

1. **According to Sheldon, 'Ectomorphic' physique refers to:**
   A. Tall and thin physique
   B. Average physique
   C. Short and obese physique
   D. None of the above
2. **According to Sheldon, 'Endomorphic' physique refers to:**
   A. Short and obese physique
   B. Average physique
   C. Tall and thin physique
   D. None of the above
3. **According to Sheldon, 'Mesomorphic' physique is used to describe:**
   A. Average physique
   B. Tall and thin physique
   C. Short and obese physique
   D. None of the above
4. **According to general classification, 'Aesthetic' physique refers to:**
   A. Tall and thin physique
   B. Average physique

C. Short and obese physique
   D. None of the above
5. **The term 'Plethoric' physique refers to:**
   A. Average physique
   B. Tall and thin
   C. Short and obese physique
   D. None of the above
6. **The term 'Athletic' physique refers to:**
   A. Short and obese physique
   B. Average physique
   C. Tall and thin physique
   D. None of the above
7. **Who classified the general body built?**
   A. Sheldon
   B. Saller
   C. Martin
   D. None of the above
8. **Mesocephalic shape of the head implies:**
   A. Average shape of head
   B. Broad and short head
   C. Long and narrow head
   D. None of the above
9. **Dolichocephalic shape of the head implies:**
   A. Long and narrow head
   B. Broad and short head
   C. Average shape head
   D. None of the above
10. **Brachycephalic shape of the implies:**
    A. Broad and short head
    B. Average shape head
    C. Long and narrow head
    D. None of the above
11. **Mesoprosopic facial form means:**
    A. Average or normal facial form
    B. Broad and short facial form
    C. Long and narrow facial form
    D. None of the above
12. **Euryprosopic facial form means:**
    A. Long and narrow facial form
    B. Broad and short facial form
    C. Average and normal facial form
    D. None of the above
13. **Leptoprosopic facial form means:**
    A. Average and normal facial form
    B. Broad and short facial form
    C. Long and narrow facial form
    D. None of the above
14. **Assessment of facial symmetry is used to determine:**
    A. Disproportions of the face in the transverse plane
    B. Disproportions of the face in the vertical plane
    C. Both A and B
    D. None of all
15. **Gross facial asymmetry occurs as a result of:**
    A. Periodontal diseases
    B. Dental caries
    C. Congenital defects
    D. None of the above
16. **Facial profile helps in diagnosing:**
    A. Gross deviation in maxillo-mandibular relationship
    B. Gross deviations in maxilla
    C. Gross deviations in mandible
    D. None of the above
17. **Straight facial profile is generally seen in which type of malocclusion:**
    A. Class I
    B. Class II
    C. Class III
    D. None of the above
18. **Convex facial profile is seen in which type of malocclusion:**
    A. Class I malocclusion
    B. Class II malocclusion
    C. Class III malocclusion
    D. None of the above
19. **Concave facial profile is seen in which type of malocclusion:**
    A. Class I malocclusion
    B. Class II malocclusion
    C. Class III malocclusion
    D. None of the above
20. **Facial divergences refer to:**
    A. Anterior or posterior inclination of the lower face relative to the forehead
    B. Anterior inclination of the lower face relative to the forehead
    C. Posterior inclination of the lower face relative to the forehead
    D. All of the above
21. **Anterior facial divergence is generally seen in which type of malocclusion:**
    A. Class I malocclusion
    B. Class II malocclusion
    C. Class III malocclusion
    D. None of the above
22. **In which type of malocclusion is posterior facial divergence generally seen?**
    A. Class I malocclusion
    B. Class II malocclusion
    C. Class III malocclusion
    D. None of the above
23. **Straight or orthognathic face is generally seen in:**
    A. Class I malocclusion
    B. Class II malocclusion
    C. Class III malocclusion
    D. None of the above
24. **Openbite refers to malocclusion in which plane:**
    A. Transverse plane
    B. Sagittal plane
    C. Vertical plane
    D. None of the above
25. **Deepbite refers to malocclusion in which plane:**
    A. Transverse plane
    B. Sagittal plane
    C. Vertical plane
    D. None of the above
26. **Crossbite is a malocclusion occurring in which plane:**
    A. Vertical plane
    B. Transverse plane
    C. Sagittal plane
    D. None of the above

27. **Scissorsbite is a malocclusion occurring in which plane:**
    A. Sagittal plane
    B. Vertical plane
    C. Transverse plane
    D. None of the above
28. **Angle's class I malocclusion occurs in which plane:**
    A. Transverse plane
    B. Sagittal plane
    C. Vertical plane
    D. None of the above
29. **Angle's class II malocclusion occurs in which plane:**
    A. Sagittal plane
    B. Vertical plane
    C. Transverse plane
    D. None of the above
30. **Angle's class III malocclusion occurs in which plane:**
    A. Vertical plane
    B. Transverse plane
    C. Sagittal plane
    D. None of the above
31. **Mentolabial sulcus is:**
    A. A concavity seen below the lower lip
    B. A convexity seen below the lower lip
    C. Combination of A and B
    D. None of the above
32. **Deep mentolabial sulcus is generally seen in:**
    A. Class II division 1 malocclusion
    B. Class II division 2 malocclusion
    C. Combination of A and B
    D. None of the above
33. **Shallow mentolabial sulcus is generally seen in:**
    A. Bimaxillary protrusion
    B. Bimaxillary retrusion
    C. Combination of A and B
    D. None of the above
34. **Hyperactive mentalis muscle activity is usually seen in:**
    A. Class II division 1 malocclusion
    B. Class II division 2 malocclusion
    C. Combination of A and B
    D. None of the above
35. **Prominent chin is generally a feature of:**
    A. Class I malocclusion
    B. Class II malocclusion
    C. Class III malocclusion
    D. None of the above
36. **Recessive chin is a feature of:**
    A. Class I malocclusion
    B. Class II malocclusion
    C. Class III malocclusion
    D. None of the above
37. **Nasolabial angle refers to:**
    A. Angle between lower border of the nose and a line connecting intersection of nose and upper lip with the tip of the lip
    B. Angle between lower border of the nose and a line connecting intersection of nose and lower lip with the tip of the lip
    C. Combination of A and B
    D. None of the above
38. **Increased nasolabial angle is seen in:**
    A. Patients with retrognathic maxilla or retroclined maxillary anteriors
    B. Patients with prognathic maxilla
    C. Combination of A and B
    D. None of all
39. **Decreased nasolabial angle is seen in:**
    A. Patients with retrognathic maxilla or retroclined maxillary anteriors
    B. Patients with prognathic maxilla
    C. Combination of A and B
    D. None of all
40. **Normal nasolabial angle is:**
    A. 110°
    B. 90-110°
    C. 112°
    D. 113°
41. **Potentially incompetent lips are lips that fail to form a lip seal due to:**
    A. Proclined upper incisors
    B. Retroclined upper incisors
    C. Retroclined lower incisors
    D. Proclined lower incisors
42. **Abnormal labial frenum may cause:**
    A. Maxillary anterior proclination
    B. Midline diastema
    C. Spacing in the arches
    D. Combination of all
43. **Blanch test is used for:**
    A. Diagnosing midline diastema
    B. To evaluate the presence of abnormal labial frenum attachment
    C. Both A and B
    D. None of all
44. **Orthodontic diagnosis deals with:**
    A. Placing of brackets
    B. Recognition of various characteristics of malocclusion
    C. Distinguishing what type of elastics are to be placed
    D. All of the above
45. **Orthodontic diagnostic aids are of how many types:**
    A. One
    B. Two
    C. Three
    D. Four
46. **Case history involves:**
    A. Eliciting and recording relevant information from patient and the parent
    B. Only the name of the patient
    C. Eliciting relevant information from the patient
    D. All of the above
47. **Specialised radiographs in orthodontic diagnosis:**
    A. Cephalometric radiographs
    B. Occlusal intraoral films
    C. Selected lateral jaw views
    D. All of the above
48. **Importance of recording patient's name is:**
    A. To know the cast
    B. For communication and identification
    C. To know the age
    D. To know the race

49. Age and sex of the patient:
    A. Are recorded as diagnostic aids
    B. Help in the treatment planning
    C. Help in the identification and communication with the patient
    D. None of the above
50. The patient's chief complaint:
    A. Establishes the reason for seeking orthodontic care
    B. Establishes the needs of the patient
    C. Establishes the mindset of the patient
    D. All of the above
51. Recording the medical history of the patient:
    A. Is not important
    B. Only matters for those with blood dyscrasias and epilepsy
    C. Is important and should be fully recorded
    D. None of the above
52. How is the antero-posterior jaw relationship determined using two finger methods:
    A. By using the index and middle finger
    B. By using the thumb and the index
    C. By using the middle and ring finger
    D. None of the above

Ans: 1. A  2. D  3. A  4. C  5. A  6. B  7. A  8. A  9. A  10. A  11. A  12. B  13. C  14. C  15. C  16. A  17. A  18. B  19. C  20. D  21. C  22. B  23. A  24. C  25. C  26. B  27. C  28. B  29. A  30. C  31. A  32. A  33. A  34. A  35. C  36. B  37. A  38. A  39. B  40. B  41. A  42. B  43. C  44. B  45. B  46. D  47. D  48. B  49. B  50. D  51. C  52. A

## MODEL ANALYSIS AS A DIAGNOSTIC AID

1. Analysis used to assess the need of extraction:
   A. Arch Perimeter Analysis
   B. Nance Carey's Model Analysis
   C. Both A and B
   D. Bolton's Model Analysis
2. Which are the model analysis used to assess the need of Arch expansion:
   A. Pont's Analysis
   B. Linder Harth Analysis
   C. Korkhaus Analysis
   D. All of the above
3. Which model analysis is used to assess the Tooth Material Excess:
   A. Korkhaus Analysis
   B. Nance Carey's Analysis
   C. Bolton's Analysis
   D. All of the above
4. Which model analysis is used in Mixed Dentition:
   A. Mixed Dentition Analysis
   B. Bolton's Analysis
   C. Korkhaus Analysis
   D. All of the above
5. Which model analysis used to assess both the need of extraction as well as the expansion:
   A. Ashley Howe's Analysis
   B. Pont's Analysis
   C. Linder Harth's Analysis
   D. All of the above
6. Arch Perimeter analysis is used to assess the need of extraction in which arch:
   A. Maxillary Arch only
   B. Mandibular Arch only
   C. In both arches
   D. None of the above
7. Which model analysis is used to assess the need of extraction in Maxillary arch:
   A. Nance Carey's model analysis
   B. Arch Perimeter analysis
   C. Pont's Analysis
   D. All of the above
8. Nance Carey's model analysis is used to assess the need of extraction in which arch:
   A. Maxillary Arch only
   B. Mandibular Arch only
   C. In both Arches
   D. None of the above
9. In Nance Carey's Analysis if the discrepancy is 2.5 mm or less what does it indicate:
   A. It indicates a non-extraction case where in minimal tooth material excess
   B. It advises the extraction of 1st Premolar
   C. It advises extraction of 2nd Premolar
   D. All of the above
10. According to Nance Carey's Analysis if the discrepancy shows 2.5-5 mm what does it suggest:
    A. Suggestive of Extraction of 1st premolar
    B. Suggestive of Extraction of 2nd Premolar
    C. Suggestive of Proximal stripping
    D. None of the above
11. According to Nance Carey's Analysis if the discrepancy is more than 5 mm then:
    A. Suggestive of Extraction of 1st Premolar
    B. Suggestive of Extraction of 2nd Premolar
    C. Suggestive of Proximal Stripping
    D. None of the above
12. How do we calculate the discrepancy in Nance Carey's Analysis:
    A. A.L – A.W
    B. A.W – A.L
    C. A.L – T.T.M
    D. Both A and C
13. How do we calculate the discrepancy in Nance Carey's Analysis:
    A. Arch length – Arch Width
    B. Arch Width – Arch length
    C. Arch length – Total tooth material
    D. Both A and C

14. **Determination of Arch Width/Total Tooth Material is done by:**
    A. Measuring distal width of the teeth anterior to the 1st Premolar at the maximum contour using Bow Divider
    B. Measuring distal width of the teeth posterior to the 1st Molar at the maximum contour using Bow Divider
    C. Measuring distal width of the teeth anterior to 2nd Permanent Molar at the maximum contour using Bow Divider
    D. Measuring distal width of the teeth posterior to 2nd Molar at the maximum contour using Bow Divider

15. **Determination of arch length in Nance Carey's analysis is done by using:**
    A. 0.012 inch soft round brass wire
    B. Bow Divider
    C. Soft round stainless steel wire
    D. All of the above

16. **In Nance Carey's Analysis in case of proclined anterior teeth determination of arch length using soft brass wire is done by passing the brass wire:**
    A. Along the cingulum of anterior teeth
    B. Labial to anterior teeth
    C. Lingual to anterior teeth
    D. On the Incisal edges

17. **According to Nance Carey's Analysis in case of retroclined anterior teeth determination of arch length is done by using soft brass wire:**
    A. Along the cingulum of anterior teeth
    B. Labial to anterior teeth
    C. Lingual to anterior teeth
    D. On the Incisal edges

18. **According to Nance Carey's Analysis in case of well aligned anterior teeth the arch length is determined by passing the brass wire:**
    A. Along the cingulum of anterior teeth
    B. Labial to anterior teeth
    C. Lingual to anterior teeth
    D. On the Incisal edges

19. **According to Nance Carey's analysis extraction of 1st Premolar is indicated, when arch length—tooth material discrepancy is about:**
    A. 0-2.5 mm    B. 2.5-5 mm
    C. 5-10 mm    D. None of the above

20. **According to Nance Carey's Analysis extraction of 2nd Premolar is indicated, when arch length—tooth material discrepancy is about:**
    A. 0-2.5 mm
    B. 2.5-5 mm
    C. 5-10 mm
    D. None of the above

21. **According to Nance Carey's Analysis is proximal stripping indicated, when arch length—tooth material discrepancy is about:**
    A. 0-2.5 mm    B. 2.5-5 mm
    C. 5-10 mm    D. None of the above

22. **In Arch Perimeter Analysis, if the discrepancy is 2.5 mm or less what does it indicate:**
    A. It indicates a non-extraction case where in minimal tooth material excess
    B. It advises the extraction of 1st Premolar
    C. It advises extraction of 2nd Premolar
    D. All of the above

23. **According to Arch Perimeter Analysis, if the discrepancy shows 2.5-5 mm what does it suggest:**
    A. Suggestive of Extraction of 1st premolar
    B. Suggestive of Extraction of 2nd Premolar
    C. Suggestive of Proximal stripping
    D. None of the above

24. **According to Arch Perimeter Analysis, if the discrepancy is more than 5 mm then:**
    A. Suggestive of Extraction of 1st Premolar
    B. Suggestive of Extraction of 2nd Premolar
    C. Suggestive of Proximal Stripping
    D. None of the above

25. **How do we calculate the discrepancy in Arch Perimeter:**
    A. A.L – A.W
    B. A.W – A.L
    C. A.L – T.T.M
    D. Both A and C

26. **How do we calculate the discrepancy in Arch Perimeter:**
    A. Arch length – Arch Width
    B. Arch Width – Arch length
    C. Arch length – Total tooth Material
    D. Both A and C

27. **Determination of Arch Width/Total Tooth Material is done by:**
    A. Measuring distal width of the teeth anterior to the 1st Premolar at the maximum contour using Bow Divider
    B. Measuring distal width of the teeth posterior to the 1st Molar at the maximum contour using Bow Divider
    C. Measuring distal width of the teeth anterior to 2nd Permanent Molar at the maximum contour using Bow Divider
    D. Measuring distal width of the teeth posterior to 2nd Molar at the maximum contour using Bow Divider

28. **Determination of Arch Perimeter is done by using:**
    A. 0.012 inch soft round brass wire
    B. Bow Divider
    C. Soft round stainless steel wire
    D. All of the above

29. **In Arch Perimeter analysis, in case of proclined anterior teeth determination of arch length using soft brass wire is done by passing the brass wire:**
    A. Along the cingulum of anterior teeth
    B. Labial to anterior teeth
    C. Lingual to anterior teeth
    D. On the Incisal edges

30. According to Arch Perimeter analysis, in case of retroclined anterior teeth determination of arch length is done by using soft brass wire:
    A. Along the cingulum of anterior teeth
    B. Labial to anterior teeth
    C. Lingual to anterior teeth
    D. On the Incisal edges
31. According to Arch Perimeter analysis, in case of well aligned anterior teeth the arch length is determined by passing the brass wire:
    A. Along the cingulum of anterior teeth
    B. Labial to anterior teeth
    C. Lingual to anterior teeth
    D. On the Incisal edges
32. According to Arch Perimeter analysis, extraction of 1st Premolar is indicated, when arch length—tooth material discrepancy is about:
    A. 0-2.5 mm      B. 2.5-5 mm
    C. 5-10 mm       D. None
33. According to Arch Perimeter analysis, extraction of 2nd Premolar is indicated, when arch length—tooth material discrepancy is about:
    A. 0-2.5 mm      B. 2.5-5 mm
    C. 5-10 mm       D. None of the above
34. According to Arch Perimeter analysis, proximal stripping is indicated, when arch length—tooth material discrepancy is about:
    A. 0-2.5 mm      B. 2.5-5 mm
    C. 5-10 mm       D. None of the above
35. Who and When proposed the Analysis called Pont's analysis:
    A. Pont in 1909  B. Pont in 1907
    C. Pont in 1908  D. Pont in 1906
36. Pont's Analysis helps in determining:
    A. Whether the dental arch is narrow or wide
    B. Need for lateral arch expansion
    C. How much expansion is possible in premolar and molar region
    D. All of the above
37. Determination of sum of Incisors in Pont's analysis is done by:
    A. Measuring mesial distal width of four Maxillary incisors and values are summed up
    B. Measuring mesial distal width of four Mandibular incisors and values are summed up
    C. Measuring mesial distal width of maxillary anteriors and values are summed up
    D. Measuring mesial distal width of mandibular anteriors and values are summed up
38. SI in Pont's Analysis stands for:
    A. Sum of lateral Incisors
    B. Sum of Incisors of Maxillary teeth
    C. Sum of Incisors of mandibular teeth
    D. All of the above
39. MPV in Pont's Analysis stands for:
    A. Measured 1st Premolar Value
    B. Measured 2nd Premolar Value
    C. Measured Premolar Value
    D. All of the above
40. MPV in Pont's Analysis is determined by:
    A. Placing the tip end of divider at distal pit of 14 and another at the distal pit of 24
    B. Placing the tip end of divider at Mesial Pit of 14 and another at mesial pit of 24
    C. Placing the tip end of divider at distal pit of 15 and another at distal pit of 25
    D. Placing the tip end of divider at mesial pit of 15 and another at mesial pit of 25
41. CPV in Pont's Analysis stands for:
    A. Computer Premolar Value
    B. Calculated Premolar Value
    C. Calculated 1st Premolar value
    D. Calculated 2nd Premolar Value
42. MMV in Pont's Analysis stands for:
    A. Mesial Molar Value
    B. Measured Molar Value
    C. Measured 1st Molar Value
    D. Measured 2nd Molar Value
43. CMV in Pont's Analysis stands for
    A. Calculated Molar value
    B. Calculated 1st molar value
    C. Calculated 2nd Molar value
    D. Calculated 3rd molar value
44. The Measured Molar Value in Pont's analysis is determined by:
    A. Placing the divider at the mesial pit of 16 to the mesial pit of 26
    B. Placing the divider at the distal pit of 16 to the distal pit of 26
    C. Placing the divider at the mesial pit of 36 to the mesial pit of 46
    D. Placing the divider at the distal pit of 36 to the distal pit of 46
45. In Pont's analysis CPV is determined by the following forrmula:
    A. $CPV = \dfrac{SI \times 100}{8}$      B. $CPV = \dfrac{SI \times 100}{80}$
    C. $CPV = \dfrac{SI \times 100}{85}$     D. $CPV = \dfrac{SI \times 100}{800}$
46. Calculated Molar Value in Pont's analysis is determined by the formula:
    A. $CMV = \dfrac{SI \times 100}{64}$      B. $CMV = \dfrac{SI \times 100}{63}$
    C. $CMV = \dfrac{SI \times 100}{65}$      D. $CMV = \dfrac{SI \times 100}{62}$
47. How much expansion is needed in premolar region in Pont's Analysis is determined by the formula:
    A. CPV – MPV      B. CPV – CMV
    C. MPV – CPV      D. CMV – CPV
48. How much expansion in the molar region in Pont's Analysis is determined by the formula:
    A. CMV – MMV      B. MMV – CMV
    C. CMV – CPV      D. MMV – MPV

49. **What is the difference between Pont's Analysis and Linder Harth Model Analysis:**
    A. In calculated premolar value in Linder Harth Analysis is 85 instead of 80 as in Pont's Analysis
    B. In calculated premolar value in Pont's Analysis is 85 instead of 80 as in Linder Harth Analysis
    C. Both are same, no difference
    D. None of the above

50. **Linder Harth's Model Analysis helps in determining:**
    A. Whether the dental arch is narrow or wide
    B. Need for lateral arch expansion
    C. How much expansion is possible in premolar and molar region
    D. All of the above

51. **Determination of sum of Incisors in Linder Harth's Model Analysis is done by:**
    A. Measuring mesio-distal width of four Maxillary incisors and values are summed up
    B. Measuring mesio-distal width of four Mandibular incisors and values are summed up
    C. Measuring mesio-distal width of maxillary anteriors and values are summed up
    D. Measuring mesio-distal width of mandibular anteriors and values are summed up

52. **SI in Linder Harth's Model Analysis stands for:**
    A. Sum of lateral Incisors
    B. Sum of Incisors of Maxillary teeth
    C. Sum of Incisors of mandibular teeth
    D. All of the above

53. **MPV in Linder Harth's Model Analysis stands for:**
    A. Measure 1st Premolar Value
    B. Measure 2nd Premolar Value
    C. Measured Premolar Value
    D. All of the above

54. **MPV in Linder Harth's Model Analysis is determined by:**
    A. Placing the tip end of divider at distal pit of 14 and another at the distal pit of 24
    B. Placing the tip end of divider at mesial pit of 14 and another at mesial pit of 24
    C. Placing the tip end of divider at distal pit of 15 and another at distal pit of 25
    D. Placing the tip end of divider at mesial pit of 15 and another at mesial pit of 25

55. **CPV in Linder Harth's Model Analysis stands for:**
    A. Computer Premolar Value
    B. Calculated Premolar Value
    C. Calculated 1st Premolar Value
    D. Calculated 2nd Premolar Value

56. **MMV in Linder Harth's Model Analysis stands for:**
    A. Mesial Molar Value
    B. Measured Molar Value
    C. Measured 1st Molar Value
    D. Measured 2nd Molar Value

57. **CMV in Linder Harth's Model Analysis stands for**
    A. Calculated Molar value
    B. Calculated 1st Molar value
    C. Calculated 2nd Molar value
    D. Calculated 3rd Molar value

58. **The Measured Molar Value in Linder Harth's Model Analysis is determined by:**
    A. Placing the divider at the mesial pit of 16 to the mesial pit of 26
    B. Placing the divider at the distal pit of 16 to the distal pit of 26
    C. Placing the divider at the mesial pit of 36 to the mesial pit of 46
    D. Placing the divider at the distal pit of 36 to the distal pit of 46

59. **According to Linder Harth's Model Analysis, CPV is determined by the following formula:**
    A. $CPV = \dfrac{SI \times 100}{8}$
    B. $CPV = \dfrac{SI \times 100}{80}$
    C. $CPV = \dfrac{SI \times 100}{85}$
    D. $CPV = \dfrac{SI \times 100}{800}$

60. **According to Linder Harth's Model Analysis, CMV is determined by the formula:**
    A. $CMV = \dfrac{SI \times 100}{64}$
    B. $CMV = \dfrac{SI \times 100}{63}$
    C. $CMV = \dfrac{SI \times 100}{65}$
    D. $CMV = \dfrac{SI \times 100}{62}$

61. **How much expansion is needed in premolar region in Linder Harth's Model Analysis is determined by the formula:**
    A. CPV – MPV
    B. CPV – CMV
    C. MPV – CPV
    D. CMV – CPV

62. **How much expansion in the molar region in Linder Harth's Model Analysis is determined by the formula:**
    A. CMV – MMV
    B. MMV – CMV
    C. CMV – CPV
    D. MMV – MPV

63. **Is there any difference between Korkhaus Analysis and Pont's Analysis:**
    A. Yes
    B. No
    C. Maybe
    D. May not be

64. **Is there any difference between Korkhaus Analysis and Linder Harth Analysis:**
    A. Yes
    B. No
    C. Maybe
    D. May not be

65. **Korkhaus Analysis helps in determining:**
    A. Whether the dental arch is narrow or wide
    B. Need for lateral arch expansion
    C. How much expansion is possible in premolar and molar region
    D. All of the above

66. **Determination of sum of Incisors in Korkhaus Analysis is done by:**
    A. Measuring mesio-distal width of 4 Maxillary incisors and values are summed up
    B. Measuring mesio-distal width of 4 Mandibular incisors and values are summed up
    C. Measuring mesio-distal width of maxillary anteriors and values are summed up

D. Measuring mesio-distal width of mandibular anteriors and values are summed up

67. **SI in Korkhaus Analysis stands for:**
    A. Sum of lateral Incisors
    B. Sum of Incisors of Maxillary teeth
    C. Sum of Incisors of mandibular teeth
    D. All of the above

68. **MPV in Korkhaus Analysis stands for:**
    A. Measure 1st Premolar Value
    B. Measure 2nd Premolar Value
    C. Measured Premolar Value
    D. All of the above

69. **MPV in Korkhaus Analysis is determined by:**
    A. Placing the tip end of divider at distal pit of 14 and another at the distal pit of 24
    B. Placing the tip end of divider at mesial pit of 14 and another at mesial pit of 24
    C. Placing the tip end of divider at distal pit of 15 and another at distal pit of 25
    D. Placing the tip end of divider at mesial pit of 15 and another at mesial pit of 25

70. **CPV in Korkhaus Analysis stands for:**
    A. Computer Premolar Value
    B. Calculated Premolar Value
    C. Calculated 1st Premolar value
    D. Calculated 2nd Premolar Value

71. **MMV in Korkhaus Analysis stands for:**
    A. Mesial Molar Value
    B. Measured Molar Value
    C. Measured 1st Molar Value
    D. Measured 2nd Molar Value

72. **CMV in Korkhaus Analysis stands for**
    A. Calculated Molar value
    B. Calculated 1st molar value
    C. Calculated 2nd Molar value
    D. Calculated 3rd molar value

73. **The Measured Molar Value in Korkhaus Analysis is determined by:**
    A. Placing the divider at the mesial pit of 16 to the mesial pit of 26
    B. Placing the divider at the distal pit of 16 to the distal pit of 26
    C. Placing the divider at the mesial pit of 36 to the mesial pit of 46
    D. Placing the divider at the distal pit of 36 to the distal pit of 46

74. **According to Korkhaus Analysis, CPV is determined by the following formula:**
    A. $CPV = \dfrac{SI \times 100}{8}$
    B. $CPV = \dfrac{SI \times 100}{80}$
    C. $CPV = \dfrac{SI \times 100}{85}$
    D. $CPV = \dfrac{SI \times 100}{800}$

75. **According to Korkhaus Analysis, CMV is determined by the formula:**
    A. $CMV = \dfrac{SI \times 100}{64}$
    B. $CMV = \dfrac{SI \times 100}{63}$
    C. $CMV = \dfrac{SI \times 100}{65}$
    D. $CMV = \dfrac{SI \times 100}{62}$

76. **How much expansion is needed in premolar region in Korkhaus Analysis is determined by the formula:**
    A. CPV – MPV
    B. CPV – CMV
    C. MPV – CPV
    D. CMV – CPV

77. **How much expansion in the molar region in Korkhaus Analysis is determined by the formula:**
    A. CMV – MMV
    B. MMV – CMV
    C. CMV – CPV
    D. MMV – MPV

78. **What is the difference between Korkhaus Analysis and Linder Harth Model Analysis:**
    A. In calculated premolar value in Linder Harth Analysis is 85 instead of 80 as in Pont's Analysis
    B. In calculated premolar value in Pont's Analysis is 85 instead of 80 as in Linder Harth Analysis
    C. Both are same no difference
    D. None of the above

79. **How do we determine Oral ratio in Bolton's Analysis**
    A. $\text{Overall ratio} = \dfrac{\text{sum of mandibular 12}}{\text{sum of maxillary 12}} \times 100$
    B. $\text{Overall ratio} = \dfrac{\text{sum of maxillary 12}}{\text{sum of mandibular 12}} \times 100$
    C. $\text{Overall ratio} = \dfrac{\text{sum of mandibular 6}}{\text{sum of maxillary 6}} \times 100$
    D. $\text{Overall ratio} = \dfrac{\text{sum of mandibular 11}}{\text{sum of maxillary 11}} \times 100$

80. **If the ratio is less than 91.3% in Bolton's Analysis what does it indicate:**
    A. Indicates Maxillary tooth material excess
    B. Indicates Mandibular tooth material excess
    C. Both A and B
    D. None of the above

81. **If the ratio is less than 77.2% in Bolton's Analysis what does it indicate:**
    A. Maxillary tooth material excess
    B. Mandibular tooth material excess
    C. Both A and B
    D. None of the above

82. **According to Bolton's analysis if the ratio is more than 91.3% what does it indicate:**
    A. Maxillary tooth material excess
    B. Mandibular tooth material excess
    C. Both A and B
    D. None of the above

83. **According to Bolton's Analysis if the ratio is more than 77.2% what does it indicate:**
    A. Maxillary tooth material excess
    B. Mandibular tooth material excess

C. Both A and B
D. None of the above

84. **Sum of Maxillary 6 in Bolton's Analysis is determined by the formula:**
    A. $\text{Sum of Maxillary 6} - \dfrac{\text{sum of mandibular 6}}{77.2} \times 100$
    B. $\text{Sum of Mandibular 6} - \dfrac{\text{sum of mandibular 6}}{77.2} \times 10$
    C. $\text{Sum of Maxillary 6} - \dfrac{\text{sum of mandibular 6}}{77.2} \times 10$
    D. $\dfrac{\text{sum of mandibular 6}}{77.2} + \text{sum of Maxillary 6} \times 100$

85. **Sum of Mandibular 6 in Bolton's Analysis is determined by the formula:**
    A. $\text{Sum of Mandibular 6} - \dfrac{\text{Sum of maxillary 6}}{100} \times 77.2$
    B. $\text{Sum of MandibularIlary 6} + \dfrac{\text{Sum of mandibular 6}}{77.2} \times 77.2$
    C. $\text{Sum of MandibularIlary 6} + \dfrac{\text{Sum of mandibular 6}}{77.2} \times 77.2$
    D. $\text{Sum of Mandibular 6} \times \dfrac{\text{Sum of mandibular 6}}{77.2} \times 77.2$

86. **According to Bolton's Analysis sum of maxillary 12 is determined by the formula:**
    A. $\text{Sum of Maxillary 12} - \dfrac{\text{Sum of mandibular 12}}{91.3} \times 100$
    B. $\text{Sum of Maxillary 12} + \dfrac{\text{Sum of mandibular 12}}{91.3} \times 100$
    C. $\text{Sum of Mandibular 12} - \dfrac{\text{Sum of maxillary 12}}{77.2} \times 100$
    D. $\text{Sum of Mandibular 12} - \dfrac{\text{Sum of mandibular 12}}{77.2} \times 100$

87. **According to Bolton's Analysis the sum of mandibular 12 is determined by the formula:**
    A. $\text{Sum of Mandibular 12} - \dfrac{\text{Sum of maxillary 12}}{100} \times 91.3$
    B. $\text{Sum of Mandibular 12} + \dfrac{\text{Sum of maxillary 12}}{77.2} \times 100$
    C. $\text{Sum of Mandibular 12} - \dfrac{\text{Sum of maxillary 12}}{91.3} \times 100$
    D. $\text{Sum of Mandibular 12} - \dfrac{\text{Sum of mandibular 6}}{77.2} \times 100$

88. **In Bolton's Analysis Sum of Mandibular 12 teeth is measured by:**
    A. Mesiodistal width of all the teeth mesial to 37 is measured and summed up
    B. Mesiodistal width of all the teeth mesial to 36 is measured and summed up
    C. Mesiodistal width of all the teeth mesial to 38 is measured and summed up
    D. None

89. **Which model analysis is used to know how much stripping to be done to relieve the crowding:**
    A. Nance Carey's
    B. Peck and Peck
    C. Bolton's analysis
    D. Both A and B

90. **Mixed Dentition Analysis the formula used is:**
    A. $Y1 = \dfrac{x^1 \times y^2}{x^2}$
    B. $Y1 = \dfrac{x^2 \times y^2}{x^1}$
    C. $Y1 = \dfrac{x^1 \times x^2}{y^2}$
    D. None of the above

91. **In mixed dentition analysis Y1 stands for:**
    A. Width of unerupted tooth whose measurement is to be determined
    B. Width of unerupted tooth on the radiograph
    C. Width of a tooth that has erupted on the cast
    D. Width of a tooth that has erupted measured on the radiograph

92. **In mixed dentition analysis Y2 stands for**
    A. Width of unerupted tooth whose measurement is to be determined
    B. Width of unerupted tooth on the radiograph
    C. Width of a tooth that has erupted on the cast
    D. Width of a tooth that has erupted measured on the radiograph

93. **In mixed dentition analysis x1 stands for:**
    A. Width of unerupted tooth whose measurement is to be determined
    B. Width of unerupted tooth on the radiograph
    C. Width of a tooth that has erupted, measured on the cast
    D. Width of a tooth that has erupted measured on the radiograph

94. **In mixed dentition analysis x2 stands for:**
    A. Width of unerupted tooth whose measurement is to be determined
    B. Width of unerupted tooth on the radiograph
    C. Width of a tooth that has erupted on the cast
    D. Width of a tooth that has erupted, measured on the radiograph

95. **According to Ashley Howe's Analysis if the ratio is between 34-44%, then what does it indicate:**
    A. Extraction case
    B. Non-extraction case
    C. Borderline case
    D. None of the above

96. **According to Ashley Howe's analysis if the ratio is 44% or more, then what does it indicate:**
    A. Extraction case
    B. Non-extraction case
    C. Borderline case
    D. None of the above

97. **According to Ashley Howe's analysis if the ratio is less than 37%, then what does it indicate:**
    A. Extraction case
    B. Non-extraction case
    C. Borderline case
    D. None of the above

98. In Ashley Howe's analysis, expansion is possible if:
    A. P.M.B.A.W is greater than P.M.D
    B. P.M.B.A.W is lesser than P.M.D
    C. P.M.B.A.W is equal to P.M.D
    D. None of the above

99. In Ashley Howe's analysis, expansion is not possible if:
    A. P.M.B.A.W is greater than P.M.D
    B. P.M.B.A.W is lesser than P.M.D
    C. P.M.B.A.W is equal to P.M.D
    D. None of the above

Ans: 1. C  2. D  3. C  4. A  5. A  6. A  7. B  8. B  9. A  10. B  11. A  12. D  13. D  14. A  15. A  16. A
17. B  18. D  19. C  20. B  21. A  22. A  23. B  24. A  25. D  26. D  27. A  28. A  29. A  30. B  31. D  32. C
33. B  34. A  35. A  36. D  37. A  38. B  39. C  40. A  41. B  42. B  43. A  44. A  45. B  46. A  47. A  48. A
49. A  50. D  51. A  52. B  53. C  54. A  55. B  56. B  57. A  58. B  59. C  60. A  61. A  62. A  63. A  64. A
65. D  66. A  67. B  68. C  69. A  70. B  71. B  72. A  73. A  74. B  75. A  76. A  77. A  78. D  79. A  80. A
81. A  82. B  83. B  84. A  85. A  86. A  87. A  88. A  89. D  90. A  91. A  92. B  93. C  94. D  95. C  96. B
97. A  98. A  99. B

## CEPHALOMETRICS IN ORTHODONTICS

1. **Cephalometrics in orthodontics is used for:**
   A. Orthodontic diagnosis
   B. To evaluate the pre-treatment dental and facial relationship of a patient
   C. To evaluate change during orthodontic treatment
   D. All of the above

2. **Types of cephalograms are:**
   A. Lateral cephalogram
   B. Frontal cephalogram
   C. Occlusal cephalogram
   D. Both A and B

3. **Lateral cephalogram provides**
   A. A Lateral view of skull
   B. An antero-posterior view of the skull
   C. Both A and B
   D. None of the above

4. **Frontal cephalogram provides**
   A. An antero-posterior view of the skull
   B. A lateral view of skull
   C. Both A and B
   D. None of the above

5. **Uses of cephalometric analysis in orthodontics are**
   A. Diagnostic purpose to assess whether malocclusion dental or skeletal in origin
   B. It enables clinician to know accurately the extent to which patient deviates from described norms
   C. To monitor the changes occurring due to growth or treatment or their combination
   D. All the above

6. **Cephalostat consists of**
   A. Two ear rods
   B. One ear rods
   C. Four ear rods, two on each side
   D. None of the above

7. **Functions of ear rods in cephalostat is**
   A. To prevent the movement of the lead in the horizontal plane
   B. To prevent the movement of the lead in the vertical plane
   C. Both A and B
   D. None of the above

8. **The distance between the X-ray source and the mid-sagittal plane of the patient in cephalometric radiograph should be**
   A. 5 feet           B. 6 feet
   C. 7 feet           D. 8 feet

9. **Cephalometric tracing in orthodontics is made on**
   A. The frosted surface of acetate tracing sheet
   B. The plane paper
   C. The white paper
   D. None of the above

10. **Which of the following is hard tissue landmark in cephalometrics?**
    A. Condylion
    B. Posterior nasal spine
    C. Gonion
    D. All of the above

11. **Basion in cephalometrics refers to**
    A. Lowest point on the anterior margin of the foramen magnum in the midline
    B. Lowest point on the posterior margin of the foramen magnum in the midline
    C. Highest point on the anterior margin of the foramen magnum in the midline
    D. Highest point on the posterior margin of the foramen magnum in the midline

12. **Condylion in cephalometrics refers to**
    A. Superior most point of the Head of the condyle of the mandible
    B. Inferior most point of the lead of the condyle of the mandible
    C. Superior most point of the neck of condyle of the mandible
    D. Inferior most point of the neck of the condyle of the mandible

13. **Se in cephalometrics refers to**
    A. Mid-entrance point of sella turcica
    B. Midpoint of sella turcica
    C. Mid-inferior point of sella turcica
    D. None of the above

14. Sella in cephalometrics refers to
    A. Midpoint of sella turcica
    B. Mid-entrance point of sella turcica
    C. Either A or B
    D. None of the above
15. ptm in cephalometrics refers to
    A. Intersection of the inferior border of the formen rotundum with the posterior wall of the pterygo-maxillary fissure
    B. Intersection of the superior border of the foramen rotundum with the posterior wall of the pterygo-maxillary fissure
    C. Intersection of anterior border of the foramen rotundum with the posterior wall of the pterygo-maxillary fissure
    D. Intersection of posterior border of the foramen rotundum with the posterior wall of pterygo-maxillary fissure
16. The hard tissue landmark porion (Po) in cephalometrics refers to
    A. Midpoint on the upper edge of the forms acusticus externus located by means of the metal rods in cephalometrics
    B. The most prominent point in the midline
    C. Midpoint on the lower edge of the porus acusticus externus located by means of the metal rods in the cephalometer
    D. None of the above
17. The hard tissue landmark, PNS, in cephalometrics refers to
    A. Intersection of a continuation of the anterior wall of the pterygopalatine fossa and the floor of the nose
    B. Tip of bony anterior nasal spine in midline
    C. Continuation of the posterior wall of the pterygopalatine fossa
    D. All of the above
18. The hard tissue landmark, ANS, in cephalometrics refers to
    A. Intersection of a continuation of the anterior wall of the pterygopalatine fossa and the floor of the nose
    B. Tip of bony anterior nasal spine in midline
    C. Continuation of the posterior wall of the pterygopalatine fossa
    E. All of the above
19. The hard tissue landmarks, ANS, in cephalometrics stands for
    A. Anterior nasal spine
    B. Andrew's nasal spine
    C. Angle's nasal spine
    D. Anterior nasal superioral
20. The hard tissue landmarks, PNS, in cephelometrics stands for
    A. **Posterior nasal spine**
    B. Anterior nasal spine
    C. Andrew's nasal spine
    D. All of the above
21. The hard tissue landmark, Po, in cephalometrics stands for
    A. **Porion**            B. Posonion
    C. Prosthion             D. Point A
22. The hard tissue landmarks, Pr, in cephalometrics stands for
    A. Poroin                B. Posonion
    C. **Prosthion**         D. Point A
23. The hard tissue landmark, S, in cephalometrics stands for
    A. **Sella**             B. Se
    C. Superior              D. Spine
24. The hard tissue landmark, Go, in cephalometrics stands for
    A. **Gonion**            B. Gnathion
    C. Gonon                 D. Gnton
25. The hard tissue landmarks, Cd, in cephalometrics stands for
    A. **Condylion**         B. Condyon
    C. Codyon                D. Codylion
26. The hard tissue cephalometric point, prosthion refers to
    A. **Lowermost anterior point of alveolar process of pre-maxilla in the midline between two central incisors**
    B. Lowermost anterior point of alveolar process between two central incisors in mandible
    C. Both A and B
    D. None of the above
27. The hard tissue cephalometric point 'Orbitale' refers to
    A. **Lowest point on the inferior bony margin of the orbit**
    B. Point on the superior bony margin of the orbit
    C. Point on the anterior bony margin of the orbit
    D. None of the above
28. The hard tissue cephalometrics point, Nasion refers to
    A. **Most anterior point of frontonasal suture in the midline**
    B. Most posterior point of frontonasal outline in the midline
    C. Somewhere in the frontonasal outline in the midline
    D. None of the above
29. The hard tissue cephalometric point, Point A refers to
    A. **The deepest point on the curved bony outline between the ANS and Pr**
    B. Point on the curved bony outline near ANS
    C. Point on the curved bony outline near Pr
    D. None of the above
30. The hard tissue cephalometrics point, point B refers to
    A. **Deepest point of curvature on the contour of mandibular alveolar process in the midline between intradentale and pogonion**

B. Deepest point on the curved bony outline between ANS and prosthion
C. Lowermost anterior part of alveolar process of mandible in midline
D. None of the above

31. The hard tissue cephalometric point, Intradentale (Id) refers to
    A. Highest anterior point of the alveolar process of mandible between two central incisors in midline
    B. Lower most anterior point of alveolar process of pre-maxilla in the midline between two maxillary central incisors
    C. Point near the periapical area
    D. None of the above

32. APOcc, in cephalometrics stands for
    A. Anterior point of occlusion
    B. Posterior point of occlusion
    C. Anterior occlusal plane
    D. Anterior prominent occlusion

33. PPOcc, in cephalometric refers for
    A. Anterior point of occlusion
    B. Posterior point of occlusion
    C. Anterior occlusal plane
    D. Anterior prominent occlusion

34. The hard tissue cephelometric point, Anterior part of occlusion refers to
    A. Anterior point for occlusal plane in the midpoint in the incisors overbites in the occlusion
    B. It is a constructed cephalometric point
    C. It is abbreviated as APOcc and is a unilateral, derivated cephalometric point
    D. All of the above

35. Which of the following is an anatomic, bilateral hard tissue cephalometric landmark in orthodontic
    A. Nasion            B. Point A
    C. Point B           D. Articulare

36. Which of the following is an anatomic, unilateral cephalometric landmark in the midline
    A. N                 B. ANS
    C. Pr                D. All of the above

37. Which of the following is a soft tissue cephalometric landmark
    A. N                 B. ANS
    C. n                 D. Id

38. Cephalometric plane includes
    A. Horizontal cephalometric planes
    B. Vertical cephalometric planes
    C. Oblique cephalometric planes
    D. All of the above

39. Soft tissue cephalometric landmarks include
    A. Tip of the nose (no)   B. Subspinale (Ss)
    C. Subnasale (Sn)         D. All of the above

40. Horizontal cephalometric reference planes are
    A. S-N plane         B. Se-N plane
    C. F-H plane         D. All of the above

41. Vertical cephalometric reference planes are
    A. N-A plane         B. N-B plane
    C. N-Pog plane       D. All of the above

42. Significance of S-N plane
    A. represents the anterior-posterior extent of anterior cranial base
    B. Assessment of growth pattern
    C. It represents the anterior-posterior extent of posterior cranial base
    D. All of the above

43. Which of the following planes is used to assess the extent of anterior cranial base
    A. S-N               B. Se-N
    C. F-H plane         D. Both A and B

44. Which of the following planes used in assessing horizontal growth pattern
    A. F-H plane         B. APOcc-PPOcc
    C. Both A and B      D. None of the above

45. F H plane is also called as
    A. Frankfort horizontal plane
    B. Frankfort vertical plane
    C. Frankfort oblique plane
    E. All of the above

46. E-plane is also called as
    A. Esthetic plane    B. External plane
    C. Both A and B      D. None of the above

47. Normal facial angle is about
    A. 82-95 degree      B. 70-82 degree
    C. 95-110 degree     D. 120-130 degree

48. Increased facial angle indicates
    A. Skeletal class III malocclusion
    B. Skeletal class II malocclusion
    C. Skeletal class I malocclusion
    D. All of the above

49. Decreased facial angle indicates
    A. Skeletal class III malocclusion
    B. Skeletal class II malocclusion
    C. Skeletal class I malocclusion
    D. All of the above

50. Facial angle signifies
    A. antero-posterior positioning of the mandible to the upper face
    B. antero-posterior position of the maxilla to the upper face
    C. Maxillomandible relationship
    D. All of the above

51. Angle of convexity in cephalometric analysis helps in
    A. Determining convexity of the skeletal profile
    B. Determining concavity of the skeletal profile
    C. Both A and B
    D. None of the above

52. The average value of angle of convexity is
    A. 8.5-10 degree     B. 3.5-5.5 degree
    C. 0.0-3.0 degree    D. 3.8-5.9 degree

53. Increased angle of convexity in Down's cephalometric analysis indicates
    A. Prominent maxillary base relative to mandible
    B. Recessive maxillary base relative to mandible
    C. Both A and B      D. None of the above

54. Decreased angle of convexity indicates
    A. Prognathic profile    B. Retrognathic profile
    C. Orthognathic profile  D. None of the above
55. A-B plane angle signifies
    A. Indication of maxillomandibular relationship to the facial plane
    B. Indication of maxilla to the mandible
    C. Maxillomandibular relationship
    D. All of the above
56. Increased A-B plane angle indicates
    A. Class III malocclusion
    B. Class II malocclusion
    C. Class I malocclusion
    D. All of the above
57. Decreased A-B plane angle in Down's analysis indicates
    A. Class III malocclusion
    B. Class II malocclusion
    C. Class I Malocclusion
    D. All of the above
58. Mandibular plane angle in Down's cephalometric analysis helps in
    A. Horizontal growth pattern
    B. Vertical growth pattern
    C. Both A and B
    D. None of the above
59. The normal value of mandibular plane angle in Down's cephalometric analysis is about
    A. 17-28 degree    B. 29-30 degree
    C. 31-45 degree    D. 46-75 degree
60. Increased mandibular plane angle in Down's cephalometric analysis indicates
    A. Vertical growth pattern
    B. Horizontal growth pattern
    C. Both A and B
    D. None of the above
61. Decreased mandibular plane angle in Down's cephalometric analysis indicates
    A. Vertical growth pattern
    B. Horizontal growth pattern
    C. Both A and B
    D. None of the above
62. Y-axis in Down's cephalometric analysis helps in
    A. Diagnosing horizontal pattern
    B. Assessing vertical growth pattern
    C. Both A and B
    D. None of the above
63. The normal value of Y-axis in Down's cephalometric analysis is about
    A. 53-66 degree    B. 66-70 degree
    C. 71-86 degree    D. 87-99 degree
64. The increased Y-axis angle in Down's cephalometric analysis indicates
    A. Vertical growth pattern
    B. Horizontal growth pattern
    C. Both A and B
    D. None of the above
65. The decreased Y-axis angle in Down's cephalometric analysis indicates
    A. Vertical growth pattern
    B. Horizontal growth pattern
    C. Both A and B
    D. None of the above
66. What are skeletal parameters of Down's analysis?
    A. SNA Angle    B. SNB Angle
    C. ANB Angle    D. Facial Angle
67. The normal value of cant of occlusal plane in Down's analysis is
    A. 1.5-14 degrees
    B. 14-28 degrees
    C. 28-32 degrees
    D. 33-46 degrees
68. Increased value of cant of occlusal plane in Down's analysis is
    A. Vertical growth pattern
    B. Horizontal growth pattern
    C. Both A and B
    D. None of the above
69. Decreased value of cant of occlusal plane in Down's analysis is
    A. Vertical growth pattern
    B. Horizontal growth pattern
    C. Both A and B
    D. None of the above
70. The normal range of interincisal angle is
    A. 130-150 degrees    B. 150-175 degrees
    C. 180-195 degrees    D. None of the above
71. Increased inter-incisal angle in Down's analysis indicates
    A. Class II malocclusion
    B. Bimaxillary protrusion
    C. Both a and b
    D. None of the above
72. Decreased inter-incisal angle in Down's analysis indicates
    A. Class II malocclusion
    B. Bimaxillary protrusion
    C. Both A and B
    D. None of the above
73. Incisor occlusal plane angle is formed by
    A. Intersection between long axis of lower incisor and the occlusal plane
    B. Intersection between long axis of lower central incisor and the occlusal plane
    C. Intersection between long axis of lower canine and the occlusal plane
    D. Intersection between long axis of upper central incisor and the occlusal plane
74. The normal value of incisal occlusal plane angle is:
    A. 3.5-20 degrees    B. 21-35.5 degrees
    C. 36-43.5 degrees   D. 44-55.5 degrees
75. Increased incisal occlusal plane angle in Down's analysis indicates:
    A. Incisor retroclination
    B. Incisor proclination

C. Incisor rotations
D. Incisor transposition

76. **Decreased incisal occlusal plane angle in Down's analysis indicates:**
    A. Incisor retroclination
    B. Incisor proclination
    C. Incisor rotations
    D. Incisor transposition

77. **Upper incisor to A-Pog line is linear measurement between:**
    A. The incisal edge of the maxillary central incisor and the line joining point A to Pogonion
    B. The incisal edge of lower central incisor and the line joining pont A to pogonion
    C. the incisal edge of the maxillary lateral incisor and the line joining point A to pogonion
    D. the incisal edge of mandibular lateral incisor and the line joining point A to pogonion

78. **Upper incisor to A-Pog line is a**
    A. linear measurement
    B. angular measurement
    C. linear and angular measurement
    D. none of the above

79. **The normal value of upper incisor to A-Pog line is:**
    A. -1 to 5 mm
    B. 3 to 9 mm
    C. 9 to 12 mm
    D. 12 to 15 mm

80. **Increased measurement of maxillary incisor to A-Pog line indicates:**
    A. Upper incisor proclination
    B. Upper incisor retroclination
    C. Lower incisor proclination
    D. Lower incisal retroclination

81. **Decreased measurement of upper incisor to A-Pog line indicates:**
    A. Upper incisor proclination
    B. Upper incisor retroclination
    C. Lower incisor proclination
    D. Lower incisal retroclination

82. **SNA angle is used to assess:**
    A. The degree of maxillary prognathism
    B. The degree of mandibular prognathism
    C. Relationship of maxilla to the cranial base
    D. Both A and C

83. **Decreased SNA angle indicates:**
    A. Maxilla lies more posteriorly in relation to the cranial base
    B. Maxilla lies more anteriorly in relation to the cranial base
    C. Maxillary retrognathism
    D. **Both A and C**

84. **Increased SNA angle indicates**
    A. Maxilla lies more anterior
    B. Maxilla lies more posterior in relation to the cranial base
    C. Maxillary prognathism
    D. Both A and C

85. **SNB angle defines**
    A. Anteroposterior position of the mandible in relation to anterior cranial base
    B. Anteroposterior position of maxilla in relation to anterior cranial base
    C. Maxillomandibular relationship in relation to cranial base
    D. All of the above

86. **Decreased SNB angle indicates**
    A. Mandibular retrognathism
    B. Mandibular prognathism
    C. Mandible displacement
    D. All of the above

87. **Increased SNB angle indicates**
    A. Mandibular retrognathism
    B. Mandibular prognathism
    C. Mandible displacement
    D. All of the above

88. **ANB angle in cephalometrics defined as**
    A. Anteroposterior position of the mandible in relation to anterior cranial base
    B. Anteroposterior position of the maxilla to anterior cranial base
    C. The mutual relationship in sagittal plane of the maxillary and mandibular bases
    D. All of the above

89. **Decreased ANB angle indicates**
    A. Class III skeletal tendency
    B. Class II skeletal tendency
    C. Class I skeletal tendency
    D. Skeletal bimaxillary protrusion

90. **Increased ANB angle indicates**
    A. Class III skeletal tendency
    B. Class II skeletal tendency
    C. Class I skeletal tendency
    D. Skeletal bimaxillary protrusion

91. **Mandibular plane angle is used to assess**
    A. Vertical growth pattern of an individual
    B. Horizontal growth pattern of an individual
    C. Growth pattern of an individual
    D. All of the above.

92. **The normal mandibular plane angle in Steiner's analysis is**
    A. 33 degrees
    B. 30 degrees
    C. 29 degrees
    D. 32 degrees

93. **Increased mandibular plane angle in Steiner's cephalometric analysis indicates**
    A. Vertical growth pattern
    B. Horizontal growth pattern
    C. Both A and B
    D. None of the above

94. **Decreased mandibular plane angle in Steiner's cephalometric analysis indicates**
    A. Vertical growth pattern
    B. Horizontal growth pattern
    C. Both A and B
    D. None of the above

95. Upper incisor to NA angle is formed by
    A. The long axis of upper central incisors and the line joining nasion to point A
    B. The long axis of upper lateral incisors and the line joining nasion to point B
    C. The long axis lower central incisors and the line joining nasion to point A
    D. The long axis of lower lateral incisors and the line joining nasion to point A

96. The normal angle of upper incisor to NA angle is
    A. 20 degrees        B. 25 degrees
    C. 22 degrees        D. 18 degrees

97. Increase in upper incisor to NA angle indicates
    A. Proclined upper incisors
    B. Retroclined upper incisors
    C. Proclined lower incisors
    D. Retroclined lower incisors

98. Decreased upper incisor to NA angle indicates
    A. Proclined upper incisors
    B. Retroclined upper incisors
    C. Proclined lower incisors
    D. Retroclined lower incisors

99. Upper incisor to NA linear is a measurement between
    A. Labial surface of upper central incisors and the line joining nasion to point A
    B. Labial surface of upper lateral incisors and the line joining nasion to point A
    C. Labial surface of lower central incisors and the line joining nasion to point A
    D. Labial surface of lower lateral incisors and the line joining nasion to point A

100. Upper incisor to NA linear helps in determining
    A. Upper incisor position
    B. Lower incisor position
    C. Both A and B
    D. None of the above

101. The normal value of upper incisor to NA linear is
    A. 2 mm        B. 3 mm
    C. 4 mm        D. 5 mm

102. Lower incisor to NB angle is formed by
    A. Between the NB plane and the long axis of lower incisors
    B. Between the NA plane and the long axis of lower incisor
    C. Between NB plane and the long axis of upper incisors
    D. Between NB plane and the long axis of upper canine

103. The normal value of upper incisor to NB plane angle is
    A. 15 degree        B. 20 degree
    C. 25 degree
    D. 30 degree

104. Increased lower incisor to NB plane angle indicates
    A. Proclination of lower incisors
    B. Retroclination of lower incisors
    C. Rotation of lower incisors
    D. Rotation of upper incisors

105. Decreased lower incisor to NB plane angle indicates
    A. Proclination of lower incisors
    B. Retroclination of lower incisors
    C. Rotation of lower incisors
    D. Rotation of upper incisors

106. Tweed's Triangle makes use of which of the following plane angles?
    A. FMPA
    B. IMPA
    C. FMIA
    D. All of the above

107. FMPA in Tweed's cephalometric analysis stands for
    A. Frankfort mandibular plane angle
    B. Incisor mandibular plane angle
    C. Frankfort mandibular incisor plane angle
    D. All of the above

108. IMPA in Tweed's cephalometric analysis stands for
    A. Frankfort mandibular plane angle
    B. Incisor mandibular plane angle
    C. Frankfort mandibular incisor plane angle
    D. All of the above

109. FMIA in Tweed's cephalometric analysis stands for
    A. Frankfort mandibular plane angle
    B. Incisor mandibular plane angle
    C. Frankfort mandibular incisor plane angle
    D. All of the above

110. The normal value of FMPA in Tweed's cephalometric analysis is
    A. 16-35 degree
    B. 35-43 degree
    C. 45-63 degree
    D. 64-74 degree

111. Decreased FMPA in Tweed's cephalometric analysis indicates
    A. Horizontal growth pattern
    B. Vertical growth pattern
    C. Both A and B
    D. None of the above

112. Increased FMPA in Tweed's cephalometric analysis indicates
    A. Horizontal growth pattern
    B. Vertical growth pattern
    C. Both A and B
    D. None of the above

113. IMPA in Tweed's cephalometric analysis is
    A. 85-95 degree        B. 95-105 degree
    C. 105-125 degree      D. 125-135 degree

114. Decreased IMPA angle in Tweed's cephalometric analysis indicates
    A. Lower incisor proclination
    B. Lower incisor rotation
    C. Lower incisor retroclination
    D. Upper incisor proclination

115. Decreased IMPA angle in Tweed's cephalometric analysis indicates
    A. Lower incisor proclination
    B. Lower incisor rotation

C. Lower incisor retroclination
D. Upper incisor proclination

116. **The normal value of FMIA in Tweed's triangle is**
    A. 60-75 degree
    B. 75-85 degree
    C. 85-95 degree
    D. 95-105 degree

117. **Decreased FMIA in Tweed's triangle indicates**
    A. Lower incisor proclination
    B. Lower incisor rotation
    C. Lower incisor retroclination
    D. Upper incisor proclination

118. **Who described Wit's appraisal**
    A. Jacobson
    B. Rakosi
    C. Rickett's
    D. Down's

119. **In Wit's appraisal, if the point BO is located behind the point AO, it denotes**
    A. Skeletal class II jaw dysplasia
    B. Skeletal class III disharmonies
    C. Skeletal class I jaw dysplasia
    D. All of the above

120. **If the point BO is ahead than the point AO in Wit's appraisal, it denotes**
    A. Skeletal class II jaw dysplasia
    B. Skeletal class III disharmonies
    C. Skeletal class I jaw dysplasia
    D. All of the above

121. **Wit's Analysis was developed in**
    A. University of New York
    B. University of Bristol
    C. University of Witwatersrand
    D. None of the above

122. **Wit's analysis was developed primarily to study the**
    A. Inter-relationship of maxilla and mandible antero-posteriorly
    B. Relationship of maxilla to the anterior cranial base
    C. Relationship of mandible to the posterior cranial base
    D. None of the above

123. **Who discovered the X-ray**
    A. Roentgen
    B. Herbert Hofrath
    C. Pacini
    D. Rickett's

124. **In which year Roentgen discovered X-ray**
    A. 1931
    B. 1890
    C. 1895
    D. 1995

125. **Cephalometric means**
    A. Cephalo means head
    B. Metric means measurement
    C. Both A and B
    D. None of the above

126. **Soft tissue nasion is abbreviated as**
    A. N
    B. n
    C. N1
    D. N2

127. **Soft tissue pogonion is abbreviated as**
    A. S Pog
    B. S1 Pog
    C. SPOG
    D. Spog

128. **Prosthion is abbreviated as**
    A. PR
    B. Pr
    C. Pr
    D. Pros

129. **Steiner's analysis is a cephalometric analysis introduced by**
    A. Cecil C Roth
    B. Cecil C Steiner
    C. Steiner John
    D. Steff

130. **In which year Cecil C Steiner introduced Steiner's analysis**
    A. 1940
    B. 1930
    C. 1953
    D. 1960

131. **Rakosi Y-axis is the measured angle between**
    A. S-Gn
    B. N-S-Gn
    C. N-Gn
    D. Gn-S-Ar

**Ans:** 1. D  2. D  3. A  4. A  5. D  6. A  7. A  8. A  9. A  10. D  11. A  12. A  13. A  14. A  15. A  16. A  17. A  18. B  19. A  20. A  21. A  22. C  23. A  24. A  25. A  26. A  27. A  28. A  29. B  30. A  31. A  32. A  33. B  34. D  35. D  36. D  37. C  38. D  39. D  40. D  41. D  42. A  43. D  44. C  45. A  46. A  47. A  48. A  49. B  50. A  51. C  52. A  53. A  54. A  55. A  56. A  57. B  58. C  59. A  60. A  61. B  62. C  63. A  64. A  65. B  66. D  67. A  68. A  69. B  70. A  71. A  72. B  34. B  74. A  75. A  76. B  77. A  78. A  79. A  80. A  81. B  82. D  83. D  84. D  85. A  86. A  87. B  88. C  89. A  90. B  91. D  92. C  93. A  94. B  95. A  96. C  97. A  98. B  99. A  100. A  101. C  102. A  103. C  104. A  105. B  106. D  107. A  108. B  109. C  110. A  111. A  112. B  113. A  114. C  115. A  116. A  117. C  118. A  119. A  120. B  121. C  122. A  123. A  124. C  125. C  126. B  127. A  128. B  129. B  130. C  131. B

## MATURITY INDICATORS

1. **The following are biologic indicators of maturity except**
    A. Dental age
    B. Chronological age
    C. Skeletal age
    D. Sexual age

2. **Chronological age is unreliable guide for assessing a child's maturational status because**
    A. There is wide individual variation in terms of timing, duration and velocity of growth
    B. Boys and girls of same age may differ in their maturity status
    C. Children of the same age may vary on their maturity status
    D. All of the above

3. **All the following are ideal requirements of a maturity indicator except**
    A. Radiation exposure should be minimal
    B. Criteria should be different for boys and girls
    C. The stages of maturity should be well defined and easily identifiable
    D. It should be cost-effective

4. Skeletal maturity can be assessed using all the following except
   A. Chest radiograph
   B. Hand-wrist radiographs
   C. Cervical certebra on lateral cephalogram
   D. Water's Projection
5. Skeletal age for accesing biologic maturity is useful
   A. In childhood
   B. For adolescence only
   C. Throughout the post-natal growth period
   D. From birth to early adolescence
6. Sexual age as a biologic indicator of maturity is useful
   A. Only for adolescent growth
   B. Only for childhood growth spurts
   C. Throughout post-natal growth period
   D. None of the above
7. Dental age can be assessd by
   A. Eruption status of primary and permanent dentition
   B. By assessing calcification of crowns and teeth on radiographs
   C. By assessing development of roots of erupted and unerupted tooth
   D. All of the above
8. Dental age maturity indicators are useful
   A. From birth to late adolescence
   B. From birth to early adolescence
   C. Throughout post-natal growth period
   D. Upto 21 years of age
9. Morphologic age is based on
   A. Height gained
   B. Weight gained by individuals
   C. Height and weight gained
   D. Facial features
10. Morphologic age as a maturity indicator is useful
    A. From birth to adolescence
    B. From birth to early adolescence
    C. From late infancy to early adulthood
    D. From adolescence to late adulthood
11. Hand-wrist region consists of a total of
    A. 51 bones
    B. 29 bones
    C. 27 bones
    D. 13 bones
12. Numerous bones in the hand-wrist area develop from a total of
    A. 51 separate growth centres
    B. 29 growth centres
    C. 27 growth centres
    D. 15 growth centres
13. Hand-wrist radiographs provide useful means of assessing skeletal maturity because
    A. Development of these numerous small bones in the area from the appearance of calcification centers to complete ossification occurs throughout the entire post-natal growth period
    B. Different ossification centers in hand and wrist appears and mature at different times
    C. The appearance and progression of ossification of various ossification centers follow a predictable and scheduled pattern which can be standardized
    D. All of the above
14. The long bones of hand-wrist region are
    A. Trapezium and trapezoid
    B. Capitates and hamate
    C. Radius and ulna
    D. All of the above
15. The skeleton of hand-wrist region is made up of the following groups of bones except
    A. Distal ends of radius and ulna
    B. Carpals and metacarpals
    C. Phalanges
    D. Proximal ends of radius and ulna
16. Carpal bones are arranged in
    A. Two rows: left and right
    B. Two rows: proximal and distal
    C. Three rows: left, right and center
    D. None of the above
17. Proximal row of carpal bones is made of
    A. Scaphoid, lunate
    B. Trapezium and trapezoid
    C. Triquetrum and pisiform
    D. Both A and C
18. The distal row of carpal bones is made of
    A. Trapezium and trapezoid
    B. Capitates and hamate
    C. Pisiform and hamular process
    D. Both A and B
19. How many carpal bones are there in hand-wrist skeleton?
    A. 9 carpal bones
    B. 5 carpal bones
    C. 8 carpal bones
    D. 10 carpal bones
20. How many metacarpal bones are there in hand-wrist skeleton?
    A. 5 metacarpal bones
    B. 8 metacarpal bones
    C. 10 metacarpal bones
    D. 2 metacarpal bones
21. How many long bones are there in hand-wrist skeleton?
    A. 5 long bones
    B. 8 long bones
    C. 3 long bones
    D. 2 long bones
22. Each carpal bone ossifies from how many centers?
    A. 4 primary and 1 secondary centers
    B. 1 primary center
    C. 2 primary centers
    D. 2 secondary centers
23. Metacarpal bones of hand are conventionally numbered in
    A. From proximal to distal order
    B. Ulno-radial order (from medial to lateral)
    C. Radio-ulnar order (from lateral to medial side)
    D. All of the above
24. The metacarpal bones of hand are conventionally numbered so that
    A. The thumb has the first metacarpal bone while the little finger has fifth

B. The little finger has the first metacarpal bone while the thumb has the fifth
C. Both A and B
D. None of the above

25. Each metacarpal bone ossifies from
    A. 1 primary center
    B. 2 primary centers
    C. 1 primary center and 1 secondary center
    D. 2 secondary centers

26. Which of the following statements about metacarpal bones is false?
    A. Each metacarpal bone has a distal head, a shaft and a proximal base
    B. The rounded head of metacarpal bones articulates with the proximal phalanges
    C. Bases of metacarpal bones articulates with the distal row of carpal bones
    D. Their shafts articulate with proximal row of carpal bones

27. Which of the following statements is true?
    A. Each metacarpal bone ossifies from one primary centre in shaft and one secondary centre on its distal end except first metacarpal bone (thumb) where the secondary center appears at the proximal end
    B. Each metacarpal bone ossifies from one primary centre in shaft and one secondary centre on its proximal end except first metacarpal bone (thumb) where the secondary center appears at the distall end
    C. All metacarpal bones ossify from one primary center in shaft and one secondary center on distal end
    D. All metacarpal bones ossify from one primary center in shaft and one secondary center on proximal end

28. The phalanges are the small bones that form the skeleton of the fingers and there are a total of
    A. 15 phalanges    B. 14 phalanges
    C. 5 phalanges     D. 10 phalanges

29. Each digit of the hand has how many phalanges?
    A. 3 phalanges except thumb which has 2 phalanges
    B. 3 phalanges except thumb which has 1 phalange
    C. All digits have 3 phalanges each
    D. All digits have 2 phalanges each except thumb which has 3 phalanges

30. The phalanges of each digit are termed
    A. Left, right and center
    B. Head, shaft and base
    C. Proximal, middle and distal
    D. None of the above

31. The phalanges are ossified from
    A. 1 primary center for shaft and one distal epiphysis
    B. 1 primary center for shaft and a second proximal epiphysial center
    C. 2 primary centers
    D. 1 primary and 2 secondary centers

32. Ossification of the primary centre (shaft) of the phalanges begins
    A. Post natally around 2 years of life
    B. Prenatally
    C. Postnatally
    D. Postnatally around 3 years of life

33. The epiphysial centres, the secondary centers of the phalanges appears
    A. Prenatally
    B. At birth
    C. Postnatally at 1 year of life
    D. Postnatally around 2-4 years of life

34. Which of the following statements is false regarding ossification of phalanges?
    A. In the first stage, epiphysis and diaphysis and phalanx are equal
    B. The epiphysis caps the diaphysis by covering it like a Cao
    C. The diaphysis caps the epiphysis
    D. Fusion occurs between the epiphysis and the diaphysis at the end stage

35. Sesamoid bone is a
    A. Long bone of hand
    B. One of Carpal bone
    C. Small modular bone
    D. One of Metacarpal bone

36. Sesamoid is situated
    A. Embedded within the tendons on the region of the thumb
    B. Within tendons between fore fingers and middle finger
    C. Embedded within tendons in region of little finger
    D. Between little finger and ring finger

37. Ossification of ulnar sesamoid begins
    A. At birth
    B. Prenatally
    C. At onset of pubertal growth spurt
    D. Postnatally at 3 years of age

38. Which is the recent method of skeletal maturity of indicator gaining popularity?
    A. Hand-wrist radiographs
    B. Cervical vertebrae assessment on lateral cephalogram
    C. Pelvic radiographs
    D. All of the above

39. Following are the methods to assess skeletal age using hand-wrist radiographs except
    A. Grave and Brown method
    B. Greenwich and Pyle method
    C. Lamparski method
    D. Ringer's method

40. An atlas containing ideal skeletal age pictures of hand-wrist for different chronological ages of males and females are used in
    A. Greenwich and Pyle method
    B. Ringer's method

C. Fishman's method
D. Hog and Taranger method

41. In Bjork, Grave and Brown method skeletal development is divided into
    A. 11 stages     B. 5 stages
    C. 15 stages    D. 9 stages

42. Initial mineralization of ulnar sesamoid occurs at which stage of Bjork, Grave and Brown method?
    A. Stage 4     B. Stage 9
    C. Stage 5     D. Stage 7

43. The last stage (stage 9) of Bjork, Grave and Brown method signifies the end of skeletal growth and is characterized by
    A. Fusion of epiphysis and diaphysis of ulna
    B. Fusion of epiphysis and diaphysis of the radius
    C. Ossification of ulnar sesamoid
    D. Ossification of hook and hamate

44. In Bjork, Grave and Brown method, which stage signifies the end of pubertal growth spurt?
    A. Stage 9     B. Stage 4
    C. Stage 7     D. Stage 6

45. Leonard S. Fishman proposed his method of skeletal maturity indicators in the year
    A. 1982     B. 1985
    C. 1989     D. 1990

46. How many skeletal maturity indicators (SMIs) are there in Fishman's method?
    A. 10     B. 11
    C. 9      D. 12

47. In Fishman's method, stages of bone maturation used is
    A. Epiphysis is equal in width to diaphysis
    B. Appearance of adductor sesamoid and thumb
    C. Capping of epiphysis and fusion of epiphysis
    D. All of the above

48. In Fishman's method the following bones of hand-wrist radiographs are used to assess SMIs except
    A. Proximal, middle and distal phalanges of third finger
    B. Middle phanlage of fifth finger
    C. Middle phalange of index finger
    D. Sesamoid bone of radius

49. In Fishman's method, appearance of adductor sesamoid occurs at
    A. SMI 4     B. SMI 11
    C. SMI 9     D. SMI 7

50. SMI 11 of Fishman's method signifies
    A. Fusion of epiphysis of ulna
    B. Fusion of epiphysis and diaphysis of the radius
    C. Fusion of epiphysis and diaphysis of middle phalange of third finger
    D. Capping of epiphysis in middle phalange of third finger

51. Singer's method was developed in the year
    A. 1989     B. 1982
    C. 1980     D. 1990

52. How many developmental stages are there in Singer's method?
    A. 6      B. 9
    C. 11     D. 12

53. Which stage of Singer's method signifies prepubertal growth period?
    A. Stage 3     B. Stage 6
    C. Stage 2     D. Stage 4

54. Which stage of Singer's method signifies pubertal onset?
    A. Stage 3     B. Stage 6
    C. Stage 4     D. Stage 2

55. Growth modification procedures are best carried out in which stage of Singer's method?
    A. Stage 1 (early)
    B. Stage 3 (pubertal onset)
    C. Stage 4 (pubertal)
    D. Stage 2 (prepubertal stage)

56. Sesamoid begins to ossify at which stage of Singer's method?
    A. Stage 1 (early)
    B. Stage 3 (pubertal onset)
    C. Stage 4 (pubertal)
    D. Stage 2 (prepubertal stage)

57. Ideally orthodontic therapy should be completed and patient should be in retention period in which stage of Singer's method?
    A. Stage 4     B. Stage 5
    C. Stage 6     D. Stage 3

58. In Hagg and Taranger method, all of the following are assessed except
    A. Ulnar sesamoid
    B. Middle and distal phalanges of the third finger
    C. The distal epiphysis of ulna
    D. The distal epiphysis of the radius

59. Onset of peak height velocity is signified by
    A. Ossification of sesamoid bone
    B. Fusion of epiphysis and metaphysis of radius
    C. Capping epiphysis on etaphysis of middle phalange of third finger
    D. All of the above

60. Major disadvantage of hand-wrist radiographs for assessing skeletal maturity
    A. They are not accurate
    B. Need additional radiation exposure to orthodontic patients
    C. Hand-wrist is far away from jaws which is in the site of orthodontic correction
    D. Both B and C

61. Who first developed a method for skeletal maturity assessment using cervical vertebrae?
    A. Hassel and Farman     B. Lamparski
    C. San Roman             D. Tarranger

62. Cervical vertebrae maturity indicators method is gaining popularity in the recent years because
    A. Cervical vertebrae maturation can be assessed on lateral cephalograms which is regularly used in orthodontics

- B. Does not need additional radiation exposure to patient
- C. High correlation has been reposted between cervical vertebrae maturation and skeletal maturation of hand-wrist
- D. All of the above

63. **Hassel and Farman's cervical vertebrae maturation method has how many stages of development?**
    A. 9
    B. 6
    C. 11
    D. 5

64. **In Hassel and Farman's method the cervical vertebrae studied are**
    A. C1, C2 and C3
    B. C2, C3 and C4
    C. C3, C4 and C5
    D. C2 and C3

65. **In Hassel and Farman's method, which of the following morphologic characteristics of the cervical vertebrae are taken into account for assessing skeletal maturity?**
    A. Shape of the vertebral bodies
    B. Height of vertebral bodies
    C. Concavity, if the lower border of the cervical bodies
    D. All of the above

66. **As the skeletal maturity increases, the shape of cervical bodies change in the following way**
    A. Wedge shaped to rectangular and then to square shaped
    B. Wedge shaped to square shaped and later to rectangular
    C. Square shaped to rectangular and then to wedge shaped
    D. Rectangular to square shaped and then to wedge shaped at last

67. **As the skeletal maturity increases, the vertical dimension of the cervical vertebrae bodies**
    A. Decreases
    B. Increases
    C. Remains same
    D. None of the above

68. **As the skeletal maturity increases, the concavity of the lower borders of the cervical vertebral bodies C2, C3, C4 becomes**
    A. Accentuated
    B. Diminished
    C. Remains same
    D. Convex

69. **The cervical vertebrae attain maturity at which stage of Hassel and Farman method?**
    A. 6
    B. 4
    C. 5
    D. 3

70. **Peak of velocity is reached at which stage of Hassel and Farman cervical vertebrae maturation method?**
    A. 3
    B. 4
    C. 5
    D. 6

**Ans:** 1. B  2. D  3. B  4. D  5. C  6. A  7. D  8. B  9. A  10. C  11. B  12. A  13. D  14. C  15. D  16. B  17. D  18. D  19. C  20. A  21. D  22. B  23. C  24. A  25. C  26. D  27. A  28. B  29. A  30. C  31. B  32. D  33. D  34. C  35. C  36. A  37. C  38. B  39. C  40. A  41. D  42. A  43. B  44. D  45. A  46. B  47. D  48. C  49. A  50. B  51. C  52. A  53. C  54. A  55. D  56. B  57. B  58. C  59. A  60. D  61. A  62. D  63. B  64. B  65. D  66. A  67. B  68. A  69. C  70. A

## 5. BIOMECHANICS

### BIOLOGY OF TOOTH MOVEMENT

1. **Physiological tooth movement includes**
    A. Pre-eruptive tooth movement
    B. Eruptive tooth movement
    C. Post-eruptive tooth movement
    D. All of the above

2. **Posteruptive tooth movement is a compensatory movement for**
    A. Proximal wears only
    B. Occlusal wear only
    C. Both A and B
    D. None of the above

3. **Which of the below is not a theory of tooth eruption**
    A. Blood eruption theory
    B. Root growth theory
    C. Blood flow theory
    D. Hammock ligament therapy

4. **Hammock ligament theory was proposed by**
    A. Bien
    B. Sicher
    C. Oppenheim
    D. Schwarz

5. **Which theory is most accepted among tooth eruption theories?**
    A. Blood pressure theory
    B. Root growth
    C. Hammock ligament
    D. Periodontal ligament traction

6. **Frontal or direct resorption occurs**
    A. As a result of mild orthodontic forces
    B. Occurs on the pressure side of tooth movement
    C. Does not cause resorption of root
    D. All of the above

7. **When a force is applied to tooth**
    A. Areas of pressure are created
    B. Areas of tension are created
    C. Bone resorption and deposition occurs
    D. All of the above

8. **Tooth movement occurs due to**
    A. Osteoblastic activity only
    B. Osteoclastic activity only
    C. Both A and B
    D. None of the above

9. **Frontal resorption occurs as a result of**
    A. Mild orthodontic forces
    B. Excessive orthodontic forces

C. Compression on pressure side of tooth movement
D. All of the above
10. Periodontal ligament deprives of nutritional supply and showing regressive changes with cell free areas is called
   A. Direct resorption
   B. Frontal resorption
   C. Hyalinization
   D. Undermining resorption
11. Undermining or rearward resorption occurs as a result of
   A. Changes following mild forces
   B. Changes following moderate forces
   C. Changes following extreme forces
   D. None of the above

Ans: 1. D  2. C  3. C  4. B  5. D  6. D  7. D  8. C  9. A  10. C  11. C

## MECHANICS OF TOOTH MOVEMENT

1. In orthodontics, forces are commonly expressed in
   A. Newtons (N)
   B. Grams (g)
   C. Gram millimeters (gm.mm)
   D. All of the above
2. An object can have a center of mass
   A. Anywhere on universe
   B. On earth
   C. In a gravity free environment
   D. In oral cavity
3. When all points on a body moves to the same amount in the same direction, such a movement is called as
   A. Translation
   B. Bodily movement
   C. Tipping
   D. Both A and B
4. A tooth in the oral cavity can have a
   A. Center of resistance
   B. Center of mass
   C. Center of rotation
   D. Both A and C
5. The center of resistance is a point at which
   A. The resistance to tooth movement is concentrated
   B. The resistance to tooth movement is equally distributed
   C. The resistance to gravity is situated
   D. A or B
6. Location of the center of resistance of a tooth depends on
   A. Root length
   B. Morphology and of roots
   C. Level of alveolar bone support
   D. All of the above
7. Force can be defined as
   A. Load applied to an object from infinity
   B. Load applied to an object that will tend to move it to a different position in the space
   C. Load applied from an object that will tend to move it to infinity
   D. Both B and C
8. The center of resistance of a single rooted tooth with normal alveolar bone level is situated at about
   A. Two third the distance from CEJ to root apex
   B. Middle third of the root
   C. One fourth to one third the distance from CEJ to the root apex
   D. At root apex of tooth
9. When alveolar bone height is decreased the center of resistance of the tooth
   A. Shifts more apically
   B. Shifts more coronally
   C. Remains unchanged
   D. At middle third of the root
10. The center of resistance in case of multirooted teeth is located at
    A. At the center of furcation
    B. 1-2 mm apical to the furcation
    C. 1-2 mm coronal to the furcation
    D. At one third to one fourth the distance from CEJ to root apex
11. The center of resistance for maxilla is about
    A. 5-10 mm inferior to the orbitale
    B. Between roots maxillary molars
    C. The center of maxillary arch
    D. 1-2 mm apical to furcation of maxillary molar
12. Center of resistance of a tooth can be described in
    A. Vertical plane
    B. Horizontal plane
    C. Sagittal plane
    D. All three planes of space
13. A force is applied through the tooth's center of resistance, brings about
    A. Tipping moving of the tooth
    B. Controlled tipping of that tooth
    C. Translation/bodily movement of that tooth
    D. Rotation of the tooth
14. A single force that does not act through the center of resistance brings about
    A. Rotation of the tooth
    B. Translation/bodily movement of the tooth
    C. Controlled tipping of the tooth
    D. Medial movement of the tooth
15. A movement of force
    A. The tendency to translate
    B. Movement of a body through space
    C. Is a measure of the tendency to rotate
    D. Tendency to rotate
16. Center of resistance of the body is located
    A. Always within the body
    B. Either internal or external to the body

C. Can be at infinity
D. B and C

17. **Center of rotation can be defined as**
    A. A Point at which resistance of the body is concentrated
    B. A point at which rotation of the body is concentrated
    C. An arbitrary point about which a body appears to have rotated as determined from its initial and final position
    D. A point at which movement of body is concentrated

18. **Which of the following statements is false**
    A. Center of rotation is constant for a tooth
    B. Location of center of rotation varies depending on how far the force is applied from the center of resistance
    C. Center of rotation is different for different type of tooth movement
    D. None of the above

19. **The center of rotation**
    A. Is same as center of resistance
    B. Can coincide with center of resistance
    C. Can approach but can never reach the center of resistance
    D. B or C

20. **Center of rotation can be located**
    A. Internal to the body always
    B. External to the body always
    C. At center of resistance
    D. Either internal or external to the body

21. **Center of rotation in bodily tooth movement is at**
    A. Infinity
    B. Apex of root
    C. Middle 3rd of root
    D. Incisal edge

22. **Center of rotation in uncontrolled tipping is at**
    A. Infinity
    B. Near but not at the center of resistance
    C. Root apex
    D. Outside the tooth

23. **In controlled tipping the center of rotation is located**
    A. Outside the tooth
    B. At infinity
    C. At infinity
    D. At root apex

24. **Center of rotation during intrusion and extrusion is**
    A. Outside the tooth
    B. At infinity
    C. At middle 3rd of root
    D. At CEJ

25. **The moment of force (Mf) is determined by multiplying the magnitude of the force (F) with**
    A. The distance from the force
    B. The perpendicular distance of the line of action of force to the center of resistance
    C. The perpendicular distance of the line of action of force to the center of rotation
    D. The parallel distance from the center of resistance

26. **The unit of measurement of moment of force is**
    A. Newtons
    B. Grams
    C. Gram millimeters
    D. Gram/millimeter

27. **Which of the following is the correct formula?**
    A. $Mf = F$
    B. $Mf = F \times d$
    C. $F = Mf \times d$
    D. None of the above

28. **A force couple is**
    A. A pair of concentrated forces having equal magnitude and opposite direction with parallel but noncollinear line of action
    B. Consists of three forces of equal magnitude acting in three planes of space
    C. A pair of forces of equal magnitude acting in same direction
    D. A and C

29. **A force couple brings about**
    A. A bodily tooth movement
    B. Pure rotation
    C. Tipping movement
    D. Intrusion of tooth

30. **Most of the tooth movements occurring in routine orthodontic treatment are**
    A. Pure translation
    B. Pure rotation
    C. Combination of translation and rotation
    D. Tipping movements

31. **In orthodontics, the term "rotation" is used to describe movement of tooth**
    A. Around a faciolingual axis
    B. Around the long axis of the tooth
    C. Around the mesiodistal axis
    D. Around buccolingual axis

32. **In orthodontics, movement of tooth around a faciolingual axis is called as**
    A. Tipping
    B. Torquing
    C. Rotation
    D. Bodily movement

33. **Movement of tooth around mesiodistal axis is called as**
    A. Tipping
    B. Torquing
    C. Rotation
    D. Translation

34. **Tipping can be of**
    A. 3 types, controlled, uncontrolled, upright
    B. 2 types, mesial and distal
    C. 2 types, right and left
    D. 2 types, uncontrolled and controlled

35. **When a single force is applied at the crown of a tooth, it brings about**
    A. Controlled tipping
    B. Uncontrolled tipping
    C. Tooth movement
    D. Rotation

36. **In uncontrolled tipping**
    A. Crown of the tooth moves in the direction of the force and the root in the opposite direction
    B. Root of the tooth moves in the direction of force and the crown in the opposite direction
    C. Crown and root both move in the direction of force
    D. Crown and root move opposite to the direction of force

37. During uncontrolled tipping, stresses in the periodontal ligament are
    A. Uniformly distributed all around the tooth
    B. Concentrated near apex
    C. Concentrated near cervical areas
    D. Not uniform and are concentrated near apex and cervical area
38. Uncontrolled tipping is
    A. Often undesirable
    B. Very difficult to achieve
    C. Most desirable type of tooth movement
    D. A and B
39. In controlled tipping
    A. Crown moves in the direction of force and root in opposite direction
    B. Crown moves in the direction of force but root does not move
    C. Both crown and root move in the same direction of force
    D. Root moves in the direction of force

Ans: 1. B  2. C  3. D  4. D  5. A  6. D  7. B  8. C  9. A  10. B  11. A  12. D  13. C  14. A  15. C  16. A  17. C  18. A  19. C  20. D  21. A  22. B  23. D  24. A  25. B  26. C  27. B  28. A  29. B  30. C  31. B  32. B  33. A  34. D  35. B  36. A  37. D  38. A  39. B

## 6. PREVENTIVE AND INTERCEPTIVE ORTHODONTICS

### PREVENTIVE ORTHODONTICS

1. Preventive orthodontics is undertaken:
    A. Before development of a malocclusion
    B. After the malocclusion has already manifested
    C. After the eruption of 3rd molars
    D. All of the above
2. Extraction of supernumerary teeth before they displace other teeth is a
    A. Interceptive procedure
    B. Preventive procedure
    C. Corrective procedure
    D. Surgical procedure
3. Which of the following is a preventive orthodontic procedure
    A. Occlusal equilibration
    B. Extraction of supernumerary teeth
    C. Prevention of damage to occlusion
    D. All of the above
4. Which procedure is undertaken as a part of preventive orthodontic procedure
    A. Parent education
    B. Caries control
    C. Management of abnormal frenal attachment
    D. All of the above
5. Preventive dentistry should ideally begin
    A. Before birth of the child
    B. After the birth of child
    C. During mixed dentition period
    D. During permanent dentition period
6. If the child is bottle, fed the mother is advised to use
    A. Physiologic nipple
    B. Conventional nipple
    C. Artificial nipple
    D. All of the above
7. Physiologic nipple permits
    A. Sucking of milk resembling normal functional activity
    B. Easy passage of milk into child's oral cavity
    C. Dental caries prevention
    D. All of the above
8. Classical example of natural space maintainer is
    A. Deciduous dentition
    B. Deciduous molars
    C. Permanent molars
    D. Permanent dentition
9. Application of topical fluorides and pit and fissure sealants
    A. Helps in preventing caries
    B. Is a common preventive orthodontic procedure
    C. Both A and B
    D. All of the above
10. Approximation of maxillary central incisors can be prevented by
    A. Abnormal labial frenum attachment
    B. Mesiodens
    C. Deciduous incisors
    D. Both A and B
11. Enamel pearls may cause
    A. Occlusal interference
    B. Premature contact
    C. Both A and B
    D. None of the above
12. Delay in eruption of teeth may be caused due to
    A. Fibrosis of gingiva
    B. Cyst and tumors
    C. Overhanging restorations in deciduous teeth
    D. All of the above
13. Ankylosed teeth show
    A. Absence of periodontal ligament
    B. Do not get resorbed
    C. Prevents eruption of suceedaneous teeth
    D. All of the above
14. Blanch test is used to diagnose
    A. Mouth breathing
    B. Tongue tie
    C. Frenal attachment
    D. Abnormally thick maxillary labial frenum attachment

15. Lowered tongue position and difficulty in speech can be due to
    A. Ankyloglossia
    B. Abnormal labial frenum in maxillary arch
    C. Occlusal interference
    D. Geographic tongue
16. Milwaukee brace is used for
    A. Correction of class II malocclusion
    B. Correction of scoliosis
    C. For TMJ stabilization
    D. Correction of class III malocclusion
17. Hitchcock Raymond C Thurrow and Hinrichsen are recognized for
    A. Space maintainers
    B. Acrylic partial dentures
    C. Complete dentures
    D. None of the above
18. A space maintainer should be
    A. Simple in construction
    B. Not exert excessive stress on adjoining teeth
    C. Not come in way of other functions
    D. All of the above
19. Example of a removable space maintainer
    A. Acrylic partial denture
    B. Full or complete denture
    C. Removable distal shoe space maintainer
    D. All of the above
20. Esthetic anterior space maintainer was first described by
    A. Hitchcock, Raymond, and Hinrichsen
    B. Hitchcock, steffen and R.C Thurrow
    C. Steffen, Miller and Johnson
    D. Raymond, Hinrichsen and Johnson
21. The most common space maintainer used in dental practice is
    A. Crown and loop
    B. Lingual arch
    C. Transpalatal arch
    D. Band and loop
22. Space maintainer of choice when there is a carious tooth adjacent to the space
    A. Acrylic partial denture
    B. Lingual arch
    C. Band and loop
    D. Crown and loop
23. Selection of a crown and loop space maintainer depends on the
    A. Carious extent of adjacent tooth to the space
    B. Periodontal support of the adjacent tooth to the space
    C. Shape of palate
    D. Both B and C
24. The most effective space maintainer in lower arch is
    A. Acrylic partial denture
    B. Distal shoe appliance
    C. Lingual arch
    D. Band and loop
25. Nance holding arch derives its support from
    A. Anterior teeth
    B. Permanent 1st molars
    C. Anterior palate
    D. Soft palate
26. Space maintainer of choice when one side of the arch is intact and several primary teeth on the other side are missing is
    A. Lingual arch
    B. Transpalatal arch
    C. Nance palatal arch
    D. Distal shoe space maintainer
27. Intra alveolar appliance is a synonym for
    A. Palatal arch appliance
    B. Lingual arch appliance
    C. Distal shoe appliance
    D. Transpalatal arch appliance
28. Appliance used to guide 1st permanent molar in case of early loss of 2nd primary molar is
    A. Crown and loop
    B. Band and loop
    C. Modification of crown and loop
    D. Intra alveolar appliance
29. The most common distal shoe appliance used in practice is
    A. Nance distal shoe     B. Roche's distal shoe
    C. Both A and b
    D. None of the above
30. Intragingival extension is a feature of
    A. Palatal arch appliance
    B. Modification of Roche's distal shoe
    C. Lingual arch
    D. Crown and band
31. Esthetic anterior space maintainer was first described in the year
    A. 1970     B. 1979
    C. 1980     D. 1971
32. Crown and bar space maintainer is a modification of
    A. Crown and loop     B. Bar and loop
    C. Band and loop      D. Band and bar
33. Which of the following is a cantilever type of space maintainer
    A. Distal shoe         B. Nance palate arch
    C. Transpalatal arch   D. Band and bar
34. Nursing bottle syndrome control can be achieved by
    A. Educating young mothers about the syndrome
    B. Using conventional nipple
    C. By Fluoride
    D. Usage of pacifiers
35. Bitewing radiograph aids in diagnosis of
    A. Root caries         B. Occlusal caries
    C. Proximal caries     D. Any of the above
36. In cleft palate patients who require obturation of palatal cleft the space maintainer of choice is
    A. Crown and loop      B. Band and loop
    C. Transpalatal arch
    D. Removable space maintainer

37. According to Hinrichsen a distal shoe appliance comes under
   A. Class I fixed space maintainer
   B. Class II fixed space maintainer
   C. Class III fixed space maintainer
   D. Class IV fixed space maintainer

38. In a deeply locked permanent 1st molar the preferred treatment would be
   A. Distal shoe or intra alveolar appliance
   B. Slicing the distal surface of primary 2nd molar
   C. Extraction of 1st molar and guiding 2nd molar
   D. Any of the above

Ans: 1. A 2. B 3. D 4. D 5. A 6. A 7. A 8. A 9. C 10. D 11. C 12. D 13. D 14. D 15. A 16. B 17. A 18. D 19. D 20. A 21. A 22. A 23. C 24. D 25. C 26. B 27. C 28. D 29. B 30. B 31. D 32. D 33. A 34. A 35. C 36. D 37. B 38. B

## INTERCEPTIVE ORTHODONTICS

1. Interceptive Orthodontics is undertaken
   A. Before the birth of child
   B. After the birth of child
   C. Before development of malocclusion
   D. When malocclusion in developing or developed

2. Which of this does not constitute a interceptive orthodontic procedure
   A. Parent and patient education
   B. Serial extraction
   C. Space maintenance
   D. Space regaining

3. The term serial extraction was first used by
   A. Kjellgren
   B. Nance
   C. Dewey
   D. Raymond. C. Thurrow

4. The term planned and progressive extraction was used by
   A. Nance in USA
   B. Nance in Sweden
   C. Kjellgren in USA
   D. Kjellgren in Sweden

5. Nance popularized the serial extraction and termed it as planned and progressive extraction in the year
   A. 1940
   B. 1929
   C. 1970
   D. 1979

6. Active supervision of teeth by extraction was termed by
   A. Kjellgren in 1929
   B. Nance in 1940
   C. Hotz in 1970
   D. Hitchcock in 1959

7. Planned and progressive extraction is related to
   A. Wilkinson's extraction
   B. Serial extraction
   C. Supernumerary tooth extraction
   D. Any of the above

8. Serial extraction is indicated in
   A. Absence of physiologic spacing
   B. Malposition or impacted teeth
   C. Lower anterior flaring
   D. All of the above

9. Serial extraction is contraindicated in
   A. Absence of physiologic spacing
   B. Ankylosis of one or more teeth
   C. Ectopic eruption
   D. Midline diastema

10. According to most authors serial extraction is carried when space needed is
    A. 5-7 mm
    B. 3-4 mm
    C. 10-12 mm
    D. 8-9 mm

11. The most common model analysis in lower arch prior to serial extraction procedure is
    A. Carey's analysis
    B. Ashley Howe's analysis
    C. Peck and Peck analysis
    D. Radiographic method of analysis

12. The most common analysis in upper arch prior to serial extraction procedure is
    A. Arch perimeter analysis
    B. Bolton's analysis
    C. Carey's analysis
    D. Ashley Howe's analysis

13. In Dewel's method, the first tooth to be extracted is
    A. Deciduous central incisor or A
    B. Deciduous lateral incisor or B
    C. Deciduous canine or C
    D. Deciduous first molar or D

14. In Dewel's method, the second tooth to be extracted is
    A. Deciduous first molar or D
    B. Deciduous central incisor or A
    C. Deciduous lateral incisor or B
    D. Deciduous canine or C

15. In Dewel's method the third tooth to be extracted is
    A. Deciduous central incisor
    B. Permanent first molar
    C. Permanent first premolar
    D. Permanent canine

16. In Dewel's method the extraction of first tooth is carried out at
    A. 8-9 years
    B. 6-7 years
    C. 5-6 years
    D. 11-12 years

17. In modified Dewel's method which tooth is enucleated at the time of extraction of first deciduous molars
    A. Permanent first premolar
    B. Permanent canine
    C. Permanent lateral incisor
    D. Deciduous canine

18. Modified Dewel's method is carried out in the case of
    A. Mandibular arch where canine erupt before first premolar
    B. Maxillary arch where canine erupt after first premolar
    C. Maxillary arch where canine erupt before first premolar
    D. Mandibular arch where canine erupt after first premolar
19. The first tooth to be extracted in Tweed's method
    A. Deciduous first molar
    B. Deciduous second molar
    C. Deciduous canine
    D. Permanent first premolar
20. The second tooth to be extracted in Tweed's technique of serial extraction
    A. Permanent first molars
    B. Deciduous first molars
    C. Permanent first premolars
    D. Deciduous canines
21. The third tooth to be extracted in Tweed's method
    A. Deciduous canines
    B. Permanent first molars
    C. Deciduous first molars
    D. Permanent first premolars
22. According to Tweed the first tooth should be extracted during the age of
    A. 7 years
    B. 6 years
    C. 8 years
    D. 10 years
23. Best time to correct anterior crossbite
    A. 6 years
    B. 7 years
    C. First time it is seen
    D. After eruption of all anterior teeth
24. Anterior crossbite is a condition in which one or more maxillary anterior teeth are
    A. In lingual relation to mandibular teeth
    B. In vertical relation to mandibular teeth
    C. In horizontal relation to mandibular teeth
    D. Any of the above
25. In anterior crossbite the overjet is
    A. Greater than 7-8 mm
    B. Greater than 5-6 mm
    C. Reversed
    D. 1-2 mm
26. Single tooth anterior crossbite usually occurs due to
    A. Functional placement of mandible in a forward direction
    B. Over retained deciduous teeth
    C. Mesiodens
    D. Supernumerary teeth
27. Dento alveolar crossbite can be best treated by
    A. Tongue blades
    B. Catlan's appliance
    C. 'Z' spring with posterior bite plane
    D. Any of the above
28. Functional anterior crossbite is seen in
    A. Class I malocclusion
    B. Class II division 2 malocclusion
    C. Class III malocclusion
    D. Pseudo Class III malocclusion
29. Functional crossbite occurs due to
    A. Supernumerary teeth
    B. Occlusal prematurities
    C. Early loss of permanent first molars
    D. Over retained deciduous teeth
30. Functional crossbite is best treated by
    A. Catlan's appliance
    B. Elimination of occlusal prematurities
    C. Removal of over retained deciduous teeth
    D. All of the above
31. Skeletal anterior crossbite can occur due to
    A. Maxillary skeletal retrognathism
    B. Maxillary skeletal prognathism
    C. Mandibular skeletal retrognathism
    D. Combination of all of the above
32. Skeletal anterior crossbite can occur due to
    A. Mandibular skeletal prognathism
    B. Maxillary skeletal prognathism
    C. Mandibular skeletal retrognathism
    D. Combination of all of the above
33. Skeletal anterior crossbites are best treated by
    A. 'Z' spring with posterior bite plane
    B. Catlan's appliance
    C. Growth modification procedures during growth
    D. Any of the above
34. The most common habit frequently practiced by children which brings about damaging effect on dentoalveolar structure is
    A. Digit sucking
    B. Tongue thrusting
    C. Mouth breathing
    D. Lip biting
35. Presence of digit or thumb sucking habit is considered normal upto
    A. 6 years the time of eruption of permanent molars
    B. 5 years
    C. 7 years
    D. 2 ½ - 3 years
36. Tongue thrust can cause
    A. Open bite
    B. Maxillary Anterior proclination
    C. Mandibular anterior proclination
    D. Any of the above
37. Educating the patient on correct method of swallowing can prevent
    A. Thumb sucking habit
    B. Digit sucking habit
    C. Lip biting habit
    D. Tongue thrusting habit
38. Mouth breathing can be of
    A. Functional or non-functional
    B. Anterior or posterior
    C. Obstructive or non-functional
    D. Obstructive or habitual

39. Obstructive mouth breathing can be due to
    A. Nasal polyps
    B. Nasal tumours
    C. Deviated nasal septum
    D. All of the above
40. Habitual mouth breathing occurs due to
    A. Nasal polyps
    B. Enlarged adenoids
    C. Persistence of habit even after removal of nasal obstruction
    D. Nasal tumours
41. Habitual oral breathing is best treated by
    A. Oral screen
    B. Catalan's appliance
    C. Night guard
    D. Anterior bite plane
42. Mirror test is used in diagnosing
    A. Lip biting
    B. Thumb sucking
    C. Tongue thrusting
    D. Mouth breathing
43. Water test is helpful in diagnosis of
    A. Mouth breathing
    B. Lip biting
    C. Thumb sucking
    D. Lateral tongue thrust
44. Rhinomanometry is used in
    A. Diagnosis of mouth breathing
    B. Treatment of thumb sucking
    C. Treatment of mouth breathing
    D. Diagnosis of thumb sucking
45. Which of the following is an interceptive orthodontic procedure?
    A. Space maintenance
    B. Space regaining
    C. Caries control
    D. Care of deciduous teeth
46. Which of the following is used for space regaining?
    A. Gerber appliance
    B. Crown and loop
    C. Roche's distal shoe
    D. Transpalatal arch
47. Clenching of teeth by the patient while counting to ten is the best exercise for
    A. Buccinators muscle
    B. Masseter muscle
    C. Mentalis muscle
    D. Muscularis oris
48. Stretching of upper lip to maintain lip seal is an important therapeutic measure in patients having
    A. Short hypertonic lip
    B. Short hypotonic lip
    C. Long hypertonc lip
    D. Hyperactive mentalis muscle
49. Button pull exercise is done for
    A. Lips
    B. Tongue
    C. Cheeks
    D. Teeth
50. Tug of war exercise is a good exercise for
    A. Masseter muscle
    B. Buccinators muscle
    C. Tongue
    D. Lips
51. One elastic swallow exercise is for
    A. To prevent tongue thrusting
    B. To prevent lip biting
    C. To prevent bruxism
    D. To correct improper positioning of tongue
52. Hold pull exercise is helpful in
    A. Preventing tongue thrusting
    B. Proper positioning of tongue
    C. Stretching the lingual frenum
    D. Lip seal
53. One elastic swallow and two elastic swallow are exercises for
    A. Lips
    B. Tongue
    C. Cheeks
    D. Preventing bruxism
54. Father of serial extraction is
    A. Kjellgren
    B. Tweed
    C. Nance
    D. Dewel

Ans: 1. D  2. C  3. A  4. A  5. A  6. C  7. B  8. D  9. D  10. A  11. A  12. A  13. C  14. A  15. C  16. A  17. A  18. A  19. A  20. C  21. A  22. C  23. C  24. A  25. C  26. B  27. D  28. D  29. B  30. B  31. A  32. A  33. C  34. A  35. D  36. D  37. D  38. D  39. D  40. C  41. A  42. D  43. A  44. A  45. B  46. A  47. B  48. B  49. A  50. D  51. D  52. C  53. B  54. C

## ORAL HABITS AND THEIR MANAGEMENT

1. Habit can be defined as
    A. Learned patterns of muscular contraction
    B. Fixed or constant practice established frequent repetition
    C. Learned patterns of muscular contraction which are complex in nature
    D. All of the above
2. According to Finn, habit is
    A. An act which is socially unacceptable
    B. Learned patterns of muscular contraction
    C. Both of the above
    D. None of the above
3. According to Moyer habit is
    A. Learned patterns of muscular contraction
    B. **Learned patterns of muscular contraction which are complex in nature**

C. An act which is socially unacceptable
D. Fixed or constant practice established by frequent repetition

4. Which statement is true?
   - All oral habits exert abnormal forces on the teeth.
   - Deleterious oral habits contribute directly or indirectly to the occurrence of different types of malocclusion.
   A. First statement is true
   B. Second statement is true
   C. Both statements A and B are true
   D. Both statements A and B are false

5. William James classified habits into
   A. Useful and harmful habits
   B. Empty and meaningful habits
   C. Compulsive and non-compulsive habits
   D. Pressure and non-pressure habits

6. William James described useful and harmful habits in the year
   A. 1926        B. 1927
   C. 1923        D. 1925

7. Klien classified habits into
   A. Useful and harmful
   B. Unintentional and intentional
   C. Compulsive and non-compulsive
   D. Pressure and non-pressure

8. Klien described empty and meaningful habits in the year
   A. 1971        B. 1972
   C. 1968        D. 1969

9. According to Klien an unintentional habit is also called as
   A. Compulsive habit    B. Empty habit
   C. Meaningful habit    D. Pressure habit

10. Klien described meaningful habit also as
    A. Intentional habit   B. Compulsive habit
    C. Pressure habit      D. All of the above

11. Finn described habit as
    A. Useful and harmful
    B. Unintentional and intentional
    C. Compulsive and non-compulsive
    D. Pressure and non-pressure

12. Useful habits include
    A. Correct tongue posture
    B. Proper respiration
    C. Deglutition
    D. All of the above

13. Which is not an "empty habit"?
    A. Chin propping
    B. Abnormal pillowing
    C. Combination of A and B
    D. Deglutition

14. Habits which are easily learned and dropped from child's behavioral pattern as he matures are called as
    A. Compulsive habits
    B. Non-compulsive habits
    C. Pressure habits
    D. Harmful habits

15. Sucking during infancy is an example for
    A. Harmful habits
    B. Empty habits
    C. Unintentional habits
    D. Physiologic habits

16. A best example of pathologic habits is
    A. Mouth breathing due to enlarged adenoids
    B. Bruxism
    C. Chin propping
    D. Nail biting

17. "Thumb sucking is placement of one thumb or one or more fingers in varying depth into the mouth" was defined by
    A. Gellin      B. Moyers
    C. Finn        D. Klein

18. "Repeated and forceful sucking of thumb with associated strong facial and lip contraction" was put forth by
    A. Moyer       B. Klein
    C. Finn        D. Gellin

19. Sucking can be classified as
    A. Useful and harmful
    B. Empty and meaningful
    C. Nutritive and non-nutritive
    D. All of the above

20. Nuk Sauger Nipple is an example of
    A. Conventional nipple
    B. Non physiologic nipple
    C. Physiologic nipple
    D. Combination of A and B

21. The term Non-nutritive sucking habits was first described by
    A. Johnson and Larson    B. Moyers and Finn
    C. William James         D. Normaa Kingsley

22. Johnson and Larson described non nutritive sucking theory in the year
    A. 1990        B. 1994
    C. 1993        D. 1989

23. Cook classified thumb sucking into
    A. Alpha group     B. Beta group
    C. Gamma group     D. All of the above

24. In alpha group of cook's classification of thumb sucking, there is
    A. Only buccal wall contraction
    B. Strong buccal wall contraction and a negative pressure
    C. Alternative positive and negative pressure
    D. All of the above

25. In beta group of Cook's classification of thumb sucking, there is
    A. Alternative positive and negative pressure
    B. Only buccal wall contraction
    C. Strong buccal wall contraction and negative pressure
    D. None of the above

26. In Gamma group of Cook's classification of thumb sucking, there is
    A. Only buccal wall contraction
    B. Alternative positive and negative pressure
    C. Strong buccal wall contraction and negative pressure
    D. Combination of A and B
27. Subtelny classified thumb sucking into
    A. Type A, B, C, D
    B. Level I,II,III,IV
    C. Division I,II,III,IV
    D. Class I,II,III,IV
28. Psychoanalytic theory was described by
    A. Sigmund Freud
    B. Scars and Wire
    C. Benjamin
    D. Sheldon
29. Sigmund Freud described psychoanalytical theory in the year
    A. 1895
    B. 1905
    C. 1915
    D. 1925
30. Who advocated that non-nutritive sucking develop from an inherent psychosexual drive
    A. Benjamin
    B. Sears and wise
    C. Sheldon
    D. Sigmund Freud
31. Oral drive theory was given by
    A. Sears and wise
    B. Benjamin
    C. Sheldon
    D. Sigmund Freud
32. Oral drive theory was given in the year
    A. 1982
    B. 1992
    C. 2002
    D. 1892
33. Who proposed that non-nutritive sucking is the result of prolongation of nursing and not the frustration of wearing
    A. Benjamin
    B. Sears and Wise
    C. Moyer's
    D. Sigmund Freud
34. Sucking increases the erotogenesis of the mouth. Who gave this theory?
    A. Sigmund Freud
    B. Benjamin
    C. Pear and Wine
    D. Palermo
35. Oral gratification theory was proposed by
    A. Sheldon
    B. Benjamin
    C. Pear and wine
    D. Palermo
36. Oral gratification theory was proposed in the year
    A. 1932
    B. 1962
    C. 1992
    D. 1902
37. Learning theory was proposed by
    A. Palermo
    B. Sheldon
    C. Benjamin
    D. Pear and Wire
38. Learning theory was putforth in the year
    A. 1956
    B. 1966
    C. 1976
    D. 1986
39. Which theory regards thumb sucking as a learned pattern with no underlying psychological basis?
    A. Oral gratification Theory
    B. Learning theory
    C. Oral drive theory
    D. None of the above
40. Trident condition factors of thumb sucking are
    A. Duration
    B. Frequency or indulgence
    C. Intensity of force
    D. All of the above
41. Prolonged digit sucking can produce effects on
    A. Maxilla
    B. Mandible
    C. Interarch relationship
    D. All of the above
42. Effects of thumb sucking on maxilla include
    A. Increased SNA angle and maxillary arch length
    B. Increased clinical crown length of maxillary incisors
    C. Counter clockwise rotation of occlusal plane
    D. All of the above
43. Effects of thumb sucking on mandible includes
    A. Retroclination of mandibular incisors
    B. Decreased SNB angle
    C. Both A and B
    D. None of the above
44. Management of thumb sucking habit includes
    A. Psychologic approach-behaviour modification
    B. Reminder therapy
    C. Appliance therapy
    D. All of the above
45. Which of the following agents are used for management of thumb sucking habit by chemical method?
    A. Cayenne pepper
    B. Quinine
    C. Asafetida and Ginger garlic paste
    D. All of the above
46. Fixed appliance in management of thumb sucking habit include
    A. Palatal arch with cribs
    B. Palatal arch with rakes or spurs
    C. Quad helix
    D. All of the above
47. When quad helix is placed as habit breaking appliance for thumb sucking, which part of the appliance act as a reminder?
    A. Anterior helices
    B. Posterior helices
    C. Palatal bridge
    D. Retentive arms
48. Which statement is correct?
    I. Tongue thrusting always causes proclination of anteriors and anterior open bite.
    II. Tongue thrusting is abnormal tongue activity in which tongue is thrust between upper and lower teeth during swallowing.
    A. I statement is true
    B. II statement is false
    C. II statement is true
    D. Both statements are true
49. Etiologic classification of tongue thrusting includes
    A. Physiologic and habitual
    B. Functional and anatomic
    C. Both A and B
    D. None of the above
50. Physiologic tongue thrust occurs due to
    A. Repeated placement of tongue

B. Macroglossia
   C. Normal tongue thrust swallow of infancy
   D. Attempt to establish oral seal during swallowing
51. Backland classified tongue thrusting into
   A. Anterior and posterior tongue thrust
   B. Simple and complex
   C. Both of the above
   D. None of the above
52. Moyer classified tongue thrust into
   A. Simple, complex and retained infantile swallow
   B. Anterior and posterior
   C. Physiologic and habitual
   D. Functional and anatomic
53. Which one of the etiological factors leads to tongue thrusting?
   A. Genetic factors
   B. Persistence infantile swallow pattern
   C. Both A and B
   D. None of the above
54. Mechanical restriction factors causing tongue thrust include
   A. Macroglossia
   B. Enlarged adenoids
   C. Constricted dental arches
   D. All of the above
55. Neurological disturbances causing tongue thrust include
   A. Hyposensitive palate
   B. Moderate motor disability and loss of precision in oral function
   C. Disruption of tactile sensory control and coordination of swallowing
   D. All of the above
56. Extraoral features of tongue thrust includes
   A. Incompetent lips
   B. Increased anterior facial height
   C. Decreased nasolabial angle
   D. All of the above
57. Which of the below does not attribute to intraoral features of tongue thrusting?
   A. Maxillary anterior proclination
   B. Decreased nasolabial angle
   C. Generalized spacing between teeth
   D. Proclination of mandibular anteriors
58. Tongue thrust can be self correcting by the age of
   A. 5-6 years        B. 7-8 years
   C. 4-5 years        D. None of the above
59. Which of the following exercise helps on management of tongue thrusting habit
   A. Whistling
   B. Reciting the count from 60-69
   C. Gargling and Yawning
   D. All of the above
60. Orthodontic trainer helps in management of
   A. Lip biting
   B. Tongue thrusting
   C. Digit sucking
   D. All of the above
61. Appliance used in treatment of tongue thrust is
   A. Habit breaking appliance with tongue crib
   B. Nance palatal arch appliance
   C. Oral screen and Fixed rake or crib
   D. All of the above
62. Sim and Finn classified mouth breathing as
   A. Obstructive and habitual
   B. Obstructive, habitual and anatomic
   C. Habitual and anatomic
   D. Physiologic and pathologic
63. Anatomic mouth breathers have
   A. Obstruction to normal flow of air through nasal passage
   B. Developed the habit even after the obstruction has been removed
   C. Short upper lip that does not permit full closure without on due effect
   D. All of the above
64. Intranasal defects causing mouth breathing
   A. Deviated nasal septum
   B. Nasal polyps
   C. Thick nasal septum
   D. All of the above
65. Playing a wind instrument may be an useful interceptive orthodontic procedure in the management of
   A. Lip biting        B. Bruxism
   C. Tongue thrusting  D. All of the above
66. Lip habits include
   A. Lip sucking       B. Lip wetting
   C. Lip biting        D. All of the above
67. Clinical features of lip biting habit include
   A. Abrasion or cuts on lips
   B. Proclination of maxillary anteriors
   C. Retroclination of mandibular anteriors
   D. All of the above
68. Management of lip biting includes
   A. Elimination of cause
   B. Correction of malocclusion
   C. Appliance therapy
   D. All of the above
69. Clinical features of cheek biting habit include
   A. Ulcer at level of occlusion
   B. Open bite
   C. Individual tooth malposition
   D. All of the above
70. Management of nail biting habit involves
   A. Scolding
   B. Nagging
   C. Treating the basic emotional factors causing the habit
   D. All of the above
71. Who defined "bruxism" as the "habitual grinding of teeth when the individual is not chewing or swallowing'?
   A. Rubina
   B. Ramfjord

C. William James
D. Moyer

72. Occupational factors contributing to bruxism
    A. Anxiety
    B. Rage
    C. Compulsive over achievers
    D. Occlusal discrepancies

73. Management of bruxism includes
    A. Occlusal adjustments
    B. Occlusal splints
    C. Psychotherapy and Acupuncture technique
    D. All of the above

74. Bruxism treatment can be achieved by
    A. Orthodontic correction
    B. Electrical methods
    C. Drugs such as ethyl chloride and Psychotherapy
    D. All of the above

Ans: 1. D  2. A  3. B  4. B  5. A  6. C  7. B  8. A  9. B  10. A  11. C  12. D  13. D  14. B  15. D  16. A  17. A  18. A  19. C  20. C  21. A  22. C  23. D  24. A  25. C  26. B  27. A  28. A  29. B  30. D  31. A  32. A  33. B  34. A  35. A  36. A  37. A  38. A  39. B  40. D  41. D  42. D  43. C  44. D  45. D  46. D  47. A  48. D  49. C  50. C  51. A  52. A  53. C  54. D  55. D  56. D  57. B  58. B  59. D  60. D  61. D  62. B  63. C  64. D  65. C  66. D  67. D  68. D  69. D  70. D  71. B  72. C  73. D  74. D

## 7. TREATMENT PLANNING

### ORTHODONTIC TREATMENT PLANNING

1. Whenever extractions are planned in a class I skeletal or dental pattern, it is vitally important that extractions are done in
    A. In both upper and lower arches
    B. In upper arch only
    C. In lower arch only
    D. In right quadrant of either upper or lower arches

2. In most class II malocclusion cases, it is possible to reduce the abnormal upper proclination and also to discourage the forward development of the upper arch by extraction of teeth only in
    A. Lower arch
    B. Upper arch
    C. Neither upper or lower arches
    D. Either right or left quadrant of lower arch

3. In Angle's class III malocclusion it is beneficial to avoid
    A. Extraction in upper arch
    B. Extraction in lower arch
    C. Extraction in either right or left quadrant of lower arch
    D. Neither in upper nor in lower arches

4. The anchorage demand for an individual patient depends on the following factors, except
    A. Number of teeth being moved
    B. Type of teeth movement
    C. Duration of treatment
    D. Number of activation of appliance

5. Selection of appliance depends on the following factors, except
    A. Growth potential
    B. Oral hygiene maintenance
    C. Type of tooth movement
    D. Cast of the patient

6. The potential for relapse is increased by the presence of certain factors which are listed as follows, except
    A. Stretched periodontal ligament
    B. Unstable occlusion
    C. Continuation of growth pattern
    D. Centric relation

7. Which of the following condition does NOT require space for orthodontic correction
    A. Correction of crowding
    B. Rotation
    C. Correction of proclined teeth
    D. Correction of midline diastema

8. At what age orthodontic treatment can be started
    A. 2 months
    B. 2 years
    C. 4 years
    D. 6 years

9. How do we manage a case of 3 years old with missing 51?
    A. Functional space maintainer
    B. Lingual arch space maintainer
    C. Band and bar space maintainer
    D. Crown and bar space maintainer

10. Midline distema of 2.5 mm width in a 50 years old women can be best treated by
    A. Orthodontic approach
    B. Prosthodontic approach
    C. Conservative approach
    D. Periodontal approach

11. The growth status of the individual for carrying out appropriate treatment procedure should be determined prior to
    A. Treatment planning
    B. Retention
    C. Both A and B
    D. None of the above

12. In the fabrication of an appliance for minor tooth movement which of the following will not be considered important while arranging for anchorage?
    A. The natural tendency for tooth movement in the arch
    B. Lip posture and function
    C. Occlusal interlock
    D. The pressure required to move teeth

13. Which of the following affect the outcome of the treatment of class II division 2 malocclusion most?
    A. Incompetent lips
    B. Class II skeletal relation
    C. Low FH angle
    D. Abnormal oral habit
14. After comprehensive orthodontic treatment, for the reorganization of the PDL, full time retention with a removable appliance should be given for
    A. 2-6 months
    B. 3-4 months
    C. 9-12 months
    D. 12-24 months
15. The optimum time for treatment of a malocclusion is
    A. Between age 5 and 8 years
    B. Between 8 and 10 years
    C. Between 10 and 12 years
    D. At any age depending on the problem involved
16. Retention period in orthodontics is necessary because
    A. The ligaments in the gingiva must be stabilized
    B. The teeth will become mobile if retention is not completed
    C. Both of the above
    D. Neither of the above
17. Which of the following is essential for tooth movement to occur?
    A. A cellular cementum
    B. Vital pulp
    C. Vital periodontal ligament
    D. Vital dentin
18. The goals of orthodontics are
    A. Acceptable facial esthetics
    B. Attainment of normal function
    C. Best possible occlusal relationsip
    D. All of the above
19. Relapse occurs most frequently with which type of tooth movement?
    A. Extrusion
    B. Tipping
    C. Rotation
    D. Translation
20. Transient malocclusions are
    A. Age related
    B. Self correcting
    C. Normal in adult occlusion
    D. Both A and B
21. Age can be expressed in
    A. Neural age
    B. Mental age
    C. Nutritional age
    D. Both A and B
22. Neural tissue reaches complete maturity at the age of
    A. 18 years
    B. 15-16 years
    C. 10-12 years
    D. 6-7 years
23. What is the benefit of treating malocclusion at an early age?
    A. Dentofacial growth is active at an early age
    B. Minimum psychological disturbances to cope with
    C. Natural tendencies of growth pattern can be used to guide erupting teeth
    D. All of the above

Ans: 1. A  2. B  3. A  4. D  5. D  6. D  7. D  8. D  9. A  10. C  11. A  12. A  13. B  14. B  15. D  16. A  17. C  18. D  19. C  20. D  21. D  22. D  23. D

## ANCHORAGE IN ORTHODONTICS

1. Definition of anchorage is given by:
    A. Graber
    B. White and Gardner
    C. Both A and B
    D. None
2. Intra-oral sources of anchorage are
    A. Teeth
    B. Alveolar bone
    C. Musculature
    D. All of the above
3. Extra-oral sources of anchorage are
    A. Cranial bones
    B. Facial bones
    C. Basal jaw bones
    D. Both A and B
4. The following is an example of intra-maxillary anchorage
    A. Class I elastics
    B. Class II elastics
    C. Class III elastics
    D. Box elastics
5. The following is an example of inter-maxillary anchorage
    A. Class I elastics
    B. Class II elastics
    C. Class III elastics
    D. Both B and C
6. Cross elastic is an example of
    A. Reciprocal anchorage
    B. Inter-maxillary anchorage
    C. Stationary anchorage
    D. Both A and B
7. Bilateral symmetrical expansion is a type of
    A. Reciprocal anchorage
    B. Inter-maxillary anchorage
    C. Stationary anchorage
    D. Simple anchorage
8. Correction of midline diastema is an example of
    A. Reciprocal anchorage
    B. Inter-maxillary anchorage
    C. Stationary anchorage
    D. Simple anchorage
9. Correction of single tooth crossbite is an example of
    A. Reciprocal anchorage
    B. Inter-maxillary anchorage
    C. Stationary anchorage
    D. Simple anchorage
10. Inter-maxillary anchorage is the anchorage in which
    A. The resistance units are situated within the same jaw
    B. Resistance units in one jaw are used to effect tooth movement in the other jaw
    C. Combination of A and B
    D. None of the above
11. Lip bumper is an example of
    A. Muscular anchorage

B. Reciprocal anchorage
C. Stationary anchorage
D. Extraoral anchorage

12. **Retraction of a premolar using a molar tooth is**
    A. **Primary anchorage**
    B. Multiple anchorage
    C. Compound anchorage
    D. Reinforced anchorage

13. **Compound anchorage is regularly used in**
    A. **Fixed mechanotherapy**
    B. Myofunctional orthodontics therapy
    C. Removable orthodontic therapy
    D. All of the above

14. **Transpalatal arch is**
    A. **Reinforced anchorage**
    B. Reciprocal anchorage
    C. Compound anchorage
    D. Stationary anchorage

15. **Anchorage planning depends on which of the following factors:**
    A. Number of teeth to be moved
    B. Type of teeth to be moved
    C. Type of tooth movement
    D. All of the above

16. **In maximum anchorage cases**
    A. No more than 25% of extraction space should be lost by forward movement of anchor teeth
    B. 75% or more of the extraction space is needed for the retraction of the anteriors
    C. Both A and B
    D. None of the above

17. **In maximum anchorage cases**
    A. Mesial movement of posteriors is not advised
    B. Distal movement of anteriors is not advised
    C. Combination of A and B
    D. None of the above

18. **Which type of anchorage is not critical**
    A. Maximum anchorage
    B. Minimum anchorage
    C. Moderate anchorage
    D. None of the above

19. **Anchor loss refers to**
    A. Unwanted movement of anchor teeth
    B. Desired movement of anchor teeth
    C. Loss of anchor teeth
    D. None of the above

20. **More the number of teeth to be moved**
    A. Less the anchorage needed
    B. Greater is the demand of anchorage
    C. Not related to anchorage
    D. None of the above

21. **Anchorage during orthodontic therapy is mainly obtained from**
    A. Intraoral and extraoral sources
    B. Intraoral sources only
    C. Cranium only
    D. Alveolar bone

22. **'Anchorage in the site of delivery from which force is exerted' was defined by**
    A. Graber
    B. White and Gardiner
    C. Newton
    D. Robert J Nicoli

23. **Greater resistance to displacement is offered when force exerted to move teeth is**
    A. Perpendicular to that of their axial inclination
    B. Parallel to that of their axial inclination
    C. Opposite to that of their axial inclination
    D. All of the above

24. **Ankylosed teeth**
    A. Are not to be used as anchor teeth
    B. Serve as excellent anchors
    C. Are easy to move
    D. Directly fused to PDL

25. **Hard palate and lingual surface of mandible in the region of roots**
    A. Used to augment intra-maxillary anchor
    B. Used to augment inter-maxillary anchor
    C. Both A and B
    D. None of the above

26. **Extraoral source of anchorage include**
    A. Cranium
    B. Back of neck
    C. Facial bone
    D. All of the above

27. **Anchorage from cranium is obtained by**
    A. Occipital bone
    B. Parietal bone
    C. Frontal bone
    D. All of the above

28. **Anchorage derived from back of the neck is**
    A. **Mainly from neck or cervical region**
    B. Cranial bone
    C. Clavicles
    D. All of the above

29. **Head gear that derives anchorage from forehead and chin is called as**
    A. Cervical head gear
    B. Occipital head gear
    C. Reverse head gear
    D. All of the above

30. **Simple anchorage in an appliance is obtained by engaging**
    A. Greater number of teeth than are to be moved in same dental arch
    B. Lesser number of teeth than are to be moved in same dental arch
    C. Equal number of teeth than are to be moved in same dental arch
    D. All of the above

31. **A classical example of simple anchorage**
    A. Pushing palatally placed premolar with rest of the teeth in dental arch as anchor
    B. Closure of midline diastema
    C. Correction of single tooth crossbite
    D. All of the above

32. **Resistance offered by two malposed units in the same dental arch applying equal and opposite forces is an example of**
    A. Simple anchorage
    B. Stationary anchorage
    C. Reciprocal anchorage
    D. All of the above

33. **Example of reciprocal anchorage**
    A. Closure of midline diastema by movement of two central incisors towards each other

B. Single tooth crossbite correction using intermaxillary elastics
C. Dental arch expansion using coffin spring
D. All of the above

34. **Lip bumper to distalize molars is an example of**
    A. Extraoral anchorage
    B. Intraoral anchorage
    C. Intramaxillary anchorage
    D. Muscular anchorage

35. **Closure of midline diastema is an example of**
    A. Intermaxillary anchorage
    B. Stationary anchorage
    C. Intramaxillary anchorage
    D. Both B and C

36. **Baker's anchorage is also known as**
    A. Intra-maxillary anchorage
    B. Intraoral anchorage
    C. Extraoral anchorage
    D. Inter-maxillary anchorage

37. **Class II and class III elastic traction used during orthodontic therapy is an example for**
    A. Inter-maxillary anchorage
    B. Baker's anchorage
    C. Both A and B
    D. None of the above

38. **Single tooth anchorage is also called**
    A. Primary anchorage
    B. Reciprocal anchorage
    C. Stationary anchorage
    D. Compound anchorage

39. **Resistance provided by more than one tooth with greater alveolar support to move teeth with lesser support is termed as**
    A. Multiple anchorage
    B. Reinforced anchorage
    C. Stationary anchorage
    D. Compound anchorage

40. **Reinforced anchorage uses**
    A. Extraoral sources
    B. Intraoral sources
    C. Combination of A and B
    D. None of the above

41. **Upper anterior inclined plane and transpalatal arch connecting left and right maxillary molars are examples of**
    A. Multiple anchorage
    B. Reinforced anchorage
    C. Both A and B
    D. Stationary anchorage

42. **Modification of anterior inclined plane is**
    A. Baller's appliance
    B. Sved appliance
    C. Activator
    D. All of the above

43. **Anchorage loss is termed as**
    A. Unwanted movement of anchor units
    B. Favourable movement of anchor units
    C. Space closed by anchor units
    D. All of the above

44. **In maximum anchorage case**
    A. ¼th of extraction space can be lost by movement of anchor units
    B. ½th of extraction space can be lost by movement of anchor units
    C. ⅔rd of extraction space can be lost by movement of anchor units
    D. Whole extraction space can be lost by movement of anchor units

45. **Anchorage demand of an extraction case can be of three types of anchorage namely**
    A. Maximum/critical, moderate, minimum
    B. Simple, stationary, reinforced
    C. Single, compound, multiple
    D. None of the above

46. **In moderate anchorage of an extraction case**
    A. ¼ – ½ of extraction space closure is permitted by movement of anchor teeth
    B. Less than ¼th of extraction space closure is permitted
    C. Whole extraction space closure may be permitted
    D. All of the above

47. **In minimum anchorage case**
    A. More than half of extraction space closure is permitted
    B. Less than half of extraction space closure is permitted
    C. ¼th of extraction space closure is permitted
    D. ½th of extraction space closure is permitted

48. **Two finger springs incorporated into a removable orthodontic appliance to close midline diastema is an example of**
    A. Stationary anchorage
    B. Reciprocal anchorage
    C. Multiple anchorage
    D. Reinforced anchorage

49. **Class I elastic traction during fixed orthodontic therapy is an example of**
    A. Intramaxillary anchorage
    B. Reciprocal anchorage
    C. Reinforced anchorage
    D. Multiple anchorage

50. **Chin cup with occipital head gear as anchor units serve the purpose of**
    A. Restriction of mandibular growth
    B. Protraction of mandible
    C. Protraction of maxilla
    D. Restriction of maxillary growth

**Ans:** 1. C  2. D  3. D  4. A  5. D  6. D  7. A  8. A  9. A  10. B  11. A  12. A  13. A  14. A  15. D  16. C  17. A  18. B  19. A  20. B  21. A  22. B  23. C  24. B  25. C  26. D  27. D  28. A  29. C  30. A  31. A  32. C  33. D  34. D  35. D  36. D  37. C  38. A  39. D  40. C  41. C  42. B  43. A  44. A  45. A  46. A  47. A  48. B  49. A  50. A

## METHODS OF GAINING SPACE

1. **Creation of space in the dental arch may be required to correct certain features of malocclusion such as:**
   A. Crowding
   B. Overjet reduction
   C. Leveling of the curve of spee
   D. All of the above

2. **Creation of space in the dental arch may be required to correct certain features of malocclusion such as:**
   A. Correction of incisor inclination
   B. Correction of incisor angulations
   C. Leveling of the curve of spee
   D. All of the above

3. **Various methods of gaining space in orthodontics includes:**
   A. Proximal stripping
   B. Uprighting of molars
   C. Proclination of anterior teeth
   D. All of the above

4. **What are the various methods of gaining space in orthodontics?**
   A. Expansion of the dental arches
   B. Extraction of certain teeth
   C. Distalization of molars
   D. All of the above

5. **Synonyms of proximal stripping includes:**
   A. Proximal slicing of a tooth/teeth
   B. Reproximation of a tooth/teeth
   C. Slenderization /disking of a tooth / teeth
   D. All of the above

6. **Indications of proximal stripping include:**
   A. To relieve mandibular anterior crowding
   B. Mild tooth material excess according to Bolton's analysis
   C. Both A and B
   D. None of the above

7. **Proximal stripping is contraindicated in patient with:**
   A. Dental caries
   B. Large pulp chamber
   C. Severe affected teeth
   D. All of the above

8. **An advantage of proximal stripping is it:**
   A. Avoids extraction in borderline cases
   B. To prevent dental caries
   C. Both A and B
   D. None of the above

9. **Disadvantage of proximal stripping include:**
   A. Patient may experience sensitivity of teeth
   B. Altered morphology of teeth
   C. Highest incidence of caries
   D. All of the above

10. **According to Peck and Peck analysis, proximal stripping is indicated if:**
    A. Mesiodistal dimension of tooth is less than labiolingual dimension
    B. Labiolingual dimension is less than mesiodistal dimension
    C. Both A and B
    D. None of the above

11. **According to Bolton's analysis, proximal stripping is indicated when there is:**
    A. An excess tooth material compatible to arch length in either of the arches
    B. An excess tooth material comparable to arch length in only maxillary arch
    C. An excess tooth material comparable to arch length in only mandibular arch
    D. All of the above

12. **Proximal stripping can be done using:**
    A. Abrasive strips
    B. Long thin tapered fissured bur
    C. Safe-sided carborundum disk
    D. All of the above

13. **When is the best time for molar distalization:**
    A. During mixed dentition period before the eruption of second permanent molar
    B. During mixed dentition period
    C. At 10-12 years of age
    D. Both A and C

14. **An advantage of molar distalization includes :**
    A. It avoids extraction of teeth
    B. It prevents arch collapse
    C. Combination of A and B
    D. None of the above

15. **Lokar distalizing appliance is a:**
    A. Intra-oral distalization appliance
    B. Extra-oral distalization appliance
    C. Both A and B
    D. Removable orthodontic appliance

16. **Which of the following is an intra-oral distalization appliance?**
    A. Veltri bilateral sagittal screw
    B. Monolateral sagittal screw
    C. Fast appliance
    D. All of the above

17. **The following are intra-oral molar distalization appliances except:**
    A. Lip bumpers    B. Jasper jumper
    C. First class appliance   D. None of the above

18. **Which of the following is the intra-oral distalization appliance?**
    A. Magnets
    B. Open coil spring appliance
    C. Pendulum appliance
    D. All of the above

19. **Which of the following is an intra-oral distalization appliance?**
    A. Schwartz appliance
    B. Sagittal appliance
    C. Willson's distalizing arch
    D. All of the above

20. **Which of the following is an extra-oral distalizing appliance?**
    A. Head gears    B. Distal jet appliance

C. Chin cup appliance
D. All of the above

21. **Uprighting of molar is:**
    A. A method of gaining space to relieve crowding in the arches
    B. Done when tilted molars due to early loss of deciduous second molar or extraction of permanent second premolar
    C. Combination of A and B
    D. None of the above

22. **Uprighting of molars can be done using:**
    A. **Uprighting spring**    B. Open coil spring
    C. Closed coil spring    D. All of the above

23. **Tilted molars can cause:**
    A. Crowding in the arch   B. Spacing in the arch
    C. Both A and B    D. None of the above

24. **Correction of rotated teeth helps in:**
    A. Relieving crowding in the arches
    B. Prevention of dental caries
    C. Prevention of periodontal disease
    D. All of the above

25. **Correction of rotated posterior teeth is best done by:**
    A. Fixed mechanotherapy using a force couple
    B. Removable orthodontic appliance
    C. Myofunctional orthodontic appliance
    D. All of the above

26. **Who first described the distal jet as a fixed lingual appliance that required no compliance from the patient?**
    A. Carano    B. Testa
    C. Carano and Testa    D. Willson

27. **Distal jet appliance consist of:**
    A. Unilateral piston and tube arrangement
    B. **Bilateral piston and tube arrangement**
    C. Neither A nor B
    D. Combination of A and B

28. **How do we activate the distal jet appliance?**
    A. By pushing the collar distally which later compress the coil spring
    B. By pushing the collar mesially which later compress the coil spring
    C. Neither A nor B
    D. Combination of A and B

29. **What is the schedule of activation of distal jet?**
    A. Once every 3-4 weeks during distalization
    B. Once every 4-6 weeks during distalization
    C. Once every 1-2 weeks during distalization
    D. Once every 7-8 weeks during distalization

30. **What is the time duration required to produce translator movement of the maxillary molar using distal jet?**
    A. 2-4 months    B. 2-5 months
    C. 4-6 months    D. 4-8 months

31. **Why distal jet appliance is referred to as piston and tube arrangement?**
    A. It consist of a tube which is embedded in the acrylic plate of a bayonet wire inserted into the lingual sheath on the first molar bands extends into the tube much like a piston
    B. It consist of piston and tube
    C. Both A and B
    D. None of the above

32. **Which type of spring is used for distal jet?**
    A. Closed coil spring
    B. Superelastic nickel-titanium open coil spring
    C. Uprighting spring
    D. Rotating spring

33. **Distal jet appliance derive the anchorage from**
    A. Molar teeth
    B. Premolar
    C. Molars and premolars
    D. **Palate with the use of acrylic button**

34. **Upon completion of distalization of the molars, how does the distal jet appliance can be converted to a palatal holding arch?**
    A. By removal of the coil spring (peeling it off the tube with utility pliers)
    B. Locking the activation collar over the junction of the tube and piston
    C. Mesial set screw is locked onto the tube
    D. All of the above

35. **Upon completion of distalization of the molars, how does the distal jet appliance can be converted to a palatal holding arch?**
    A. The distal jet is locked onto the piston
    B. Supporting wire is sectioned from the premolars
    C. Nance button is sectioned with a dental hand piece of a bur
    D. All of the above

36. **Who introduced the pendulum appliance?**
    A. Hilgers
    B. Casino
    C. Testa
    D. None of the above

37. **Pendulum appliance is used mainly for:**
    A. Class II correction in the noncompliant patient to expand the maxilla and simultaneously rotate and distalize the maxillary first molars
    B. Class III correction
    C. Both A and B
    D. None of the above

38. **Pendulum appliance:**
    A. Was introduced by Hilgers
    B. Was used for class II correction in the non-compliant patient to expand the maxilla and simultaneously rotate and distalize the maxillary first molars
    C. It requires minimum patient cooperation
    D. All of the above

39. **Distalization spring in pendulum appliance is made of:**
    A. 0.032" beta-titanium wire
    B. 0.031" beta-titanium wire
    C. 0.030" beta-titanium wire
    D. 0.029" beta-titanium wire

40. **How much force is produced from pendulum appliance?**
    A. 230 g/side B. 231 g/side
    C. 229 g/side D. 230.8 g/side

41. **How many activations pendulum appliance required?**
    A. It requires only a one time activation of 60-70°
    B. It requires only a one time activation of 40-60°
    C. It requires only a one time activation of 10-20°
    D. It requires only a one time activation of 90°

42. **What is the function of a loop in the spring of pendulum appliance?**
    A. For expansion
    B. Prevent any tendency for the maxillary molar to move lingually into a crossbite
    C. Both A and B
    D. None of the above

43. **What are the common features among distal jet, pendulum and Jones jig appliance?**
    A. All three consist of acrylic button in their design
    B. All three are used for distalization
    C. All three are intra-oral distalizing appliance
    D. All of the above

44. **Acrylic palatal button is anchored to which tooth in Jones jig appliance?**
    A. Palatal aspect of band of first premolar and first molars
    B. Buccal aspect of band of 1st premolar and 1st molars
    C. Either A or B
    D. Neither A or B

45. **Acrylic palatal button is anchored to which tooth in distal jet appliance?**
    A. Palatal aspect of band of first premolar and first molars
    B. Buccal aspect of band of first premolar and first molars
    C. Either A or B
    D. Neither A or B

46. **Acrylic palatal button is anchored to which tooth in pendulum appliance?**
    A. Palatal aspect of band of first premolar and first molars
    B. Buccal aspect of band of first premolar and first molars
    C. Either A or B
    D. Neither A or B

47. **Who and when Herbst appliance developed?**
    A. Herbst in 1900 B. Herbst in 1901
    C. Herbst in 1902 D. Herbst in 1903

48. **Slenderization is carried out to:**
    A. Reduce mesio-distal width of the teeth
    B. Reduce labio-lingual width of teeth
    C. Both of the above
    D. None of the above

49. **Reproximation is carried out routinely in:**
    A. Lower anteriors
    B. Upper anteriors
    C. Buccal segment of upper arch
    D. Buccal segment of lower arch

50. **Proximal stripping is indicated when Carey's analysis shows discrepancy of:**
    A. 0 – 1 mm B. 0 – 2.5 mm
    C. 2.5 – 5 mm D. More than 5 mm

51. **In proximal stripping the enamel thickness is reduced maximum up to:**
    A. 60 % B. 40 %
    C. Not more than 50 % D. 70 %

52. **Proximal stripping is carried out by:**
    A. Metallic abrasive strips
    B. Safe sided carborundum discs
    C. Long thin tapered fissure burs
    D. All of the above

53. **The major drawback of slenderization**
    A. Increased susceptibility to caries
    B. Sensibility
    C. Periodontal problem
    D. Tooth mobility

54. **Increased susceptibility to caries following slenderization is best treated by:**
    A. Composite restoration B. Crown
    C. Fluoride program D. All of the above

55. **One of the older non invasive method of gaining space is:**
    A. Proximal stripping B. Arch expansion
    C. Extraction D. Distalization

56. **Expansion as a method of gaining space can be best considered in patients with:**
    A. Constricted maxillary arch
    B. Broad maxillary arch
    C. Retrognathia maxilla
    D. Any of the above

57. **Extraction undertaken as a part of orthodontic treatment is called:**
    A. Balanced extraction
    B. Serial extraction
    C. Therapeutic extraction
    D. Wilkinson's extraction

58. **Most frequently sacrificed tooth as part of orthodontic treatment is:**
    A. First premolar
    B. Second premolar
    C. Lateral incisor
    D. Third molar

59. **Space gained by extraction of premolar can be utilized for correction of:**
    A. Anterior segment of arch
    B. Posterior segment of arch
    C. Both A and B
    D. None of the above

60. **Advanced method of gaining space in recent times is:**
    A. Extraction of premolars
    B. Expansion

C. Proximal stripping
D. Distalisation

61. **Ideal time for distalisation is**
    A. During mixed dentition period
    B. During mixed dentition after eruption of 1st permanent molar
    C. During mixed dentition after eruption of second permanent molar
    D. During mixed dentition before eruption of second permanent molar

62. **Which of the below cannot be used for distalisation?**
    A. Open coil spring
    B. Closed coil spring
    C. Jack screw incorporated into baseplate
    D. Intraoral magnets

63. **Space gaining can be accompanied by**
    A. Uprighting of molars
    B. De-rotation of posterior teeth
    C. Proclination of anterior teeth
    D. All of the above

64. **Which of the below is not a space gaining technique?**
    A. Uprighting of molars
    B. De-rotation of anterior teeth
    C. Proclination of anterior teeth
    D. Slenderization

65. **Proclination of anteriors can be undertaken when:**
    A. Less or minimal effect on soft tissue profile of the patient
    B. Spacing in the arches
    C. Patient is cooperative
    D. Any of the above

66. **Correction of many malocclusions requires:**
    A. Teeth and time
    B. Space and time
    C. Teeth and space
    D. None of the above

67. **Space can be obtained:**
    A. By only 1 method
    B. By many methods
    C. Only by extractions
    D. None of the above

68. **Proximal stripping and distalization are:**
    A. Methods of gaining space
    B. Methods of slicing the tooth for esthetics
    C. Involves pushing the tooth only
    D. Tooth space gainer and reducing the tooth

69. **Proclination of anteriors:**
    A. Cause mandibular retrognathism
    B. Create space
    C. Solves crowding
    D. Cause maxillary prognatism

70. **Extraction in orthodontics:**
    A. Create disturbance in dentition
    B. Cause space formation
    C. Cause tooth retraction
    D. Cause teeth to be lost without any effect on malocclusion

71. **Proximal stripping means:**
    A. Slice the tooth B – L
    B. Slice the tooth M – L
    C. Slice the tooth both bucco – lingual and M – L
    D. All of the above

72. **Slenderization refers to:**
    A. Reproximation, disking and proximal slicing
    B. Reproximation, slicing the whole tooth and cutting the tooth
    C. Reproximation only
    D. Disking but not proximal slicing

73. **Reproximation refers to:**
    A. Lower anteriors only
    B. Lower anteriors and upper anteriors only
    C. On any tooth surface
    D. Only on molars

74. **Space required in case of proximal stripping:**
    A. 0 – 0.5 mm
    B. 0 – 2.5 mm
    C. 0.5 – 2.5 mm
    D. 0.8 – 2.5 mm

75. **Analysis of proximal stripping is named as:**
    A. Bolton's analysis
    B. Boulber's analysis
    C. Boucher's analysis
    D. Bolder's analysis

76. **Proximal stripping should be carried out in patient:**
    A. Young patients without caries
    B. Increased risk of pulpal exposure
    C. Higher caries index
    D. None of the above

77. **In case of borderline cases in proximal stripping it is better:**
    A. To slice mesially only
    B. To slice buccally only
    C. To slice both mesial and buccal only
    D. To avoid extraction in borderline cases

78. **Broadening the contact area:**
    A. Useful as it eliminates small contact points
    B. Useless as it decreases tooth surface area
    C. Should not be carried out as risk of pulpal exposure
    D. Good as increases surface area and cause rotation

79. **Diagnostic aids for proximal stripping:**
    A. Arch perimeter analysis
    B. Bolton's analysis
    C. Both A and B
    D. None of the above

80. **Arch perimeter analysis is:**
    A. Same as Carey's analysis
    B. Not same as Carey's analysis
    C. Same as Bolton's analysis
    D. Different criteria taken into consideration

81. **Amount of proximal stripping:**
    A. 50 % dentin
    B. 50 % dentin and enamel
    C. 50 % enamel
    D. 100 % enamel

82. **Proximal stripping cause:**
    A. Plaque accumulation

B. Caries susceptibility
C. Sensitivity   D. All of the above

83. **Proximal stripping is carried out by:**
    A. Use of metallic abrasive strips
    B. Safe sided carborundum discs
    C. Long thin tapered fissure burs
    D. All of the above

84. **Expansion is indicated in case of:**
    A. Constricted maxillary arch
    B. Unilateral or bilateral cross bite
    C. Both A and B
    D. All of the above

85. **Expansion can be:**
    A. Skeletal or dentoalveolar
    B. Single tooth
    C. Whole arch
    D. One segment

86. **Expansion can be brought about by:**
    A. Jack screw and springs
    B. Nance holding arch
    C. Sagittal appliance
    D. All of the above

87. **Skeletal expansion means:**
    A. Dento alveolar expansion
    B. No skeletal change
    C. Only dental expansion
    **D. Splitting of mid palatal suture**

88. **Extraction in orthodontic treatment is:**
    A. Therapeutic extraction
    B. Normal extraction
    C. Premolar extraction
    D. Molars and lower incisors only

89. **Distalization is:**
    A. Moving the molars in a distal direction
    B. Extracting the tooth which is distally placed
    C. Moving anteriors in a distal direction
    D. None of the above

90. **Distalization can be brought by:**
    A. By extraoral method
    B. Intraoral method
    C. Both extraoral and intraoral method
    D. Neither extraoral nor intraoral

91. **Extraoral method of distalization:**
    A. Head gears   B. Sagittal appliance
    C. None of the above   D. All of the above

92. **Head gears consist of:**
    A. Face bow with inner and outer bow
    B. Inner bow only
    C. Outer bow only
    D. Face bow without inner and outer bow

93. **Distalization is advantageous because:**
    A. No need for patient cooperation
    B. Has not to be worn continuously
    C. Both A and B
    D. All of the above

94. **Intraoral appliance are:**
    A. Sagittal appliance
    B. Nance holding appliance
    C. Open coils and pendulum appliance
    D. All of the above

95. **Pendulum appliance:**
    A. Extra oral method
    B. Intra oral method
    C. Modified nance button
    D. B and C only

96. **Pendulum appliance consists of:**
    A. Helix and sleeves
    B. Helix only
    C. Sleeves only
    D. None of the above

Ans: 1. **D**  2. **D**  3. **D**  4. **D**  5. **D**  6. **C**  7. **D**  8. **A**  9. **D**  10. **A**  11. **A**  12. **D**  13. **D**  14. **C**  15. **A**  16. **D**
17. **D**  18. **D**  19. **D**  20. **C**  21. **C**  22. **A**  23. **C**  24. **D**  25. **A**  26. **C**  27. **B**  28. **A**  29. **B**  30. **C**  31. **A**  32. **B**
33. **D**  34. **D**  35. **D**  36. **A**  37. **A**  38. **D**  39. **A**  40. **A**  41. **A**  42. **C**  43. **D**  44. **A**  45. **A**  46. **A**  47. **A**  48. **A**
49. **A**  50. **B**  51. **C**  51. **D**  52. **D**  53. **A**  54. **C**  55. **A**  56. **A**  57. **C**  58. **A**  59. **C**  60. **D**  61. **D**  62. **B**  63. **D**
64. **B**  65. **A**  66. **B**  67. **B**  68. **A**  67. **B**  70. **B**  71. **A**  72. **A**  73. **C**  74. **B**  75. **A**  76. **A**  77. **D**  78. **A**  79. **C**
80. **A**  81. **B**  82. **D**  83. **D**  84. **C**  85. **A**  86. **D**  87. **D**  88. **A**  89. **A**  90. **C**  91. **A**  92. **A**  93. **C**  94. **D**  95. **D**
96. **A**

## ARCH EXPANSION IN ORTHODONTICS

1. **Who is regarded as the "Father of expansion appliances"?**
   A. Emesson C Angel   B. Walter Coffin
   C. Andrew Hass   D. Issacson

2. **Who developed the appliance called "Coffin Spring"?**
   A. Emesson C Angel
   B. Walter Coffin
   C. Andrew Hass
   D. Issacson

3. **Rapid maxillary expansion is also called as:**
   A. Palatal expansion
   B. Split palate
   C. Both A and B
   D. None of the above

4. **Indications of rapid maxillary expansion are:**
   A. Posterior cross-bite caused due to either maxillary deficiency or mandibular excess
   B. Class III malocclusion of dental or sleletal cause
   C. Cleft palate patient's with collapsed maxillary arch
   D. All of the above

5. **What is the effect of RME on maxillary skeletal base?**
   A. Triangular or fan shaped opening of the mid-palatal suture
   B. Maximum opening of the mid-palatal suture in the maxillary incisor region
   C. Minimum opening of the mid-palatal suture in the region of the palate
   D. All of the above

6. **According to Korbs, what are the effects of RME on the maxillary skeletal base:**
   A. In sagittal plane, maxilla rotates in a downward and forward direction
   B. In coronal plane, the two halves of the maxilla rotate away from each other
   C. Both A and B
   D. None of the above

7. **What are the effects of RME on maxillary anterior teeth?**
   A. Proclination of maxillary incisors
   B. Rotations of maxillary incisors
   C. Results in midline diastema
   D. Spacing in the maxillary anterior region

8. **What are the effects of RME on maxillary posterior teeth?**
   A. Buccal tilting of maxillary posterior teeth
   B. Some extent of extension of maxillary posterior teeth
   C. Both A and B
   D. None of the above

9. **What are the effects of RME on mandible?**
   A. Downward and backward rotation of mandible due to extension of posterior teeth
   B. Upward and forward rotation of mandible due to extension of maxillary posterior teeth
   C. Both A and B
   D. None of the above

10. **What are the effects of RME on alveolar bone?**
    A. Alveolar bone bends bucally due to the compression of periodontal ligament fibers
    B. Alveolar bone bends palatally due to the compression of periodontal ligament fibers
    C. Both A and B
    D. None of the above

11. **What are the effects of RME on cranial bones of sutures?**
    A. Displacement of parietal bone
    B. Displacement of occipital bone
    C. Both A and B
    D. None of the above

12. **What are the effects of RME on nasal cavity?**
    A. Increased intra-nasal space
    B. Decreased intra-nasal space
    C. Both A and B
    D. None of the above

13. **How much expansion can be achieved with RME?**
    A. Up to 10 mm   B. Up to 15 mm
    C. Up to 20 mm   D. Up to 25 mm

14. **What is the rate of expansion with RME**
    A. 0.2-0.5 mm/day   B. 0.0-0.5 mm/day
    C. 1.0-2.0 mm/day   D. 3.0-4.0 mm/day

15. **What type of expansion can be achieved by removable expansion appliance?**
    A. Distal expansion
    B. Skeletal expansion only when used in deciduous or mixed dentition
    C. Both A and B
    D. Skeletal expansion even when used in adults

16. **An example for tooth borne expansion appliances is:**
    A. Issacson type   B. Hyrax
    C. Both A and B   D. Hass appliance

17. **An example for tooth and tissue borne expansion appliance is:**
    A. Issacson type   B. Has appliance
    C. Derichsweiler type   D. Both B and C

18. **Derischsweiler type of expansion appliance consists of molar bands on:**
    A. Molars and premolars
    B. First permanent molar and first permanent premolar on either side of maxillary arch
    C. First permant molar and first permanent premolar in the mandibular arch
    D. First permanent molar and permanent canine

19. **How do we activate Issacson type of expansion appliance?**
    A. By closing the nut so that the spring gets compressed
    B. By opening the nut
    C. Either by closing or opening the nut
    D. None of the above

20. **What is Timm's schedule of activation of expansion screw for the patient's aged up to 15 years?**
    A. 90 degrees, 2 times in a day
    B. 45 degrees, 2 times in a day
    C. 90 degrees, 4 times in a day
    D. 45 degrees, 4 times in a day

21. **What is the Timm's schedule of activation of expansion screw for the patient's aged above 15 years?**
    A. 90 degrees, 2 times in a day
    B. 45 degrees, 2 times in a day
    C. 90 degrees, 4 times in a day
    D. 45 degrees, 4 times in a day

22. **The amount of force used in slow arch expansion is:**
    A. 2-4 pounds   B. 10-20 pounds
    C. 5-10 pounds   D. 10-15 pounds

23. **The amount of force used in RME is:**
    A. 2-4 pounds   B. 10-20 pounds
    C. 5-10 pounds   D. 10-15 pounds

24. **Tissue response in slow arch expansion is:**
    A. Physiologic
    B. Traumatic
    C. Either physiologic or traumatic
    D. None of the above

25. **Tissue response in RME is:**
    A. Physiologic
    B. Traumatic

C. Either physiologic or traumatic
D. None of the above

26. **Frequency of activation in slow arch expansion is:**
    A. Less frequent
    B. More frequent
    C. One time activation only
    D. None of the above

27. **Frequency of activation of appliance in RME is:**
    A. Less frequent
    B. More frequent
    C. One time activation only
    D. None of the above

28. **Post-treatment stability is greater in which type of expansion?**
    A. Slow arch expansion
    B. Rapid maxillary expansion
    C. Both A and B
    D. None of the above

29. **Chance of trauma is more in which type of expansion?**
    A. Slow arch expansion
    B. Rapid maxillary expansion
    C. Both A and B
    D. None of the above

30. **Loss of periodontal attachment is not generally seen in which type of expansion?**
    A. Slow arch expansion
    B. Rapid maxillary expansion
    C. Both A and B
    D. None of the above

31. **Loss of periodontal attachment is seen to some extent in which type of expansion?**
    A. Slow arch expansion      B. RME
    C. Both A and B             D. None of the above

32. **What types of appliances are used as slow arch expansion?**
    A. Functional appliance
    B. Only fixed appliance
    C. Only removable appliance
    D. Can be removable or fixed

33. **Chances of relapse is more followed by which type of expansion?**
    A. Slow maxillary expansion
    B. Rapid maxillary expansion
    C. Both A and B
    D. None of the above

34. **In which type of expansion, the chances or relapse is less?**
    A. Slow maxillary expansion
    B. Rapid maxillary expansion
    C. Both A and B
    D. None of the above

35. **Coffin spring is a:**
    A. Removable orthodontic expansion appliance
    B. Fixed orthodontic expansion appliance
    C. Functional orthodontic appliance
    D. Semi-fixed expansion appliance

36. **Coffin spring is a removable orthodontic expansion appliance which brings about:**
    A. Slow dentoalveolar expansion
    B. Rapid dentoalveolar expansion
    C. Rapid skeletal expansion
    D. All of the above

37. **The design of coffin spring is:**
    A. Omega shaped       B. U shaped
    C. Oval shaped        D. None of the above

38. **What thickness of hard round stainless steel wire is used to fabricate coffin spring?**
    A. 0.5 mm             B. 1.25 mm
    C. 1.0 mm             D. 1.50 mm

39. **The coffin spring is activated by**
    A. Pulling the two sides apart manually
    B. By using three pong plier by bending the omega wire at the center of the base
    C. Either A or B
    D. By compressing omega shaped wire

40. **The quad helix appliance consist of:**
    A. 4 helices          B. 8 helices
    C. 2 helices          D. 6 helices

41. **Quad helix is activated by using:**
    A. Three pong plier   B. Universal plier
    C. Light wire plier   D. Adam's plier

42. **What is the portion of wire between two anterior helices in Quad helix appliance called as?**
    A. Anterior bridge    B. Posterior bridge
    C. Palatal bridge     D. Lingual bridge

43. **What is the portion of wire between the anterior helices and posterior helices called as?**
    A. Anterior bridge    B. Posterior bridge
    C. Palatal bridge     D. Lingual bridge

44. **The Quad helix appliance can be activated at**
    A. Center of anterior bridge
    B. Center of palatal bridge
    C. Both A and B       D. None of the above

45. **If the Quad helix appliance is activated at the center of anterior bridge, this brings about:**
    A. Anterior expansion
    B. Posterior expansion
    C. There is dimensional expansion
    D. Lateral expansion

46. **If the Quad helix appliance is activated at the center of palatal bridge, this brings about:**
    A. Anterior expansion
    B. Posterior expansion
    C. There is dimensional expansion
    D. Lateral expansion

47. **Rapid maxillary expansion can be used:**
    A. At any age
    B. Before fusion of mid palatal suture
    C. After 30 years of age
    D. Between 14-18 years of age

48. **The following is used for slow expansion of arch:**
    A. Hass appliance     B. Coffin spring
    C. Hyrax              D. Issacson's appliance

**49.** The following appliance is used for RME:
A. Hyrax
B. Coffin spring
C. Jaw screw
D. None of the above

**50.** Retention followed by RME should be:
A. Not less than 3-6 months
B. 2-5 months
C. 5-6 months
D. Only one month

Ans: 1. A  2. B  3. C  4. D  5. D  6. C  7. C  8. A  9. C  10. A  11. C  12. A  13. C  14. C  15. C  16. C
17. D  18. B  19. B  20. A  21. D  22. A  23. B  24. A  25. B  26. A  27. B  28. A  29. B  30. A  31. B  32. C
33. B  34. A  35. A  36. A  37. A  38. B  39. A  40. A  41. A  42. A  43. C  44. C  45. A  46. D  47. A  8. B
49. A  50. A

## EXTRACTION IN ORTHODONTICS

1. **Extraction of teeth in conjunction to orthodontic treatment is necessary in order to:**
   A. To relieve crowding in the arches especially when jaws are not large enough to accommodate all the teeth
   B. To achieve proper sagittal inter-arch relationship
   C. Just as a procedure of orthodontics
   D. Both A and B

2. **The decision of extraction is based on the following factors:**
   A. Patient's age
   B. Sex of the patient
   C. The amount of space needed for tooth alignment
   D. Both A and C

3. **The decision to opt for extraction should only be made:**
   A. After careful clinical evaluation
   B. After model analysis done
   C. After cephalometric tracing
   D. All of the above

4. **Injudicious extraction of teeth can cause:**
   A. Arch collapse
   B. Deep overbite
   C. Spacing of tissue damage
   D. All of the above

5. **Who was the major proponent of "No extraction philosophy"?**
   A. Edward H Angle
   B. Calvin Case
   C. John Humber
   D. All of the above

6. **Who reintroduced the concept of extraction as a part of orthodontic treatment?**
   A. Calvin Case
   B. Charles Tweed
   C. Angle
   D. John Hunter

7. **In which year Charles Tweed reintroduced the concept of extraction as a part of orthodontic treatment?**
   A. 1950
   B. By late 1940
   C. By late 1941
   D. By late 1942

8. **Who supported the concept of extracting teeth for relieving crowding in the arches and to achieve post treatment stability of occlusion?**
   A. Calvin Case
   B. Charles Tweed
   C. John Hunter
   D. Both A and C

9. **In Angle's Class II division 1 malocclusion with proclined maxillary anteriors and well aligned lower anteriors, extraction of teeth is done in which arch?**
   A. Only in maxillary arch
   B. Only in mandibular arch
   C. Both the arches
   D. Neither maxillary nor mandibular arches

10. **In the correction of Angle's Class II division 1 malocclusion where there is lower arch crowding or when molars are not in full Class II occlusion, it may be:**
    A. Necessary to extract teeth in both the arches
    B. Necessary to extract teeth only in maxillary arch
    C. Necessary to extract teeth only in mandibular arch
    D. All of the above

11. **What is the necessity of extraction in Angle's Class II division 1 malocclusion where there is lower arch crowding?**
    A. To achieve proper sagittal inter-arch relationship
    B. To relieve crowding
    C. Both A and B
    D. None of the above

12. **What is the necessity of extraction of teeth in Angle's Class II division 1 malocclusion with well aligned lower arch?**
    A. To achieve proper sagittal inter-arch relationship
    B. To relieve crowding
    C. To relieve lower anterior rotation
    D. All of the above

13. **Why extraction of teeth in upper arch is avoided in Angle's Class III malocclusion management?**
    A. It may impair the forward development of the maxilla
    B. It may impair the forward development of the mandible
    C. Both A and B
    D. None of the above

14. **It is generally preferable to extract teeth in which of the arches in the management of Angle's Class III malocclusion?**
    A. Only in the lower arch
    B. Only in the upper arch
    C. In both arches
    D. None of the above

15. Which of the following factors are to be considered in the selection of teeth to be extracted?
    A. Condition of teeth
    B. Severity of crowding
    C. Position of teeth
    D. All of the above
16. Which are the following factors to be considered for choosing of teeth in extraction?
    A. Age of patient
    B. Carious status of the teeth
    C. General health status of the dentition
    D. All of the above
17. The tooth most rarely extracted as a part of orthodontic treatment is:
    A. Maxillary central incisors
    B. Maxillary third molars
    C. Mandibular third molar
    D. Maxillary and mandibular premolars
18. Most commonly extracted teeth for orthodontic purpose are:
    A. Maxillary first molars
    B. Maxillary and mandibular premolars
    C. Mandibular incisors
    D. Maxillary incisors
19. Which of the following is an indication of extraction of maxillary central incisor?
    A. Periapical infection
    B. Periodontal abscess
    C. Severe internal resorption
    D. None of the above
20. Indications of maxillary central incisors are:
    A. Unfavourably impacted
    B. Severely fractured
    C. Grossly decayed
    D. All of the above
21. Which tooth exhibits greatest variation next to third molar in form, number and eruption pattern?
    A. Maxillary central incisor
    B. Maxillary lateral incisor
    C. Mandibular central incisor
    D. Mandibular lateral incisor
22. The usual reasons for removal of maxillary lateral incisor:
    A. Severely malposition
    B. Missing one lateral incisor on one side
    C. Malformation of tooth
    D. All of the above
23. Indications of lower incisor extraction:
    A. When a lower incisor is completely excluded from the arch with good alignment of the remaining teeth
    B. In some cases of Class III malocclusion
    C. Lower incisor with poor periodontal support
    D. All of the above
24. What are the reasons for favouring first premolar extraction for orthodontic treatment?
    A. First premolar extraction provides maximum space which can be utilized for the retraction of proclined anteriors
    B. First premolar extraction provides maximum space which can be utilized for the correction of anterior and posterior crowding
    C. The extraction of first premolar leaves behind a posterior segment that has adequate anchorage potential for the retaraction of the anteriors
    D. All of the above
25. Indications of the first premolar extraction are:
    A. Moderate severe crowding of anteriors
    B. Moderate to severe crowding of posterior
    C. Moderate to severe proclination of anterior
    D. All of the above
26. Which of the following statement is true regarding first premolar extraction?
    A. First premolars are extracted as a part of serial extraction
    B. First premolars extractions provides very minimum space
    C. First premolars are always extracted to relieve crowding
    D. Second premolars extractions are preferred to that of first premolars
27. The most commonly extracted teeth next to first premolar for orthodontic treatment is:
    A. Upper second premolars
    B. Lower second premolars
    C. Both A and B
    D. Mandibular incisors
28. Which of the following statement is false regarding extraction of second premolar?
    A. Extraction of second premolars is preferred when space required for the correction of malocclusion is minimized
    B. Second premolars are extracted when anchorage demand is minimum
    C. Premature loss deciduous second molar may cause mesial migration of first molar leaving inadequate space for second premolar eruption, in such cases, second premolar may erupt completely out of the arch and may be indicated for extraction
    D. Second premolars are always extracted as a part of orthodontic treatment
29. Indications of extractions of second premolar:
    A. Unfavourably impacted second premolar
    B. Grossly decayed second premolar
    C. In open bite cases
    D. All of the above
30. Which is the key tooth in Angle's classification of malocclusion?
    A. Mandibular first permanent molar
    B. Maxillary first permanent molar
    C. Maxillary canine
    D. Mandibular canine
31. Contraindication of extraction of first permanent molars:
    A. Extraction of first molar does not provide adequate space for the relief of anterior crowding

B. First molar can lead to deepening of the bite
C. Both A and B
D. None of the above

32. **Indications of first permanent molars are:**
    A. Grossly decayed first permanent molar
    B. In open bite cases
    C. Both A and B
    D. None of the above

33. **At what age Wilkinson advocated extraction of first permanent molar?**
    A. 8.5-9.5 years
    B. 8-9 years
    C. 7-8 years
    D. 9.5-10.5 years

34. **What are the benefits of first permanent molar extraction in Wilkinson's method of extraction?**
    A. To prevent third molar impaction
    B. To relieve crowding in the arch
    C. It helps in decresing the incidence and occurrence of dental caries
    D. All of the above

35. **Drawback of Wilkinson's method of extraction**
    A. It relieves crowding in the arches only to a certain extent
    B. Extraction of permanent first molar results in lack of anchorage for orthodontic therapy
    C. Both A and B
    D. None of the above

36. **Indication of extraction of second permanent molar:**
    A. To prevent third molar impaction
    B. To relieve impaction of second molar
    C. To relieve lower incisor crowding
    D. All of the above

37. **Indications of extraction of second permanent molar are:**
    A. In open bite cases
    B. For distalization of first molars
    C. Both A and B
    D. None of the above

38. **What are the different extraction procedures?**
    A. Balanced extraction
    B. Compensatory extraction
    C. Enforced extraction
    D. All of the above

39. **Compensatory extraction refers to:**
    A. Extraction of tooth in the opposite jaw to the same teeth group
    B. The extraction of a tooth in the same jaw to the same teeth group
    C. The extraction of a tooth in the contralateral side to the same teeth group
    D. None of the above

40. **According to balanced extraction, if the tooth 14 (FDI notation) is missing, which tooth is extracted?**
    A. 24  B. 34
    C. 44  D. None of the above

41. **If the tooth 14 (FDI notation) is missing which tooth is extracted in compensatory method of extraction?**
    A. 24  B. 34
    C. 44
    D. None of the above

42. **What are the indications of enforced method of extraction in orthodontics?**
    A. Grossly decayed tooth
    B. Fractured tooth
    C. Impacted and periodontally compromised teeth
    D. All of the above

43. **Phased extraction refers to:**
    A. The tooth in one arch is extracted few months earlier than in the other arch
    B. The tooth in one arch is extracted a few months later then in the other arch
    C. Combination of A and B
    D. None of the above

**Ans:** 1. D  2. D  3. D  4. D  5. A  6. B  7. B  8. A  9. A  10. A  11. C  12. A  13. A  14. A  15. D  16. D
17. A  18. B  19. C  20. D  21. B  22. D  23. D  24. D  25. D  26. A  27. C  28. D  29. D  30. D  31. C  32. C
33. A  34. D  35. C  36. D  37. C  38. D  39. A  40. A  41. C  42. D  43. A

## 8. ORTHODONTIC INSTRUMENTS

### ORTHODONTIC INSTRUMENTS

1. **Which of the following instruments is used for placing the elastic ring separator?**
   A. Separator placing pliers
   B. Light wire pliers
   C. Mathew hemostat
   D. Howe pliers

2. **Which of the following instrument is used for placing the Kesling metallic ring separator?**
   A. Separator placing pliers
   B. Light wire pliers
   C. Mathew hemostat
   D. Howe pliers

3. **Which of the following instrument is used for bracket positioning?**
   A. Boon's gauge
   B. Bracket positioning height gauge
   C. Direct bonding bracket holder
   D. All of the above

4. **Which of the following pliers are used for contouring the band in band application procedure?**
   A. Band forming pliers   B. Band contouring pliers
   C. Band pincliable pliers
   D. Band crimping pliers

5. **Utility and speciality pliers are**
   A. Three prong pliers
   B. Weingart pliers
   C. Mathew hemostat
   D. All of the above
6. **Wire forming pliers are**
   A. Bird beak pliers
   B. Clasp forming pliers
   C. Both A and B
   D. None of the above
7. **Which of the following pliers is used for debonding of brackets at the end of active orthodontic treatment?**
   A. Debonding pliers anterior
   B. Posterior debonding plier
   C. Both A and B
   D. None of the above
8. **Which of the following pliers is used for debanding procedure?**
   A. Straight band remover
   B. Curved band remover
   C. Both A and B
   D. None of the above
9. **3D modular orthodontic instruments include**
   A. Howe pliers
   B. Light wire pliers
   C. Belzer wire pliers
   D. All of the above
10. **3D modular orthodontic instruments include**
    A. Lingual arch forming pliers
    B. Jaw pliers
    C. Band pusher
    D. All of the above
11. **3D modular orthodontic instruments are**
    A. Angle wire bending pliers
    B. Band director
    C. Modular omega pliers
    D. All of the above
12. **3D modular orthodontic instruments are**
    A. Angle wire bending pliers
    B. Modular omega pliers
    C. Both A and B
    D. None of the above
13. **Which of the following instruments is used for placing the brass wire separator for the separation of teeth during banding procedures?**
    A. Separator placing pliers
    B. Light wire pliers
    C. Combination of A and B
    D. None of the above
14. **Markings in bracket positioning orthodontic instruments are**
    A. 3.5 mm, 4.0 mm, 4.5 mm, 5.0 mm
    B. 3.0 mm, 4.0 mm, 4.5 mm, 5.0 mm
    C. 4.5 mm, 5.0 mm, 5.5 mm, 6.0 mm
    D. 2.5 mm, 3.5 mm, 4.5 mm, 5.5 mm
15. **Light wire pliers is also known as:**
    A. Bird beak pliers
    B. Very light wire pliers
    C. Wire forming pliers
    D. All of the above
16. **Light wire pliers is used for**
    A. Placement of separators such as Kesling and Brass wire separator
    B. Adjusting and activating the 3D appliances
    C. Adjusting 0.05 inch expanders on all 3D appliances
    D. All of the above
17. **De La Rosa pliers is used for**
    A. Fabrication of arch wire
    B. Helps to accentuate the curvature of arch wire
    C. Both A and B    D. None of the above
18. **Loop forming pliers is used for**
    A. Fabrication of different types of bows
    B. Fabrication of different types of springs
    C. Fabrication of canine retractors
    D. All of the above
19. **What is the special feature of Nance loop forming plier that permits fabrication of varying sized loops?**
    A. The pliers has 4 distinct step formations in its design
    B. The pliers has 3 distinct step formations in its design
    C. The pliers has 2 distinct step formations in its design
    D. The pliers has 6 distinct step formations in its design
20. **Three prong pliers is used for**
    A. Activation of quad helix
    B. Activation of 'W' appliance
    C. Activation of coffin spring
    D. All of the above
21. **Weingart pliers is used for**
    A. Holding the arch wire
    B. Carrying the arch wire
    C. Placing the arch wire
    D. All of the above
22. **The various designs of Weingart pliers are**
    A. Standard tip Weingart pliers
    B. Standard size Weingart pliers
    C. Heavy tip Weingart pliers
    D. All of the above
23. **The various designs of distal end cutter include**
    A. Micro distal end cutter with safety hold
    B. Distal end cutter with safety hold
    C. Both A and B
    D. None of the above
24. **Distal end cutter is used for**
    A. To cut the excess arch wire distal to the molar band
    B. To cut the ligature tag
    C. To cut elastic modules
    D. All of the above
25. **Which feature of distal end cutter prevents getting tissue injury and accidental swallowing of the cut piece of wire when the arch wire is cut using distal end cutter?**
    A. Safety hold mechanism
    B. Safety mechanism
    C. Combination of A and B
    D. None of the above

26. **Pin and ligature cutter is used for**
    A. To cut the terminal ends of lock pins in Begg technique
    B. To cut excessive ends of ligature wire
    C. Both A and B
    D. None of the above
27. **Anterior debonding pliers is used for**
    A. Debonding maxillary anterior brackets
    B. Debonding mandibular anterior brackets
    C. Both A and B
    D. None of the above
28. **Posterior debonding pliers is used for**
    A. Debonding maxillary posterior brackets
    B. Debonding mandibular posterior brackets
    C. Both A and B    D. None of the above
29. **What are the key features of angulated debonding pliers over debonding pliers?**
    A. An extra width of 6mm
    B. Shank is angulated which helps in accessibility
    C. Both A and B
    D. None of the above
30. **Howe plier is used for**
    A. Carrying of 3D appliances to the arch
    B. Rotating, tipping and torquing 3D appliances
    C. Both A and B
    D. None of the above
31. **Lingual arch forming pliers is used for**
    A. Rotating the 3D quad helix appliance
    B. Torquing the 3D quad helix appliance
    C. Both A and B
    D. None of the above
32. **Jaw pliers in orthodontics is used for**
    A. Tightening wire from 3D posts for any loose fit
    B. Adjusting quad helix appliance
    C. Adjusting 3D activators
    D. All of the above
33. **Angle wire bending pliers is used for**
    A. Adjusting the 3D appliance
    B. Activating the 3D appliance
    C. Both A and B
    D. None of the above
34. **Modular omega pliers is used for**
    A. Adjusting the expansion of omega loop on the 3D maxillary biometric distalizing arch
    B. For the contraction of omega loop on the 3D biometric distalizing arch
    C. Both A and B
    D. None of the above
35. **Which of the following statements is true regarding sterilization of orthodontic appliances?**
    A. Use soap and water to clean pliers
    B. Put orthodontic instruments in glutaraldehyde solution
    C. Brush the pliers
    D. Always use distilled water or surgical milk for pre-cleaning of orthodontic instruments
36. **What are the reasons for dull cutting edges of orthodontic pliers?**
    A. Pliers left too long in ultrasonic cleaner
    B. Bending and cutting specifications are not followed
    C. Pliers used to cut or bend a heavier wire than its standards
    D. All of the above
37. **What are the reasons for discoloration of orthodontic pliers?**
    A. Pliers were in touch with water
    B. Chemicals and minerals in tap water are the reason for discoloration of the pliers
    C. Both A and B
    D. None of the above
38. **What are the reasons for getting orthodontic pliers rusted?**
    A. Pliers were in touch with water
    B. Chemicals and minerals in tap water
    C. Combination of A and B
    D. None of the above
39. **Which of the orthodontic instrument has working portions at both ends?**
    A. Bracket positioning height gauge
    B. Ligature director
    C. Both A and B
    D. None of the above
40. **Which of the following pliers is used for placing dumb-bell shaped separator?**
    A. Light wire pliers
    B. Separator placing pliers
    C. Combination of A and B
    D. None of the above

Ans: 1. A  2. B  3. D  4. B  5. D  6. C  7. C  8. C  9. D  10. D  11. D  12. C  13. B  14. A  15. A  16. D
17. C  18. D  19. A  20. A  21. D  22. D  23. C  24. A  25. A  26. C  27. C  28. C  29. C  30. C  31. C  32. D
33. C  34. C  35. D  36. D  37. C  38. A  39. C  40. D

## 9. PRECLINICAL ORTHODONTICS

### PRECLINICAL ORTHODONTICS

1. **Basically orthodontic wires are used for:**
    A. To fabricate active component of orthodontic appliances such as bows, springs and canine retractors, that apply tooth moving forces
    B. To fabricate retentive component of orthodontic appliances such as clasps-that hold the appliance in contact with teeth
    C. Both A and B
    D. None of the above
2. **Following are basic types of bends that are used to fabricate orthodontic appliances, except**
    A. Right angled bend    B. Loops and helices

C. Curves
D. None of the above

3. **Right angled bend is formed by**
   A. Placing the thumb as close to beaks as possible and wire is pushed over the round beak of the 139 plier
   B. Placing the thumb as close to beaks as possible and wire is pushed over Weingart pliers
   C. Placing the thumb as close to beaks as possible and wire is pushed over band contouring pliers
   D. Placing the thumb as close to beaks as possible and wire is pushed over hard wire cutter

4. **Armamentarium required to perform preclinical wire bending procedure are**
   A. Universal plier
   B. Adam's plier
   C. 201 Three prong plier/3 beak/3jaw plier
   D. All of the above

5. **Universal pliers is called so because**
   A. It can be used for fabricating many of the wire components such as bows, clasps, springs and wire components of myofunctional orthodontic appliance
   B. It can be used for fabricating many of the arch wires
   C. It can be used for activating quad helix appliance
   D. It can be used for activation 'W' arch appliance

6. **Loops in the universal pliers are**
   A. Each loop has progressively increasing diameter throughout its length
   B. Each loop has progressively decreasing diameter throughout its length
   C. Both A and B
   D. None of the above

7. **Small sized loop in the universal pliers is used for fabricating**
   A. Springs such as finger spring and "Z" spring
   B. Arch wires
   C. Large diameter helices
   D. None of the above

8. **The medium sized loop part of the working end of universal pliers is used in fabrication of**
   A. Bows
   B. Canine retractors
   C. Both A and B
   D. None of the above

9. **The working end of Adam's pliers consists of**
   A. 2 halves          B. 3 halves
   C. 4 halves
   D. 5 halves

10. **Both the halves of working end of an Adam's pliers are**
    A. Both the halves are smooth, shiny and similar in shape and design
    B. Both the halves are very rough, dull and dissimilar in shape and design
    C. Both A and B
    D. None of the above

11. **Adam's pliers are used for**
    A. Fabrication of Adam's clasp and all its modifications
    B. Fabrication of "C" clasp and all its modifications
    C. Fabrication of Pin clasp and all its modifications
    D. Fabrication of Jackson's clasp and all its modifications

12. **201 Three prong pliers/3 beak/3jaw pliers has**
    A. 2 beaks          B. 3 beaks
    C. 4 beaks          D. 4 beaks

13. **201 Three prong pliers/3 beak/3jaw pliers is used for**
    A. Activation quad helix appliance
    B. Activation of labial bows
    C. Activation of canine retractors
    D. Activation of springs

14. **Optical pliers bends the wire by**
    A. By simply squeezing the wire
    B. By opening the beaks of the pliers
    C. Both A and B
    D. None of the above

15. **Bird beak pliers has**
    A. A round beak and a flat beak
    B. Both beaks are round
    C. Both beaks are flat
    D. None of the above

16. **Hard round stainless steel wire is cut using**
    A. Light wire pliers
    B. Hard wire cutter
    C. Pin and ligature cutter
    D. None of the above

17. **Both halves/ beaks of the hard wire cutter is**
    A. Both the halves are symmetrical in shapes and design
    B. Both the halves are non symmetrical in shapes and design
    C. Both A and B
    D. None of the above

18. **Precautions during cutting the hard round stainless steel wire using hard wire cutter are following except**
    A. Always hold the cutter away from the face while cutting
    B. Always incline the cutter towards a rough surface of the floor
    C. Don't face the discarding part of the wire towards glass floor/ or any polished surface because the discarded piece of wire may get reflected and may cause injury
    D. Always hold the cutter towards the face while cutting

Ans: 1. C   2. D   3. A   4. D   5. A   6. A   7. A   8. C   9. A   10. A   11. A   12. B   13. A   14. A   15. A   16. B   17. A   18. D

# 10. ORTHODONTIC APPLIANCES

## GENERAL PRINCIPLES OF ORTHODONTIC APPLIANCES

1. Which of the following statement is not true?
   A. Mechanical appliances exert mild pressure on a tooth or a group of teeth and their supportive structures
   B. Myofunctional appliances are loose fitting appliances that harness the natural forces of the orofacial musculature
   C. Orthodontic appliances exert strong forces on groups of teeth
   D. Myofuctional appliances transmit, eliminate or guide the natural perioral muscle forces on the dentition

2. Orthodontic appliances may be classified as
   A. Removable or fixed only
   B. Mechanical or myofunctional only
   C. Active or passive only
   D. Combination of A, B and C

3. **Myofunctional appliances**
   A. Usually contain active components
   B. Harness natural forces from perioral structures
   C. Fixed only
   D. Not loose fitting

4. **Examples of passive fixed appliances are**
   A. Fixed lingual bonded retainers, distal band and spur
   B. Begg's retainer
   C. Hawley's appliance
   D. Frankel's functional regulator

5. Which of the following is used for maintaining the position of teeth after premature extraction of deciduous teeth?
   A. Distal shoe space maintainer
   B. Kesling tooth positioner
   C. Molar band
   D. None of the above

6. What is done to enhance stability of the orthodontic correction?
   A. Prolong active orthodontic therapy
   B. Removable retainers given at the end of treatment
   C. Both A and B
   D. None of the above

7. In active fixed appliances, active tooth movement is carried out by
   A. Arch wire
   B. Elastic band
   C. Open and closed coiled spring
   D. Combination of all the above

8. Which of the following can be used in active removable orthodontic appliance?
   A. Expansion screws
   B. Kesling tooth positioned
   C. Springs and bows
   D. Both A and C

9. Passive removable orthodontic appliances are designed
   A. To bring about movement in a tooth or a group of teeth
   B. To maintain teeth in their current position
   C. To harness natural forces from perioral musculature
   D. None of the above

10. Which of the following statement is not true?
    A. Removable orthodontic appliances can be fitted by the patient
    B. Removable orthodontic appliances can be removed by the patient
    C. Removable orthodontic appliances can be further classified as active and passive
    D. Oral hygiene maintenance is difficult with removable orthodontic appliance

11. Fixed orthodontic appliances includes those appliances
    A. Which the patient can remove
    B. Which the patient cannot remove
    C. Which maintain teeth in a fixed position
    D. None of the above

12. Passive removable appliances
    A. Are designed to achieve tooth movement
    B. Are designed to maintain teeth in their present position
    C. Have active component incorporated in their design
    D. None of the above

13. Myofunctional orthodontic appliances can
    A. Engage both the arches
    B. Harness and transmit natural forces of the circumoral musculature to the teeth or alveolar bone
    C. Can be either or removable
    D. All of the above

14. Which are the requirements considered for orthodontic treatment?
    A. Biologic requirements
    B. Mechanical requirements
    C. Esthetic requirements
    D. All of the above

15. The mechanical requirements of orthodontic appliances include
    A. Forces delivered should be continuous and controlled
    B. Forces delivered should be in alternative pattern
    C. Forces delivered should be in the desired direction
    D. Both A and C

16. Which of the following statement is **not** true?
    A. Finger pressure brings about tooth movement
    B. Orthodontic forces applied are continuous, mild
    C. Orthodontic forces are of high magnitude
    D. None of the above

17. Which of the following statement is not true?
    A. Myofunctional orthodontic appliances engage both arches
    B. Myofunctional appliances are only removable

C. Myofunctional appliances harness and transmit natural forces of the circumoral musculature to the teeth and for alveolar bone
D. Myofunctional appliances hold the mandible away from its resting position

18. Begg's retainer is a
    A. Passive removable orthodontic appliance
    B. Active removable orthodontic appliance
    C. Passive fixed orthodontic appliance
    D. Active fixed orthodontic appliance

19. Distal shoe space maintainer is
    A. An active fixed orthodontic appliance
    B. An active removable orthodontic appliance
    C. A passive removable orthodontic appliance
    D. A passive fixed orthodontic appliance

20. Frankel's regulator is an example of
    A. Fixed orthodontic appliance
    B. Mechanical orthodontic appliance
    C. Functional orthodontic appliance
    D. Orthopedic orthodontic appliance

21. Oral screen is an example of
    A. Fixed orthodontic appliance
    B. Mechanical orthodontic appliance
    C. Functional orthodontic appliance
    D. Orthopedic orthodontic appliance

22. An example of fixed passive orthodontic appliance is
    A. Frankel's regulator
    B. Begg's retainer
    C. Lingual canine to canine retainer
    D. Hawley retainer

23. Which of the following can be used as a semi-fixed/fixed orthodontic appliance?
    A. Lip bumper
    B. Frankel's regulator
    C. Oral screen
    D. None of the above

24. Which of the following apply heavy orthodontic forces?
    A. Removable appliances
    B. Fixed appliances
    C. Functional appliances
    D. Orthopedic appliances

25. Orthopedic appliances bring about heavy orthodontic forces
    A. To bring about skeletal changes
    B. To bring about teeth movement
    C. Both A and B
    D. Neither A, nor B

26. Which of the following is a Biologic requirement of orthodontic appliance?
    A. Appliance should deliver continuous and controlled forces
    B. Appliances should be esthetically acceptable to the patient
    C. Appliances should withstand routine masticatory forces
    D. Appliances should not disintegrate in the oral environment

27. Which of the following is a mechanical requirement of orthodontic appliance?
    A. It shouls not have a detrimental impact on the teeth and/or periodontium
    B. Anchor units should remain in their original position
    C. Appliance should deliver controlled forces of desired intensity in the desired direction
    D. It should not produce any allergic or toxic reactions

28. Advantage of removable orthodontic appliance over fixed orthodontic appliance is
    A. Removable orthodontic appliance is easy to clean and allows better maintaining of oral hygiene
    B. Removable orthodontic appliance allows multiple movement of multiple teeth
    C. Treatment duration of removable orthodontic appliance is less than fixed orthodontic appliance
    D. Tooth movement is more precise than fixed orthodontic appliance

29. Disadvantages of fixed orthodontic appliance include
    A. Prolonged chair side time
    B. Patient cooperation is vitally important
    C. Multiple tooth movements cannot be carried out at a time
    D. Multiple rotations are different to treat

30. Patient cooperation is least needed in
    A. Removable orthodontic appliance
    B. Fixed orthodontic appliance
    C. Functional orthodontic appliance
    D. Orthopedic orthodontic appliance

31. Orthopedic orthodontic appliance brings about
    A. Skeletal changes only
    B. Dental changes i.e. tooth movement only
    C. Both skeletal changes and also tooth movement
    D. None of the above

Ans: 1. C  2. D  3. B  4. A  5. A  6. C  7. D  8. D  9. B  10. D  11. B  12. B  13. D  14. D  15. D  16. C  17. B  18. A  19. D  20. C  21. C  22. C  23. A  24. D  25. A  26. D  27. C  28. A  29. A  30. B  31. C

## REMOVABLE ORTHODONTIC APPLIANCES

1. What type of tooth movement is achieved in removable orthodontic appliance
   A. Bodily movement   B. Tipping
   C. Simple rotation
   D. Both B and C

2. What are retentive components of removable orthodontic appliances
   A. Wires           B. Retentive tag
   C. Clasps          D. Bows

3. What are active components of removable orthodontic appliances
   A. Springs         B. Bows

C. Retractors   D. All of the above
4. What is the other name for c-clasp
   A. Jackson clasp   B. Three quarter clasp
   C. Circumferential clasp   D. Both B and C
5. Which undercut does the c-clasp utilizes
   A. Mesiocervical undercut
   B. Buccocervical undercut
   C. Distocervical undercut
   D. None of the above
6. What is major disadvantage of c-clasp
   A. It cannot be used in partially erupted teeth
   B. It cannot be fabricated on deciduous molar
   C. It does not provide adequate retention as Adam clasp
   D. All of the above
7. What are the other names for Jackson clasp
   A. Full clasp   B. U-clasp
   C. Both of the above   D. None of the above
8. Which clasps are most commonly used
   A. U-clasp   B. Adams clasp
   C. C-clasp   D. Schwarz clasp
9. What are the other names of Adam's clasp
   A. Universal clasp
   B. Liverpool clasp
   C. Modified arrowhead clasp
   D. All of the above
10. Who introduced Adam's clasp
    A. Crozat   B. Schwartz
    C. Phillips C Adams   D. Robin
11. Bridge of Adam's clasp is fabricated of what angulations?
    A. 90 degrees   B. 60 degrees
    C. 30 degrees   D. 45 degrees
12. What is major advantage of Adam's clasp?
    A. Fabricated on both deciduous and permanent teeth
    B. It can be used in partially or fully erupted teeth
    C. Excellent retentive property and it does not require special pliers for fabrication
    D. All of the above
13. What is the use of triangular clasp?
    A. Additional retention
    B. It is used as accessory clasp
    C. Both of the above
    D. None of the above
14. What is the other name of Schwarz clasp?
    A. Head clasp
    B. Arrowhead clasp
    C. Arrow clasp
    D. All of the above
15. Adam's clasp is the modification of which clasp?
    A. C-clasp   B. Triangular clasp
    C. Schwarz clasp   D. Ball end clasp
16. Which is modified version of Adam's clasp?
    A. Pin clasp   B. Resta clasp
    C. Visick clasp   D. All of the above
17. Which clasp is used in anterior segment?
    A. Adam's clasp   B. South end clasp
    C. Both A and B   D. None of above
18. Which clasp is used as accessory clasp?
    A. Ball end clap   B. Triangular clasp
    C. C-clasp   D. Both A and B
19. Short labial bow is extended from which tooth to which tooth?
    A. Canine to canine   B. Premolar to premolar
    C. Incisors   D. None of above
20. How do you activate the short labial bow?
    A. Compression of 'U' loop
    B. Opening the 'U' loop
    C. Twisting the 'U' loop
    D. All of the above
21. Split labial bow is commonly used in
    A. Closure of midline diastema
    B. Closure of space distal to central incisors
    C. Closure of space in the mandibular anterior segment
    D. Retraction of maxillary incisors
22. How do you activate reverse labial bow?
    A. Closing the 'U' loop
    B. Opening of the 'U' loop
    C. Both A and B
    D. None of the above
23. What gauge is used in fabrication of Roberts's retractor?
    A. 0.9 mm   B. 0.7 mm
    C. 0.5 mm   D. 0.6 mm
24. Mill's retractor is also called as
    A. It is in the shape of a Mill
    B. Extensive labial bow
    C. Both A and B
    D. None of the above
25. What gauge is used for labial bow with apron spring?
    A. 0.2 mm
    B. 0.9-1 mm and 0.4 mm wire
    C. 0.3 mm
    D. 0.1 mm
26. How do you activate labial bow with apron spring?
    A. Opening the apron spring
    B. Bending of apron spring towards the teeth
    C. Both A and B
    D. None of the above
27. Keeping the principles of spring, when diameter of wire is increased, force increases by
    A. 8 times   B. 20 times
    C. 16 times   D. 32 times
28. What formula is used for spring in relation to diameter and strength of wire?
    A. $F = D/9/L^9$
    B. $F = D1/L1$
    C. $F = D^4/L^3$
    D. $F = D^8/L^8$
29. Keeping the principles of spring, when length of wire is increased, force reduces by
    A. 3 times   B. 2 times
    C. 8 times   D. 10 times

30. What is the amount of force delivered by springs depending on root surface area?
    A. 6 gm/cm
    B. 9 gm/cm
    C. 20 gm/cm
    D. 10 gm/cm
31. What type of tooth movement is achieved in a finger spring?
    A. Mesiolabial tooth movement
    B. Mesiodistal tooth movement
    C. Distolabial tooth movement
    D. Labiolingual tooth movement
32. What gauge is used in springs?
    A. 0.2 mm
    B. 0.5 or 0.6 mm
    C. 0.3 mm
    D. 0.2 mm
33. How do you activate the finger spring?
    A. Closing the helix
    B. Opening the helix or moving the active arm towards the tooth
    C. Moving the active arm away from the tooth
    D. None of the above
34. How do you activate the z-spring?
    A. By closing simultaneously both helices by 8 mm
    B. By opening simultaneously both helices by 2-3 mm
    C. Both A and B
    D. None of the above
35. What type of tooth movement is achieved by Z spring?
    A. Labial movement of incisors
    B. Correctional deep bite
    C. Both of above
    D. None of the above
36. What type of tooth movement is achieved by T-spring?
    A. Distal movement of premolar and canines
    B. Buccal movement of premolars and canines
    C. Lingual movement of premolars and canines
    D. Mesial movement of premolars and canines
37. How do you activate the T-spring?
    A. It is activated by cutting one free arm of T
    B. It is activated by pulling the free end of T
    C. Both A and B
    D. None of the above
38. What hard round stainless steel wire gauge is used in mattress-spring?
    A. 0.7 mm
    B. 0.6 mm
    C. 0.5 mm
    D. 0.9 mm
39. What type of tooth movement is achieved by 'U' loop canine retraction?
    A. Labial movement of canine
    B. Movement of canine in distal direction
    C. Mesial movement of canine
    D. Lingual movement of canine
40. How do you activate 'U' loop canine retractor?
    A. Compressing the loop
    B. By cutting the free end of active arm by 2 mm
    C. Both of above
    D. None of above
41. How do you activate helical canine retractor?
    A. Opening the helix by 9 mm
    B. Opening the helix
    C. By cutting 2 mm from the end of active arm
    D. Both B and C
42. How do you activate the buccal self supported canine retractor?
    A. Opening the helix by 1 mm
    B. Closing the helix by 1 mm at 4 times
    C. Either by closing the helix or by opening the helix
    D. None of the above
43. What is the minimal thickness of base of base plate?
    A. 0.0-1.0 mm
    B. 1.5-2 mm
    C. 4 mm
    D. 0.1-0.9 mm
44. Anterior bite plane is used to correct the following?
    A. Scissors bite
    B. Deep bite
    C. Open bite
    D. Cross bite
45. Sved bite plane is modification of the following?
    A. Lower anterior inclined bite plane
    B. Upper anterior inclined bite plane
    C. Both of A and B
    D. None of the above
46. Finger spring is also called as
    A. Double cantilever spring
    B. Single cantilever spring
    C. One helix spring
    D. None of the above
47. Z-spring is also called as
    A. Helical spring
    B. Double cantilever spring
    C. Cantilever spring
    D. Simple cantilever spring
48. C in c-clasp means
    A. Circular
    B. Circumferential
    C. Conical
    D. None of the above
49. What thickness of wire is used for fabrication of Adam's clasp for anterior teeth?
    A. 0.5 mm
    B. 0.6 mm
    C. 0.7 mm
    D. 0.9 mm
50. What thickness of wire is used for fabrication of Adam's clasp for posterior teeth?
    A. 0.5 mm
    B. 0.6 mm
    C. 0.7 mm
    D. 0.9 mm
51. Long labial bow extends from
    A. Right 2nd premolar to left 2nd premolar
    B. 1st premolar to 1st premolar
    C. Right 1st premolar to left 2nd premolar
    D. left 1st premolar to right 2nd premolar
52. How do you activate the long labial bow?
    A. By compressing the 'U' loop by 1-2 mm and reducing the acrylic plate behind incisors
    B. By compressing the loop by 1-2 mm
    C. Both the above
    D. None of the above

53. **How do you activate split labial bow?**
    A. By compressing the 'U' loop of the bow by 1 mm
    B. By compressing the 'U' loop by 1-2 mm
    C. By compressing the 'U' loop of the bow by 4 mm
    D. By compressing the 'U' loop by 3 mm
54. **Modified split labial bow is used for**
    A. Closure of space between central and lateral incisors
    B. Closure of space distal to canine
    C. Closure of midline diastema
    D. All of the above
55. **What gauge of hard round stainless steel wire is used for fabrication of labial bow?**
    A. 0.5 mm/24 gauge
    B. 0.7 mm/22 gauges
    C. 0.6 mm/23 gauge
    D. 0.8 mm/21 gauge
56. **What type of tooth movement is achieved by mattress spring?**
    A. Lingual movement of upper teeth
    B. Labial movement of upper teeth
    C. Mesial movement of upper teeth
    D. Distal movement of upper teeth
57. **What thickness of hard round wire is used to fabricate 'U' loop canine retractor?**
    A. 0.5 mm
    B. 0.6 or 0.7 mm
    C. 0.8 mm
    D. 0.9 mm
58. **How do you activate the palatal canine retractor?**
    A. Activated by opening the helix by 1 mm
    B. Activated by opening the helix by 4 mm
    C. Activated by opening the helix by 2 mm
    D. Activated by opening the helix by 5 mm

**Ans:** 1. D  2. C  3. D  4. D  5. B  6. C  7. C  8. B  9. D  10. C  11. D  12. D  13. C  14. B  15. C  16. B  17. C  18. D  19. A  20. A  21. D  22. B  23. C  24. B  25. B  26. B  27. C  28. C  29. C  30. C  31. B  32. B  33. B  34. B  35. A  36. B  37. B  38. B  39. B  40. A  41. D  42. B  43. B  44. B  45. B  46. B  47. B  48. B  49. C  50. C  51. B  52. C  53. B  54. C  55. B  56. B  57. B  58. C

## FIXED ORTHODONTIC APPLIANCES AND TECHNIQUES

1. **Following are the steps in banding except**
    A. Separation of teeth
    B. Selection of band material
    C. Pinching of band
    D. Curing the bands
2. **Which one of the following is a passive component of fixed appliances?**
    A. Buccal tube      B. Springs
    C. Separations      D. Arch wres
3. **Which one of the band size is indicated for canine?**

    | Band Thickness | Band Width |
    |---|---|
    | A. 0.004 | 0.150 |
    | B. 0.003 | 0.150 |
    | C. 0.003 | 0.125 |
    | D. 0.005 | 0.180 |

4. **Which type of bracket does not permit tipping of teeth?**
    A. Ribbon arch bracket
    B. Metallic bracket
    C. Edgewise type of bracket
    D. Weldable and bondable bracket
5. **Ceramic brakets were introduced in which year**
    A. 1960      B. 1970
    C. 1980      D. 1990
6. **Metallic brackets have the following advantages except**
    A. They resist deformation
    B. They corrode
    C. They exhibit least friction
    D. They can be recycled
7. **Buccal tube can be**
    A. Round and squarish
    B. Round and rectangular
    C. Round and rhomboidal
    D. Round and trapezoidal
8. **What is ligation?**
    A. The process of welding arch wire to bracket
    B. The process of attaching of wire to bracket
    C. The process of securing arch wire to bracket
    D. The process of bonding arch wire to bracket
9. **The diameter of ligature arch wire is**
    A. 0.008 to 0.0010      B. 0.009 to 0.0011
    C. 0.008 to 0.0011      D. 0.009 to 0.010
10. **Lock pins are made of**
    A. Copper      B. Brass
    C. Stainless steel      D. Bronze
11. **Which of the arch wire exhibit superior elastic properties?**
    A. Stainless steel wire
    B. Pure gold wire
    C. Multi-stranded wire
    D. Titanium based arch wire
12. **Elastic deflection is also known as**
    A. Resilience      B. Spring back property
    C. Formability      D. Stiffness
13. **Which among the following material is not used in manufacturing arch wires?**
    A. Stainless steel      B. Nickel titanium alloys
    C. Bronze material      D. Beta titanium
14. **Austentic stainless steel wire is also known as**
    A. 15/5 stainless steel      B. 16/6 stainless steel
    C. 17/7 stainless steel      D. 18/8 stainless steel

15. **Nickel titanium alloys were introduced to orthodontic community by**
    A. Williams R Buchler   B. Anderson
    C. Goldberg   D. Burrstone
16. **Which of the wires exhibit increased flexibility?**
    A. Multistranded arch wire
    B. Optiflex arch wire
    C. Mitinol arch wire
    D. Austhentic arch wire
17. **Which one of the following elastics is used for correction of anterior open bite?**
    A. Cross bite elastic   B. Box elastic
    C. Class III elastic   D. Class II elastic
18. **Elastic chains are made of**
    A. Polyglyconate   B. Rubber
    C. Latex   D. Polyerythene
19. **All these are springs used to bring about tooth movement except**
    A. Torquing spring   B. Tipping spring
    C. Uprighting spring   D. Closed coil spring
20. **Kesling separator consists of**
    A. Two coils and one arm
    B. One coil and two arms
    C. Two coils and two arms
    D. One coil and one arm
21. **Who devised the orthodontic appliance to expand the dental arch?**
    A. Pierre Fauchard
    B. Edward H Angle
    C. Edgewise
    D. Charles H Tweed
22. **Orthodontic management malocclusion using Begg's appliance involves how many stages of treatment?**
    A. 2   B. 3
    C. 4   D. 5
23. **Pre-adjusted edgewise appliance is also known as**
    A. Straight wire appliance
    B. Lingual technique
    C. Begg technique
    D. Edgewise technique
24. **What is the significance of leveling and alignment?**
    A. Bracket alignment in buccal and lingual space
    B. Bracket alignment in vertical and lingual space
    C. Bracket alignment in occlusal and vertical space
    D. Bracket alignment in vertical and horizontal space
25. **The following are the various designs for loops in the design of orthodontic appliance except**
    A. T-Loop   B. Key Hole loop
    C. Dumbbell Loop   D. Omega Loop
26. **Torquing implies root movement in**
    A. Buccolingual direction
    B. Mesiodistal direction
    C. Only buccal direction
    D. Only lingual direction
27. **The mehod of fixing attachments directly to the teeth is called as**
    A. Banding   B. Bonding
    C. Soldering   D. Welding
28. **Which of the cements can be used for cementation of bands on to the teeth?**
    A. Zinc Phosphate
    B. Zinc Oxide Eugenol
    C. Reinforced Zinc Oxide Eugenol
    D. Resin luting cement
29. **To which depth is enamel etched during bonding?**
    A. 15-20 microns   B. 20-25 microns
    C. 25-30 microns   D. 30-35 microns
30. **Which among the following is not a disadvantage of bonding?**
    A. Bonded attachement are weaker than banded attachment and hence are more prone to band failure
    B. Bonding involve etching of enamel with acid which may lead to enamel loss
    C. The risk of caries under loose bands is eliminated
    D. Enamel fracture can occur during debonding
31. **In Begg fixed appliance, the brackets used are**
    A. Ribbon arch bracket
    B. Metallic bracket
    C. Weldable bracket
    D. Bondable bracket
32. **Examples of lingual attachments include the following, except**
    A. Lingual button   B. Lock pin
    C. Eyelets   D. Ball and hook
33. **Lock pins are small pins that are used to**
    A. Lock the arch wire to brackets
    B. Secure the arch wire to brackets
    C. Attach the arch wire to brackets
    D. Cement the arch wire to brackets
34. **Which component acts as handle on the teeth**
    A. Lingual cleaks   B. Brackets
    C. Buccal tube   D. Arch wires
35. **The most important disadvantage of fixed appliance**
    A. Very costly
    B. Cannot be removed by patient at will
    C. Oral hygiene maintenance is difficult
    D. Increased number of visits
36. **Advantage of fixed appliance over removable appliance is it**
    A. Can not be removed by patient at will
    B. More than one type of tooth movement at same time
    C. Patient cooperation is dispensed
    D. All of the above
37. **Simplest type of tooth movement**
    A. Torquing   B. Uprighting
    C. Derotation   D. Tipping
38. **Tipping in a tooth movement in which**
    A. Movement is produced by application of a single force
    B. Crown move in the direction of force
    C. Root move in the opposite direction
    D. All of the above
39. **Extrusion refer to**
    A. Lateral movement of teeth along their long axis

B. Horizontal movement of teeth along their long axis
C. Vertical movement of teeth along their long axis
D. All of the above

40. **Banding is indicated**
    A. In case of posterior teeth where moisture control is a problem for bonding
    B. In tooth that require buccal as well as lingual attachement
    C. When bands are likely to resist heavy force as in case of extra oral device
    D. In porcelain or gold restoration of crown
    E. All of the above

41. **A well pinched band is one that has**
    A. Adequate retention even without use of cement
    B. Can be removed easily from the tooth
    C. Does not require cementation
    D. All of the above

42. **Cementation of band is done to**
    A. Eliminate space between band and tooth
    B. Prevent caries
    C. Prevent cariogenic from seep and stagnate
    D. All of the above

43. **Acid etch technique was introduced by**
    A. Buonocore         B. Jon Golberg
    C. CJ Burstone       D. MF Tolass

44. **Acid etch technique was introduced in the year**
    A. 1955              B. 1965
    C. 1975              D. 1985

45. **Advantages of bonding over banding**
    A. Esthetically superior and oral better hygiene
    B. Faster to band than to pinch bands
    C. Easier to bond the band in case of partially erupted and fractured teeth
    D. All of the above

46. **Which one of the following constitute active components of fixed appliances?**
    A. Arch wires        B. Springs
    C. Elastics          D. All of the above

47. **Disadvantages of bonding over banding**
    A. Bonded attachments are weaker than banded attachments
    B. Enamel loss
    C. Increased risk of demineralization
    D. All of the above

48. **Ceramic brackets are made up of**
    A. Aluminium oxide   B. Zirconium oxide
    C. Both A and D      D. None of the above

49. **Plastic brackets are made up of**
    A. Polycarbonate     B. Aluminium oxide
    C. Zirconium oxide
    D. All of the above

50. **Lock pins are used in**
    A. Vertical slots of brackets
    B. Horizontal slots of brackets
    C. Rebond arch brackets
    D. Both A and C

51. **Buccal tube with double or triple tube serve the purpose of**
    A. Increasing the bulk of the material to resist occlusal force
    B. Esthetics
    C. Additional arch wire and facebow insertion
    D. None of the above

52. **Nitinol was invented by**
    A. Williams R Butchler   B. Jon Golberg
    C. CJ Burstone           D. Anderson

53. **NITINOL stands for**
    A. Nickel Titanium Naval orthodontic laboratory
    B. Nickel Titanium Naval ordinance laboratory
    C. Nickel Titanium Naval orthodontic law
    D. Nickel Titanium Naval ordinance law

54. **Disadvantage of NITINOL is**
    A. Resistance to taking a bend
    B. No loops and helices can be formed
    C. It cannot be soldered or weldered
    D. All of the above

55. **Beta-titanium was introduced by**
    A. John Golberg
    B. CJ Burstone
    C. Anderson
    D. Both A and C

56. **Cobalt Chromium Nickel alloys are available commercially as**
    A. Elgiloy           B. Optiflex
    C. TMA wire          D. Nitinol

57. **Separators serve the purpose of**
    A. Breaking tight interdental contact
    B. Easy placement of bands
    C. Avoiding distortion of bands
    D. All of the above

58. **Who devised the first appliance to expand dental arch?**
    A. John Golberg
    B. CJ Burstone
    C. Anderson
    D. Pierre Fauchard

59. **Difficult tooth movement to achieve with with ribbon arch appliance**
    A. Buccolingual
    B. Incisolingual
    C. Rotation control
    D. Mesiodistal tiping

**Ans:** 1. D  2. A  3. B  4. C  5. C  6. B  7. B  8. C  9. B  10. B  11. D  12. A  13. C  14. D  15. B  16. A  17. B  18. D  19. B  20. B  21. A  22. B  23. A  24. D  25. C  26. A  27. B  28. A  29. B  30. C  31. A  32. B  33. B  34. B  35. C  36. D  37. D  38. D  39. C  40. E  41. A  42. D  43. A  44. A  45. D  46. D  47. D  48. C  49. A  50. D  51. C  52. A  53. B  54. D  55. D  56. A  57. A  58. D  59. D

# FUNCTIONAL APPLIANCES

1. Most of the functional appliances are normally designed to correct
   A. Skeletal Class I relationship
   B. Skeletal Class II relationship
   C. Skeletal Class III relationship
   D. All of the above

2. An example for removable tooth borne functional appliance includes
   A. Activator
   B. Herbst appliance
   C. Jasper jamper
   D. All of the above

3. An example of removable tissue borne functional appliance is
   A. Activator
   B. Frankel appliance
   C. Jasper jamper
   D. All of the above

4. An example of fixed tooth borne appliance is
   A. Activator
   B. Frankel appliance
   C. Herbst appliance
   D. All of the above

5. Mode of action of functional appliances includes
   A. A forced mandibular posture which transmit forces to the teeth and jaws
   B. Bite planes which produce differential eruption
   C. Both A and B
   D. None of the above

6. Following are the advantages of fuctional appliances except
   A. Functional appliances are effective in vertical control of increased overbite
   B. Functional appliances can be used in the mixed dentition
   C. Functional appliances requires minimal chair side adjustment
   D. Functional appliances can also be used in older adult patients

7. Following are the disadvantages of fuctional appliances except
   A. The success of functional appliances therapy solely depends on patient cooperation
   B. Precise tooth movement is not possible with functional appliances
   C. Treatment duration of functional appliances is often prolonged
   D. Functional appliances can be used in the mixed dentition

8. Effect of functional appliance on dentititon includes
   A. Intrusion of maxillary incisors
   B. Protrusion of mandibular incisors
   C. Both A and B
   D. None of the above

9. Effect of functional appliance on skeletal structure includes
   A. Functional appliances are designed to stimulate the growth in the condylar region
   B. They can do procedure change in the direction of growth of the jaws
   C. They can also bring about downward and forward remodeling of the glenoid fossa
   D. All of the above

10. Effect of functional appliance on muscles includes
    A. They are designed to facilitate improvement of toxicity of orofacial musculature
    B. They produce downward and forward remodeling of the glenoid fossa
    C. They can change the direction of growth of the jaws
    D. All of the above

11. Who designed the activator?
    A. Viggo Anderson    B. EH Angle
    C. Farrar            D. Hunter

12. Activator is also known as
    A. Monoblock appliance B. Andreson appliance
    C. Both A and B      D. None of the above

13. Which of the following is not a modification of activator?
    A. The propulsor
    B. Kawetzky modification
    C. Wanderer's modification
    D. Monoblock appliance

14. The dental changes produced by activator include
    A. Overjet reduction
    B. Overbite reduction
    C. Upward and forward eruption of the lower molars
    D. All of the above

15. The skeletal changes produced by the activator include
    A. Downward and forward growth of the mandible
    B. Point A can move distally with the incisor roots
    C. Both A and B
    D. None of the above

16. Which of the following is not an indication of activator appliance?
    A. Class I malocclusion with deep bite
    B. Class II malocclusion with open bite
    C. Class II division 1 malocclusion
    D. Nail biting habit

17. Following are the contraindications of activator except
    A. Crowded arch
    B. Extreme vertical mandibular growth
    C. Severe proclined lower incisor
    D. Class I malocclusion with deep bite

18. Advantages of activator include
    A. Treating mixed and deciduous dentition is possible
    B. Tissue injury is very less
    C. Helps to eliminate abnormal habits
    D. All of the above

19. Disadvantages of activator include
    A. Fully rely on patient cooperation
    B. Bulky and uncomfortable
    C. Little or no response in older patients
    D. All of the above
20. Which of the following is not a patient instructions after delivering the activator?
    A. The patient is asked to wear the activator atleast 10-12 has in a day
    B. Patient is instructed to clean the appliance with a little of toothpaste and a toothbrush using cold water
    C. Patient is asked to keep the appliance in the mouth or in the box and not elsewhere
    D. Patient is also instructed to keep the appliance near pets
21. Where Bionator appliance was developed?
    A. Germany      B. France
    C. Switzerland  D. England
22. Who developed the appliance Bionator?
    A. Wilhelm Balter  B. Coffein
    C. Pierre Robin    D. Hapul
23. In which year Wilhem Balter developed Bionator appliance?
    A. Early 1950   B. Late 1980
    C. Early 1850
    D. None of the above
24. Standard Bionator is used for
    A. Treatment of Class II division 1 malocclusion
    B. Treatment of Class I malocclusion having constricted arches
    C. Both A and B
    D. None of the above
25. Which of the following is a wire component of standard Bionator?
    A. Maxillary wire
    B. Mandibular wire
    C. Interocclusal wire
    D. Vestibular wire
26. Which of the following is not a acrylic component of standard Bionator?
    A. Palatal arch
    B. Maxillary acrylic part
    C. Interocclusal acrylic part
    D. Mandibular acrylic part
27. Class III or reverse Bionator is used for
    A. Angle's Class III malocclusion caused due to mandibular prognathism
    B. Angle's Class II malocclusion
    C. Angle's Class I malocclusion
    D. All of the above
28. Which of the following is a acrylic component of Class III Bionator?
    A. Interocclusal acrylic part
    B. Palatal arch wire
    C. Vestibular wire
    D. Mandibular wire
29. Which of the following is not a wire component of Class III Bionator?
    A. Maxillary acrylic part
    B. Partial wire
    C. Vestibular view
    D. Both B and C
30. What are the differences between standard and Class III Bionator?
    A. Palatal arch wire is placed in opposite direction in Class III Bionator
    B. No acrylic component in Class II bionator
    C. Both A and B
    D. None of the above
31. Which of the following is not a type of Frankel I appliance?
    A. FR- Ig   B. FR- Ia
    C. FR- Ib   D. FR- Ic
32. Which of the following is not a Frankel appliance?
    A. FR-3abc  B. FR-1a
    C. FR-II    D. FR-IV
33. FR-Ia is indicated in
    A. Angle's Class I malocclusion with deep bite
    B. Angle's Class I malocclusion with cross bite
    C. Angle's Class I malocclusion with scissors bite
    D. All of the above
34. FR-Ib appliance of Frankel is indicated in
    A. Angle's Class II division 1 malocclusion where the overjet is more than 7 mm
    B. Angle's Class II division 1 malocclusion where the overjet does not exceeds 5 mm
    C. Angle's Class II division 2 malocclusions
    D. All of the above
35. FR-Ic appliance of Frankel is indicated in
    A. Angle's Class II division 1 malocclusion where the overjet is more than 7 mm
    B. Angle's Class II division 1 malocclusion where the overjet does not exceeds 5 mm
    C. Angle's Class II division 2 malocclusion
    D. All of the above
36. FR-II appliance of Frankel is not indicated in
    A. Angle's Class III malocclusion
    B. Angle's Class II division 1 malocclusion
    C. Angle's Class II malocclusion
    D. Both B and C
37. FR-III appliance of Frankel is not indicated in
    A. Angle's Class III malocclusion
    B. Angle's Class II division 1 malocclusion
    C. Angle's Class II malocclusion
    D. Both B and C
38. FR-IV appliance of Frankel is indicated in
    A. For treating bimaxillary proclination
    B. For treating open bite
    C. Both A and B
    D. None of the above
39. Who developed oral screen?
    A. Newell    B. Pierre Robin
    C. Hapul     D. Andersen

40. **Which year Newell developed oral screen?**
    A. 1910
    B. 1810
    C. 1912
    D. 2000
41. **Indications of oral screen are**
    A. Oral habits
    B. In cases of mild proclinations of maxillary anterior teeth
    C. Both A and B
    D. None of the above
42. **Which of the following is a modification of oral screen?**
    A. Double oral screen
    B. Hotz modification
    C. Oral screen with holes
    D. All of the above
43. **Uses of lip bumper include**
    A. To treat lip sucking habit
    B. To treat lip biting habit
    C. Used as a molar anchorage
    D. All of the above
44. **Lip bumper should be worn**
    A. 24 hours a day
    B. 10 hours a day
    C. 2 hours a day
    D. 12 hours a day
45. **Who introduced the Herbst appliance?**
    A. Emil Herbst
    B. Angle
    C. Case
    D. Ferrer
46. **Indications of Herbst appliance includes**
    A. Dental Class II malocclusion
    B. Deep bite with retroclined mandibular incisors
    C. Skeletal Class II mandibular deficiency
    D. All of the above
47. **Contraindications of Herbst appliance includes**
    A. Dental open bite
    B. Skeletal open bite
    C. Cases prone to root resorption
    D. All of the above
48. **Disadvantages of Herbst appliance are**
    A. High cost
    B. Associated with more chances of breakage
    C. Less patient acceptance
    D. All of the above
49. **Who introduced Twin Block appliance?**
    A. William Clark
    B. Twin
    C. Pancharg
    D. Andersen
50. **In which year William Clark developed Twin Block appliance?**
    A. 1970
    B. 1870
    C. 1977
    D. 1777
51. **Which of the following is not a disadvantage of Jasper jumper appliance?**
    A. It is more susceptible for breakage
    B. Lack of force when the mouth is held open slightly such as in sleeping mouth breathing
    C. Both A and B
    D. Ease of insertion of activation

**Ans:** 1. B  2. A  3. B  4. C  5. C  6. D  7. D  8. C  9. D  10. A  11. A  12. C  13. D  14. D  15. C  16. D  17. D  18. D  19. D  20. D  21. A  22. A  23. A  24. C  25. D  26. A  27. A  28. A  29. A  30. A  31. A  32. A  33. A  34. B  35. A  36. A  37. A  38. C  39. A  40. C  41. C  42. D  43. D  44. A  45. A  46. D  47. D  48. D  49. A  50. C  51. D

## DENTOFACIAL ORTHOPEDICS

1. **Following are the three basic types of orthodontic appliances that can be used for modifying the growth of maxilla and/or mandible, except**
    A. Orthopedic appliances
    B. Functional appliances
    C. Inter-arch elastic traction
    D. Space maintainers
2. **Orthodontic force, which when applied brings about**
    A. Dental change
    B. Skeletal change
    C. Both A and B
    D. None of above
3. **Orthopedic force, which when applied brings about**
    A. Dental change
    B. Skeletal change
    C. Both A and B
    D. None of above
4. **Orthodontic force is**
    A. Light forces (50-100 gms)
    B. Heavy forces (300-500 gms)
    C. Both A and B
    D. None of above
5. **Orthopedic force is**
    A. Light forces (50-100 gms)
    B. Heavy forces (300-500 gms)
    C. Both A and B
    D. None of above
6. **Head-gears are mainly used in**
    A. The management of skeletal class II malocclusion by growth modifications
    B. For distalization of molars
    C. Both A and B
    D. None of the above
7. **Which of the following is the anchor unit of the head-gear?**
    A. Face bow

B. J hook
C. Force generating unit
D. Head cap/neck strap

8. Which of the following is the force delivering unit of head-gear?
   A. Face bow or J hook
   B. Head cap
   C. Neck strap
   D. All of the above

9. Followings are the parts of face bow of the head-gear orthopedic appliance except
   A. Outer bow
   B. Inner bow
   C. Junction
   D. Outer wire joint

10. Outer bow of the face bow of the head-gear orthopedic appliance is made of
    A. A round stainless steel wire of 0.051" or 0.062"
    B. A round stainless steel wire of 0.7" or 0.9"
    C. 1"-3.0"
    D. 4.0"-5.0"

11. Inner bow of the face bow of the head gear is made of
    A. 0.045"
    B. 1.25"
    C. Both of A and B
    D. None

12. Head gear appliance derives anchorage from
    A. Bones of skull
    B. Bones of back of neck
    C. Both A and B
    D. None of the above

13. Following are the indications of head gear therapy except
    A. Variety of skeletal class II problems
    B. For distalization of maxillary molars
    C. To reinforce intraoral anchorage
    D. For distalization of mandibular molars

14. Usually at what age the head gear therapy is given in females?
    A. 8.5-10.5 years    B. 14.5-17.5 years
    C. 19.5-23.5 years   D. 24.5-28.5 years

15. Usually at what age the head gear therapy is given in males?
    A. 9.5-11.5 years    B. 8.5-10.5 years
    C. 14.5-17.5 years   D. 24.5-28.5 years

16. Followings are the types of head gear except
    A. Cervical head gear    B. Occipital head gear
    C. High pull head gear   D. Pulling head gear

17. Cervical head gear derives anchorage from
    A. Back of the neck    B. Front of the neck
    C. Forehead            D. All of the above

18. What kind of force is produced from cervical head gear?
    A. Mesial and superior force
    B. Distal and superior force
    C. Distal and inferior force
    D. Mesial and inferior force

19. Cervical headgear produces
    A. Distal movement of maxilla
    B. Distal movement of maxillary molars
    C. Extrusion of molars
    D. All of the above

20. Which of the following statement is true
    A. Cervical headgear should be used only in patients with flat mandibular and occlusal planes in which an increase in facial height is desired
    B. Cervical headgear derives anchorage from front of the neck
    C. Cervical headgear produces intrusion of molars
    D. Cervical headgear produces a mesial and superior force

21. Cervical headgear are contraindicated in
    A. Patient with open bite
    B. High angle cases
    C. Both A and B    D. None of the above

22. Which type of headgear has better patient compliance?
    A. Cervical headgear
    B. Occipital headgear
    C. High pull headgear
    D. All of the above

23. Why cervical headgear has better patient compliance than over any of other types of headgear
    A. Due to its simple design
    B. Cervical headgear assembly having only one strap
    C. Both A and B
    D. None of the above

24. Disadvantage of cervical headgear includes
    A. It produces intrusion of molars
    B. It produces bite closure
    C. It produces opening of bite by rotating mandible downward and backward
    D. All of the above

25. Occipital headgear derives anchorage from
    A. Anterior to occipital bone
    B. Posterior to occipital bone
    C. From occipital region of the head
    D. None of the above

26. Occipital headgear is used in the correction of
    A. Anterior-posterior maxillary excess
    B. Vertical maxillary excess
    C. Horizontal maxillary excess
    D. Both A and B

27. **Vertical pull headgear derives anchorage from**
    A. Parietal region
    B. Occipital region
    C. Frontal region
    D. All of the above
28. **Vertical pull headgear produces**
    A. Intrusion and distalization of maxillary molar
    B. Extrusion and distalization of maxillary molar
    C. Rotation of maxillary molar
    D. All of the above
29. **Face mask is also called as**
    A. Reverse pull headgear
    B. Protraction headgear
    C. Both A and B
    D. None of the above
30. **Face mask is used in the treatment of patients with**
    A. Class III malocclusion
    B. Class II malocclusion
    C. Class I malocclusion
    D. All of the above
31. **Following are the parts of the face mask except**
    A. Forehead cap
    B. Chin cup
    C. Metal frame work
    D. Arch wire
32. **Which of the following is not a type of face mask**
    A. Delarie type of face mask
    B. Tubinger type of face mask
    C. Petit type of face mask
    D. Henrry type of face mask
33. **Which type of face mask has least patient acceptance**
    A. Delarie type of face mask
    B. Tubinger type of face mask
    C. Petit type of Face mask
    D. All of the above
34. **Which type of face mask has least metal frame work of the face in their design?**
    A. Delarie type of face mask
    B. Tubinger type of face mask
    C. Petit type of face mask
    D. Face masking device
35. **What is common in all three types of face mask?**
    A. Metal frame work
    B. Forehead cap
    C. Chin cup
    D. All of the above
36. **Chin cup assembly consists of**
    A. Chin cup–covers chin
    B. Head cap–covers the head
    C. Elastic strap–connects chin cup with head cap
    D. All of the above
37. **Which of the following is not a type of chin cup appliance**
    A. Occipital pull chin cup
    B. Vertical pull chin cup
    C. Both A and B
    D. None of the above
38. **Which type of chin cup is most commonly used**
    A. Occipital pull chin cup
    B. Vertical pull chin cup
    C. Horizontal pull chin cup
    D. Oblique pull chin cup
39. **Which of the following is not the effect of chin cup appliance**
    A. Lingual tipping of lower incisors
    B. Improvement in skeletal and soft tissue profile
    C. Remodelling of the mandible and a decrease in mandibular plane angle or gonial angle
    D. Redirection of mandibular growth in a upward and forward direction
40. **Chin cup appliance is indicated in**
    A. Patient with a mild skeletal prognathism of the mandible
    B. In the case of decreased facial height
    C. Patient who has aligned or protrusive but not retroclined mandibular incisors
    D. All of the above
41. **Orthopedic appliance wear usually recommended for how many hours in a day**
    A. 10-12 Hours
    B. Whole day
    C. 6-8 Hours
    D. 2-3 Hours
42. **Orthopedic appliance wear usually recommended for what time in a day**
    A. During evening and night
    B. During morning and afternoon
    C. Any time during day
    D. None of the above
43. **Force generating unit of the headgear may be in the form of**
    A. Springs
    B. Elastics
    C. Other stretchable material
    D. All of the above
44. **Which form of force generating unit is most commonly used for headgear therapy**
    A. Springs
    B. Elastics
    C. Other stretchable material
    D. All of the above
45. **Where both terminal ends of inner bow of face bow of the headgear is inserted**
    A. Rectangular buccal-tube
    B. Round buccal-facebow-tube
    C. Kept free
    D. Soldered to premolar brackets
46. **Outer bow of facebow can be**
    A. Short
    B. Medium
    C. Long
    D. All of the above
47. **What is the purpose of having bayonet bends mesial to the buccal tube of first permanent molar?**
    A. To prevent the inner bow from sliding too far distally through the buccal tube

B. To prevent the outer bow from sliding too far distally through the buccal tube
C. To prevent the inner bow from sliding too far mesially through the buccal tube
D. None of the above

48. Where center of resistance of maxilla is located
    A. Between the roots of the premolar teeth
    B. Between the roots of the molar teeth
    C. Between the roots of the second molar teeth
    D. None of the above

**Ans:** 1. D  2. A  3. B  4. A  5. B  6. C  7. D  8. A  9. D  10. A  11. C  12. C  13. D  14. A  15. A  16. D  17. A  18. C  19. D  20. A  21. C  22. A  23. C  24. C  25. C  26. D  27. A  28. A  29. C  30. A  31. D  32. D  33. A  34. C  35. D  36. D  37. D  38. A  39. D  40. D  41. A  42. A  43. D  44. A  45. B  46. D  47. A  48. A

## 11. CORRECTIVE ORTHODONTICS

### MANAGEMENT OF CLASS I MALOCCLUSION

1. The most commonly encountered problem in Class I malocclusion is
   A. Bimaxillary protrusion
   B. Proclination
   C. Crowding of maxillary and mandibular arches
   D. All of the above

2. If there is harmonious relationship of the underlying skeletal structures and malocclusion is restricted to the dental malrelations only, then the malocclusion is
   A. Class I malocclusion
   B. Class II division 1 malocclusion
   C. Class II division 2 malocclusion
   D. Class III malocclusion

3. In general the problems associated with Class I malocclusion are primarily of
   A. Skeletal in origin
   B. Dental in origin
   C. Both of the above
   D. None of the above

4. Periodontal complications are very frequently seen in
   A. Class I malocclusion
   B. Class II division 1 malocclusion
   C. Class II division 2 malocclusion
   D. Class III malocclusion

5. The two most commonly occuring forms seen in Class I malocclusion is
   A. Bimaxillary proclination and crowding
   B. Crowding and Spacing
   C. Anterior crossbite and crowding
   D. None of the above

6. Bimaxillary protrusion is commonly seen in
   A. Afro-Asian population
   B. Afro-Carribean population
   C. Asians population
   D. Chinese population

7. Class I skeletal cases having a severe arch length discrepancy may be treated in preadolescent stages by
   A. Fixed orthodontics
   B. Serial extraction
   C. Expansion
   D. All of the above

8. True skeletal protrusion is best treated by
   A. Fixed appliance
   B. Removable appliance
   C. Subapical osteotomy with concomitant extraction of first premolar
   D. All of the above

9. Crowding occurs due to
   A. Decrease in arch length
   B. Increase in tooth length
   C. Both A and B
   D. None of the above

10. Crowding manifests due to
    A. Presence of supernumerary teeth
    B. Over retained deciduous teeth
    C. Abnormalies in size and shape of teeth
    D. All of the above

11. For every 1mm of crowding, the space needed for correction and alignment is
    A. 1.5 mm
    B. 1.25 mm
    C. 1 mm
    D. 2 mm

12. Rotations can be
    A. Mesolingual
    B. Distobuccal
    C. Distolingual
    D. All of the above

13. Tooth movement around their long axes is called as
    A. Tipping
    B. Bodily movement
    C. Rotation
    D. None of the above

14. Mild rotation can be treated by
    A. NiTi arch wires
    B. Stainless steel round wire
    C. Stainless steel rectangular wire
    D. Stainless steel square wire

15. Surgical correction in Class I malocclusion can be done for patients exhibiting
    A. Tissue dental protrusion
    B. Bimaxillary protrusion
    C. True skeletal protrusion
    D. Any of the above

16. For alignment of mild crowding, space may be created by
    A. Proximal stripping
    B. Expansion of the arch
    C. Derotation of adjacent posterior teeth
    D. All of the above

Ans: 1. D   2. A   3. B   4. A   5. A   6. B   7. B   8. D   9. C   10. D   11. C   12. D   13. C   14. A   15. C   16. D

## MANAGEMENT OF CLASS II MALOCCLUSION

1. Which is the most difficult malocclusion to treat
    A. Class I with bimaxillary protrusion
    B. Class II malocclusion
    C. Class III skeletal malocclusion
    D. All of the above

2. Treatment of Class II malocclusion mainly depends on
    A. Adequate knowledge of normal growth pattern
    B. Cephalometric analysis
    C. Treatment planning
    D. All of the above

3. Angle divided the Class II malocclusion as
    A. Class II division 2
    B. Class II division 1
    C. Both of the above
    D. None of the above

4. If molar relation is Class II with proclination of upper anteriors, the resultant malocclusion is
    A. Class II division 2
    B. Class II division 1
    C. Class II subdivision
    D. Class I subdivision

5. If molar relation is Class II with retroclined upper centrals overlapped by upper laterals, the malocclusion is
    A. Class II division 1 malocclusion
    B. Class II division 2 malocclusion
    C. Class III subdivision malocclusion
    D. None of the above

6. Patient with Class II malocclusion exhibits
    A. Straight profile
    B. Concave profile
    C. Convex profile
    D. Orthognatic profile

7. (I) In Class II malocclusion division 1, proclination in upper anteriors is present.
   (II) The lower anterior teeth contacts the palatal surface of upper teeth
    A. I statement is true    B. II statement is true
    C. Both statements are true
    D. Both statements are false

8. Curve of Spee in Class II malocclusion is
    A. Increased
    B. Decreased
    C. Straight
    D. None of the above

9. Short hypotonic upper lip is a feature of
    A. Class I malocclusion
    B. Class II malocclusion
    C. Class III malocclusion
    D. None of the above

10. Lip trap is a feature of
    A. Class I malocclusion
    B. Class II malocclusion
    C. Class III malocclusion
    D. None of the above

11. In Von-der-Lindon's classification, Class II division 2 type A
    A. Upper central and lateral incisors are retroclined
    B. Upper central incisors are retroclined and overlapped by laterals
    C. Upper central and lateral incisors are retroclined and overlapped by canines
    D. None of the above

12. In Von-der-Lindon's classification of Class II division 2 type B
    A. Upper central and lateral incisors are retroclined
    B. Upper central incisors are retroclined and overlapped by laterals
    C. Upper central and lateral incisors are retroclined and overlapped by canines
    D. None of the above

13. In Von-der-Lindon's classification of Class II division 2 type C
    A. Upper central and lateral incisors are retroclined
    B. Upper central incisors are retroclined and overlapped by laterals
    C. Upper central and lateral incisors are retroclined and overlapped by canines
    D. None of the above

14. Abnormal skeletal relationship of maxilla and mandible in Class II malocclusion are
    A. Maxillary protrusion   B. Mandibular retrusion
    C. Both A and B           D. None of the above

15. Abnormal buccinator activity is found in
    A. Class II division 1 malocclusion
    B. Class II division 2 malocclusion
    C. Class I malocclusion
    D. Class III malocclusion
16. Prenatal factors in etiology of Class II malocclusion include
    A. Hereditary
    B. Teratogenesis
    C. Irradiation
    D. All of the above
17. Well aligned deciduous dentition leads to
    A. Well aligned permanent dentition
    B. Spacing in permanent dentition
    C. Crowding in permanent dentition
    D. None of the above
18. Post-natal factors in etiology of Class II malocclusion is
    A. Traumatic injury to mandible and TMJ
    B. Long time radiation therapy
    C. Habits such as thumb sucking or mouth breathing
    D. All of the above
19. Which of the following is a treatment objective of Class II malocclusion?
    A. Reduction of overjet
    B. Reduction of overbite and crowding
    C. Crowding of local irregularities
    D. All of the above
20. Treatment of skeletal Class II malocclusion is done by
    A. Growth modification
    B. Camouflage
    C. Surgical correction
    D. All of the above
21. Growth modification in Class II division 1 is undertaken during
    A. Mixed dentition period
    B. Early permanent dentition period prior to cessation of growth
    C. Both A and B
    D. None of the above
22. Most important prerequisite in treatment of Class II division 1 malocclusion include
    A. Diagnosis
    B. Cephalometric analysis
    C. Growth modification
    D. All of the above
23. The appliance which best treats Class II division 1 malocclusion at the end of growth period is
    A. Herbst appliance
    B. Activator
    C. Jasper Jumper
    D. Both A and C
24. Class II division 1 malocclusion is best treated during mixed dentition period by
    A. Activator
    B. Functional regulator
    C. Both A and B
    D. Herbst appliance
25. The main aim of fixed functional appliance treatment of Class II division 1 is to
    A. Correct maxillary prognathism
    B. Correct mandibular prognathism
    C. Correct maxillary retrognathism
    D. Correct mandibular retrognathism
26. Correction of maxillary prognathism in Class II division 1 malocclusion is achieved by
    A. Myofunctional appliances
    B. Orthopedic appliances
    C. Both A and B
    D. None of the above
27. Which teeth are extracted in class III surgical case?
    A. Upper first premolars only
    B. Lower first premolars only
    C. Lower second premolars only
    D. Upper first premolars and lower second premolars
28. Common feature of class II division 1 malocclusion is
    A. Crossbites
    B. Deep bite
    C. Bimaxillary protrusion
    D. Rotations
29. The initial stage in correction of class II division 1 malocclusion should be focused on
    A. Management of functional disturbance
    B. Management of deep bite
    C. Management of bimaxillary protrusion
    D. None of the above
30. Extraoral forces using headgear in treatment of class II division 1 is most effective in
    A. Correction of mandibular prognathism
    B. Restriction of maxillary retrognathism
    C. Correction of maxillary prognathism
    D. Combination of the above
31. Myofunctional appliances when given in class II division 1 malocclusion results in
    A. Correction of maxillary retrognathism
    B. Restriction of the growth of maxilla
    C. Correction of mandibular prognathism
    D. Correction of mandibular retrognathism
32. In class II division 2 the patient presents with a face form of
    A. brachycephalic
    B. dolicocephalic
    C. mesocephalic
    D. combination of the above
33. Traumatic deep bite is usually seen in
    A. Class I malocclusion
    B. Class II division 2 malocclusion
    C. Class III true malocclusion
    D. Class III pseudomalocclusion

34. In class II division 2 malocclusion the upper arch is
    A. Broad and U-shaped
    B. Narrow and V-shaped
    C. Broad and V-shaped
    D. Narrow and U-shaped

35. Patient with class II division 2 malocclusion usually presents with
    A. Round Face
    B. Oval face
    C. Squarish face
    D. None of the above

36. The main treatment aspect in class II division 2 malocclusion is
    A. Correction of incisal relationship
    B. Relief of crowding and local irregularities
    C. Correction of buccal segment relationship
    D. All of the above

37. Characteristic feature of Class II division 2 malocclusion is
    A. Deep anterior overbite
    B. Retroclination
    C. Both A and B
    D. None of the above

38. Deep anterior overbite and retroclination in Class II divison 2 malocclusion is treated by
    A. Reduction in incisal overbite
    B. Alteration of incisal inclination
    C. Both A and B
    D. Proclination of lower jaw

39. Orthognathic surgery for treatment of Class II division 1 malocclusion should be undertaken
    A. Only after cessation of growth
    B. Before cessation of growth
    C. Early permanent dentition period
    D. None of the above

40. Surgical approaches for correction of maxillary prognathism
    A. Total maxillary retro positioning
    B. Partial maxillary retro positioning
    C. Both A and B
    D. None of the above

41. Surgical approach for correction of mandibular retrognathism is
    A. L- osteotomy
    B. C- osteotomy
    C. Bilateral saggital split osteotomy
    D. All of the above

42. Major disadvantage of saggital split osteotomy in correction of Class II division 1 malocclusion is
    A. Damage to lingual nerve
    B. Damage to long buccal nerve
    C. Damage to optic nerve
    D. Both A and B

43. Torquing spring when used to correct Class II division 2 malocclusion brings
    A. Movement of upper incisors roots lingually
    B. Movement of upper incisors crown bucally
    C. Both A and B
    D. None of the above

44. Which of the following may be used to correct anterior deep bite in Class II malocclusion
    A. Anterior bite planes
    B. Reverse curve of spee wires
    C. Anchor bends in arch wires
    D. All of the above

45. The teeth most frequently extracted in Class II division 2 malocclusion during fixed orthodontic therapy is
    A. First premolar only
    B. Second premolar only
    C. Lower second premolar and upper first premolar only
    D. Any of the above

46. Distalisation of maxillary molars as a part of orthodontic camouflage is done
    A. Prior to eruption of second molars
    B. In late mixed dentition period
    C. Mild class II division 1 cases
    D. All of the above

47. Most Class II division 1 malocclusion exhibit
    A. Bimaxillary protrusion
    B. Deep bite
    C. Abnormal muscle activity
    D. All of the above

48. Lip trap with short upper lip may cause
    A. Proclination of lower anteriors
    B. Retroclination of upper anteriors
    C. Proclination of upper anteriors
    D. All of the above

49. Hyperactive mentalis muscle is a common finding of
    A. Class I malocclusion with bimaxillary protrusion
    B. Class II division 1 malocclusion
    C. Class II division 2 malocclusion
    D. Class III malocclusion

50. Class II division 1 malocclusion can be associated with
    A. Proclined lower anteriors sometimes
    B. Proclined lower anteriors always
    C. Retroclined upper anteriors sometimes
    D. Any of the above combination

Ans: 1. B  2. D  3. C  4. B  5. B  6. C  7. A  8. A  9. B  10. B  11. A  12. B  13. C  14. C  15. A  16. D  17. C  18. D  19. D  20. D  21. C  22. A  23. D  24. C  25. D  26. C  27. B  28. A  29. A  30. C  30. D  31. A  32. B  33. B  34. A  35. C  36. D  37. C  38. C  39. A  40. C  41. D  42. D  43. C  44. D  45. A  46. D  47. C  48. B  49. B  50. A

## MANAGEMENT OF CLASS III MALOCCULUSION

1. Malocclusion which is easy to diagnose and pose a challenge to treat is
   A. Class I malocclusion
   B. Class II division 1 malocclusion
   C. Class III division 2 malocclusion
   D. Class III malocclusion

2. The most common problem associated after the treatment of Class III malocclusion is
   A. Restricted mandibular growth
   B. Restricted maxillary growth
   C. Mandibular retrognathism
   D. High tendency relapse

3. Progressive type of malocclusion is
   A. Class I
   B. Class III
   C. Class II
   D. Combination of A and B

4. Class III malocclusion
   A. Pose therapeutic challenge to orthodontist
   B. Has high tendency of relapse following treatment
   C. Is easy to diagnose
   D. Is difficult to treat
   E. All of the above

5. Edge to edge relation is a feature of
   A. Class I malocclusion
   B. Class III malocclusion
   C. Class II division 1 malocclusion
   D. Class II division 2 malocclusion

6. Narrow and short upper arch and broad lower arch is found in
   A. Class I malocclusion
   B. Class II malocclusion
   C. Class I with bimaxillary malocclusion
   D. Class III malocclusion

7. Crowded upper arch and spaced lower arch is usually found in
   A. Class I malocclusion
   B. Class III malocclusion
   C. Class II division 1 malocclusion
   D. Class II division 2 malocclusion

8. Class III malocclusion usually presents with
   A. Straight to concave profile
   B. Prominent chin
   C. Posterior crossbites
   D. All of the above

9. Gonial angle in Class III malocclusion is
   A. Acute            B. Obtuse
   C. 90 degrees       D. Any of the above

10. Class III malocclusion presents with
    A. Class III canine relationship
    B. Reverse overjet
    C. Labially inclined lower incisors and lingually inclined upper incisors
    D. All of the above

11. Skeletal Class III malocclusion occurs due to
    A. A short or retrognathic maxilla
    B. A long or prognathic mandible
    C. Combination of A and B
    D. None of the above

12. Malocclusion which have a strong genetic background is
    A. Class III malocclusion
    B. Class II division 1
    C. Class II division 2
    D. Class I

13. Class III skeletal imbalance occurs due to
    A. Large mandible and short maxilla
    B. Too small maxilla relative to mandible
    C. Retropositioned maxilla
    D. All of the above

14. Class III malocclusion can be classified into
    A. Dental or skeletal
    B. True or pseudo
    C. Both of the above
    D. None of the above

15. (I) Unfavourable incisal guidance leads to pseudo Class III.
    (II) Pseudo Class III, if unattended, can lead to a true skeletal Class III
    A. Statement I is true
    B. Statement I is false
    C. Statement II is true
    D. Both the statements are true

16. Treatment of Class III malocclusion in preadolescent child can be attempted by
    A. Frankel III appliance
    B. Chin cup
    C. Anterior facemask
    D. All of the above

17. 3D expansion screws when used in Class III malocclusion brings about
    A. Forward placement of maxilla
    B. Lateral expansion of maxilla
    C. Expansion in all three directions
    D. All of the above

18. Activator of choice in treatment of Class III malocclusion
    A. Reduced activator   B. Propulsor
    C. Reverse activator
    D. Palate free activator

19. Choice of Frankel appliance in treatment of Class III malocclusion is
    A. FR 1              B. FR 1 C
    C. FR 2              D. FR 3

20. Frankel 3 appliance when used to treat Class III malocclusion brings about
    A. Growth of maxilla
    B. Growth of mandible
    C. Restrict growth of maxilla
    D. Restrict growth of mandible
21. FR3 to treat Class III malocclusion is indicated when
    A. Maxillary skeletal retrusion is present
    B. Mandibular prognathism is present
    C. Both of the above
    D. None of the above
22. Vertical and anteroposterior deficiency of maxilla with normal mandible is seen in
    A. Pierre Robin syndrome
    B. Cleidocranial dystosis
    C. Cleft lip and palate
    D. All of the above
23. Chin cup when used to treat Class III malocclusion change the direction of growth of mandible in the direction
    A. Forward and upward
    B. Downward and backward
    C. Forward and downward
    D. Backward and forward
24. Pressure from chin cup tends to
    A. Tip the mandibular incisors labially
    B. Tip the maxillary incisors lingually
    C. Tip the mandibular incisors lingually
    D. Tip the maxillary incisors labially
25. Recent advancement in treating Class III malocclusion includes
    A. Chin cup
    B. Anterior facemask
    C. 3D screws
    D. RME with anterior facemask
26. Anterior facemask used to treat Class III malocclusion provide mainly
    A. Anterior and/or downward rotation of maxilla
    B. Posterior and/or upward rotation of mandible
    C. Both of the above
    D. None of the above
27. Which of the following can be used with anterior facemask in treating Class III malocclusion to bring a synergistic action?
    A. FR 3
    B. Chin cup
    C. 3D screws
    D. Rapid maxillary expander
28. Dental compensation in skeletal Class III cases is achieved by
    A. Proclining lower incisor only
    B. Retroclining lower incisors
    C. Proclining lower and upper incisors
    D. Retroclining lower and proclining upper incisors
29. Mid saggital suture opening after RPE is assessed by
    A. OPG
    B. Lateral Cephalogram
    C. Periapical
    D. Upper occlusal radiograph
30. Treatment of Class III malocclusion in adolescent is limited to
    A. Orthodontic camouflage
    B. Orthodontic decompensation
    C. Both of the above
    D. None of the above
31. Class III elastics is placed between
    A. Upper canine to lower molar
    B. Upper canine to upper molar
    C. Upper molar to lower canine
    D. Lower canine to lower molar
32. Class III malocclusion treatment involves extraction of
    A. Upper first premolars and lower first premolars
    B. Upper first premolars
    C. Lower first premolars and second premolars
    D. Upper second premolars and lower first premolars
33. Class III malocclusion treatment during adulthood is best achieved by
    A. Orthodontic camouflage only
    B. Orthognathic surgery
    C. Orthopedic appliance
    D. All of the above
34. Commonly used procedure in surgical management of Class III malocclusion is
    A. Sagittal split osteotomy in mandible
    B. Lefort I down fracture in maxilla
    C. Both of the above
    D. None of the above
35. Pseudo Class III is best treated by
    A. Removal of occlusal prematurity
    B. 3D expansion screws
    C. Orthopedic appliance
    D. All of the above
36. Non surgical management for Class III malocclusion includes
    A. Anterior vertical elastics
    B. Posterior bite blocks
    C. High pull headgear
    D. All of the above
37. Who was the first person to perform a surgery on a prognathic jaw?
    A. Hulliken
    B. Babcock
    C. Blair
    D. All of the above

38. Habsburg jaw is usually referred to
    A. Dominant protrusive maxilla
    B. Dominant protrusive mandible
    C. Retrusive maxilla
    D. Retrusive mandible
39. Modified Tandem Appliance is used to treat
    A. Class I
    B. Class II division 1
    C. Class II division 2
    D. Class III
40. Multilooped edgewire technique in treatment for severe Class III malocclusion uses
    A. Extraction of maxillary third molar
    B. Extraction of mandibular third molar
    C. Extraction of maxillary first molar
    D. Extraction of mandibular first molar
41. Orthopedic appliances used to treat class III malocclusion in pre-adolescent are
    A. Chin-cup appliance
    B. Anterior face mask with RME
    C. High pull headgear
    D. Both A and B
42. Orthopedic appliances used to treat class III malocclusion in adolescent are
    A. Chin-cup appliance
    B. Anterior face mask with RME
    C. High pull headgear
    D. All of the above
43. Orthopedic appliances used to treat class III malocclusion in adults are
    A. Chin-cup appliance
    B. Anterior face mask with RME
    C. High pull headgear
    D. None of the above
44. Functional appliances used in the management of class III malocclusion in pre-adolescent are
    A. Frankel III appliance
    B. Frankel II appliance
    C. Activator
    D. Lip Bumper
45. Functional appliance used in the management of class III malocclusion in adolescents is
    A. Class III bionator
    B. Frankel II appliance
    C. Activator
    D. Lip Bumper
46. How do we manage class III malocclusion in adults?
    A. Orthognathic surgery
    B. Removable orthodontic appliance
    C. Orthopedic appliances
    D. None of the above
47. How do we manage class III malocclusion in adolescent using fixed orthodontic appliances?
    A. Fixed orthodontic appliance with class III intermaxillary elastics
    B. Dental camouflage using fixed mechanotherapy
    C. Both A and B
    D. None of the above
48. Skeletal class III malocclusion caused due to severe mandibular prognathism can be treated by
    A. Mandibular set back procedure
    B. Le-Fort I osteotomy
    C. Both A and B
    D. None of the above
49. Skeletal class III malocclusion caused due to maxillary retrognathism can be treated by
    A. Mandibular set back procedure
    B. Le-Fort I osteotomy
    C. Both A ande B
    D. None of the above
50. Posterior cross bite in class III malocclusion can be treated by
    A. RME
    B. Anterior bite plane
    C. Both A and B
    D. None of the above

Ans: 1. D  2. D  3. B  4. E  5. B  6. D  7. B  8. D  9. B  10. D  11. C  12. A  13. D  14. C  15. D  16. D  17. C  18. C  19. D  20. A  21. A  22. C  23. B  24. C  25. C  26. A  27. D  28. C  29. D  30. C  31. C  32. C  33. B  34. A  35. A  36. D  37. A  38. B  39. D  40. B  41. D  42. D  43. D  44. A  45. A  46. A  47. C  48. A  49. B  50. A

## MANAGEMENT OF MIDLINE DIASTEMA

1. Midline diastema is spacing between:
    A. Two permanent maxillary central incisors
    B. Permanent upper central and lateral incisors
    C. Two deciduous maxillary central incisors
    D. Deciduous upper central and lateral incisors
2. (I) Midlin diastema is easy to treat.
   (II) It is very easy to retain.
    A. Transient malocclusion
    B. Developmental disturbances
    C. Pathological factors and Iatrogenic factors
    D. All of the above
3. Midline diastema is easy to treat.It is very easy to retain:
    A. First statement is true
    B. Second statement is true
    C. Both statements are true
    D. Both statements are false
4. Tooth material discrepancy causing midline diastema can be attributed to:
    A. Microdontia

B. Congenitally missing laterals
C. Mesiodens
D. All of the above

5. Oral habits in the aetiology of midline diastema:
   A. Thumb sucking habit
   B. Tongue thrusting habit
   C. Mouth breathing habit
   D. All of the above

6. Pathological conditions causing midline diastema:
   A. Cystic lesions      B. Midline tumours
   C. Odontomes           D. All of the above

7. Causes of midline diastema can be:
   A. Hereditary factors
   B. Racial predisposition
   C. Transient malocclusion
   D. All of the above

8. Ugly duckling stage is also known as:
   A. Transient malocclusion
   B. Self correcting malocclusion
   C. Iatrogenic induced malocclusion
   D. Both A and B

9. Midline diastema seen in ugly duckling stage is :
   A. Self correcting
   B. Transient
   C. Seen in 8-9 years of age
   D. All of the above

10. Midline diastema in ugly duckling stage is corrected by:
    A. Eruption of lateral incisors
    B. Eruption of permanent maxillary canines
    C. Eruption of permanent maxillary laterals
    D. Eruption of permanent maxillary second molar

11. Midline spacing in deciduous dentition:
    A. Occurs as a part of generalised spacing
    B. Is normal
    C. Helps in accommodating large sized permanent teeth
    D. All of the above

12. Iatrogenic midline diastema occurs as a result of:
    A. Orthodontic treatment procedures
    B. Rapid maxillary expansion
    C. Opening of intermaxillary suture
    D. All of the above

13. Prognostic sign during rapid maxillary expansion:
    A. Midline diastema appearance
    B. Spacing between teeth
    C. Crowding between teeth
    D. All of the above

14. Most common etiological cause of midline diastema:
    A. Thumb sucking habit
    B. Mouth breathing habit
    C. Genetic factors
    D. Abnormal labial frenum

15. Midline diastema due to abnormal labial frenum is diagnosed by:
    A. Cotton test
    B. Water test
    C. Blanch test
    D. Mirror test

16. Clinical features of midline diastema include:
    A. Localised papillary gingivitis in relation to permanent central incisors
    B. Unaesthetic appearance during conversation and smiling
    C. Hampered phonation and escape of saliva during speech
    D. All of the above

17. Blanching present in oral cavity indicates:
    A. Midline diastema
    B. Presence of thick and fleshy frenum
    C. Both A and B
    D. None of the above

18. Presence of notch like radiolucent area in the interdental region between 2 permanent maxillary central incisors in the midline indicates:
    A. Presence of mesiodens
    B. Presence of cyst in midline
    C. Presence of abnormal frenal attachment
    D. Any of the above

19. First phase of treatment in midline diastema:
    A. Conservative treatment
    B. Active orthodontic therapy
    C. Removable orthodontic appliance
    D. Removal of cause of midline diastema

20. Treatment of midline diastema due to presence of oral habits should be aimed at:
    A. Active orthodontic therapy
    B. Removable orthodontic appliance
    C. Elimination of oral habits
    D. All of the above

21. Midline diastema due to abnormal labial frenum should be treated by:
    A. Midline elastics
    B. Removable orthodontic appliance
    C. Frenectomy
    D. Split labial bow

22. Secondary phase of treatment in midline diastema:
    A. Elimination of habit
    B. Frenectomy
    C. Treatment of midline pathologies
    D. Active orthodontic therapy

23. The main disadvantage of using split labial bow in treatment of midline diastema is:
    A. Opening of space in premolar region
    B. Opening of space between central and lateral incisors

C. Both A and B
D. None of the above

24. **Split labial bow to treat midline diastema should extend upto:**
    A. Distal surface of canines on opposite sides
    B. Distal surface of lateral incisors on opposite sides
    C. Distal surface of central incisors on opposite sides
    D. Combination of the above

25. **Removable orthodontic appliance used in treatment of midline diastema incorporates:**
    A. Finger spring
    B. Split labial bow
    C. Modified split labial bow
    D. All of the above

26. **The third phase of treatment of midline diastema include:**
    A. Elimination of oral habits
    B. Removal of any midline pathologies
    C. Active orthodontic therapy
    D. Retaining the corrected midline diastema

27. **Fixed orthodontic appliance in treatment of midline diastema includes:**
    A. Closed coil spring
    B. E-chain
    C. Elastic thread and M spring
    D. All of the above

28. **"M spring" used in treatment of midline diastema is activated by:**
    A. Closing the three helices of the spring
    B. Closing the two helices of the spring
    C. Opening the three helices of the spring
    D. Opening the two helices of the spring

29. **Conservative approach of treating midline diastema is attempted if:**
    A. Space is upto 3-4 mm
    B. Space is upto 0-2 mm
    C. Space is upto 4-5 mm
    D. All of the above

30. **Conservative treatment of midline diastema includes;**
    A. Closure of space by removable orthodontic appliance
    B. Closure of space by fixed orthodontic appliance
    C. Closure space by composite build up
    D. Closure of space by fixed prosthesis

31. **Midline diastema needs:**
    A. Short term retention
    B. No retention
    C. Long term retention
    D. Any of the above

32. **Prosthetic treatment of midline diastema is done:**
    A. In case of microdontic tooth
    B. Missing tooth
    C. Peg shaped laterals
    D. All of the above

**Ans:** 1. A  2. D  3. A  4. D  5. D  6. D  7. D  8. D  9. D  10. B  11. D  12. D  13. A  14. D  15. C  16. D  17. B  18. C  19. D  20. C  21. C  22. D  23. B  24. C  25. D  26. D  27. D  28. A  29. B  30. C  31. C  32. D

## MANAGEMENT OF OPEN BITE

1. **Open bite is a malocclusion occurring in**
    A. Sagittal plane
    B. Transverse plane
    C. Vertical plane
    D. All of the above

2. **Lack of vertical overlap between maxillary and mandibular dentition is know as**
    A. Cross bite
    B. Open bite
    C. Deep bite
    D. None of the above

3. **Etiologic factors of open bite include**
    A. Unfavorable growth patterns
    B. Digit sucking habits
    C. Tongue and orofacial muscle activity
    D. All of the above

4. **Etiology of open bite**
    A. Imbalance between jaw posture
    B. Occlusal and eruptive forces
    C. Hereditary
    D. All of the above

5. **Absence of vertical overlap between upper and lower anteriors is known as**
    A. Anterior cross bite
    B. Anterior open bite
    C. Anterior deep bite
    D. None of the above

6. **Anterior open bite can be**
    A. Skeletal
    B. Dental
    C. Both A and B
    D. None of the above

7. **Etiology of anterior open bite can be**
    A. Multifactorial
    B. Local factors only
    C. Hereditary
    D. Non hereditary

8. **Thumb sucking habit in the etiology of open bite is due to**
    A. Posture of thumb positioning
    B. Intensity
    C. Frequency of sucking
    D. All of the above

9. **The greatest focus on possible etiologic factors can be attributed to**
    A. Tongue thrust
    B. Nasopharyngeal airway obstruction with mouth breathing
    C. Increased tongue size
    D. Abnormal skeletal growth pattern

10. **Features of skeletal anterior open bite include**
    A. Increased lower anterior facial height
    B. Decreased upper anterior facial height
    C. Both A and B
    D. None of the above

11. **Increased anterior and decreased posterior facial height is a feature of**
    A. Anterior skeletal cross bite
    B. Posterior skeletal cross bite
    C. Posterior skeletal open bite
    D. Anterior skeletal open bite

12. **Skeletal anterior open bite is characterized by**
    A. Long and narrow face
    B. Steep mandibular plane angle
    C. Small mandibular plane angle and Steep anterior cranial base
    D. All of the above

13. **Cephalometric analysis of anterior skeletal open bite reveals**
    A. Downward and forward rotation of mandible
    B. Upward tipping of maxillary skeletal base
    C. Vertical maxillary increase
    D. All of the above

14. **Dental anterior open bite is characterized by**
    A. Proclined upper anterior teeth
    B. Upper and lower which fail to overlap each other
    C. Narrow maxillary arch
    D. All of the above

15. **Anterior open bite is best treated by**
    A. Removal of cause
    B. Myofunctional therapy
    C. Orthodontic therapy and Surgical correction
    D. All of the above

16. **Anterior open bite can be treated in mixed dentition stages by**
    A. Vertical pull headgear with chin cup
    B. Orthodontic correction
    C. Surgical correction
    D. None of the above

17. **Myofunctional therapy in treatment of skeletal anterior open bites includes**
    A. FR IV
    B. Modified activator
    C. Vertical pull headgear with chin cup
    D. All of the above

18. **Mild to moderate open bite can be treated by fixed orthodontics by using**
    A. Class I elastics
    B. Class II elastics
    C. Class III elastics
    D. Box elastics

19. **Box elastics in treatment of open bite is**
    A. Elastics stretched in upper anteriors and lower anteriors separately
    B. Stretched between upper and lower anteriors
    C. Stretched between upper and lower molar
    D. All of the above

20. **Severe form of skeletal open bite can be treated by**
    A. Surgical correction
    B. Box elastics
    C. Myofunctional therapy
    D. Removal of the cause

21. **Skeletal open bite in adults are treated by**
    A. Removing the cause
    B. Myofunctional therapy
    C. Orthodontic therapy in conjuction with box elastics
    D. Surgical correction

22. **Posterior open bite is a condition characterized by lack of contact between posteriors when**
    A. Teeth are in centric occlusion
    B. Teeth are in centric relation
    C. Either of the above
    D. None of the above

23. **Fish mouth appearance is a characteristic feature of**
    A. Anterior cross bite    B. Anterior open bite
    C. Anterior deep bite    D. All of the above

24. **Surgical correction of open bite in adults is done by**
    A. Lefort I osteotomy    B. Lefort II osteotomy
    C. Lefort III osteotomy    D. All of the above

25. **Posterior open bite can be caused due to**
    A. Lateral tongue thrust
    B. Ankylosed/ submerged posterior teeth that fail to reach occlusal plane
    C. Both A and B
    D. None of the above

26. **Open bite can be treated by**
    A. Intrusion of posterior teeth
    B. Extrusion of posterior teeth
    C. Both A and B
    D. None of the above

27. **Incomplete overbite is a condition characterized by**
    A. Presence of overjet but not vertical overlap
    B. Confined to tooth and alveolar process
    C. More than 1mm of space is seen between the incisors
    D. All of the above

28. **Open bite tendency is also known as**
    A. Incomplete overbite
    B. Simple open bite
    C. Complete open bite
    D. Iatrogenic open bite

29. **Simple open bite is a condition in which**
    A. Problem confined to teeth and alveolar process
    B. More than 1mm of space is seen between the incisors
    C. Posterior teeth are in occlusion
    D. All of the above

30. Iatrogenic open bite is
    A. Caused by orthodontic treatment
    B. Open up to molars
    C. Characterized by absence of vertical overlap
    D. Both B and C
31. Open bite can be classified into
    A. Single and multiple
    B. Anterior and posterior
    C. Local and generalized
    D. All of the above
32. Open bite can be divided into
    A. Unilateral or bilateral
    B. Anterior or posterior
    C. Skeletal or dental
    D. All of the above
33. Posterior open bite caused due to submerged/ankylosed teeth is treated by
    A. Forced extrusion of antagonistic teeth
    B. Restoring the normal occlusal level using crowns on submerged teeth
    C. Surgical correction   D. Both A and B
34. Simple posterior open bite is best treated by
    A. Bionator
    B. Modified activator with flanges to prevent lateral tongue thrust
    C. Removal of ankylosed teeth
    D. All of the above
35. Posterior open bite is classified into
    A. Unilateral or bilateral  B. Skeletal or dental
    C. Both A and B            D. None of the above

Ans: 1. C  2. B  3. D  4. D  5. B  6. C  7. A  8. D  9. B  10. C  11. D  12. D  13. D  14. D  15. D  16. A  17. D  18. D  19. B  20. A  21. D  22. A  23. B  24. A  25. C  26. C  27. A  28. A  29. D  30. A  31. B  32. D  33. D  34. D  35. A

## MANAGEMENT OF DEEP BITE

1. The condition deep bite is referred to as
    A. Increased overbite   B. Decreased overbite
    C. Over bite            D. None of the above
2. Deep bite may be
    A. Dental or skeletal
    B. Complete or incomplete
    C. Both A and B
    D. None of the above
3. Corrections of deep bite involves
    A. Intrusion of maxillary and mandibular anteriors
    B. Extrusion of maxillary and mandibular posteriors
    C. Both A and B
    D. None of the above
4. Deep bite can be corrected by using
    A. Removable orthodontic appliances
    B. Fixed orthodontic appliances
    C. Myofunctional appliances
    D. All of the above
5. How do we correct deep bite using removable orthodontic appliances?
    A. By using anterior bite plane
    B. By using posterior bite plane
    C. Both A and B
    D. None of the above
6. How do we treat deep bite using myofunctional appliances?
    A. Using activator
    B. Bionator
    C. Oral screen
    D. Both A and B
7. Incomplete overbite refers to
    A. Lower incisors fails to occlude with upper incisors
    B. Lower incisors fails to occlude with mucosa of the palate
    C. Both A and B
    D. None of the above
8. Complete over bite refers to
    A. Lower incisors contact the palatal surface of upper incisors
    B. Lower incisors contact the palatal tissue when the teeth are in occlusion
    C. Both A and B
    D. None of the above
9. Dental deep bite is seen in
    A. Angle's class II division 2 malocclusion
    B. Angle's class II division 1 malocclusion
    C. Angle's class III malocclusion
    D. All of the above
10. Skeletal deep bite is seen in
    A. Skeletal class II division 1 malocclusion
    B. Skeletal class II division 2 malocclusion
    C. Skeletal class III malocclusion
    D. All of the above
11. Extra-oral features of dental deep bite include
    A. Decreased lower facial height
    B. Increased lower facial height
    C. Normal lower facial height
    D. None of the above
12. Intra-oral features of dental deep bite include
    A. Increased over bite
    B. Decreased over bite
    C. Normal over bite   D. None of the above

13. Cephalometric findings of deep bite is
    A. Increased interincisal angle
    B. Decreased interincisal angle
    C. Normal interincisal angle
    D. None of the above
14. Extra-oral features of skeletal deep bite include
    A. Decreased lower facial height
    B. Increased lower facial height
    C. Normal lower facial height
    D. None of the above
15. Diagnosis of deep bite made from
    A. Clinical examination
    B. Study models
    C. Cephalograms
    D. All of the above
16. What is the amount of force used to intrude the lower incisors
    A. 12.5 gm / tooth
    B. 15 – 20 gm / tooth
    C. 0 – 8 gm / tooth
    D. 30 – 40 gm / tooth
17. What is the amount of forced used to intrude upper incisors
    A. 12.5 gm / tooth        B. 15 – 20 gm / tooth
    C. 0 – 8 gm / tooth       D. 30 – 40 gm / tooth
18. Hawley's retainer with anterior bite plane is generally used in
    A. Correction of deep bite in Angle's class I malocclusion
    B. Correction of deep bite in Angle's class II division 2 malocclusion
    C. Correction of deep bite in Angle's class II division 1 malocclusion
    D. All of the above
19. Flat anterior bite plane is used in the
    A. Correction of deep bite in Angle's class I malocclusion
    B. Correction of deep bite in Angle's class II division 1 malocclusion
    C. Correction of deep bite in Angle's class II division 2 malocclusion
    D. All of the above
20. Inclined anterior bite plane is used in the
    A. Correction of deep bite in Angle's class I malocclusion
    B. Correction of deep bite in Angle's class II division 1 malocclusion
    C. Correction of deep bite in Angle's class II division 2 malocclusion
    D. All of the above
21. Thickness of anterior bite plane used in the correction of deep bite should be of
    A. 1.5 – 2.0 mm in thickness
    B. 2.0 – 4.0 mm in thickness
    C. 6.0 – 8.0 mm in thickness
    D. 10.0 – 13.0 mm in thickness
22. Mode of action of inclined anterior bite plane is the management of deep bite in
    A. Forward mandibular posture
    B. Reciprocal backward force in the maxillary appliance from the masticatory force
    C. Extrusion of lower posteriors
    D. All of the above
23. Fixed orthodontic appliance can be used to correct deep bites using
    A. Intrusion arch wires    B. Utility arches
    C. RCS                     D. All of the above
24. Utility arches with fixed appliances brings about
    A. Incisor protrusions     B. Intrusion of incisors
    C. Retraction of incisors  D. All of the above
25. How do we activate utility arches in the correction of deep bite?
    A. By giving a " V " bend in the buccal segment of the wire mesial to molar
    B. By giving a " V " bend in the labial segment of the wire mesial to canine
    C. By just bending the wire any where between the canine and molar
    D. None of the above
26. RCS (Reverse Curvature Spring) can also be used in the management of deep bite which when used brings about
    A. Intrusive force in the anterior teeth
    B. An eruptive force on the posterior teeth
    C. Both A and B
    D. None of the above
27. Is over correction required in the deep bite cases?
    A. Yes                     B. No
    C. Maybe                   D. None of the above
28. How much retention time is usually recommended followed by deep bite correction?
    A. Continuously for the period of minimum 4 – 6 months
    B. Continuously for the period of minimum 2 – 3 months
    C. Continuously for the period of minimum 1 – 2 months
    D. None of the above

Ans: 1. A  2. C  3. C  4. D  5. A  6. D  7. A  8. C  9. A  10. B  11. A  12. A  13. A  14. A  15. D  16. A  17. B  18. A  19. C  20. B  21. A  22. D  23. D  24. D  25. A  26. C  27. A  28. A

## MANAGEMENT OF CROSS BITE

1. **Malocclusion in which the mandibular teeth are in abnormal buccolingual relation to maxillary teeth is**
   A. Deep bite
   B. Cross bite
   C. Open bite
   D. None of the above

2. **Cross bite is classified into**
   A. Anterior or posterior
   B. Dental or skeletal
   C. Single tooth or multi teeth and functional cross bite
   D. All of the above

3. **Anterior cross bite is classified into**
   A. Single tooth or segmental
   B. Skeletal or dental
   C. Both A and B
   D. None of the above

4. **Posterior cross bite is classified into**
   A. Unilateral
   B. Bilateral
   C. Single tooth cross bite
   D. All of the above

5. **Posterior cross bite are classified into**
   A. Unilateral or bilateral
   B. Skeletal or dental
   C. Both A and B
   D. None of the above

6. **According to extent of cross bite it can be divided into**
   A. Simple posterior cross bite
   B. Buccal non occlusion
   C. Lingual non occlusion
   D. All of the above

7. **Scissor bite is also termed as**
   A. Telescopic bite
   B. Buccal non occlusion
   C. Both A and B
   D. None of the above

8. **Anterior cross bite is a condition in which**
   A. Mandibular anteriors overlap maxillary anteriors
   B. Maxillary anteriors overlap mandibular anteriors
   C. No overlap between upper and lower anteriors
   D. Any of the above

9. **Anterior cross bite is also known as**
   A. Reverse overjet
   B. Reverse bite
   C. Under bite
   D. All of the above

10. **Etiology of anterior cross bite can be**
    A. Dental
    B. Skeletal
    C. Functional
    D. All of the above

11. **Abnormal axial inclination of maxillary incisors in dental anterior cross bite may occur due to**
    A. Trauma to primary teeth or permanent tooth bud
    B. Over retained primary tooth
    C. Labially positioned supernumerary tooth and lip biting habit
    D. All of the above

12. **Abnormal axial inclination of maxillary incisors is caused due to**
    A. Inadequate arch length which causes lingual eruption of permanent tooth
    B. Repaired cleft lip
    C. Over retained primary tooth
    D. All of the above

13. **Skeletal factors causing anterior cross bite**
    A. Excessive mandibular growth
    B. Genetics or inherited
    C. Retrognathic maxilla in case of cleft palate
    D. All of the above

14. **Buccal cusps of one or more maxillary posterior teeth occluding lingual to buccal cusps of mandibular teeth is referred to as**
    A. Lingual non occlusion
    B. Lingual occlusion
    C. Buccal non occlusion
    D. Buccal occlusion

15. **Buccal cusp of maxillary tooth placed lingual to the lingual cusp of mandibular posterior teeth is referred to as**
    A. Buccal occlusion
    B. Buccal non occlusion
    C. Lingual non occlusion
    D. Lingual occlusion

16. **Single tooth cross bite is**
    A. Dental in origin
    B. Functional in origin
    C. Skeletal in origin
    D. All of the above

17. **In dental crossbite in centric occlusion molar and canine relationships will be**
    A. Class I
    B. Class II
    C. Class III
    D. All of the above

18. **In true skeletal cross bite the molar and canine relationship will be**
    A. Class I
    B. Class II
    C. Class III
    D. None of the above

19. **Lateral cephalogram advised to treat cross bite aids in**
    A. Differentiating between skeletal and dental
    B. Knowing axial inclination of incisor relation to the skeletal
    C. Both A and B
    D. None of the above

20. **Factors to be considered in diagnosis of cross bite**
    A. Number of teeth involved
    B. Location of teeth in cross bite
    C. Functional path of closure and molar and canine relationship
    D. All of the above

21. **Factors to be considered in treatment of anterior cross bite**
    A. Availability of mesiodistal space to correct the inlocked tooth

B. Sufficient over bite
   C. Position of tooth
   D. All of the above
22. **Correction of anterior cross bite can be achieved by**
   A. Occlusal equilibration
   B. Inclined planes
   C. Fixed planes and Tongue blade therapy
   D. All of the above
23. **Functional cross bite occurs due to**
   A. Presence of occlusal interference
   B. Premature loss of deciduous molar
   C. Insufficient overbite
   D. Both A and B
24. **Functional cross bite may lead to**
   A. Class I malocclusion
   B. Class II true malocclusion
   C. Pseudo Class III malocclusion
   D. All of the above
25. **Skeletal cross bite can be caused due to**
   A. Mouth breathing    B. Thumb sucking
   C. Trauma at birth    D. All of the above
26. **Correcting of anterior cross bite in pre-adolescent age group is done by**
   A. Tongue blade
   B. Catlan's appliance
   C. Removable orthodontic appliance with "z" spring and Frankel III Appliance
   D. All of the above
27. **Correction of anterior cross bite in adolescent and adults is by**
   A. ROA with mini expansion screw
   B. ROA with medium expansion screw
   C. Fixed orthodontic appliances
   D. All of the above
28. **Developing anterior cross bite can be best treated by**
   A. Tongue blade therapy
   B. Removable orthodontic appliance with finger spring
   C. Both A and B
   D. Fixed orthodontic appliance
29. **Which of the following is an indication for Catlan's Appliance**
   A. Sufficient space in the arch for alignment of maxillary teeth in cross bite
   B. Crowded lower anterior teeth
   C. Periodontal problems in lower arch
   D. Malaligned lower incisors
30. **Chin cup appliance for treatment of anterior cross bite is used in patients with**
   A. Retrognathic maxilla
   B. Excessive mandibular growth
   C. Prognathic mandible
   D. Prognathic maxilla
31. **Chin cup appliance tends to rotate the mandible**
   A. Posterior and inferiorly
   B. Anteriorly and superiorly
   C. Anteriorly and inferiorly
   D. Posteriorly and superiorly
32. **Frankel's appliance of choice to correct a developing class 3 skeletal jaw with anterior cross bite**
   A. FR- I          B. FR-III
   C. FR -II         D. FR-IV
33. **Removable orthodontic appliance with mini screw can be used to correct anterior cross bite involving**
   A. Any one side of the arch
   B. Full arch
   C. All upper anteriors
   D. Up to 2 teeth
34. **Correction of posterior cross bite can be achieved by**
   A. ROA with expansion screw
   B. ROA with coffin spring
   C. Quad helix appliance
   D. All of the above
35. **Single tooth posterior cross bite can be best treated by**
   A. Box elastics        B. Cross elastics
   C. Straight elastics   D. Class I elastics
36. **Coffin spring used to treat cross bite can bring**
   A. Single tooth cross bite correction
   B. Single tooth posterior cross bite correction
   C. Slow and bilateral symmetric expansion
   D. All of the above
37. **Cross elastic is stretched from**
   A. Palatal surface of maxillary posterior teeth to buccal surface of mandibular teeth
   B. Anterior teeth to posterior in same arch
   C. Maxillary canine to mandibular molar
   D. Maxillary molar to mandibular canine
38. **Unfavorable sequelae of posterior cross bite**
   A. Abnormal wear of dentition
   B. Interference with normal growth and development of dental arches
   C. Pain due to muscle spasm
   D. All of the above
39. **Midline shift present in both centric and rest position indicates**
   A. True skeletal cross bite
   B. True skeletal deep bite
   C. True skeletal open bite
   D. Pseudo class III malocclusion
40. **Appliances for unilateral contraction of maxillary arch**
   A. Removable plates
   B. W arch appliance
   C. Coffin spring and Quad helix
   D. All of the above

41. Cross bite is abnormal occlusion occurring in
    A. Transverse plane
    B. Sagittal plane
    C. Vertical plane
    D. All of the above
42. Cross bite can occur due to
    A. Retarded development of maxilla in sagittal as well as transverse direction
    B. Narrow upper arch resulting from decreased growth stimulation in midpalatal suture
    C. Collapse of maxillary arch as in cleft palate and unilateral hypo or hyperplastic growth of any of the jaws
    D. All of the above
43. Retarded development of maxilla in sagittal as well as transverse direction can cause
    A. Anterior cross bite      B. Posterior cross bite
    C. Both A and B              D. Open bite
44. The inclined plane to treat cross bite should be at an angle of
    A. 30 degree
    B. 45 degree
    C. 60 degree                 D. 75 degree
45. Skeletal anterior cross bite can occur as a result of
    A. Retarded maxillary growth
    B. Backward placed maxilla
    C. Excessively growing mandible
    D. All of the above
46. Skeletal posterior cross bite are usually characterized by
    A. Narrow upper arch
    B. Narrow lower arch
    C. Broad upper arch          D. Straight upper arch
47. Maxillary incisors in cross bite have
    A. Greater than normal labial inclination
    B. Smaller than normal labial inclination
    C. Greater than normal lingual inclination
    D. Smaller than normal lingual inclination
48. Mandibular incisors in cross bite have
    A. Greater than normal lingual inclination
    B. Greater than normal labial inclination
    C. Lesser than normal labial inclination
    D. Lesser than normal lingual inclination
49. Brodie Syndrome is
    A. Scissor bite of first premolar of patient with class II division 1 malocclusion
    B. Scissor bite of all teeth in patient with class II division 2 malocclusion
    C. Scissor bite of first premolar of patient with true class III malocclusion
    D. Scissor bite of all teeth in patient and pseudo class III malocclusion
50. Most patients having unilateral posterior cross bite shifts their mandible
    A. Toward the side with cross bite when closing into Centric occlusion
    B. Toward the opposite side of cross bite when closing into Centric occlusion
    C. Toward the side with cross bite when closing into Centric relation
    D. Toward the opposite side of cross bite when closing into Centric relation

Ans: 1. B  2. D  3. C  4. D  5. C  6. D  7. C  8. A  9. D  10. D  11. D  12. D  13. D  14. C  15. C  16. A
17. A  18. C  19. C  20. D  21. D  22. D  23. D  24. C  25. D  26. D  27. D  28. A  29. A  30. B  31. A  32. B
33. D  34. D  35. B  36. C  37. A  38. D  39. A  40. D  41. A  42. D  43. C  44. B  45. D  46. A  47. A  48. A
49. A  50. A

## MANAGEMENT OF CLEFT LIP AND PALATE

1. The word "cleft" literally means:
    A. Gap or crack
    B. Cliff
    C. Valley
    D. None of the above
2. Orofacial clefts are:
    A. Congenital defects
    B. Caused by smoking during pregnancy
    C. Induced by gynaecologist during delivery
    D. Caused by deficiency of protein
3. Cleft lip is also known as:
    A. Lip of camel
    B. Harelip
    C. Sorcerer's lip
    D. None of the above
4. Cleft may occur:
    A. In isolation
    B. As part of a syndrome
    C. Resulting from a nutritional deficiency
    D. Both A and B
5. Management of cleft lip requires;
    A. Orthodontist only
    B. Oral and maxillofacial surgeon only
    C. Paediatrician only
    D. Multidisciplinary approach
6. Cleft lip and palate is associated with:
    A. Impaired facial appearance only
    B. Impaired speech and hearing

C. Impaired occlusion, mastication and deglutition
D. All of the above

7. **Cleft lip arises from failure of fusion:**
   A. Between medial nasal processes
   B. Between medial nasal processes and maxillary process
   C. Of palatine shelves
   D. Of nasal plate and primary palate

8. **Cleft palate arises from failure of fusion between**
   A. Palatine shelves
   B. Nasal septum
   C. Primary palate
   D. All of the above

9. **Veau's classification of cleft lip and palate is:**
   A. Embryological
   B. Morphological
   C. Symbolic classification using a stripped 'Y'
   D. According to etiology

10. **Classification by the International Confederation for Plastic and Reconstructive Surgery is divided:**
    A. 2 groups          B. 3 groups
    C. 4 groups          D. 9 groups

11. **Veau's classification describes how many types of clefts?**
    A. Two               B. Three
    C. Four              D. Seven

12. **The symbolic stripped 'Y' classification was proposed by:**
    A. Veau
    B. Kernahan
    C. International Confederation for Plastic and Reconstructive Surgery
    D. Davis And Ritchie

13. **Velocardiofacial syndrome means:**
    A. Velo = cycle, cardia = heart, facies = face
    B. Velum = palate, cardia = heart, facies = face
    C. Velo = cleft, cardia = heart, facies = face
    D. Velo = harelip, cardia = heart, facies = face

14. **Which of the following may not be a causative factor of clefts?**
    A. Exposure to radiation
    B. Stress
    C. Vitamin deficiencies
    D. Surgery

15. **Increased maternal age:**
    A. Increases the risk of clefting
    B. Decreases the risk of clefting
    C. Has no effect on clefting
    D. Is directly proportional to the risk of cleft palate only

16. **What is the structure that is least affected by clefts?**
    A. Upper lip         B. Lower lip
    C. Alveolar ridge    D. Hard and soft palate

17. **Clefting anterior to the incisive foramen is defined as:**
    A. The cleft of primary palate
    B. The cleft of secondary palate
    C. Complete cleft
    D. Isolated cleft palate

18. **Clefting posterior to the incisive foramen is defined as:**
    A. The cleft of primary palate
    B. The cleft of secondary palate
    C. Complete cleft
    D. Isolated cleft palate

19. **A complete cleft palate constitutes cleft of**
    A. Vermillion border of lip, hard palate and soft palate
    B. Soft palate and hard palate
    C. Soft palate, hard palate and uvula
    D. Incisive foramen, soft palate and hard palate

20. **Mildest form of cleft palate is:**
    A. Cleft of soft palate
    B. Cleft of hard palate
    C. Bifid uvula
    D. Cleft of incisive foramen

21. **Which of the following is not an associated problem of cleft lip with cleft palate?**
    A. Midline diastema
    B. Ear problems
    C. Speech difficulties
    D. Impaired facial aesthetics

22. **Which of the following is not a dental problem associated with cleft lip with cleft palate?**
    A. Presence of supernumerary teeth
    B. Ectopically erupting teeth
    C. Midline diastema
    D. Crowding

23. **Most clefts of alveolus and palate show:**
    A. Class I malocclusion
    B. Class II division 1 malocclusion
    C. Class II division 2 malocclusion
    D. Class III malocclusion

24. **Which of the following statements is true?**
    A. Babies with cleft lip and palate cannot swallow normally if fed towards the hypopharynx
    B. Structural defects of cleft lip and palate prevent positive oral pressure
    C. Cleft palate patients are predisposed to middle ear infection
    D. Babies should only be breast fed

25. **Which of the following statements is not true?**
    A. In cleft palate middle ear becomes a closed space
    B. In cleft palate, there is excessive drainage from middle ear
    C. In cleft palate, there is accumulation of serous fluid in the middle ear

D. Chronic otitis media causes hearing impairment in patients with cleft palate

26. Valopharyngeal mechanism is responsible for:
    A. Gag reflex
    B. Controlling distribution of escaping air between oropharynx and nasopharynx
    C. Action of soft palate as a valve
    D. Both B and C

27. The management of cleft lip and cleft palate:
    A. Starts at birth till 18 years of age
    B. Starts at 4 months till 16 years of age
    C. Starts at 5 years till 18 years of age
    D. Starts at 6 years till 11 years of age

28. The management of cleft lip and palate can be divided into how many stages?
    A. 3 stages
    B. 4 stages
    C. 5 stages
    D. 6 stages

29. To which dentition stage does stage 2 treatment of cleft palate correspond to?
    A. Predentate period
    B. Primary dentition stage
    C. Mixed dentition stage
    D. Permanent dentition stage

30. Treatment done during the permanent dentition stage at 12-18 years of age:
    A. Stage 1
    B. Stage 2
    C. Stage 3
    D. Stage 4

31. Treatment carried out from 6 to 11 years of age corresponds with:
    A. Stage 1
    B. Stage 2
    C. Stage 3
    D. Stage 4

32. When is the firsts stage of management of cleft lip and palate?
    A. From birth to 18 months
    B. From 18 months to 5 years
    C. From 6 years to 11 years
    D. As from 4 weeks

33. What is the purpose of extra oral strapping?
    A. To hide the defect caused by the cleft
    B. To aid nasal breathing
    C. To reposition the premaxillary portion of the jaw
    D. All of the above

34. At which stage is mechanotherapy carried out?
    A. Stage 1
    B. Stage 2
    C. Stage 3
    D. Stage 4

35. At which stage is orthodontic treatment of the most limited advantage?
    A. Predentate period
    B. Primary dentition stage
    C. Mixed dentition stage
    D. Permanent dentition stage

36. At what age is secondary alveolar bone graft usually carried out?
    A. At birth
    B. At 3 months
    C. At 9-18 months
    D. At 9-10 years

37. At which age is lip repair carried out?
    A. At birth
    B. At 3 months
    C. At 9-18 months
    D. At 9-10 years

38. At which age is repair of cleft palate started?
    A. At birth
    B. At 3 months
    C. At 9-18 months
    D. At 9-10 years

39. Most of orthodontic cases showing a severe class III skeletal pattern requires:
    A. Orthodontic treatment only
    B. Orthognathic surgeries only
    C. Bone grafting only
    D. All of the above

40. Which of the following statements is not true?
    A. Maxillary obturator is an intra oral prosthetic device
    B. Maxillary obturator improves the aesthetic appearance of the orofacial cleft patient
    C. Maxillary obturator causes maxillary arch to collapse
    D. Maxillary obturator reduces feeding deficiencies

41. Who suggested the rule of 10?
    A. Veau
    B. Millard
    C. Kernahan
    D. Davis and Rithchie

42. Early repair of cleft palate:
    A. Facilitates normal speech
    B. Facilitates hearing
    C. Improves swallowing
    D. All of the above

43. Which of the following statements is true?
    A. After orthodontic treatment, cleft palate patient should not be put on a retention phase
    B. Surgical procedures carried out on cleft palate patient act as retention
    C. Presence of scar tissue after surgery of cleft palate acts as retention.
    D. Inadequate bone support is a reason for prolonged retention

44. What are the reasons for prolonged retention phase after orthodontic treatment of orofacial cleft?
    A. Inadequate bone support
    B. Absence of some teeth
    C. Presence of stretched scar tissue
    D. All of the above

45. Which of the following statement is false?
    A. Cleft lip with or without cleft palate is more common than isolated cleft palate
    B. Isolated cleft palate is observed to be more common in males than females

C. Unilateral clefts are more common as compared to that of bilateral clefts
D. Cleft lip with or without cleft palate is more common in female than in male

46. Overall incidence of cleft lip and palate in humans appears to be:
    A. 1 in 100 live births
    B. 1 in 200 live births
    C. 1 in 700 live births
    D. 1 in 1400 live births

47. An example of a syndrome associated with cleft lip and cleft palate is:
    A. Turner's syndrome
    B. Kleinfelter's syndrome
    C. Pierre Robin syndrome
    D. Apert's syndrome

48. What percentage of cleft lip with or without cleft palate is genetic in origin?
    A. 80%
    B. 60%
    C. 50%
    D. 40%

49. The following environmental factors have been suggested to be causative factors of formation of cleft lip and palate, except
    A. A defective vascular supply to the area involved during critical time of embryonic development
    B. Mechanical disturbance in which size of tongue prevents union of parts
    C. Excessive concentration of circulating substances such as alcohol, certain drugs and toxins
    D. Oral submucous fibrosis

50. What is the chance of having a child with a cleft in case if parents have a cleft?
    A. 2-5%
    B. 4-10%
    C. 15-20%
    D. 20-30%

Ans: 1. A   2. A   3. B   4. D   5. D   6. D   7. B   8. D   9. B   10. B   11. C   12. B   13. B   14. D   15. A   16. B
17. A   18. B   19. C   20. C   21. A   22. C   23. D   24. C   25. B   26. D   27. B   28. A   29. B   30. D   31. C   32. A
33. C   34. D   35. B   36. D   37. B   38. C   39. D   40. C   41. B   42. D   43. D   44. D   45. D   46. C   47. D   48. D
49. D   50. A

## 12. SURGICAL ORTHODONTICS

### SURGICAL ORTHODONTICS

1. Following are the minor surgical procedures in conjunction with orthodontic treatment except
    A. Frenectomy
    B. Distraction Osteogenesis
    C. Circumferential supracrostal fibrotomy
    D. Corticotomy

2. Following are the major surgical orthodontic procedures in conjunction with orthodontic treatment except
    A. Orthognathic surgeries
    B. Transplantation
    C. Distraction osteoporosis
    D. Rapid maxillary expansion

3. Frenectomy is indicated in all of the following conditions except
    A. Abnormal thick labial frenum attachment causing midline diastema
    B. Abnormal thick lingual frenum causing ankylossia
    C. Thick fibrous labial frenum which impedes stabilization of upper complete denture
    D. Midline diastema during ugly duckling stage

4. The surgical procedure "pericision" is also called as
    A. Circumferential infracrestal fibrotomy
    B. Circumferential supracrestal fibrotomy
    C. Circumferential gingivectomy
    D. Circumferential alveolar fibrotomy

5. Circumferential supracrestal fibrotomy is done to prevent relapse of
    A. Rotation of teeth       B. Spacing
    C. Open bite               D. Crowding

6. Circumferential supracrestal fibrotomy procedure involves
    A. Surgical excision of hyperplastic gingival
    B. Surgical lysis of gingival and transeptal fibres
    C. Surgical excision of fibrous frenum
    D. Surgical excision of high frenum

7. Indications of traction in conjunction with orthodontic treatment include
    A. Ankylosed teeth
    B. Therapeutic extraction of permanent teeth
    C. Removal of supranumerary teeth
    D. All of above

8. The most common impacted tooth next to third molars is
    A. Maxillary lateral incisors
    B. Canines (maxillary)
    C. Premolars (maxillary)
    D. Mandibular canines

9. Before surgical exposure the impacted tooth is localized by
    A. Two radiographs taken at different angulations (SLOB) technique
    B. More than 1 radiographic technique

C. Both A and B
D. None of the above

10. **Corticotomy refers to**
    A. Involves surgical cutting of vertical cortex
    B. Involves the sectioning of the dentoalveolar region into multiple small units
    C. Vertical cuts are given on either side of each tooth parallel and away from roots nad these apical ends of vertical cuts at joined by a horizontal cut
    D. Both B and C

11. **Orthognathic surgery is indicated in**
    A. Adult patient with severe skeletal discrepancies
    B. Children 10 years of age
    C. Adolescent patient with mild skeletal discrepancy
    D. Adult patient with severe malocclusion

12. **Steps involved in orthognathic surgeries include**
    A. Patient evaluation and presurgical orthodontics
    B. Final planning of surgery with
    C. Surgery and stabilization and posterior surgical orthodontics
    D. All of the above

13. **While evaluating the patient for orthognathic surgeries anterioposterior cephalogram helps in**
    A. To access the impacted teeth
    B. To access the facial asymmetry
    C. Ankylosed teeth
    D. None of the above

14. **While evaluating the patient for orthognathic surgeries, lateral cephalogram is useful in**
    A. To determine facial asymmetry
    B. In determining the nature and extend of skeletal discrepancy
    C. To determine dental abnormalities
    D. Presence of impacted teeth

15. **Decompensation refers to**
    A. Repositioning the teeth properly over the dental bone
    B. Alignment of crowded teeth
    C. Repositioning the teeth properly over the skeletal bone without consideration of bite relationship to the opposing arch
    D. All of the above

16. **The following are orthognathic surgical procedure for mandible except**
    A. Bilateral sagittal split osteotomy
    B. Vertical ramus osteotomy
    C. Lefort I osteotomy
    D. Mandibular subapical osteotomy

17. **The following orthognathic surgical procedures are for maxilla except**
    A. Segmental maxillary osteotomy
    B. Anterior maxillary subapical set back
    C. BSSO
    D. Lefort I osteotomy

18. **Following are the orthognathic surgical procedures to treat mandibular excess except**
    A. Vertical ramus osteotomy
    B. Segmental maxillary osteotomy
    C. BSSO
    D. Mandibular subapical osteotomy

19. **"BSSO" stands for**
    A. Biomechanical surgical septal osteotomy
    B. Bimaxillary saggital split osteotomy
    C. Bilateral sagittal split osteotomy
    D. None of the above

20. **Following is the most popular method for treating both mandibular deficiency and excess**
    A. Lefort I osteotomy
    B. Vertical ramus osteotomy
    C. BSSO
    D. Mandibular subapical osteotomy

21. **Who popularized the transoral vertical osteotomy**
    A. Obswequer
    B. Caldwell and lettermon in 1950
    C. Trainer
    D. Httnsuck

22. **Who first described the BSSO orthognathic surgical procedure**
    A. Letterman
    B. Obswequer
    C. Caldwell
    D. Dalpont

23. **Modification of BSSO technique was given by**
    A. Obswequer
    B. Letterman
    C. Dalpont, Hunsuck and Epker
    D. Trainer

24. **Following are the orthognathic surgical procedures for treatment of mandibular deficiency except**
    A. BSSO with mandibular advancement
    B. Mandibular total subapical osteotomy
    C. Anterior maxillary subapical set back
    D. Vertical Z and C osteotomy

25. **Following is the most common orthognathic surgical procedure to correct maxillary abnormality**
    A. Vertical 'C' and 'L' osteotomy
    B. Lefort I osteotomy (total maxillary osteotomy)
    C. BSSO
    D. Anterior maxillary subapical set back

26. **Following is the orthognathic surgical procedure for treatment of maxillary excess in anterior posterior dimension**
    A. Anterior maxillary subapical set back
    B. Lefort I osteotomy
    C. Both A and B
    D. None of the above

27. **Following orthognathic surgical procedure is used for vertical maxillary excess**
    A. Lefort I osteotomy with maxillary impaction
    B. Segmental maxillary osteotomy
    C. Both A and B
    D. None of above

28. **Skeletal discrepancy with maxillary deficiency can be treated by**
    A. BSSO
    B. Lefort I osteotomy with maxillary advancement

C. Segmental maxillary osteotomy
D. Transoral vertical osteotomy

29. **Skeletal discrepancy with transverse deficiency of maxilla can be treated by**
    A. Rapid maxillary expansion
    B. Modification of Lefort I osteotomy
    C. Both A and B
    D. None of above

30. **Cosmetic surgeries include the following except**
    A. Rhinoplasty
    B. Genioplasty
    C. Vertical osteotomy
    D. Molar augmentation

31. **Distraction osteogenesis includes**
    A. Cutting osteotomy to separate the segments of bone
    B. Application of traction appliances
    C. Incremental separation of bone segments to facilitate bone formation
    D. All of the above

32. **Distraction osteogenesis can be used in**
    A. Maxilla only
    B. Mandible only
    C. Maxilla and mandible
    D. TMJ

33. **Distraction osteogenesis can be used to treat**
    A. Skeletal discrepancy with deficiencies only
    B. Skeletal discrepancy with jaw excesses
    C. Both for jaw deficiencies and excesses
    D. None of the above

34. **Presurgical orthodontics is aimed at**
    A. Done before orthognathic surgery
    B. Correcting the dental compensation that has occurred in resposnse to skeletal deformity
    C. Done after orthognathic surgical procedure
    D. Both A and B

35. **After presurgical orthodontic tooth movement**
    A. The skeletal discrepancy is accentuated
    B. The skeletal discrepancy gets corrected
    C. Dental malocclusion gets corrected
    D. All of the above

36. **The orthognathic surgical technique preferred when extreme mandibular advanced greater than 10 – 15 mm required**
    A. Lefort I osteotomy
    B. Vertical 'L' or 'C' osteotomy
    C. BSSO with advancement
    D. All of the above

37. **Lefort II osteotomy can be used to treat skeletal discrepancies of maxilla in**
    A. Sagittal plane     B. Transverse plane
    C. Vertical plane
    D. All 3 planes of space

**Ans:** 1. B  2. B  3. D  4. B  5. A  6. B  7. D  8. B  9. C  10. D  11. A  12. D  13. B  14. B  15. C  16. C  17. C  18. B  19. C  20. C  21. B  22. B  23. C  24. C  25. B  26. C  27. C  28. B  29. C  30. C  31. D  32. C  33. A  34. D  35. A  36. B  37. D

## 13. RETENTION AND RELAPSE

### RETENTION AND RELAPSE

1. **Teeth return to their original position after orthodontic treatment because of**
   A. Periodontal influence
   B. Occlusal forces and soft tissue forces
   C. Continuing dentofacial growth
   D. All of the above

2. **Loss of any correction achieved by orthodontic treatment is reffered to as**
   A. Retention
   B. Relapse
   C. Orthodontic correction
   D. Orthodontic migration

3. **Retention is acquired due to**
   A. Gingival and periodontal tissues which require time for reorganization after appliance removal
   B. Pressure from soft tissues which produce relapse tendency
   C. Growth of dentofacial structures
   D. All of the above

4. **Relapse after orthodontic treatment occurs by**
   A. Elastic recoil of gingival fibers
   B. Cheek/lip/tongue pressures
   C. Differential jaw growth
   D. All of the above

5. **According to Kingsley, which of the below factor is key factor in determining the stability of newly moved teeth**
   A. Proper occlusion
   B. Elastic recoil of gingival fibers
   C. Cheek/lip/tongue pressures
   D. All of the above

6. **The occlusion school of thought was proposed by**
   A. Alex Lundstrom     B. Mc Couley
   C. Nance              D. Kingsley

7. **Destabilizing factors of retention**
   A. Persistant etiology     B. Erupting 3rd molar
   C. Stretched fibers        D. All of the above

8. **The apical base school of retention was formulated by**
   A. Alex Lundstrom
   B. Mc Couley
   C. Nance
   D. All of the above

9. According to Alex Lundstrom, which factor is the key in retention
   A. Occlusion
   B. Apical base
   C. Mandibular incisor
   D. Muscle balance
10. Which of the below should not be altered to minimize retention according to Mc Couley
    A. Intercanine width
    B. Intermolar width
    C. Both A and B
    D. None of the above
11. Who believed that arch length should not be increased to a major extent to avoid relapse
    A. Mac Couley
    B. Nance
    C. Alex Lundstrom
    D. Kingsley
12. Mandibular incisor school of thought was proposed by
    A. Grieves and Tweed
    B. Mc Couley, Nance and Alex Lundstrom
    C. Kingsley
    D. None of the above
13. According to Grieves and Tweed, mandibular incisors are the key factors to
    A. Retention
    B. Relapse
    C. Arch lengthening
    D. None of the above
14. Mandibular incisor school of retention states that
    A. Mandibular incisors should be placed upright or slightly retroclined over basal bone
    B. Mandibular incisors should be proclined over basal bone
    C. Mandibular incisors do not play any role in retention
    D. All of the above
15. Musculature school of retention was proposed by
    A. Mc Couley
    B. Rojers
    C. Alex Lundstrom
    D. Kingsley
16. According to Rojers, what plays an important role in retention
    A. Muscles of orofacial region
    B. Occlusion
    C. Apical base
    D. Mandibular incisors
17. Relapse occurs due to
    A. Pdl traction
    B. Bone changes
    C. Persistent etiology
    D. All of the above
18. Relapse due to growth related changes occurs in
    A. Class ll malocclusion
    B. Class lll malocclusion
    C. Open bite
    D. All of the above
19. Supra-alveolar gingival fibers require how many weeks for reorganization after active orthodontic therapy
    A. 10 weeks
    B. 20 weeks
    C. 30 weeks
    D. 40 weeks
20. Full time retention after comprehensive orthodontic therapy is needed for
    A. 4-5 months
    B. No full time retention is needed
    C. 3-4 months
    D. 1-2 months
21. Basic theorems of retention was summarized by
    A. Riedel
    B. Moyers
    C. Nance
    D. Alex Lundstrom
22. The 10th theorem of retention was included by
    A. Riedel
    B. Moyers
    C. Nance
    D. Alex Lundstrom
23. According to theorem 3 of retention, malocclusion should be overcorrected
    A. As a safety factor
    B. To prevent relapse
    C. To decrease the period of retention
    D. All of the above
24. According to theorem 4 of retention, elimination of the cause of malocclusion will
    A. Avoid the need for fixed therapy
    B. Decrease the treatment duration
    C. Prevent relapse
    D. Increase retention
25. Theorem 10 of retention states that
    A. Many treated malocclusions require permanent retaining devices
    B. Was added by Moyers
    C. Both A and B
    D. None of the above
26. Keys to eliminate lower retention was proposed by
    A. Moyers
    B. Alex Lundstrom
    C. Raleigh Williams
    D. Nance
27. According to Raleigh Williams, to avoid relapse, the incisal edges should be placed
    A. At the A-p line
    B. 1mm in front of A-p line
    C. Both A and B
    D. None of the above
28. Types of retention includes
    A. Natural or no retention
    B. Limited or short term retention
    C. Prolonged or permanent retention
    D. All of the above
29. Upper anteriors crossbite correction with adequate overbite requires
    A. No retention
    B. Self retentive
    C. Requires retention of 3-6 months
    D. Both A and B
30. Upper anteriors crossbite correction with no adequate overbite requires
    A. No retention
    B. Self retentive
    C. Both A and B
    D. Retention of 3-6 months

31. **Permanent retention may be indicated in**
    A. Mandibular expansion cases
    B. Midline diastema
    C. Cleft palate cases
    D. All of the above
32. **Retention appliance is**
    A. Passive orthodontic appliance
    B. Stabilizes the teeth in newly aligned position
    C. Is a removable type only
    D. Both A and B
33. **Requirements of retention appliance**
    A. Should be easily cleanable
    B. Should be inconspicuous
    C. Should be strong enough to achieve the objectives of retention
    D. All of the above
34. **Charles Hawley designed Hawley retainer in the year**
    A. 1910
    B. 1920
    C. 1930
    D. 1940
35. **Hawley retainer**
    A. Was designed by Charles Hawley
    B. Most routinely used
    C. Is a fixed retainer
    D. Both A and B
36. **Hawley retainer**
    A. Was designed in the year 1920
    B. Is most routinely used
    C. Is a removable type
    D. All of the above
37. **Removable retainers include**
    A. Hawley retainer
    B. Essix retainer
    C. Tooth positioners
    D. All of the above
38. **Fixed retainers include**
    A. Bonded canine to canine retainer
    B. Banded canine to canine retainer
    C. Band and spur
    D. All of the above
39. **Drawback of standard Hawley retainer is**
    A. Difficult to fabricate
    B. That it is active always
    C. Opening of premolar extraction space
    D. All of the above
40. **Prevention of wedging effect on extraction site by Hawley retainer can be attempted by**
    A. Short labial bow
    B. Long labial bow
    C. High labial bow
    D. Either of the above
41. **Tooth positioner as a retainer was described by**
    A. Kesling          B. Moyers
    C. Alex Lundstrom   D. Charles Hawley
42. **Spring aligner or clip or retainer is usually used to retain the correction of**
    A. Maxillary anteriors
    B. Mandibular anteriors
    C. Midline diastema
    D. Anterior crossbite
43. **Kesling tooth positioner was developed in the year**
    A. 1945            B. 1935
    C. 1925            D. 1905
44. **Wrap around retainer is**
    A. An extended version of spring aligner
    B. Used in periodontally weak dentition
    C. The labial and lingual surfaces of all teeth embedded in a strip of acrylic
    D. All of the above
45. **Band and spur retainer is used for**
    A. Stabilizing the de-rotated tooth
    B. Stabilizing the midline diastema correction
    C. Stabilizing crossbite correction
    D. None of the above
46. **Begg's retainer was designed by**
    A. P.R Begg of Austria
    B. P.R Begg of America
    C. P.R Begg of Australia
    D. P.R Begg of France
47. **Retainer of choice in stabilizing lower incisors after orthodontic correction is**
    A. Spring aligner
    B. Banded canine to canine retainer
    C. Bonded canine to canine retainer
    D. Wrap around retainer
48. **Use of head gears or functional appliances to correct class II malocclusion is indicated**
    A. If the active treatment is completed at an early age
    B. Continued growth after active phase of treatment
    C. Both A and B
    D. None of the above
49. **Mild class III cases are best retained by**
    A. Reverse activator    B. FR-III
    C. Class III bionator
    D. All of the above
50. **Limited or short term retention is required in**
    A. Class I non extraction cases
    B. Deep bites
    C. Class II division 1 and division 2 malocclusion cases treated by extraction
    D. All of the above

Ans: 1. D  2. B  3. D  4. D  5. A  6. D  7. D  8. D  9. B  10. C  11. B  12. A  13. A  14. A  15. B  16. A  17. D  18. D  19. D  20. A  21. A  22. B  23. A  24. C  25. C  26. C  27. C  28. D  29. D  30. D  31. D  32. D  33. D  34. B  35. D  36. D  37. D  38. D  39. C  40. B  41. A  42. B  43. A  44. D  45. A  46. C  47. C  48. C  49. D  50. D

# 14. LABORATORY PROCEDURES IN ORTHODONTICS

## ORTHODONTIC STUDY MODEL

1. The anatomic portion of study model
   A. Is that part of the study model which is the actual impression of the dental arch and its surrounding structure?
   B. Is that part of the study model which shows the occlusion?
   C. Is that part of the study model that consist of plaster base?
   D. Both 'A' and 'B'

2. The artistic is that part of the study model
   A. That helps in depicting the actual orientation and occlusion
   B. That consist of a plaster base that supports the anatomic portion
   C. That reproduces the teeth and alveolar structures and surrounding soft tissue
   D. None of the above

3. The maxillary impression should cover
   A. The soft palate
   B. The hard palate
   C. The posterior palatal seal
   D. Both A and B

4. What is the most common impression material used in orthodontics
   A. Impression compound
   B. Agar-agar
   C. Alginate
   D. Zinc oxide eugenol

5. During procedure of impression making the patient should be seated
   A. In a horizontal position
   B. In a vertical position
   C. At a 45 degree angulation
   D. In a supine position

6. The base of the mandibular orthodontic cast should be
   A. Parallel to the occlusal plane
   B. Perpendicular to the occlusal plane
   C. 45 degree angulation to the floor
   D. 45 degree angulation to the base of the cast

7. The back of the mandibular cast should be trimmed
   A. Perpendicular to the occlusal plane
   B. Perpendicular to the base
   C. Perpendicular to long axis of last erupted tooth
   D. None of the above

8. Which of the following statements is NOT true?
   A. Maxillary back surface is trimmed before mandibular back surface
   B. Mandibular back surface is trimmed before maxillary back surface
   C. The upper and lower models are occluded together and the maxillary back surface is trimmed
   D. Maxillary back surface is trimmed after mandibular back surface is trimmed

9. Which of the following statements is true?
   A. Base of maxillary cast should be trimmed parallel to back of mandibular cast
   B. Base of maxillary cast should be trimmed parallel to base of mandibular cast
   C. Base of maxillary and mandibular cast should be parallel to each other
   D. Both B and C

10. Which of the following is NOT a purpose of orthodontic models?
    A. Fabrication of removable orthodontic appliance (ROA) on models
    B. Repair of ROA
    C. Indirect banding procedure
    D. Placement of Elastic modules to secure the arch wire in the slot of brackets

11. Following are the sequential steps involved in the fabrication of orthodontic study models; Except
    A. Step I-Case history
    B. Step II- Disinfection of the impression
    C. Step III- Cast the impression
    D. Step –IV –Basing and trimming the cast.

12. How much clearance should exist between teeth and the tray to accommodate the impression material
    A. 7.3 mm
    B. 8.0 mm
    C. 3.0 mm
    D. 10.0 mm

13. Disinfection of impression is done by
    A. Soaking the impression in solution such as biocide
    B. Soaking the impression in soap water for half an hour
    C. Soaking the impression in spirit for 10 minutes
    D. Keep the impression in boiler for 20 minutes

14. Why impression is rinsed in water after the disinfection?
    A. To clear of any residual disinfectant
    B. To clear of food particles
    C. To clear of blood
    D. All of the above

15. Casting the impression for the fabrication of orthodontic study model is done by
    A. Using finely mixed dental powder
    B. Using finely mixed dental stone
    C. Both A and B
    D. None of the above

16. How many steps are involved in the trimming of the orthodontic study models
    A. 8 steps
    B. 9 steps
    C. 10 steps
    D. 15 steps

17. In step 1, of trimming of orthodontic study models, the base of the mandibular cast trimmed in such a way that, it should be
    A. Parallel to the Occlusal plane
    B. Perpendicular to the Occlusal plane
    C. Both A and B
    D. None of the above

18. In step 2 of trimming of orthodontic study models, the back of the mandibular cast trimmed so that it is
    A. Parallel to the base of the mandibular cast
    B. Perpendicular to the base and a line drawn between two central incisors
    C. 5 mm of plaster should be left distal to the most posterior part
    D. Both A and C
19. In step of trimming of orthodontic study model, back of the upper cast is trimmed so that
    A. Maxillary back is in flush with the mandibular back
    B. Maxillary back is perpendicular to the mandibular back
    C. Both A and B
    D. None of the above
20. In which step of trimming of orthodontic study model, the base of the maxillary cast should be trimmed in such a way that it is parallel to the base of mandibular cast
    A. Step 2
    B. Step 3
    C. Step 6
    D. Step 5
21. In which step of trimming of orthodontic study models, the buccal cuts are made on the mandibular cast 5-6 mm away from the buccal surface of the posterior teeth
    A. Step 3            B. Step 4
    C. Step 5            D. Step 6
22. The buccal cuts to the back of orthodontic study models are to be made of
    A. 40 degrees        B. 65 degrees
    C. 90 degrees        D. 60 degrees
23. Step 6 of trimming of orthodontic study model involves
    A. Trimming the anterior segment of lower cast
    B. Trimming the anterior segment of upper cast
    C. Both A and B
    D. None of the above
24. The posterior cuts of the lower models to the back of the models are made at
    A. 100 degrees
    B. 110 degrees
    C. 115 degrees
    D. 120 degrees
25. The buccal cuts to the back of orthodontic study models used to be made of
    A. 60 degrees
    B. 65 degrees
    C. 70 degrees
    D. 90 degrees
26. In maxillary cast, the anterior cuts to the back of the cast are made at
    A. 30 degrees
    B. 40 degrees
    C. 50 degrees
    D. 60 degrees
27. The posterior cuts of the upper cast are made in such a way that they are
    A. In flush with the posterior cuts of the mandibular cast
    B. In parallel with the anterior cut of the maxillary cast
    C. Both A an B
    D. None of the above
28. Step 5, finishing and polishing, of trimming of orthodontic study model involves
    A. The artistic portion of the study model is polished using the grained sand paper to obtain a smooth finish
    B. The casts are soaked in soap solution for about an hour
    C. While finishing and polishing of the models, care should be taken not to disturb the acute angles of the artistic portion
    D. All of the above
29. Orthodontic study model are stored in
    A. Anywhere
    B. In special racks designed for this purpose
    C. In the cupboard
    D. In glove box
30. Following are the uses of orthodontic study models except
    A. They are used in direct banding procedures
    B. They are used in indirect banding procedure
    C. They are used in fabrication of removable orthodontic appliance
    D. All of the above
31. Gnathostatic study models are the orthodontic study models in which
    A. Base of the mandibular cast is trimmed to correspond to the Frankfort horizontal plane
    B. Base of maxillary cast is trimmed to correspond to the Frankfort horizontal plane
    C. Both A and B
    D. None of the above
32. Storage of orthodontic study models includes
    A. The finished orthodontic study models are labeled with patient's name, reference number and date on the back of both upper and lower casts
    B. The study models are usually stored in special racks designed for this purpose
    C. It is advisable to always pick and return the upper and lower models together to avoid damage to the anatomic portion
    D. All of the above
33. Followings are the type of orthodontic study models except
    A. Orthodontic study model
    B. Gnathostatic study model
    C. Digital study model
    D. Digito-M and l study model
34. In a well fabricated set of study models the ratio of the anatomic portion to artistic portion is
    A. 2:1               B. 3:1

C. 4:1
D. 1:1

35. Width of posterior cuts of the mandibular cast in step 7 of trimming of orthodontic study models should be of
    A. 2-8 mm
    B. 10-12 mm
    C. 13-15 mm
    D. 20-30 mm

36. During impression making procedure for the fabrication of orthodontic study models the patient is made to sit in a vertical position to avoid
    A. Entry of the impression material into the pharynx
    B. Patient will be more comfortable in such a situation
    C. Trauma to the hard tissue
    D. Trauma to the soft tissue

**Ans:** 1. D  2. B  3. D  4. C  5. C  6. A  7. A  8. A  9. D  10. D  11. A  12. C  13. A  14. A  15. B  16. C
17. A  18. D  19. A  20. B  21. C  22. D  23. A  24. C  25. B  26. A  27. A  28. D  29. B  30. A  31. B  32. D
33. D  34. B  35. C  36. A

## WELDING AND SOLDERING

1. **Soldering is defined as a process of joining metals by use of filler metal which has**
   A. Fusion temperature more than 450 degrees
   B. Fusion temperature lower than the metals to be joined
   C. Fusion temperature equal to the metals to be joined
   D. Either of the above

2. **Brazing is defined as a process of joining metals by use of filler metal which has**
   A. Fusion temperature exceeding 450 degrees
   B. Fusion temperature lower than the metals to be joined
   C. Fusion temperature equal to the metals to be joined
   D. Either of the above

3. **Soldering and Brazing**
   A. Signify the same procedure
   B. Vary in fusion temperature of filler metals to be joined
   C. Both of the above
   D. None of the above

4. **The flow of rotten filler metals in between the metals to be joined is by**
   A. Magnetic attraction
   B. Pressure
   C. Capillary attraction
   D. Either of the above

5. **Dental solders are**
   A. Filler metals to join two or more metallic parts
   B. Has fusion temperature less than that of metals to be joined
   C. Both of the above
   D. None of the above

6. **Dental solder should have**
   A. Excellent tarnish and corrosion resistance
   B. Fusion temperature 50 to 100 degrees less than the parts being joined
   C. Free flow
   D. Strength equal to the metals being joined
   E. All of the above

7. **Dental solder should be**
   A. Persistent to tarnish and corrosion
   B. Matching the colour of metal parts to be soldered
   C. 50 to 100 degrees less than the temperature soldered of metals being soldered
   D. All of the above

8. **Dental solders is composed of**
   A. Gold
   B. Silver
   C. Copper
   D. All of the above

9. **Copper component in dental solder gives**
   A. Black appearance to the solder
   B. White appearance to the solder
   C. Yellow appearance to the solder
   D. Crystal appearance to the solder

10. **Nickel component in dental solder gives**
    A. White colour to the solder
    B. Yellow colour to the solder
    C. Black colour to the solder
    D. Either of the above

11. **"Flux" in Latin means**
    A. Magnetic attraction
    B. Flow
    C. Pressure
    D. Capillary attraction

12. **The success of good soldered joint depends on**
    A. How good the dental solder flows over the parts
    B. Constituents of dental solder to be joined
    C. Flux
    D. Antiflux

13. **Oxidized layer in the metallic surfaces to be joined is removed by**
    A. Flux
    B. Antiflux
    C. Dental solder
    D. All of the above

14. **Oxidized layer in the metallic surfaces to be joned has to be removed**
    A. For flux to wet the metallic surfaces
    B. For antiflux to wet the metallic surfaces
    C. For dental solders to wet the metallic surfaces
    D. None of the above

15. Flux
    A. Dissolves any surface impurities on metals to be joined
    B. Prevents oxidization of the metals
    C. Reduces the melting point of dental solder
    D. All of the above
16. Dental flux contains
    A. Borax glass
    B. Boric acid
    C. Silica
    D. All of the above
17. The main component of dental flux is
    A. Boric acid
    B. Borax glass
    C. Silica
    D. Fluoride
18. The major component in fluoride flux is
    A. Boric acid
    B. Potassium fluoride
    C. Both of the above
    D. None of the above
19. Material used to restrict or confine the flow of molten solder over the metals being joined is
    A. Antiflux     B. Flux
    C. Fluoride flux     D. All of the above
20. Examples of commonly used Antiflux are
    A. Lead pencil markings
    B. Graphite lines
    C. Iron rouge
    D. All of the above
21. Soldering process rquires
    A. Dental solders
    B. Flux
    C. Antiflux
    D. All of the above
22. In dental practice, soldering is carried by
    A. Investment soldering
    B. Free hand soldering
    C. Both of the above
    D. None of the above
23. Investment soldering is carried out when
    A. Contact area between metallic parts being joined is large
    B. Metallic parts need adequate stability
    C. Precision is needed to join the metals
    D. All of the above
24. Soldering method most commonly carried out by orthodontist is
    A. Investment
    B. Freehand
    C. Both A and B
    D. None of the above
25. The parts to be joined during soldering are mostly stabilized by
    A. Plaster
    B. Orthophosphate cement
    C. Sticky wax
    D. Both A and B
26. The space between the metals to be joined should be
    A. 0.5 mm
    B. 0.1 mm
    C. 1.0 mm
    D. 2.0 mm
27. Quenching the soldered assembly immediately after introduction of heat is to
    A. Limit the flow of flux
    B. Limit the flow of antiflux
    C. Limit the flow of solder
    D. Limit the spread of heat
28. Factor considered during soldering is
    A. Reducing flame of soldering torch
    B. Limit the spread of heat by using wet cotton and asbestos
    C. Antiflux to be used to prevent excessive spread of solder
    D. All of the above
29. Welding is a process of joining two metals by
    A. Filler metal with temperature above 450 degrees
    B. Filler metal with temperature below 450 degrees
    C. Filler metal with temperature equal to 450 degrees
    D. Directly under pressure
30. Cold welding is done by
    A. Hammering
    B. Pressure
    C. Either of the above
    D. By introduction of heat
31. Heat welding is done by
    A. Heat of sufficient intensity to melt the metals being joined
    B. By introduction of filler materials
    C. By hammering
    D. All of the above
32. Welding used to join orthodontic component is termed as
    A. Free hand soldering
    B. Cold welding
    C. Hot welding
    D. Spot welding
33. Best example for cold welding is
    A. Welding of buccal tube to molar band
    B. Welding of lip bumper to molar band
    C. Gold foil filling
    D. Either of the above

34. **Spot welding is preferred over soldering because**
    A. It is very easy
    B. Less chairside time
    C. Physical properties of metals being joined is preserved
    D. No stabilization is required

35. **Basic principles involved in spot welding**
    A. Dental solders
    B. Heat
    C. Pressure
    D. Both B and C

36. **Spot welding requires**
    A. Step down transformer
    B. Low voltage and high amperage current
    C. 2 copper electrodes
    D. All of the above

37. **Electrodes use in spot welding is made up of**
    A. Stainless steel
    B. Copper
    C. Nickel
    D. Titanium

38. **Passage of current at the weld spot should be**
    A. 1/20th of a second
    B. 1/30th of a second
    C. 1/10th of a second
    D. Less than 1/10th of a second

39. **Weld decay occurs due to**
    A. Plasticity of the metal
    B. Stainless steel electrodes
    C. Precipitation of carbides from the metal
    D. All of the above

40. **Welding of stainless steel depends largely on**
    A. Current flow through the circuit
    B. Time during which current is allowed to flow
    C. Mechanical pressure applied welding heads
    D. All of the above

41. **A good spot weld joint depends on**
    A. Total contact of metals joined
    B. Maintaining the electrode pressure for a few seconds
    C. A broad electrode for thin material
    D. All of the above

42. **Surface of each electrode in spot welder should be**
    A. Flat
    B. Smooth
    C. Perpendicular to its long axis
    D. All of the above

43. **An important component of most removable and functional orthodontic appliance is**
    A. Bows
    B. Springs
    C. Clasps
    D. Acrylic base plates

44. **Base plate used in orthodontic appliance is fabricated from**
    A. Heat cure acrylic resins
    B. Cold cure acrlic resins
    C. Methyl methacylate
    D. None of the above

45. **Acrylization in fabrication of orthodontic appliance is done by**
    A. Heat cure acrylic resins
    B. Self cure acrylic resins
    C. Cold cure acrylic resins
    D. Both B and C

46. **Acrylization using cold cure resins can be done by**
    A. Salt and pepper method
    B. Single mix method
    C. Both B and C
    D. None of the above

47. **Disadvantage of salt and pepper method is**
    A. Difficulty in obtaining uniform thickness
    B. Time consuming
    C. Possess high risk of porosity
    D. All of the above

48. **Thermoplastic sheets used to fabricate base plate are warmed on biostar machine upto temperature of**
    A. 220 degrees
    B. 420 degrees
    C. 320 degrees
    D. 110 degrees

49. **Advantage of using thermoplastic sheets in fabrication of base plate**
    A. Cost effective
    B. Less porosity
    C. Uniform thickness of base plate
    D. All of the above

50. **The cast to be acrylized is soaked in water because**
    A. To increase the strength of base plate
    B. To reduce porosity
    C. To prevent liquid monomer from being absorbed into dry plaster
    D. To easily remove the appliance from the cast after acrylization

**Ans:** 1. B  2. A  3. C  4. C  5. C  6. E  7. D  8. D  9. C  10. A  11. B  12. A  13. B  14. C  15. D  16. D  17. B  18. C  19. A  20. D  21. D  22. C  23. D  24. B  25. D  26. A  27. D  28. D  29. D  30. C  31. A  32. D  33. C  34. C  35. D  36. D  37. B  38. D  39. C  40. D  41. D  42. D  43. D  44. C  45. D  46. C  47. D  48. A  49. C  50. C

## 15. RECENT ADVANCES IN ORTHODONTICS

### ADULT ORTHODONTICS

1. **Reasons for increase in adult patient seeking orthodontic treatment in today practice**
   A. Esthetics conscious society
   B. Increased public awareness
   C. Increased social acceptance
   D. All of the above

2. **Orthodontic tooth movement impeded by certain drugs such as**
   A. Antipyretics
   B. Inhibitor of bone resorption to treat osteoporosis, e.g. calcitonin, biphosphates.
   C. Potent prostaglandin inhibitors, e.g. Indomethacin
   D. B and C

3. **Root resorption is one of the common problem while treating adult patient especially in which type of 100th movement**
   A. Bodily movement    B. Intrusive
   C. Extrusive          D. Rotation

4. **What are types of orthodontic treatment in adults?**
   A. Adjunctive orthodontic treatment
   B. Comprehensive orthodontic treatment
   C. Surgical orthodontic treatment
   D. All of the above

5. **Adjunctive orthodontic treatment refers to**
   A. Movement of teeth to facilitate other dental procedures necessary to control disease and restore function.
   B. Adjunctive orthodontic treatment requires less time as compared comprehensive orthodontic treatment
   C. Both A and B
   D. None of the above

6. **Comprehensive orthodontic treatment refers**
   A. Orthodontic treatment requires less time
   B. Complete treatment to achieve the best balance between dental and facial esthetics ideal occlusal relationships and dentoalveolar stability.
   C. Both A and B
   D. None of the above

7. **Surgical orthodontic treatment includes the following phases**
   A. Presurgical
   B. Surgical
   C. Post surgical
   D. All of the above

8. **Generally the duration of comprehensive orthodontic treatment is**
   A. 8 – 2 months       B. 8 – 16 months
   C. 7 – 24 months      D. 4 – 6 months

9. **Generally duration of adjunctive treatment is**
   A. 8 – 12 months      B. More than 12 months
   C. 6 months or more
   D. More than 24 months

10. **Following are examples of adjunctive orthodontic treatment in adults except**
    A. Opening for insertion of single tooth implant
    B. Elimination of interproximal black space
    C. Full fledged orthodontic treatment with or without extraction
    D. Parallel the abutment

11. **Comprehensive orthodontic treatment patient is usually carried out in**
    A. 6 – 7 years        B. 7 – 9 years
    C. Young adults
    D. Older individual

12. **Orthodontic treatment can be carried out in**
    A. Only in children
    B. Only in adolescent
    C. Any age
    D. Only in older individual

13. **Aim of adjunctive orthodontic treatment in adult patient with anterior diastemas requiring composite build up is**
    A. To close the space
    B. Orthodontic tooth movement can simplify restorative procedures and greatly improve esthetics
    C. Space redistribution by orthodontic tooth movement improve access and permits placement of well adapted and contoured restoration.
    D. All of the above

14. **Presence of open gingival embrassures between incisor tooth creates esthetically unpleasing " black spaces". Such poor embrassure form may be created due to**
    A. Presence of interdental calculus
    B. Roots of incisors are divergent
    C. Abnormal crown shape with incisal edge much wider than cervical portion
    D. Both B and C

15. **The following is a prosthodontic indication of adjunctive orthodontic treatment in adults**
    A. Paralleling the abutment teeth
    B. Space opening for insertion of single tooth implant
    C. Uprighting of tilted teeth and regaining of space prior to prosthetic replacement of missing teeth
    D. All of the above

16. **Before placement of crown and bridge prosthesis it is essential to achieve parallelism of abutment teeth because**
    A. It increases retention of the prosthesis
    B. Occlusal forces are better distributed when abutment teeth are upright and parallel with each other
    C. Esthetics is improved
    D. Patient comfort is increased

17. **In diabetic patients orthodontic treatment**
    A. Is absolutely contraindicated
    B. Can be done if diabetis is under control and periodontium is healthy
    C. Can be done below the age of 40
    D. None of the above

18. Severe skeletal discrepencies in adult patients can be treated with
    A. Dental camouflage
    B. Orthognathic surgery
    C. Myofunctional appliances
    D. Orthopedic appliances
19. Orthodontist may have to alter the position of bracket placement while treating an adult patient due to
    A. Loss of alveolar bone height that shifts the center of resistance of the tooth more apically
    B. Loss of alveolar bone height that shifts the center of resistance of the tooth more coronally
    C. Position of bracket placement need not be altered in adults
    D. Both A and C
20. While treating adult orthodontic patients with multiple missing teeth anchorage can be gained by
    A. Teeth
    B. Ridge
    C. Mini-implants
    D. All of the above

Ans: 1. D  2. D  3. B  4. D  5. C  6. B  7. D  8. B  9. C  10. C  11. C  12. C  13. C  14. D  15. D  16. B  17. B  18. B  19. D  20. C

## IMPLANTS IN ORTHODONTICS

1. The importance of implant in orthodontics is
    A. Its ability to treat hypodontia
    B. It acts as anchorage
    C. Can be used for space closure
    D. All of the above
2. Which of the following statements is NOT true ?
    A. Implants can be used to study bone growth
    B. Endosseous implants are ankylosed in alveolar bone
    C. Implants cannot be used for orthodontic treatment
    D. Combinative therapy of implant placement and orthodontics give a better result
3. Success of implant is compromised by
    A. Midline diastema
    B. Tongue tie
    C. Smoking
    D. Leukoplakia
4. Which of the following statements is NOT true ?
    A. Aggressive periodontal disease compromises success of an implant
    B. There is no contra-indication of implants
    C. Poor oral hygiene compromises success of implant
    D. Smoking reduces osseointegration of implant
5. Which material has best osseointegration properties?
    A. Pure titanium
    B. Pure gold
    C. Pure stainless steel
    D. Pure nickel
6. What are the requirements to implant bone?
    A. Good periodontal health
    B. Adequate bone volume
    C. Adequate oral hygiene
    D. All of the bone
7. What age is considered safer for implant?
    A. 6 years
    B. 10-12 years
    C. 16 years
    D. 18 years
8. What are the methods of ridge mapping?
    A. Use of calipers to pierce the mucosa and measure bone width
    B. Impression making
    C. Elevation of flap
    D. Intra-oral periapical radiograph
9. What implants have the highest success rates?
    A. Maxillary implants
    B. Mandibular implants
    C. Anterior maxillary implants
    D. Upper canine implants

Ans: 1. D  2. C  3. C  4. B  5. A  6. D  7. D  8. A  9. B

## INVISALIGN

1. Who introduced the Invisalign?
    A. E H Angle
    B. Cruz
    C. Align technologies
    D. None of the above
2. In which year align technologies introduced invisalign
    A. 1990
    B. 1999
    C. 1980
    D. 1993
3. Invisalign can be used to correct the following types of malocclusions except
    A. Malocclusions with mild crowding
    B. Malocclusions with mild spacing
    C. In case of mild relapse
    D. Severe skeletal class III malocclusions
4. A typical invisalign treatment requires
    A. 20-30 aligners
    B. 50-80 aligners
    C. 90-110 aligners
    D. 120-130 aligners
5. Benefits of invisalign are
    A. Easier cleaning

B. Invisible thus no unwarranted attention to your mouth
C. No brackets
D. All of the above

6. Contra-indications of invisalign are following except
   A. Malocclusions with severe crowding
   B. Skeletal malocclusions
   C. Severe skeletal class II divisions I malocclusions
   D. Malocclusions with mild spacing

7. Which of the following appliance is more esthetic
   A. Fixed orthodontic appliance with metal brackets
   B. Fixed orthodontic appliance with gold brackets
   C. Invisalign
   D. Functional appliances

8. Invisalign is
   A. Fixed
   B. Semi-fixed
   C. Removable
   D. Semi-removable

9. What is the maximum tooth movement potential with one invisalign aligner
   A. 0.025 mm/aligner
   B. 0.2 m/aligner
   C. 1 mm/aligner
   D. 2 mm/aligner

10. Models for invisalign are made by the process called
    A. Steriography
    B. Stereolithiography
    C. Sterography
    D. Steroanginography

Ans: 1. C  2. B  3. D  4. A  5. D  6. D  7. C  8. C  9. A  10. B

## LASERS IN ORTHODONTICS

1. Which of the following is *NOT* an advantage of Lasers?
   A. Reduces the risk of post-operative infections.
   B. Reduces the risk of blood – borne transmission of diseases.
   C. Less damage occurs to adjacent tissues.
   D. Hinders the area of operation

2. Which of the following is *NOT* a soft tissue laser?
   A. $CO_2$
   B. He-Ne
   C. Nd-YAG
   D. Er: YAGEr

3. Which of the following is an hard tissue laser?
   A. Cr:YSGG
   B. Ruby
   C. Argon
   D. Rhodium

4. An example of soft tissue laser in Gas state;
   A. Nd:YAG
   B. Ruby
   C. Rhodium
   D. $CO_2$

5. Which of the following soft tissue lasers are in solid state?
   A. He-Ne
   B. Argon
   C. Nd:YAG
   D. Rhodium

6. He-Ne is
   A. Soft tissue laser
   B. Hard tissue laser
   C. Neither soft nor hard tissue lasers
   D. Both soft and hard tissue lasers

7. Rhodium is an soft tissue laser and is in
   A. Solid state
   B. Liquid state
   C. Gas state
   D. All of the above

8. $CO_2$ Laser operates with
   A. 10600 nm wavelength
   B. 20000 nm wavelength
   C. 1830 nm wavelength
   D. 2560 nm wavelength

9. Which of the following statement is TRUE regarding $CO_2$ laser
   A. It does not contact the tissue during the cutting phase
   B. It is well absorbed by water
   C. It operates with 10600 nm wavelength
   D. All of the above

10. Erbium laser has a wavelength of
    A. 2790 to 2940 nm
    B. 10600 nm
    C. 5000 nm to 8000 nm
    D. 12000 nm to 15000 nm

11. Erbium laser is useful in
    A. Caries removal
    B. Tooth preparation
    C. Bone ablation
    D. All of the above

12. Diode laser has a wavelength of
    A. 812 nm to 980 nm
    B. 10600 nm
    C. 2790 nm to 2940 nm
    D. 5000 nm to 8000 nm

13. Which of the following statement is TRUE regarding diode laser
    A. It is a solid active semiconductor
    B. It can be used often without anesthesia to perform very precise anterior soft tissue esthetic surgery
    C. It can deliver energy in both continuous as well as in pulsed mode
    D. All of the above

14. Argon laser has a wavelength of
    A. 488 nm
    B. 514 nm
    C. Both (A) and (B)
    D. None of the above

15. Which of the following statement is FALSE regarding Argon laser
    A. Argon laser delivers energy either continuous or gated pulse mode

B. It is well absorbed in pigmented tissue and hemoglobin
C. It is useful as good haemostatic activity and in acute inflammatory soft tissue lesions
D. All of the above

16. Nd: YAG laser has wavelength of
    A. 1064 nm
    B. 10600 nm
    C. 514 nm
    D. 488 nm

17. Frenectomy by Laser has the following advantages Except
    A. Painless and bloodless procedure
    B. Recurrence can be prevented
    C. Facilitates the diastema closure
    D. Moves the maxillary permanent central incisors and there by closes the midline diastema

18. Application of Laser in patient with separators reduces
    A. The level of pain threshold
    B. Increases patient compliance
    C. Both (A) and (B)
    D. Neither (A) nor (B)

19. Which of the following statement is TRUE regarding Nd: YAG Laser
    A. It can be easily absorbed by pigmented tissue
    B. It delivers the energy in free running pulse mode
    C. It is useful in periodontal surgery
    D. All of the above

20. Exposure of impacted tooth by laser provides
    A. Good accessibility
    B. Decreases the risk of bond failure
    C. Painless procedure
    D. All of the above

21. Application of laser in bonding orthodontic bracket
    A. Takes only few seconds that is approximately (3-5) seconds
    B. It reduces the chair time
    C. Increases the efficiency of bonding
    D. All of the above

22. Lasers can be used for
    A. Debonding of metal brackets
    B. Debonding of ceramic brackets
    C. Both (A) and (B)
    D. Neither (A) nor (B)

23. Which of the following statement is FALSE regarding management of apthous ulcer by laser during orthodontic treatment
    A. Helps in reducing the pain
    B. Promotes healing
    C. Both (A) and (B)
    D. Neither (A) nor (B)

24. Lasers in orthodontics used for
    A. Caries control
    B. Controlling growth of facial structures
    C. Ablation of surface enamel for orthodontic bracket placement
    D. All of the above

**Ans:** 1. D  2. D  3. A  4. D  5. C  6. A  7. B  8. A  9. D  10. A  11. D  12. A  13. D  14. C  15. D  16. A  17. D  18. C  19. D  20. D  21. D  22. C  23. D  24. D

# Index

Page numbers followed by *f* refer to figure and *t* refer to table.

## A

Abrasive strip
   double sided 240
   single-sided 240
Abutment teeth, paralleling of 482
Ackerman-profit classification 85, 86*f*
   advantages of 87
   disadvantages of 87
Acrylic
   base material 310, 461*f*
   component 351-354, 356, 462, 461, 464
   plate 248*f*
Acrylization 310
Adam's clasp 14, 299, 299*f*, 300, 301*f*, 302, 411*f*, 461, 463*f*
   advantages of 300
   disadvantages of 300
   double 301*f*
   modifications of 300, 301*f*
   parts of 300*f*
Adam's pliers 279, 280, 283, 301
   consists 280
   parts of 280*f*
Adenoid 128
   facies 221
Adolescent growth spurt 23, 24*f*
Adult orthodontic treatment, types of 482*t*
Aesthetic component 115, 117
Alginate impression trays 470*f*
Alloy arch wire exhibit 322
Alveolar
   bone 232
      height 480
   process 49
American Association of Orthodontists 10
Amniotic lesions 94
Anchor unit 363, 364
Anchorage
   demand 236
   planning 235, 480
   sources of 231, 231*t*
   system, design of 370
Andresen's concepts 15
Andrew's six keys of occlusion 67
Angle's class
   I malocclusion, extraoral features of 78
   II division 1 malocclusion, extraoral features of 391
   II malocclusion
      classification of 390
      management of 326*f*
Angle's classification 80
Ankyloglossia 91, 447*f*
Ankylosed
   mandibular deciduous second molar 102*f*
   primary teeth, surgical removal of 447
Ankylosis 96, 102
Anodontia, partial 377, 379*f*
Anthropoid spaces 56
Anthropometry 20
Antiflux 474
Apatite crystals 499
Aphthous ulcer, management of 502, 503*f*
Appliance, removable
   functional 346
   habit breaking 201*f*, 214
Apron spring 304, 307*f*, 309
Arch
   curvatures 61
   deficiency 198
   dimension 91
   expansion 240, 245, 253
      slow 250, 251
   length 379
      determination of 136
      tooth material discrepancy 256*f*, 406
   perimeter analysis 136, 239
   width, determination of 136
   wire 321, 336, 338, 340, 423, 426*f*
      classification of 322*f*, 322*t*
      fabrication 339
      insertion 338*f*
Argon laser 500
Arm, circumferential 298, 302
Armamentarium 135, 278*f*, 279
Arrow-pin clasp 298
Arter orthodontic treatment 459
Ashley Howe's analysis 138, 139*t*
Austenitic
   active alloy 323
   wire 323
Australian austenitic arch wire 321
Auxiliary wires 360

## B

Ballard's classification 83, 85
Ballard's skeletal class malocclusion 84, 84*f*
Band
   cementation of 330
   completed 331
   contouring plier 266, 267
   custom-made 329
   cutting scissors 266, 267, 267*f*, 331
   director 273
   material, contoured 331
   pinchable pliers 266, 267, 268*f*
   pusher 266
   remover 272, 274*f*
   scaler/pusher 273
   seater 266, 268, 269*f*
Base plate, modification of 316
Begg's appliance 339
Begg's retainer 16, 462, 464*f*
Begg's technique 16, 340
   stages of 340
Belzer wire cutter 273
Benjamin's theory 210
Bennett's class malocclusion 85
Bennett's classification 85
Bilaminar disk 35
   formation of 36*f*
Bilaminar embryonic disc, formation of 36*f*
Bimaxillary protrusion 126*f*, 383, 385, 385*f*, 479
   management of 383
   treatment of 385-387
Bimaxillary retrusion 387
   management of 387
   treatment of 387
Bionator 15, 351, 424
   functional appliance 16
   uses of 353
Bird beak pliers 266, 270, 321
Birth injury 89
Bisphosphates 480
Bite
   anterior open 326*f*, 456*f*
   correction of deep 426*f*
Bite plane 316
   anterior 316, 422, 423, 424, 424*f*
   anterior inclined 316, 317
   posterior 317
   types of anterior 423

Biting habits 207
Bjork, Grave and Brown method 165
Blanch test 407, 408*f*
Blastocyst 36*f*
   formation 35
Blood
   flow theory 176
   vessels 176
Bolton's analysis 139, 239
Bondable brackets 334, 334*f*, 340
Bondable buccal tubes 334, 339, 340
Bondable lingual button 331*f*
Bonded canine-to-canine retainer 466*f*
Bonded rapid maxillary expansion 248
Bonded retainer, fixed 411*f*
Bone 38
   adaptation 460
   basal 232
   bending 177
   deposition 48*f*
   formation
      modes of 24
      trajectorial theory of 32
   growth 25
   remodeling 25, 47, 47*f*
      of palate 48*f*
      secondary 174
   secondary displacement of 26*f*
   segments, separation of 457*f*
   transformation, Wolff's law of 33
Boon's gauge 266, 268, 269*f*
Borax glass 474
Boric acid 474
Brachycephalic 121, 391
   head 121, 122*f*
Brass wire
   separator 319-321
   soft 320
British Society of Orthodontists 1
Bruxism 225
   etiology 225
   treatment 225
   types 225
Buccal
   cervical margin 299
   cusps 67*f*
   displacement 72
      of canine 73*f*
   inclination 72
   interdental arm 298
   nonocclusion 429, 430*f*
   occlusion 116
   segment relationship 397
      anteroposterior 117
   self-supported canine retractor 314, 315*f*
   shield 353, 354
   surface 67*f*, 435*f*
   tube 334, 340
      classification of 335
      welding 331
Buccopharyngeal membrane 37*f*

Bud stage 52
Butler's field theory 112, 112*f*

## C

Calcitonin 480
Calcium metabolism 480
Canine 54, 259
   erupting 407*f*
   extension 353
      wire 354
   guidance 65
   lateral 375
   lingual eruption of 99*f*
   primary 448*f*
   protected occlusion 63
   relationship 76, 393, 402
      class I 76, 76*f*, 385*f*, 392
      class II 76
      class III 77, 403
   retractor 312
      classification of 313*t*
      loop 312, 313
      types of 315*t*
   simon law of 83
   teeth, missing 118
   to canine
      lingual retainer 384*f*
      retainer, banded 465, 465*f*
Capsular matrix 27, 31
Carey's analysis 135
Caries, increased predisposition to 483
Carpal bones 164
Cartilage 38
   in mandibular development, secondary 42
Cartilaginous theory 26
Casting impressions 350
Catalan's appliance 432, 432*f*
Cell
   ball of 35*f*
   reduced 480
Cellular elements 176
Cellular hyperplasia 18
Central incisor, distally inclined 73*f*
Cephalic
   examination 121
   index 121*t*, 122
Cephalogram
   anteroposterior 452
   lateral 142, 421, 444
   types of 142
Cephalometric
   analyses 13, 142, 147, 222
   evaluation 451
   findings 383, 387, 421
   landmarks 143
   planes 145, 147*f*
   radiograph 132
   reference planes 145, 147
   roentgenography 12*f*
   types 142
   uses 142
   X-ray tracing techniques 143

Cephalometry 11, 11*t*
Ceramic brackets 333, 333*f*, 481, 482*f*
Cerebral
   hemisphere theory 31
   palsy 89, 92
Cervical
   headgear 366, 367*f*
   region 233
   vertebrae 170*t*, 362
      maturation of 170*f*
      maturity indicator 169
      skeletal maturity indicator 169
      vertebral maturation method 169*f*
Chain theory, reflex 31
Cheek-biting habit 224
   treatment 224
Childhood growth spurt 23
Chin 49
   cup 370, 371
      appliance 363, 372, 372*f*, 432, 433*f*
      custom fabrication of 372
      fabrication of 371
      types of 371
   position 125, 125*t*
   prominence 125, 125*t*, 455*f*
   recessive 127*f*
Circumoral musculatures 202
Clasp 13, 298, 461
   circumferential 298, 298*f*, 299
   forming pliers 266, 269, 270*f*
   types of 14, 64
   wire 302
Cleansing electrodes 473
Cleft deformity 440
Cleft lip 92, 108, 437-439
   bilateral 92*f*, 437*f*
   management of 442
   stages of 442
   treatment of 443
   unilateral 437
   with cleft palates, unilateral 437*f*
Cleft palate 92, 92*f*, 108, 437, 439-441
   cases, retention in 466
   isolated 437*f*
   management of 442
   stages of 442
   treatment of 443
   unilateral 441
Cleidocranial
   dysostosis 93
   dysplasia 108
   dystosis 92
Cobalt-chromium-nickel alloy 322
Coffin spring 14, 252*f*
Coil spring 324, 325
   closed 323, 324, 325*f*
Coiled portion of Z-spring 280
Cold welding 473
Competent lip 126, 127, 127*f*
Composite restoration, after 410*f*
Concave facial profile 123*f*, 402
Concave inner surfaces 280, 282

Concave opposite beak 281
Condylar cartilage 42
Condylar guidance 65
Condylar mandibular growth, reflection of 46
Condylar process 42
Congenital
　defects 92
　syphilis 93
Congenitally missing
　lateral incisors 111*f*
　maxillary lateral incisors 488
　teeth 92, 97, 390
Convex
　facial profile 123*f*, 385*f*, 391, 391*f*
　nose 125*f*
Cook's classification 209
Copper electrodes 473
Coronoid cartilage 42
Coronoid process 42, 43, 48
Corticotomy 449, 451*f*
Cosmetic surgeries 456
Cotton test 130*f*, 131, 222
Cranial
　base 41, 44, 45
　bones and sutures, adjacent 246
　nerve 38
　vault 41, 44, 45, 45*t*
Craniofacial
　complex 44
　development 26
　disorders 108
　growth 30, 478
　　completed 45*t*
　skeletal growth 346
Craniomandibular disorders 466
Craniometry 20
Cranium 233
Crest of curvature 66
Crile needle holder 270
Crossbite 117, 325, 326, 430
　after correction of 435*f*
　anterior 93, 428, 428*f*, 433*f*
　bilateral posterior 429, 429*f*
　classification of 428
　　anterior 428
　　posterior 429
　correction of 326
　　anterior 430-432
　elastic 325, 326
　functional 428, 430, 431*f*
　　anterior 199, 200, 200*f*, 200*f*
　management of 428, 431*t*
　posterior 391, 402*t*, 428*f*, 429, 434
　segmental
　　anterior 428, 428*f*
　　posterior 429, 429*f*
　simple posterior 429, 430*f*
　tendency 348
　treatment of 200*t*
　　anterior 404
　　posterior 404

types of
　anterior 200, 200*t*
　posterior 429
unilateral 429
　posterior 75, 429
Crown
　angulations 68, 68*f*
　completion 51, 53
　inclination 68
　　of teeth 68*f*
　lengthening procedure 504, 505*f*
　of central and lateral incisors, anterior 68
Crozat clasp 14, 302, 302*f*
Crystal lattice, part of 177
Cumulative curve 21
Curve bend 278
Curve of Spee 65, 66*f*, 69*f*, 391
Curve of Wilson 66, 66*f*
Cusp
　centric holding 64, 64*f*
　embrasure occlusion 65, 65*f*
　fossa occlusion 65, 65*f*
　supporting 64, 64*f*
Cuspid 51, 52
　guidance 65
Cyst of
　face 92
　palate 92

## D

De La Rosa pliers 266, 269, 271*f*
Debanding plier 266, 272, 273
　anterior 274*f*
Deciduous canine 113*f*
　extraction of 197
　premature loss of 193
Deciduous dentition 3, 56*f*
　care of 187
　chronology of 51*t*
　stage 54, 55*f*
Deciduous first molar
　extraction of 198
　premature loss of 187, 193
Deciduous left central incisor 375
Deciduous molar 298
　second 375
　　premature loss of 193
Deciduous teeth 91, 187, 199
　acting 187*f*
　ankylosis of 187
　management of ankylosed 187
　premature loss of 96, 98, 100*t*, 187, 374, 375
　proximal caries of 186*f*
　retention of 96, 98, 374
Deep bite 56, 75*f*, 342*f*, 420
　management of 420
　types of 420
Deglutition 32
Deleterious oral habits 206
Delta clasp 298

Dental
　abnormalities, number of 92*f*
　aesthetic index 115, 118
　age 163
　analysis 157
　anterior open bite 413*f*, 414, 414*f*
　　treatment of 415, 416*t*
　arch 8*f*, 239
　　maxillary arch, V-shaped 392
　　occlusal of 422*f*
　　relationship, sagittal 256
　calculus 393
　camouflage 480
　caries 1, 96, 100
　　extensive 93
　class III malocclusion 400, 401, 401*t*, 402
　compensation 452, 452*f*
　crossbite 428, 430, 430*f*
　crowding 375
　deep bite 420, 420*f*
　follicle 172
　health component 115, 116*t*
　parameters 148
　problems 441
　proclination 451*f*
　restoration, improper 102*t*
　science dentistry 7
　solder 474, 475*f*
　status 227
Dentition 91
　and occlusion, development of 51
　development of 51
　late mixed 4
　stage, mixed (6–12 years) 57
Dentoalveolar
　anterior crossbite 199, 200
　procedures 447
　segment, anterior 454
Dentofacial anomalies, management of 5
Dentures, removable partial 482
Depression
　side, triangular 283
　triangular 282
Derichsweiler expansion appliance 14
　parts of 248*f*
Dewel's method 197, 197*f*, 198
Dewey's classification 80
Diastema 118
　anterior 310
　closure of midline 410*f*, 482
　midline 406, 406*f*, 407, 407*f*
　of hereditary origin, midline 406*f*
　treatment of midline 409, 410
Diode laser 500
Distal displacement 72
Distal end
　cutter 266, 272, 273*f*
　of bones of forearm 164
Distal extension 301*f*
Distal jet appliance 242
Distal shoe 191

Disto-occlusion 82f
Distraction osteogenesis 456, 457
Dizygotic twins 106f, 107, 107f, 108, 108f
Dolichocephalic 121, 391
    facial form 221
    head 121, 122f
Down's analysis 147, 148t, 151f
Down's cephalometric analysis 147
Down's syndrome 108
Dumb bell separator 319
    shaped elastic 320, 321f
Duyzing clasp 298

### E

Ectodermal dysplasia 90f
Ectopic maxillary canine 112
Edentulous spaces 479
Edge wire technique 16
Edgewise appliance 9, 10f, 338
Edgewise brackets 334, 338
Elastics 324, 340, 370
    chain 327t, 328
    ligature 328, 329
    module 328
    of latex 324
    ring 319
        separator 319, 320, 320f
    swallow 203
    thread 328 328f
Elastomeric links 328
Electrodes, selection of 473
Embryo, period of 35
Embryologic classification 439
Enamel
    etching 335, 336f
    for orthodontic bracket placement 502
    formed, amount of 51
Endochondral ossification 24
Endocrine imbalance 89
Endodontic indications 483
Endomorphic physique 110
Endosseous implants 488
Endotracheal tube 505
Enlow's counterpart principle 30
Enmass retraction 341
Epiblast layer, midline of 36f
Epigenetic factors, local 31
Epilepsy 121
Eruptive path, abnormal 96, 102
Esophageal stage 32
Esthetic
    harmony 2
    requirements 295
Ethmoidal-maxillary suture 46
Euryprosopic face 122f
Exhibits adequate strength 322
Expansion appliance, isaacson type of 249f
Expansion screw 248
Extraction procedures 195

Extraoral
    anchorage 235, 235f
    bone grafts 487
    distalization appliances 243
    elastics 326
    examination 121, 213
    features 78, 80, 217, 383, 387, 391, 421
    force appliances 3
    habit 201f
    methods 130
    orthopedic force 365
    sources 233
    strapping 443, 443f
Eyelet clasp 298

### F

Fabrication 303, 306, 310, 313, 314, 431
Face bow 363, 364f
    fitting 363
    parts of 364f
Face mask 235f, 369, 369f, 327f, 404, 432, 433
    components of 370
    delaire type of 370, 371f
    parts of 371
    petit type of 370, 371f
    protraction 363, 369
    therapy 369
    Tübinger type of 370, 371f
    types of 370
Face, development of 38
Facial
    angle 149f
        planes of 147
    asymmetry 122, 452
    bones 233
    clefts 108
    discrepancy 452f
    divergence 110, 122, 123f, 124, 124t, 391
        anterior 123f, 401, 402
        posterior 110, 123f, 391
        straight 123f
    esthetics 483
        evaluation of 451
    examination 121
    form 110, 122, 122t, 221, 391
    height, lower 348f, 391
    nerve 38
    profile 110, 122, 123f, 123t, 391, 392
    prominences 39
    proportions, evaluation of 124, 125f
    structure
        derivation of 39t
        growth of 502
    symmetry 110
Fetal posture during gestation, abnormal 94
Fetus, period of 35
Fibroids, maternal 94
Finger
    spring 310, 310f

    fabrication of 310
    helix of 310
    parts of 310
    touching wire 283
First permanent molars, emergence of 57
Fishman's skeletal maturity indicators 166, 167f, 168t
Fishman's system 166
Fluid dynamic theory 176
Fluoride fluxes 474
Flush terminal plane 57
Force
    delivering unit 363
    duration of 362
    generating unit 364
Fractures of maxilla, treatment of 10
Frankel appliance 15, 16, 353
    types of 353
Frankel hypothesizes 355
Frankfort mandibular plane angle 160
Frenal attachments 126
Frenectomy 446, 447f, 501
Frenum attachment, abnormal 406
    management of 188
Friction mechanics 341
Frontal cephalogram 142, 142f
Frontal cranial bones 362
Frontal dynamism 131
Frontoethmoidal suture 46
Frontomaxillary suture 46
Frontonasal buttress/pillar 33

### G

Gait 121
Gardiner's classification 90
Gardner's syndrome 108
Genetic
    factors, intrinsic 31
    theory 26
Genioplasty 457f
Genital curve 22
Genome 105
Gerber's space regainer 202, 202f, 477
German measles 89
Gingiva 128, 129f
    by laser, depigmentation of 504, 504f
Gingival
    arm 321
    recontouring, subsequent 488
    tissue, treatment of 223
Glass slab 278, 279
Glossopharyngeal nerve 38
Gnathostatic models, trimming of 470
Gold 322, 474
    alloy 321
Graber's classification 89
Graphite lines 474
Greulich and Pyle method 165
Grewe's method 198
Growth 18
    basic tenets of 21
    centers 24, 163

cephalocaudal gradient of 22, 22f
factors 19
fields 24
hormones 19
modification 365
pattern, abnormal 414f
rhythm 23
sites 24
spurts 23, 24
Guiding cusp 64f
Gum pad 54f
   stage 53, 54
Gummy smile 221

## H
Habitual tongue thrust 215
Hamate, hook of 164
Hand
   and wrist, anatomy of 163
   wire cutter 283
Hard palate 20, 33, 232f
Hard round stainless steel wire 303
Hard stainless steel wire 299, 301, 314
Hard tissue
   cephalometric landmarks 144f
   landmarks 144
Hard wire cutter 279, 281
   parts of 282f
Hass expansion appliance 14
Hawley's retainer 11f, 16, 411f, 422f, 461-463, 463f
   design of 461
   modifications of 462
   parts of 461
Hay fever 121
Head
   brachycephalic, shape of 110
   shape of 122, 122f, 391
Headgear 363, 364, 366
   derive anchorage 233f
   therapy 365, 366
   types of 366
Heat 473, 475
Helical
   canine retractor 313, 314f
      parts of 313
   coil spring 312
   spring 313f
Herbst appliance 15, 16, 359, 359f
Herbst bite jumping 359
Herren's modification 15
Hinge 279, 280, 281, 282
   movement 280
   portion 281
Hollow tube waveguide 497
Holly Broadbent's contribution 12
Hook pin 340
Hotz modifications 357
Howe pliers 266, 272, 275f
Human dental tissues 499
Hutchinson's incisors 93
Hyalinization 174, 175
   tissue, formation of 176

Hyalinized areas, formation of 175
Hyperactive mentalis muscle activity 126f
Hyperemia 173
Hyperparathyroidism 94
Hyperthyroidism 94
Hypertrophy 221
Hypobranchial eminence 40
Hypoparathyroidism 94
Hypothyroidism 94
Hypotonic lips 202
Hyrax maxillary expander 477

## I
Implant placement
   prohibit 487
   single 488
Implantation, sites of 20
Incisal segments, spacing in 118
Incisor
   central 51, 52, 54, 407f, 410f
   crowding, lower 262
   lateral 51, 52, 54, 375
   left lateral 375f
   lower central 151
   mandibular plane angle 153, 153f, 160
   occlusal plane 153
      angle 151, 152f
      angle, planes of 151
      increased 153
   overbite, correction of 404
   relationship 56, 61, 75, 391
      class II 76
      class II division 1 76
      class II division 2 392
      class III 76, 76f
      classification of 75
      correction of 397
      edge-to-edge 82f
      severity of 390
   retraction 341
   retroclination of upper 452f
   retroclined
      lower 452f
      upper 348
   rotations of central 96f
   severe proclined lower 348
   teeth, missing 118
   upper 348f, 452f
      lateral 92
Infantile
   growth spurt 23
   open bite 54
Infectious diseases 89
Inflammatory soft tissue lesions, acute 501
Interarch malocclusions 73
Interincisal angle 151
   increased 422f
Intermaxillary
   anchorage 234
   elastics 9f, 324

International Confederation for Plastic and Reconstructive Surgery 439
International Dental Congress in Berlin 359
Interstitial fluid 176
Intra-alveolar space maintainer 191
Intra-arch malocclusion 72
Intramaxillary anchorage 234
Intranasal defects 221
Intraoral
   anchorage 234
   distalization appliances 243
   elastics 370
      slot for 371f
   examination 126, 213
   features 217, 383, 387, 391, 421
   methods 130
   sources teeth 231
Intrauterine
   fetal posture 390
   position, abnormal 92
Intrusive tooth movement 183f
Invisalign aligners 492, 493
Invisalign system 492
Invisalign technique 16, 492
Isaacson expansion appliance 248
Issacson's expansion appliances 14

## J
Jack expansion screw 14
Jackson clasp 299, 299f
Jackson triad 2f
Jasper jumper 16, 360
   appliance 360f
Jaw
   anteroposterior 365
   development, abnormalities of 92
   growth of 29
   involved 234
   pliers 273
   position, edge-to-edge class I 219
   positioning 219
   protruded, lower 349
   relationship, anteroposterior 123
Johnson and Larson's classification 209
Joint, selection of 475

## K
Kawetzky modification 15
Kernahan's stripped 'Y' classification 439, 439f
Kesling metallic ring 319, 321
   separator, parts of 321
Kesling tooth position 16, 464, 465f
Korkhaus analysis 138

## L
Labial bow
   extensive 306
   long 14, 304, 305
   reverse 14, 304, 306, 307f
   short 14, 304
   types of 308t

Labial frenum
  abnormal 96, 100
  attachment 128f
  normal attachment of 128f
Labial wire
  lower 354, 356
  upper 354, 356
Labiolingual crown inclination 68
Laser
  advantages of 501
  application of 502, 505f
  beam delivery system 497, 497f
  energy 499f
  in orthodontics 495, 501
  on tissue, action of 498f
  physics 495
  resonator 497
  safety 505
  tissue interaction 497
  treatment 495
  types of 500, 500t
  unit 497f
    components of 496
Le Fort I osteotomy 455, 455f, 456f
Leeway space 60
Leong's premolar/dens evaginatus 99f
Leptoprosopic
  face 122f
  facial form 402
Light wire pliers 266
Lingual
  appliance 344
  arch 273, 477
  bonded
    canine, fixed 295f
    retainer, fixed 486f
  button, classification of 330
  cleat, types of 330
  eyelet 330, 332, 332f
  frenectomy 446
  holding arch, lower 191
  nonocclusion 429, 430f
  orthodontic 16, 478
    technique 481
  pad, lower 353
  sheath, types of 330
  shield, lower 354
  spring, lower 353, 354, 354f
  wire, upper 353, 354, 356
Lip 125, 391
  biting 223, 356
    habit 224f, 357f
  bumper 219, 232f, 236f, 295f, 357, 357, 358f
    appliances 224f
  competent 110
  forms of 127t
  habits 223
    classification 223
    management 224
  incompetant 126, 127, 221, 391
  pads 353, 354

support wire of 353
  upper 356
placement 212
  lingual, lower 212
seal exercises 355
sucking 223
  habit 212f, 224f
wetting 223
Lischer's classification 81
Lower anterior inclined plane 432
Lower facial height 348, 421f
Lower incisors, proclination of 348f, 452f
Lower lingual holding arch 192
Lower lip sucking habit 224f
Lower posterior teeth, mesial movement of 397
Lymphoid curve 22

# M

Macrodontic
  left permanent central incisors 375
  maxillary central incisors 431f
  right maxillary central incisor 98f
  right permanent central incisors 375
  teeth 374
Macroglossia 92, 377
Macroskeletal unit 27
Madibular impression 470
Malocclusion 1, 115, 297
  Angle's class 78, 80
    division 1 78
    I 78, 82f, 125f, 228, 228f, 256, 256f, 257, 258, 326f
    II 78, 82f
    II division 1 78, 229
    II division 2 80, 420f
    III 80, 110, 228, 229f, 256, 259f, 326f, 401
  angle's classification of 77
  class I 198, 380
  class II 390
  class II
    division 1 108, 368f, 391
    division 2 109, 391, 392
  class III 111, 400, 466
    type 1 82f
  classification of 9, 71
    class II 390
  deflective 64
  Dewey's class I
    type 1 81f
    type 2 81f
    type 3 81f
    type 4 81f
    type 5 82
  Dewey's class III
    type 2 82
    type 3 82f
  genetic basis of 107
  heritability of 107
  in identical twins, class II division 2 109f

interception of class II 200
intra-arch 71
management of
  class I 374
  class II 390, 399
  class III 400
mandible deficiency, class II 454f
of dental origin 4
of skeletal origin 4
of teeth, treatment of 10
pseudo class III 80, 400
severe skeletal class II division 1 256f, 393, 396
severity of 118
traits 106
treatment of class III 401
true class III 400
with rotation, treatment of class I 380
Mandible 20, 41, 44, 47
  angle of 48
  body of 48
  clockwise rotation of 414f
  development of 41
  mandibular growth of 348
  ossification of 42f
  posterior body of 453
  trajectories of 33
Mandibular
  12 teeth, sum of 139
  6 teeth, sum of 139
  abnormalities, correction of 453, 454
  acrylic part 352
  anterior 325
    crowding 376f
    crowding, severe 198
    overlap maxillary anterior 428f
    proclination 385
    retrusion of 404f
    teeth, severe rotation of 382f
  arch 60, 65f, 67f, 111f, 339, 375
    eruption sequence for 61
  central incisors, eruption of 55f
  condyle 48
  deciduous
    canine, premature loss of 198
    second molar, premature loss of 100f
  deficiency 454
  excess 452, 453
  first permanent molar, mesiobuccal developmental groove of 68f
  growth, extreme vertical 348
  incisor 259, 459
  irregularity, anterior 118
  lateral incisor, gemination of 99f
  lateral sulcus 54f
  molars 326f
  overjet, anterior 118
  posterior
    bite plane 317, 317f
    crowns 68
  process 39

prognathism 110
retrognathism 390, 391, 391*f*
segment, anterior 453*f*
subapical osteotomy 453
   anterior 454
teeth 435*f*
   incisal edges of 67*f*
third molars 133*f*
total subapical osteotomy 454, 455*f*
Marginal gingivitis 129*f*
Martensitic
   active alloy 323
   stabilized alloy 323
Masseter muscle 202
Mastication 31
   control of 31
Masticatory
   forces 424*f*
   function, reduced 483
**Matrix theory, functional 27**
Maxilla 20, 41, 43, 211
   counter-clockwise rotation of 414*f*
   development of 41
   eruption sequence in 61
   fractures of 10
   growth of 348
   horizontal trajectories of 33
   primary displacement of 26*f*
   resistance of 365, 365*f*
   rotation of 421
   trajectories of 33
   with interpositional bone grafting 456*f*
Maxillary
   12 teeth, sum of 139
   6 teeth, sum of 139
   abnormalities 455*f*
   acrylic part 352
   and mandibular processes 39*f*
   anterior 316*f*, 317, 391
      crowding 376f
      extrusion of 422
      proclination 258, 385
      protrusion of 404*f*
      region 379*f*
      region, spacing in 379
      retraction of 393
      segment 393, 455*f*
      teeth 246
      teeth, incisal edges of 67*f*
   arch 65*f*, 111*f*, 259*f*, 339, 393
      shape of 391
      U-shaped 392*f*
   bite plane, posterior 435
   canine, impacted 449*f*
   central incisor 257, 301*f*, 410*f*, 502
      impacted 450
      mesiolabial rotation of 382
   deficiency 93, 201*f*, 369*f*, 452, 456, 456*f*, 457
      anteroposterior 456*f*
   excess 414*f*, 455
      sagittal 455*f*

expansion 250
   rapid 223, 245, 246, 248, 251*t*, 404, 407, 408
   slow 251*t*
expansion appliance
   acrylic bonded rapid 433*f*
   fixed rapid 247
   removable rapid 247
   types of rapid 247
first molar 365
   permanent, mesiobuccal cusp of 68*f*
height, increase in 47
impression 470
labial frenectomy 446
lateral incisors 99, 257
lateral sulcus 54*f*
lingual wire 354
molar 366*f*
   palatal surface of 326
   resistance of 365*f*, 366
osteotomy
   segmental 455, 456*f*
   total 455*f*
overjet, anterior 118
palatal arch with crib, removable 214*f*
posterior
   bite plane 317, 317*f*
   crowns 68
   teeth 67*f*, 246
process 39
prognathism 390, 391, 391*f*
setback 455
sinus 43, 47
skeletal base 246
subapical setback, anterior 455, 455*f*
tuberosity 26*f*, 47, 369
width, increase in 47
Mayne's space maintainer 190
Meckel's cartilage 41, 42
Mental
   nerves 42*f*
   region 42, 43
Mentalis muscle activity 124
Mentolabial sulcus 124, 125*f*, 125*t*, 126*f*, 391
   deep 110, 126*f*, 391, 392*f*
   normal depth of 126*f*
Mershoon band pusher 268
Mesial
   displacement 72
   inclination 72
Mesiodens 375
Mesiodistal
   crown angulations 68
   tip 68
Mesio-occlusion 81
Mesocephalic 121, 391
   head 121, 122*f*
Mesoprosopic face 122*f*
Metabolic disturbances 89
Metacarpal bones 164

Metal
   brackets 332, 333*f*, 482
   framework 370, 371
   handle 282
   strips, joining of 473
Metallic
   abrasive strip 240
      double-sided 240
      single sided 240
   scale 279
   tubes 309
Metals, joining 474
Microdontia 92, 377, 430
Microdontic
   second molar 113, 113*f*
      right maxillary 98*f*
   teeth 407*f*
Microglossia 92
Microskeletal unit 27
Microstomia 91
Midline diastema 407, 408, 408*t*
Mid-palatine suture and maxilla, anatomy of 245
Midsagittal plane 83, 84*f*
Mill's retractor 14, 304, 306, 307*f*
Milwaukee brace 188, 189
Mirror test 22*f*, 130*f*, 131
Mock surgery 453
Modular orthodontic instruments 267, 272
Molar
   band 248*f*, 339
      material 331
      palatal surface of 477*f*
   buccal tube 273*f*
   changes 348
   distalisation of 202*f*, 240, 243, 250
      advantages of 243
   expansion
      of first 262
      of third 262, 448
      upper 348
   first 51, 54
   lower 348*f*
   mesial drifting of 82*f*
   relation, anteroposterior 118
   relationship 56, 61, 67, 68, 68*f*, 77, 391, 397, 402
      class I 77, 385*f*
      class II 77, 392
      class III 77, 403*f*
      correction of 404
   retraction of 366*f*
   rotation 250
   second 54
   submerged primary 112
   uprighting of 243
   value 137
Monogenic traits 105
Monozygotic twins 107, 108
Moon's molar 98
Moss's functional matrix model 28

Mouth breathing 222, 356, 414, 430
    cause of 220
    correction of 222
    habit 219, 356
        classification of 219
Moyer's classification 216, 233t
Mulberry molars 93, 98
Multistrand arch wires 322
Muscle 38
    exercises 202
    in speech 32
Muscular
    anchorage 235
    effect 347
    forces 460
Myofunctional
    appliances 294
    orthodontic appliance 4f
        components of 279

# N

Nail-biting habit 224, 225f
    management 224
Nance Carey's analysis 239
Nance loop-forming pliers 269, 271f
Nance method 198
Nance palatal arch
    appliance 219
        acrylic buttons of 220f
    space maintainer 192, 192f
Narrow maxillary arch 92
Nasal
    breathing 221
    cavity 47, 247
    deformity 442
    floor, resorption of 48f
    obstruction 221
    placodes, formation of 39f
    process
        lateral 39
        medial 39
    septal theory 26
    septum 40f, 46
    spine
        anterior 144
        posterior 145
Nasolabial angle 125, 125t, 127f, 391
Nasomaxillary complex 44, 45
    secondary displacement of 46f
Natal teeth 54f
Neck, back of 233
Neural
    crest cells 36, 37f
        migration of 37f
    curve 22
    tube, formation of 37f
Neuroepithelial trophism 31
Neurological disturbances 217
Neuromuscular
    system 91
    trophism 31
Neurovisceral trophism 31

Neutron-occlusion 81
Nickel 342, 474
    titanium alloy 322, 324, 325f
Nongingival smile line 488
Nonlatex 324
Non-nutritive sucking 209
    habit 209
Non-supporting cusp 64f
Non-syndromic clefts 440
Nose
    shape of 124, 125f
    size of 124
    straight 125f
Nostrils
    shape of 124, 125f
    width of 124
Nutrition 19
Nutritional deficiencies 94
Nutritive sucking 208

# O

Occipital pull
    chin cup 372f
    headgear 235f, 366, 367, 369f
Occlusal
    arm 321
    contacts 65f
        anterior centric 65
        centric 64
    interdental arm 298
    interferences, correction of 200
    plane 69
        cant of 152f
        curve of 65
    prematurities, treatment of 188
    radiograph 438f, 444
    rest 354
        lower 356
    splints 226
Occlusion
    centric relation 63
    development of 53
Oligodontia 377
Open bite 94f, 201
    anterior 75f, 218f, 391, 413, 413f, 415, 417f
    appliance 352
        components of 352
    bilateral posterior 75f, 417, 417f
    bionator 352f
    classification of 413
    correction of anterior 404
    malocclusions, classification of 413
    management of 413, 418t
    mild anterior 218f
    posterior 417
    treatment of posterior 416t, 418
    unilateral posterior 417
    vertical anterior 118
Optiflex arch wire 322
Oral
    cavity 293

drive theory 210
gratification theory 210
habits 206, 390
    abnormal 199, 407
    correction of deleterious 199
    management of 188, 206
mucosa 207
screen, double 358f
stage 32
Orbital plane 84f
Orofacial growth 31
Oropharyngeal development 37f
Orthodontic 105, 113, 231, 255, 461, 473
    adult 4, 478
    anchorage 487
    Angle's contribution to 9t
    appliance 2, 219, 253, 293, 294, 320, 398f
        components of fixed 319
        components of removable 297
        expansion 14, 14t
        fabricate active components of 277
        fabricate retentive components of 277
        fixed 3, 3f, 222, 224, 293, 294, 294f, 295f, 328, 343f, 358f, 380, 385f, 404f, 409, 409f, 410f, 415-417, 426, 434, 435, 435f, 444f, 485f
        functional 14, 16t, 294
        myofunctional 14, 16t, 416, 423, 424
        removable 3, 3f, 13, 220f, 293, 294, 294f, 377f, 380, 383f, 387, 396f, 408, 431-433
        with 3D screw, removable 434
        with canine retractor, removable 377f
        with coffin spring, removable 434, 435f
        with expansion screw, removable 387, 434
        with finger springs, removable 410f
        with Z spring, removable 377f
    bonding 334
        classification of 334
    branches of 2
    correction 226
    diagnosis 120, 135
    evolution of term 7t
    expansion 488
    extraction, slow 483
    force 173, 174, 362, 478
        mild 173
        optimum 174
        types of 184, 184f
    instruments 266
        maintenance of 274
        sterilization of 275
    interceptive 2, 195
    intervention, timing of 3
    invisible 478
    laser in 495

management 489
preclinical 277
preventive 2, 186
procedures 186
    surgical 446, 484
removable 297
retention in 16
scope of 4
soldering in 476f, 477
study model
    portions of 468
    uses of 472
surgical 446, 478
techniques, fixed 16, 16t
therapy 255
tooth movement 172, 176f, 480
trainer 219, 220f
treatment 2f, 5, 120, 135, 293, 465, 466, 478, 480, 481, 481f, 483, 484, 485f, 493, 502
    active 294
    adjunctive 481, 482
    adult 480, 481
    appliance, fixed 423
    in adults, types of 481
    index of 115, 116t
    plan 227, 493
    purposes 447
    surgical 484
welding applications in 475f
wire 277, 278, 281
Orthogenetic surgery 478
Orthognathic surgery 450, 479
    steps in 450
Orthopantomogram 90f
Orthopedic
    appliance 3, 362, 416, 432
        therapy 362
    force 362
    orthodontic appliances 294
Osamu's invisible retainer 464, 465f
Osteogenesis imperfecta 108
Osteogenic space expansion 489
Osteotomey
    bilateral sagittal split 453, 454
    technique 489f
        bilateral sagittal split 453
Overbite 116, 391, 393
    complete 420, 420f
    incomplete 420
    reduction of 341, 393
Ovum, period of 35

# P

Palatal
    arch 352
        wire 352
    bow 353
    canine retractor 314, 314f
    expansion 245
    growth 48f
    remodeling 47
    wire 354, 356

Palate
    defects, soft 442f
    development of 38
    free activator 15
    ossification of 40
Palatine shelves 40f
Palatomaxillary suture 46
Parietal bones 233
Peer assessment rating 115
Peg-shaped lateral incisors 99f
Peg-shaped teeth 92
Pendulum appliances 242
Periodontal
    bone defects 479
    disease 1, 480
    ligament 182
        complex 172
        traction 459
    tissue, treatment of 223
Periodontium, reduced 480
Periosteal matrix 28
Permanent canines, eruption of 59
Permanent dentition 52, 57f, 60, 61
    chronology of 52
    early 4
Permanent first premolar 387f
Permanent incisors, eruption of 58
Permanent lateral incisor, gemination of left 375f
Permanent left canine 375
Permanent lower canine, left 428f
Permanent maxillary central incisor 97f, 406f
Permanent molars, management of first 188
Permanent second
    molars, ruption of 60
    premolar 387
        eruption of right 375
Permanent teeth 56, 56t
    delayed eruption of 96, 98, 101f
    eruption of 91
Phalanges, ossification of 165f
Pharyngeal
    arches, derivatives of 38t
    stage 32
Phenotype 105
Phonetic method 129
Phosphoric acid 336f
Physiologic
    nipple 209
    tongue thrust 215
    tooth movement 172
Piezoelectric theory 177
Plastic brackets 333, 333f
Pliers
    beak of 278
    position of 283
Polycarbonate 333
Polygenic inheritance 106
Pont's analysis 137
Poor bone density 488

Poor facial appearance 1
Poor oral hygiene maintenance 1
Poor periodontal health 319
Posteruptive tooth movement 172
Postsurgical orthodontics 456
Postsurgical scar tissue 126
Pre-eruptive tooth movement 172
Premaxilla, development of 92
Premolar
    bands 248f
    basal arch width 138
    dimension 138
    extraction of
        first 136, 198, 261f
        second 136, 260, 262
    extraction, first 261
    first 260
    infraversion of 74f
    teeth
        missing 118
        removal of 454
        roots of 365f
    value 137
Prenatal
    development 35
    environmental factors 93
    factors 390
    growth 19, 35
    history 121
Prenormal occlusion 74f
Presurgical orthodontic 451, 452
Primary teeth, removal of retained 447
Prognathic mandible 402
Prominent chin 127f, 402t
Prophylactic
    brushes 336f
    paste 336f
Prosthesis, fixed 409, 411
Prosthodontic indications 482
Proximal stripping 199, 239
    methods of 240, 241f
Pseudo-class III malocclusion, treatment of 404
Pseudoelastic effect 322, 323
Psychological stress 19
Psychosocial problems 1, 442
Pterygoid
    buttress/pillar 33
    muscle 202
    response 355
Pterygomaxillary fissure 145
Pterygopalatine 369
    suture 46
Pull chin cup 370, 372f

# Q

Quad helix appliance 251, 252f, 434
    fixed 435f
    parts of 252f

# R

Ramus 48
    osteotomy 453, 453f

Rapid maxillary expansion 245
Reciprocal anchorages 234*f*
Redundant gingival tissue 502
Relapse, causes of 459
Resistance, center of 365
Respiration 32
    assessment of 130, 130*f*
Resta clasp 302, 303*f*
Restorative treatment 226
Retainers, classification of 461
Retentive arm 298, 301, 303-305, 310, 311, 313, 321
Retrognathic maxilla 403, 403*f*
Rheumatic fever 121
Rhythm generation theory 32
Ribbon arch
    appliance 9, 338
    brackets 334
Ridge expansion 488
Robert's retractor 14, 304, 306, 307*f*
Rochette temporary bridges 488
Roo*t*
    completion 53
    formation 53
    forms of 232*f*
    resorption 480
        mild 481*f*
    size of 232
    torque 183*f*
Rubella infection, maternal 93
Rweed's triangle 160*f*

## S

Safety pin, double 340
Samarium cobalt magnet 328
Scammon's growth 23
    curve 22, 23*f*
Schwartz clasp 14, 301, 302, 302*f*
Scissor bite 387, 388, 391, 429
    management of 388
    treatment of 388*f*
Sella-gnathion plane 150
Servosystem theory 28, 29
    of growth 29*f*
Servosystem, components of 29
Seudoelastic effect 322
Shallow mentolabial sulcus 126*f*, 385*f*, 402
Shear cusp 64*f*
Sheldon's classification of physique 121*t*
Silver 474
Simon's classification 83
    of malocclusion 83
Singer's method 166
Skeletal
    age 163
    analysis 154
    anterior
        crossbite 200
        open bite 413*f*, 414*f*, 415, 415*f*
    class I malocclusion 72*f*, 83
    class II jaw dysplasias 161
    class II malocclusion 85, 391
    class III malocclusion 85, 400, 400*f*, 401, 401*t*, 402, 403
    crossbite 76*f*, 428, 430, 431*f*
    deep bite 421
    discrepancy 452
    growth 355
    malocclusion 74, 76*f*
        classification of 74
        in sagittal planes 74
        in transverse plane 75
        in vertical plane 75
        interception of 200
    maturity 170*t*
        using cervical vertebrae 170*f*
    open bite 414*f*, 415
        treatment of 418
    parameters 147, 148, 151*f*
    relationship 227
        abnormal 390
        vertical 124, 124*f*
    structures 38, 91
    unit 27
Skull 44
    development of 41
Soldered buccal tube 301*f*
Soldering
    procedure, steps in 475*f*, 476
    steps in 475
Speech 32
    difficulties 442
    disturbance 218
Sphenoethmoid suture 46
Sphenoid synchondrosis 45
Sphenooccipital synchondrosis 46
Split labial bow 14, 304, 306, 306*f*
Spot welding 473
    procedure of 473
Springs, types of 309*t*, 323, 324*t*
Stainless steel 322
    wire 311
Stamp cusp 64, 64*f*
Standard bionator 351
Steiner's analysis 154
Steiner's dental analysis 157*t*
Steiner's lip analysis 157
Steiner's skeletal
    analysis 154*t*
    parameters 156*f*
Subtelny classification 209
Sucking
    habits, classification of non-nutritive 210*t*
    reflex 207
Supernumerary teeth, extraction of 188
Supracrestal fibrotomy, circumferential 447, 447*f*
Surgical orthodontics, field of 478
Swallowing 32
    patterns 130
Symphyseal cartilage 42
Synchondroses 45
Syndromic cleft cases 440
Synthetic polyurethane material 328
Systemic health 479

## T

Talon's cusp 98, 99*f*
Teeth
    after prophylaxis 336*f*
    anterior 66, 407*f*
    bonding 334
    condition of 256
    controlled force on 493
    derotation of 384
        posterior 243
    gemination of 374
    hypoplasia of 94*f*
    in crossbite, upper 312
    intrusion of supraerupted 483
    irregularities of 10
    lower 344*f*
    malocclusion of 10
    malposed 479
    missing 96, 430
    natal 54
    neonatal 54
    number of 91
    opposing 67
    position of 257
    posterior 66
        crossbite, segmental 436
    requires application, derotation of rotated 383
    retention of 10
    rotated anterior 243*t*
    rotated posterior 243*t*
    rotation of 92
    separation of 329
    0 in primary 56
    supernumerary 92, 93*f*, 96, 374, 375, 430
    support of 480
    transplantation of 449
    trauma to 1
    type of 237
    upper 344*f*, 349
Temporary rochette bridge 488
Temporomandibular joint 1, 43, 480
    injury 89
Teratogenesis 390
Therapeutic extraction 264
    of mesiodens 407
    of permanent teeth 447
Therapeutic occlusion 63
Thermoelastic effect 323
Third molars, role of 460
Three-prong pliers 266, 270, 272*f*
Thumb
    digit sucking habit 413
    pads of 283
    sucking 207, 209, 210, 211*f*, 212*f*, 356, 377, 390, 430
        classification of 209

habit 188*f*, 201*f*, 208*f*, 209, 357*f*, 379
habit causing midline diastema 407*f*
maxillary cast of 213*f*
Tin 474
Tip-edge
brackets 334
techniques 324
Tissue
analysis, soft 157
cephalometric landmarks
hard 144*t*
soft 145*t*, 146*f*
damage, soft 321
degeneration, type of 175
landmarks, soft 145
nasion, soft 145
procedures, soft 446
retraction 489*f*
soft 91
temperature 499*f*
Tissue-borne functional appliances, removable 346
Tongue 126, 202, 207
blade therapy 199*f*, 431, 432
crib, fixed 416*f*
development of 40
examination 218
guard 219
holds exercise 203
posture at rest 218
tag 219
thrusting 217, 218, 356, 377
habit 201*f*, 207, 214, 218*f*, 357*f*
habit, anterior 414, 416*f*
self-correcting 218
with malocclusion 218
tie 447*f*
Tonsils 128
Tooth 51
anatomic position of 232
anterior crossbite, single 428*f*, 431*f*
axial inclination of 232
bodily movement of 183*f*
borne
appliances, removable 346
functional appliances, fixed 346
contacts, intra-arch 61
crossbite 433*f*
multiple 326*f*
single 428, 434*f*
development, stages of 52, 53*f*

eruption 172
exposure 450*f*
of impacted 448, 501, 501*f*
extracted 197
guidance 65, 219
implant, insertion of single 482
in oral cavity 179
material
discrepancy 379
total 138
movement 175, 183, 228, 481*f*, 488
biology of 172
direction of 310
duration of 237, 361
eruptive 172
mechanics of 179, 480
piezoelectric theory of 177*f*
potential 492
theories of 176
type of 181, 237
number of 111, 430
anomalies 96
posterior crossbite, single 429
rotation, single 384*f*
scissor bite, single 75*f*
separation 321*f*
shape of 91
abnormal 112
anomalies of 96-98, 98*t*, 430
size of 91, 111
anomalies of 96, 97, 430
surgical exposure of 449
whitening by laser 504, 504*f*
Torque springs 323, 340
Total tooth material 136, 256
Transpalatal arch 193, 193*f*, 236, 477
functions of 193
Trauma 89
from occlusion 64
increased predisposition to 483
Traumatic injury 390
Traumatic occlusion 63
Trigeminal nerve 38
T-spring, parts of 311, 312
Tweed's method 198
Tweed's triangle 157, 160*t*
Twin-block appliance 15, 16, 360, 360*f*
Two-finger test 123

U

U loop canine retractor, parts of 313
Ugly duckling stage 59, 59*f*, 407*f*

Ulnar sesamoid
bone 164
ossification onset of 165*f*
Unesthetic gingival level discrepancies 482
Upper posterior teeth, mesial movement of 397

V

Vagus nerve 38
Van Limborgh's compromise theory 30
Veau's classification 439
Vital staining 20
Von-der-Linden's classification 390

W

Water test 130*f*, 131, 222
Weingart pliers 266, 271, 273*f*, 321, 329
beaks of 273*f*
Weldable buccal tubes 334, 340
Weldable lingual
button 331
cleat 332
sheath 332*f*
Welding buccal tube 331*f*
Wilkinson's extraction 262, 264
drawbacks of 262
Wilson distalizing arch 242
Wire
appliances, fixed straight 444*f*
component 351-352, 461, 462, 464
of frankel II appliances 353
of frankel III appliance 356
cutting instruments 266, 272
forming pliers 266, 268
technique, straight 294
Wit's appraisal 161, 161*f*
Wunderer's modification 15

Z

Zinc 474
Z-spring 311, 311*f*
fabrication of 311
helices of 311
parts of 311
Zygoma 47
enlargement of 47*f*
Zygomatic arches 33
Zygomaticomaxillary suture 46
Zygomaticotemporal suture 46